Emergency Care

ninth
edition

Emergency Care

BRADY

Daniel Limmer

Michael F. O'Keefe

Harvey D. Grant

Robert H. Murray, Jr.

J. David Bergeron

ninth edition

Contributors
Beth Lothrop Adams
Bob Elling
David M. Habben
Fitzgerald Petersen

Additional Contributions
James B. Miller, NREMT-P, US Army
EMT Program Manager

Medical Editor
Edward T. Dickinson, M.D., FACEP

MILITARY EDITION

Prentice Hall

BRADY/PRENTICE HALL HEALTH
Upper Saddle River, NJ 07458

Publisher: *Julie Alexander*

Executive Editor: *Greg Vis*

Managing Development Editor: *Lois Berlowitz*

Project Editor: *Josephine Cepeda*

Director of Production and Manufacturing: *Bruce Johnson*

Managing Production Editor: *Patrick Walsh*

Manufacturing Manager: *Ilene Sanford*

Production Liaison: *Julie Boddorf*

Production Editor: *Lisa Garboski*

Managing Photography Editor: *Michal Heron*

Photographers: *Michael Gallitelli, Michal Heron, Richard Logan, Stephen Ogilvy*

Photo Research: *Romy Charlesworth, Michal Heron*

Creative Director: *Marianne Frasco*

Cover Design Coordinator: *Maria Guglielmo*

Cover Designer: *LaFortezza Design Group*

Interior Designer: *Amy Rosen*

Marketing Manager: *Tiffany Price*

Marketing Coordinator: *Cindy Frederick*

Composition: *The Clarinda Company and Carlisle Communications*

Prentice-Hall International (UK) Limited, *London*
Prentice-Hall of Australia Pty. Limited, *Sydney*
Prentice-Hall Canada, Inc., *Toronto*
Prentice-Hall Hispanoamericana, S.A., *Mexico*
Prentice-Hall of India Private Limited, *New Delhi*
Prentice-Hall of Japan, Inc., *Tokyo*
Prentice-Hall Singapore Pte. Ltd.
Editora Prentice-Hall do Brasil, Ltda., *Rio de Janeiro*

Cover photograph courtesy of James Miller.

NOTICE ON CARE PROCEDURES

It is the intent of the authors and publisher that this textbook be used as part of a formal EMT-Basic education program taught by qualified instructors and supervised by a licensed physician. The procedures described in this textbook are based upon consultation with EMT and medical authorities. The authors and publisher have taken care to make cer-tain that these procedures reflect currently accepted clinical practice; however, they cannot be consid-ered absolute recommendations.

The material in this textbook contains the most cur-rent information available at the time of publication. However, federal, state, and local guidelines con-cerning clinical practices, including without limita-tion, those governing infection control and univer-sal precautions, change rapidly. The reader should note, therefore, that the new regulations may require changes in some procedures.

It is the responsibility of the reader to familiarize himself or herself with the policies and procedures set by federal, state, and local agencies as well as the institution or agency where the reader is employed. The authors and the publisher of this textbook and the supplements written to accompa-ny it disclaim any liability, loss or risk resulting directly or indirectly from the suggested procedures and theory, from any undetected errors, or from the reader's misunderstanding of the text. It is the read-er's responsibility to stay informed of any new changes or recommendations made by any federal, state, and local agency as well as by his or her employing institution or agency.

NOTICE ON GENDER USAGE

The English language has historically given prefer-ence to the male gender. Among many words, the pronouns "he" and "his" are commonly used to describe both genders. Society evolves faster than language, and the male pronouns still predominate in our speech. The authors have made great effort to treat the two genders equally, recognizing that a sig-nificant percentage of EMTs are female. However, in some instances, male pronouns may be used to describe both males and females solely for the pur-pose of brevity. This is not intended to offend any readers of the female gender.

NOTICE RE "STREET SCENES" AND OTHER SCENARIOS AND CASE STUDIES

The names used and situations depicted in "Street Scenes" and other scenarios and case studies throughout this text are fictitious.

Published in cooperation with Pearson Custom Publishing.
A Pearson Education Company.

10 9 8 7 6 5 4 3 2
ISBN 0-536-63074-7

To Sarah Katherine, my little Miss Magic
D. L.

To my parents, Mike and Noreen,
my first and best teachers.
M. O'K.

BRIEF CONTENTS

BRIEF CONTENTS *Continued*

DETAILED CONTENTS

Module 1 PREPARATORY

Chapter One Introduction to Emergency Medical Care 2

Chapter Two The Well-being of the EMT-Basic 14

Chapter Three Medical/Legal and Ethical Issues 32

Module 3   PATIENT ASSESSMENT

Module 6   INFANTS AND CHILDREN

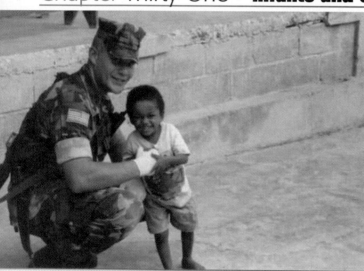

Module 7 OPERATIONS

Chapter Thirty-Two   Ambulance Operations   686

Chapter Thirty-Three   Gaining Access and Rescue Operations   718

Chapter Thirty-Four   Special Operations   740

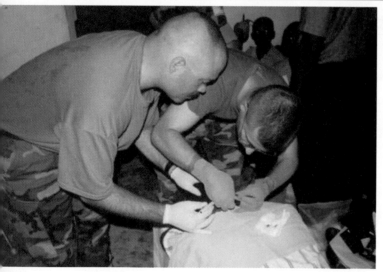

PHOTO SCANS

FOREWORD TO SPECIAL MILITARY EDITION

Since the beginning of our nation, medics and corpsmen have performed a vital role in support of our military operations, and in support of our military. From the Revolutionary War through the Civil War and the wars of this last century, preserving and restoring the fighting strength of our soldiers, sailors and airmen has been a critical task.

Military medical corpsmen and combat medics receive the same training as their civilian counterparts, but must also possess some specialized skills and abilities. Sometimes these skills are different for military situations; sometimes they are applied differently. Our medics and corpsmen must have all the skills necessary to save and preserve life.

While practicing medicine has changed tremendously in the last half-century, what hasn't changed is our commitment to properly prepare our medics to provide the best care to our armed forces anywhere in the world. Training in the age of worldwide communications and global connectivity may take new forms, but our goal of maintaining the highest possible standards of care is timeless.

There is an extremely proud history of service by medics and corpsmen of all branches of the military throughout our nation's history, and I encourage and support any effort to increase and maintain their readiness, here and around the world.

Kevin C. Kiley
Major General, Medical Corps
United States Army

LETTER TO STUDENTS

Congratulations. You are about to begin your training to become an Emergency Medical Technician-Basic, or EMT-B—a career that you are sure to find challenging and rewarding. The knowledge you will gain in this course will prepare you for important responsibilities, and the skills you learn will save lives. We hope that the *Emergency Care* textbook—plus the free *Electronic Extras CD* included—provides you with a solid foundation upon which to develop your hands-on skills as an EMT-B.

DOT's EMT-BASIC CURRICULUM

Your EMT-B course is most likely based on guidelines set by the U.S. Department of Transportation (DOT). This is not to say that there is one universal EMT-B course. Using the DOT curriculum as a foundation, physicians and instructors in your local EMS system have designed your course to meet specific training needs of your community. The basic training is the same, but there are differences in each state as to what materials are presented. The U.S. DOT's 1994 EMT-Basic Curriculum forms the basis of *Emergency Care.*

The intent of the DOT curriculum is for students to follow a particular sequence in learning the knowledge and skills of an EMT-B. After completing CPR, students begin the course with the preparatory module. This covers some of the foundation material students will need to know in order to understand later topics. Airway management, because of its importance, comes next. Then students learn how to assess patients. At this point, either trauma or medical emergencies could follow. The curriculum puts medical emergencies first, but instructors may alter this to meet local needs and suit local resources. The last two sections of the curriculum are on pediatrics and operations. The problems of infants and children are near the end, not because they are any less important than those of adults, but because at this point the students will have the background needed to understand the differences between adults and children.

Alternative Methods of Care

As you read through the textbook, you will find alternative methods of care cited. There are some procedures that vary so much that only the most common methods in use are discussed. For such cases, you will be directed to follow local protocols.

Why is there no one method of providing care for certain illnesses and injuries? In some cases, more than one procedure works. Your EMS system may have tested only one procedure and decided that it was efficient, easy to learn, and simple to use. A different EMS system may have tested a second method and had the same results. You will be trained to use the methods in which your own local EMS system has confidence based upon its own rigorous testing.

One thing is certain. Not all the methods you learn in your training will stay the same during your career as an EMT. *You must keep up to date with local procedures.* Your instructor will tell you how continuing education programs for EMT-Bs are presented in your locality. Find out what prehospital emergency care journals and videos may be recommended by your EMS system, and make use of state or local newsletters that are available to help the EMT-B stay current.

Interventions

Today's EMT-B assesses patients and provides treatment based on that assessment. The number of interventions, or treatments, available today for the EMT-B to help patients has never been greater.

This text will prepare you to administer medications such as oral glucose and activated charcoal to patients who need them. You will also be taught to assist patients in taking some of their own medications. You will come across patients who have prescribed nitroglycerin for chest pain, inhalers for breathing problems, and epinephrine auto-injectors for allergic reactions. Assisting your patients in taking these medications will make them more comfortable, reduce pain, and may save their lives.

As an EMT-B, you will also be called upon to use several important devices. Perhaps the most noteworthy is the automated external defibrillator, or AED. This truly lifesaving device applies an electrical shock to the chest of a person whose heart has stopped. You will also use the pneumatic anti-shock garment and the flow-restricted, oxygen powered ventilation device.

PREFACE

Emergency Care has set the standard for EMT-B training texts for over 30 years. The famous "yellow book" has been used by over 1.6 million students to pass the National Registry and state exams. More than any other text, this book has defined the field. The thoroughly revised Ninth Edition continues this tradition of excellence, reflecting the latest techniques and innovations in emergency patient care and including the latest advances in instructional technology.

The authors have based *Emergency Care* on the U.S. DOT 1994 EMT-Basic National Standard Curriculum; everything in the 1994 curriculum is addressed in the text. In addition, the text and the accompanying CD-ROM were developed taking into account the years of experience that the authors, with the input of countless instructors and students, have had with the DOT curriculum since its publication. The result is a proven text with outstanding readability and a level of detail that more instructors have found appropriate for their classrooms than any other.

The content of the Ninth Edition is summarized below:

Module 1, PREPARATORY: CHAPTERS 1-5

This first module sets a framework for all the modules that follow by introducing some essential concepts, information, and skills. The EMS system and the role of the EMT-B within the system are introduced. Issues of EMT-B safety and well-being and legal and ethical issues are covered. Basic anatomy and physiology and techniques of safe lifting and moving are also included in this first module.

Module 2, AIRWAY MANAGEMENT: CHAPTER 6

There is only one chapter in Module 2, but it may be considered the most important module in the text, because no patient will survive without an open airway. Basic airway management techniques are covered in detail.

Module 3, ASSESSMENT: CHAPTERS 7-15

The ability to perform a rapid but accurate assessment, treat for life-threatening conditions, and initiate transport to the hospital within optimum time limits are the essence of the EMT-B's job. In this module, all of the steps of the assessment and their application to different types of trauma and medical patients, plus the skills of measuring vital signs, taking a patient history, communication, and documentation, are explained and illustrated.

Module 4, MEDICAL EMERGENCIES: CHAPTERS 16-25

The Medical Emergencies module begins with a chapter on pharmacology in which the medications the EMT-B can administer or assist with under the 1994 curriculum are introduced. The module continues with chapters on respiratory, cardiac, diabetic, allergy, poisoning and overdose, environmental, behavioral, and obstetric/gynecological emergencies. It ends with a new chapter on caring for patients with multiple medical complaints.

Module 5, TRAUMA: CHAPTERS 26-30

The Trauma module begins with a chapter on bleeding and shock; continues with chapters on soft-tissue injuries, musculoskeletal injuries, and injuries to the head and spine; and ends with a new chapter on caring for multiple-trauma patients.

Module 6, INFANTS AND CHILDREN: CHAPTER 31

The difference between treating adult and pediatric patients often lies in understanding the physical and psychological differences in infants and children compared to adults. This module explores these special aspects of pediatric care as well as medical conditions and injury patterns that are especially common to or critical for infants and children.

Module 7, OPERATIONS: CHAPTERS 32-34

This module deals with nonmedical operations and special situations, including ambulance operations, motor-vehicle collision rescues, and multiple-casualty and hazardous materials incidents.

Module 8, ADVANCED AIRWAY MANAGEMENT (ELECTIVE): CHAPTER 35

In some states and regions, EMT-Bs will be trained to perform invasive airway management procedures, including orotracheal intubation and, in children, nasogastric intubation. Module 8 is included as an elective to cover these advanced airway management skills.

Special Section, MILITARY EMS: CHAPTER 36

This chapter is intended to make military medics aware of the history, special needs, and techniques of military emergency care.

APPENDICES AND BCLS REVIEW

There are four appendices to this textbook, covering advanced life support assist skills, stress, and the National Registry of Emergency Medical Technicians skill sheets. There is also a review of the basic cardiac life support course, which is a prerequisite to the EMT-Basic course.

INNOVATIONS STUDENTS NEED— FEATURES OF THE BOOK AND THE COMPANION CD-ROM

The features of the Ninth Edition of *Emergency Care* and its accompanying *Electronic Extras CD* have been designed to address the needs of students training to become EMT-Bs. Some features—like the "Patient Assessment" and "Patient Care" sections and Scans—are hallmarks of *Emergency Care* and have been used successfully in several editions. Other new or revised features—like the Street Scenes and Topic Overview—have been added based on the comments of instructors and students who have used the book in the past and were kind enough to provide us with their suggestions.

Here's what we have found about what students need most in their studies—and here's how this latest revision of *Emergency Care* meets those needs:

Students want material to be relevant to real life. Only work in the field provides *real* life experience, but case-based learning is an effective way of integrating concepts with practice in the classroom.

- **New! Word on the Street.** Each chapter opens with a brief anecdote, where experienced EMTs share their insights, wisdom, and experiences.
- **New! Street Scenes.** Each chapter concludes with a case study that applies information from the chapter to a life-like scenario. The Street Scenes case study begins, then stops to ask students questions; to make decisions; to figure out what to do next. As the case study continues, the story answers the questions by explaining what the EMTs would really do.
- **An Electronic Edge.** More case studies, plus on-the-scene action video footage and photos of trauma injuries, are found on the *Electronic Extras CD*.

Students prefer material in easy-to-read, easy-to-locate "chunks." So do we! Whether it's a mnemonic device like SAMPLE or a quick-reference *Scan* page that summarizes a skill, *Emergency Care* is designed to make important information accessible.

- **Scans.** Key information and step-by-step procedures are summarized and presented for easy reference in illustrated Scans.

Medication Scans give you all the information you need in order to administer or help administer medications. Procedure Scans list and describe the steps in performing particular procedures.

- **Study Guides.** Sprinkled throughout the text, these summarize key points or mnemonic devices.
- **Special Notes.** "Pediatric Notes" and "Geriatric Notes" in many chapters describe what is unique in dealing with infants, children, or older adults and how you should deal with those differences. "Safety Notes" appear throughout the book as needed to point out situations where you need to take special care.

Patient assessment practice is essential. Because today's EMTs must assess patients accurately in order to perform their jobs well, training must contain a strong focus on this important skill.

- **Patient Care and Patient Assessment sections.** These segments describe the assessment and treatment you should provide for particular types of patients, disorders, or injuries. Patient Assessment typically lists the important signs and symptoms. Patient Care lists the key steps of EMT-B emergency care.
- **An Electronic Edge.** Video Activities on the *Electronic Extras CD* emphasize patient assessment with actual video footage and interactive exercises.

Good documentation skills require practice, practice, practice. One of the most common problems students encounter when they begin work on the street is documentation of calls.

- **Documentation Tips.** The Ninth Edition continues the use of the popular Documentation Tips throughout the text, with new examples added to the end of every medical, trauma, and pediatric chapter.
- **New! Sample Documentation.** After the chapter on documentation (Chapter 15), each Street Scenes case study concludes with a filled-out run sheet for the call.
- **An Electronic Edge.** The video activities on the *Electronic Extras CD* include documentation practice.

Retention improves when students have a broader framework in which to place newly learned information. When students first grasp a general overview, they are better prepared to synthesize details.

- **New! Topic Overview.** The chapter opens with a list of the key topics to be covered in the chapter.
- **DOT Objectives.** This list of cognitive, affective, and skills objectives opens each chapter and represents what is required by the U.S. DOT's National Standard. Includes page references to the chapter for quick review.

Sometimes students want to know more than what's in the DOT.

- **FYIs.** These popular "For Your Information" sections include material that is intended to broaden your knowledge of a chapter topic but it is not essential to an understanding of your job as an EMT-B.
- **New! How and Why.** This feature, posted throughout the text, brings to your attention extra information related to the topic at hand. In-depth expansions on these notes can be found on your *Electronic Extras CD.*
- **New! Web Medic.** The internet can be a large, confusing place for students. We will show them the right places to go for the best information. Each chapter has recommended web sites for your students to check out, located on the *Emergency Care* Companion Website so that URLs can be updated as needed.
- **An Electronic Edge.** Spanish phrases are included in audio format on the *Electronic Extras CD!*

Quality review material means better grades. Most students believe there is never too much opportunity for review and practice. We agree.

- **In-text Chapter Review.** Each chapter concludes with a Summary, a list of Key Terms (and definitions), Review Questions, and an Application Question.
- **An Electronic Edge.** Chapter Quizzes, Puzzles, Case Studies, and Patient Assessment activities are included on the CD for further practice.

- **On the Companion Website.** Even more chapter questions, anatomy review material, and interactive case studies can be found here.
- **National Registry Skill Sheets.** The practical skill sheets used at the EMT-Basic level by the National Registry of Emergency Medical Technicians are included in Appendix C as a tool to aid skill practice. The skill sheets also allow the instructor the opportunity to use a formal evaluation instrument when evaluating student performance. Preceding the skill sheets are instructions provided to the candidate prior to practical testing. This information should allay student fears and uncertainties about what criteria will be tested on the practical examination.

OUR GOAL: IMPROVING FUTURE TRAINING AND EDUCATION

Some of the best ideas for better training and education methods come from instructors who can tell us what areas of study caused their students the most trouble. Other sound ideas come from practicing EMT-Bs who let us know what problems they faced in the field. We welcome any of your suggestions. If you are an EMS instructor who has an idea on how to improve this book, the companion CD, or EMT-Basic training in general, please write to us at:

Brady/Prentice Hall Health
c/o EMS Editor
Pearson Education
One Lake Street
Upper Saddle River, NJ 07458

If you have access to a computer with a modem, you can also reach us through the following addresses:

danlimmer@earthlink.com
mikeokvt@aol.com

Visit Brady's Web Site
http://www.bradybooks.com

ACKNOWLEDGMENTS

PROGRAM DEVELOPMENT

Medical Editor

Edward T. Dickinson, MD, FACEP, and NREMT-P is Medical Editor for the *Emergency Care* program and was invaluable to the preparation of this edition. Ed is thorough, knowledgeable, and conscientious. His experience on the street as a firefighter and paramedic combined with his insights and knowledge as a physician makes Ed a highly regarded team member. His contributions as editor, writer, and friend are greatly appreciated.

Contributors

There are many contributors to this edition. We thank everyone who shared experiences in the "Word on the Street" feature. Please see the list of "Word on the Street" contributors that appears later in this Acknowledgments section.

Andrew Stern, NREMT-P, Paramedic/Flight Medic, and educator spent a considerable amount of time creating realistic "Street Scenes" and, with the aid of Hugh Skerker, documentation examples for you to learn from. Michael Grill, NREMT-P and educator, Sierra Vista (AZ) Fire Department also contributed to our "Street Scenes." Jo Anne Schultz contributed ideas for our "How and Why?" feature. Stephanie Kraus searched for and compiled web sites we highlight in our "Web Medic" feature.

Many people have contributed to past editions of *Emergency Care*. The contributions to prior editions have helped shape future editions. Many of those contributions are still a part of what you read today. Continued thanks go to Beth Lothrop Adams, Bob Elling, David M. Habben, and Fitzgerald Petersen for their contributions of chapters and ideas. Their attention to detail and currency are greatly appreciated.

Beth Lothrop Adams (MA, RN, NREMT-P) is ALS Coordinator at the Commonwealth Prehospital Education at The George Washington University in Fairfax, Virginia. Bob Elling (MPA, REMT-P) is Faculty, American College of Prehospital Medicine. Bob is an especially important member of our group, since he is co-author of the Workbook that accompanies *Emergency Care*. David M. Habben (NREMT-P) is EMS Instructor/Consultant, Boise, Idaho. Fitzgerald Petersen is a Firefighter/EMT-P with the Salt Lake County Fire Department in Salt Lake City, Utah. Our continued thanks also to Rick Buell, Jon Politis, Andy Stern, and Owen Traynor, MD, for their contributions.

We would like to thank Jim Miller, US Army EMT Program Manager, for his work and vision toward making this book a reality. His work on the package that accompanies *Emergency Care* and his contribution of military material to our program is greatly appreciated.

Brady/Prentice Hall Health

There have been considerable changes at Brady/Prentice Hall Health since our last edition. This "changing of the guard" has brought a new team together. We find ourselves wishing to thank those who are now with us and those who are not but who have contributed so much to the book over previous editions.

The current team at Brady is led by publisher Julie Alexander, who has taken the helm of an organization recently reorganized as Prentice Hall Health. We thank Julie for her support during the revision process. Lois Berlowitz, Senior Managing Editor for Brady, has been a tireless advocate for us and our project over the years. This has been and will always be appreciated.

We would especially like to thank Jo Cepeda, our developmental editor. We have all been fortunate to work with Jo on this—and other—projects. Her experience, dedication, magnificent eye for detail, and support for us on the main text and supplements have been invaluable to us all in this revision. Special thanks also to Michel Heron, who provided an unprecedented level of talent and dedication to the photo program in this book. Her work in this and previous editions has been critical to *Emergency Care's* success.

Once a book is written, it must be produced and printed. This is a colossal task and fortunately for us we have a great production team. Pat Walsh leads a team that includes Marianne Frasco from Design and Ilene Sanford from Manufacturing. Julie Boddorf is also a seasoned veteran who has produced many books with us. Her role as Production Manager for this project is deeply appreciated. Finally, Lisa Garboski, our Production Editor, possesses a dedication and tenacity that proved vital to producing this text.

The sales and marketing staff get this book into your hands. Thanks go to Leslie Cavaliere, Tiffany Price, and Cindy Frederick. The sales team, lead by Judy Stamm, also deserves our appreciation for their work and continued feedback that help our book to thrive.

We have many old friends, some of whom have left Brady or changed jobs during this edition. The work you have done with us and the effort and dedication you have provided over the editions will not be forgotten: Susan Katz, Carol Sobel, Sandy Breuer, and Judy Streger fall into this category. Thank you.

WORD ON THE STREET CONTRIBUTORS

James B. Allen, BS, NREMT-P
Past President, NAEMT
Captain, Clinton Fire & Rescue
Clinton, MS

Brenda M. Beasley, RN, BS, EMT-P
EMS Program Director
Calhoun State Community College
Decatur, AL

Dawson Blackmore, Jr., EMT-I
EMS Instructor
West Haven, CT

Ken Bouvier, NREMT-I
Hazardous Materials Specialist
New Orleans, LA

Will Chapleau, EMT-P, RN, TNS
Assistant EMS Coordinator
Good Samaritan Hospital
Downers Grove, IL

Richard A. Cherry, MS, NREMT-P
Clinical Assistant Professor of Emergency Medicine
Director of Paramedic Training
SUNY Upstate Medical University
Syracuse, NY

Harold C. Cohen, PhD, EMT-P
Battalion Chief
Baltimore County Fire Department
Baltimore, MD

Heather Davis, MS, NREMT-P
Clinical Coordinator
UCLA-DFA Paramedic Education
Inglewood, CA

Kate Dernocoeur, BS, EMT-P
Lowell, MI

Edward T. Dickinson, MD, NREMT-P, FACEP
Assistant Professor
Director of EMA Field Operations
Department of Emergency Medicine
University of Pennsylvania School of Medicine
Philadelphia, PA

Bob Elling, MPA, REMT-P
Faculty
American College of Prehospital Medicine
Schenectady, NY

Michael Grill, NREMT-P
Sierra Vista Fire Department
Sierra Vista, AZ

Jeff Grunow, MSN, NREMT-P
Director, Prehospital Education
Carolinas Medical Center
Charlotte, NC

Eric W. Heckerson, RN, MA, EMT-P
EMA Coordinator
Mesa Fire Department
Mesa, AZ

Thom Hillson, EMT-P
Field Supervisor
Lakeside, CA

Linda Honeycutt, EMT-P, I/C
EMS Programs Coordinator
Providence Hospital and Medical Centers
Novi, MI

Daniel Paul Layne I, MICP
Mobile Intensive Care Paramedic

Cissy Matthews, EMT-P
College of the Mainland
Texas City, TX

Scott J. Meagher, NREMT-P, REMT-B I/C
Safety Program Consultants, Inc.
Taunton, MA

Cynthia Osborne, EMT-P, IC
Assistant Professor
Dona Ana Branch Community College
New Mexico State University

David Page
Emergency Health Services Department
Inver Hills Community College
St. Paul, MN

Mike Smith, MICP
Vice President
Emergency Medical Training Associates
University Place, WA

David Spiro, BA, EMT-P
Organ Recovery/Placement Coordinator
Finger Lakes Donor Recovery Network
Rochester, NY

Andrew Stern, NREMT-P, MPA, MA
Senior Paramedic/Flight Medic
Town of Colonie Emergency Medical Services
Colonie, NY

Charles Stewart, MD, FACEP
Colorado Springs, CO

Matthew R. Streger, MPA, NREMT-P
Deputy Commissioner
Cleveland Emergency Medical Services
Cleveland, Ohio

Paul A. Werfel, NREMT-P
Director, Paramedic Program
Clinical Instructor in Health Sciences
State University of New York
Stony Brook, NY

REVIEWERS

We wish to thank the following reviewers for providing invaluable feedback and suggestions in preparation of the Ninth Edition of *Emergency Care*.

Frank Amato
Assistant Professor
EMT Department Chairman
Indian River Community College
Fort Pierce, FL

Debbie Harris
Director of EMS
Fire and Law Enforcements
Wayne Community College
Goldsboro, NC

Jon F. Levine
Bureau Chief
Boston Emergency Medical Service
Boston, MA

Kathleen A. Riker
Director
Burlington County First Aid Academy
Hainesport, NJ

Holly A. Weber
Co-Director
Stonehearth Open Learning Opportunities
Conway, NH

Brian J. Wilson, NREMT-P
Director of Education
Texas Technical University
El Paso, TX

We also wish to thank the EMS professionals listed below who reviewed the Eighth Edition of *Emergency Care*. They helped to make this program a successful teaching tool.

Marianne J. Barry, MA, EMT-P
Allied Health/Emergency Medical Technology
Lee College
Baytown, TX

F. Anne Beckle, BA, EMT-B
Wyoming Ambulance and EMS Association
Cheyenne, WY

Ken Beers
Program Coordinator/Lecturer
Emergency Medical Services Programs
Monroe Community College
Rochester, NY

Linda Caroll Brumfield, RN, MICN
County of Los Angeles-DHS
Emergency Medical Services Agency
Commerce, CA

Terry Burkley, EMT-P
Methodist Medical Center
Dallas, TX

Nadja Vawryk Button, MS, EMT-P
Etters, PA

Stephen Collins, BS, EMT-P
Instructor—South Tech Fire Academy
Boynton Beach, FL

Patrick R. Coonan, Ed.D, RN, CEN, EMT-CC
Associate Vice President of Patient and Health Services
Episcopal Health Services
Uniondale, NY

Henry B. Dunham, III, EMT-CC, NREMT, CIC
Training Coordinator
Southern Columbia County Ambulance, NY

Lorraine M. Giordano, MD, FACEP
Medical Director
Fire Department
New York, NY

Mike Kennamer
Director of EMS Education
Northeast Alabama State Community College
Rainsville, AL

Kathryn M. Lewis, RN, BSN, PhD
Department Chair
Emergency Medical Technology/Fire Science
Phoenix College
Phoenix, AZ

Steve Moffitt
Alabama Fire College
Program in Emergency Medicine
Shelton State Community College
Tuscaloosa, AL

Joseph E. Peters, Jr. NREMT-P, I/C
Department of EMT
University of Texas Health Science Center
San Antonio, TX

Monte Posner, BS, MSW, EMT-D
Executive Director
Training Institute for Medical Emergencies & Rescue
Staten Island, NY

Thomas J. Rahilly, MS, EMT-CC
Chief Instructor
Nassau County, NY EMS Academy

Captain Michael W. Robinson, MA, NREMT-P
EMS Training Administrator
Baltimore County Fire Department
Towson, MD

Kelly J. Schreiner, NREMT-P
Basic Curriculum Coordinator
Creighton University
Omaha, NE

Michael Tretola, BS, EMT-P
Administrative Coordinator
EMS Institute/Department of Emergency Medicine
Catholic Medical Center of Brooklyn and
Queens, Inc., NY

Douglas H. Warren
Executive Director
Lowcountry Regional EMS Council
Charleston, SC

Paul A. Werfel
Paramedic Program Director
School of Health Technology and Management
Department of Emergency Medicine
State University of New York at Stony Brook

MILITARY REVIEW BOARD

We also wish to thank the members of our Military Review Board for their expert review of the chapter on Military EMS.

Robert A. De Lorenzo, MD, FACEP
Lieut. Colonel, Medical Corps, U.S. Army, Department of Emergency Medicine, Brooke Army Medical Center, Ft. Sam Houston, TX
Associate Clinical Professor of Military and Emergency Medicine, Uniformed Services University of the Health Sciences, Bethesda, MD

Richard Ellis, MSgt, USAF
USAF Emergency Medical Services Program Manager
Sheppard Air Force Base, TX

Jerry L. Mothershead, MD, FACEP
CDR, MC, USN
Special Advisor for Prehospital Care and Emergency Medical Services
Navy Bureau of Medicine and Surgery
Washington, D.C.

Les Painter
HMC (SW/FMF)
Bureau of Medicine and Surgery
Washington, D.C.

PHOTO ACKNOWLEDGMENTS

All photographs not listed below were photographed on assignment for Brady Prentice Hall/Pearson Education.

Charles Stewart MD: 27-06, 27-08a, 27-09a, 27-09b, 27-10a, 27-10b, 27-12a, 27-12b, 27-25b, CO-28, 29-07

Custom Medical Stock/Keith: CO-24

David Handschuh: 3-01, 3-03, 5-04, CO-14, 29-22, CO-30, CO-31, CO-32, CO-34, 34-13

Eddie Sperling: 7-04, 7-08, 7-10, 13-10

In the Dark Photography/Craig Jackson: 1-01, 2-11, 3-07, CO-06, 7-01, 10-01, 13-08, 14-03, 31-09, CO-33

Masterfile/Mark Tomalty: Chapter Feature road

Medichrome/Tom Tracy: CO-12, Chapter Review

Photo Researchers: CO-4 Biophoto Associates, 4-16 Ken Edwards/Science Source, 10-05b Science Photo Library, 18-02b Simon Fraser/Science Photo Library, 18-04b Dr. E. Walker/Science Photo Library, 18-09 Science Photo Library, 22-10a Alan & Sandy Carey, 22-10b C.K. Lorenz, 22-10c Phil A. Dotson, 22-10d Science Photo Library, 26-02a, 26-02b CNRI Science Photo Library, 26-11 Dr. P. Marazzi/Science Photo Library, 27-28 Western Opthalmic Hospital/ Science Photo Library, 31-11 Science Photo Library, 31-12 Biophoto Associates/Science Photo Library

Ralph T. Hutchings: Scan 4-1a-f

Robert Bennett: 7-06

Shout Pictures/John Callan: CO-27

Sygma/Charles H. Porter IV: 2-06

The Stock Market: Chris Collins CO-03, Phillip Wallick CO-07, David Woods CO-10, Lightscapes, Inc. CO-18, Marco Cristofori CO-23, Denis Scott CO-29

Stone/Getty CO-20, CO-26

WorkbookStock/Helen Ashford CO-22

Companies

We wish to thank the following companies for their cooperation in providing us with photos:

Laerdal, Inc.
Medtronic Physio-Control
Redmond, WA

Organizations

We wish to thank the following organizations for their assistance in creating the photo program for the Ninth Edition.

Chief Gustave Pappas
Fire Department New York
Bureau of Training
Bayside, NY

Chief Brian Gorski, Captain Paul Dezzi
Sarasota County Fire Department
Sarasota, FL

Conrad T. Kearns, EMTP
Pinellas County EMS
Largo, FL

Sunstar Ambulance Service, Pinellas County, FL

Technical Advisors

Thanks to the following people for providing technical support during the photo shoots:

Captain Paul Dezzi, Sarasota County Fire Department

Chief Gustave Pappas, Fire Department New York, Bureau of Training

Emergency Care ninth edition

THE CONTENT YOU *TRUST*

For over 30 years, **Emergency Care** has set the standard for EMT-B training. In fact, nearly 1.6 million students have passed the National Registry and state exams using **Emergency Care**—more than any other text on the market. Brady continues this tradition of publishing excellence with the Ninth Edition—*providing the content you trust and the innovation you need.* The new edition has been revised to meet the needs of today's students—helping them to prepare for any emergency. Two new chapters have been added to help you "put it all together" for both medical and trauma emergencies. From case studies to practical field tips to outstanding multimedia support, **Emergency Care** engages students—helping them achieve career success in a demanding field.

THE INNOVATION YOU *NEED*

In today's fast-paced learning environment, training takes place beyond the printed page. **Emergency Care's** rich multimedia package expands upon the book content to provide interactive learning opportunities.

Electronic Extras **Student CD-ROM** (0-13-032421-3) includes 30 minutes of patient assessment video footage, expansions of the in-text *How and Why* student feature, vocabulary-building games and puzzles, both an English and a Spanish audio-glossary, National Registry Skill Sheets, and trauma photos.

Companion Website (www.bradybooks.com/emergencycare) contains chapter-by-chapter interactive review quizzes with immediate scoring and feedback, message boards, annotated links to appropriate EMS resources, and a Syllabus Manager for instructors.

Setting the standard for instructor's resources! *Emergency Care* **has a comprehensive Teaching/Learning Package** that includes a *Test Manager* which provides you with the capability for online testing, an improved text-specific *PowerPoint presentation,* an *Instructor's Resource Manual,* a *printed test-item-file,* and an online *Syllabus Manager* located on the Companion Website.

When it comes to EMT-B training, nothing beats *Emergency Care's* full range of multimedia support.

Companion Website

www.bradybooks.com/emergencycare

▲ **Activities** – Text-specific links and activities that correspond to end-of-chapter material in the text.

▲ **Syllabus Manager** – Online aid for instructors who wish to post course syllabi and assignments on the web for easy student access.

▲ **Links** – Annotated links to useful EMS sites.

▲ **Message boards** – Students and instructors can post messages, respond to questions, and conduct ongoing discussions.

▲ **Interactive student quizzes** provide chapter-by-chapter questions with immediate feedback to help students master the necessary concepts to be an effective EMT.

Electronic Extras Student CD-ROM

This useful multimedia tool brings an added dimension to your students' learning experience with interactive case studies, realistic patient assessment video footage, quizzes, and games.

▲ **Browser-based interface:** Allows students to access the CD using familiar commands and programs, such as Netscape or Internet Explorer. No learning curve—they can jump right in!

▲ **Patient Assessment Video:** 30-minute video segment provides valuable assessment training reinforcement with critical thinking questions and activities.

▲ **Vocabulary Games:** Engaging puzzles— including crosswords and word searches—are a fun way for students to practice their mastery of EMS language.

See why BRADY is the Leader in Technology!

Check www.bradybooks.com for the latest information on our products as well as additional content to reinforce learning.

Case Study Simulations

Interactive online case studies at www.bradybooks.com allow students to fully assess and treat the situation and patient just like in a real-life setting. Students receive points for assessing and treating correctly, and lose points for incorrect actions.

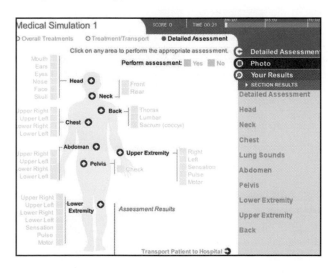

Case studies don't get any more realistic than this.

Medical Emergency Response Simulator (MERS)

Brady's *Medical Emergency Response Simulator* (ISBN 0-13-089857-0) contains over a dozen different "calls," providing you with truly interactive scenarios so your students can practice the decision making skills they need to master to become a top-notch EMT. Students can practice critical EMT skills including scene size-up, patient assessment, treatment and transport decisions, and proper call documentation. A complete product demo is available at www.bradybooks.com.

HALLMARK FEATURES

Strong Patient Assessment Coverage

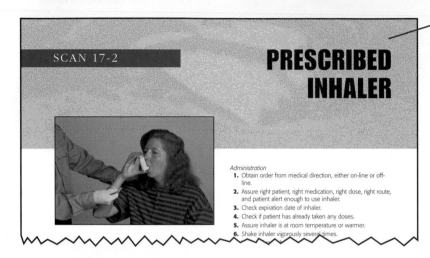

SCAN 17-2

PRESCRIBED INHALER

Administration

1. Obtain order from medical direction, either on-line or off-line.
2. Assure right patient, right medication, right dose, right route, and patient alert enough to use inhaler.
3. Check expiration date of inhaler.
4. Check if patient has already taken any doses.
5. Assure inhaler is at room temperature or warmer.
6. Shake inhaler vigorously several times.

▲ **Scans.** Key information and step-by-step procedures are summarized and presented for easy reference in illustrated Scans. Medication Scans give students all the information they need to administer or help administer medications. Procedure Scans list and describe the steps in performing particular procedures.

▲ **Patient Assessment and Patient Care.** *Patient Assessment* and *Patient Care* segments provide additional resources for students learning this difficult concept and describe the assessment and treatment you should provide for particular types of patients, disorders, or injuries. *Patient Assessment* typically lists the important signs and symptoms. *Patient Care* lists the key steps of EMT-B emergency care.

Figure 17-3 A patient with chronic obstructive pulmonary disease (COPD).

Patient CARE

Breathing Difficulty

When a patient is suffering from breathing difficulty, provide the following care:

• *Assessment.* Assess the airway during the initial assessment and then frequently throughout the call. Assist respiration with artificial ventilations and supplemental oxygen whenever the patient has or develops inadequate breathing.

• *Oxygen.* Oxygen is the main treatment for any patient in respiratory difficulty. If the patient is breathing adequately, use a nonrebreather mask at 12 to 15 liters per minute to provide oxygen.

You may hear from other EMT-Bs that oxygen must be administered to some patients with caution—or not at all. This is because of a condition sometimes called the *hypoxic drive.* (You read about hypoxic drive in Chapter 6.) This occurs in a few patients who have lung diseases such as emphysema or chronic bronchitis. For

How AND Why?

Not all inhalers are designed to help respiratory distress. Some inhalers are prescribed steroids or other medications, which will not help the patient in respiratory distress right away. Go to your Electronic Extras CD for more information.

ENRICHMENT ABOVE AND BEYOND THE D.O.T.

RESPIRATORY DISEASES

It is not necessary to diagnose a patient's condition to provide effective treatment as an EMT-B. In fact, the care for all respiratory conditions is essentially the same, as described earlier in this chapter. The information that follows on chronic obstructive pulmonary diseases (Figure 17-3) and asthma is provided to enrich your knowledge of respiratory diseases.

Chronic Obstructive Pulmonary Disease (COPD)

Emphysema—as well as chronic bronchitis, black lung, and many undetermined respiratory illnesses that cause the patient problems like those seen in emphysema—are all classified as chronic obstructive pulmonary disease (COPD).

COPD is mainly a problem of end-

in the bronchioles that normally clear away accumulations of mucus are not able to do so. The sweeping apparatus on these cells, the cilia, have been damaged or destroyed.

In emphysema, the walls of the alveoli break down, greatly reducing the surface area for respiratory exchange. The lungs begin to lose elasticity. These factors combine to allow stale air laden with carbon dioxide to be trapped in the lungs, reducing the effectiveness of normal breathing efforts.

Many COPD patients will exhibit characteristics of both emphysema and chronic bronchitis. Usually the reason a COPD patient calls the ambulance is that a recent upper respiratory infection has caused an acute worsening of the disease.

A very few COPD patients develop a hypoxic drive to trigger respirations. In patients without COPD, the brain determines when to breathe based on increased levels of carbon dioxide in the blood. Since COPD patients develop a tol-

ministration. If the patient has a possible heart attack or stroke, is developing shock, or has respiratory distress, a higher concentration of oxygen will be required in spite of the potential problems. *If oxygen is required by the COPD patient, do not withhold it.*

Constantly monitor the patient. If the patient's breathing becomes inadequate or stops, be prepared to assist respirations through artificial ventilation, and contact medical direction.

Asthma

Seen in young and old patients alike, asthma is an episodic disease (a disease that only affects the patient at irregular intervals). This is far different from chronic bronchitis and emphysema, both of which afflict the patient continually. Asthma also differs from chronic bronchitis and emphysema in that it does not produce a hypoxic drive. Although the disease is episodic, an asthma attack can be life

▲ **FYI.** Some segments of information are marked "FYI", "for your information." These include material that goes beyond the DOT objectives to broaden students' understanding of the chapter topic.

... New to this Edition

Prescribed inhalers can help patients in respiratory distress. The proper delivery of these medications is not an easy task—especially when a patient is not calm! Go to your Electronic Extras CD for more information.

▲ **How and Why?** This feature brings attention to additional background material that students will find helpful and interesting. Students can find even more information about the "Hows and Whys" on the CD-ROM that is packaged with the *Emergency Care* textbook.

▲ **Pediatric Notes** help students be prepared to deal with stressful pediatric calls by describing what is different or special in infants and children with regard to the chapter topic and giving students directions as to how they should deal with those differences.

▲ **Documentation Tips** explain or remind students of important information to write on their prehospital care reports.

▲ **Safety Notes** appear throughout the book as needed to point out situations where students need to take special precautions.

STUDENT REINFORCEMENT AT EVERY TURN

Students have found success with *Emergency Care* because we have always kept their needs paramount. The **NINTH EDITION** continues this tradition with a wide range of review content.

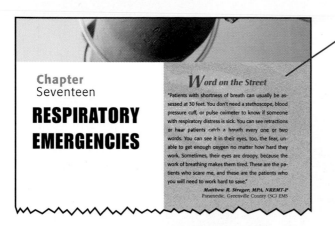

Chapter
Seventeen

RESPIRATORY EMERGENCIES

Word on the Street

"Patients with shortness of breath can usually be assessed at 30 feet. You don't need a stethoscope, blood pressure cuff, or pulse oximeter to know if someone with respiratory distress is sick. You can see retractions or hear patients catch a breath every one or two words. You can see it in their eyes, too, the fear, unable to get enough oxygen no matter how hard they work. Sometimes, their eyes are droopy, because the work of breathing makes them tired. These are the patients who scare me, and these are the patients who you will need to work hard to save."

Matthew R. Streger, MPA, NREMT-P
Paramedic, Greenville County (SC) EMS

▲ Word on the Street. Each chapter opens with a comment or insight relevant to the chapter topic from an experienced EMS provider to get students interested in the chapter material as well as to show them a real-world glimpse of the profession.

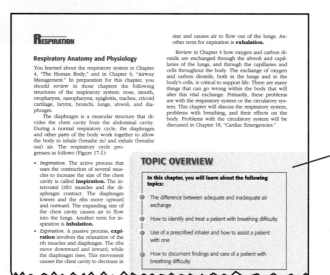

RESPIRATION

Respiratory Anatomy and Physiology

You learned about the respiratory system in Chapter 4, "The Human Body," and in Chapter 6, "Airway Management." In preparation for this chapter, you should review in those chapters the following structures of the respiratory system: nose, mouth, oropharynx, nasopharynx, epiglottis, trachea, cricoid cartilage, larynx, bronchi, lungs, alveoli, and diaphragm.

The diaphragm is a muscular structure that divides the chest cavity from the abdominal cavity. During a normal respiratory cycle, the diaphragm and other parts of the body work together to allow the body to inhale (breathe in) and exhale (breathe out) air. The respiratory cycle progresses as follows (Figure 17-1):

• *Inspiration.* The active process that uses the contraction of several muscles to increase the size of the chest cavity is called **inspiration.** The intercostal (rib) muscles and the diaphragm contract. The diaphragm lowers and the ribs move upward and outward. The expanding size of the chest cavity causes air to flow into the lungs. Another term for inspiration is **inhalation.**

• *Expiration.* A passive process, **expiration** involves the relaxation of the rib muscles and diaphragm. The ribs move downward and inward, while the diaphragm rises. This movement causes the chest cavity to decrease in

size and causes air to flow out of the lungs. Another term for expiration is **exhalation.**

Review in Chapter 4 how oxygen and carbon dioxide are exchanged through the alveoli and capillaries of the lungs, and through the capillaries and cells throughout the body. The exchange of oxygen and carbon dioxide, both in the lungs and in the body's cells, is critical to support life. There are many things that can go wrong within the body that will alter this vital exchange. Primarily, these problems are with the respiratory system or the circulatory system. This chapter will discuss the respiratory system, problems with breathing, and their effects on the body. Problems with the circulatory system will be discussed in Chapter 18, "Cardiac Emergencies."

TOPIC OVERVIEW

In this chapter, you will learn about the following topics:

● The difference between adequate and inadequate air exchange

● How to identify and treat a patient with breathing difficulty

● Use of a prescribed inhaler and how to assist a patient with one

● How to document findings and care of a patient with breathing difficulty

▲ Topic Overview. This built-in study aid contains key points from the chapter to help students anticipate chapter content and guide their reading and studies.

Street Scenes and Sample Documentation. *Street Scenes* are designed to help students integrate all the information they have learned so far. You can find the answers to the questions right inside these real-life "calls." Some chapters also include filled-out Sample Documentation with handwritten reports of the *Street Scene* for the chapter.

Study Guides. This feature provides lists, mnemonics, and summaries of key information for quick reference and review.

BUILT-IN REVIEW AND PRACTICE

CHAPTER REVIEW

SUMMARY

Respiratory emergencies are common calls that require diligent assessment, care, and emotional support. It is very important to evaluate your patient for adequate breathing throughout the call. If at any time you find breathing inadequate, you must assist ventilations. Providing artificial ventilation to a patient promptly may prevent him from slipping into respiratory arrest—and death!

For a patient who is experiencing difficulty breathing but whose breathing is adequate, administration of high-concentration oxygen by nonrebreather mask, coaching the patient in the use of a prescribed inhaler if the patient has one, placing the patient in a position of comfort, and providing reassurance are the key treatments the EMT-B can provide.

KEY TERMS

bronchoconstriction constriction, or blockage, of the bronchi that lead from the trachea to the lungs.
exhalation (EX-huh-LAY-shun) another term for expiration.
expiration (EK-spuh-RAY-shun) a passive process in which the intercostal (rib) muscles and the diaphragm relax, causing the chest cavity to decrease in size and forcing air from the lungs.

inhalation (IN-huh-LAY-shun) another term for inspiration.
inspiration (IN-spuh-RAY-shun) an active process in which the intercostal (rib) muscles and the diaphragm contract, expanding the size of the chest cavity and causing air to flow into the lungs.

REVIEW QUESTIONS

1. List the normal rates of breathing for adults, children, and infants. List the other signs of adequate breathing. (pp. 322, 323)
2. List the signs of inadequate breathing. (pp. 323–324)
3. Explain the treatment you will give, as an EMT-B, when a patient's breathing is inadequate. (pp. 324, 325)
4. List the signs and symptoms of breathing difficulty. (p. 326)
5. Explain the treatments you may give, as an EMT-B, for breathing difficulty when breathing is adequate. (p. 327)
6. Explain the steps to follow before, during, and after helping a patient to use a prescribed inhaler. (pp. 329–331)
7. List some differences between adult and infant/child respiratory systems. (p. 324)
8. List some special considerations in the assessment and treatment of infants and children with respiratory problems. (pp. 324, 325)

334 Chapter 17 • *Respiratory Emergencies*

The **Summary** provides students with a concise review of important chapter information.

Key Terms list all terms that appear in bold type in the chapter with their definitions.

Review Questions ask students to recall certain information and to apply the principles they learned.

Application Questions require students to think on a higher level and apply chapter learning to new situations. Answers to both the Review Questions and the Applications may be found on the textbook pages noted at the end of each question. Answers also appear in the *Instructor's Resource Manual*.

Web Medic. At the end of each chapter, the Web Medic opens the opportunities of the World Wide Web for students and provides ideas for further exploration of chapter-related topics.

Additional Student Resources

- *Electronic Extras CD-ROM* (0-13-032421-3) contains case studies, patient assessment video footage, quizzes, games, and more.
- **Companion Website** (www.bradybooks.com/emergencycare) This online study guide contains chapter-by-chapter review quizzes with immediate scoring and feedback, message boards, annotated links, and a Syllabus Manager for instructors.
- **Student Workbook** (0-13-031951-1) Designed to accompany *Emergency Care 9e*, this workbook includes multiple-choice, fill-in-the-blank, and labeling questions, case studies, answer key with page references, and National Registry Skill Sheets. This is the perfect accompaniment to the text for any serious student!
- **EMT-B Computerized Student Review** (0-8359-5205-3) This IBM-compatible review software covers all major DOT topics with 750 multiple choice, fill-in-the blank, and True/False questions. Each correct answer is followed by a rationale to help students understand why the answer is correct.
- **MedEMT CD-ROM** (Individual Version 0-8385-6368-6) (Institutional Version 0-8385-6402-X) This CD-ROM offers student videos and quizzes.

THE MOST COMPLETE PACKAGE AVAILABLE

- **Instructor's Resource Manual** (0-13-031952-X) Available both on disk and in print, this valuable resource contains lesson plans, lecture outlines, student activities, list of additional resources, answers to student handouts, and more.

- **Custom Test Manager** (WIN 0-13-031940-6) (MAC 0-13-0132422-1) This test bank contains 1200 text-specific questions on disk in a customizable format that allows instructors to construct and administer online tests. An electronic gradebook is also included.

- **Test Item File** (0-13-031953-8) A printed version of the test questions from the computerized test item file.

- **CD-ROM with PowerPoint slides** (0-13-091302-2) This CD-ROM contains approximately 1800 slides with text and images in PowerPoint. These slides can be customized and changed to suit individual classroom needs.

- **35-mm Slides** (0-13-091303-0) Approximately 1800 slides coordinated with the text in traditional 35-mm format.

- **Anatomy & Physiology Color Acetates** (0-8359-5203-7) This set contains 41 acetates with 88 overlays to form multiple transparent layers that allow anatomical systems to be viewed at various depths and levels.

- **MedArt** (Win 0-8385-6366-X) (Mac 0-8385- 0594-5) This CD-ROM contains EMS and medical clip art.

Emergency Care
ninth edition

**THE
ROAD
TO
SUCCESS**

Emergency Care

Care

ninth
edition

Chapter One

INTRODUCTION TO EMERGENCY MEDICAL CARE

When a person is injured or becomes ill, it rarely happens in a hospital with doctors and nurses standing by. In fact, some time usually passes between the onset of the injury or illness and the patient's arrival at the hospital, time in which the patient's condition may deteriorate, time in which the patient may even die. The modern Emergency Medical Services (EMS) system has been developed to provide what is known as "prehospital" or "out-of-hospital" care. Its purpose is to get trained personnel to the patient as quickly as possible and to provide emergency care on the scene, en route to the hospital, and at the hospital. The Emergency Medical Technician-Basic (EMT-B) is a key member of the EMS team.

As you begin to study for a career as an EMT-B, you will want to answer some basic questions, such as: What is the EMS system? How did it develop? And what will be your role in the system? This chapter will help you begin to answer these questions.

THE EMERGENCY MEDICAL SERVICES SYSTEM

How It Began

In the 1790s, the French began to transport wounded soldiers away from the scene of battle so they could be cared for by physicians. This is the earliest documented emergency medical service. No medical care was provided for the wounded on the battlefield. The idea was simply to carry the victim from the scene to a place where medical care was available.

Other wars inspired similar emergency services. For example, during the American Civil War, Clara Barton began such a service for the wounded and later helped establish the American Red Cross. During World War I, many volunteers joined battlefield ambulance corps. And during the Korean Conflict and the Vietnam War, medical teams produced further advances in field care, many of which led to advances in the civilian sector, including specialized emergency medical centers devoted to the treatment of trauma (injuries).

Non-military ambulance services began in some major American cities in the early 1900s—again as transport services only, offering little or no emergency care. Smaller communities did not develop ambulance services until the late 1940s, after World War II. Often the local undertaker provided a hearse for ambulance transport. Where emergency care was offered along with transport to the hospital, the fire service often was the responsible agency.

The importance of providing hospital-quality care at the emergency scene—that is, beginning care at the scene and continuing it, uninterrupted, during transport to the hospital—soon became apparent. The need to organize systems for such emergency prehospital care and to train personnel to provide it also was recognized.

EMS Today

During the 1960s, the development of the modern Emergency Medical Services (EMS) system began. In 1966 the National Highway Safety Act charged the United States Department of Transportation (DOT) with developing EMS standards and assisting the states to upgrade the quality of their prehospital emergency care. Most EMT-B courses today are based on models developed by the DOT.

In 1970, the National Registry of Emergency Medical Technicians was founded to establish professional standards. In 1973, Congress passed the National Emergency Medical Services Systems Act as the cornerstone of a federal effort to implement and improve EMS systems across the United States.

TOPIC OVERVIEW

In this chapter, you will learn about the following topics:

- The chain of human resources that forms the EMS system

- How the public activates the EMS system

- Your roles and responsibilities as an EMT-Basic

- The process of EMS quality improvement (QI)

✔ **Knowledge and Attitude**

1. Define Emergency Medical Services (EMS) systems. (pp. 3–4)

2. Differentiate the roles and responsibilities of the EMT-Basic from other prehospital care providers. (pp. 6–7)

3. Describe the roles and responsibilities related to personal safety. (p. 7)

4. Discuss the roles and responsibilities of the EMT-Basic towards the safety of the crew, the patient, and bystanders. (p. 7)

5. Define quality improvement, and discuss the EMT-Basic's role in the process. (pp. 9–10)

6. Define medical direction, and discuss the EMT-Basic's role in the process. (pp. 11–12)

7. State the specific statutes and regulations in your state regarding the EMS system. (p. 12)

8. Assess areas of personal attitude and conduct of the EMT-Basic. (pp. 8–9)

9. Characterize the various methods used to access the EMS system in your community. (pp. 5–6)

Since then, the states have gained more control over their EMS systems, but the federal government continues to provide guidance and support. For example, the National Highway Traffic Safety Administration (NHTSA) Technical Assistance Program has established an assessment program with a set of standards for EMS systems. The categories and standards set forth by NHTSA, summarized below, will be discussed in more detail throughout this chapter and the rest of this textbook.

- *Regulation and policy.* Each state EMS system must have in place enabling legislation (laws that allow the system to exist), a lead EMS agency, a funding mechanism, regulations, policies, and procedures.
- *Resource management.* There must be centralized coordination of resources so that all victims of trauma or medical emergencies have equal access to basic emergency care and transport by certified personnel, in a licensed and equipped ambulance, to an appropriate facility.
- *Human resources and training.* At a minimum, all transporting prehospital personnel (those who ride the ambulances) should be trained to the EMT-Basic level using a standardized curriculum taught by qualified instructors.
- *Transportation.* Safe, reliable ambulance transportation is a critical component. Most patients can be effectively transported by ground ambulances. Other patients require rapid transportation, or transportation from remote areas, by helicopter or airplane.
- *Facilities.* The seriously ill or injured patient must be delivered in a timely manner to the closest appropriate facility.
- *Communications.* There must be an effective communications system, beginning with the universal system access number (9-1-1), dispatch-to-ambulance, ambulance-to-ambulance, ambulance-to-hospital, and hospital-to-hospital communications.
- *Public information and education.* EMS personnel may participate in efforts to educate the public about their role in the system, their ability to access the system, and prevention of injuries.
- *Medical direction.* Each EMS system must have a physician as a medical director accountable for the activities of EMS personnel within that system. The medical director delegates medical practice to nonphysician providers (such as EMT-Bs) and must be involved in all aspects of the patient care system.
- *Trauma systems.* In each state, enabling legislation must exist to develop a trauma system including one or more trauma centers, triage and transfer guidelines for trauma patients, rehabilitation programs, data collection, mandatory autopsies (examination of bodies to determine cause of death), and means for managing and assuring the quality of the system.
- *Evaluation.* Each state must have a program for evaluating and improving the effectiveness of the EMS system, known as a quality improvement (QI) program, a quality assurance (QA) program, or total quality management (TQM).

With the development of the modern Emergency Medical Services (EMS) system, the concept of ambulance service as a means merely for transporting the sick and injured passed into oblivion. No longer could ambulance personnel be viewed as people with little more than the strength to lift a victim in and out of an ambulance. The hospital emergency department was extended, through the EMS system, to reach the sick and injured at the emergency scene. "Victims" became patients, receiving prehospital assessment and emergency care from highly trained professionals. The "ambulance attendant" was replaced by the Emergency Medical Technician (EMT).

A current development in some areas is use of the term "out-of-hospital care," rather than "prehospital care," as EMS personnel begin to provide primary care for some conditions and in some circumstances without transport to a hospital. However, the term "prehospital care" will be used in the remainder of this text (Figure 1-1).

Figure 1-1 New methods of delivering EMS services.

COMPONENTS OF THE EMS SYSTEM

To understand the EMS system, you must look at it from the view of the patient rather than from that of the EMT-B (Figure 1-2). For the patient, care begins with the initial phone call to the Emergency Medical Dispatcher (EMD). The EMS system responds to the call for help by sending to the scene available responders, including First Responders, EMT-Basics, and advanced life support providers (EMT-Intermediates and EMT-Paramedics). An ambulance will transport the patient to the hospital.

From the ambulance, the patient is received by the Emergency Department. There the patient receives laboratory tests, diagnosis, and further treatment. The Emergency Department serves as the gateway for the rest of the services offered by the hospital. If a patient is brought to the Emergency Department with serious injuries, care is given to stabilize the patient, and the operating room is readied to provide further life-saving measures.

Study Guide for Specialty Hospitals

✔ Trauma centers
✔ Burn centers
✔ Pediatric centers
✔ Poison control centers

Some hospitals handle all routine and emergency cases but have a specialty that sets them apart from other hospitals. One specialty hospital is the trauma center. In some hospitals, a surgery team may not be available at all times. In a trauma center, surgery teams are available 24 hours a day.

In addition to trauma centers, there are also hospitals that specialize in the care of certain conditions and patients, such as burn centers, pediatric centers, and poison control centers.

As an EMT-B, you will become familiar with the hospital resources available in your area. Many EMS regions have specific criteria for transporting patients with special needs. It is important to weigh the condition of the patient against the additional transport time that may be required to take him to a specialized facility. On-line medical direction (see page 11) may be available to help with this decision.

First Responders, EMT-Bs, and dispatchers are key members of the prehospital EMS team. Many others make up the hospital portion of the EMS system. They include physicians, nurses, physician's assistants, respiratory and physical therapists, technicians, aides, and others.

On-line medical direction (see page 11)

How and Why?

Many years ago, the "dispatcher" was an untrained person (sometimes the local mortician) who simply answered the phone. Today the emergency medical dispatcher (EMD) is a trained professional who provides emergency medical advice, including CPR instructions, over the phone. Go to your Electronic Extras CD to find out more about the EMD.

Accessing the EMS System

Many localities have a **9-1-1 system** for telephone access to report emergencies. A dispatcher answers the call, takes the information, and alerts EMS or the fire or police departments as needed. Still other localities are in the process of implementing the system. Since the number 9-1-1 is designed to be a national emergency number, there will be a time when 9-1-1 may be dialed from any phone in the country to be connected to the appropriate emergency center.

Some communications centers have enhanced 9-1-1. This system has the capability of automati-

| Patient | A citizen calls 9-1-1. | 9-1-1 dispatcher | First Responders |

Figure 1-2 The chain of human resources that make up the EMS system.

cally identifying the caller's phone number and location. If the phone is disconnected or the patient loses consciousness, the dispatcher will still be able to send emergency personnel to the scene.

Some communities do not have 9-1-1 systems. In these locations, a standard seven-digit telephone number must be dialed to reach ambulance, fire, or police services. Dialing 9-1-1 where a 9-1-1 system is not in operation will usually connect the caller to an operator who will attempt to route the call to the appropriate dispatch center. This adds an extra step and extra time to the process, so it is important to make sure that the emergency numbers in use in a local area are prominently displayed on all telephones.

Another development in the communication and dispatch portion of the EMS system is the training and certification of Emergency Medical Dispatchers (EMDs). These specially trained dispatchers not only obtain the appropriate information from callers, they also provide medical instructions for emergency care. These include instructions for CPR, artificial ventilation, bleeding control, and more. Research has consistently pointed to the importance of early access and prompt initiation of emergency care and CPR. The Emergency Medical Dispatcher is one example of the EMS system providing emergency care at the earliest possible moment.

Levels of EMS Training

There are four general levels of EMS training and certification (described below). These levels vary from place to place. Your instructor will explain any variations that may exist in your region or state.

- *First Responder.* This level of training is designed for the person who is often first at the scene. Many police officers, firefighters, and industrial health personnel are certified EMS First Responders. The emphasis is on activating the EMS system and providing immediate care for life-threatening injuries,

controlling the scene, and preparing for the arrival of the ambulance.

- *EMT-Basic.* In most areas, the EMT-Basic, or EMT-B, is considered the minimum level of certification for ambulance personnel. Certification as an EMT-B requires successful completion of the U.S. DOT's EMT-Basic National Standard Training Program or its equivalent and approval by a state emergency medical services program or other authorized agency. The curriculum for the EMT-B deals with the assessment and care of the ill or injured patient. EMT-Basic is the level of certification for which this textbook and the course you are now taking are intended to help you prepare.

HOW AND WHY?

In your career, you will work with EMS First Responders, EMT-Intermediates, and EMT-Paramedics. Go to your Electronic Extras CD to find out how similar or how different their knowledge and training is from yours.

- *EMT-Intermediate.* This EMT has passed specific additional training programs in order to provide some level of advanced life support, such as the initiation of IV (intravenous) lines, advanced airway techniques, and administration of some medications beyond those the EMT-B is permitted to administer. In some states, this level includes those EMTs who are given the title of Shock-Trauma Technician or Critical Care Technician.

- *EMT-Paramedic.* Paramedic training includes or equals the U.S. DOT's National Standard Paramedic Curriculum. Paramedics can generally perform relatively invasive field care, including insertion of endotracheal tubes, initiation of IV lines, administration of a variety of medications, interpretation of electrocardiograms, and cardiac defibrillation. Although some of these kinds of procedures are now

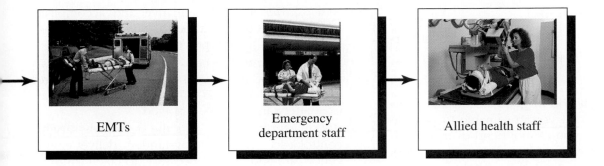

EMTs   Emergency   Allied health staff
              department staff

performed by basic- and intermediate-level EMTs in many areas, the EMT-P may perform such procedures on a more advanced level.

Roles and Responsibilities of the EMT-B

As an EMT-B, you will be responsible for a wide range of activities. In addition to patient assessment and emergency care, your responsibilities will include preparation, a safe response to the scene, safe transportation to the hospital, and transferring the patient to hospital personnel for continuity of care. The following are specific areas of responsibility for the EMT-B.

- *Personal safety.* It is not possible to help a patient if you are injured before you reach him or while you are providing care, so *your first responsibility is to keep yourself safe.* Safety concerns include dangers from other human beings, animals, unstable buildings, fires, explosions, and more. Though emergency scenes are usually safe, they also can be unpredictable. You must take care at all times to stay safe.

- *Safety of the crew, patient, and bystanders.* The same dangers you face will also be faced by others at the scene. As a professional, you must be concerned with their safety as well as your own.

- *Patient assessment.* As an EMT-B, one of your most important functions will be assessment of your patient, or finding out enough about what is wrong with your patient to be able to provide the appropriate emergency care. Assessment always precedes emergency care.

- *Patient care.* The actual care required for an individual patient may range from simple emotional support to life-saving CPR and defibrillation. Based on your assessment findings, patient care is an action or series of actions that your training will prepare you to take in order to help the patient deal with and survive his illness or injury.

- *Lifting and moving.* Since EMT-Bs are usually involved in transporting patients to the hospital, lifting and moving patients are important tasks. You must perform them without injury to yourself and without aggravating or adding to the patient's existing injuries.

- *Transport.* It is a serious responsibility to operate an ambulance at any time, but even more so when there is a patient on board. Safe operation of the ambulance, as well as securing and caring for the patient in the ambulance, will be important parts of your job as an EMT-B.

- *Transfer of care.* Upon arrival at the hospital, you will turn the patient over to hospital personnel. You will provide information on the patient's condition, your observations of the scene, and other pertinent data so that there will be continuity in the care of the patient. Although this part of patient care comes at the end of the call, it is very important. You must never abandon care of the patient at the hospital until transfer to hospital personnel has been properly completed.

- *Patient advocacy.* As an EMT-B, you are there for your patient. You are an advocate, the person who speaks up for your patient and pleads his cause. It is your responsibility to address the patient's needs and to bring any of his concerns to the attention of the hospital staff. You will have developed a rapport with the patient during your brief but very important time together, a rapport that gives you an understanding of his condition and needs. As an advocate, you will do your best to transmit this knowledge in order to help the patient continue through the EMS and hospital system. In your role as an advocate you may perform a task as important as reporting information that will enable the hospital staff to save the patient's life—or as simple as making sure a relative of the patient is notified. Acts that may seem minor to you may often provide major comfort to your patient.

Traits of a Good EMT-B

There are certain physical traits and aspects of personality that are desirable for an EMT-B.

Physical Traits

Physically, you should be in good health and fit to carry out your duties. If you are unable to provide needed care because you cannot bend over or catch your breath, then all your training may be worthless to the patient who is in need of your help.

You should be able to lift and carry up to 125 pounds. Practice with other EMT-Bs is essential so that you can learn how to carry your share of the combined weight of patient, stretcher, linens, blankets, and portable oxygen equipment. For such moves, coordination and dexterity are needed, as well as strength. You will have to perform basic rescue procedures, lower stretchers and patients from upper levels, and negotiate fire escapes and stairways while carrying patients.

Your eyesight is very important in performing your EMT-B duties. Make certain that you can clearly see distant objects as well as those close at hand. Both types of vision are needed for patient assessment, reading labels, controlling emergency scenes, and driving. Should you have any eyesight problems, they must be corrected with prescription eyeglasses or contact lenses.

Be aware of any problems you may have with color vision. Not only is this important to driving, but it could also be critical for patient assessment. Colors seen on the patient's skin, lips, and nail beds often provide valuable clues to the patient's condition.

You should be able to give and receive oral and written instructions and communicate with the patient, bystanders, and other members of the EMS system. Eyesight, hearing, and speech are important to the EMT-B; thus, any significant problems must be corrected if you are going to be an EMT-B.

Personal Traits

Good personality traits are very important to the EMT-B (Figure 1-3). You should be:

- *Pleasant* to inspire confidence and help to calm the sick and injured.
- *Sincere* to be able to convey an understanding of the situation and the patient's feelings
- *Cooperative* to allow for faster and better care, establish better coordination with other members of the EMS system, and bolster the confidence of patients and bystanders
- *Resourceful* to be able to adapt a tool or technique to fit an unusual situation

- *A self-starter* to show initiative and accomplish what must be done without having to depend on someone else to start procedures
- *Emotionally stable* to help overcome the unpleasant aspects of an emergency so that needed care may be rendered and any uneasy feelings that exist afterwards may be resolved
- *Able to lead* in order to take the steps necessary to control a scene, organize bystanders, deliver emergency care and, when necessary, to take charge
- *Neat and clean* to promote confidence in both patients and bystanders and to reduce the possibility of contamination
- *Of good moral character and respectful of others* to allow for trust in situations when the patient cannot protect his own body or valuables and so that all information relayed is truthful and reliable
- *In control of personal habits* to reduce the possibility of rendering improper care and to prevent discomfort to the patient. This includes never consuming alcohol within eight hours of duty and not smoking when providing care. (Remember: smoking can contaminate wounds and it is a danger around oxygen delivery systems.)
- *Controlled in conversation and able to communicate properly* in order to inspire confidence and avoid inappropriate conversation that may upset or anger the patient or bystanders or violate patient confidentiality
- *Able to listen to others* to be compassionate and empathetic, to be accurate with interviews, and to inspire confidence

Figure 1-3 A professional appearance inspires confidence.

Education

An EMT-B must also maintain up-to-date knowledge and skills. Since ongoing research in emergency care causes occasional changes in procedure, some of the information you receive while you are studying to become an EMT-B will become out of date during your career. There are many ways to stay current.

One way to stay current is through refresher training. Most areas require recertification at regular intervals. Refresher courses present material to the EMT-B who has already been through a full course but needs to receive updated information. Refresher courses are usually shorter than original courses. They are required at two- to four-year intervals.

Continuing education is another way to stay current. This type of training supplements the EMT-B's original course. It should not take the place of original training. For example, you may wish to learn more about pediatric or trauma skills or driving techniques. You can obtain this education in conferences and seminars, and through lectures, classes, videos, or demonstrations.

It is important for you to realize that training is a constant process that extends long past your original EMT-B course.

National Registry of Emergency Medical Technicians

The National Registry of Emergency Medical Technicians (NREMT), as part of its effort to establish and maintain national standards for EMTs, provides registration to First Responders, EMT-Basics, EMT-Intermediates, and EMT-Paramedics. Registration is obtained by successfully completing NREMT practical and written examinations. Holding an NREMT registration may help in reciprocity (transferring to another state or region). It is usually considered favorably when you apply for employment, even in areas where NREMT registration is not required.

Many states use the National Registry examinations as their certification exams. If your state or region does not use the registry exam, ask your instructor how you can sit for the examination. Upon passing the exam and obtaining registry, you will be entitled to wear the NREMT-Basic patch (Figure 1-4).

The National Registry is also active in EMS curriculum development and other issues that affect EMS today. For information, contact:

National Registry of Emergency Medical Technicians
6610 Busch Boulevard, P.O. Box 29233
Columbus, OH 43229
614-888-4484

Figure 1-4 The NREMT-Basic patch.

Quality Improvement

Quality improvement is an important concept in EMS. It consists of continuous self-review with the purpose of identifying aspects of the system that require improvement. Once a problem is identified, a plan is developed and implemented to prevent further occurrences of the same problem. As implied by the name, quality improvement is designed and performed to assure that the public receives the highest quality prehospital care.

A sample quality improvement review might go as follows:

As part of a continuous review of calls, the Quality Improvement (QI) committee has reviewed all of your squad's run reports that involve trauma during one particular month. The committee has noted that the time spent at the scene of serious trauma calls was excessive. (You will learn later that time at the scene of serious trauma should be kept to a minimum, because the injured patient must be transported to the hospital for care that cannot be provided in the field.)

The QI committee has brought this fact to the attention of the medical director and the leadership of the ambulance squad. As a result, better protocols have been instituted. Monthly squad training is developed that covers topics such as how to identify serious trauma patients and then requires skill practice to reinforce techniques of trauma care. (Later in the year, the QI committee will review the same criteria to assure that the extra training has been effective in improving the areas that were found to be deficient.)

During the review, the QI committee has also identified calls during which the crews followed procedures and performed well. A letter has been sent to these EMT-Bs commending them for their efforts.

As an EMT-B, you will have a role in the quality improvement process. In fact, a dedication to quality can be one of the strongest assets of an EMT-B.

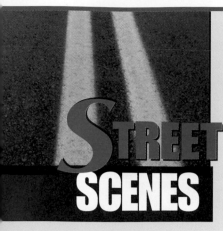

As a new EMT, you are assigned to Station 2 to ride with Susan Miller, a seasoned EMS veteran with seven years on the job. You have heard that she is a good EMT, and you remember that she helped teach some of your skill sessions. She was a good instructor—patient, understanding, and considerate.

When you arrive at the station, you find out she has been delayed and you will be riding with Chuck Hartley instead. When you are introduced to Chuck, you see that his uniform is unkempt. He tells you to sit until he needs you.

Your first call of the day is a 70-year-old female with abdominal pain. As you approach the ambulance, Chuck tells you to get in the back. He'll let you know when you can help. After assuring scene safety, you both enter the patient's home. Chuck doesn't bother to introduce himself and proceeds to ask the patient, "What's wrong, Hon?" She describes her symptoms. Chuck tells you to put her on a nasal cannula. As you hook up the O_2, Chuck says in a loud voice, "Didn't you learn anything in EMT class? That liter flow rate is too high."

As the patient is being loaded onto the stretcher, she tries to tell Chuck something that she obviously believes is urgent. Chuck tells her that if it's that important, she can tell the doctor at the hospital.

STREET SCENE QUESTIONS

1. What would have been a more appropriate action for Chuck when the shift started?

2. What behavior characteristics of Chuck's would be considered unprofessional?

3. What would you expect from someone providing initial field training?

The transport of the day's first patient was uneventful. When you return to the station, Susan Miller has arrived. This time when you are intro-

---

There are several ways you can work toward quality care. These include:

- *Keeping carefully written documentation.* Call reviews are based on the prehospital care reports that you and other crew members write. If a report is incomplete, it is difficult for a QI team to assess the events of a call. If you are ever involved in a lawsuit, an inaccurate or incomplete report may also be a cause for liability. Be sure the reports you write are neat, complete, and accurate.

- *Becoming involved in the quality process.* As you gain experience, you may wish to volunteer for assignment to the QI committee. In addition, quality improvement has a place on every call. An individual ambulance crew can perform a critique after each call to determine things that went well and others that may need improvement. Have another EMT-B or advanced EMT look over your report before turning it in to assure that it is accurate and complete.

- *Obtaining feedback from patients and the hospital staff.* This may be done informally or, in some cases, formally. Your organization may send a letter to patients that asks for comments on the care they were given while under your care. Hospital staff may be able to provide information that will help strengthen your care-giving skills.

- *Maintaining your equipment.* It will be difficult to provide quality care with substandard, damaged, or missing equipment. While the ingenuity of EMT-Bs should never be underestimated, it would be impossible to administer oxygen or provide cardiac defibrillation without proper, functional equipment. Check and maintain equipment regularly.

- *Continuing your education.* An EMT-B who was certified several years ago and has never attended subsequent training will have a problem providing quality care. Seldom-used skills deteriorate without practice. Procedures change. Without some form of regular continuing education, it will be difficult to maintain standards of quality.

Quality improvement is another name for providing the care that you would want to have provided to yourself or a loved one in a time of emergency. That is the best care possible. Maintaining continuous high quality is not easy; it requires constant attention and a sense of pride and obligation. Striving for quality—both in the care you personally give to patients and as a collective part of an ambuduced, you notice that her uniform is pressed and neat. She asks you about your background and when you finished training. She remembers you from class, she says. Then she tells you there are some things you both need to do. "First, let's go to the ambulance and check the equipment. Next, I want to explain how we operate on calls. You need to know what equipment we always take to the patient and responsibilities of the crew members."

Just as you are completing your orientation, a call comes in for a 55-year-old male with chest pain. While en route, Susan briefly goes over the routine that she and her partner use. She asks you to take the automatic defibrillator. When you enter the patient's house, Susan introduces herself and the members of the crew. She asks the patient: "Sir, why did you call 9-1-1?" He tells you that he had chest pain but he took a nitroglycerin tablet and now most of the pain is gone. He apologizes for calling.

While you get the vital signs, Susan tells the patient that he did just the right thing by calling EMS. He is reassured and agrees to be transported for further evaluation.

STREET SCENE QUESTIONS

4. What did Susan Miller do that was appropriate and professional?

5. How was Susan's behavior beneficial to you as a new EMT?

6. What personal traits are the professional standards for EMTs?

During the trip to the hospital Susan continues to reassure the patient. In fact, she tells you to talk to the patient about his medical history. When you arrive at the hospital, Susan sees that the oxygen tank is getting low, so she asks you to switch "bottles" before moving the patient, but you forget to turn off the tank being replaced. Susan turns it off, sets it aside, looks you in the eyes, and gives you a smile. You both know that you will not forget the next time.

After the call, Susan gives a short critique and discusses the prehospital care report. When you call back in service, you realize that to be a good EMT you not only need to have good technical skills but, just as important, you also must act as a professional with your patients and with your colleagues.

lance squad—is to uphold the highest standards of the EMS system.

Medical Direction

Each EMS system has a **Medical Director,** a physician who assumes the ultimate responsibility for **medical direction,** or oversight of the patient-care aspects of the EMS system. The Medical Director also oversees training, develops **protocols** (lists of steps for assessment and interventions to be performed in different situations), and is a crucial part of the quality improvement process. An EMT at a basic or advanced level is operating as a **designated agent** of the physician. This means that, as an EMT-B, your authority to give medications and provide emergency care is actually an extension of the Medical Director's license to practice medicine.

The physician obviously cannot physically be at every call. This is why EMS systems develop **standing orders.** The physician has issued a policy or protocol that authorizes EMT-Bs and others to perform particular skills in certain situations. An example may be the administration of glucose. Glucose is very beneficial to certain diabetic patients who are experiencing a medical emergency. The Medical Di-

rector issues a standing order that allows EMT-Bs to give glucose in certain circumstances without speaking to the Medical Director or another physician. This kind of "behind the scenes" medical direction is called *off-line medical direction.*

Certain other procedures that are not covered by standing orders or protocols require the EMT-B to contact the on-duty physician by radio or telephone prior to performing a skill or administering a medication. For example, EMT-Bs carry a medication called "activated charcoal." This medication is beneficial to many but not all poisoning victims. Prior to administering activated charcoal, you may be required to consult with the on-duty physician. You would use a radio or cellular phone from the ambulance to provide patient information to the physician. After receiving your information, the physician would instruct you on how to proceed with care, including whether and how much activated charcoal to give. Orders from the on-duty physician given by radio or phone are called *on-line medical direction.* On-line medical direction may be requested at any time you feel that medical advice would be beneficial to patient care.

Protocols and procedures for on-line and off-line medical direction vary from system to system. Your instructor will inform you what your local policies are. Always follow your local protocols.

Special Issues

In the coming weeks and through the chapters that follow in this textbook, you will be studying to become an EMT-Basic. As part of your course, your instructor will advise you on local issues and administrative matters, such as a course description, class meeting times, criteria including physical and mental requirements for certification as an EMT-B, as well as specific statutes and regulations regarding EMS in your state, region, or locality.

The Americans with Disabilities Act (ADA) has set strict guidelines preserving the rights of Americans with disabilities. If you have a disability or have questions about the ADA, ask your instructor for more information.

CHAPTER REVIEW

SUMMARY

The EMS system has been developed to provide prehospital as well as hospital emergency care. The EMS system includes the 9-1-1 or other emergency access system, dispatchers, First Responders, EMTs, the hospital emergency department, physicians, nurses, physician's assistants, and other health professionals.

The EMT-B's responsibilities include safety; patient assessment and care; lifting, moving, and transporting patients; transfer of care; and patient advocacy. An EMT-B must have certain personal and physical traits to assure the ability to do the job.

Education (including refresher training and continuing education), quality improvement procedures, and medical direction are all essential to maintaining high standards of EMS care.

KEY TERMS

designated agent an EMT-B or other person authorized by a Medical Director to give medications and provide emergency care. The transfer of such authorization to a designated agent is an extension of the Medical Director's license to practice medicine.

medical direction oversight of the patient care aspects of an EMS system by the Medical Director. Off-line medical direction consists of standing orders issued by the Medical Director that allow EMTs to give certain medications or perform certain procedures without speaking to the Medical Director or another physician. On-line medical direction consists of orders from the on-duty physician given directly to an EMT-B in the field by radio or telephone.

Medical Director a physician who assumes ultimate responsibility for the patient care aspects of the EMS system.

9-1-1 system a system for telephone access to report emergencies. A dispatcher takes the information and alerts EMS or the fire or police departments as needed. Enhanced 9-1-1 has the additional capability of automatically identifying the caller's phone number and location.

protocols lists of steps, such as assessment and interventions, to be taken in different situations. Protocols are developed by the Medical Director of an EMS system.

quality improvement a process of continuous self-review with the purpose of identifying and correcting aspects of the system that require improvement.

standing orders a policy or protocol issued by a Medical Director that authorizes EMT-Bs and others to perform particular skills in certain situations.

REVIEW QUESTIONS

1. What are the components of the Emergency Medical Services system? (pp. 5–6)
2. What are some of the special designations that hospitals may have? List them. Then name the special centers you have in your region. (p. 5)
3. What are the four national levels of EMS training and certification? (pp. 6–7)
4. What are the roles and responsibilities of the EMT-B? (p. 7)
5. What are desirable personal and physical attributes of the EMT-B? (pp. 8–9)
6. What is the definition of the term "quality improvement"? (pp. 9–10)
7. What is the difference between on-line and off-line medical direction? (p. 11)

APPLICATIONS

- What qualities would you like to see in an EMT-B who is caring for you? How can you come closer to being this kind of EMT-B? (pp. 8–10)

- You are devoting a considerable amount of time to becoming an EMT-B. How do you plan to refresh your knowledge and stay current once you are out of the classroom? (p. 9)

WEB MEDIC

Visit Brady's *Emergency Care* website for direct weblinks. At **www.bradybooks.com/emergencycare**, you will find information related to Chapter 1 topics:

- National EMT organizations
- Medical direction
- Reciprocity
- Future of EMS

Chapter
Two

THE WELL-BEING OF THE EMT-BASIC

Word on the Street

"In over 25 years in EMS, the thing that is painfully obvious to me is the fact that we make a great effort to protect ourselves from infectious diseases, blood spatters, and hazardous materials. All the while, the most insidious and widespread problem out there for EMS practitioners, their families, and friends is the inability to leave EMS at the station. This eventually gets to the point of sacrificing close and meaningful relationships in our zeal for professional gratification. You need to make sure to take care of yourself while you are taking care of others."

Paul A. Werfel NREMT-P, Director, Paramedic Program, and Clinical Instructor in Health Sciences, State University of New York at Stony Brook

Learning how to safeguard your well-being as an EMT-Basic is critical. During your EMS service, you will be exposed to all kinds of stress, including that which accompanies death and dying. You will also sometimes be exposed to infectious diseases and dangerous situations.

It is important to use the proper equipment and strategies to help you stay physically safe and emotionally well. Remember: If the EMT-B becomes a victim, he is of little or no use to a patient and even may put other rescuers in jeopardy. Ways to safeguard your well-being include taking body substance isolation (BSI) precautions before treating a patient, understanding and dealing with the stress that normally accompanies critical incidents, and ensuring scene safety.

PERSONAL PROTECTION

Body Substance Isolation (BSI) Precautions

Diseases are caused by **pathogens,** organisms that cause infection, such as viruses and bacteria. Pathogens may be spread through the air or by contact with blood and other body fluids. *Bloodborne pathogens* can be contracted by exposure to the patient's blood and sometimes other body fluids, especially when they come in contact with an open wound or sore on the EMT-B's hands, face, or other exposed parts including mucous membranes, such as those in the nose, mouth, or eyes. Even minor breaks in the skin, such as those found around fingernails, can be enough for a pathogen to enter your body. *Airborne pathogens* are spread by tiny droplets sprayed during breathing, coughing, or sneezing. These particles can be absorbed through your eyes or when you inhale.

Since it is impossible for an EMT-B or other health-care professional to identify patients who carry infectious diseases just by looking at them, all body fluids must be considered infectious and appropriate precautions taken for all patients at all times.

Equipment and procedures that protect you from the blood and body fluids of the patient—and the patient from your blood and body fluids—are referred to as **body substance isolation (BSI) precautions**. BSI precautions also are referred to as infection control. For each situation you encounter, it is important to apply the appropriate precautions. Taking too few will clearly increase your risk of exposure to disease. Too many can potentially alienate the patient and reduce your effectiveness.

The Occupational Safety and Health Administration (OSHA) has issued strict guidelines about precautions against exposure to bloodborne pathogens. Under the OSHA guidelines, employers and employees share responsibility for these precautions. Employers must develop a written exposure control plan and must provide emergency care providers training, immunizations, and proper **personal protective equipment (PPE)** to prevent transmission of disease. (Most volunteer organizations provide these services for their members.) The employee's responsibility is to participate in the training and to follow the exposure control plan.

There is also a requirement for all agencies to have a written policy in place in the event of an

TOPIC OVERVIEW

In this chapter, you will learn about the following topics:

- Body substance isolation (BSI) precautions, or how to protect yourself from transmitted diseases

- The impact that dying patients have on you and others

- The kinds of stress caused by involvement in EMS and how they can affect you, your fellow EMT-Bs, and your family and friends

- How to identify potential hazards and maintain scene safety

DOT OBJECTIVES

✔ Knowledge and Attitude

1. List possible emotional reactions that the EMT-Basic may experience when faced with trauma, illness, death, and dying. (pp. 24–25)

2. Discuss the possible reactions that a family member may exhibit when confronted with death and dying. (p. 25)

3. State the steps in the EMT-Basic's approach to the family confronted with death and dying. (pp. 25–26)

4. State the possible reactions that the family of the EMT-Basic may exhibit due to their outside involvement in EMS. (pp. 23–24)

5. Recognize the signs and symptoms of critical incident stress. (p. 24)

6. State possible steps the EMT-Basic may take to help reduce or alleviate stress. (p. 24)

7. Explain the need to determine scene safety. (pp. 26–27)

8. Discuss the importance of body substance isolation (BSI). (pp. 15–16)

9. Describe the steps the EMT-Basic should take for personal protection from airborne and bloodborne pathogens. (pp. 15–16, 18, 23)

10. List the personal protective equipment necessary for each of the following situations: (pp. 16–17)
- Hazardous materials
- Rescue operations
- Violent scenes
- Crime scenes
- Exposure to bloodborne pathogens
- Exposure to airborne pathogens

11. Explain the rationale for serving as an advocate for the use of appropriate protective equipment. (p. 17)

✔ Skills

1. Given a scenario with potential infectious exposure, the EMT-Basic will use appropriate personal protective equipment. At the completion of the scenario, the EMT-Basic will properly remove and discard the protective garments.

2. Given the above scenario, the EMT-Basic will complete disinfection/cleaning and all reporting documentation.

---

exposure to infectious substances. Any contact such as a needle-stick or contact with a potentially infectious fluid must be documented. Refer to your local policy for reporting an exposure incident. Most plans call for baseline testing of the exposed person immediately following the exposure and periodic follow-up testing. Additionally, federal legislation has made it possible for emergency care providers to be notified if a patient with whom they have had potentially infectious contact turns out to be infected by a disease or virus such as tuberculosis (TB), hepatitis B, or HIV (the virus associated with AIDS).

While BSI issues may seem intimidating—especially if you are just beginning your training—remember that it is possible, by following the proper precautions, to have a long and safe career in EMS free from infection and disease.

Personal Protective Equipment

Protect yourself from all possible routes of **contamination,** or introduction of disease or infectious materials. Follow BSI guidelines and wear the appropriate personal protective equipment on every call (Figure 2-1).

Protective Gloves

Latex, vinyl, or other synthetic gloves should be used whenever there is the potential for contact with blood and other body fluids. This includes actions such as controlling bleeding, suctioning, artificial ventilation, and CPR. Make sure that you have the

gloves on before you come in contact with a patient. Do not wait. You might get distracted and forget the gloves or you may accidentally become contaminated. Be sure to change gloves between patients.

Some EMT-Bs and patients are allergic to latex. The allergic reactions can be serious. Vinyl and other non-latex gloves are available. If your patient is known to be allergic to latex, use non-latex gloves. (You also will find that many other medical supplies such as oxygen masks, tubing, and some tapes contain latex. Be aware of the potential problems these may cause and use substitute materials when appropriate and possible.)

Figure 2-1 Always wear BSI equipment to prevent exposure to contagious disease.

A different type of glove must be worn when you clean the ambulance and soiled equipment. This glove should be heavyweight and tear-resistant. The force and type of movements involved in cleaning can cause lightweight gloves to rip, exposing your hands to contamination.

Note

Even though you wear protective gloves while you are with a patient, hand washing must be performed immediately after each call. There may have been microscopic holes or tiny tears in the gloves through which infectious agents have reached your hands. Additionally, items you touched while you were wearing gloves (clipboard, door handle, equipment), may still have body fluids on them. Touching them again without gloves can cause contamination. Frequent, careful, methodical hand washing (Figure 2-2) will help to reduce exposure to yourself, your crew, and your next patient.

Eye Protection

The mucous membranes surrounding the eyes are capable of absorbing fluids. Wear eye protection to prevent splashing, spattering, or spraying fluids from entering the body through these membranes. Protective eyewear should provide protection from the front and the sides. There are various types of eyewear on the market. Goggles provide acceptable protection but can fog and become uncomfortable. Goggles are not necessary because acceptable substitutes are available. If you wear prescription eyeglasses, clip-on side protectors are available. Some companies offer protective eyewear that resembles eye glasses. These are much easier than goggles to use and carry, and they do not fog up or cause excessive perspiration.

Masks

In cases where there will be blood or fluid spatter, wear a surgical-type mask. In cases where tuberculosis (a disease that is carried by fine particles in the air) is suspected, an N-95 or a high efficiency particulate air (HEPA) respirator approved by the National Institute for Occupational Safety and Health (NIOSH) is the standard (Figure 2-3). In some jurisdictions, when a patient is suspected of having an infection spread by droplets (such as measles), a surgical-type mask may be placed on the patient if he is alert and cooperative.

Warning

When you cover a patient's mouth and nose with a mask of any kind, use caution. The mask reduces your ability to visualize and protect the airway. Monitor respirations and be prepared to remove the mask and use suction to clear the airway if necessary.

Gowns

A gown is worn to protect clothing and bare skin from spilled or splashed fluids. Arterial (spurting) bleeding is an indication for a gown. Childbirth and patients with multiple injuries also often produce considerable amounts of blood. Any situation that would call for the use of a gown would also require gloves, eye protection, and a mask.

It is a good idea not only to use personal protective equipment yourself but also to be an advocate for its use; that is, to encourage members of your crew and others to use appropriate protective equipment. In addition to the moral and ethical obligation to do so, you will be helping to keep your crew in good health.

Figure 2-2 Careful, methodical hand washing is effective in reducing exposure to contagious disease.

Figure 2-3 Wear a NIOSH-approved respirator when you suspect a patient may have tuberculosis.

Always properly remove and discard protective garments after use, carry out disinfection and cleaning operations, and complete all reporting documentation regarding infection control. You will learn more about these procedures in Chapter 32, "Ambulance Operations."

Note:

When you finish your EMT-B training and begin in the field, you will observe differences in the methods and levels of BSI precautions taken by those around you. You will likely notice that some EMTs don gloves and protective eyewear before exiting the ambulance and wear them throughout the call. Others will go through an entire call without even wearing gloves.

In the 1980s an increased emphasis was placed on BSI. Diseases such as AIDS and hepatitis brought a startling reality to the health-care professions. As a result, gloves, protective eyewear, and masks were used with increasing frequency. These items were worn as a "precaution," even when not technically necessary.

Today, providers have a more realistic attitude about BSI. Think back to your last physical examination, for example. Your physician most likely examined your eyes and ears, palpated your abdomen, and performed other examinations without gloves. Why is this? Because it is not necessary to wear gloves, if your skin and the skin of your patient is intact. Additionally, wearing gloves while you exit the ambulance, carry equipment, and enter a scene may cause the gloves to rip before you reach the patient, rendering them ineffective.

Common sense should be the rule. To protect yourself from disease:

- Follow BSI guidelines as outlined in this chapter and in the rules and policies of your organization.
- Always have BSI equipment immediately available on your person and in your kits.
- If in doubt, wear gloves. This applies to incidents such as motor-vehicle collisions where there is broken glass. Even if you do not see blood at the scene, remember it can still be present but hidden under clothes. In contrast, if your skin is intact and your patient has no open wounds, you will not need gloves unless the patient's condition changes.

DISEASES OF CONCERN

The communicable diseases we are most concerned with are caused by blood-borne and airborne pathogens, such as viruses, bacteria, and other harmful organisms. Bloodborne pathogens are contracted by exposure to an infected patient's blood, especially exposure through breaks in the non-infected person's skin. Airborne pathogens are spread by tiny droplets sprayed when a patient breathes, coughs, or sneezes. These droplets are inhaled or are absorbed through the non-infected person's eyes, mouth, or nose.

Although there are many communicable diseases, three are of particular concern: hepatitis B, tuberculosis, and HIV/AIDS.

- *Hepatitis* is an infection that causes an inflammation of the liver. It comes in at least four forms: hepatitis A, B, C, and Delta. Hepatitis A is acquired primarily through contact with stool. The other forms are acquired through contact with blood and other body fluids. The virus that causes hepatitis is especially hardy. Hepatitis B has been found to live for many days in dried blood spills, posing a risk of transmission long after many other viruses would have died. For this reason, it is critical for you to assume that any body fluid in any form, dried or otherwise, is infectious until proven otherwise. Hepatitis B can be deadly. The virus (HBV) kills up to 200 health-care workers every year in the United States, more than any other occupationally acquired infectious disease. There is no cure, but an effective vaccine is available. (See "Immunizations" in the next section.)

- *Tuberculosis (TB)* is an infection that sometimes settles in the lungs and can be fatal. It was thought to be largely eradicated but in the late 1980s, it made a comeback. TB is highly contagious. Unlike many other infectious diseases, it can spread through the air. Health-care workers and others can become infected even without any direct contact with a carrier. Because it is impossible for the EMT-B to determine why a patient has a productive cough, it is safest to assume that it could be the result of TB and that you should take the necessary respiratory precautions. This is especially true in institutions such as nursing homes or homeless shelters where there is an increased risk of TB.

- *AIDS* is the name for a set of conditions that result when the immune system has been attacked by HIV (human immunodeficiency virus) and rendered unable to combat certain infections adequately. Although advances are being made in the treatment of HIV/AIDS, no cure has been discovered at the time of publication of this text. However, HIV/AIDS presents far less risk to health-care workers than hepatitis and TB, because the virus does not survive well outside the human body. This limits the routes of exposure to direct contact with blood by way of open wounds, intravenous drug use, unprotected sexual contact, or blood transfusions. Puncture wounds into which HIV is introduced, such as with an accidental needle stick, are also potential routes of infection. However, less than half of one percent of such incidents result in infection, according to the U. S. Occupational Safety and Health Administration (OSHA), compared to 30% for the hepatitis B virus (HBV). The difference is due to the quantity and strength of HBV compared to HIV.

Hepatitis B, TB, and HIV/AIDS are the communicable diseases of greatest concern because they are life-threatening. However, there are many communicable diseases to which emergency response and other health-care personnel may be exposed. Table 2-1 lists common communicable diseases, their modes of transmission, and their incubation periods (the time between contact and first appearance of symptoms).

TABLE 2-1 Communicable Diseases

Disease	Mode of Transmission	Incubation
AIDS (acquired immune deficiency syndrome)	HIV-infected blood via intravenous drug use, unprotected sexual contact, blood transfusions, or (rarely) accidental needle sticks. Mothers also may pass HIV to their unborn children.	Several months or years
Chickenpox (varicella)	Airborne droplets. Can also be spread by contact with open sores.	11 to 21 days
German measles (rubella)	Airborne droplets. Mothers may pass the disease to unborn children.	10 to 12 days
Hepatitis	Blood, stool, or other body fluids, or contaminated objects.	Weeks to months, depending on type
Meningitis, bacterial	Oral and nasal secretions.	2 to 10 days
Mumps	Droplets of saliva or objects contaminated by saliva.	14 to 24 days
Pneumonia, bacterial and viral	Oral and nasal droplets and secretions.	Several days
Staphylococcal skin infections	Direct contact with infected wounds or sores or with contaminated objects.	Several days
Tuberculosis (TB)	Respiratory secretions, airborne or on contaminated objects.	2 to 6 weeks
Whooping cough (pertussis)	Respiratory secretions or airborne droplets.	6 to 20 days

INFECTION CONTROL AND THE LAW

Scientists have identified the main culprits in the transmission of many deadly infectious diseases—blood and body fluids. EMT-Bs and other health-care workers have been recognized as having a higher-than-usual exposure and, therefore, a higher risk of contracting these unwanted infections.

Congress and federal agencies have responded by taking several steps to ensure the safety of people who are in high-risk positions. In particular, the Occupational Safety and Health Administration (OSHA) of the U. S. Department of Labor, and the Centers for Disease Control and Prevention (CDC) of the U. S. Department of Health and Human Services, have issued standards and guidelines for the protection of workers whose jobs may expose them to infectious diseases. The Ryan White CARE Act establishes procedures by which emergency response workers may find out if they have been exposed to life-threatening infectious diseases. These legal protections are described in more detail in the next sections.

Occupational Exposure to Bloodborne Pathogens

In 1992, the OSHA standard on bloodborne pathogens took effect. It mandates measures employers of emergency responders must take to protect employees who are likely to be exposed to blood and other body fluids. One of the basic principles behind the standard is that infection control is a joint responsibility between employer and employee. The employer must provide training, protective equipment, and vaccinations to employees who are subject to exposure in their jobs. In return, employees must participate in an infection exposure control plan that includes training and proper workplace practices.

Without the active participation of both the employer and the employee, any workplace infection control program is destined to fail. Be sure your system has an active and up-to-date infection exposure control plan and that you and your fellow EMT-Bs follow it carefully at all times. Consult with your state OSHA representative to make sure that specific hazards are identified and corrected.

Contact the U. S. Department of Labor to request the booklet "Occupational Exposure to Bloodborne Pathogens: Precautions for Emergency Responders— OSHA 3106 1998," an overview of the standard. For details regarding how to develop an infection control plan, request Title 29 Code of Federal Regulation 1910.1030 for the complete text of the standard and all requirements regarding occupational exposure to bloodborne pathogens. Critical elements of the standard are summarized below:

• *Infection exposure control plan.* Each emergency response employer must develop a plan that identifies and documents job classifications and tasks in which there is the possibility of exposure to potentially infectious body fluids. The plan must outline a schedule of how and when the bloodborne pathogen standards will be implemented. It also must include identification of the methods used for communicating hazards to employees, post-exposure evaluation, and follow-up.

• *Adequate education and training.* EMT-Bs must be provided with training that includes general explanations of how diseases are transmitted, uses and limitations of practices that reduce or prevent exposure, and procedures to follow if exposure occurs.

• *Hepatitis B vaccination.* Employers must make the hepatitis B vaccination series available free of charge and at a reasonable time and place.

• *Personal protective equipment* must be of a quality that will not permit blood or other infectious materials to pass through or reach an EMT-B's work clothes, street clothes, undergarments, skin, eyes, mouth, or other mucous membranes. This equipment must be provided by the employer to the EMT-B at no cost and includes but is not limited to protective gloves, face shields, masks, protective eyewear, gowns and aprons, plus bag-valve masks, pocket masks, and other ventilation devices.

• *Methods of control.* Engineering controls remove potential infectious disease hazards or separate the EMT-B from exposure. Examples include pocket masks, disposable airway equipment, and puncture-resistant needle containers. Work practice controls improve the manner in which a task is performed to reduce risk of exposure. Examples include the proper and safe use of personal protective equipment; proper handling, labeling, and disposal of contaminated materials; and proper washing and decontamination practices.

• *Housekeeping.* Clean and sanitary conditions of the emergency response vehicles and work sites are the responsibility of both the EMT-B and the employer. Procedures include the proper handling and proper decontamination of work surfaces, equipment, laundry, and other materials.

• *Labeling.* The standard requires labeling of containers used to store, transport, or ship blood and other potentially infectious materials, including the use of the biohazard symbol (Figure 2-4).

Figure 2-4 The biohazard symbol must be included with warning labels for containers used to ship blood or other potentially infectious materials.

• *Post-exposure evaluation and follow-up.* EMT-Bs must immediately report suspected exposure incidents—including mucous membrane or broken-skin contact with blood or other potentially infectious materials—that result from the performance of an employee's duties. (See Figure 2-5 for a model plan based on the Ryan White CARE Act, which is described below.)

Ryan White CARE Act

In 1994, the CDC issued the final notice for the Ryan White Comprehensive AIDS Resources Emergency (CARE) Act Regarding Emergency Response Employees. This federal act, which applies to all 50 states, mandates a procedure by which emergency response personnel can seek to find out if they have been exposed to potentially life-threatening diseases while providing patient care. Emergency response personnel referred to in this act include firefighters, law enforcement officers, EMTs, and other individuals such as First Responders who provide emergency aid on behalf of a legally recognized volunteer organization.

CDC has published a list of potentially life-threatening infectious and communicable diseases to which emergency response personnel can be exposed. The list includes airborne diseases such as TB, bloodborne diseases such as hepatitis B and HIV/AIDS, and uncommon or rare diseases such as diphtheria and rabies.

The Ryan White CARE Act requires every state's public health officer to designate an official within every emergency response organization to act as a "designated officer." The designated officer is responsible for gathering facts surrounding

INFECTIOUS DISEASE EXPOSURE PROCEDURE

Figure 2-5 Under the Ryan White CARE Act, there is a procedure for finding out and following up if you have been exposed to a life-threatening disease.

possible emergency responder airborne or bloodborne infectious disease exposures. Take time to learn who is the designated officer within your organization.

Two different notification systems for infectious disease exposure are defined in the act:

• *Airborne disease exposure.* You will be notified by your designated officer when you have been exposed to an airborne disease.

• *Bloodborne or other infectious disease exposure.* You may submit a re-

quest for a determination as to whether or not you were exposed to bloodborne or other infectious disease.

The difference between the two procedures results from the differences in how an exposure is most likely to be detected. With an airborne disease such as TB, you may not realize that the patient you have cared for and transported was infected. However, a disease like TB will be diagnosed at the hospital. Therefore, the Ryan White Act states that for airborne diseases like TB, the hospital will notify the designated officer who will notify you.

A bloodborne disease such as hepatitis B or HIV/AIDS may or may not be diagnosed at the hospital, but you will know if you have had contact with a patient's blood or body fluids. If so, you can submit a request to your designated officer who will gather the information necessary to request a determination from the hospital on whether you have been exposed and then will notify you of the result.

In either case, once you have been notified of an exposure, your employer will refer you to a doctor or other health-care professional for evaluation and follow-up.

Consider how the Ryan White CARE Act would apply in the following example of exposure to an airborne pathogen:

As an EMT-B, you treat and transport a patient who complains of weakness, fever, and chronic cough. The next day you receive a phone call from your organization's designated officer, who informs you that you have been exposed to a patient with TB. The designated officer helps you arrange an appointment with a doctor who can determine if you have contracted the disease and arrange for early treatment if you have.

According to CDC guidelines, exposure to airborne pathogens may occur when you share "air space" with a tuberculosis patient. So, if a medical facility diagnoses that patient as having the airborne infectious disease, it must notify the designated officer within 48 hours. The designated officer must then notify the emergency care workers of disease exposure. Finally, the employer must schedule a post-exposure evaluation and follow-up.

Consider another example, this one an incident in which exposure to a bloodborne pathogen occurs:

As an EMT-B, you are called to treat an unconscious woman. During the scene size-up you put on disposable gloves, mask, gown, and eye shield. The patient is lying on the kitchen floor. Pink, frothy sputum trickles from her mouth. Breathing is labored. A hypodermic needle lies beside her. While you are suctioning the patient, your eye shield slips and fluids from her mouth splash into your eyes. You report the incident immediately after the call is completed. Your designated officer follows up, and you learn that you have not been exposed to a life-threatening bloodborne disease.

Under CDC guidelines, after contact with the blood or body fluids of a patient you have transported, you may submit a request for a determination to your designated officer. The designated officer must then gather information about the possible exposure. If the information indicates a possible exposure, the officer forwards the information to the medical facility where the patient is being treated. If the

patient can be identified, medical records are reviewed to determine if the patient has a life-threatening disease. The medical facility then must notify your designated officer of their findings in writing within 48 hours after receiving the officer's request. The designated officer must notify you, and you will be directed by your employer to a health-care professional for a post-exposure evaluation and follow-up as appropriate.

It is important to note that the Ryan White Act does not empower hospitals to test patients for bloodborne diseases at the request of the emergency worker or designated officer. Rather, they can only review the patient's medical records to see if evidence of a bloodborne or other disease exists. Thus a patient could be infected, but if the records reveal no testing or known indication of the presence of such an infection, the hospital can only report that "no evidence of bloodborne infection could be detected."

Note: If you are actually exposed to a bloodborne pathogen (e.g., a needle stick or splashing of fluids to a mucous membrane), you must seek medical attention immediately. It is important that you receive care for the wound, obtain baseline blood work including determining hepatitis B immunity, evaluate the need for a tetanus shot, and document the incident for worker's compensation or insurance. You may also be asked to consider taking the drug AZT and another drug or combination of drugs to attempt to counteract the effects of HIV if it is present. This is a personal issue and a very serious decision. It is important to know that current research indicates that waiting 48 hours for the requested Ryan White information to determine if the patient whose blood you were exposed to may be HIV-infected will reduce the effectiveness of the drugs. Each situation is different. You will wish to seek the advice of the attending physician where you are being treated as well as of your medical director.

Tuberculosis Compliance Mandate

Thousands of new cases of TB are reported in the U. S. each year. Hundreds of health-care workers have been infected or

exposed. Of particular concern are the rising cases of multi-drug resistant TB (MDR-TB). In 1994 CDC issued guidelines for treating a suspected or confirmed TB patient, "Guidelines for Preventing the Transmission of *Mycobacterium Tuberculosis* in Health Care Facilities." OSHA stated they would enforce those guidelines as if they were OSHA rules.

Study the guidelines as summarized below. Learn to recognize situations in which the potential of exposure to TB exists. Those at greatest risk of contracting and transmitting TB are people who have suppressed immune systems, including people with HIV/AIDS and elderly patients such as those living in nursing homes. Patients who have TB may have the following signs and symptoms: productive cough (coughing up mucus or other fluid) and/or coughing up blood, weight loss and loss of appetite, lethargy and weakness, night sweats, and fever. *It is safest to assume that any person with a productive cough may be infected with TB.*

When the potential exists for exposure to exhaled air of a person with suspected or confirmed TB, OSHA requires that you wear a NIOSH-approved N-95 or high efficiency particulate air (HEPA) respirator. You are required to wear an N-95 or HEPA respirator when:

• You are caring for patients suspected of having TB. High-risk areas include correctional institutions, homeless shelters, long-term care facilities for the elderly, and drug treatment centers.

• Transporting an individual from such a setting in a closed vehicle. If possible, keep the windows of the ambulance open and set the heating and air conditioning system on the non-recirculating cycle.

• Performing high-risk procedures such as endotracheal suctioning and intubation.

Remember to take all recommended infection control precautions, including hand washing and using personal protective equipment and barrier devices such as pocket masks or bag-valve masks for rescue breathing. Properly dispose of contaminated equipment and materials, and decontaminate all surfaces, clothing, and equipment.

Immunizations

Immunizations against many diseases are available. Most people receive tetanus immunizations either routinely or after certain injuries. There is currently an immunization available to prevent hepatitis B. It will be provided by your EMS agency, usually through a local physician or your medical director.

While there is no current immunization against tuberculosis, a test called a *purified protein derivative (PPD) test* can detect exposure. EMT-Bs are often given this test during routine or employment screening physicals. If the test determines that you have been exposed to tuberculosis, seek treatment and follow-up from a doctor or other health-care professional. EMS workers should be checked for exposure to TB on a regular basis (usually yearly).

Some EMS agencies and medical facilities may require immunizations for measles and other common communicable diseases. Consult your instructor, your medical director, or your personal physician for more information on your current status and local protocols for immunizations.

EMOTION AND STRESS

Causes of Stress

Emergencies are stressful. That is their nature. While most EMS calls are considered "routine," some calls seem to have a higher potential for causing excess stress on EMS providers (Figure 2-6). They include the following:

- *Multiple-casualty incidents (MCIs).* A **multiple-casualty incident** is a single incident in which there are multiple patients. Examples range from a motor-vehicle crash in which two drivers and a passenger are injured to a hurricane that causes the injury of hundreds of people.
- *Calls involving infants and children.* Involving anything from a serious injury to sudden infant death syndrome (SIDS), these calls are known to be particularly stressful to all health-care providers.
- *Severe injuries.* Expect a stress reaction when your call involves injuries that cause major trauma or distortion to the human body. Examples include amputations, deformed bones, deep wounds, and violent death.

- *Abuse and neglect.* Cases of abuse and neglect occur in all social and economic levels of society. You may be called to treat infant, child, adult, or elder abuse victims.
- *Death of a coworker.* A bond is formed among members of the public services. The death of another public-safety worker—even if you do not know that person—can cause a stress response.

Stress may be caused by a single event or it may be the cumulative result of several incidents. Remember that any incident may affect you and coworkers differently. Two EMT-Bs on the same call may have opposite responses. Try never to make negative judgments about another person's reaction.

Stress may also stem from a combination of factors, including problems in your personal life. One common cause of stress is people who "just don't understand" the job. For example, your EMS organization may require you to work on weekends and holidays. Time spent on call may be frustrating to friends and family members. They may not understand why you cannot participate in certain social activities or why you cannot leave a certain area. You might get frustrated too, because you cannot plan around the unpredictable nature of emergencies. Then, after a very trying or exciting call, for instance, you may wish to share your feelings with a friend or someone you love. You find instead that the person

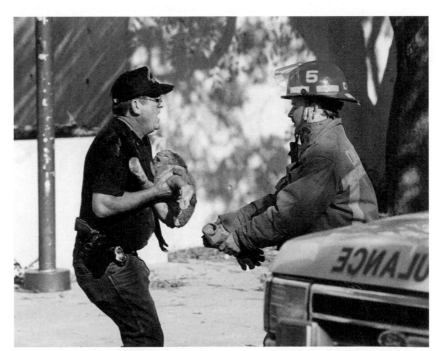

Figure 2-6 Emergencies are often stressful for EMS providers.

does not understand your emotions. This can lead to feelings of separation and rejection, which are highly stressful.

Signs and Symptoms of Stress

There are two types of stress: eustress and distress. Eustress is a positive form of stress that helps people work under pressure and respond effectively. Distress is negative. It can happen when the stress of a scene becomes overwhelming. As a result, your response to the emergency will not be effective. Distress also can cause immediate and long-term problems with your health and well-being.

The signs and symptoms of stress include irritability with family, friends, and coworkers; inability to concentrate; changes in daily activities, such as difficulty sleeping or nightmares, loss of appetite, and loss of interest in sexual activity; anxiety; indecisiveness; guilt; isolation; and loss of interest in work.

Dealing with Stress

Life-Style Changes

There are several ways to deal with stress. They are called "life-style changes":

- *Develop more healthful and positive dietary habits.* Avoid fatty foods and increase your carbohydrate intake. Also reduce your consumption of alcohol and caffeine, which can have negative effects, including an increase in stress and anxiety and disturbance of sleep patterns.

- *Exercise.* When performed safely and properly, exercise helps to "burn off" stress. It also helps you deal with the physical aspects of your responsibilities, such as carrying equipment and performing physically demanding emergency procedures.

- *Devote time to relaxing.* Try relaxation techniques, too. These techniques, which include deep-breathing exercises and meditation, are valuable stress reducers.

In addition to the changes you can make in your personal life to help reduce and prevent stress, there also are changes you can make in your professional life. If you are in an organization with varied shifts and locations, consider requesting a change to a different location that offers a lighter call volume or different types of calls. You may also want to change your shift to one that allows more time with family and friends.

There are many types of help available for EMT-Bs and others experiencing stress. Seek them out. It is not a sign of weakness. There are many professionals who can help you deal with stress, and much of the care may be covered by health insurance policies or employee assistance programs.

Critical Incident Stress Management

Critical incident stress management (CISM) refers to a comprehensive plan to deal with the stresses you face as an EMT. There are two basic CISM techniques: the critical incident stress debriefing and the defusing.

The **critical incident stress debriefing (CISD)** is a process in which a team of trained peer counselors and mental health professionals meet with rescuers and health-care providers who have been involved in a major incident (Figure 2-7). The meetings are generally held within 24 to 72 hours after the incident. The goal is to assist emergency-care workers in dealing with the stress related to that incident.

The CISD is an open discussion of the feelings experienced during and after the call. Participants are encouraged to talk about any fears or reactions they have had. It is critical that the CISD does not become a method of investigation of the events of the call. Everything discussed at the meetings is confidential and all participants are asked not to disclose information once the meeting is over. Any breach in the confidentiality of the discussion prevents others from

Figure 2-7 Critical incident stress management usually includes a debriefing 24 to 72 hours after an incident.

sharing information that can help them. After the open discussion, the CISD team offers suggestions on how to deal with and overcome the stress. It is important once again to state that stress after a major incident is normal and should be expected. The CISD process can help to accelerate the recovery process.

Sometimes a "defusing session" is held within the first few hours after a critical incident. While CISD includes all personnel involved in the incident, a defusing session is usually limited to a small group, often the people who were most directly involved with the most stressful aspects of the incident. It provides them an opportunity to vent their feelings and receive information about the stress they may feel before the larger group meets.

After a CISD, follow-up is essential. A member of the peer team should contact all CISD attendees within 24 hours to offer support and referrals. No two emergency-care workers will perceive, experience, or recover from critical incident stress in the same way. The process of overcoming the stress will be different from person to person. Resources must be available immediately as well as long after the incident, including "anniversary dates"—anniversaries of stressful events.

Comprehensive critical stress management goes beyond the CISD session to include pre-incident stress education, on-scene peer support, one-on-one support, disaster support services, spouse and family support, community outreach programs, and other health and welfare programs such as wellness programs. Remember, stress is a normal and perhaps an inevitable response to a critical incident. Learn to recognize the signs and symptoms and find out where to turn for help in your area.

Understanding Reactions to Death and Dying

As an EMT-B, you will undoubtedly be called to patients who are in various stages of a terminal illness. Understanding what the families and the patients go through can help you deal with the stress they feel as well as your own.

When a patient finds out that he is dying, he goes through emotional stages, each varying in duration and magnitude, sometimes overlapping, and all affecting both the patient and the family.

- *Denial or "Not me."* The patient denies that he is dying. This puts off dealing with the inevitable end of the process.
- *Anger or "Why me?"* The patient becomes angry at his situation. This anger is commonly vented upon family members and EMS personnel.
- *Bargaining or "Okay, but first let me . . ."* In the mind of the patient bargaining seems to postpone death, even for a short time.

- *Depression or "Okay, but I haven't . . ."* The patient is sad, depressed, and despairing, often mourning things not accomplished, dreams that will not come true. He retreats into a world of his own, unwilling to communicate with others.
- *Acceptance or "Okay, I'm not afraid."* The patient may come to accept death, although he does not welcome it. Often, the patient may come to accept the situation before family members do. At this stage, the family may need more support than the patient.

Not all patients go through all these stages. Some may seem to be in more than one stage at the same time. Some reactions may not seem to fit any of the described stages. Those who die rapidly are likely not to have such a predictable response to their own mortality. However, a general understanding of the process can help you to communicate with patients and families effectively.

As an EMT-B, you will also encounter sudden, unexpected death, for example as a result of a motor-vehicle collision. In cases of sudden death, family members are likely to react with a wide range of emotion.

There are several steps or approaches that you can take in dealing with the patient and family members confronted with death or dying:

- *Recognize the patient's needs.* Treat the patient with respect and do everything you can to preserve the patient's dignity and sense of control. For example, talk directly to the patient. Avoid talking about the patient to family members in the patient's presence as if the patient were incompetent or no longer living. Be sensitive to how the patient seems to want to handle the situation. For example, allow or encourage the patient to share feelings and needs, rather than cutting off such communications because of your own embarrassment or discomfort. Respect the patient's privacy if he does not want to communicate personal feelings.
- *Be tolerant of angry reactions from the patient or family members.* There may be feelings of helpless rage about the death or prospect of death. The anger is not personal. It would be directed at anyone in your position.
- *Listen empathetically.* You cannot "fix" the situation, but just listening with understanding and patience will be very helpful.
- *Do not falsely reassure.* Avoid saying things like "Everything will be all right," which you, the patient, and the family all know is not true. Offering false reassurance will only be irritating or convey the impression that you do not really understand.

- *Offer as much comfort as you realistically can.* Comfort both the patient and the family. Let them know that you will do everything you can to help or to get them whatever help is available from other sources. Use a gentle tone of voice and a reassuring touch, if appropriate.

SCENE SAFETY

Hazardous Materials Incidents

Many chemicals are capable of causing death or life-long complications even if they are only briefly inhaled or in contact with a person's body. Many of these materials are commercially transported, often by truck or rail. Such materials are also often stored in warehouses and used in industry. When there is an accident or when containers begin to leak, a **hazardous-material incident** may occur, which will pose serious dangers for you as an EMT-B as well as for others who are in the vicinity. When you face an emergency involving such materials, remember—you will not be able to help anyone if you are injured. Exercise caution.

The primary rule is to maintain a safe distance from the source of the hazardous material. Make sure your ambulance or other emergency vehicle is equipped with binoculars. They will help you identify placards, which are placed on vehicles, structures, and storage containers when they hold hazardous materials (Figure 2-8). These placards use coded colors and identification numbers that are listed in the *North American Emergency Response Guidebook* published by the U. S. Department of Transportation, Transport Canada, and the Secretariat of Communications and Transportation of Mexico.

Figure 2-8 Placards with coded colors and identification numbers must be used on vehicles and containers to identify hazardous materials.

This reference book should be placed in every vehicle that responds to or may respond to a hazardous-material incident. It provides important information about the properties of the dangerous substance as well as information on safe distances, emergency care, and suggested procedures in the event of spills or fire. (The *Emergency Response Guidebook* is also available on the internet at hazmat.dot.gov/gydebook.htm.)

Your most important role at the scene of a hazardous-material incident includes recognizing potential problems, taking initial actions for your personal safety and the safety of others, and notifying an appropriately trained hazardous-materials response team. Do not take any actions other than those aimed at protecting yourself, patients, and bystanders at the scene. An incorrect action can cause a bigger problem than the one that already exists.

The hazardous-materials response team is made up of specially trained technicians who will coordinate the safe approach and resolution of the incident. Each wears a special suit that protects the skin. A self-contained breathing apparatus (SCBA) is also required because of the strong potential for poisonous gases, dust, and fumes at a hazardous-material incident. You will generally not be required to wear personal protective equipment of this sort unless you have been specially trained to be part of a hazardous-materials response team. Instead, you will remain at a distance until the team has made the scene safe.

As an EMT-B, you should not be treating patients until after they have undergone **decontamination** (cleansing of dangerous chemicals and other materials). If you take a contaminated patient into your ambulance, it will be considered contaminated and cannot be used again until it is thoroughly decontaminated. Furthermore, should you bring a contaminated patient to the emergency department of a hospital, you could effectively close that hospital down. (See Chapter 34, "Special Operations," for more information on hazardous-materials incidents.)

Rescue Operations

Rescue operations include rescuing or disentangling victims from fires, auto collisions, explosions, electrocutions, and more. As with hazardous materials, it is important to evaluate each situation and ensure that appropriate assistance is requested early in the call. Depending on the emergency, you may need the police, fire department, power company, or other specialized personnel. Never perform acts that you are not properly trained to do. Do your best to secure the scene. Then stand by for the specialists. (You will learn more about rescue operations in

Chapter 33, "Gaining Access and Rescue Operations.")

As you work in rescue operations or on patients during a rescue operation, you will need personal protective equipment that includes turnout gear (coat, pants, and boots), protective eyewear, helmet, and puncture-proof gloves.

Violence

As an EMT-B, you will be called to scenes involving violence. Your first priority—even before patient care—is to be certain that the scene is safe. Dangerous persons or pets, people with weapons, intoxicated people, and others may present problems you are not prepared to handle. Learn to recognize those occasions. If the dispatcher knows that violence is or potentially may be present, he will advise you not to approach the scene until it is safe. The dispatcher may name a certain location where you should wait, or stage, a location that is far enough from the scene to be safe but near enough that you can respond as soon as the scene has been secured. Remember, it is the responsibility of the police to secure a scene and make it safe for you to perform your EMS duties.

Three words sum up the actions required to respond to danger: plan, observe, and react.

Plan

Many EMT-Bs work together to prevent dangerous accidents and know what to do as a team when danger strikes. Scene safety begins long before the actual emergency. Plan to be as safe as possible under all circumstances. Factors to be addressed include the following:

- *Wear safe clothing.* Nonslip shoes and practical clothing will not only help you provide emergency care more efficiently, but they also help you to respond to danger without unnecessary restrictions. For personal protection, have reflective clothing available if you will be near traffic or in areas where it is important for you to be visible. Some

HOW AND WHY?

According to the CDC's National Center for Injury Prevention and Control, approximately 1.5 million women and 834,700 men are raped and/or physically assaulted by an intimate partner every year. That's over 6,000 per day, or 4 every minute. Go to your Electronic Extras CD to find out more about domestic violence.

EMT-Bs wear body armor (bullet-proof vests) when working in high-risk areas or situations.

- *Prepare your equipment so it is not cumbersome.* You will be carrying your first-response kit into emergencies. If it is too heavy or bulky, it will take your attention away from the careful observation of the scene as you approach and slow you down if retreat becomes necessary. Many practical containers of reasonable size and weight are available.

- *Carry a portable radio whenever possible.* A radio allows you to call for help if you are separated from your vehicle.

- *Decide on safety roles.* If there will be more than one EMT-B on any call, tasks should be split up. For example, one EMT-B can obtain vital signs while another applies oxygen. One role that is frequently under-used is that of observer. The EMT-B directly involved in patient care should always be aware of, but will have trouble constantly monitoring, the surroundings. The EMT-B who is not directly involved with patient care will be better able to actively observe for such things as weapons, mechanisms of injury, medications, and other important information.

Observe

Remember that it is always better to prevent a dangerous situation than to deal with one. If you observe or suspect danger, call the police. Do not enter the scene until they have secured it.

Observation begins early in the call. Observe the neighborhood as you look for house or building numbers. As you near the scene, turn off your lights and sirens to avoid broadcasting your arrival and attracting a crowd.

As you approach an emergency scene, notice what is going on. Emergencies are very active events. In situations where you notice an unusual silence, a certain amount of caution is advisable (Figure 2-9). In addition, observe for the following:

- *Violence.* Any indication that violence has occurred or may take place is significant. Signs include broken glass or overturned furniture, arguing, threats, or other violent behavior.

- *Crime scenes.* Try not to disturb a crime scene except as necessary for patient care. Make every effort to preserve evidence. You will learn more about these aspects of emergency care at a crime scene in Chapter 3, "Medical/Legal and Ethical Issues."

- *Alcohol or drug use.* When people are under the influence of alcohol and other drugs, their behavior may be unpredictable. You also may be mistaken for the police because you drove up in a vehicle with lights and sirens.

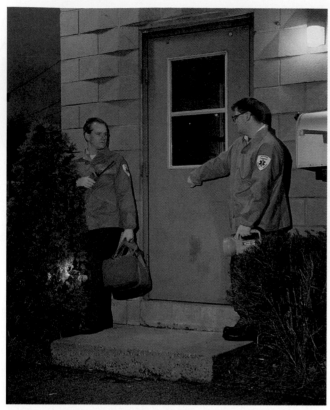

Figure 2-9 As a safety precaution, do not stand directly in front of a door when knocking or ringing the bell.

- *Weapons.* If anyone at the scene (other than the police) is in possession of a weapon, your safety is in danger. Even weapons that are only in view of a hostile person are a potential problem. Remember that almost any item may be used as a weapon. Weapons are not limited to knives and guns. If you observe or suspect the presence of any kind of weapon, notify the police immediately.
- *Family members.* Emotional or overwrought family members are often capable of violence or unpredictable behavior. Even though you are there to take care of a loved one, the violence may be directed at you.
- *Bystanders.* Many people gather at the scene of an accident (or anywhere an emergency vehicle parks). Sometimes you will find a bystander or group of bystanders beginning to show aggressive behavior. If this happens, call for the police. In some settings, it may be necessary to place the patient in the ambulance and leave the scene rather than wait for the police.
- *Perpetrators.* A perpetrator of a crime may still be on the scene—in sight or in hiding. Do not enter a crime scene or a scene of violence until police have secured it and told you it is safe to do so.

- *Pets.* While most domestic animals are not dangerous in ordinary circumstances, the presence of an animal at the emergency scene poses problems. Even friendly animals may become defensive when you begin to treat the owner. Animals also can be very distracting, interfere with patient care, and cause falls while you are lifting and moving the patient. No matter what the pet owner says ("He won't hurt you. He's very friendly."), it is usually best to have pets placed securely in another room.

Keep in mind that the vast majority of EMS calls will go by uneventfully. As an EMT-B, you are a vital part of the EMS system. Nothing in this text is intended to create fear or paranoia. However, when a call does pose some kind of threat, you must be prepared to recognize the subtle and not-so-subtle signs that can warn you before danger strikes.

React

Observation has provided the critical information needed about the danger. The next step is knowing how to react. The three Rs of reacting to danger are retreat, radio, and reevaluate.

It is not part of your responsibilities as an EMT-B to subdue a violent person or wrestle a weapon away from anyone. A clear and justified course of action is to *retreat* from such dangers. Note that some ways of retreating are safer than others:

- *Flee.* Get far enough away so you will have time to react should the danger begin to move toward your new position. Place two major obstacles between you and the danger. If the dangerous person gets through one of the obstacles, you have a built-in buffer with the second.
- *Get rid of any cumbersome equipment.* In the event you must flee from the scene, do not get bogged down by your equipment. Discard all of it if this will enhance your ability to get away. Use equipment to your benefit. For example, if you are being pursued, wedge your stretcher in a doorway to slow down the aggressor.
- *Take cover and conceal yourself* (Figure 2-10). Taking cover is finding a position that protects your body from projectiles, such as behind a brick wall. Concealing yourself is hiding your body behind an object that cannot protect you, such as a shrub. Find a position that will both conceal and protect you.

When fleeing danger, your best option is to use distance, cover, and concealment to protect yourself. Do not return to the scene until the police have secured it.

The second R of reacting to danger is *radio*. The portable radio is an important piece of safety equip-

Figure 2-10a Concealing yourself is placing your body behind an object that can hide you from view.

Figure 2-10b Taking cover is finding a position that both hides you and protects your body from projectiles.

ment. Use it to call for police assistance and to warn other responding units of the danger. Speak into it clearly and slowly. Advise the dispatcher of the exact nature and location of the problem. Specify how many people are involved and whether or not weapons were observed. Remember, the information you have about the scene must be shared as soon as possible to prevent others from encountering the same danger.

Finally, the third R of reacting to danger is *reevaluate*. Do not reenter a scene until it has been secured by the police (Figure 2-11). Even then, be aware that where violence has been, it may begin again. Emergencies are situations packed with stress for families, patients, responders, and bystanders. Maintain a level of alert observation throughout the call. Occasionally you may find weapons or drugs while you are assessing the patient. If that happens, stop what you are doing and radio the police immediately. After the call, document the situation on your run report. Occasionally, the danger may cause delays in reaching the patient. Courts have held this delay acceptable, provided there has been a real and documented danger.

Figure 2-11 Never enter a scene that is potentially violent until the police have secured it and told you it is safe.

STREET SCENES

While en route to a motor-vehicle collision, the dispatcher gives your responding ambulance an update. "Ambulance Charlie 7, you have one patient with bad facial injuries." After judging the scene safe to enter, you immediately start to assess the patient. Just as you open the airway and your partner provides oxygen, the paramedic unit arrives and takes over care of the patient.

As you are finishing loading the patient into the back of the paramedic's ambulance, one of them asks where your gloves are. You don't think much of it and start to clean up your equipment. As you get into the ambulance, your partner tells you that not only is it against the ambulance service's standard operating procedure for you not to wear gloves on this type of call, but it is foolish. You reluctantly agree to tell your supervisor.

Later, you enter the supervisor's office, you describe the call, the amount of blood, and then tell her that you had not worn any protective gloves. You also point out that you may have had a partially healed cut on your hand. She tells you that you are out-of-service.

STREET SCENE QUESTIONS

1. Why wear protective gloves on this type of call?
2. What is the impact of an occupational exposure on you, your family, and your fellow EMS workers?
3. What can you expect after exposure?

Your supervisor explains that you need to go to the emergency department for an occupational evaluation. There is a pre-arrangement with the hospital, and they will have a member of their infection control staff go through your evaluation and counseling.

When you get to the hospital the infection control nurse interviews you and asks many specific questions about the call, your health, and what type of immunizations you have had. She examines your hands for breaks in the skin, and a number are identified. When the interview is over it is recommended that you get some base-line blood tests; one is for HIV. All of a sudden you realize how serious this situation is. It is recommended that you take some medications, and you are given information on precautions that you need to take when having intimate relations with your spouse. It hits you again how serious this has become.

STREET SCENE QUESTIONS

4. How will stress be a factor in your life for the next few months?
5. How important is handwashing?
6. What type of BSI precautions should EMTs always be ready to use on all EMS calls?

You try to take your mind off the situation, but you can't. It affects your sleep. You are irritable around your family. When you try to talk to your partner, you find you're too embarrassed.

Quite sometime later, the infection control nurse tells you that your latest blood tests are back. They're all negative. A personal tragedy has been avoided. As you start to leave her office, the nurse tells you to remember—gloves and handwashing are very important. With a big smile, you look back and say: "I GET IT!"

CHAPTER REVIEW

SUMMARY

Safeguarding your well-being as an EMT-Basic is critical. One way is to protect yourself from bloodborne and airborne pathogens with the appropriate personal protective equipment (PPE) and other infection-control procedures. Another is to make lifestyle changes that help to reduce the stress associated with treating angry, scared, violent, seriously injured, and ill patients. Finally, you can ensure your personal safety by consistently being alert to the potential for danger at every emergency call.

KEY TERMS

body substance isolation (BSI) a form of infection control based on the presumption that all body fluids are infectious.

contamination the introduction of dangerous chemicals, disease, or infectious materials.

critical incident stress debriefing (CISD) a process in which teams of professional and peer counselors provide emotional and psychological support to EMS personnel who are or have been involved in a critical (highly stressful) incident.

decontamination the removal or cleansing of dangerous chemicals and other dangerous or infectious materials.

hazardous-materials incident the release of a harmful substance into the environment.

multiple-casualty incident (MCI) an emergency involving multiple patients.

pathogens the organisms that cause infection, such as viruses and bacteria.

personal protective equipment (PPE) equipment that protects the EMS worker from infection and/or exposure to the dangers of rescue operations.

REVIEW QUESTIONS

1. Name some of the causes of stress for an EMT-B and explain some ways the EMT-B can alleviate job-related stress. (pp. 23–26)
2. Describe the purpose and process of a critical incident stress debriefing (CISD). (pp. 24–25)
3. What are the stages of grief? Why should the EMT-B deal with these emotions? (pp. 25–26)

4. List the types of personal protective equipment used in body substance isolation (BSI). Identify a condition or patient with which each one should be used. (pp. 15–18)

APPLICATIONS

• You are called to an unknown emergency at a tavern. As you approach the scene, you see a man lying supine in the parking lot, apparently bleeding profusely. Two other men are scuffling, and one seems to have a gun. What actions must you take? (pp. 27–29)

WEB MEDIC

Visit Brady's *Emergency Care* website for dilrect weblinks. At **www.bradybooks.com/ emergencycare**, you will find information related to the following Chapter 2 topics:

• Allergies to latex
• Stress and EMS

Chapter
Three

MEDICAL/LEGAL AND ETHICAL ISSUES

*W*ord on the Street

"Most people outside of EMS have never been deposed or had to testify at a trial. It is said that there are two types of motorcyclists: those who have crashed and those who will. EMS is no different in this regard. There are EMS folks who have been called to court and those who will be. We operate on a legal platform that is dynamic, changing from one day to the next. Ignorance is not an excuse. Expect to be called to court and document accordingly. Use your integrity when dealing with patients, and protect it at all costs—it is the only thing you ever really own."

Paul A. Werfel   NREMT-P, Director, Paramedic Program, and Clinical Instructor in Health Sciences, State University of New York at Stony Brook

Every time you respond to a call, you will be faced with some aspect of medical/legal or medical/ethical issues. The issue may be as simple as making sure that the patient will accept help or as complex as a terminally ill patient who refuses all care. You may also be faced with decisions such as "Should I stop and help even though I am off-duty?" "Can I get sued if I stop to help outside of my ambulance district?" Understanding of medical, legal, and ethical issues is an essential foundation for all emergency care. This knowledge may also reduce or prevent the legal liability that you may face as a result of calls.

SCOPE OF PRACTICE

The EMT-Basic is governed by many medical, legal, and ethical guidelines. This collective set of regulations and ethical considerations may be referred to as a **scope of practice,** which defines the scope, or extent and limits, of an EMT-B's job. The skills and medical interventions (what you do to help the patient) that may be performed by an EMT-B are defined by legislation. This legislation varies from state to state. Sometimes different regions within the same state may have different rules and guidelines for their EMT-Bs.

For example, an EMT-B in one area may be able to perform certain basic procedures and levels of care. In the adjoining region, EMT-Bs may provide that care and in addition perform special advanced procedures. Your duty is to provide for the well-being of the patient by rendering necessary and legally allowed care as defined under the scope of practice in your area.

Falling within your scope of practice are certain ethical responsibilities. The primary ethical consideration is to make patient care and well-being a priority, even if this requires some personal sacrifice. For example, there may be times when a patient feels cold, even in a hot climate. You may want to turn on the air conditioner in the ambulance, but you refrain out of consideration for your patient. Actions such as this may seem small but mean a lot to the patient.

To be an effective EMT-B, you must maintain your skills and knowledge. This includes practicing until you have obtained confidence and mastery of the skills. After that, continuing education and recertification are necessary to maintain mastery. Every patient deserves the best care.

Emergency care can be improved on a crew and squad level as well as on an individual level. After a call, constructively critique both yourself and the crew. Accept suggestions from others to improve your skills, communication, and patient outcome. Participation in this kind of mutual critique is part of the process known as *quality improvement*. It should be practiced with the aim of maintaining the standards you would wish to have provided for yourself or someone in your family.

During the rest of this chapter, you will learn about some specific aspects of the scope of practice.

PATIENT CONSENT AND REFUSAL

Consent

Consent, or permission from the patient, is required for any treatment or action by the EMT-B. Most patients or their families will have called for your assistance and will readily accept it. A simple statement, such as "I'm Karla Maguire, an EMT-B from the ambulance. I'd like to help you, okay?" is enough to request consent. Most patients will respond positively. Expressed consent must be obtained from every conscious, mentally competent adult before providing care and transportation.

TOPIC OVERVIEW

In this chapter, you will learn about the following topics:

- The scope of practice of an EMT-Basic
- How a patient may consent to or refuse emergency care
- What it means to have a duty to act
- The legal concepts of negligence and abandonment
- The responsibilities of an EMT at a crime scene

DOT OBJECTIVES

✔ **Knowledge and Attitude**

1. Define the EMT-Basic scope of practice. (p. 33)

2. Discuss the importance of do not resuscitate (DNR) orders (advance directives) and local or state provisions regarding EMS application. (pp. 35, 37–38)

3. Define consent and discuss the methods of obtaining consent. (pp. 33–34)

4. Differentiate between expressed and implied consent. (p. 34)

5. Explain the role of consent of minors in providing care. (p. 34)

6. Discuss the implications for the EMT-Basic in patient refusal of transport. (pp. 34–35)

7. Discuss the issues of abandonment, negligence, and battery and their implications to the EMT-Basic. (pp. 38–39)

8. State the conditions necessary for the EMT-Basic to have a duty to act. (pp. 38–39)

9. Explain the importance, necessity, and legality of patient confidentiality. (p. 39)

10. Discuss the considerations of the EMT-Basic in issues of organ retrieval. (pp. 39–40)

11. Differentiate the actions that an EMT-Basic should take to assist in the preservation of a crime scene. (pp. 40, 42)

12. State the conditions that require an EMT-Basic to notify local law enforcement officials. (pp. 35, 40, 42)

13. Explain the role of EMS and the EMT-Basic regarding patients with DNR orders. (pp. 35, 37–38)

14. Explain the rationale for the needs, benefits, and usage of advance directives. (pp. 35, 37–38)

15. Explain the rationale for the concept of varying degrees of DNR. (pp. 35, 37–38)

The principle of consent may seem simple, but it often brings up complex issues in patient care. There are three types of consent: expressed, implied, and consent to treat minors or incompetent patients.

Expressed Consent

The consent given by adults who are of legal age and mentally competent to make a rational decision in regard to their medical well-being is **expressed consent.** It must be obtained from all patients who are physically or mentally able to give it. Expressed consent must be informed consent. That is, patients must understand the risks associated with the care they will receive. It is not only a legal requirement but also sound emotional care to explain all procedures to the patient.

Implied Consent

In the case of an unconscious patient, consent may be assumed. The law states that rational patients would consent to treatment if they were conscious. This is known as **implied consent.** In this situation, the law allows EMT-Bs and other health-care providers to provide treatment, at least until the patient becomes conscious and able to make rational decisions.

Children and Mentally Incompetent Adults

Children and mentally incompetent adults are not legally allowed to provide consent or refuse medical care and transportation. For these patients, their parents and guardians have the legal authority to give consent, so it must be obtained before care can be given. There are times, however, when care may be given without this direct consent from a parent or guardian.

In cases of life-threatening illness or injury when a parent or guardian is not present, care may be given based on implied consent. The law provides that it is reasonable to believe that a responsible parent or guardian would consent to care if he were present. In some states, statutes allow emancipated minors—those who are married or of a certain age—to provide consent. Find out the laws where you will practice as an EMT-B in reference to consent of minors.

When a Patient Refuses Care

You may think that all patients who need medical care will accept it. Most do. However, you will find that some patients who require treatment and transportation to the hospital will refuse care. There are many reasons for this including denial, fear, failing to understand the seriousness of the situation, intoxication, and others.

While patients generally have the right to refuse care, it is your responsibility as an EMT-B to be sure that the patient is fully informed about his situation and the implications of refusing care.

In order for a patient to refuse care or transport several conditions must be fulfilled:

- *Patient must be legally able to consent.* He must be of legal age or an emancipated minor.
- *Patient must be mentally competent and oriented.* He must not be affected by any disease or condition that would impair judgment. These conditions include unstable vital signs and altered mental status.

How and Why?

Patients and their families are more likely than ever to have prepared a written statement detailing the patient's own preference for future medical care. To find out more about advance directives, go to your Electronic Extras CD.

- *Patient must be fully informed* and understand the risks associated with refusing treatment and/or transport.
- *Patient must sign a "release" form.* Such a form is designed to release the ambulance squad and individuals from **liability** (legal responsibility) arising from the patient's informed refusal.

Even carefully following the steps outlined above will not guarantee that you will be free from liability if a patient refuses care or transport. Leaving a patient who will not accept care or transport is a leading cause of lawsuits against EMS agencies and providers, even though it was the patient who refused. Occasionally the patient's condition deteriorates to the point of unconsciousness, which leaves the patient unable to summon help, leading to a severely worsened condition or even death.

In addition to the liability factor, there is also an ethical issue. You would undoubtedly feel guilty if a patient was found unconscious or deceased after refusing care and you felt that transportation would have prevented the circumstance.

If in doubt, do everything possible to persuade the patient to accept care and transport. Take all possible actions to persuade a patient who you feel should go to the hospital but refuses. These actions may include:

- *Spend time speaking to the patient.* Use principles of effective communication. It may take reasoning, persistence, "dealing" ("We'll call a neighbor to take care of your cat, but then you go to the hospital"), or other strategies.
- *Inform the patient of the consequences* of not going to the hospital, even if they are not pleasant.
- *Consult medical direction.* If you are in a residence, use the patient's phone to contact medical direction. If the on-line doctor is willing, let him speak to the patient when all else fails.
- *Contact family members* to help convince the patient. Often family members can provide reasons for the patient to go to the hospital. An offer from a loved one to meet the patient at the hospital may be very helpful.
- *Call law enforcement personnel* if necessary. Police may be able to order or "arrest" the patient who refuses care to force him to go to the hospital. This is done under the premise that the patient is temporarily mentally incompetent as demonstrated by refusing care that might save his life.
- *Try to determine why the patient is refusing care.* Often the patient has a fear of the hospital, procedures, prolonged hospitalization, or even death.

Refusal to go to the hospital may be a form of denial, or unwillingness to accept the idea of being ill. If you identify the cause of the refusal, you may be able to develop a strategy to persuade the patient to accept your care and transportation to the hospital.

Bear in mind, however, that you do not have the right in most cases to force a competent patient to go to the hospital against his will. Subjecting the patient to unwanted care and transport has actually been viewed as assault or battery in court.

If all efforts fail and the patient does not accept your care or transportation, it becomes vital to document the attempts you made—to make your efforts a part of the official record—in order to prevent liability. Write into your records every step you took to persuade the patient to accept care or to go to the hospital. Include the names of any witnesses to your attempts and the patient's refusal. (A sample EMS patient refusal procedures checklist is shown in Figure 3-1.)

In all cases of refusal, you should advise the patient that he should call back at any time if he has a problem or wishes to be cared for or transported. It is advisable to call a relative or neighbor who can stay with the patient in case problems develop. Leave phone stickers with emergency numbers so the patient will be able to call for help if necessary. You should also recommend that the patient or a relative call the family physician to report the incident and arrange for follow-up care. Document all actions you have taken for the patient.

While there may be patients who legitimately refuse care (for minor wounds, unfounded calls, and the like) a patient with any significant medical condition should be transported and seen at a hospital.

Do Not Resuscitate Orders

It will only be a matter of time before you come upon a patient who has a **do not resuscitate (DNR) order** (Figure 3-2). This is a legal document, usually signed by the patient and his physician, which states that the patient has a terminal illness and does not wish to prolong life through resuscitative efforts. A DNR order is called an **advance directive,** because it is written and signed in advance of any event where resuscitation might be undertaken. It is more than the expressed wishes of the patient or family. It is an actual, legal document.

There are varying degrees of DNR orders, expressed through a variety of detailed instructions that may be part of the order. Such an instruction might stipulate, for example, that resuscitation be attempted only if cardiac or respiratory arrest is observed, but

EMS PATIENT REFUSAL CHECKLIST

PATIENT's NAME: _____ AGE: _____

LOCATION OF CALL: _____ DATE: _____

AGENCY INCIDENT #: _____ AGENCY CODE: _____

NAME OF PERSON FILLING OUT FORM: _____

I. ASSESSMENT OF PATIENT (Check appropriate response for each item)

1. Oriented to:
   Person? ☐ Yes ☐ No
   Place? ☐ Yes ☐ No
   Time? ☐ Yes ☐ No
   Situation? ☐ Yes ☐ No

2. Altered level of consciousness? ☐ Yes ☐ No

3. Head injury? ☐ Yes ☐ No

4. Alcohol or drug ingestion by exam or history? ☐ Yes ☐ No

II. PATIENT INFORMED (Check appropriate response for each item)

☐ Yes ☐ No   Medical treatment/evaluation needed

☐ Yes ☐ No   Ambulance transport needed

☐ Yes ☐ No   Further harm could result without medical treatment/evaluation

☐ Yes ☐ No   Transport by means other than ambulance could be hazardous in light of patient's illness/injury

☐ Yes ☐ No   Patient provided with Refusal Information Sheet

☐ Yes ☐ No   Patient accepted Refusal Information Sheet

III. DISPOSITION

☐ Refused all EMS assistance

☐ Refused field treatment, but accepted transport

☐ Refused transport, but accepted field treatment

☐ Refused transport to recommended facility

☐ Patient transported by private vehicle to_____

☐ Released in care or custody of self

☐ Released in care or custody of relative or friend

   Name: _____ Relationship: _____

☐ Released in custody of law enforcement agency

   Agency: _____ Officer: _____

☐ Released in custody of other agency

   Agency: _____ Officer: _____

IV. COMMENTS: _____

_____

_____

_____

Figure 3-1 Certain procedures should be followed when a patient refuses care or transport. The above checklist is from Spokane County Emergency Medical Services, Washington State.

PREHOSPITAL DO NOT RESUSCITATE ORDERS

<u>ATTENDING PHYSICIAN</u>

In completing this prehospital DNR form, please check part A if no intervention by prehospital personnel is indicated. Please check Part A and options from Part B if specific interventions by prehospital personnel are indicated. To give a valid prehospital DNR order, this form must be completed by the patient's attending physician and must be provided to prehospital personnel.

A) _____ **Do Not Resuscitate (DNR):**
No Cardiopulmonary Resuscitation or Advanced Cardiac Life Support be performed by prehospital personnel

B) _____ **Modified Support:**
Prehospital personnel administer the following checked options:
_____Oxygen administration
_____Full airway support: intubation, airways, bag/valve/mask
_____Venipuncture: IV crystalloids and/or blood draw
_____External cardiac pacing
_____Cardiopulmonary resuscitation
_____Cardiac defibrillator
_____Pneumatic anti-shock garment
_____Ventilator
_____ACLS meds
_____Other interventions/medications (physician specify)
_____

Prehospital personnel are informed that (print patient name)_____
should receive no resuscitation (DNR) or should receive Modified Support as indicated. This directive is medically appropriate and is further documented by a physician's order and a progress note on the patient's permanent medical record. Informed consent from the capacitated patient or the incapacitated patient's legitimate surrogate is documented on the patient's permanent medical record. The DNR order is in full force and effect as of the date indicated below.

_____   _____

Attending Physician's Signature   _____

_____   _____

Print Attending Physician's Name   Print Patient's Name and Location
                                          (Home Address or Health Care Facility)

_____

Attending Physician's Telephone

_____   _____

Date   Expiration Date (6 Mos from Signature)

Figure 3-2   Example of a do not resuscitate (DNR) order.

not attempted if the patient is found already in arrest (to avoid the possibility of resuscitating a patient who may already have sustained brain damage).

Many states also have laws governing living wills, which are statements signed by the patient, usually regarding use of long-term life-support and comfort measures such as respirators, intravenous feedings, and pain medications. Other states require naming a *proxy*—a person whom the signer of the document names to make health-care decisions in case he is unable to make such decisions for himself.

Living wills and health-care proxies usually pertain to situations that will occur in the hospital rather than in the prehospital situation.

Become familiar with the laws regarding DNR orders, living wills, and health-care proxies for your region or state and the laws and rules governing their implementation. It is important to know the forms and policies before you go to the call, since often the patient is in cardiac arrest (heart and breathing have stopped) or near death. These are stressful times for the family and for you, occasions when the window of time for making a resuscitation decision may be only a few moments.

A legal DNR order prevents unwanted resuscitation and awkward situations. In most cases, the oral requests of a family member are not reason to withhold care. If the family requests you to not resuscitate the patient, and if there are no legal DNR orders available, it is a legal and ethical dilemma that is usually best resolved by providing care. It is better to be criticized or sued for attempting to save a life than for letting a patient die.

OTHER LEGAL ASPECTS

Negligence

To the layperson, negligence means that something that should have been done was not done or was done incorrectly. The legal concept of negligence in emergency care is not that simple. A finding of **negligence,** or failure to act properly, requires that *all* of the following circumstances be proved:

- *The EMT had a duty to the patient* (duty to act—see the next section).
- *The EMT did not provide the standard of care* (committed a breach of duty). This may include the failure to act; that is, he did not provide needed care as would be expected of an EMT-B in your locality. Failure to act is a major cause of legal actions against EMS systems or EMTs.
- *By not providing the standard of care, the EMT caused harm to the patient.* This harm can be physical or psychological.

Negligence is the basis for a large number of lawsuits involving prehospital emergency care. If the above circumstances are proved, the EMT may be required to pay damages if the harm to the patient is considered by the court to be a loss that requires reimbursement (compensable). The negligent EMT may be required to pay for medical expenses, lost wages (possibly including future earnings), pain and suffering, and various other factors as determined by the court.

Two of the most common and significant causes of lawsuits against EMTs are patient refusal and ambulance collisions (Figure 3-3). In patient refusal situations, EMTs are sued because the patient's condition deteriorated after the ambulance left the scene. This makes it critical to follow your agency's guidelines when a patient refuses care.

Figure 3-3 Ambulance collisions are a leading cause of injury, death, and legal liability to EMTs.

Collisions are dangerous in any vehicle. When an ambulance is involved, collisions become serious because of the size and weight of the vehicle, the number of occupants (including the patient), and the nature of emergency driving. It is important to remember that most collisions are preventable. (This is why they are no longer referred to as "accidents.") Emergency driving must be done responsibly.

Lawsuits against EMT-Bs are actually quite rare, especially when compared to the number of calls that are dispatched each day in this country. While liability and negligence should be important considerations, you should not live or work in fear of a lawsuit. When you perform proper care that is within your scope of practice and is properly documented, you will prevent most, if not all, legal problems.

Duty to Act

An EMT-B in certain situations has a **duty to act,** or an obligation to provide emergency care to a patient. An EMT-B who is on an ambulance and is dispatched to a call clearly has a duty to act. If there is no threat to safety, the EMT-B must provide care. This duty to act continues throughout the call.

If an EMT-B has initiated care, then leaves a patient without assuring that the patient has been turned over to someone with equal or greater medical training, **abandonment** exists.

The duty to act is not always clear. It depends on your state and local laws. In many states, an off-duty EMT-B has no legal obligation to provide care. However, you may feel a moral or ethical obligation to act. An example of this would be if you observe a motor-vehicle collision while off duty. You may feel morally bound to provide care, even if no legal obligation exists. If you are off duty, begin care, and then leave before other trained personnel arrive, you may still be considered to have abandoned the patient.

Other situations are even more confusing. If you are an EMT-B in an ambulance, but you are out of your jurisdiction, the laws are again often unclear. In general, if you follow your conscience and provide care, you will incur less liability than if you do not act. Always follow your local protocols and laws. Your instructor will provide information about local issues.

Good Samaritan Laws

Good Samaritan laws have been developed in all states to provide immunity to individuals trying to help people in emergencies. Most of these laws will grant immunity from liability if the rescuer acts in good faith to provide care to the level of his training and to the best of his ability. These laws do not prevent someone from initiating a lawsuit, nor will they protect the rescuer from being found liable for acts of gross negligence and other violations of the law.

You must familiarize yourself with the laws that govern your state. Good Samaritan laws may not apply to EMT-Bs in your locality. In some states, the Good Samaritan laws only apply to volunteers. If you are a paid EMT-B, different laws and regulations may apply.

Some states have specific statutes that authorize, regulate, and protect EMS personnel. Typically, to be protected by such laws, you must be recognized as an EMT in the state where care was provided. Some states have specific licensing and certification requirements that must be met for recognition under Good Samaritan laws.

Confidentiality

When you act as an EMT-B, you obtain a considerable amount of information about a patient. You also are allowed into homes and other personal areas that are private and contain much information about people.

Any information you obtain about a patient's history, condition, or treatment is considered confidential and must not be shared with anyone else. This principle is known as **confidentiality.** Such infor-

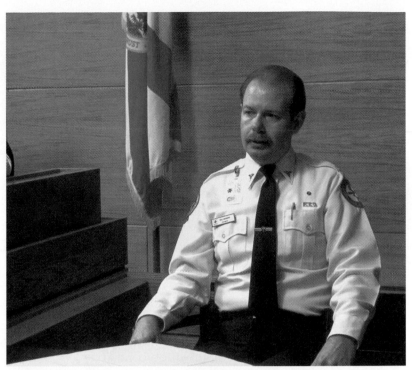

Figure 3-4 An EMT-Basic may be required to testify in court in a variety of legal settings.

mation may be disclosed only when a written release is signed by the patient. Your organization will have a policy on this. Patient information should not be disclosed based on verbal permission, nor should information be disclosed over the telephone.

However, you may be subpoenaed, or ordered into court by a legal authority, where you may legally disclose patient information (Figure 3-4). If you have a question about the validity of a legal document, contact a supervisor or your agency's attorney for advice.

Patient information also may be shared with other health-care professionals who will have a role in the care of the patient or in quality improvement. It is appropriate to turn over information about the patient to the nurse and physician at the receiving hospital. This is necessary for continuity in patient care. It may also be necessary and permissible to supply certain patient-care information for insurance billing forms.

Special Situations

A patient may wear a medical identification device (Figure 3-5). This device is worn to alert EMT-Bs and other health-care professionals that the patient has a particular medical condition. If the patient is found unconscious, the device provides important medical information. The device may be a necklace, bracelet,

Figure 3-5 Example of a medical identification device (front and back).

or card and may indicate a number of conditions including:

- Heart conditions
- Allergies
- Diabetes
- Epilepsy

You may respond to calls where a patient is critically injured, perhaps near death, and is an organ donor. An **organ donor** is a patient who has completed a legal document that allows for donation of organs and tissues in the event of his death. Many people have benefited from the donation of organs by persons who have completed this paperwork (Figure 3-6).

You may find that the patient is an organ donor when told so by a family member. Often a patient may have an organ donor card on him. The back of the patient's driver's license may also contain an indication that the patient wishes to donate organs upon his death.

The emergency care of a patient who is an organ donor must not differ from the care of a patient who is not a donor. All emergency care measures must be taken. If a patient is recognized as an organ donor, contact medical direction. The on-line physician may order you to perform CPR on a patient when you might normally not resuscitate due to fatal injuries.

The oxygen delivered to body cells by CPR will help preserve the organs until they can be harvested for implantation in another person.

Crime Scenes

A **crime scene** is defined as the location where a crime has been committed or any place that evidence relating to a crime may be found (Figure 3-7). Many crime scenes involve crimes against people. These crimes cause injuries that are often serious. Once police have made the scene safe, the priority of the EMT-B at a crime scene is to provide patient care.

While you are providing care at the crime scene, there are actions that you can take to help preserve evidence. To preserve evidence, you must first know what evidence is, as described below.

- *Condition of the scene.* The way you find the scene is important evidence to the police. Should you arrive first, make a mental note of the exterior of the scene. Remember how you gained access. Doors found ajar, pry marks, and broken windows are signs of danger for you and important evidence for the police. Make a note of whether the lights were on or off and the condition of the TV and radio.
- *The patient.* The patient himself provides valuable information. The position the patient is found in, condition of clothing, and injuries are all valuable pieces of evidence.
- *Fingerprints and footprints.* Fingerprints are perhaps the most familiar kind of evidence. They may be obtained from almost any surface. It is important for you to avoid unnecessarily touching anything at the scene in order to preserve prints. Since

**Valley General Hospital
Permission For
Organ Donation/Anatomical Gift
By An Individual Prior To Death**

PATIENT IDENTIFICATION PLATE

I, _____ , currently residing at _____

_____ , being eighteen (18) years of age or older, do hereby make the

following organ donation/anatomical gift to take effect upon my death:

1.　　I give, if medically acceptable:

☐ My body
☐ Any needed organs or parts
☐ The following organs or parts: _____

_____

_____

2.　　I make this gift to Valley General Hospital or to physicians or institutions designated by them for
　　　the following purposes:

☐ Any purpose authorized by law
☐ Transplantation
☐ Therapy
☐ Medical Research and/or Education

3.　　I acknowledge that I have read this document in its entirety and that I fully understand it and that
　　　all blank spaces have either been completed or crossed off prior to my signing.

4.　　I understand that Valley General Hospital and its authorized designees will rely upon this consent.

SIGNATURE	DATE	WITNESS TO SIGNATURE (PRINT NAME and ADDRESS BELOW)	DATE

PRINT NAME

ADDRESS

TELEPHONE NUMBER

WITNESS TO SIGNATURE
(PRINT NAME and ADDRESS BELOW)　　　　DATE

Figure 3-6　　Example of an organ donor form.

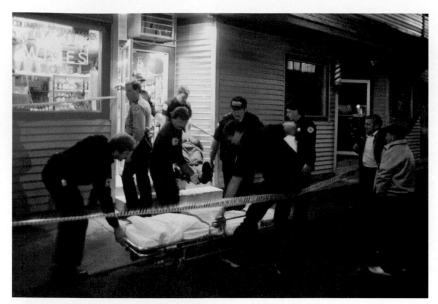

Figure 3-7 Example of a crime scene.

you will be wearing gloves at most scenes, you will not leave your fingerprints on objects. If you touch these objects, however, you may smudge fingerprints that were left by someone else.

- *Microscopic evidence.* Microscopic evidence is a wide range of evidence that is usually invisible to the naked eye. It consists of small pieces of evidence such as dirt and carpet fibers. To the eye, there may be no way to distinguish one from another. Under the microscope, scientists can develop valuable information. From just a few fibers, the materials and sometimes the brand name of carpets or clothes can be determined. Traces of blood may be enough to determine blood type or to be used for DNA comparison.

To preserve evidence at the crime scene, the following actions will be helpful to the police. Remember that your first priority is always patient care.

- *Remember what you touch.* It may be necessary to move the patient or furniture to begin CPR or other patient care. This cannot be avoided, but it is helpful to tell the police what you have touched or moved. Once you leave, if they find furniture moved or blood stains in two locations, they may think that a scuffle took place when in fact it did not. If you are forced to break a window to get to the patient and do not tell the police, they will think that a breaking-and-entering has occurred.

- *Minimize your impact on the scene.* If you are forced to move the patient or furniture to begin care, move as little as possible. Do not wander through the house or go to areas where it is not necessary to go. Avoid using the phone, which will

prevent the police from using the "redial" button to determine who the victim called last. Do not use the bathroom since this may also destroy evidence.

- *Work with the police.* The police may require you to provide a statement about your actions or observations at the scene. While it may not be possible to make notes while patient care is going on, after you arrive at the hospital make notes about your observations and actions at the scene.

You may also wish to critique the scene—both with your crew and, if possible, with the police. Invite a member of your local or state police department to your agency for an in-service drill on crime scenes. Evidence recovery methods and procedures vary from area to area. The police officer who comes to your station will brief you on local procedures.

Interestingly enough, police are often as unfamiliar with EMS procedures as you are with evidence procedures. The police may ask you to delay your work at the scene so they can take photographs or interview the patient. They may do this because they do not understand—as you will learn in later chapters—that in the case of serious injury, the time that elapses before on-scene care and transport to the hospital must be kept to a minimum for the patient to have the best chance of survival. Education and critiques can be beneficial to both EMT-Bs and police officers.

Special Crimes and Reporting

Many states require EMT-Bs and other health-care professionals to report certain types of incidents. Many areas have hotlines for reporting crimes such as child, elder, or domestic abuse. This may be mandatory in your area. Failure to report certain incidents may actually be a crime. There is also a strong moral obligation to report these crimes. Many states offer immunity from liability for people who report incidents such as these in good faith.

Other crimes may also require reports. Violence (such as gunshot wounds or stabbings) and sexual assaults often fall into this category. If you are required by law to report such incidents, you are usually exempt from confidentiality requirements in making these reports.

You may also be required to notify police of other situations, such as cases where restraint may be necessary, intoxicated persons found with injuries, or mentally incompetent people who have been injured.

STREET SCENES

It is a hot summer day when you receive a call for a 37-year-old woman with general body weakness. After your initial assessment, you ask the patient about her medical history. She informs you that she has AIDS. You continue to take vital signs, find it appropriate to provide oxygen, and package her for transport. Your partner makes the radio report to the hospital, and you notice that he makes no reference to AIDS. When you arrive at the hospital, your partner gives the patient report in the hallway leading to the examination room. He provides all the patient information but does not tell the doctor the patient reported she has AIDS until he can do it discreetly in the room.

STREET SCENE QUESTIONS

1. Was it appropriate not to include the information that the patient had AIDS during the radio report to the hospital?
2. What is the obligation of these EMTs concerning the confidentiality of patient information?
3. Would you have handled the transfer of information differently?

After the call was over, you discuss with your partner issues of confidentiality. He tells you that he felt the fact the patient had AIDS did not need to be part of the radio report. He was concerned that it might breach the patient's confidentiality if it was said over the radio. But your partner was quick to add that AIDS was definitely a pertinent part of the medical history and he made sure it was conveyed in a discreet manner at the hospital.

STREET SCENE QUESTIONS

4. Would it be appropriate to tell all the hospital staff so they would know to take BSI precautions?

As you and your partner further discuss the issue, you tell him that alerting the hospital staff so they would know to use BSI precautions would be appropriate. He responds by telling you that all emergency medical personnel, whether EMS or in-hospital, should be taking infection control precautions. However, this should not be a reason for being careless with patient information and possibly breaching a patient's confidentiality.

STREET SCENE QUESTIONS

5. Should the information that this patient has AIDS be shared with other EMS providers in case they get a call for this patient?
6. What are the principles for confidentiality that EMTs should always maintain?

As you pull into the garage, you suggest to your partner that you should alert the other crews about this patient having AIDS. Your partner tells you that this would be a breach of the patient's confidentiality. It would be very inappropriate to do this. He reminds you that patient information is always to be kept confidential, unless it needs to be shared for the purpose of giving care. "For example," he says, "the patient's information on the report to the hospital included the fact that she told us she had AIDS. Also, the physician needed to know because it was part of the medical history that we obtained. Unless there is another reason to share this information that I haven't thought of, no one else needs to hear from us that this patient has AIDS. Confidentiality is an EMS standard that pertains to the history, condition, and treatment of all the patients we see." As he gets out of the ambulance at the station, he adds: "Remember, confidentiality is a professional responsibility."

CHAPTER REVIEW

SUMMARY

Medical, legal, and ethical issues are a part of every EMS call. A number of such issues involve consent, the permission a patient, or patient's parent or guardian, gives for care or transport. Consent may be expressed or implied. If a competent patient refuses care or transport, you should make every effort to persuade him, but you cannot force him to accept care or go to the hospital.

Negligence is failing to act properly when you have a duty to act. As an EMT-B, you have a duty to act whenever you are dispatched on a call. You may have a legal or moral duty to act even when off duty or outside your jurisdiction. Abandonment is leaving a patient after you have initiated care and before you have transferred the patient to a person with equal or higher training. Confidentiality is the obligation not

to reveal personal information you obtain about a patient except to other health-care professionals involved in the patient's care, under court order or when the patient signs a release. As an EMT-B, you may be sued or held legally liable on any of these issues. However, EMT-Bs are rarely held liable when they have acted within their scope of practice and have carefully documented the details of the call.

Special situations include patients who are organ donors (care of the patient takes precedence; follow the advice of medical direction) and patients who wear medical identification devices. At a crime scene, care of the patient takes precedence over preservation of evidence, but you should make every effort not to disturb the scene unnecessarily and to report your actions and observations to the police.

KEY TERMS

abandonment leaving a patient after care has been initiated and before the patient has been transferred to someone with equal or greater medical training.

confidentiality the obligation not to reveal information obtained about a patient except to other health-care professionals involved in the patient's care, or under subpoena, or in a court of law, or when the patient has signed a release of confidentiality.

consent permission from the patient for care or other action by the EMT-B.

crime scene the location where a crime has been committed or any place that evidence relating to a crime may be found.

do not resuscitate (DNR) order a legal document, usually signed by the patient and his physician, which states that the patient has a terminal illness and does not wish to prolong life through resuscitative efforts.

duty to act an obligation to provide care to a patient.

expressed consent consent given by adults who are of legal age and mentally competent to make a rational decision in regard to their medical well-being.

Good Samaritan laws a series of laws, varying in each state, designed to provide limited legal protection for citizens and some health-care personnel when they are administering emergency care.

implied consent the consent it is presumed a patient or patient's parent or guardian would give if they could, such as for an unconscious patient or a parent who cannot be contacted when care is needed.

liability being held legally responsible.

negligence a finding of failure to act properly in a situation in which there was a duty to act, needed care as would reasonably be expected of the EMT-B was not provided, and harm was caused to the patient as a result.

organ donor a person who has completed a legal document that allows for donation of organs and tissues in the event of death.

scope of practice a set of regulations and ethical considerations that define the scope, or extent and limits, of the EMT-B's job.

REVIEW QUESTIONS

1. Define *scope of practice, negligence, duty to act, abandonment,* and *confidentiality.* (pp. 33, 38–39)

2. List several steps that must be taken when a patient refuses care or transportation. (pp. 34–35)

3. List several types of evidence and ways you may act to preserve it at a crime scene. (pp. 40, 42)

APPLICATIONS

• You are called to the scene of a motor-vehicle collision. An eight-year-old child has been struck by a vehicle and fortunately has sustained only slight injuries. Who can give consent for her care? How might you obtain consent? (p. 34)

WEB MEDIC

Visit Brady's *Emergency Care* website for direct weblinks. At **www.bradybooks.com/ emergencycare**, you will find information related to the following Chapter 3 topics:

• Good Samaritan laws

• Advance directives

• Organ donation

Chapter
Four

THE HUMAN BODY

As an EMT-Basic, you will be called when a person has some problem with his body. The problem may be a traumatic injury, or it may be a medical problem such as chest pain. In any case, your assessment of the patient's condition will be based on your knowledge of the **anatomy,** or structure, of the body. You will also be required to know some of the body's functions, referred to as **physiology.** Your knowledge will not only help you assess the patient, it also will allow you to communicate your findings with other EMS personnel and hospital staff accurately and efficiently.

ANATOMICAL TERMS

The body is made up of a number of regions (Figure 4-1). Certain terms are used to describe directions and positions of the body.

Directional Terms

There must be a standardized method of referring to places on the body when describing illness or injury. For this reason, standardized anatomical directional terms are used (Figure 4-2). For example, the directions left and right always refer to the *patient's* left and right.

All descriptions of the body start with the assumption that the body is in anatomical position, even if the patient is not in that position when found. **Anatomical position** is best described as a person standing, facing forward, with his palms forward (Figures 4-1 and 4-2). The importance of always referring to this standardized position is that all healthcare providers, anywhere, will use the same anatomical starting point when describing the body and will understand each other's references.

Also, think of the body as if it has been divided into planes. A **plane** is a flat surface, the kind that would be formed if you sliced straight through a department store dummy or an imaginary human body. Cutting through from top to bottom, you could slice the body either into right and left halves or into front and back halves.

The **midline** of the body is created by drawing an imaginary line down the center of the body, passing between the eyes and extending down past the umbilicus (belly button, or navel) (refer again to Figure 4-2). Slicing through the imaginary body at the midline divides the body into right and left halves.

The term **medial** refers to a position closer to the midline, and the term **lateral** refers to a position farther away from the midline. For example, you would say: "The bridge of the nose is medial to the eyes." You also can say that an arm has a medial side (close to the body) and a lateral side (the outer arm, away from the body).

The term **bilateral** refers to "both sides" of anything. Patients may have diminished lung sounds on both sides when you listen with a stethoscope. This would be reported as "The patient has diminished lung sounds bilaterally." Or, in a patient with chest pain, you might report that "The patient has pain in her chest that radiates bilaterally to the shoulders."

The **mid-axillary line** extends vertically from the mid-armpit to the ankle. (The anatomical term for the armpit is *axilla,* so *mid-axillary* means "middle of the armpit.") This line divides the body into front and back halves. The term for the front is **anterior.** The term for the back is **posterior.** For example, you would say: "The patient has wounds to the posterior arm and the anterior thigh." A synonym for anterior is **ventral** (referring to the front of the body). A synonym for posterior is **dorsal** (referring to the back of the body or back of the hand or foot).

The terms **superior** and **inferior** refer to vertical, or up-and-down, directions. Superior means above; inferior means below. An example of this would be "The nose is superior to the mouth."

The terms **proximal** and **distal** are relative terms. Proximal means closer to the torso (the trunk

TOPIC OVERVIEW

In this chapter, you will learn about the following topics:

- The terms used to describe regions of the body

- The terms used for anatomic reference and description

- The structure and function of major body systems

DOT OBJECTIVES

✔ **Knowledge and Attitude**

1. Identify the following topographic terms: medial, lateral, proximal, distal, superior, inferior, anterior, posterior, midline, right and left, mid-clavicular, bilateral, mid-axillary. (pp. 47–48)

2. Describe the anatomy and function of the following major body systems: respiratory (pp. 54–56), circulatory (pp. 56–60), musculoskeletal (pp. 49, 52–54), nervous (p. 60), and endocrine (p. 63). (Scan 4-1, pp. 65–72; Scan 4-2, pp. 73–74)

of the body, or the body without the head and the extremities). Distal means farther away from the torso. For example, think of an elbow. It is proximal to the hand, because it is closer to the torso than the hand. The elbow also is distal to the shoulder, since the elbow is farther away from the torso than the shoulder. The terms are usually used when describing locations on extremities. For example, to be sure circulation has not been cut off after splinting an arm or leg, you must feel for a distal pulse. This is a pulse found in an extremity, a pulse point that is farther away from the torso than the splint.

Two other terms you may sometimes hear are **palmar** (referring to the palm of the hand) and **plantar** (referring to the sole of the foot).

The **mid-clavicular line** runs through the center of a clavicle (collarbone) and the nipple below it. Since there are two clavicles, there are two mid-clavicular lines. When you use a stethoscope to listen for breath sounds, you will place the stethoscope at the mid-clavicular lines to listen to each side of the chest and assess the function of both lungs.

When describing the abdomen, which contains many vital organs, it is helpful to divide it into four parts, or quadrants. This can be done by drawing horizontal and vertical lines through the navel. The **abdominal quadrants** would be the right upper quadrant, the left upper quadrant, the right lower quadrant, and the left lower quadrant (Figure 4-3). These are often abbreviated as, respectively, RUQ, LUQ, RLQ, and LLQ.

Positional Terms

There are five positions for which you will also need to know the names: supine, prone, recovery, Fowler's, and Trendelenburg:

A **supine** patient is lying on his back. A **prone** patient is lying on his abdomen. A person may also be lying on his side, a position known as the **recovery position,** because it is the position a patient is placed in when recovering from respiratory or cardiac arrest. It is also the preferred position for any unconscious non-trauma patient, because it is a position in which fluids or vomitus can drain from the mouth and be less likely to be aspirated (inhaled) into the lungs. Because the patient is lying on his side, this position is also called the *lateral recumbent position* (Figure 4-4).

When patients are transported on a stretcher, there are several positions that they may be placed in. In the **Fowler's position,** the patient is seated. This is usually accomplished by raising the head end of the stretcher so the body is at a 45°-to-60° angle. The patient may be sitting straight up or leaning slightly back. If leaning back in a semi-sitting position, this is sometimes called *semi-Fowler's* (Figure 4-5). In a Fowler's position, the legs may be straight out or bent.

In the **Trendelenburg position,** the patient is lying with the head slightly lower than the feet (Figure 4-6). This may be accomplished by having the

Figure 4-1 Body regions.

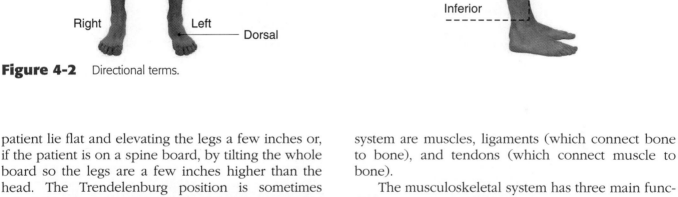

Figure 4-2 Directional terms.

patient lie flat and elevating the legs a few inches or, if the patient is on a spine board, by tilting the whole board so the legs are a few inches higher than the head. The Trendelenburg position is sometimes called the *shock position*, because it is used to treat patients in shock (those who have no possibility of head injury. Patients with head injuries must remain supine with the head and feet on the same level).

BODY SYSTEMS

Musculoskeletal System

Unlike many other systems, the **musculoskeletal system** extends into all parts of the body. The skeleton consists of the skull and spine, ribs and sternum, shoulders and upper extremities, pelvis and lower extremities (Figure 4-7). Interacting with the skeletal

system are muscles, ligaments (which connect bone to bone), and tendons (which connect muscle to bone).

The musculoskeletal system has three main functions:

• To give the body shape
• To protect vital internal organs
• To provide for body movement

Skull

To list the parts of the skeleton from top to bottom, you would begin with the skull (Figure 4-8). The **skull** is the bony structure of the head. A main function of the skull is to enclose and protect the brain. The **cranium** consists of the top, back, and sides of the skull. The face is the front of the skull.

The bones of the anterior cranium connect to facial bones, including the **mandible** (lower jaw), **maxillae** (fused bones of the upper jaw), **zygomatic**

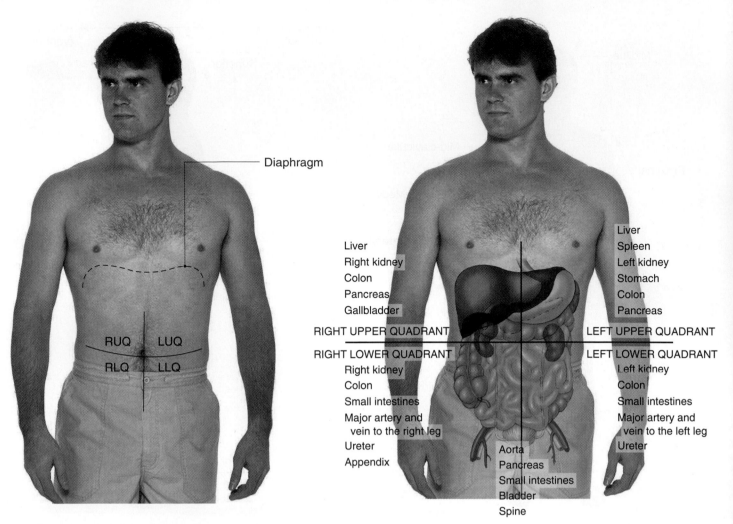

Diaphragm

RUQ | LUQ
RLQ | LLQ

Liver
Right kidney
Colon
Pancreas
Gallbladder

RIGHT UPPER QUADRANT

RIGHT LOWER QUADRANT

Right kidney
Colon
Small intestines
Major artery and
  vein to the right leg
Ureter
Appendix

Liver
Spleen
Left kidney
Stomach
Colon
Pancreas

LEFT UPPER QUADRANT

LEFT LOWER QUADRANT

Left kidney
Colon
Small intestines
Major artery and
  vein to the left leg
Ureter

Aorta
Pancreas
Small intestines
Bladder
Spine

Figure 4-3 Abdominal quadrants.

Supine

Prone

Lateral recumbent position

Figure 4-4 Anatomical postures.

Figure 4-5 Semi-Fowler's position.

Figure 4-6 Trendelenburg position.

Skull

Cervical spine (neck)
Acromion process
Manubrium
Sternum (breast bone)

Xiphoid process
Thoracic spine
Costal cartilage
Lumbar spine

Ilium

Pelvis

Femur head
Acetabulum
Pubis

Clavicle (collarbone)
Scapula
(shoulder blade)

Ribs
Humerus
Elbow

Ulna
Radius

Sacral
spine

Coccyx (tail bone)
Carpals (wrist)
Metacarpals (hand)
Phalanges (fingers)
Femur (thigh bone)
Patella (knee cap)
Tibia
Fibula
Tarsals (ankle)
Metatarsals (foot)
Phalanges (toes)
Calcaneus (heel)

Medial malleolus
Lateral malleolus

Figure 4-7 The skeleton.

51

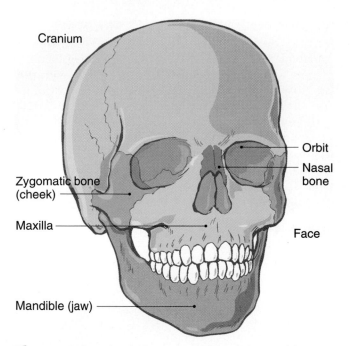

Figure 4-8   The skull consists of the cranium and face.

Figure 4-9   The five divisions of the spine.

bones (cheekbones), and the **nasal bone** (which provides some of the structure of the nose). These bones form the facial structures. Some of these structures consist of multiple bones, such as the **orbits,** which surround the eyes, and the zygomatic arches, which form the structures of the cheeks.

Spinal Column

The spinal column is an essential part of the anatomy. Not only does it provide structure and support for the body, it also houses and protects the spinal cord.

The spinal column (also referred to simply as the spine), consists of 33 **vertebrae,** the separate bones of the spine. Like building blocks, vertebrae are stacked one upon the other to form the spinal col-umn. Vertebrae are open in the middle, somewhat like donuts, creating a hollow center for the spinal cord. Since the spinal cord is essential for movement, sensation, and vital functions, injuries to the spine have the potential to damage the cord, possibly resulting in paralysis or death. For this reason, you will see references throughout this text to "taking spinal precautions" for some patients.

The five divisions of the spine are listed in Table 4-1 and shown in Figure 4-9.

The anatomy of the body allows some vertebrae to be injured more easily than others. Since the head is large and heavy, resting on the slender neck, incidents such as car crashes may cause the head to whip back and forth or strike an object such as the windshield. This frequently causes injuries to the cervical spine. An injury to the spinal cord at this level may be fatal because control of the muscles of breathing, such as the diaphragm and the

TABLE 4-1   The Divisions of the Spine

Division	Corresponding Anatomy	Number of Vertebrae
Cervical	Neck	7
Thoracic	Thorax, ribs, upper back	12
Lumbar	Lower back	5
Sacral	Back wall of pelvis	5
Coccyx	Tailbone	4

muscles between the ribs, arise from the spinal cord in the cervical region. The lumbar region is also subject to injury because it is not supported by other parts of the skeleton. The thoracic spine, to which the ribs are attached, and the sacral spine and coccyx, which are supported by the pelvis, are less easily injured.

Thorax

The **thorax** is the chest. The bones of the thorax form an internal space called the *thoracic cavity.* This cavity contains the heart, lungs, and major blood vessels. An important function of the thorax is to protect these vital organs. This is accomplished by the 12 pairs of ribs that attach to the 12 thoracic vertebrae of the spine. In the front, 10 of these pairs of ribs are attached to the **sternum** (breastbone) and two are called floating ribs since they have no anterior attachment. You will remember the sternum from your CPR training. This flat bone is divided into three sections: the **manubrium** (superior portion), the body (center portion), and the **xiphoid process** (inferior tip).

Pelvis

The pelvis is commonly referred to as the hip, although the hip is actually the joint where the femur (thigh bone) and pelvis join. The pelvis contains bones that are fused together. The **ilium** is the superior bone that contains the iliac crest, which is the wide bony wing that can be felt near the waist. The **ischium** is the inferior, posterior portion of the pelvis. The **pubis** is formed by the joining of the bones of the anterior pubis. The pelvis is joined posteriorly to the sacral spine.

The hip joint consists of the **acetabulum** (the socket of the hip joint) and the ball at the proximal end of the femur.

Lower Extremities

The pelvis and hip joint, described above, may be considered part of the lower extremities. Moving downward from the hip, the large thigh bone is the **femur.** Progressing down the leg, the **patella,** or kneecap, sits anterior to the knee joint. The knee connects with the femur superiorly and with the bones of the lower leg, the tibia and fibula, inferiorly.

The **tibia** is the medial and larger bone of the lower leg, also referred to as the shin bone. The **fibula** is the lateral and smaller bone of the lower leg.

The ankle connects the tibia and fibula with the foot. Two distinct landmarks are the **lateral malleolus** (at the lower end of the fibula) and the **medial malleolus** (at the lower end of the tibia). These are the protrusions that you see on the lateral and medial aspects of your ankles. The ankle consists of bones called **tarsals.** The foot bones are called **metatarsals.** The heel bone is called the **calcaneus.** The toe bones are the **phalanges.**

Upper Extremities

Each shoulder consists of several bones: the clavicle, the scapula, and the proximal humerus. The **clavicle,** or collarbone, is located anteriorly. The **scapula,** or shoulder blade, is located posteriorly. The **acromion process** of the scapula is the highest portion of the shoulder. It forms the **acromioclavicular joint** with the clavicle and is a frequent area of shoulder injury.

The upper arm and forearm consist of three bones connected at the elbow. The bone between the shoulder and the elbow is the **humerus.** The **radius** and **ulna** are the two bones between the elbow and the hand. The radius is the lateral bone of the forearm. It is always aligned with the thumb. (The radial pulse is taken over the radius.) The ulna is the medial forearm bone.

The wrist consists of several bones called **carpals.** The bones of the hand are the **metacarpals.** The finger bones, like the toe bones, are called **phalanges.**

By this point in the chapter, you are realizing the importance of anatomical terms such as *superior, inferior, medial, lateral, anterior,* and *posterior!* These terms will be used throughout the text, and you will need to use them correctly to properly document and report your patient's injuries and complaints.

Joints

Joints are formed when bones connect to other bones. There are several types of joints, including ball-and-socket joints and hinge joints. The hip is an example of a ball-and-socket joint, in which the ball of the femur rotates in a round socket in the pelvis. The elbow is an example of a hinge joint in which the angle between the humerus and ulna—which are connected by ligaments—bends and straightens, as the name suggests, like a hinge.

Muscles

Like the skeleton, the muscles protect the body, give it shape, and allow for movement. There are three types of muscle (Figure 4-10): voluntary muscle, involuntary muscle, and cardiac muscle.

Figure 4-10 Three types of muscle.

cle is extremely sensitive to decreased oxygen supply and can tolerate interruption of blood supply only for very short periods. The heart muscle has its own blood supply through the coronary artery system.

The heart also has a property called **automaticity.** This means that the heart has the ability to generate and conduct electrical impulses on its own. The heartbeat (contraction) is controlled by these electrical impulses.

Respiratory System

The purpose of the respiratory system is to move oxygen (O_2) into the bloodstream through inhalation and pick up carbon dioxide (CO_2) to be excreted through exhalation. To review the anatomy (structure) of the respiratory system, follow the path of air through the system from the mouth and nose to its final destination in the bloodstream.

Respiratory Anatomy

There are a number of structures that make up the respiratory system (Figure 4-11). Air enters the body through the mouth and nose. It moves through the **oropharynx** (the area directly posterior to the mouth) and the **nasopharynx** (the area directly posterior to the nose). The **pharynx** is the area that includes both the oropharynx and the nasopharynx.

Air then proceeds on a path toward the lungs. A leaf-shaped structure called the **epiglottis** closes to prevent foods and foreign objects from entering the trachea during swallowing. The **larynx,** also known as the voice box, contains the vocal cords. The **cricoid cartilage** is a ring-shaped structure that forms the lower portion of the larynx.

The **trachea,** or windpipe, is the tube that carries inhaled air from the larynx down toward the **lungs.** At the level of the lungs, the trachea splits (bifurcates) into two branches called the **bronchi.** One "mainstem" bronchus goes to each lung. Inside each lung, the bronchi continue to branch and split and the air passages get smaller and smaller. Eventually, each branch ends at a group of **alveoli.** The alveoli are the small sacs within the lungs where gas exchange takes place with the bloodstream.

The **diaphragm** is the muscular structure that divides the chest cavity from the abdominal cavity.

Voluntary muscle, or skeletal muscle, is under conscious control of the brain via the nervous system. Attached to the bones, the voluntary muscles form the major muscle mass of the body. They are responsible for movement. Voluntary muscle can contract upon voluntary command of the individual. For example, if you want to, you can reach to pick up an item or walk away. These are examples of voluntary muscle use.

Involuntary muscle, or smooth muscle, is found in the gastrointestinal system, lungs, blood vessels, and urinary system and controls the flow of materials through these structures. Involuntary muscles respond automatically to orders from the brain. You do not have to consciously think about using them to breathe, digest food, or perform other functions that occur under their control. In fact, we have no direct control over involuntary muscles. Involuntary muscles do respond to stimuli such as stretching, heat, and cold.

Cardiac muscle is found only in the heart. It is a specialized form of involuntary muscle. Cardiac mus-

HOW AND WHY?

Did you know that much of our sensory data is dependent on the gravitational force of the Earth? Go to your Electronic Extras CD for information on how NASA and space travel are helping us understand how our bodies work.

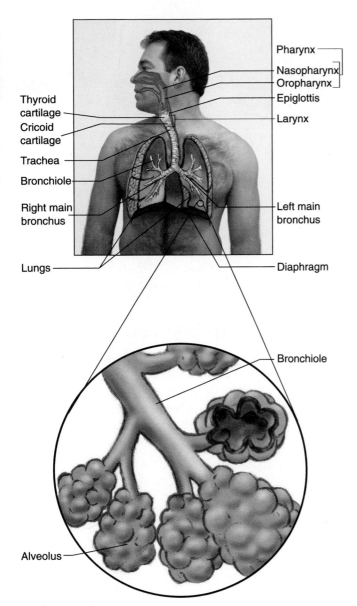

Thyroid cartilage
Cricoid cartilage
Trachea
Bronchiole
Right main bronchus
Lungs

Pharynx
Nasopharynx
Oropharynx
Epiglottis
Larynx
Left main bronchus
Diaphragm

Bronchiole
Alveolus

Figure 4-11   The respiratory system.

During a normal respiratory cycle, the diaphragm and other parts of the body work together to allow the body to inhale and exhale. The role of the diaphragm and other muscles in the respiratory cycle is described below.

Physiology
Inhalation is an active process. The intercostal (rib) muscles and the diaphragm contract. The diaphragm lowers, and the ribs move upward and outward. This expands the size of the chest cavity, causing air to flow into the lungs.

Exhalation is a passive process during which the intercostal muscles and the diaphragm relax. The ribs move downward and inward, while the diaphragm rises. This movement causes the chest cav-

ity to decrease in size and causes air to flow out of the lungs.

Air moves into the lungs through the series of air passages (known as the *airway*), which were described in the anatomy section above. During inhalation, air is moved into the alveoli. These small sacs in the lungs are where gas exchange with the blood takes place. The alveoli are very small. The blood vessels that pass by the alveoli are the smallest type of vessel, capillaries. Oxygen is transferred from the air in the alveoli to the bloodstream through the very thin walls of the alveoli and the capillaries. At the same time carbon dioxide, a waste product of the body's cells, moves from the bloodstream into the alveoli.

Oxygenated blood is carried from the lungs to the heart so it can be pumped into the circulatory system of the body. As the blood leaves the heart, it travels through a branching series of arteries that gradually become smaller and smaller until they are capillaries. Capillaries are found throughout the body. Through the capillary walls, gases are exchanged with all the tissues of the body. Oxygen carried by the blood is given up to the cells. Waste carbon dioxide is picked up from the cells and returned through veins to the heart and then the lungs where it moves from the bloodstream into the alveoli and out of the body through exhalation.

This exchange of gases, both in the lungs and at the body's cells, is critical to support life.

Breathing (the process of inhaling and exhaling air) may be classified as adequate or inadequate. Simply stated, adequate breathing is sufficient to support life. Inadequate breathing is not. Adequate and inadequate breathing, and how you as an EMT-B should assess and care for breathing problems, will be discussed in detail in Chapter 17, "Respiratory Emergencies."

Pediatric Notes

There are a number of special aspects of the respiratory anatomy of infants and children (Figure 4-12). In general, all structures in a child are smaller and more easily obstructed than in an adult. Their tongues take up proportionally more space in the pharynx than do an adult's. The trachea is relatively narrower than in adults and, therefore, more easily obstructed by swelling or foreign matter. The trachea is also softer and more flexible in infants and children, so more care must be taken during any procedure when pressure might be placed on the neck, such as in applying a cervical collar or during procedures to place a tube in the trachea. The cricoid cartilage is less developed and less rigid in infants and children. Because the chest wall is softer, infants and children tend to rely more on the diaphragm

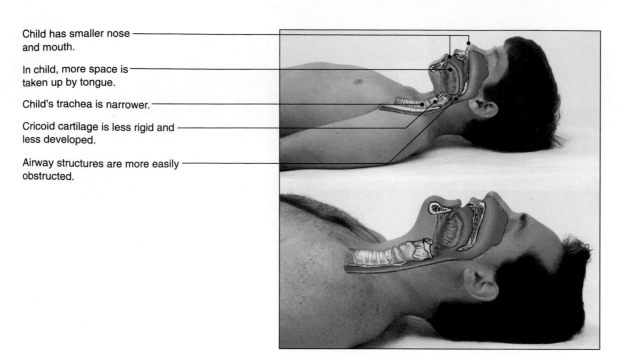

Child has smaller nose and mouth.

In child, more space is taken up by tongue.

Child's trachea is narrower.

Cricoid cartilage is less rigid and less developed.

Airway structures are more easily obstructed.

Figure 4-12 Comparison of child and adult respiratory systems.

when they are having breathing difficulty. This causes a visible "seesaw" breathing pattern in which the chest and abdomen alternate movement.

Special procedures that take into account the respiratory anatomy of infants and children will be discussed in later chapters on the airway and the respiratory system.

Cardiovascular System

The **cardiovascular system** consists of the heart and the blood vessels through which blood is circulated throughout the body. It is also called the **circulatory system.**

Anatomy of the Heart

The human heart is a muscular organ about the size of your fist, located in the center of the thoracic cavity (Figure 4-13). The heart has four chambers: two upper chambers called **atria** and two lower chambers called **ventricles.**

The atria both contract at the same time. When they contract, blood is forced into the heart's lower chambers, the ventricles. Both ventricles contract simultaneously to pump the blood out of the heart. The path the blood takes on its journey through the body is as follows: right atrium to right ventricle to lungs to left atrium to left ventricle to body, then back to the right atrium to start its journey all over again. Below, this path of the circulatory system is described in a little more detail:

- *Right atrium.* The **venae cavae** (the superior vena cava and the inferior vena cava) are the two large

veins that return blood to the heart. The right atrium receives this blood and, upon contraction, sends it to the right ventricle.

- *Right ventricle.* The right ventricle receives blood from the chamber above it, the right atrium. When the right ventricle contracts, it pumps this blood out to the lungs via the pulmonary arteries. Remember, this blood is very low in oxygen and is carrying waste carbon dioxide that was picked up as the blood circulated through the body. While this blood is in the lungs, the carbon dioxide is excreted (taken out of the blood and when the person exhales, carried out of the body), and oxygen is obtained (taken into the blood from air the person has inhaled). The oxygen-rich blood is now returned to the left atrium via the pulmonary veins.

- *Left atrium.* The left atrium receives the oxygen-rich blood from the lungs. When it contracts, it sends this blood to the left ventricle.

- *Left ventricle.* The left ventricle receives oxygen-rich blood from the chamber above it, the left atrium. When it contracts, it pumps this blood into the **aorta,** the body's largest artery, for distribution to the entire body. Since the blood must reach all parts of the body, the left ventricle is the most muscular and strongest part of the heart.

Between each atrium and ventricle is a one-way valve to prevent blood in the ventricle from being forced back up into the atrium when the ventricle contracts. The pulmonary artery has a one-way valve

From body
Superior vena cava

To lung
Right pulmonary
artery (branches)

From lung
Right pulmonary
vein (branches)

Right atrium

Coronary sinus

Tricuspid valve

Epicardium (outer layer)

Right ventricle

Inferior vena cava

Aorta

To lung
Left pulmonary
artery (branches)

From lung
Right pulmonary
vein (branches)

Left atrium

Bicuspid valve

Left ventricle

Interventricular
septum
Myocardium
(heart muscle)

Apex

Descending aorta

From body

To body

Figure 4-13   Cross-section of the heart.

so that blood in the artery does not return to the right ventricle. The aorta also has a one-way valve to prevent backflow to the left ventricle. This system of one-way valves keeps the blood moving in the correct direction along the path of circulation.

The contraction, or beating, of the heart is an automatic, involuntary process. The heart has its own natural "pacemaker" and a system of specialized muscle tissues that conduct electrical impulses that stimulate the heart to beat. This network is called the **cardiac conduction system** (Figure 4-14). Regulation of rate, rhythm, and force of heartbeat comes, in part, from the cardiac control centers of the brain. Nerve impulses from these centers are sent to the pacemaker and conduction system of the heart. These nerve impulses and chemicals (epinephrine, for example) released into the blood control the heart's rate and strength of contractions.

Circulation of the Blood

When the blood leaves the heart, it travels throughout the body through several types of blood vessels. Blood vessels are described by their function, location, and whether they carry blood away from or to the heart.

The kind of vessel that carries blood away from the heart is called an **artery.** There are several arteries that are important to know:

- *Coronary arteries.* The **coronary arteries** (Figure 4-15) branch off from the aorta and supply the heart muscle with blood. Although the heart has blood constantly moving through it, it receives its own blood supply from the coronary arteries. Damage or blockage to these arteries usually results in chest pain.

- *Aorta.* The aorta is the largest artery in the body. It begins at its attachment to the left ventricle, travels

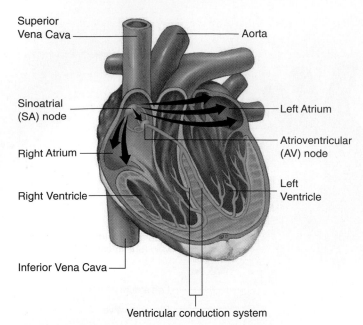

Superior Vena Cava

Aorta

Sinoatrial (SA) node

Left Atrium

Atrioventricular (AV) node

Right Atrium

Left Ventricle

Right Ventricle

Inferior Vena Cava

Ventricular conduction system

Figure 4-14 The cardiac conduction system.

superiorly, then arches inferiorly in front of the spine through the thoracic and abdominal cavities. At the level of the navel, it splits into the iliac arteries.

- *Pulmonary artery*. The **pulmonary artery** begins at the right ventricle. It carries oxygen-poor blood to the lungs. You may notice that this is an exception to the rule (arteries carry oxygen-rich blood, and veins carry oxygen-poor blood). It does, however, follow the rule that arteries carry blood away from the heart while veins carry blood to the heart.

Right Coronary Artery

Left Coronary Artery

Anterior Descending Branch

Figure 4-15 The coronary arteries.

- *Carotid artery*. The **carotid artery** is the major artery of the neck. You will be familiar with this vessel from your CPR class. It is the artery that is palpated during CPR pulse checks for adults and children. It carries the main supply of blood for the head. There is a carotid artery on each side of the neck. Never palpate both at the same time because of the danger of interrupting the supply of blood to the brain.

- *Femoral artery*. The **femoral artery** is the major artery of the thigh. You can relate the name "femoral" to the bone in the thigh, the femur. Pulsations for this artery can be felt in the crease between the abdomen and the groin. This artery is the major source of blood supply to the thigh and leg.

- *Brachial artery*. The **brachial artery** is in the upper arm. It is the pulse checked during infant CPR. Its pulse can be felt anteriorly in the crease over the elbow and along the medial aspect of the upper arm. It is also the artery that is used when determining blood pressure with a blood pressure cuff and a stethoscope.

- *Radial artery*. This artery travels through and supplies the lower arm. The **radial artery** is the artery felt when taking a pulse at the thumb side of the wrist. Again, you can relate the name "radial" to the radius, a bone in the forearm which the radial artery is near.

- *Posterior tibial artery*. This artery is often used when determining the circulatory status of the lower extremity. The **posterior tibial artery** may be palpated on the posterior aspect of the medial malleolus.

- *Dorsalis pedis artery*. The **dorsalis pedis artery** lies on the top (dorsal portion) of the foot, lateral to the large tendon of the big toe.

Arteries begin with large vessels, like the aorta. They gradually branch to smaller and smaller vessels. The smallest branch of an artery is called an **arteriole.** These small vessels lead to the capillaries. **Capillaries** are tiny blood vessels found throughout the body. As explained earlier, the capillaries are where gases, nutrients, and waste products are exchanged between the body's cells and the bloodstream. From the capillaries the blood begins its return journey to the heart by entering the smallest veins. One of these small veins is called a **venule.** (See Figure 4-16.)

The kind of vessel that carries the blood from the capillaries back to the heart is called a **vein.** Remember that the blood flow from the heart started in the largest arteries and moved into smaller and smaller arteries until it reached the capillaries. The blood takes an opposite course through the veins. The

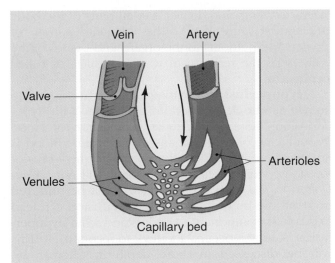

Figure 4-16 Arteries, capillaries, and veins.

From the heart, oxygen-rich blood is carried out into the body by arteries. The arteries gradually branch into smaller arteries called arterioles. The arterioles gradually branch into tiny vessels called capillaries.

In the capillaries, the blood gives up oxygen and nutrients, which move through the thin walls of the capillaries into the body's cells. At the same time, carbon dioxide and other wastes move in the opposite direction, from the cells and through the capillary walls, to be picked up by the blood.

On its return journey to the heart, the oxygen-poor blood, now carrying carbon dioxide and other wastes, flows from the capillaries into small veins called venules which gradually merge into larger veins.

blood travels from the smaller to the larger vessels on its return trip to the heart. Immediately after leaving the capillaries, the blood enters **venules,** the smallest veins. From the venules, the veins get gradually larger, eventually reaching the venae cavae.

There are two **venae cavae.** The superior vena cava collects blood that is returned from the head and upper body. The inferior vena cava collects blood from the portions of the body below the heart. The superior and inferior venae cavae meet to return blood to the right atrium, where the process of circulation begins again.

The **pulmonary vein** carries oxygenated blood from the lungs to the left atrium of the heart. This is an exception to the rule that veins carry oxygen-poor blood. It does follow the rule that arteries carry blood away from the heart while veins return blood to the heart.

Composition of the Blood

The blood is made up of several components: plasma, red and white blood cells, and platelets (Figure 4-17).

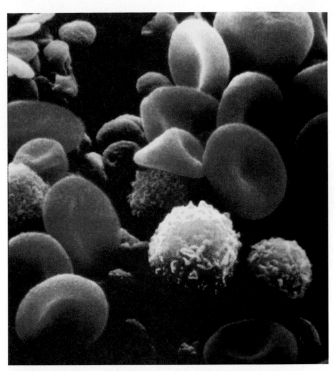

Figure 4-17 Blood consists of plasma, red and white blood cells, and platelets.

- *Plasma.* **Plasma** is a watery, salty fluid that makes up over half the volume of the blood. The red and white blood cells and platelets are carried in the plasma.
- *Red blood cells* are also called RBCs, erythrocytes, or red corpuscles. Their primary function is to carry oxygen to the tissues and carbon dioxide away from the tissues. These cells also provide the red color to the blood.
- *White blood cells* are also called WBCs, leukocytes, or white corpuscles. They are involved in destroying microorganisms (germs) and producing substances called antibodies, which help the body resist infection.
- *Platelets.* **Platelets** are membrane-enclosed fragments of specialized cells. When these fragments are activated, they release chemical factors needed to form blood clots.

HOW AND WHY?

Sickle-cell anemia affects red blood cells. One African American in 12 carries the sickling trait, although it is now known to be present in people of Mediterranean, Middle Eastern, and East Indian ancestry. To learn more, go to your Electronic Extras CD.

Pulse

A **pulse** is formed when the left ventricle contracts, sending a wave of blood through the arteries. The pulse is felt by compressing an artery over a bone. This allows you to feel the wave of blood, or pulse, as it comes through the artery.

Earlier in this chapter, several arteries were named. Among them were the primary arteries where a pulse is taken for vital signs or CPR: the carotid, brachial, and radial arteries. You will also use the pulses at the ankles and feet (posterior tibial and dorsalis pedis) to check for adequate circulation to the lower extremities.

The points where a pulse can be felt may also be used for control of bleeding. Pressure applied to the brachial and femoral arteries can be used to control bleeding to the arm and leg respectively. You will learn about these techniques in Chapter 26, "Bleeding and Shock."

The radial, brachial, posterior tibial, and dorsalis pedis pulses are called **peripheral pulses** because they can be felt on the periphery, or outer reaches, of the body. The carotid and femoral pulses are called **central pulses** because they can be felt in the central part of the body. Because they are larger vessels closer to the heart, the carotid and femoral pulses can be felt even when peripheral pulses are too weak to be felt.

Providing chest compressions during CPR is dangerous if the heart is beating, however weakly. This is why the carotid pulse, rather than a peripheral pulse, is used to determine pulselessness, the sign that CPR compressions should begin. If a peripheral pulse site were felt when the heartbeat was weak but still present, the EMT-B might make an incorrect and potentially harmful decision to begin CPR.

Blood Pressure

The force blood exerts against the walls of blood vessels is known as **blood pressure.** Usually, it is arterial blood pressure (pressure in an artery) that is measured.

Each time the left ventricle of the heart contracts, it forces blood out into circulation. The pressure created in the arteries by this blood is called the **systolic** blood pressure. When the left ventricle of the heart is relaxed and refilling, the pressure remaining in the arteries is called the **diastolic** blood pressure. The systolic pressure is reported first, the diastolic second, as in "120 over 80," which is written as "120/80."

Perfusion

The movement of blood through the heart and blood vessels is called *circulation*. In healthy individuals, circulation is adequate. That is, there is enough blood within the system and there is a means to pump and deliver it to all parts of the body efficiently (Figure 4-18). The adequate supply of oxygen and nutrients to the organs and tissues of the body, with the removal of waste products, is called **perfusion.**

Hypoperfusion (inadequate perfusion), also known as **shock,** is a serious condition. With hypoperfusion, there is inadequate circulation of blood through one or more organs or structures. Blood is not reaching and filling all the capillary networks of the body, which means that oxygen will not be delivered to, and waste products will not be removed from, all the body's tissues. Hypoperfusion can lead to death. It is important to understand what hypoperfusion is, how it occurs, and how to recognize it. This will be discussed in more depth in Chapter 26, "Bleeding and Shock."

Nervous System

The **nervous system** (Figure 4-19) is the system of brain, spinal cord, and nerves, which transmits impulses and governs sensation, movement, and thought. It controls the voluntary and involuntary activity of the body. It consists of the central and peripheral nervous systems.

The **central nervous system** is composed of the brain and the spinal cord. The brain could be likened to a powerful computer that receives information from the body and, in turn, sends impulses to different areas of the body to respond to the changes in and outside the body. The spinal cord rests within the spinal column and stretches from the brain to the lumbar vertebrae. Nerves branch from each part of the cord and reach throughout the body.

The **peripheral nervous system** consists of two types of nerves, sensory and motor. The sensory nerves pick up information from throughout the body and transmit it to the spinal cord and brain. If you touch something hot, your sensory nerves transmit this to the brain so action may be taken. The motor nerves carry messages from the brain to the body. In the example given above, the brain would send a message to the part of the body that has just touched the hot item to pull away.

The **autonomic nervous system** is the division of the peripheral nervous system that controls involuntary motor functions and affects such things as digestion and heart rate.

Skin

The skin performs a variety of functions, including protection, water balance, temperature regulation, excretion, and shock absorption.

MAJOR ARTERIES

MAJOR VEINS

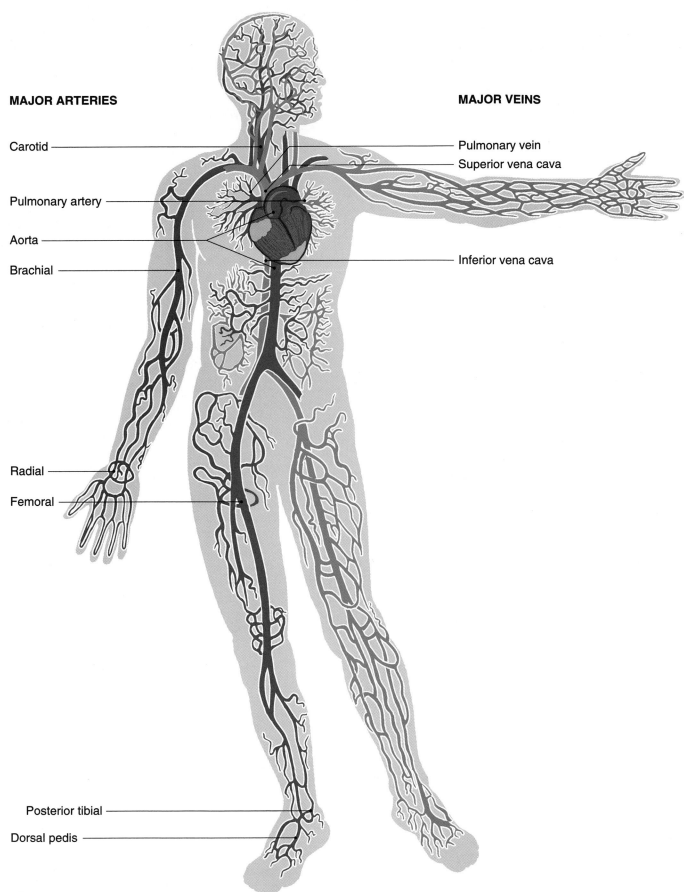

Carotid

Pulmonary artery

Aorta

Brachial

Radial

Femoral

Pulmonary vein

Superior vena cava

Inferior vena cava

Posterior tibial

Dorsal pedis

Figure 4-18 The circulatory system.

THE NERVOUS SYSTEM

CENTRAL NERVOUS SYSTEM
Controls all basic bodily functions, and responds to external changes

PERIPHERAL NERVOUS SYSTEM
Provides a complete network of motor and sensory nerve fibers connecting the central nervous system to the rest of the body

Figure 4-19   The nervous system.

- *Protection.* The skin serves as a barrier to keep out microorganisms, debris, and unwanted chemicals. Underlying tissues and organs are protected from environmental contact. This helps preserve the chemical balance of body fluids and tissues.
- *Water balance.* The skin helps prevent water loss and stops environmental water from entering the body.
- *Temperature regulation.* Blood vessels in the skin can dilate (increase in diameter) to carry more blood to the skin, allowing heat to radiate from the body. When the body needs to conserve heat, these vessels constrict (decrease in diameter) to prevent heat loss. The sweat glands found in the skin produce perspiration, which will evaporate and help cool the body. The fat that is part of the skin serves as a thermal insulator.
- *Excretion.* Salts and excess water can be released through the skin.
- *Shock (impact) absorption.* The skin and its layers of fat help protect the underlying organs from minor impacts and pressures.

The skin has three major layers: the epidermis, dermis, and subcutaneous layer (Figure 4-20). The outer layer of the skin is called the **epidermis.** It is composed of four layers (strata) everywhere except at the palms of the hands and soles of the feet. These two regions have five skin layers. The outermost layers of the epidermis are composed of dead cells, which are rubbed off or sloughed off and replaced. The pigment granules of the skin and living cells are found in the deeper layers. The cells of the innermost layer actively divide, replacing the dead cells of the outer layers. Note that the epidermis contains no blood vessels or nerves. Except for certain types of burns and injuries due to cold, injuries of the epidermis present few problems in EMT-level care.

The layer of skin below the epidermis is the **dermis,** which is rich with blood vessels, nerves, and specialized structures such as sweat glands, sebaceous (oil) glands, and hair follicles. Specialized nerve endings are also found in the dermis. They are involved with the senses of touch, cold, heat, and pain. Once the dermis is opened to the outside world, contamination and infection become major problems. These wounds can be serious, accompanied by profuse bleeding and intense pain.

The layers of fat and soft tissue below the dermis are called the **subcutaneous layers.** Shock absorption and insulation are major functions of this layer. Again, there are the problems of tissue and bloodstream contamination, bleeding, and pain when these layers are injured or exposed.

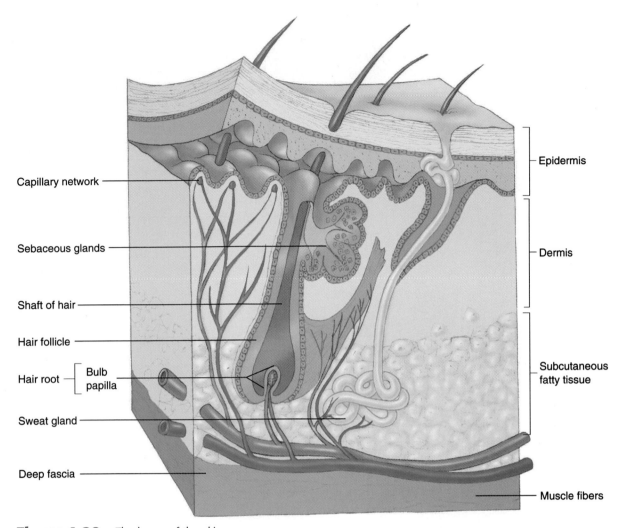

Capillary network

Sebaceous glands

Shaft of hair

Hair follicle

Hair root { Bulb
papilla

Sweat gland

Deep fascia

Epidermis

Dermis

Subcutaneous
fatty tissue

Muscle fibers

Figure 4-20 The layers of the skin.

Endocrine System

The endocrine system (Figure 4-21) produces chemicals called *hormones,* which help to regulate many body activities and functions. You will later learn about a chemical called **insulin.** It is a hormone that is critical in the use of glucose, a sugar that fuels the body. **Epinephrine** is another example of a substance secreted by the endocrine system. Epinephrine (sometimes called adrenaline) helps us to respond to stressful situations.

The endocrine system is complex and interacts with many other body systems.

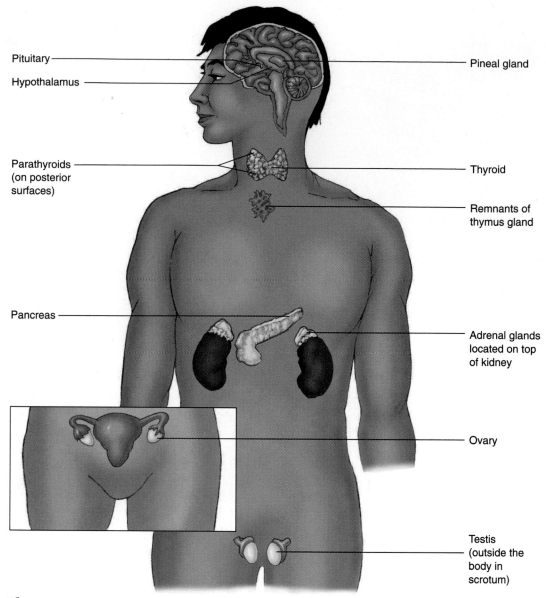

Figure 4-21 The endocrine system.

Pituitary

Hypothalamus

Pineal gland

Parathyroids (on posterior surfaces)

Thyroid

Remnants of thymus gland

Pancreas

Adrenal glands located on top of kidney

Ovary

Testis (outside the body in scrotum)

LOCATING BODY ORGANS AND STRUCTURES

As an EMT-B, you will find it useful to understand the position of the body's major organs and structures. There are two ways to help locate organs and structures of the body. The first is *visualizing*, or being able to picture organs and structures inside the body as you look at the external body. The second is *topography*, or external landmarks such as notches, joints, and "bumps" on bones. Some external landmarks are obvious (e.g., navel, nipples), some you know by other names but will have to learn the medical terms (e.g., the "Adam's apple," which is properly called the thyroid cartilage), and some will probably be new to you (e.g., the xiphoid process). It is important to learn where internal organs and structures are in relation to these landmarks, which you can easily see or feel from outside the body.

Scan 4–1 shows the positions of major organs and systems. Scan 4–2 shows the positions of major landmarks on the outer body (topography) and skeletal structures within the body.

MAJOR BODY ORGANS

Meninges

Frontal lobe

Pituitary gland

Sphenoidal sinus

Pons

Occipital lobe

Cerebellum

Medulla oblongata

Dura mater

Spinal cord

▲ **1** Cross-section of the brain and brain stem.

(continued)

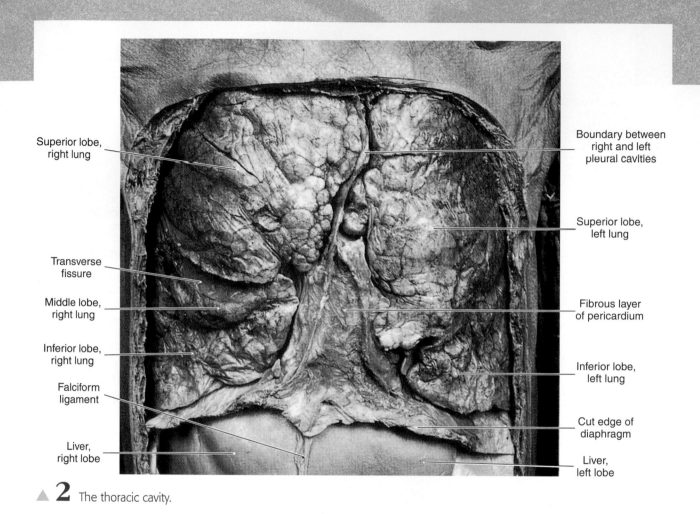

Superior lobe, right lung

Transverse fissure

Middle lobe, right lung

Inferior lobe, right lung

Falciform ligament

Liver, right lobe

Boundary between right and left pleural cavities

Superior lobe, left lung

Fibrous layer of pericardium

Inferior lobe, left lung

Cut edge of diaphragm

Liver, left lobe

▲ **2** The thoracic cavity.

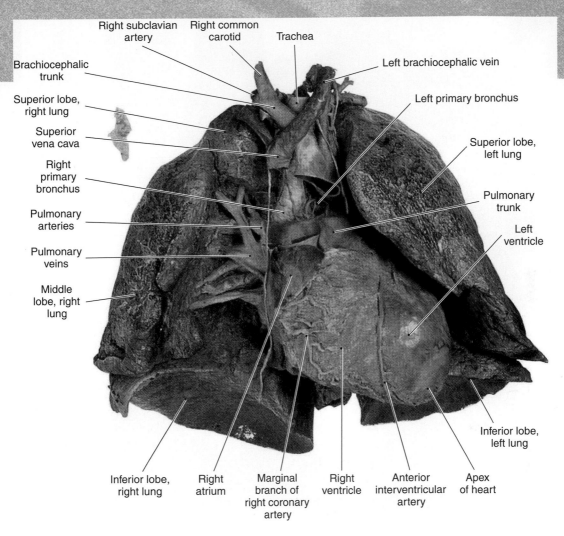

Right subclavian artery
Right common carotid
Trachea
Left brachiocephalic vein
Brachiocephalic trunk
Superior lobe, right lung
Left primary bronchus
Superior vena cava
Superior lobe, left lung
Right primary bronchus
Pulmonary trunk
Pulmonary arteries
Left ventricle
Pulmonary veins
Middle lobe, right lung
Inferior lobe, left lung
Inferior lobe, right lung
Right atrium
Marginal branch of right coronary artery
Right ventricle
Anterior interventricular artery
Apex of heart

▲ **3** Lungs, heart, and great vessels.

(continued)

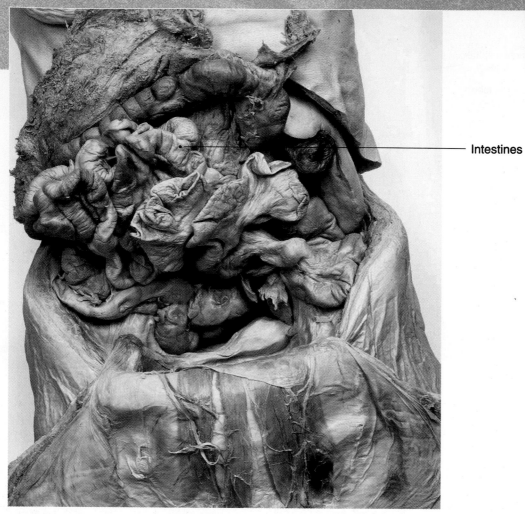

Intestines

▲ **4** Abdominal cavity.

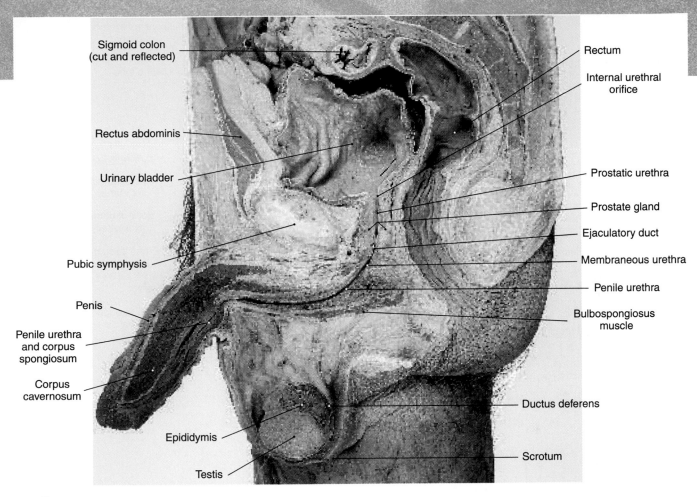

Sigmoid colon
(cut and reflected)

Rectus abdominis

Urinary bladder

Pubic symphysis

Penis

Penile urethra
and corpus
spongiosum

Corpus
cavernosum

Epididymis

Testis

Rectum

Internal urethral
orifice

Prostatic urethra

Prostate gland

Ejaculatory duct

Membraneous urethra

Penile urethra

Bulbospongiosus
muscle

Ductus deferens

Scrotum

▲ **5** Cross-section of the male reproductive system.

(continued)

Sigmoid colon
(cut and reflected)

Suspensory ligament
of ovary

Uterine tube

Ovary

Fundus of
uterus

Endometrium
of uterus

Body of uterus
(myometrium)

Probe through
internal os

Urinary bladder

Pubic symphysis

Urethra

External urethral orifice

Vestibule

Fat of mons pubis

Labium minus

Labium majus

Cervix

Probe through
external os

Vagina

Rectum

Anus

▲ **6** Cross-section of the female reproductive system.

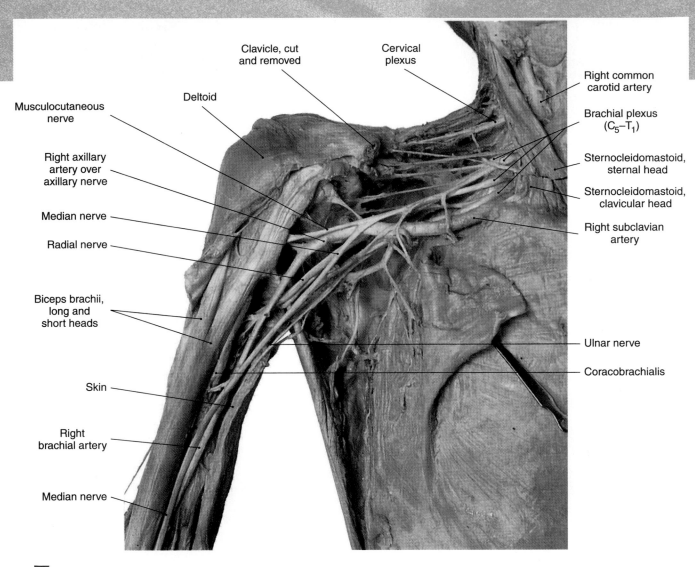

Clavicle, cut and removed

Cervical plexus

Right common carotid artery

Deltoid

Brachial plexus (C₅–T₁)

Musculocutaneous nerve

Sternocleidomastoid, sternal head

Right axillary artery over axillary nerve

Sternocleidomastoid, clavicular head

Median nerve

Right subclavian artery

Radial nerve

Biceps brachii, long and short heads

Ulnar nerve

Coracobrachialis

Skin

Right brachial artery

Median nerve

▲ **7** Right axillary region.

(continued)

Iliac
crest

Inguinal
ligament

Iliopsoas

Tensor
fasciae
latae

Sartorius

Femoral
artery

Pectineus

Adductor
longus

Rectus
femoris

Gracilis

Vastus
lateralis

▶ **8** Muscles of the lower extremity.

Vastus
medialis

Quadriceps
tendon

Patella

Patellar
ligament

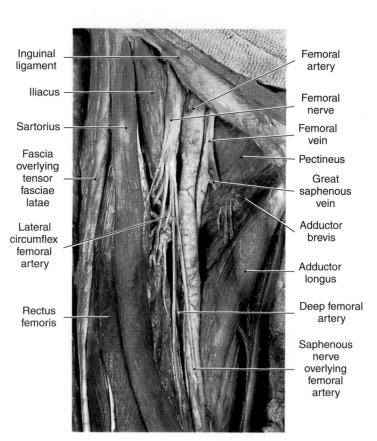

Inguinal
ligament

Femoral
artery

Iliacus

Femoral
nerve

Sartorius

Femoral
vein

Fascia
overlying
tensor
fasciae
latae

Pectineus

Great
saphenous
vein

Lateral
circumflex
femoral
artery

Adductor
brevis

Adductor
longus

Rectus
femoris

Deep femoral
artery

Saphenous
nerve
overlying
femoral
artery

▲ **9** Major blood vessels of the thigh.

TOPOGRAPHY AND SKELETON

TOPOGRAPHY OF TORSO

Suprasternal (jugular) notch

Clavicle

Sternum

Diaphragm

Umbilicus

Sternoclavicular joints

Pectoral region

Xiphoid process

Costal arch (margin)

Pubis

Scapular region

Lumbar region

Iliac crest

HEAD AND NECK TOPOGRAPHY

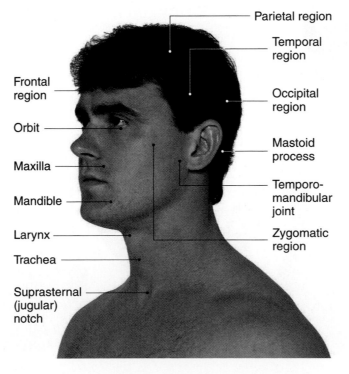

Frontal region

Orbit

Maxilla

Mandible

Larynx

Trachea

Suprasternal (jugular) notch

Parietal region

Temporal region

Occipital region

Mastoid process

Temporo-mandibular joint

Zygomatic region

(continued)

LOWER BODY TOPOGRAPHY AND SKELETON

POSTERIOR

ANTERIOR

Femoral head

Femoral neck

Shaft of femur

Lateral
femoral condyle

Medial femoral condyle

Patella

Tibia

Fibula

**LOWER
EXTREMITY**

Lateral malleolus

Medial malleolus

Calcaneus

UPPER BODY TOPOGRAPHY AND SKELETON

Humeral head

Acromioclavicular joint

Glenohumeral
joint

Shaft of humerus

Lateral
humeral
condyle

Radial
and
ulnar
styloids

Elbow

Medial
humeral
condyle

Ulnar
shaft

"Respond to Elm Street near the intersection on Central Avenue for a report of a motor-vehicle crash. Third party call from a passerby on a mobile phone. The time is now 1505 hours." Your response time is relatively fast, and you arrive before the dispatcher can provide any additional information. As you approach the scene, you see two vehicles are involved in the crash; it appears the truck rear-ended the four-door sedan. A police officer has already taken care of traffic control. You ask him, "How many patients?" and are told there are three. You find an open area to place the ambulance. Once assured that the scene is safe, you begin your assessment.

The driver of the truck is walking around the scene. The other vehicle had two occupants—a mother and her son, who was belted in the back seat. The mother is tending to the child who appears to be unresponsive. It doesn't look as if the impact speed was great, but the child hit his head fairly hard on the arm rest and you can still see the dent. A First Response unit is also on scene and they tell you they will check on the driver of the truck. You turn your attention to the child.

The mother tells you she is fine, "Just take care of my son. Peter is only six years old." You get into the vehicle next to the child and hear that he has snoring respirations. You remember that the tongue is the most likely cause, so you manually stabilize the head and neck to prevent any further injury to his head and cervical spine. As you do so, you push the patient's jaw forward to move the tongue in the direction of the mandible. It works, and the snoring sound stops. Your partner prepares for extrication to the backboard.

STREET SCENE QUESTIONS

1. As you assess your patient, how does the anatomy impact on the process?

2. What should you be alert to when examining the abdomen?

Before rotating the patient onto the backboard, you apply a cervical collar. Then you rotate Peter onto the board. Remembering that a child's head is larger in proportion to the rest of the body as compared to adults, you place a folded towel under Perer's shoulders in order to keep the patient's head in a neutral position with the airway open. Your partner calls out to Peter to see if his mental status has changed. Peter responds to painful stimuli only.

Once the patient is moved into the ambulance, you perform a head-to-toe exam. When you get to the abdomen, you palpate all four quadrants and observe a bruise, probably caused by the lap portion of the seat belt. Peter reacts, as if in pain, when you touch the left upper quadrant and you think that his spleen may have been injured.

En route to the hospital, you find the patient is breathing at a rate of 32 and has a pulse of 150. You call out to Peter, and this time he responds to your voice.

STREET SCENE QUESTIONS

3. What are the significant findings based on the assessment and your knowledge of the human body?

4. Do you have any concerns about additional injuries to this patient? If so, what are they?

You take another set of vital signs and find that the patient has an increase in pulse and respiration rates. You perform an ongoing assessment and find there is still pain in the upper left quadrant of the abdomen. As you run your hands over the patient's back, you are concerned by pain in the lumbar region of the spine, which may have been caused by the force of the crash.

Your partner tells you the ETA to the hospital is 10 minutes and notifies emergency department personnel by radio. The transmission gives an overview of the injuries and the vital signs, noting the change in the last 10 minutes. He mentions how the mental status of the patient has changed and describes the abdominal pain and location.

When the patient is being wheeled into the trauma room, they do a quick assessment and check the abdomen. The emergency department physician tells you that because of assessment findings given in the radio report, she has a surgeon on the way to check Peter. "Good job!"

CHAPTER REVIEW

SUMMARY

As an EMT-Basic, your knowledge of the anatomy, or structure, of the body and the functions, or physiology, of the body will be important in allowing you to assess your patient and communicate your findings with other EMS personnel and hospital staff accurately and efficiently.

Major body systems with which you should be familiar include the musculoskeletal system, respiratory system, cardiovascular system, nervous system, the skin, and endocrine system.

KEY TERMS

abdominal quadrants four divisions of the abdomen used to pinpoint the location of a pain or injury: the right upper quadrant (RUQ), the left upper quadrant (LUQ), the right lower quadrant (RLQ), and the left lower quadrant (LLQ).

acetabulum (AS-uh-TAB-yuh-lum) the pelvic socket into which the ball at the proximal end of the femur fits to form the hip joint.

acromioclavicular (ah-KRO-me-o-klav-IK-yuh-ler) **joint** the joint where the acromion and the clavicle meet.

acromion (ah-KRO-me-on) **process** the highest portion of the shoulder.

alveoli (al-VE-o-li) the microscopic sacs of the lungs where gas exchange with the bloodstream takes place.

anatomical position the standard reference position for the body in the study of anatomy. In this position, the body is standing erect, facing the observer, with arms down at the sides and the palms of the hands forward.

anatomy the study of body structure.

anterior the front of the body or body part.

aorta (ay-OR-tah) the largest artery in the body. It transports blood from the left ventricle to begin systemic circulation.

arteriole (ar-TE-re-ol) the smallest kind of artery.

artery any blood vessel carrying blood away from the heart.

atria (AY-tree-ah) the two upper chambers of the heart. There is a right atrium (which receives unoxygenated blood returning from the body) and a left atrium (which receives oxygenated blood returning from the lungs).

automaticity (AW-to-muh-TISS-it-e) the ability of the heart to generate and conduct electrical impulses on its own.

autonomic (AW-to-NOM-ik) **nervous system** the division of the peripheral nervous system that controls involuntary motor functions.

bilateral on both sides.

blood pressure the pressure caused by blood exerting force against the walls of blood vessels. Usually arterial blood pressure (the pressure in an artery) is measured. See also *diastolic blood pressure* and *systolic blood pressure*.

brachial artery artery of the upper arm; the site of the pulse checked during infant CPR.

bronchi (BRONG-ki) the two large sets of branches that come off the trachea and enter the lungs. There are right and left bronchi. Singular *bronchus*.

calcaneus (kal-KAY-ne-us) the heel bone.

capillary (KAP-i-lair-e) a thin-walled, microscopic blood vessel where the oxygen/carbon dioxide and nutrient/waste exchange with the body's cells takes place.

cardiac conduction system a system of specialized muscle tissues which conduct electrical impulses that stimulate the heart to beat.

cardiac muscle specialized involuntary muscle found only in the heart.

cardiovascular (KAR-de-o-VAS-kyu-ler) **system** the system made up of the heart (*cardio*) and the blood vessels (*vascular*); the circulatory system.

carotid (kah-ROT-id) **arteries** the large neck arteries, one on each side of the neck, that carry blood from the heart to the head.

carpals (KAR-pulz) the wrist bones.

central nervous system (CNS) the brain and spinal cord.

central pulses the carotid and femoral pulses, which can be felt in the central part of the body.

circulatory system See *cardiovascular system*.

clavicle (KLAV-i-kul) the collarbone.

coronary (KOR-o-nar-e) **arteries** blood vessels that supply the muscle of the heart (myocardium).

cricoid (KRIK-oid) **cartilage** the ring-shaped structure that forms the lower portion of the larynx.

dermis (DER-mis) the inner (second) layer of skin, rich in blood vessels and nerves, found beneath the epidermis.

diaphragm (DI-uh-fram) the muscular structure that divides the chest cavity from the abdominal cavity. A major muscle of respiration.

diastolic (di-as-TOL-ik) **blood pressure** the pressure in the arteries when the left ventricle is refilling.

distal farther away from the torso. See also *proximal*.

dorsal referring to the back of the body or the back of the hand or foot. A synonym for *posterior*.

dorsalis pedis (dor-SAL-is PEED-is) **artery** artery supplying the foot, lateral to the large tendon of the big toe.

epidermis (ep-i-DER-mis) the outer layer of skin.

epiglottis (EP-i-GLOT-is) a leaf-shaped structure that prevents food and foreign matter from entering the trachea.

epinephrine (EP-uh-NEF-rin) a hormone produced by the body. As a medication, it dilates respiratory passages and is used to relieve severe allergic reactions.

exhalation (EX-huh-LAY-shun) a passive process in which the intercostal (rib) muscles and the diaphragm relax, causing the chest cavity to decrease in size and air to flow out of the lungs.

femoral (FEM-o-ral) **artery** the major artery supplying the leg.

femur (FEE-mer) the large bone of the thigh.

fibula (FIB-yuh-luh) the lateral and smaller bone of the lower leg.

Fowler's position a sitting position.

humerus (HYU-mer-us) the bone of the upper arm, between the shoulder and the elbow.

hypoperfusion inadequate perfusion of the cells and tissues of the body caused by insufficient flow of blood through the capillaries. See also *perfusion*.

ilium (IL-e-um) the superior and widest portion of the pelvis.

inferior away from the head; usually compared with another structure that is closer to the head (e.g., the lips are inferior to the nose).

inhalation (IN-huh-LAY-shun) an active process in which the intercostal (rib) muscles and the diaphragm contract, expanding the size of the chest cavity and causing air to flow into the lungs.

insulin (IN-suh-lin) a hormone produced by the pancreas or taken as a medication by many diabetics.

ischium (ISH-e-um) the lower, posterior portions of the pelvis.

involuntary muscle muscle that responds automatically to brain signals but cannot be consciously controlled.

larynx (LAIR-inks) the voice box.

lateral to the side, away from the midline of the body.

lungs the organs where exchange of atmospheric oxygen and waste carbon dioxide take place.

malleolus (mal-E-o-lus) protrusion on the side of the ankle. The lateral malleolus, at the lower end of the fibula, is seen on the outer ankle; the medial malleolus, at the lower end of the tibia, is seen on the inner ankle.

mandible (MAN-di-bul) the lower jaw bone.

manubrium (man-OO-bre-um) the superior portion of the sternum.

maxillae (mak-SIL-e) the two fused bones forming the upper jaw.

medial toward the midline of the body.

metacarpals (MET-uh-KAR-pulz) the hand bones.

metatarsals (MET-uh-TAR-sulz) the foot bones.

mid-axillary (mid-AX-uh-lair-e) **line** a line drawn vertically from the middle of the armpit to the ankle.

mid-clavicular (mid-clah-VIK-yuh-ler) **line** the line through the center of each clavicle.

midline an imaginary line drawn down the center of the body, dividing it into right and left halves.

musculoskeletal (MUS-kyu-lo-SKEL-e-tal) **system** the system of bones and skeletal muscles that support and protect the body and permit movement.

nasal (NAY-zul) **bones** the nose bones.

nasopharynx (NAY-zo-FAIR-inks) the area directly posterior to the nose.

nervous system the system of brain, spinal cord, and nerves that govern sensation, movement, and thought.

orbits the bony structures around the eyes; the eye sockets.

oropharynx (OR-o-FAIR-inks) the area directly posterior to the mouth.

palmar referring to the palm of the hand.

patella (pah-TEL-uh) the kneecap.

perfusion the supply of oxygen to and removal of wastes from the cells and tissues of the body as a result of the flow of blood through the capillaries.

peripheral nervous system (PNS) the nerves that enter and leave the spinal cord and travel between the brain and organs without passing through the spinal cord.

peripheral pulses the radial, brachial, posterior tibial, and dorsalis pedis pulses, which can be felt at peripheral (outlying) points of the body.

phalanges (fuh-LAN-jiz) the toe bones and finger bones.

pharynx (FAIR-inks) the area directly posterior to the mouth and nose. It is made up of the oropharynx and the nasopharynx.

physiology the study of body function.

plane a flat surface formed when slicing through a solid object.

plantar referring to the sole of the foot.

plasma (PLAZ-mah) the fluid portion of the blood.

platelets components of the blood; membrane-enclosed fragments of specialized cells.

posterior the back of the body or body part.

posterior tibial (TIB-ee-ul) **artery** artery supplying the foot, behind the medial ankle.

prone lying face down.

proximal closer to the torso. See also *distal*.

pubis (PYOO-bis) the medial anterior portion of the pelvis.

pulmonary (PUL-mo-nar-e) **arteries** the vessels that carry blood from the right ventricle of the heart to the lungs.

pulmonary veins the vessels that carry oxygenated blood from the lungs to the left atrium of the heart.

pulse the rhythmic beats caused as waves of blood move through and expand the arteries.

radial artery artery of the lower arm. It is felt when taking the pulse at the wrist.

radius (RAY-de-us) the lateral bone of the forearm.

recovery position lying on the side. Also called *lateral recumbent position*.

red blood cells components of the blood. They carry oxygen to and carbon dioxide away from the cells.

respiratory (RES-pir-ah-tory-e) system the system of nose, mouth, throat, lungs, and muscles that brings oxygen into the body and expels carbon dioxide.

scapula (SKAP-yuh-luh) the shoulder blade.

shock See *hypoperfusion*.

sternum (STER-num) the breastbone.

subcutaneous (SUB-ku-TAY-ne-us) **layers** the layers of fat and soft tissues found below the dermis.

superior toward the head (e.g., the chest is superior to the abdomen).

supine lying on the back.

systolic (sis-TOL-ik) **blood pressure** the pressure created in the arteries when the left ventricle contracts and forces blood out into circulation.

tarsals (TAR-sulz) the ankle bones.

thorax (THOR-ax) the chest.

tibia (TIB-e-uh) the medial and larger bone of the lower leg.

torso the trunk of the body; the body without the head and the extremities.

trachea (TRAY-ke-uh) the "windpipe"; the structure that connects the pharynx to the lungs.

Trendelenburg (trend-EL-un-berg) **position** a position in which the patient's feet and legs are higher than the head. Also called shock position.

ulna (UL-nah) the medial bone of the forearm.

vein any blood vessel returning blood to the heart.

venae cavae (VE-ne KA-ve) the superior vena cava and the inferior vena cava. These two major veins return blood from the body to the right atrium. (Venae cavae is plural, vena cava singular.)

ventral referring to the front of the body. A synonym for anterior.

ventricles (VEN-tri-kulz) the two lower chambers of the heart. There is a right ventricle (which sends oxygen-poor blood to the lungs) and a left ventricle (which sends oxygen-rich blood to the body).

venule (VEN-yul) the smallest kind of vein.

vertebrae (VER-te-bray) the 33 bones of the spinal column.

voluntary muscle muscle that can be consciously controlled.

white blood cells components of the blood. They produce substances that help the body fight infection.

xiphoid (ZI-foid) **process** the inferior portion of the sternum.

zygomatic (ZI-go-MAT-ik) bones the cheekbones.

REVIEW QUESTIONS

1. Define the following anatomical terms (pp. 47–48):

medial	lateral
anterior	posterior
mid-clavicular	distal

2. List the three functions of the musculoskeletal system. (p. 49)

3. Name the five divisions of the spine and describe the location of each. (p. 52)

4. Describe the physical processes of inhalation and exhalation. (p. 55)

5. List four places a peripheral pulse may be felt. (p. 60)

6. Describe the central nervous system and peripheral nervous system. (p. 60)

7. List three functions of the skin. (p. 60)

APPLICATIONS

• As an EMT-B, you are called to respond to a teenage boy who has taken a hard fall from his dirt bike. He has a deep gash on the outside of his left arm about halfway between the shoulder and the elbow and another on the inside of his right arm just above the wrist. His left leg is bent at a funny angle about halfway between hip and knee, and when you cut away his pants leg, you see a bone sticking out of a wound on the front side. You take the necessary on-scene assessment and care steps and are on the way to the hospital in the ambulance. How do you describe your patient's injuries over the radio to the hospital staff?

WEB MEDIC

Visit Brady's *Emergency Care* website for direct weblinks. At **www.bradybooks.com/ emergencycare**, you will find information related to the following Chapter 4 topics:

• Heart

• Human anatomy

Chapter
Five

LIFTING AND MOVING PATIENTS

Speed is a major objective on many of the calls you will make as an EMT-Basic. At certain dangerous scenes, for example, you must rapidly move the patient to a safe place. When the patient has a life-threatening medical problem or a serious injury, getting him to the hospital quickly can mean the difference between life and death.

Doing things fast, however, can mean doing them wrong. You can be so focused on the need to hurry as you lift and carry the patient that you make careless moves. These can injure your patient. They can also injure you. Back injuries are serious and have the potential to end an EMS career as well as cause life-long problems. With the proper techniques, however, you can lift and move patients safely. Proper lifting and moving must be practiced on every call.

PROTECTING YOURSELF: BODY MECHANICS

Body mechanics refers to the proper use of your body to prevent injury and to facilitate lifting and moving. Consider the following before lifting any patient:

- *The object*. What is the weight of the object? Will you require additional help in lifting?
- *Your limitations*. What are your physical characteristics? Do you (or your partner) have any physical limitations that would make lifting difficult? While it may not always be possible to arrange, EMT-Bs of similar strength and height can lift and carry together more easily.
- *Communication*. Make a plan. Then communicate the plan for lifting and carrying to your partner. Continue to communicate throughout the process to make the move comfortable for the patient and safe for the EMT-Bs.

When it comes time to do the lifting, there are rules that must be followed to prevent injury. These include:

- *Position your feet properly*. They should be on a firm, level surface and positioned shoulder-width apart.
- *Use your legs,* not your back to do the lifting.
- *Never turn or twist*. Attempts to make any other moves while you are lifting are a major cause of injury.
- *Do not compensate when lifting with one hand.* Avoid leaning to either side. Keep your back straight and locked.

- *Keep the weight close to your body,* or as close as possible. This allows you to use your legs rather than your back while lifting. The farther the weight is from your body, the greater your chance of injury.
- *Use a stair chair when carrying a patient on stairs* whenever possible. Keep your back straight. Flex your knees and lean forward from the hips, not the waist. If you are walking backward down stairs, ask a helper to steady your back (Figure 5-1).

There are many kinds of patient carrying devices, including stretchers, backboards, and stair chairs. (Specifics are offered later in this chapter). When possible, it is almost always safer, as well as more efficient, to move patients over distances on a wheeled device such as a wheeled stretcher or a stair chair. These devices allow the patient to be rolled along instead of carried.

TOPIC OVERVIEW

In this chapter, you will learn about the following topics:

- How using "body mechanics" to lift and move patients can help prevent injury

- When it is proper to move a patient, and how to do so safely

- The various devices used to immobilize, move, and carry patients

✔ Knowledge and Attitude

1. Define body mechanics. (p. 81)

2. Discuss the guidelines and safety precautions that need to be followed when lifting a patient. (pp. 81–83)

3. Describe the safe lifting of cots and stretchers. (pp. 89, 92, 99)

4. Describe the guidelines and safety precautions for carrying patients and/or equipment. (pp. 81–83)

5. Discuss one-handed carrying techniques. (p. 81)

6. Describe correct and safe carrying procedures on stairs. (pp. 89, 92)

7. State the guidelines for reaching and their application. (p. 83)

8. Describe correct reaching for log rolls. (p. 84)

9. State the guidelines for pushing and pulling. (p. 83)

10. Discuss the general considerations of moving patients. (pp. 81–83)

11. State three situations that may require the use of an emergency move. (p. 84) (Scan 5-1, p. 85; Scan 5-2, p. 86; Scan 5-3, p. 87)

12. Identify the following patient carrying devices: (Scan 5-4, p. 88; Scan 5-5, pp. 90–91; Scan 5-6, pp. 93–95)

- wheeled ambulance stretcher
- portable ambulance stretcher
- stair chair
- scoop stretcher
- long spine board
- basket stretcher
- flexible stretcher

13. Explain the rationale for properly lifting and moving patients. (p. 81) (Scan 5-7, pp. 96–98; Scan 5-8, p. 100)

✔ Skills

1. Working with a partner, prepare each of the following devices for use, transfer a patient to the device, properly position the patient on the device, move the device to the ambulance, and load the patient into the ambulance:

- wheeled ambulance stretcher
- portable ambulance stretcher
- stair chair
- scoop stretcher
- long spine board
- basket stretcher
- flexible stretcher

2. Working with a partner, the EMT-Basic will demonstrate techniques for the transfer of a patient from an ambulance stretcher to a hospital stretcher.

When lifting a patient carrying device, it is best to use an even number of people. For a stretcher or backboard, one EMT-B lifts from the end near the patient's head, the other from the feet. If there are four rescuers available, one person can take each corner of a stretcher or board. If there are only three people available, never allow the third person to assist by lifting one side. This can cause the device to be thrown off balance, resulting in the stretcher tipping over and injuring the patient.

To prevent injury when lifting a patient carrying device, the general rules of body mechanics mentioned earlier apply. Two more methods also can help to prevent injury. The first is the **power lift** (Figure 5-2a). It is so named because it is used by power weight lifters. It is also known as the *squat-lift position*. In this position, you will squat rather than bend at the waist, and you will keep the weight close to your body, even straddling it if possible. When rising, your feet should be a comfortable distance apart, flat on the ground, with the weight primarily on the balls of the feet or just behind them. Your back should be locked-in. Be sure to raise your upper body before your hips. When you are lowering a patient, use the reverse order of this procedure.

The second method is the **power grip** (Figure 5-2b). Remember that your hands are often the only portion of your body actually in contact with the object you are lifting, making your grip a very impor-

HOW AND WHY?

Lifting patients onto stretchers can be very hard on your back. But did you know that being overweight is, too? Go to your Electronic Extras CD for more on how to keep your back healthy.

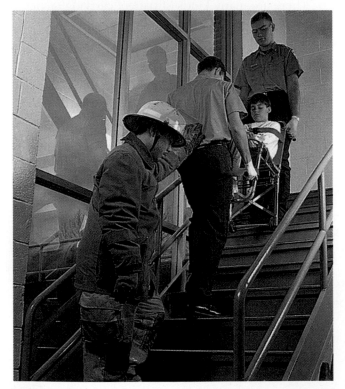

Figure 5-1 Moving a stair chair down steps.

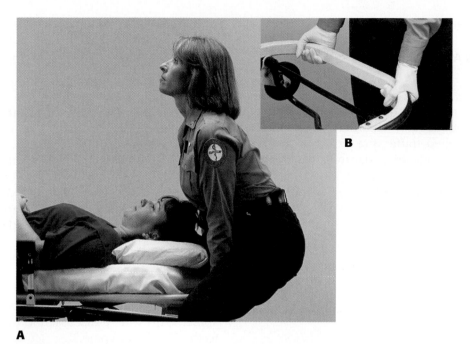

Figure 5-2 The power lift (A), and the power grip (B).

tant element in the process. As great an area of your fingers and palms as possible should be in contact with the object. All of your fingers should be bent at the same angle. When possible, keep your hands at least 10 inches apart.

There are situations in which you will find yourself reaching for patients or using a considerable amount of effort to push and pull a weight. These are moves that must be performed carefully to prevent injury. In general:

When reaching

- Keep your back in a locked-in position.
- Avoid twisting while reaching.
- Avoid reaching more than 15 to 20 inches in front of your body.
- Avoid prolonged reaching when strenuous effort is required.

When pushing or pulling

- Push, rather than pull, whenever possible.
- Keep your back locked-in.
- Keep the line of pull through the center of your body by bending your knees.
- Keep the weight close to your body.
- If the weight is below your waist level, push or pull from a kneeling position.
- Avoid pushing or pulling overhead.
- Keep your elbows bent and arms close to your sides.

PROTECTING YOUR PATIENT: EMERGENCY, URGENT, AND NON-URGENT MOVES

How quickly should you move a patient? Must you complete your assessment before moving him? How much time should you spend on spinal precautions and other patient safety measures? The answer is: it depends on the circumstances.

If the patient is in a building that is threatening to collapse or a car that is on fire, speed is the overriding concern. The patient must be moved to a safe place, probably before you have time to begin or complete an assessment, immobilize the patient's spine, or move a stretcher into position. In this situation, you would use what is known as an *emergency move.*

Sometimes the situation is such that you have time to carry out an abbreviated version of assessment and spinal immobilization. For example, consider the patient who has been trapped in wreckage, possibly incurring serious injuries. When the patient is extricated, you would place him on a spine board, working quickly to perform the proper assessments and patient care. That move to the spine board is called an *urgent move.*

Most of the time, you will be able to complete your on-scene assessment and care procedures and then move the patient onto a stretcher or other device in the normal way. This would be called a *non-urgent move.*

Emergency Moves

There are three situations that may require the use of an emergency move:

- *The scene is hazardous.* Hazards may make it necessary to move a patient quickly in order to protect you and the patient. This may occur when there is uncontrolled traffic, fire or threat of fire, possible explosions, electrical hazards, toxic gases, or radiation.
- *Care of life-threatening conditions requires repositioning.* You may have to move a patient to a hard, flat surface to provide CPR, or you may have to move a patient to reach life-threatening bleeding.
- *You must reach other patients.* When there are patients at the scene requiring care for life-threatening problems, you may have to move another patient to access them.

The greatest danger to the patient in an emergency move is that a spine injury may be aggravated. Since the move must be made immediately to protect the patient's life, full spinal precautions will not be possible. So to minimize or prevent aggravation of the injury, *move the patient in the direction of the long axis of the body when possible.* The long axis is the line that runs down the center of the body from the top of the head and along the spine.

There are several rapid moves called *drags.* In this type of move, the patient is dragged by the clothes, the feet, the shoulders, or a blanket. These moves are reserved only for emergencies, because they do not provide protection for the neck and spine. Most commonly, a long-axis drag is made from the area of the shoulders. This causes the remainder of the body to fall into its natural anatomical position, with the spine and all limbs in normal alignment.

Drags and other emergency moves known as *carries* and *assists* are illustrated in Scans 5-1, 5-2, and 5-3.

Urgent Moves

Urgent moves are required when the patient must be moved quickly for treatment of an immediate threat to life. But unlike emergency moves, urgent moves are performed with precautions for spinal injury. Examples for which urgent moves may be required include the following:

- *The required treatment can only be performed if the patient is moved.* A patient must be moved in order to support inadequate breathing or to treat for shock or altered mental status.

- *Factors at the scene cause patient decline.* If a patient is rapidly declining because of heat or cold, for example, he may have to be moved.

Moving a patient onto a long spine board, also called a *backboard*, is an urgent move used when there is an immediate threat to life and suspicion of spine injury. If the patient is supine on the ground, a log roll maneuver must be performed to move him onto his side. The spine board is then placed next to the patient's body, and he is log-rolled back onto the board. After the patient is secured and immobilized on the spine board, the board and patient are lifted together onto a stretcher and loaded into the ambulance. (When reaching across the patient to perform a log roll, remember the principles of body mechanics: Keep your back straight, lean from the hips, and use your shoulder muscles to help with the roll. (See Figure 5-3.) Log rolls and immobilization on a long spine board will be discussed in Chapter 29, "Injuries to the Head and Spine."

Another example of an urgent move is the rapid extrication procedure from a vehicle. If the patient has critical injuries, taking the time to immobilize him with a short backboard or vest while he is still in the car may cause a deadly delay. During a rapid extrication, EMT-Bs use a quicker procedure: they stabilize the spine manually as they move the patient from the car onto a long spine board. Rapid extrication will be discussed in Chapter 29, "Injuries to the Head and Spine."

Non-Urgent Moves

When there is no immediate threat to life, the patient should be moved when ready for transportation, using a non-urgent move. On-scene assessment and any needed on-scene treatments, such as splinting, should be completed first. Non-urgent moves should be carried out in such a way as to prevent injury or

Figure 5-3 When doing a log roll, keep your back straight, lean from the hips, and use your shoulder muscles.

EMERGENCY MOVES, ONE-RESCUER DRAGS

Caution: Always pull in the direction of the long axis of the patient's body. Do not pull the patient sideways. Avoid bending or twisting the patient's trunk.

▲ **CLOTHES DRAG.**

▲ **INCLINE DRAG.** Always head first.

▲ **SHOULDER DRAG.**

▲ **FOOT DRAG.** Do not bump patient's head.

▲ **FIREFIGHTER'S DRAG.** Place patient on his back and tie his hands together. Straddle him, crouch, and pass your head through his trussed arms. Raise your body, and crawl on your hands and knees. Keep the patient's head as low as possible.

▲ **BLANKET DRAG.** Gather half of the blanket material up against the patient's side. Roll him toward your knees, place the blanket under him, and gently roll him onto the blanket. During the drag, keep the patient's head as low as possible.

EMERGENCY MOVES, ONE RESCUER

 ◀ **ONE-RESCUER ASSIST.** Place patient's arm around your neck, grasping her hand in yours. Place your other arm around the patient's waist. Help patient walk to safety. Be prepared to change movement technique if level of danger increases. Be sure to communicate with patient about obstacles, uneven terrain, and so on.

 ▲ **PIGGY BACK CARRY.** ▼ Assist the patient to stand. Place her arms over your shoulder so they cross your chest. Bend over and lift patient. While she holds on with her arms, crouch and grasp each leg. Use a lifting motion to move her onto your back. Pass your forearms under her knees and grasp her wrists.

 ◀ **CRADLE CARRY.** Place one arm across patient's back with your hand under her arm. Place your other arm under her knees and lift. If patient is conscious, have her place her near arm over your shoulder. Note: This carry places a lot of weight on the carrier's back. It is usually appropriate only for very light patients.

 ◀ **PACK STRAP CARRY.** Have patient stand. Turn your back to her, bringing her arms over your shoulders to cross your chest. Keep her arms as straight as possible, her armpits over your shoulders. Hold patient's wrists, bend, and pull her onto your back.

 ◀ **FIREFIGHTER'S CARRY.** ▶ Place your feet against her feet and pull patient toward you. Bend at waist and flex knees. Duck and pull her across your shoulder, keeping hold of one of her wrists. Use your free arm to reach between her legs and grasp her thigh. Weight of patient falls onto your shoulders. Stand up. Transfer your grip on thigh to patient's wrist.

EMERGENCY MOVES, TWO RESCUERS

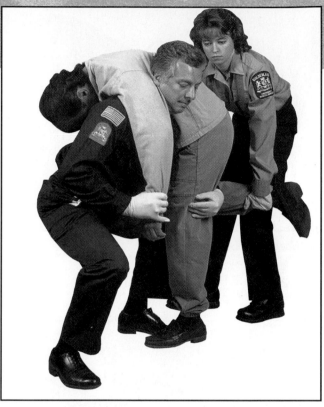

▲ **TWO-RESCUER ASSIST.** Patient's arms are placed around shoulders of both rescuers. They each grip a hand, place their free arms around patient's waist, and then help him walk to safety.

▲ **FIREFIGHTER'S CARRY WITH ASSIST.** Have someone lift patient. The second rescuer helps to position patient.

PATIENT CARRYING DEVICES

▲ Wheeled ambulance stretcher

▲ Portable stretcher

▲ Basket stretcher

▲ Scoop (orthopedic) stretcher

▲ Stair chair

▲ Flexible stretcher

additional injury to the patient and to avoid discomfort and pain.

In a non-urgent move, the patient is moved from the site of on-scene assessment and treatment (perhaps a bed or sofa, perhaps the floor or the ground outdoors) onto a patient carrying device.

Patient Carrying Devices

A patient carrying device is a stretcher or other device designed to carry the patient safely to the ambulance and/or to the hospital. The devices described below and on the following pages are pictured in Scan 5-4.

Patient carrying devices are mechanical devices, and all EMT-Bs must be familiar with how to use them. Errors in use of these devices may result in injuries to the patient and to you. For example, a stretcher that is not locked in position may collapse, and untended stretchers may simply roll away. Such incidents may be cause for a lawsuit if the patient is injured as a result of improper practices or faulty equipment. The devices must be regularly maintained and inspected. You should know the rating of each piece of equipment (how much weight it will hold safely). Have alternatives available if the patient is too heavy or too large for any device.

Wheeled Stretcher This device is commonly referred to simply as the stretcher, cot, or litter (Figure 5-4). It is the device that is in the back of all ambulances. There are many brands and types of wheeled stretcher, but their purpose is the same: to safely transport a patient from one place to another, usually in a reclining position. The head of the stretcher can be elevated, which will be beneficial for some patients, including cardiac patients, who have no suspected neck or spinal injuries.

Depending on the model, the stretcher will have variable levels. When moving the patient, the safest level is closest to the ground. Wheeling the stretcher in the elevated position raises the center of gravity, making it easier for the stretcher to tip over. The stretcher is ideal for level surfaces. Rough terrain and uneven surfaces may cause the stretcher to tip.

Make sure to use proper body mechanics while placing the stretcher into or taking it out of the ambulance. Proper body mechanics are also important while wheeling the stretcher from place to place. Remember, as discussed earlier in the chapter, odd numbers of EMT-Bs may cause the stretcher to become off-balance. When the stretcher is lifted, two EMT-Bs should lift at opposite ends of the stretcher—head and foot. The EMT-Bs should move to the sides of the stretcher to load it into the ambulance (Scan 5-5).

A stretcher can be carried by four EMT-Bs, one at each corner. This method can be useful on rough terrain because it helps keep the wheels from touching the ground and provides greater stability. It is also beneficial when carrying a patient a long distance because it divides the weight among four EMT-Bs instead of two.

The stretcher is the device that the patient will stay on during transport to the hospital. Make sure that it is always used in accordance with manufacturer's recommendations. Secure the patient to the stretcher before lifting or moving. After placing the patient into the ambulance, secure the stretcher to the ambulance. Ambulances have installed hardware for keeping the stretcher secured while the ambulance is moving. Failure to secure the stretcher properly will cause it to shift during transit, causing an unsafe condition for the EMT-Bs as well as the patient.

Stair Chair The stair chair has many benefits for moving patients from the scene to the stretcher. The first benefit, as the name implies, is that it is excellent for use on stairs. Large stretchers often cannot be carried around tight corners and up or down narrow staircases. The stair chair transports the patient in a sitting position, which greatly reduces the length of patient and device, allowing the EMT-B to maneuver around corners and through narrow spaces. It also has a set of wheels that allow the device to be rolled like a wheelchair over flat surfaces, lessening the strain on the EMT-B.

As with all devices in this chapter, there are times when the stair chair should be used and times when it should not. The device is often ideal for

Figure 5-4 A wheeled stretcher is carried on every ambulance.

LOADING THE WHEELED STRETCHER INTO THE AMBULANCE

Self-Loading Stretcher

▲ **1** Position the wheels closest to the patient's head securely on the inside floor of the ambulance.

▲ **2** Once wheels are securely on the ambulance floor, rescuer at rear of stretcher activates the lever to release wheels. (This may require a slight lift to get weight off the wheels.) The second rescuer should guide the collapsing carriage, if necessary.

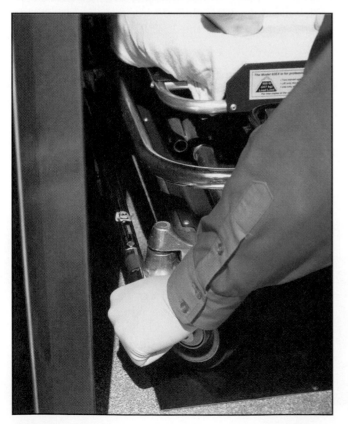

◄ **3** Secure the stretcher in front and rear.

Standard Stretcher

▲ **1** After you have moved stretcher as close to ambulance as possible, lock it in its lowest level. Then position yourselves on opposite sides, bend at the knees, and grasp the lower bar of stretcher frame.

▲ **2** Come to a full standing position with your backs straight. Take small sideways steps to move stretcher into the ambulance

◄ **3** Move stretcher into the securing device, and engage both forward and rear catches.

patients with difficulty breathing. (You will learn about this in Chapter 17, "Respiratory Emergencies.") These patients usually find that they must sit up to breathe more easily, which the stair chair allows them to do. The stair chair must not be used for patients with neck or spine injury, because these patients must be immobilized supine on a backboard to prevent further injury.

Spine Boards There are two types of spine boards, or backboards: long and short (Scan 5-6). They are used for patients who are found lying down or standing and who must be immobilized. These devices are available in traditional wood as well as in plastics that resist splintering. (Splintered boards absorb body fluids, which may harbor infection.)

Short spine boards are used primarily for removing patients from vehicles when a neck or spine injury is suspected. A short spine board can slide between the patient's back and seat back. Once secured to the short spine board and wearing a rigid cervical collar, the patient can be moved from a sitting position in the vehicle to a supine position on a long spine board. Often, a vest-type extrication device is used in place of a short spine board. (You will learn more about extrication using short spine boards and vests in Chapter 29, "Injuries to the Head and Spine.")

Other Types of Stretchers The *portable stretcher*, or folding stretcher, may be beneficial in multiple-casualty incidents (incidents with many patients). These stretchers may be canvas, aluminum, or heavy plastic and usually fold or collapse.

The *scoop stretcher*, or orthopedic stretcher, splits into two pieces vertically, allowing the patient to be "scooped" by pushing the halves together under him. The scoop stretcher does not offer any support directly under the spine, so it is not recommended for patients with suspected spinal injury. Follow your local protocols on the use of this device.

A *basket stretcher*, or Stokes stretcher, can be used to move a patient from one level to another or over rough terrain. The basket should be lined with a blanket before positioning the patient.

A *flexible stretcher*, or Reeves stretcher, is made of canvas or rubberized or other flexible material, often with wooden slats sewn into pockets and three carrying handles on each side. Because of its flexibility, it can be useful in restricted areas or narrow hallways.

Moving Patients onto Carrying Devices

There are several ways to move a patient onto a carrying device. Choose a move based on the position the patient is in when it is time to move him to a carrying device and whether or not the patient is suspected of having a spine injury.

Patient with Suspected Spine Injuries A patient with suspected spine injury must have his head, neck, and spine immobilized before being moved. After manual stabilization, place a rigid cervical collar on this patient. If he is seated in a vehicle, you will next immobilize him with a short spine board or vest and then on a long spine board (unless it is an urgent situation and you substitute the rapid extrication procedure described earlier under "Urgent Moves").

If the patient is lying down or standing, move him directly to a long spine board. The long spine board will then be placed on a wheeled ambulance stretcher for transport to the hospital. (You will learn more about manual stabilization in Chapter 8, "Initial Assessment," about cervical collars in Chapter 10, "Assessment of the Trauma Patient," and about immobilization for possible spine injury in Chapter 29, "Injuries to the Head and Spine.")

Remember that immobilization is mandatory for any patient who has any possibility of a spine injury.

Patients with No Suspected Spine Injury The extremity lift, direct ground lift, draw-sheet method, and direct carry, listed below, are methods of moving a patient to a stretcher. All are appropriate *only* for a patient with *no* suspected spine injury. See Scan 5-7 for pictures and detailed descriptions of these methods:

- An **extremity lift** is used to carry a patient with no suspected spine or extremity injuries to a stretcher or a stair chair. It can be used to lift a patient from the ground or from a sitting position.
- A **direct ground lift** is performed when a patient with no suspected spine injury needs to be lifted from the ground to a stretcher.
- The **draw-sheet method** is one of two methods (along with the direct carry method, below) that is performed during transfers between hospitals and nursing homes, or when a patient must be moved from a bed at home to a stretcher. It is used for a patient with no suspected spine injury.
- A **direct carry** is performed to move a patient with no suspected spine injury from a bed or from a bed-level position to a stretcher.

Patient Positioning

Positioning the patient during transfer to the ambulance and during transportation is a very important part of your care. Lifting, moving, and transport must be performed as an integral part of your total patient-care plan. The position in which the patient is transported depends on his medical condition and the device best designed to help this condition.

PATIENT IMMOBILIZATION DEVICES

▲ Short spine board.

▲ Patient properly secured to short spine board, front view.

◀ Side view.

(continued)

▲ Long spine board.

▲ Patient properly secured to long spine board.

▲ Vest-type extrication device.

▲ Patient properly secured to vest-type extrication device, front view.

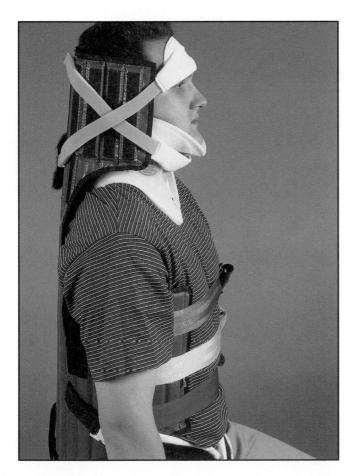

◀ Side view.

NON-URGENT MOVES, NO SUSPECTED SPINE INJURY

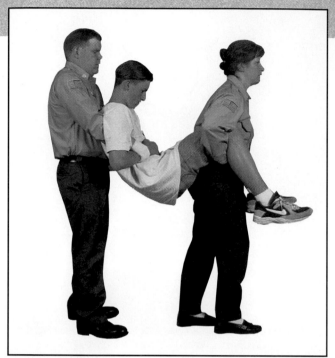

Extremity Carry

◀ The extremity carry may be used as an emergency move or a non-urgent move for patients with no suspected spine injury.

Place patient on his back with knees flexed. Kneel at patient's head. Place your hands under his shoulders. Second EMT-B kneels at patient's feet, grasps patient's wrists, and lifts patient forward. At the same time, slip your arms under patient's armpits and grasp his wrists. Second EMT-B can grasp patient's knees while facing or facing away from patient. Direct second EMT-B, so you both move to a crouch and then stand at the same time. Move as a unit when carrying a patient.

If patient is found sitting, crouch and slip your arms under patient's armpits and grasp his wrists. Second EMT-B crouches, then grasps patient's knees. Lift patient as a unit.

Draw-Sheet Method

▲ **1** Loosen bottom sheet of bed and roll it from both sides toward patient. Place stretcher, rails lowered, parallel to bed and touching side of bed. EMT-Bs use their bodies and feet to lock the stretcher against the bed.

▲ **2** EMT-Bs pull on draw sheet to move patient to side of bed. Both use one hand to support patient while they reach under him to grasp draw sheet. Then they simultaneously draw patient onto the stretcher.

Direct Ground Lift

▲ **1** Stretcher is set in its lowest position and placed on the opposite side of patient. EMT-Bs face patient, drop to one knee and, if possible, place patient's arms on his chest. Head-end EMT-B cradles patient's head and neck by sliding one arm under the neck to grasp shoulder, the other arm under patient's back. The foot-end EMT-B slides one arm under patient's knees and other arm under patient above buttocks.

▲ **2** On signal, the EMT-Bs lift patient to their knees.

NOTE: If a third rescuer is available, he should place both arms under patient's waist while the other two slide their arms up to the mid back or down to the buttocks as appropriate.

▲ **3** On signal, the EMT-Bs stand and carry patient to stretcher, drop to one knee, and roll forward to place him onto mattress.

(continued)

Direct Carry

▲ Stretcher is placed at 90° angle to bed, depending on room configuration. Prepare stretcher by lowering rails, unbuckling straps, and removing other items. Both EMT-Bs stand between stretcher and bed, facing patient.

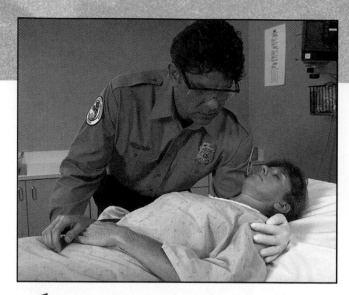

▲ **1** Head-end EMT-B cradles patient's head and neck by sliding one arm under patient's neck to grasp shoulder.

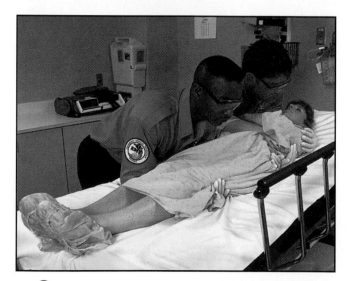

▲ **2** Foot-end EMT-B slides hand under patient's hip and lifts slightly. Head-end EMT-B slides other arm under patient's back. Foot-end EMT-B places arms under patient's hips and calves.

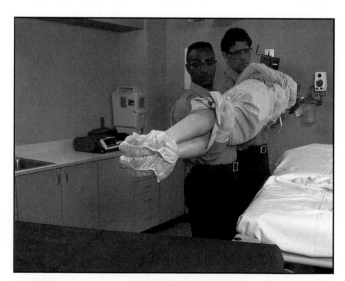

▲ **3** EMT-Bs slide patient to edge of bed and bend toward him with their knees slightly bent. They lift and curl patient to their chests and return to a standing position. They rotate, then slide patient gently onto stretcher.

Unresponsive patients with no suspected spine injury should be placed in the recovery position (Figure 5-5). The patient should be on his side to aid drainage from his mouth and, if he vomits, to help prevent his breathing the vomitus into his lungs. This can be accomplished on a wheeled stretcher. You should avoid transporting the unresponsive patient in a chair-type device since the airway cannot be properly maintained.

Many patients who have no suspected spine injuries may be transported in a position of comfort. This includes many patients with medical complaints such as chest pain, nausea, or difficulty breathing. In this situation, allow the patient to choose a position he feels comfortable in. Breathing is often aided by raising the back of the stretcher so that the patient is in a semi-sitting position, also called Fowler's or semi-Fowler's position (Figure 5-6). The position must be safe and not prohibit the proper use of any transportation device. The position of comfort must be used cautiously in case the patient vomits. Always monitor the patient's airway and level of responsiveness. Place the patient in the recovery position at the first sign of a decreased level of responsiveness.

If any patient has a suspected neck or spine injury, he must be placed on a long backboard. Pa-

Figure 5-6   For many patients, the position of comfort is a semi-sitting position.

tients with spinal injuries who are found in a sitting position, such as in a vehicle, should first be secured to a short backboard to prevent injuries while being moved.

Patients in shock for any reason require treatment for that condition (see Chapter 26, "Bleeding and Shock"). If there is no possibility of head or spine injury, elevate the patient's legs 8 to 12 inches. Do not risk harm to a spine-injured patient. For a patient with possible spinal injury, in general, you should elevate the foot end of the backboard 8 to 12 inches so that the patient's entire body is inclined with the head 8 to 12 inches lower than the feet. This is often called the Trendelenburg position (Figure 5-7).

Transferring the Patient to a Hospital Stretcher

When you arrive at the hospital, you will move the patient from the ambulance stretcher to the hospital stretcher. You will probably use a modified draw-sheet method to transfer the patient (Scan 5-8).

Figure 5-5   A patient in the recovery position.

Figure 5-7   For a patient in shock, raise the legs 8 to 12 inches when appropriate.

TRANSFER TO A HOSPITAL STRETCHER

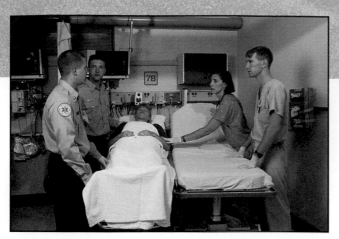

▲ **1** Position raised ambulance cot next to hospital stretcher. Hospital personnel then adjust stretcher (raise or lower the head) to receive patient.

▲ **2** You and hospital personnel gather the sheet on either side of the patient and pull it taut in order to transfer the patient securely.

▲ **3** Holding the gathered sheet at support points near patient's shoulders, mid torso, hips, and knees, you and hospital personnel slide patient in one motion onto hospital stretcher.

▲ **4** Make sure patient is centered on stretcher and stretcher rails are raised before turning him over to emergency department staff.

STREET SCENES

You are having a discussion with a group of your EMS colleagues about the role of the EMT. You focus on direct patient care and the need to do thorough assessments. Another person argues that EMS focuses on doing airway, breathing, and circulation care really well. Kim, an EMT who has been doing EMS for more time than anyone else in the room, says that EMTs must know how to do all those things well "but don't forget that moving and transporting patients is significant, too." When you hear that, you silently disagree. "That's really not an important part of patient care," you say.

Well, the discussion ends—at least for you—when dispatch sends you and your partner to a single-occupant motor-vehicle crash. When you reach the scene, the police tell you that the patient is conscious and alert but is complaining of neck pain, that the crash appears to be low impact with significant front-end damage, and that the patient was wearing a lap belt only.

You introduce yourself to the patient, who is still sitting in the driver's seat of her car, and begin your assessment. The patient states that she ran into a parked car. At impact, her head hit the steering wheel, but she denies any loss of consciousness. You continue with the initial assessment and determine the patient is alert and having no difficulty breathing. No signs of bleeding are observed.

STREET SCENE QUESTIONS

1. What device should be used to remove the patient from the vehicle?

2. What patient-care issues are important when using an extrication device?

3. What is the next thing to consider when actually moving the patient from the vehicle?

Your local protocol requires that a patient with this mechanism of injury—a car crash resulting in the head impacting the steering wheel—gets a cervical collar and a short immobilization device. Your partner, who has been stabilizing the patient's head and neck since shortly after making contact, asks the First Responder unit from the fire department for assistance and suggests to you that a quick neuro exam should be done to check for pulses, motor function, and sensation in all extremities. After the neuro exam, you size a cervical collar and apply it to the patient. You ask the patient if it is causing any additional pain, and she responds that it is uncomfortable but "no additional pain." Next, you position a vest-type extrication device behind her. As you tighten the straps to secure it in place, you ask if it is causing any difficulty with breathing. The patient responds again, "No." You then perform another quick neuro exam. Once completed, the long backboard is positioned and the patient is rotated onto it, with head and neck stabilization still being maintained. The patient is then lowered to the ground.

STREET SCENE QUESTIONS

4. What emergency-care equipment was used for this patient? Why?

5. What is the next step before moving this patient again?

6. What other safety considerations should be considered when moving the long board to the wheeled stretcher?

After the patient is properly secured to the long board, the head immobilizer is positioned, applied, and secured. You continue to talk to the patient to make sure her level of responsiveness has not changed and no breathing difficulty has developed. Another quick neuro exam is performed, with the patient having pulses, movement, and sensation in all four extremities.

The long board needs to be carried about 30 feet to the stretcher, so you and your partner decide to have someone on each corner of the long board. This will provide stability and all EMS personnel can be facing forward. The move is uneventful, and after placing the stretcher in the ambulance, you recheck the stretcher locking device. During transport to the hospital, the patient's vital signs are taken and a patient history obtained. At the hospital, the stretcher is moved from the ambulance and raised onto its wheels. You take the patient to an examination room in the emergency department and, with assistance, you move the long board to the hospital gurney.

After the call, you return to the station. The folks are still in the ready room having the same discussion about the role of an EMT. You pipe in and say, "You know, after this last call, I have to agree with Kim. EMS has a lot to do with knowing how to properly, effectively, and safely move patients."

CHAPTER REVIEW

SUMMARY

Lifting and moving patients is a task that requires planning, proper equipment, and careful attention to body mechanics in order to prevent injury to your patient and to yourself. While some may feel that this task is only secondary to patient care, it is actually a critical part.

Emergency moves are those that may aggravate spine injuries and, therefore, are reserved for life-threatening situations. Urgent moves are used when the patient must be moved quickly but there is time to provide quick, temporary spinal stabilization. Non-urgent moves are normal ways of moving a patient to a stretcher after complete on-scene assessment and any needed spinal stabilization and immobilization have been completed.

Positioning the patient for transport should take into account the patient's comfort, medical needs, and safety. Remember the importance of correct lifting and moving techniques on every call. Protect your patient and protect yourself from injury to maintain a long and positive EMS experience.

KEY TERMS

body mechanics the proper use of the body to facilitate lifting and moving and prevent injury.

direct carry a method of transferring a patient from bed to stretcher, during which two or more rescuers curl the patient to their chests, then reverse the process to lower the patient to the stretcher.

direct ground lift a method of lifting and carrying a patient from ground level to a stretcher in which two or more rescuers kneel, curl the patient to their chests, stand, then reverse the process to lower the patient to the stretcher.

draw-sheet method a method of transferring a patient from bed to stretcher by grasping and pulling the loosened bottom sheet of the bed.

extremity lift a method of lifting and carrying a patient during which one rescuer slips hands under the patient's armpits and grasps the wrists, while another rescuer grasps the patient's knees.

power grip gripping with as much hand surface as possible in contact with the object being lifted, all fingers bent at the same angle, hands at least 10 inches apart.

power lift a lift from a squatting position with weight to be lifted close to the body, feet apart and flat on the ground, body weight on or just behind balls of feet, back locked in. The upper body is raised before the hips. Also called the *squat-lift position*.

REVIEW QUESTIONS

1. Define the term *body mechanics*. Then describe several principles of body mechanics related to safe lifting and moving. (p. 81)
2. List several situations that may require an emergency move of a patient. (p. 84)
3. Describe several lifts and drags. (pp. 84–87. 92)
4. Define a long-axis drag and explain its importance. (p. 84)

APPLICATIONS

For each of the following patients, use the knowledge gained in this chapter to identify the appropriate procedure or device for lifting and moving that patient:

• A patient who has fallen 18 feet and has suspected spinal injuries (p. 84)

• A patient with chest pain (with no spine injury) who lives on the fifth floor of a building with no elevator (pp. 89–92)

• A patient who is found in an environment with a risk of immediate explosion (p. 84)

WEB MEDIC

Visit Brady's *Emergency Care* website for direct weblinks. At **www.bradybooks.com/emergencycare**, you will find information related to Chapter 5 topics:

• Back injuries in EMS

• Body mechanics

Chapter
Six

AIRWAY MANAGEMENT

*W*ord on the Street

"It was a single car roll-over, and the driver had been ejected onto the pavement. He was unconscious, cyanotic, and not breathing. His head was slightly flexed with his chin on his upper chest, so I knelt down and performed a jaw-thrust to open his airway. It must have been completely obstructed by his tongue, because he began to breathe immediately. I kept the airway open until the paramedics arrived about 5 minutes later. I had no equipment that day. But in reality, the only equipment I needed to save that person's life was my two hands and a jaw-thrust."

Edward T. Dickinson M.D., FACEP, NREMT-P

The cells of the human body must have oxygen to survive. The reason the ABCs—airway, breathing, and circulation—are so important is that they are the means by which oxygen is brought into the body and carried to the cells. If the airway (the passageways that lead from the mouth and nose to the lungs) is not open, air cannot get into the lungs. If the patient is unable to breathe, air does not get into the body even if the airway is open. If the heart is not pumping blood through the lungs to pick up oxygen and circulate it to the cells of the body, an open airway and the ability to breathe are of no use. (In fact, breathing and heartbeat are so dependent on each other that if breathing stops first, heartbeat will stop very soon, or if heartbeat stops first, breathing will stop almost at once.)

EMT-B training puts a great deal of emphasis on the airway because it is so easy and so common for a patient's airway to become occluded (blocked). It is also so easy to forget to monitor the patient's airway in the midst of an emergency when so many other details demand the EMT-B's attention.

The EMT-B's chief responsibilities (although not the only ones) are to immediately find and correct life-threatening problems—airway, breathing, and circulation problems—and to get the patient to the hospital. As a prerequisite to your EMT-B course, you took a CPR course which included providing rescue breathing, performing cardiopulmonary resuscitation (CPR), and treating airway obstructions in infants, children, and adults. You can review these topics by reading "Basic Cardiac Life Support Review" in the back of this book.

In this chapter, you will learn additional EMT-B-level skills that relate to the airway, artificial ventilation, and oxygen therapy.

RESPIRATION

Another word for breathing is **respiration.** You learned about the respiratory system in Chapter 4, "The Human Body." In preparation for this chapter, you should review the following structures of the respiratory system and be able to label them on a blank diagram of the respiratory system (Figure 6-1):

- Nose
- Mouth
- Pharynx
- Oropharynx
- Nasopharynx
- Uvula
- Epiglottis
- Larynx (voice box)
- Trachea
- Cricoid cartilage
- Bronchi (right and left mainstem)
- Carina
- Bronchioles
- Lungs
- Alveoli (alveolar sacs)
- Diaphragm

TOPIC OVERVIEW

In this chapter, you will learn about the following topics:

- Anatomy and physiology of the respiratory system

- How to recognize adequate and inadequate breathing

- How to open an airway, maintain an open airway, and ventilate a patient

- Principles and techniques of oxygen administration

- Principles and techniques of suctioning

DOT OBJECTIVES

Also review how oxygen and carbon dioxide are exchanged between the alveoli and capillaries in the lungs, and between the capillaries and the cells throughout the body.

Adequate and Inadequate Breathing

The function of the respiratory system is to enable the body to inhale (breathe in) oxygen, which is then used by all the cells and organs in the body, and to exhale (breathe out) carbon dioxide, the major waste product of respiration. If either of these vital functions is disrupted, then the patient is likely to develop the sensation of shortness of breath and be at risk for respiratory failure.

Simply stated, **respiratory failure** is the reduction of breathing to the point where oxygen intake is not sufficient to support life. When breathing stops completely, the patient is in **respiratory arrest.** Respiratory arrest can develop during heart attack, stroke, airway obstruction, drowning, electrocution, drug overdose, poisoning, brain injury, severe chest injury, suffocation, or prolonged respiratory failure.

HOW AND WHY?

Any condition that leads to inadequate oxygenation of the patient's blood can lead to respiratory arrest, including diseases or injuries to the respiratory system, abuse or overdose of drugs, and head trauma. Go to your Electronic Extras CD for more information.

● Patient ASSESSMENT

Breathing Adequacy

As an EMT-B, you must be able to determine whether or not a patient is breathing adequately so that you can manage the airway properly.

Signs of Adequate Breathing

To determine signs of adequate breathing, you should:

- *Look* for adequate and equal expansion of both sides of the chest when the patient inhales.
- *Listen* for air entering and leaving the nose, mouth, and chest. The breath sounds (when auscultated, or listened to, with a stethoscope) should be present and equal on both sides of the chest. The sounds from the mouth and nose should be typically free of gurgling, gasping, crowing, wheezing, snoring, and stridor (harsh, high-pitched sound during inhalation).
- *Feel* for air moving out of the nose or mouth.

23. Explain the rationale for basic life support artificial ventilation and airway protective skills taking priority over most other basic life support skills. (p. 105)

24. Explain the rationale for providing adequate oxygenation through high inspired oxygen concentrations to patients who, in the past, may have received low concentrations. (pp. 131–132)

✔ Skills

1. Demonstrate the steps in performing the head-tilt, chin-lift.

2. Demonstrate the steps in performing the jaw thrust.

3. Demonstrate the techniques of suctioning.

4. Demonstrate the steps in providing mouth-to-mouth artificial ventilation with body substance isolation (barrier shields).

5. Demonstrate how to use a pocket mask to artificially ventilate a patient.

6. Demonstrate the assembly of a bag-valve-mask unit.

7. Demonstrate the steps in performing the skill of artificially ventilating a patient with a bag-valve mask for one and two rescuers.

8. Demonstrate the steps in performing the skill of artificially ventilating a patient with a bag-valve mask while using the jaw thrust.

9. Demonstrate artificial ventilation of a patient with a flow-restricted, oxygen-powered ventilation device.

10. Demonstrate how to artificially ventilate a patient with a stoma.

11. Demonstrate how to insert an oro-pharyngeal (oral) airway.

12. Demonstrate how to insert a nasopharyngeal (nasal) airway.

13. Demonstrate the correct operation of oxygen tanks and regulators.

14. Demonstrate the use of a nonrebreather face mask and state the oxygen flow requirements needed for its use.

15. Demonstrate the use of a nasal cannula and state the flow requirements for its use.

16. Demonstrate how to artificially ventilate the infant and child patient.

17. Demonstrate oxygen administration for the infant and child patient.

- Check for typical skin coloration. There should be no blue or grey colorations.
- Note the rate, rhythm, quality, and depth of breathing typical for a person at rest (Table 6-1).

Signs of Inadequate Breathing

Signs of inadequate breathing include the following:

- Chest movements are absent, minimal, or uneven.
- Movement associated with breathing is limited to the abdomen (abdominal breathing).
- No air can be felt or heard at the nose or mouth, or the amount of air exchanged is below normal.
- Breath sounds are diminished or absent.
- Noises such as wheezing, crowing, stridor, snoring, gurgling, or gasping are heard during breathing.
- Rate of breathing is too rapid or too slow.
- Breathing is very shallow, very deep, or appears labored.
- Patient is cyanotic; that is, the patient's skin, lips, tongue, ear lobes, or nail beds are blue or grey. This condition is called **cyanosis.**
- Inspirations are prolonged (indicating a possible upper airway obstruction) or expirations are prolonged (indicating a possible lower airway obstruction).

- Patient is unable to speak, or the patient cannot speak full sentences because of shortness of breath.
- In children, there may be retractions (a pulling in of the muscles) above the clavicles and between and below the ribs.
- Nasal flaring (widening of the nostrils of the nose with respirations) may be present, especially in infants and children.

🔴 Patient *CARE*

Inadequate Breathing

When the patient's signs indicate inadequate breathing or no breathing (respiratory failure or respiratory arrest), a life-threatening condition exists and prompt action must be taken. The principal procedures by which life-threatening respiratory problems are treated are:

- Opening and maintaining the airway
- Providing artificial ventilation to the non-breathing patient and the patient with inadequate breathing
- Providing supplemental oxygen to the breathing patient
- Suctioning as needed

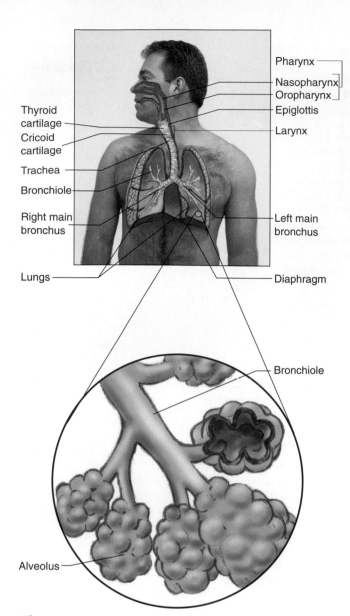

Figure 6-1 The respiratory system.

TABLE 6-1	**Adequate Breathing**
Normal Rates	
Adult–12-20 per minute	
Child–15-30 per minute	
Infant–25-50 per minute	
Rhythm	
Regular	
Quality	
Breath sounds–present and equal	
Chest expansion–adequate and equal	
Minimum effort	
Depth	
Adequate	

These procedures are discussed below and on the following pages.

OPENING THE AIRWAY

The **airway** is the passageway by which air enters or leaves the body. The structures of the airway are the nose, mouth, pharynx, larynx, trachea, bronchi, and lungs.

The procedures for airway evaluation, opening the airway, and artificial ventilation are best carried out with the patient lying supine, or flat on his back. Often you will find a patient already supine in bed. You can perform airway procedures with the patient in this position. Scan 6-1 illustrates the technique for positioning a patient found lying on the floor or ground. Patients who are found in positions other than supine or on the ground should be moved to a supine position on the floor or stretcher for evaluation and treatment.

Any movement of a trauma (injured) patient before immobilization of the head and spine can produce serious injury to the spinal cord. If injury is suspected, protect the head and neck as you position the patient. Airway and breathing, however, have priority over protection of the spine and must be assured as quickly as possible. If the trauma patient must be moved in order to open the airway or to provide ventilations, you will probably not have time to provide immobilization with a cervical collar or head immobilization device on a stretcher but, instead, will provide as much manual stabilization as possible.

Use the following as indications that head, neck, or spinal injury may have occurred, especially when the patient is unconscious and cannot tell you what happened:

• Mechanism of injury is one that can cause head, neck, or spine injury. For example, a patient who is found on the ground near a ladder or stairs may have such injuries. Motor-vehicle collisions are another common cause of head, neck, and spine injuries.

POSITIONING THE PATIENT FOR BASIC LIFE SUPPORT

▲ **1** Straighten the legs and position the closer arm above the patient's head.

▲ **2** Then grasp under the distant armpit.

▲ **3** Cradle the head and neck, and move the patient as a unit onto his side.

▲ **4** Move the patient onto his back and reposition the extended arm.

Note: This maneuver is used when the rescuer must act alone.

- Any injury at or above the level of the shoulders indicates that head, neck, or spine injuries may also be present.
- Family or bystanders may tell you that an injury to the head, neck, or spine has occurred, or they may give you information that leads you to suspect it.

As an EMT-B you must open and maintain the airway in any patient who cannot do so for himself. This includes patients who have an altered mental status (including unconsciousness) or who are in respiratory or cardiac arrest.

Most airway problems are caused by the tongue. As the head flexes forward, the tongue may slide into the airway, causing an obstruction. If the patient is unconscious, the tongue loses muscle tone and muscles of the lower jaw relax. Since the tongue is attached to the lower jaw, the risk of airway obstruction by the tongue is even greater during unconsciousness. The basic procedures for opening the airway help to correct the position of the tongue.

There are two procedures commonly recommended for opening the airway: the *head-tilt, chin-lift maneuver* and the *jaw-thrust maneuver,* the latter being recommended when head, neck, or spine injury is suspected.

Figure 6-2   Head-tilt, chin-lift maneuver, side view. Inset shows EMT's fingertips under bony area at center of patient's lower jaw.

Head-tilt, Chin-lift Maneuver

The **head-tilt, chin-lift maneuver** (Figure 6-2) provides for the maximum opening of the airway. It is useful on patients who are in need of assistance in maintaining an airway or breathing. It is one of the best methods for correcting obstructions caused by the tongue.

✋ Warning

If any indication of head, neck, or spine injury is present, DO NOT USE THE HEAD-TILT, CHIN-LIFT MANEUVER. (USE THE JAW-THRUST MANEUVER INSTEAD.) Remember that any unconscious and many conscious trauma patients may be suspected of having an injury to the head, neck, or spine.

To perform the head-tilt, chin-lift maneuver, follow the steps listed below:

1. Once the patient is supine, place one hand on the forehead and place the fingertips of the other hand under the bony area at the center of the patient's lower jaw.

2. Tilt the head by applying gentle pressure to the patient's forehead.

3. Use your fingertips to lift the chin and to support the lower jaw. Move the jaw forward to a point where the lower teeth are almost touching the upper teeth. Do not compress the soft tissues under the lower jaw, which can obstruct the airway.

4. Do not allow the patient's mouth to be closed. To provide an adequate opening at the mouth, you may need to use the thumb of the hand supporting the chin to pull back the patient's lower lip. Do not insert your thumb into the patient's mouth (to avoid being bitten).

Jaw-Thrust Maneuver

The **jaw-thrust maneuver** (Figure 6-3) is most commonly used to open the airway of an unconscious patient or one with suspected head, neck, or spine injuries. Follow the steps listed below to perform the jaw-thrust maneuver:

Note

THE JAW-THRUST MANEUVER IS THE ONLY RECOMMENDED PROCEDURE FOR USE ON UNCONSCIOUS PATIENTS OR PATIENTS WITH POSSIBLE HEAD, NECK, OR SPINE INJURIES.

1. Carefully keep the patient's head, neck, and spine aligned, moving him as a unit as you place him in the supine position.

2. Take a position at the top of the patient's head, resting your elbows on the same surface on which the patient is lying.

3. Carefully reach forward and gently place one hand on each side of the patient's lower jaw, at the angles of the jaw below the ears.

Figure 6-3 Jaw-thrust maneuver, side view. Inset shows EMT's finger position at angle of the jaw just below the ears.

4. Stabilize the patient's head with your forearms.

5. Using your index fingers, push the angles of the patient's lower jaw forward.

6. You may need to retract the patient's lower lip with your thumb to keep the mouth open.

7. Do not tilt or rotate the patient's head.

Remember

THE PURPOSE OF THE JAW-THRUST MANEUVER IS TO OPEN THE AIRWAY WITHOUT MOVING THE HEAD OR NECK.

In addition to physically opening the airway with the head-tilt, chin-lift or the jaw-thrust maneuver, it is imperative that the airway also be cleared of any secretions, blood, or vomitus. The most effective way to clear the patient's airway is with a wide-bore, rigid-tip Yankauer suction device. For this reason it is crucial that a suction unit be ready for immediate use when opening and maintaining the airway. The equipment and techniques used for suctioning will be discussed later in this chapter.

TECHNIQUES OF ARTIFICIAL VENTILATION

If you determine that the patient is not breathing or that the respiratory efforts are so minimal that respiratory arrest is imminent, you will have to provide artificial ventilation. **Ventilation** is the breathing in of air or oxygen. **Artificial ventilation** (also called **positive pressure ventilation**) is forcing air or oxygen into the lungs when a patient has stopped breathing or has inadequate breathing. There are various techniques available to you as an EMT-B with which you can provide artificial ventilations. In order of preference they are:

1. Mouth-to-mask (preferably with high-flow supplemental oxygen at 15 liters per minute)

2. Two-rescuer bag-valve mask (preferably with high-flow supplemental oxygen at 15 liters per minute)

3. Flow restricted, oxygen-powered ventilation device

4. One-rescuer bag-valve mask

No matter what method is used to ventilate the patient, you must assure that the patient is being ventilated adequately. To

Figure 6-4 Examples of barrier devices.

Figure 6-5 Only use a pocket face mask that has a one-way valve.

determine the signs of adequate artificial ventilation, you should:

- Watch the chest rise and fall with each ventilation
- See the patient's heart rate return to normal with artificial ventilation
- Assure that the rate of ventilation is sufficient—approximately 12 per minute in adults, 20 per minute in children, and a minimum of 20 per minute in infants

Inadequate artificial ventilation occurs when:

- The chest does not rise and fall with ventilations
- The patient's heart rate does not return to normal with artificial ventilations
- The rate of ventilation is too fast or too slow

Techniques used for artificial ventilation should also assure adequate isolation of the rescuer from the patient's body fluids, including saliva, blood, and vomit. For this reason, mouth-to-mouth ventilation is not recommended unless there is no alternative method of artificial ventilation available. There are a number of compact barrier devices available for personal use (Figure 6-4).

Mouth-to Mask Ventilation

Mouth-to-mask ventilation is performed using a **pocket face mask.** The pocket face mask is made of soft, collapsible material and can be carried in your pocket, jacket, or purse (Figure 6-5). Many EMT-Bs purchase their own pocket face masks for their workplace or automobile first aid kits.

Face masks have important infection control features. Your ventilations (breaths) are delivered through a valve in the mask so that you do not have direct contact with the patient's mouth. Most pocket masks have one-way valves that allow your ventilations to enter but prevent the patient's exhaled air from coming back through the valve and into contact with you.

Some pocket masks have oxygen inlets. When high-concentration oxygen is attached to the inlet, an

oxygen concentration of approximately 50% is delivered. This is significantly better than the 16% oxygen concentration (in exhaled air) delivered by mouth-to-mask ventilations without supplemental oxygen.

Most pocket face masks are made of a clear plastic. This is important because you must be able to observe the patient's mouth and nose for vomiting or secretions that need to be suctioned. You also need to observe the color of the lips, an indicator of the respiratory status of the patient. Some pocket face masks may have a strap that goes around the patient's head. This is helpful during one-rescuer CPR, since it will hold the mask on the patient's face while you are performing chest compressions. However, it does not replace the need for proper hand placement on the mask as described below.

To provide mouth-to-mask ventilation (Figure 6-6), follow these steps:

1. Position yourself at the patient's head and open the airway. It may be necessary to clear the airway of obstructions. If necessary, insert an oropharyngeal airway to help keep the patient's airway open (as described later in this chapter).

2. Connect oxygen to the inlet on the face mask. Oxygen should be run at 15 liters per minute. *If oxygen is not immediately available, do not delay mouth-to-mask ventilations.*

3. Position the mask on the patient's face so that the apex (top of the triangle) is over the bridge of the nose and the base is between the lower lip and prominence of the chin. (Center the ventilation port over the patient's mouth.)

4. Hold the mask firmly in place while maintaining the proper head tilt by:

- Placing thumbs over the top half of the mask, index and middle fingers over the bottom half
- Using the ring and little fingers to bring the jaw up to the mask

5. Take a deep breath and exhale into the mask port or one-way valve at the top of the mask port.

Figure 6-6   Mouth-to-mask ventilation.

Figure 6-7   Adult, child, and infant bag-valve-mask units.

Each ventilation should be delivered over 1½ to 2 seconds in adults, 1 to 1½ seconds in infants and children. Watch for the patient's chest to rise.

6. Remove your mouth from the port and allow for passive exhalation. Continue as you would for mouth-to-mouth ventilations or CPR.

When properly used, the pocket face mask will deliver higher volumes of air to the patient than the bag-valve-mask device.

Bag-Valve Mask

The **bag-valve mask** is a hand-held ventilation device. It may also be referred to as a bag-valve-mask unit, system, device, resuscitator, or simply BVM. The bag-valve-mask unit can be used to ventilate a non-breathing patient and is also helpful to assist ventilations in the patient whose own respiratory attempts are not enough to support life, such as a patient in respiratory failure or drug overdose. The BVM also provides an infection-control barrier between you and your patient. The use of the bag-valve mask in the field is often referred to as "bagging" the patient.

Bag-valve-mask units come in sizes for adults, children, and infants (Figure 6-7). Many different types of bag-valve-mask systems are available; however, all have the same basic parts. The bag must be a self-refilling shell that is easily cleaned and steril-

ized. (Some bag-valve-mask units are designed for single use and are then disposed of.) The system must have a non-jam valve that allows an oxygen inlet flow of 15 liters per minute. The valve should be *nonrebreathing* (preventing the patient from re-breathing his own exhalations) and not subject to freezing in cold temperatures. Most systems have a standard 15/22 mm respiratory fitting to ensure a proper fit with other respiratory equipment, face masks, and endotracheal tubes.

Warning

Many older bag-valve masks have "pop-off" valves. These valves were designed to open after certain pressures were obtained. Studies have shown that pop-off valves may prevent adequate ventilations. BVM systems with pop-off valves should be replaced. A BVM system should also have a clear face mask so that you can observe the lips for cyanosis and monitor the airway in case suctioning is needed.

The mechanical workings of a bag-valve-mask device are simple. Oxygen, flowing at 15 liters per minute, is attached to the BVM and enters the reservoir. When the bag is squeezed, the air inlet to the bag is closed, and the oxygen is delivered to the patient. BVM systems without a reservoir supply approximately 50% oxygen. Systems with an oxygen reservoir provide nearly 100% oxygen.

When the squeeze of the bag is released, a passive expiration by the patient will occur. While the

Figure 6-8 Delivering two-rescuer BVM ventilation when *no* trauma is suspected in the patient.

patient exhales, oxygen enters the reservoir to be delivered to the patient the next time the bag is squeezed. The bag itself will hold anywhere from 1,000 to 1,600 milliliters of air. According to American Heart Association guidelines, at least 700–1000 milliliters of air must be delivered to the patient. Lesser volumes may be used (400–600 milliliters) if supplemental oxygen is used and the chest rises adequately. This means that the bag-valve-mask system must be used properly and efficiently.

The most difficult part of delivering BVM artificial ventilations is obtaining an adequate mask seal so that air does not leak in or out around the edges of the mask. It is difficult to maintain the seal with one hand while squeezing the bag with the other, and one-rescuer bag-valve-mask operation is often unsuccessful or inadequate for this reason. Therefore, it is strongly recommended by the American Heart Association that BVM artificial ventilation be performed by two rescuers. In two-rescuer BVM ventilation, one rescuer is assigned to squeeze the bag while the other rescuer uses two hands to maintain a mask seal.

The two-rescuer technique can also be modified so that the jaw-thrust can be used during BVM ventilations. This technique is to be used when performing BVM ventilation on a patient with a suspected head, neck, or spine injury. Proficiency in this technique requires frequent mannikin practice. To perform BVM ventilation when trauma (injury) is not suspected (Figure 6-8) and when trauma is suspected (Figure 6-9), follow the steps listed below.

Two-Rescuer BVM Ventilation—No Trauma Suspected

1. Open the patient's airway USING THE HEAD-TILT, CHIN-LIFT MANEUVER. Suction and insert an airway adjunct as necessary.

2. Select the correct bag-valve mask size (adult, child, or infant).

3. Kneel at the patient's head. Position thumbs over the top half of the mask, index and middle fingers over the bottom half.

4. Place the apex, or top, of the triangular mask over the bridge of the patient's nose. Then lower the mask over the mouth and upper chin. If the mask has a large, round cuff surrounding a ventilation port, center the port over the patient's mouth.

5. Use ring and little fingers to bring the patient's jaw up to the mask. MAINTAIN THE HEAD-TILT, CHIN-LIFT.

6. The second rescuer should connect bag to mask, if not already done. While you maintain the mask seal, the second rescuer should squeeze the bag with two hands until the patient's chest rises. The second rescuer should squeeze the bag *once every 5 seconds for an adult, once every 3 seconds for a child or infant.*

7. The second rescuer should release pressure on the bag and let the patient exhale passively. While this occurs the bag is refilling from the oxygen source.

Two-Rescuer BVM Ventilation— Trauma Suspected

1. Open the patient's airway USING THE JAW-THRUST MANEUVER. Suction and insert an airway adjunct (see later in this chapter) as necessary.

2. Select the correct bag-valve mask size (adult, child, or infant).

3. Kneel at the patient's head. Place thumbs over the nose portion of the mask and place your index

Figure 6-9 Delivering two-rescuer BVM ventilation while providing manual stabilization of the head and neck when trauma *is* suspected in the patient.

and middle fingers over the portion of the mask that covers the mouth.

4. Use your ring and little fingers to bring the jaw upward, toward the mask, WITHOUT TILTING THE HEAD OR NECK.

5. The second rescuer should squeeze the bag to ventilate the patient as described above for the non-trauma patient.

As noted above, use of a bag-valve mask by a single rescuer is the last choice of artificial ventilation procedure behind use of a pocket face mask with supplemental oxygen, a two-rescuer bag-valve-mask procedure, and use of a flow-restricted, oxygen-powered ventilation device. You should provide ventilations with a one-rescuer bag-valve-mask procedure only when no other options are available. When using the bag-valve-mask device alone you should follow the steps listed below.

One-Rescuer BVM Ventilation

1. Position yourself at the patient's head and establish an open airway. Suction and insert an airway adjunct as necessary.

2. Select the correct size mask for the patient. Position the mask on the patient's face as described above for the two-rescuer BVM technique.

3. Form a "C" around the ventilation port with thumb and index finger. Use middle, ring, and little fingers under the patient's jaw to hold the jaw to the mask.

4. With your other hand, squeeze the bag once every 5 seconds. The squeeze should be a full one, causing the patient's chest to rise. For infants and children, squeeze the bag once every 3 seconds.

5. Release pressure on the bag and let the patient exhale passively. While this occurs the bag is refilling from the oxygen source.

If the chest does not rise and fall during BVM ventilation, you should:

1. Reposition the head.

2. Check for escape of air around the mask and reposition fingers and mask.

3. Check for airway obstruction or obstruction in the BVM system. Re-suction the patient if necessary. Consider insertion of an airway adjunct if not already done.

4. If none of the above methods work, use an alternative method of artificial ventilation, such as a pocket mask or a flow-restricted, oxygen-powered ventilation device.

The BVM may also be used during CPR. The bag is squeezed once each time a ventilation is to be delivered. In one-rescuer CPR, it is preferable to use a pocket mask with supplemental oxygen rather than a BVM system (Figure 6-10). A single rescuer would take too much time picking up the BVM and obtaining a face seal each time a ventilation is to be delivered, in addition to the normal difficulty in maintaining a seal with the one-rescuer BVM technique.

Artificial Ventilation of a Stoma Breather

The BVM can be used to artificially ventilate patients with a **stoma,** a surgical opening in the neck through which the patient breathes. Patients with stomas who are found to be in severe respiratory distress or respiratory arrest frequently have thick secretions blocking the stoma. It is recommended that you suction the stoma frequently in conjunction with BVM-to-stoma ventilations.

As with other BVM uses, a two-rescuer technique is preferred over a one-rescuer technique. To provide artificial ventilation to a stoma breather with a BVM, follow these steps:

1. Clear any mucus plugs or secretions from the stoma.

2. Leave the head and neck in a neutral position, as it is unnecessary to position the airway prior to ventilations in a stoma breather.

3. Use a pediatric-sized mask to establish a seal around the stoma.

4. Ventilate at the appropriate rate for the patient's age.

5. If unable to artificially ventilate through the stoma, consider sealing the stoma and attempting artificial ventilation through the mouth and nose. (This may work if the trachea is still connected to the passageways of mouth, nose, and pharynx. In

Figure 6-10 Two-rescuer CPR using a pocket face mask with supplemental oxygen.

some cases, the trachea has been permanently connected to the neck opening with no remaining connection to mouth, nose, or pharynx).

✋ Note

Bag-valve mask devices should be completely disassembled and disinfected after each use. Because proper decontamination is often costly and time consuming, many hospitals and EMS agencies use single-use disposable BVMs.

Flow-Restricted, Oxygen-Powered Ventilation Device

A **flow-restricted, oxygen-powered ventilation device (FROPVD)** uses oxygen under pressure to deliver artificial ventilations through a mask placed over the patient's face. This device is similar to the traditional demand-valve resuscitator but includes newer features designed to optimize ventilations and safeguard the patient (Figure 6-11). Recommended features include:

- A peak flow rate of 100% oxygen at up to 40 liters per minute
- An inspiratory pressure relief valve that opens at approximately 60 cm of water pressure
- An audible alarm when the relief valve is activated
- A rugged design and construction
- A trigger that enables the rescuer to use both hands to maintain a mask seal while triggering the device
- Satisfactory operation in both ordinary and extreme environmental conditions

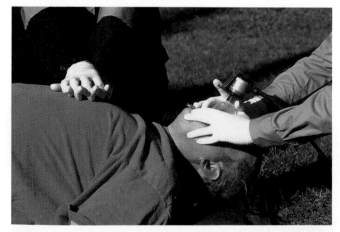

Figure 6-11 Providing ventilations with a flow-restricted, oxygen-powered ventilation device (FROPVD).

Follow the same procedures for mask seal as recommended for the BVM. Trigger the device until the chest rises and *repeat every 5 seconds.* If the chest does not rise, reposition the head, check the mask seal, check for obstructions, and consider the use of an alternative artificial ventilation procedure.

When using the FROPVD on a patient with chest trauma, be especially careful not to overinflate, as you may actually make the chest injury worse. Also, always make sure the airway is fully opened, and watch the chest rise. Make sure you are not forcing excess air to enter the stomach instead of the lungs, causing gastric distention, which could cause the patient to regurgitate and possibly compromise the airway with stomach contents.

If neck injury is suspected, have an assistant hold the patient's head manually or use your knees to prevent movement. Bring the jaw up to the mask without tilting the head or neck.

The flow-restricted, oxygen-powered ventilation device should be used only on adults unless you have a child unit and have been given special training in its use by your medical director.

AIRWAY ADJUNCTS

Once you gain access to a patient and begin your initial assessment, your first course of action is to establish an open airway. The airway must be maintained throughout all care procedures.

The most common impediment to an open airway is the tongue. When a patient becomes unconscious, the muscles relax. The tongue will slide back into the pharynx and obstruct the airway. Even though a head-tilt, chin-lift or jaw-thrust maneuver will help open the airway of a patient, the tongue may return to its obstructive position once the maneuver is released. Sometimes even when the head-tilt, chin-lift or jaw-thrust is maintained, the tongue will "fall back" into the pharynx.

Airway adjuncts, devices that aid in maintaining an open airway, may be used early in the treatment of the unresponsive patient and continue throughout your care. There are several types of airway adjuncts. In this chapter, only the devices that are a part of the standard EMT-B course—those whose main function is to keep the tongue from blocking the airway—will be discussed.

The two most common airway adjuncts for the EMT-B to use are the **oropharyngeal airway** (or oral airway) and the **nasopharyngeal airway** (or nasal airway). The structure and use of these airways can be understood by analyzing their names. *Oro* refers to the mouth, *naso* the nose, and *pharyngeal* the pharynx. Oropharyngeal airways are inserted into the mouth and help keep the tongue from falling back into the pharynx. Nasopharyngeal airways are inserted through the nose and rest in the pharynx, also helping keep the tongue from becoming an airway obstruction.

Rules for Using Airway Adjuncts

Some general rules apply to the use of oropharyngeal and the nasopharyngeal airways:

- Use an airway on all unconscious patients who do not exhibit a **gag reflex.** The gag reflex causes vomiting or retching when something is placed in the pharynx. When a patient is deeply unconscious, the gag reflex usually disappears but may reappear as a patient begins to regain consciousness. A patient with a gag reflex who cannot tolerate an oropharyngeal airway may be able to tolerate a nasopharyngeal airway.
- Open the patient's airway manually before using an adjunct device.
- When inserting the airway, take care not to push the patient's tongue into the pharynx.
- Do not continue inserting the airway if the patient begins to gag. Continue to maintain the airway manually and do not use an adjunct device. If the patient remains unconscious for a prolonged time, you may later attempt to insert an airway to determine if the gag reflex is still present.
- When an airway adjunct is in place, *you must maintain head-tilt, chin-lift or jaw-thrust and monitor the airway.*
- When an airway adjunct is in place, you must remain ready to suction the patient's airway to clear secretions as necessary.
- If the patient regains consciousness or develops a gag reflex, remove the airway immediately. Be prepared to suction the patient again.
- Use infection control practices while maintaining the airway. Wear disposable gloves. In airway maintenance, there is a chance of a patient's body fluids coming in contact with your face and eyes. Wear mask and goggles or other protective eyewear to prevent this contact.

Oropharyngeal Airways

Once a patient's airway is opened, an oropharyngeal airway can be inserted to help keep it open. An oropharyngeal airway is a curved device, usually made of plastic, that can be inserted into the patient's mouth. The oropharyngeal airway has a flange that

Figure 6-12 Oropharyngeal airways in various sizes.

will rest against the patient's lips. The rest of the device holds the tongue as it curves back to the pharynx. The proper use of an oropharyngeal airway greatly reduces the chances of the patient's airway becoming obstructed.

There are standard sizes of oropharyngeal airways (Figure 6-12). Many manufacturers make a complete line, ranging from airways for infants to large adult sizes. An entire set should be carried to allow for quick, proper selection.

The airway adjunct cannot be used effectively unless you select the correct airway size for the patient. An airway of proper size will extend from the corner of the patient's mouth to the tip of the earlobe on the same side of the patient's face. An alternative method is to measure from the center of the patient's mouth to the angle of the lower jaw bone. Do not use an airway unless you have measured it against the patient and verified it as being the proper size. If the airway is not the correct size, do not use it on the patient.

To insert an oropharyngeal airway follow the steps listed below (Scan 6-2):

1. Place the patient on his back. When caring for a medical patient with no indications of spinal injury, the neck may be hyperextended. If there are possible spinal injuries, use the jaw-thrust maneuver, moving the patient no more than necessary to ensure an open airway (the airway takes priority over the spine). Extreme care must be taken.

2. Perform a crossed-finger technique. That is, cross the thumb and forefinger of one hand and place them on the upper and lower teeth at the corner of the patient's mouth. Spread your fingers apart to open the patient's jaws.

3. Position the airway so that its tip is pointing toward the roof of the patient's mouth.

INSERTING AN OROPHARYNGEAL AIRWAY

▲ **1** Assure the oropharyngeal airway is the correct size by checking to make sure it either extends from the center of the mouth to the angle of the jaw or . . .

▲ from the corner of the patient's mouth to the tip of the earlobe.

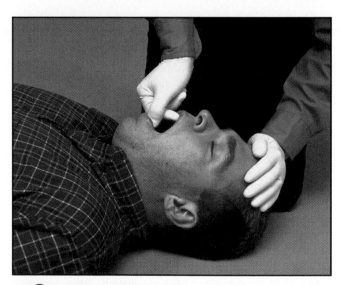

▲ **2** Use the crossed-fingers technique to open the patient's mouth.

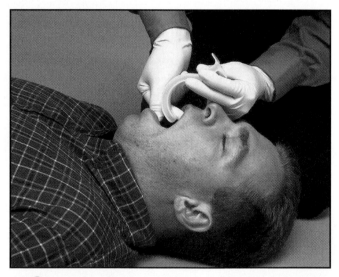

▲ **3** Insert the airway with the tip pointing to the roof of the patient's mouth.

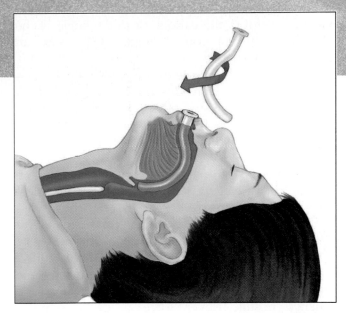

▲ **4** Rotate it 180 degrees into position. When the airway is properly positioned, the flange rests against the patient's mouth.

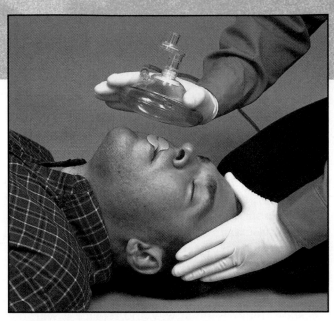

▲ **5** After proper insertion, the patient is ready for ventilation.

Warning: Monitor the patient closely. If there is a gag reflex, remove the airway adjunct at once by following the anatomical curvature. You do not need to rotate the device when removing it.

4. Insert the airway and slide it along the roof of the patient's mouth, past the soft tissue hanging down from the back (the uvula), or until you meet resistance against the soft palate. Be certain not to push the patient's tongue back into the pharynx. Any airway insertion is made easier by using a tongue blade (tongue depressor). In a few cases, you may have to use a tongue blade to hold the tongue in place. Watch what you are doing when inserting the airway. This procedure should not be performed by "feel" only.

5. Gently rotate the airway 180 degrees so that the tip is pointing down into the patient's pharynx. This method prevents pushing the tongue back. Alternatively, insert the airway with tip already pointing "down" towards the patient's pharynx, using a tongue depressor to press the tongue down and forward to avoid obstructing the airway. *This is the preferred method for airway insertion in an infant or child.*

6. Position the patient. Place the non-trauma patient in a maximum head-tilt position. If there are possible spine injuries, maintain cervical stabilization at all times during airway management.

7. Check to see that the flange of the airway is against the patient's lips. If the airway is too long or too short, remove the airway and replace it with the correct size.

8. Place the mask you will use for ventilation over the in-place airway adjunct. If no barrier device is available, provide direct mouth-to-adjunct ventilation just as you would provide mouth-to-mouth ventilation.

9. Monitor the patient closely. If there is a gag reflex, remove the airway adjunct at once by following the anatomical curvature. You do not need to rotate the device when removing it.

Note: Some EMS systems allow an oropharyngeal airway to be inserted with the tip pointing to the side of the patient's mouth. The device is then rotated 90 degrees so that its tip is pointing down the patient's pharynx. Use this approach only if it is part of the protocol of your EMS system.

Nasopharyngeal Airways

The nasopharyngeal airway has gained popularity because it often does not stimulate the gag reflex. This allows the nasopharyngeal airway to be used in patients who have a reduced level of responsiveness but still have an intact gag reflex. Other benefits include the fact that it can be used when the teeth are clenched and when there are oral injuries.

Use the soft flexible latex nasal airway and not the rigid clear plastic airway in the field. The soft ones are less likely to cause soft-tissue damage or bleeding. The typical sizes for adults are 34, 32, 30, and 28 French.

To insert a nasopharyngeal airway, follow the steps listed below (Scan 6-3):

1. Measure the nasopharyngeal airway from the patient's nostril to the earlobe or to the angle of the jaw. Choosing the correct length will assure an appropriate diameter.

2. Lubricate the outside of the tube with a water-based lubricant before insertion. Do not use a petroleum jelly or any other type of non-water-based lubricant. Such substances can damage the tissue lining of the nasal cavity and the pharynx and increase the risk of infection.

3. Gently push the tip of the nose upward. Keep the patient's head in a neutral position. Most nasopharyngeal airways are designed to be placed in the right nostril. The bevel (angled portion at the tip) should point toward the base of the nostril or toward the septum (wall that separates the nostrils).

4. Insert the airway into the nostril. Advance the airway until the flange rests firmly against the patient's nostril. Never force a nasopharyngeal airway. If you experience difficulty advancing the airway, pull the tube out and try the other nostril.

Warning

Do not attempt the use of a nasopharyngeal airway if there is evidence of clear (cerebrospinal) fluid coming from the nose or ears. This may indicate a skull fracture in the area where the airway would pass.

Oropharyngeal and nasopharyngeal airways can be a tremendous asset to the EMT-B when used properly. However, no device can replace the EMT-B. The proper use of these airways or any other device depends on the appropriate use, good judgment, and adequate monitoring of the patient by the EMT-B.

Oropharyngeal and nasopharyngeal airways prevent blockage of the upper airway by the tongue. To ensure an open airway to the level of the lungs, it is sometimes necessary to insert an endotracheal (through-the-trachea) tube. Endotracheal intubation is an advanced-life-support procedure that, in some jurisdictions, may be performed by EMT-Bs. The techniques for endotracheal intubation are discussed in Chapter 35, "Advanced Airway Management."

INSERTING A NASOPHARYNGEAL AIRWAY

▲ **1** Measure the nasopharyngeal airway from the patient's nostril to the earlobe or to the angle of the jaw.

▲ **2** Apply a water-based lubricant before insertion.

▲ **3** Gently push the tip of the nose upward, and insert the airway with the beveled side toward the base of the nostril or toward the septum (wall that separates the nostrils).

▲ **4** Insert the airway, advancing it until the flange rests against the nostril.

Warning: Do not attempt to use a nasopharyngeal airway if there is evidence of clear (cerebrospinal) fluid coming from the nose or ears. This may indicate a skull fracture in the area where the airway would pass.

    Also, never force a nasopharyngeal airway. If you experience difficulty advancing the airway, pull the tube out and try the other nostril.

SUCTIONING

The patient's airway must be kept clear of foreign materials, blood, vomitus, and other secretions. Materials that are allowed to remain in the airway may be forced into the trachea and eventually into the lungs. This will cause complications ranging from severe pneumonia to complete airway obstruction. **Suctioning** is the method of using a vacuum device to remove such materials. A patient needs to be suctioned immediately whenever a gurgling sound is heard, whether before, during, or after artificial ventilation.

Suctioning Devices

Each suction unit consists of a suction source, a collection container for materials you suction, tubing, and suction tips or catheters. Systems are either mounted in the ambulance or are portable and may be brought to the scene.

Mounted Suction Systems

Many ambulances have a suction unit mounted in the patient compartment (Figure 6-13). These units are usually installed near the head of the stretcher so they are easily used. Mounted systems, often called "on-board" units, create a suctioning vacuum produced by the engine's manifold or an electrical power source. To be effective, suction devices must furnish an air intake of at least 30 liters per minute at the open end of a collection tube. This will occur if the system can generate a vacuum of no less than 300 mm Hg (millimeters of mercury) when the collecting tube is clamped.

Portable Suction Units

There are many different types of portable suction units (Figure 6-14). They may be electrically powered (by batteries or household current), oxygen- or air-powered, or manually operated. The requirement for the amount of suction a portable unit must provide is identical to that of the fixed unit (30 liters per minute, 300 mmHg). It is important to have the ability to suction anywhere. Portable suction provides that ability.

Tubing, Tips, and Catheters

For suctioning to be effective, the proper equipment must be used. While a suction unit might be the most powerful available, it will do no good unless used with the proper attachments. Before operating a suction unit, you must have:

- Tubing
- Suction tips
- Suction catheters

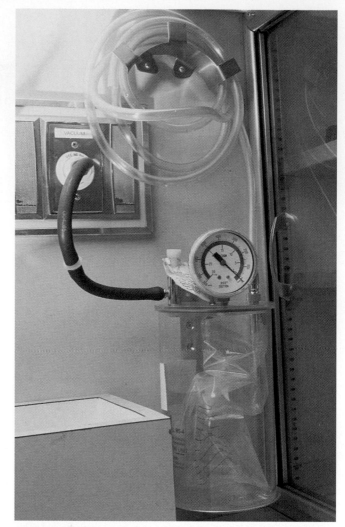

Figure 6-13 A mounted suction unit installed in the ambulance patient compartment.

- Collection container
- Container of clean or sterile water

The *tubing* attached to a suction unit must be thick-walled, non-kinking, wide-bore tubing. This is because the tubing must not collapse due to the suction, must allow "chunks" of suctioned material to pass, and must not kink, which would reduce the suction. The tubing must be long enough to reach comfortably from the suction unit to the patient.

Currently, the most popular type of *suction tip* is the rigid pharyngeal tip, also called "Yankauer" or "tonsil sucker" or "tonsil-tip" suction. This rigid device allows you to suction the mouth and pharynx with excellent control over the distal end of the device. It also has a larger bore than flexible catheters. Most successfully used with an unresponsive patient, rigid-tip suction must be used with caution especially if the patient is not completely unresponsive or may be regaining consciousness. When the tip is placed

A

B

C

Figure 6-14 (A) An oxygen-powered portable suction unit, (B) a battery-powered portable unit, and (C) a manually operated unit.

into the pharynx, the gag reflex may be activated, producing additional vomiting. It is also possible to stimulate the vagus nerve in the back of the pharynx, which can slow the heart rate. So be careful not to suction more than a few seconds at a time with a rigid tip and never lose sight of the tip.

Suction catheters are flexible plastic tubes. They come in various sizes identified by a number "French." The larger the number, the larger the catheter. A "14 French" catheter is larger than an "8 French" catheter. These catheters are usually not large enough to suction vomitus or thick secretions and may kink. Flexible catheters are designed to be used in situations when a rigid tip cannot be used. For example, a soft catheter can be passed through a tube such as a nasopharyngeal or endotracheal tube or used for suctioning the nasopharynx. (A bulb suction device may also be used to suction nasal passages.)

Another important part of a suction device is the *collection container*. All units should have a nonbreakable container to collect the suctioned materials. These containers must be easily removed and decontaminated. Remember to wear gloves, protective eyewear, and mask not only while suctioning but also while cleaning the equipment. Most newer suction devices have disposable containers to eliminate the time and risks involved in decontamination.

Suction units also must have a container of clean (preferably sterile) water nearby. This water is used to clear matter that is partially blocking the tubing. When this partial blockage of the tube occurs, place the suction tip or catheter in the container of water. This will cause a stream of water to flow through the tip and tubing, usually forcing the clog to dislodge. When the tip or tubing becomes clogged with an item that will not dislodge, replace it with a new tip or catheter.

In the event of copious, thick secretions or vomiting, consider removing the rigid tip or catheter and using the large bore, rigid suction tubing. After you are finished, place the standard tip back on for further suctioning.

Techniques of Suctioning

Although there may be some variations in suction technique (a suggested technique is shown in Scan 6-4), a few rules always apply. The first rule is *always use appropriate infection control practices while suctioning.* These practices include the use of protective eyewear, mask, and disposable gloves. Proper suctioning requires you to have your fingers around and sometimes inside the patient's mouth. Disposable gloves prevent contact between the EMT-B and the patient's bodily fluids. Protective eyewear and mask are also recommended since these fluids might splatter, or the patient may gag or cough, sending droplets to your face, eyes, and mouth.

The second rule is *never suction for longer than 15 seconds at a time,* since supplemental oxygen or ventilations cease during suctioning, keeping oxygen from the patient. If the patient produces secretions as rapidly as suctioning can remove them, suction for

SUCTIONING TECHNIQUES

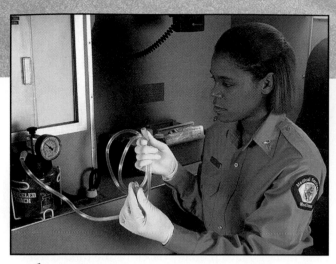

▲ **1** Turn the unit on, attach a catheter, and test for suction at the beginning of your shift.

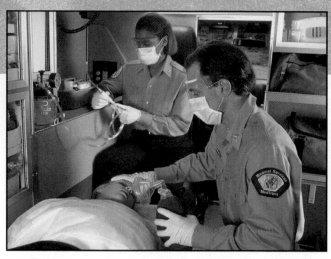

▲ **2** Position yourself at the patient's head and turn the patient to the side.

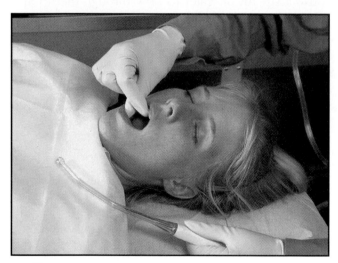

▲ **3** Open and clear the patient's mouth.

▲ **4** Place the convex side of the rigid tip against the roof of the mouth. Insert just to the base of the tongue.

▲ **5** Apply suction only after the rigid tip is in place. Do not lose sight of the tip while suctioning. Suction while withdrawing the tip.

▲ Measure a flexible catheter from the patient's earlobe to the corner of the mouth or the center of the mouth to the angle of the jaw.

15 seconds, artificially ventilate for 2 minutes, then suction for 15 seconds, and continue the sequence. Consult medical direction in this situation.

Patients who need airway control and suctioning are often unconscious and may be in cardiac or respiratory arrest. Oxygen delivery to this patient is very important. During suctioning, the ventilations or other method of oxygen delivery is discontinued to allow for the passage of the suction catheter. To prevent critical delays in oxygen delivery, limit suctioning to a few seconds, then resume ventilations or oxygen delivery.

You may **hyperventilate** a patient before and after suctioning. That is, you may ventilate a patient who is receiving artificial ventilations at a faster rate before and after suctioning to compensate for the oxygen not delivered during suctioning.

The third rule for suctioning is *place the tip or catheter where you want to begin the suctioning and suction on the way out*. Most suction tips and catheters do not produce suction at all times. You have to start the suctioning. The tip or catheter will have an open distal end where the suction is delivered. It will also have an opening, or port, in the proximal portion. When you put your finger over the proximal port, suctioning begins from the distal end.

It is not necessary to measure when using a rigid tip. Rather, you should be sure not to lose sight of the tip when inserting it. However, do measure the suction catheter in a manner similar to an oropharyngeal airway. The length of catheter that should be inserted into the patient's mouth is equal to the distance between the corner of the patient's mouth and earlobe.

Carefully bring the tip of the catheter to the area where suctioning is needed. Never "jab" or force the suction tip into the mouth or pharynx. Then place your finger over the proximal opening to begin the suctioning, and suction as you slowly withdraw the tip from the patient's mouth, moving the tip from side to side.

Suctioning is usually delivered with the patient turned on his side. This allows free secretions to flow from the mouth while suctioning is being delivered. Caution must be used in patients with suspected neck or spine injuries. If the patient is fully and securely immobilized, the entire backboard may be tilted to place the patient on his side. For the patient for whom such injuries are suspected but who is not immobilized, suction the best you can without turning the patient. If all other methods have failed, as a last resort you may turn the patient's body as a unit, attempting to keep the neck and spine in line. Suctioning should not be delayed to immobilize a patient.

The rigid suction tip or flexible catheter should be moved into place carefully and not forced. Rigid suction devices may cause tissue damage and bleeding. Never probe into wounds or attempt to suction away attached tissue with a suction device. Certain skull fractures may actually cause brain tissue to be visible in the pharynx. If this occurs, do not suction near this tissue; limit suctioning to the mouth.

Suction devices may also cause activation of the gag reflex and stimulate vomiting. In a patient who already has secretions that need to be suctioned, vomiting only makes things worse. If you advance a suction catheter or rigid suction tip and the patient begins to gag, withdraw the tip to a position that does not cause gagging and begin suctioning.

The above techniques apply to suctioning of the upper airway. Techniques for orotracheal deep suctioning to the level of the lungs—an advanced life support procedure that may be performed by EMT-Bs in some jurisdictions—are discussed in Chapter 35, "Advanced Airway Management."

OXYGEN THERAPY

Importance of Supplemental Oxygen

Oxygen administration is often one of the most important and beneficial treatments an EMT-B can provide. The atmosphere provides approximately 21% oxygen. If a person is without illness or injury, that 21% is enough to support normal functioning. However, the fact is that people EMT-Bs come in contact with are sick or injured and often require supplemental oxygen.

Conditions Requiring Oxygen
Conditions that may require oxygen include:

- *Respiratory or cardiac arrest.* CPR is only 25% to 33% as effective as normal circulation. High-concentration oxygen administration provides a better chance of survival for the patient in respiratory or cardiac arrest.
- *Heart attacks and strokes.* These emergencies result from an interruption of blood to the heart or brain. When this occurs, tissues are deprived of oxygen. Providing extra oxygen is extremely important.
- *Shock.* Since shock is the failure of the cardiovascular system to provide sufficient blood to all the vital tissues, all cases of shock reduce the amount of oxygenated blood reaching the tissues. Administration of oxygen helps the blood that does reach the tissues deliver the maximum amount of oxygen.

- *Blood loss.* Whether bleeding is internal or external, there is a reduced amount of circulating blood and red blood cells, so the blood that is circulating needs to be saturated with oxygen.
- *Lung diseases.* The lungs are responsible for turning oxygen over to the blood cells to be delivered to the tissues. When the lungs are not functioning properly, supplemental oxygen helps assure that the body's tissues receive adequate oxygen.
- *Broken bones, head injuries, and more.* There are very few emergencies where oxygen administration would not be appropriate. All our body's systems work together. An injury in one part may cause shock that affects the rest of the body.

Hypoxia

Hypoxia is an insufficiency in the supply of oxygen to the body's tissues. There are several major causes of hypoxia. Consider the following scenarios:

- *A patient is trapped in a fire.* The air that the patient breathes contains smoke and reduced amounts of oxygen. Since the patient cannot breathe in enough oxygen, hypoxia develops.
- *A patient has emphysema.* This lung disease decreases the efficiency of the transfer of oxygen between the atmosphere and the body. Since the lungs cannot function properly, hypoxia develops.
- *A patient overdoses* on a drug that has a depressing effect on the respiratory system. The patient's respirations are only 5 per minute. In this case, the victim is not breathing frequently enough to support the body's oxygen needs. Hypoxia develops.
- *A patient has a heart attack.* The lungs function properly by taking atmospheric air and turning it over to the blood for distribution. The damaged heart, however, cannot pump the blood throughout the body, and hypoxia develops.

There are many causes of hypoxia in addition to the examples named, including stroke, shock, and others. The most important thing to know is how to recognize signs of hypoxia so that it may be treated. Hypoxia may be indicated by cyanosis (blue or grey color to the skin). Additionally, when the brain suffers hypoxia, the patient's mental status may deteriorate. Restlessness or confusion may result.

As an EMT-B your concern will be to prevent hypoxia from developing or becoming worse and, when possible, to reduce the level of hypoxia. This is done with the administration of oxygen.

Oxygen Therapy Equipment

In the field, oxygen equipment must be safe, lightweight, portable, and dependable. Some field oxy-

Figure 6-15 An oxygen delivery system.

gen systems are very portable and can be brought almost anywhere. Other systems are installed inside the ambulance so that oxygen can be delivered during transportation to the hospital.

Most oxygen delivery systems contain several items (Figure 6-15): oxygen cylinders, pressure regulators, and a delivery device (nonrebreather mask or cannula). When the patient is not breathing or is breathing inadequately, additional devices (such as a pocket mask, bag-valve mask, or positive pressure ventilator) can be used to force oxygen into the patient's lungs.

Oxygen Cylinders

Outside a medical facility, the standard source of oxygen is the **oxygen cylinder,** a seamless steel or lightweight alloy cylinder filled with oxygen under pressure, equal to 2,000 to 2,200 pounds per square inch (psi) when the cylinders are full. Cylinders come in various sizes, identified by letters (Figure 6-16). Those in common use in emergency care include:

- *D cylinder* contains about 350 liters of oxygen
- *E cylinder* contains about 625 liters of oxygen
- *M cylinder* contains about 3,000 liters of oxygen

Fixed systems on ambulances (commonly called onboard oxygen) include the M cylinder and larger cylinders (Figure 6-17):

- *G cylinder* contains about 5,300 liters of oxygen
- *H cylinder* contains about 6,900 liters of oxygen

The *United States Pharmacopoeia* has assigned a color code to distinguish compressed gases. Green and white cylinders have been assigned to all grades of oxygen. Unpainted stainless steel and aluminum cylinders are also used for oxygen. Regardless of the

Figure 6-16 Left to right: jumbo D cylinder, D cylinder, and E cylinder.

Figure 6-17 Larger cylinders are used for fixed systems on ambulances.

color, always check the label to be certain you are using medical grade oxygen.

Part of your duty as an EMT-B is to make certain that the oxygen cylinders you will use are full and ready before they are needed to provide care. The length of time you can use an oxygen cylinder depends on the pressure in the cylinder and the flow rate. You cannot tell if an oxygen cylinder is full, partially full, or empty by lifting or moving the cylinder. The method of calculating cylinder duration is shown in Table 6-2.

Oxygen cylinders should never be allowed to empty below the safe residual or the tank may be permanently damaged. The safe residual for an oxygen cylinder is when the pressure gauge reads 200 psi or above. Below this point there is not enough oxygen in the cylinder to allow for proper delivery to the patient. Before the cylinder reaches the 200 psi reading, you must switch to a fresh cylinder.

Safety is of prime importance when working with oxygen cylinders. You should:

- *Always* use pressure gauges, regulators, and tubing that are intended for use with oxygen.
- *Always* use nonferrous metal oxygen wrenches for changing gauges and regulators or for adjusting

flow rates. Other types of metal tools may produce a spark should they strike against metal objects.

- *Always* ensure that valve seat inserts and gaskets are in good condition. This prevents dangerous leaks. Disposable gaskets on oxygen cylinders should be replaced each time a cylinder change is made.
- *Always* use medical grade oxygen. Industrial oxygen contains impurities. The cylinder should be labeled "OXYGEN U.S.P." The oxygen must not be more than 5 years old.
- *Always* open the valve of an oxygen cylinder fully, then close it half a turn to prevent someone else from thinking the valve is closed and trying to force it open. The valve does not have to be turned fully to be open for delivery.
- *Always* store reserve oxygen cylinders in a cool, ventilated room, properly secured in place.

TABLE 6-2 Oxygen Cylinders: Duration of Flow

SIMPLE FORMULA:

Gauge pressure in psi (pounds per square inch) minus the safe residual pressure (always 200 psi) times the constant (see list below) divided by the flow rate in liters per minute = duration of flow in minutes.

CYLINDER CONSTANTS

D = 0.16	G = 2.41
E = 0.28	H = 3.14
M = 1.56	K = 3.14

EXAMPLE

Determine the life of an M cylinder that has a pressure of 2000 psi displayed on the pressure gauge and a flow rate of 10 liters per minute.

$$\frac{(2000 - 200) \times 1.56}{10} = \frac{2808}{10} = 280.8 \text{ minutes}$$

- *Always* have oxygen cylinders hydrostatically tested *every 5 years*. The date a cylinder was last tested is stamped on the cylinder. Some cylinders can be tested every 10 years. These will have a star after the date (e.g., 4M86MM★).
- *Never* drop a cylinder or let it fall against any object. When transporting a patient with an oxygen cylinder, make sure the oxygen cylinder is strapped to the stretcher or otherwise secured.
- *Never* leave an oxygen cylinder standing in an upright position without being secured.
- *Never* allow smoking around oxygen equipment in use. Clearly mark the area of use with signs that read "OXYGEN–NO SMOKING."
- *Never* use oxygen equipment around an open flame.
- *Never* use grease, oil, or fat-based soaps on devices that will be attached to an oxygen supply cylinder. Take care not to handle these devices when your hands are greasy. Use greaseless tools when making connections.
- *Never* use adhesive tape to protect an oxygen tank outlet or to mark or label any oxygen cylinders or oxygen delivery apparatus. The oxygen can react with the adhesive and debris and cause a fire.
- *Never* try to move an oxygen cylinder by dragging it or rolling it on its side or bottom.

Pressure Regulators

The pressure in an oxygen cylinder (approximately 2000 psi in a full tank—varying with surrounding temperature) is too high to be delivered to a patient. A **pressure regulator** must be connected to the cylinder to provide a safe working pressure of 30 to 70 psi.

On cylinders of the E size or smaller, the pressure regulator is secured to the cylinder valve assembly by a yoke assembly. The yoke is provided with pins that must mate with corresponding holes in the valve assembly. This is called a *pin-index safety system*. Since the pin position varies for different gases, this system prevents an oxygen delivery system from being connected to a cylinder containing another gas.

Cylinders larger than the E size have a valve assembly with a threaded outlet. The inside and outside diameters of the threaded outlets vary according to the gas in the cylinder. This prevents an oxygen regulator from being connected to a cylinder containing another gas. In other words, a nitrogen regulator cannot be connected to an oxygen cylinder, or vice versa.

Before connecting the pressure regulator to an oxygen supply cylinder, stand to the side of the main valve opening and open (crack) the cylinder valve slightly for just a second to clear dirt and dust out of the delivery port or threaded outlet.

Note: You must maintain the regulator inlet filter. It has to be free of damage and clean to prevent contamination of and damage to the regulator.

Flowmeters

A flowmeter allows control of the flow of oxygen in liters per minute. It is connected to the pressure regulator. Most services keep the flowmeter permanently attached to the pressure regulator.

Three major types of flowmeters are available. For use in the field, the pressure-compensated flowmeter is considered to be superior to the Bourdon gauge flowmeter; however, it is more delicate than the Bourdon gauge and must be operated in an upright position. For these reasons, many EMS systems use the pressure-compensated flowmeter for fixed oxygen systems only.

- *Bourdon Gauge Flowmeter* (Figure 6-18a). This unit is a pressure gauge calibrated to indicate flow in liters per minute. The meter is fairly inaccurate at low flow rates and has often been criticized as being unstable. However, it is rugged and will operate at any angle. It is a useful gauge for most portable units.

  The major fault with this type of flowmeter is its inability to compensate for back pressure. A partial obstruction (as from kinked tubing) will be

A

B

C

Figure 6-18 (A) Bourdon gauge flowmeter (pressure gauge), (B) a pressure-compensated flowmeter, and (C) a constant flow selector valve.

reflected in a reading that is higher than the actual flow. The gauge may read 6 liters per minute and only be delivering 1 liter per minute. This type of gauge contains a filter that can become clogged, causing the gauge to read higher than the actual flow. Inspect and change the filter as recommended by the manufacturer.

- *Pressure-Compensated Flowmeter* (Thorpe tube-type flowmeter, Figure 6-18b). This meter is gravity dependent and must be in an upright position to deliver an accurate reading. The unit has an upright, calibrated glass tube in which there is a ball float. The float rises and falls according to the amount of gas passing through the tube. This type of flowmeter indicates the actual flow at all times, even though there may be a partial obstruction to gas flow (as from a kinked delivery tube). If the tubing collapses, the ball will drop to show the lower delivery rate. This unit is not practical for many portable delivery systems. Recommended use is for larger (M, G, and H) oxygen cylinders.

- *Constant Flow Selector Valve* (Figure 6-18c). This type of flowmeter is gaining in popularity. It has no gauge. It allows for the adjustment of flow in liters per minute in stepped increments (2, 4, 6, 8 . . . to 15 liters or more per minute). It can be accurately used with the nasal cannula or nonrebreather mask and with any size oxygen cylinder. It is rugged and will operate at any angle.

    When using this type of flowmeter, make certain that it is properly adjusted for the desired flow and monitor it to make certain that it stays properly adjusted. All types of meters should be tested for accuracy as recommended by the manufacturer.

Humidifiers

A **humidifier** can be connected to the flowmeter to provide moisture to the dry oxygen coming from the supply cylinder (Figure 6-19). Oxygen without humidification can dry out the mucous membranes of the patient's airway and lungs. In most short-term use, the dryness of the oxygen is not a problem; however, the patient is usually more comfortable when given humidified oxygen. This is particularly true if the patient has COPD or is a child.

A humidifier is usually no more than a nonbreakable jar of water attached to the flowmeter. Oxygen passes (bubbles) through the water to become humidified. As with all oxygen delivery equipment, the humidifier must be kept clean. The water reservoir can become a breeding ground for algae, harmful bacteria, and dangerous fungal organisms. Always use fresh water in a clean reservoir for each shift. Sterile single-patient-use humidifiers are available and preferred.

Figure 6-19 A simple oxygen humidifier.

In many EMS systems humidifiers are no longer used because they are not indicated for short transports and because of the infection risk. The devices may be beneficial on long transports and on certain pediatric patients with signs of inadequate breathing.

Hazards of Oxygen Therapy

Although the benefits of oxygen are great, oxygen must be used carefully. The hazards of oxygen therapy may be grouped into two categories: non-medical and medical.

Non-medical hazards are extremely rare and can be avoided totally if oxygen and oxygen equipment are treated properly. They include:

- The oxygen used in emergency care is stored under pressure, usually 2,000 to 2,200 pounds per square inch (psi) or greater in a full cylinder. If the tank is punctured, or a valve breaks off, the supply tank can become a missile (damaged tanks have been able to penetrate concrete walls).

Imagine what would happen in the passenger compartment of an ambulance if such an accident occurred.

- Oxygen supports combustion, causing fire to burn more rapidly. It can saturate towels, sheets, and clothing, greatly increasing the risk of fire.
- Under pressure, oxygen and oil do not mix. When they come into contact, a severe reaction occurs which, for our purposes, can be termed an explosion. This is seldom a problem, but it can easily occur if you lubricate a delivery system or gauge with petroleum products, or allow contact with a petroleum-based adhesive (e.g., adhesive tape).

The medical hazards of oxygen rarely affect the patients treated by the EMT-B. There are certain patients who, when exposed to high concentrations of oxygen for a prolonged time, may develop negative side effects. These situations are rare in the field:

- *Oxygen toxicity or air sac collapse.* These problems are caused in some patients whose lungs react unfavorably to the presence of oxygen and also may result from too high a concentration of oxygen for too long a period of time. The body reacts to a sensed "overload" of oxygen by reduced lung activity and air sac collapse. Like the other conditions listed here, these are extremely rare in the field.
- *Infant eye damage.* This condition may occur when premature infants are given too much oxygen. These infants may develop scar tissue on the retina of the eye. Oxygen by itself does not cause this condition but it is the result of many factors. Oxygen should never be withheld from any infant with signs of inadequate breathing.
- *Respiratory depression or respiratory arrest.* Patients in the end stage of chronic obstructive pulmonary disease (COPD) may over time lose the normal ability to use the body's blood carbon dioxide levels as a stimulus to breathe. When this occurs, the COPD patient's body may use low blood oxygen as the factor that stimulates him to breathe. Because of this so-called hypoxic drive, EMTs have for years been trained to administer only low concentrations of oxygen to these patients for fear of increasing blood oxygen levels and wiping out their "drive to breathe." It is now widely believed that more harm is done by withholding high-concentration oxygen than could be done by administering it.

As an EMT-B you will probably never see oxygen toxicity or any other adverse conditions that can result from oxygen administration. The time required for such conditions to develop is too long to cause any problems during emergency care in the field. The bottom line is: NEVER WITHHOLD HIGH CONCENTRATION OXYGEN FROM A PATIENT WHO NEEDS IT!

Administering Oxygen

Scans 6-5 and 6-6 will take you step by step through the process of administering oxygen and discontinuing the administration of oxygen. Do not attempt to learn on your own how to use oxygen delivery systems. You should work with your instructor and follow your instructor's directions for the specific equipment you will be using.

Oxygen is administered to assist in the delivery of artificial ventilations to nonbreathing patients, as was discussed earlier in this chapter under "Techniques of Artificial Ventilation." Oxygen is also very commonly administered to breathing patients for a variety of conditions. A number of oxygen-delivery devices and systems are used. Each has benefits and drawbacks. A device that is good for one patient may not be ideal for another. The goal is to use the oxygen delivery device that is best for each patient.

For the patient who is breathing adequately and requires supplemental oxygen due to potential hypoxia, there are various oxygen delivery devices available. In general, however, the nonrebreather mask and the nasal cannula are the two devices most commonly used by the EMT-B to provide supplemental oxygen (Table 6-3).

Nonrebreather Mask

The **nonrebreather mask** (Figure 6-20) is the EMT-B's best way to deliver high concentrations of oxygen to a breathing patient. This device must be placed properly on the patient's face to provide the necessary seal to ensure high-concentration delivery. The reservoir bag must be inflated before the mask is placed on the patient's face.

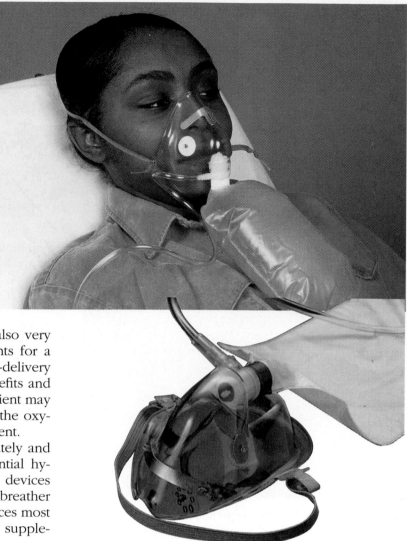

Figure 6–20 Nonrebreather mask.

To inflate the reservoir bag, use your finger to cover the exhaust port or the connection between the mask and the reservoir. The reservoir must always contain enough oxygen so that it does not

TABLE 6-3 Oxygen Delivery Devices			
Nonrebreather mask	12–15 liters per minute	80%–90%	Delivery system of choice for patients with signs of inadequate breathing and patients who are cyanotic, cool, clammy, short of breath, or suffering chest pain, suffering severe injuries, or displaying an altered mental status.
Nasal cannula	1–6 liters per minute	24%–44%	Appropriate for patients who cannot tolerate a mask.

PREPARING THE OXYGEN DELIVERY SYSTEM

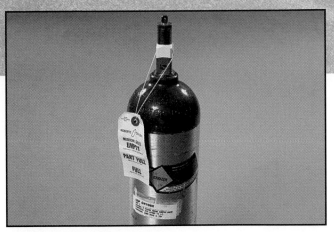

▲ **1** Select desired cylinder. Check label, "Oxygen U.S.P."

▲ **2** Place the cylinder in an upright position and stand to one side.

▲ **3** Remove the plastic wrapper or cap protecting the cylinder outlet.

▲ **4** Keep the plastic washer (some set ups).

(continued)

▲**5** "Crack" the main valve for one second.

▲**6** Select the correct pressure regulator and flowmeter. Pin yoke is shown on the left, threaded outlet on the right.

▲**7** Place the cylinder valve gasket on the regulator oxygen port.

▲**8** Make certain that the pressure regulator is closed.

▲ **9** Align pins (left), or thread by hand (right).

▲ **10** Tighten T-screw for pin yoke and . . .

▲ Tighten a threaded outlet with a nonferrous wrench.

▲ **11** Attach tubing and delivery device.

ADMINISTERING OXYGEN

▲ **1** Explain to the patient the need for oxygen.

▲ **2** Open the main valve and adjust the flowmeter.

▲ **3** Place oxygen delivery device on the patient.

▲ **4** Adjust the flowmeter.

▲ **5** Secure the cylinder during transfer.

Discontinuing Oxygen

▲ **1** Remove the delivery device.

▲ **2** Close the main valve.

▲ **3** Remove the delivery tubing.

▲ **4** Bleed the flowmeter.

deflate by more than one third when the patient takes his deepest inspiration. This can be maintained by the proper flow of oxygen (15 liters per minute). Air exhaled by the patient does not return to the reservoir (is not rebreathed). Instead, it escapes through a flutter valve in the face piece.

This mask will provide concentrations of oxygen ranging from 80% to 100%. The minimum flow rate is 8 liters per minute. Depending on the manufacturer and the fit of the mask, the maximum flow can range from 12 to 15 liters per minute. New design features allow for one emergency port in the mask so that the patient can still receive atmospheric air should the oxygen supply fail. This feature keeps the mask from being able to deliver 100% oxygen but is a necessary safety feature. The mask is excellent for use in patients with inadequate breathing or who are cyanotic (blue or grey), cool, clammy, short of breath, or suffering chest pain, or displaying an altered mental status.

Nonrebreather masks come in different sizes for adults, children, and infants.

Nasal Cannula

A **nasal cannula** (Figure 6-21) provides low concentrations of oxygen (between 24% and 44%). Oxygen is delivered to the patient by two prongs that rest in the patient's nostrils. The device is usually held to the patient's face by placing the tubing over the patient's ears and securing the slip-loop under the patient's chin.

Patients who have chest pain, signs of shock, hypoxia, or other more serious problems need a higher concentration than can be provided by a cannula. However, some patients will not tolerate a mask-type delivery device because they feel "suffocated" by the mask. For the patient who refuses to wear an oxygen face mask, the cannula is better than no oxygen at all. The cannula should be used only when a patient will not tolerate a nonrebreather mask.

When a cannula is used, the liters per minute delivered should be no more than 4 to 6. At higher flow rates the cannula begins to feel more uncomfortable, like a windstorm in the nose, and dries out the nasal mucous membranes.

SPECIAL CONSIDERATIONS

There are a number of special considerations in airway management:

- *Facial injuries.* Take extra care with the airway when there have been facial injuries. Because the blood supply to the face is so rich, blunt injuries to the face frequently result in severe swelling or bleeding that may block or partially block the airway. Frequent suctioning may be required. Insertion of an airway adjunct or endotracheal tube may be necessary.

- *Obstructions.* Many suction units are not adequate for removing solid objects like teeth and large particles of food or other foreign objects. These must be removed using manual techniques for clearing airway obstructions, such as abdominal thrusts, chest thrusts, or finger sweeps, which you learned in your basic life support course and which are reviewed in "Basic Cardiac Life Support Review" at the back of this book. You may need to log roll the patient into a supine position to clear the oropharynx manually.

- *Dental appliances.* Dentures should ordinarily be left in place during airway procedures. Partial dentures may become dislodged during an emergency. Leave a partial denture in place if possible, but be prepared to remove it if it endangers the airway.

Figure 6-21 Nasal cannula.

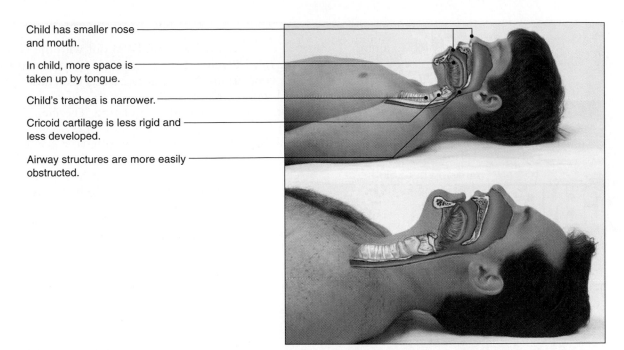

Child has smaller nose and mouth.

In child, more space is taken up by tongue.

Child's trachea is narrower.

Cricoid cartilage is less rigid and less developed.

Airway structures are more easily obstructed.

Figure 6–22 Comparison of child and adult respiratory passages.

Pediatric Notes

There are several special considerations that you must take into account when managing the airway of an infant or child (Figure 6-22):

Anatomic Considerations

- The mouth and nose are smaller and more easily obstructed than in adults.
- In infants and children the tongue takes up more space proportionately in the mouth than in adults.
- The trachea (windpipe) is softer and more flexible in infants and children.
- The trachea is narrower and is easily obstructed by swelling.
- The chest wall is softer, and infants and children tend to depend more on their diaphragm for breathing.

Management Considerations

- Open the airway gently. Infants can be placed in a neutral neck position and children only require slight extension of the neck. Do not overextend the neck, because it may collapse the trachea.
- When ventilating, avoid excessive pressure and volume. Use only enough to make the chest rise.
- Use properly sized face masks when providing ventilations to assure a good mask seal.
- Flow-restricted, oxygen-powered ventilation devices are contraindicated (should not be used) in infants and children, unless you have a child unit and have been properly trained in its use.
- Use pediatric-sized nonrebreather masks and nasal cannulas when administering supplemental oxygen.
- Infants and children are prone to gastric distention during ventilations or respiratory distress, which may impair adequate ventilations. (See gastric tube insertion in Chapter 35, "Advanced Airway Management.")
- An oral or nasal airway may be considered when other measures fail to keep the airway open.
- In suctioning infants and children, use a rigid tip but be careful not to touch the back of the airway.

STREET **SCENES**

"**D**ispatch to ambulance one-five," your radio blurts out. You respond, "Go ahead, Dispatch." Dispatch tells you that you have a priority-one response to a child, age unknown, choking, at 155 Baldwin Street, cross street of Third Avenue. Sonya, your partner, drives and while en route, you make sure that you have a plan. Sonya will take the lead. When she pulls up to the scene, a frantic person is waving his arms. He tells you the child is inside and not breathing.

STREET SCENE QUESTIONS

1. What is your first priority when starting to assess this patient?

2. What type of emergency care should you be prepared to give?

3. What equipment should you have taken into the house to make sure you are properly prepared for this call?

As you enter the house, you immediately see a child about 2 years old, cyanotic, being held by a frantic mother. You take the child and try to open the airway—always your first priority. You hear some air movement, but it appears that the child has an obstruction. The mother tells you he was eating breakfast when he started to cough. After your partner performs a few abdominal thrusts, the child expels a piece of food.

You already have the BVM out with the connective tube attached to the reservoir, so you start to assist ventilations. Your partner takes the child's pulse and reports that it is 60. You both realize that is too low, and you continue ventilating. The child has a gag reflex, so you don't attempt an oropharyngeal airway. You make sure that you have a good airway seal and you squeeze the bag slowly looking for chest rise. Your partner reminds you to pause between ventilations. You count quietly in order to keep track of the rate.

STREET SCENE QUESTIONS

4. What is the best way to determine if the ventilations are adequate?

5. What additional assessment should be done on this patient?

Your partner comments that there is good chest rise and the child is less cyanotic. "Good technique," she observes, "The pulse rate is now 110." The child starts to get restless and pushes the face mask away. You remove the mask but continue to give oxygen by blow-by. As you package the patient, you reassure the mother. En route to the hospital, you reassess the patient. His color is good, and his pulse rate is 120. He responds well to his mother and calms down quite a bit.

At the hospital, you discuss the call with your partner. She says that it was important to start ventilations quickly. When the heart doesn't get enough oxygen, it will start to slow, so giving 100% oxygen is important to bringing the heart rate back up. As you are leaving the emergency department to return to service, the doctor stops you and says the child is doing well.

CHAPTER REVIEW

SUMMARY

The airway is the passageway by which air enters the body during respiration, or breathing. A patient cannot survive without an open airway. Maintaining an open airway is the first priority of emergency care.

Respiratory failure is inadequate breathing, breathing that is insufficient to support life. A patient in respiratory failure or respiratory arrest (complete stoppage of breathing) must receive artificial ventilations.

Airway adjuncts—the oropharyngeal and nasopharyngeal airway—can help keep the airway open during artificial ventilation. It may also be necessary to suction the airway or to use manual techniques to remove fluids and solids from the airway before, during, or after artificial ventilation.

Oxygen can be delivered to the nonbreathing patient as a supplement to artificial ventilation. Oxygen can also be administered as therapy to the breathing patient whose breathing is inadequate or who is cyanotic (grey or blue), cool and clammy, short of breath, suffering chest pain, suffering severe injuries, or displaying an altered mental status.

KEY TERMS

airway the passageway by which air enters or leaves the body. The structures of the airway are the nose, mouth, pharynx, larynx, trachea, bronchi, and lungs.

artificial ventilation forcing air or oxygen into the lungs when a patient has stopped breathing or has inadequate breathing.

bag-valve mask (BVM) a hand-held device with a face mask and self-refilling bag that can be squeezed to provide artificial ventilations to a patient. Can deliver air from the atmosphere or oxygen from a supplemental oxygen supply system.

cyanosis (SIGH-uh-NO-sis) a blue or grey color resulting from lack of oxygen in the body.

flowmeter a valve that indicates the flow of oxygen in liters per minute.

flow-restricted, oxygen-powered ventilation device (FROPVD) a device that uses oxygen under pressure to deliver artificial ventilations. Its trigger is placed so that the rescuer can operate it while still using both hands to maintain a seal on the face mask. Has automatic flow restriction to prevent overdelivery of oxygen to the patient.

gag reflex vomiting or retching that results when something is placed in the back of the pharynx. This is tied to the swallow reflex.

head-tilt, chin-lift maneuver a means of correcting blockage of the airway by the tongue by tilting the head back and lifting the chin. Used when no trauma, or injury, is suspected.

humidifier a device connected to the flowmeter to add moisture to the dry oxygen coming from an oxygen cylinder.

hyperventilate (HI-per-VEN-ti-late) to provide ventilations at a higher rate than normal.

hypoxia (hi-POK-se-uh) an insufficiency of oxygen in the body's tissues.

jaw-thrust maneuver a means of correcting blockage of the airway by moving the jaw forward without tilting the head or neck. Used when trauma, or injury, is suspected to open the airway without causing further injury to the spinal cord in the neck.

nasal cannula (NAY-zul KAN-yuh-luh) a device that delivers low concentrations of oxygen through two prongs that rest in the patient's nostrils.

nasopharyngeal (NAY-zo-fah-RIN-jul) **airway** a flexible breathing tube inserted through the patient's nose into the pharynx to help maintain an open airway.

nonrebreather mask a face mask and reservoir bag device that delivers high concentrations of oxygen. The patient's exhaled air escapes through a valve and is not rebreathed.

oropharyngeal (OR-o-fah-RIN-jul) **airway** a curved device inserted through the patient's mouth into the pharynx to help maintain an open airway.

oxygen cylinder a cylinder filled with oxygen under pressure.

pocket face mask a device, usually with a one-way valve, to aid in artificial ventilation. A rescuer breathes through the valve when the mask is placed over the patient's face. Also acts as a barrier to prevent contact with a patient's breath or body fluids. Can be used with supplemental oxygen when fitted with an oxygen inlet.

positive pressure ventilation See *artificial ventilation*.

pressure regulator a device connected to an oxygen cylinder to reduce cylinder pressure to a safe pressure for delivery of oxygen to a patient.

respiration (RES-pir-AY-shun) breathing.

respiratory (RES-pir-uh-tor-e) **arrest** when breathing completely stops.

respiratory failure the reduction of breathing to the point where oxygen intake is not sufficient to support life.

stoma a permanent surgical opening in the neck through which the patient breathes.

suctioning (SUK-shun-ing) use of a vacuum device to remove blood, vomitus, and other secretions or foreign materials from the airway.

ventilation the breathing in of air or oxygen or providing breaths artificially.

REVIEW QUESTIONS

1. Name the main structures of the airway. (p. 106)
2. Explain why care for the airway is the first priority of emergency care. (p. 106)
3. Name the signs of adequate breathing and of inadequate breathing. (pp. 106–107)
4. Explain when the head-tilt, chin-lift maneuver should be used and when the jaw-thrust maneuver should be used to open the airway—and why. (pp. 110–111)
5. Name the techniques of artificial ventilation in the recommended order of preference. (p. 111)
6. Explain how airway adjuncts and suctioning help in airway management and artificial ventilation. (pp. 116–117, 122)
7. Name patient problems that would benefit from administration of oxygen and explain how to decide whether a nonrebreather mask or nasal cannula should be used to deliver oxygen to a patient. (pp. 126–127, 132, 138)

APPLICATIONS

- On arrival at the emergency scene, you find an adult female patient with gurgling sounds in the throat and inadequate breathing slowing to almost nothing. How do you proceed to protect the airway and support the patient's breathing?

WEB MEDIC

Visit Brady's *Emergency Care* website for direct weblinks. At **www.bradybooks.com/emergencycare**, you will find information related to the following Chapter 6 topics:

- Oxygen safety equipment

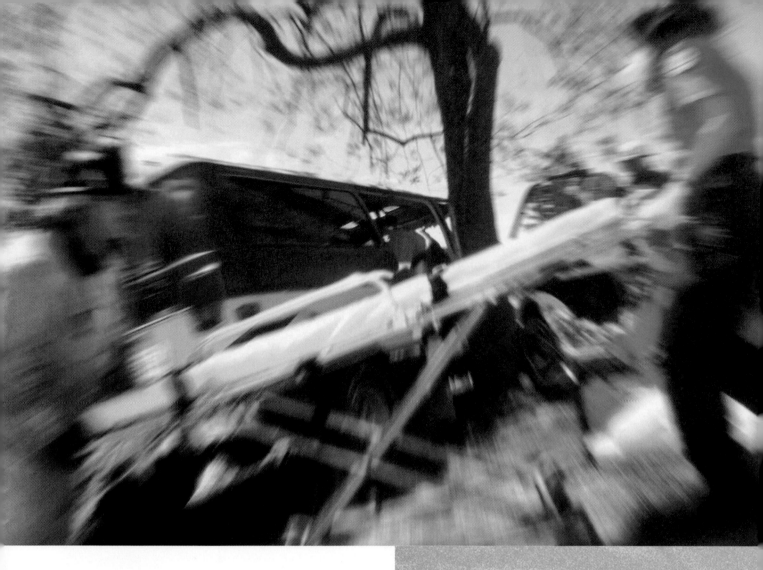

Chapter
Seven

SCENE SIZE-UP

Scene size-up sets a foundation for the remainder of the patient assessment process, as well as the rest of the call. What potential hazards does this scene present? Do I have the personal protective equipment I may need? What is the likely mechanism of injury or the nature of the patient's illness? Will we need additional assistance? These are questions you will ask as you size up the scene and prepare for the safe and effective care of your patient.

SCENE SIZE-UP

Scene size-up is the first part of the patient assessment process. It begins as you approach the scene, surveying it to determine if there are any threats to your own safety or to the safety of your patients or bystanders, to determine the nature of the call, and to decide if you will need additional help (Scan 7-1).

Study Guide for Scene Size-up

✔ Scene safety
   • Personal safety, including BSI precautions
   • Patient safety
   • Bystander safety
✔ Mechanism of injury or nature of illness
✔ Number of patients
✔ Additional resources

However, scene size-up is not confined to the first part of the assessment process. These considerations should continue throughout the call. Since emergencies are dynamic, always changing events, you may find, for example, that patients, family members, or bystanders who were not a problem initially may become increasingly hostile later in the call or that vehicles or structures that seemed stable suddenly shift and pose a danger.

After your initial scene size-up, you will become more directly involved in patient assessment and care. However, it is a good idea to remember the key size-up elements throughout the call to prevent dangerous surprises later.

You can obtain important information from just a brief survey of the scene. For example, you might see a downed electrical wire at the scene of a vehicle collision, a potentially deadly situation for you as the EMT-B, your pa-

tient, and bystanders. Further observations of the scene are likely to reveal more important information about the mechanism of injury. For example, damage to the steering wheel or windshield would be a strong indicator of potential chest, head, or neck injury caused by driver impact with those surfaces.

Just as important as your observations will be the actions you take to obtain needed assistance and prevent further injury. For example, if there were two patients at a collision, you would request that a second ambulance be dispatched to the scene—more if you discovered that there were additional passengers. If at that scene there also was a downed wire, which poses a danger of fire, you would notify the fire department as well as the power company and the police department. And you would take steps to keep bystanders clear of traffic, the collision, and the patients.

Scene Safety

The only predictable thing about emergencies is that they are often unpredictable and can pose many dangers if you are not careful.

Before you arrive on scene, the dispatcher may relay important information to you. A well-trained emergency medical dispatcher (EMD) uses a set of questions to determine information that may affect you directly. For example, if the caller tells the EMD

TOPIC OVERVIEW

In this chapter, you will learn about the following topics:

- How to identify hazards at a scene

- How to determine if a scene is safe to enter

- Mechanism of injury and how it relates to patient condition

- When additional assistance will be needed at a scene

DOT OBJECTIVES

✔ Knowledge and Attitude

1. Recognize hazards or potential hazards. (pp. 145–146) (Scan 7-1, p. 147)

2. Describe common hazards found at the scene of a trauma and a medical patient. (pp. 145–146) (Scan 7-2, p. 148)

3. Determine if the scene is safe to enter. (pp. 146, 149-150)

4. Discuss common mechanisms of injury or nature of illness. (pp. 151, 153–154, 156–157) (Scan 7-3, p. 152)

5. Discuss the reason for identifying the total number of patients at the scene. (pp. 157–158)

6. Explain the reason for identifying the need for additional help or assistance. (pp. 157–158)

7. Explain the rationale for crew members to evaluate scene safety prior to entering. (p. 145)

8. Serve as a model for others, explaining how patient situations affect your evaluation of mechanism of injury or illness. (pp. 151, 153–154, 156–157)

✔ Skills

1. Observe various scenarios and identify potential hazards.

---

of particular hazards, you could call for additional specialized assistance immediately. You will learn more about the questions an EMD asks in Chapter 32, "Ambulance Operations."

Often you will arrive at a scene where there are police, fire, and even other ambulances already present. In a situation like this, do not assume that the scene is safe because others have taken care of any hazards. Always perform your own size-up, no matter who arrives first. Scan for scene hazards, infection-control concerns, mechanisms of injury, and number of patients. The scene size-up begins even before the ambulance comes to a stop. Observe the scene while you approach and again before you exit the vehicle.

The following are scene size-up considerations you should keep in mind when you approach a crash or hazardous material emergency:

As you near the collision scene
- Look and listen for other emergency service units approaching from side streets.
- Look for signs of a collision-related power outage, such as darkened areas which suggest that wires are down at the collision scene.
- Observe traffic flow. If there is no opposing traffic, suspect a blockade at the collision scene.
- Look for smoke in the direction of the collision scene—a sign that fire has resulted from the collision.

When you are within sight of the scene
- Look for clues to escaped hazardous materials, such as placards, a damaged truck, escaping liquids, fumes, or vapor clouds. If you see anything suspicious, stop the ambulance immediately and consult your hazardous-materials reference book or hazardous-materials team, if one is available. (See more below under "Establishing the Danger Zone.")
- Look for collision victims on or near the road. A person may have been thrown from a vehicle as it careened out of control, or an injured person may have walked away from the wreckage and collapsed on or near the roadway.

- Look for smoke not seen at a distance.
- Look for broken utility poles and downed wires. At night, direct the beam of a spotlight or handlight on poles and wire spans as you approach the scene. Keep in mind that wires may be down several hundred feet from the crash vehicles.
- Be alert for persons walking along the side of the road toward the collision scene. Curious onlookers (excited children in particular) are often oblivious to vehicles approaching from behind.
- Watch for the signals of police officers and other emergency service personnel. They may have information about hazards or the location of injured persons.

How AND Why?

To identify a downed power line, look at the next pole down the line. Count the number of power lines at the top crossarm. If the number of lines at the top of the damaged pole is the same, then the scene is safe from that hazard. Go to your Electronic Extras CD for more tips on scene safety.

As you reach the scene
- Sniff for odors such as gasoline or diesel fuel or any unusual odor that may signal a hazardous material release.

Establishing the Danger Zone

A **danger zone** exists around the wreckage of every vehicle collision, within which special safety precautions must be taken. The size of the zone depends on the nature and severity of collision-produced hazards (Scan 7-2). An ambulance should never be parked within the danger zone. Follow these guidelines in establishing the danger zone:

- *When there are no apparent hazards,* consider the danger zone to extend at least 50 feet in all

SCENE SIZE-UP

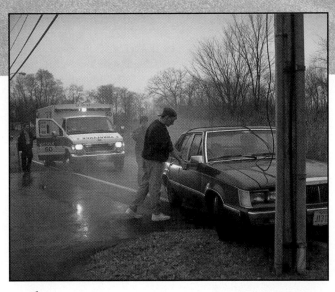

▲ **1** Determine scene safety. Look for possible threats to safety of crew, patient, and bystanders.

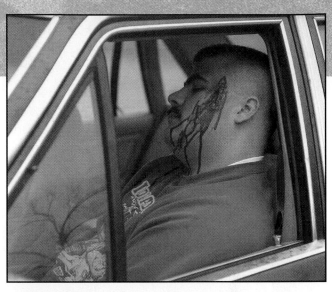

▲ **2** Determine the mechanism of injury or the nature of the patient's illness.

▲ **3** Determine the number of patients. Be alert for patients in addition to the first patient you see at the scene.

▲ **4** Request additional help if necessary.

ESTABLISHING THE DANGER ZONE

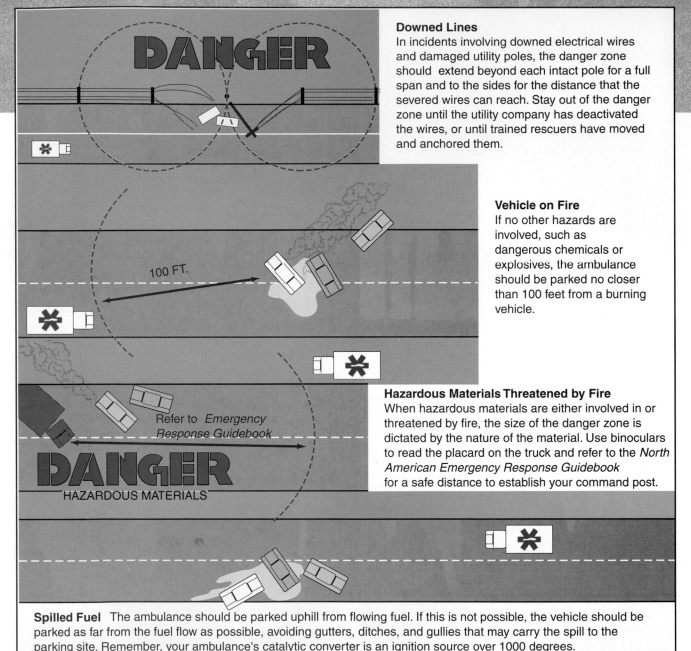

Downed Lines
In incidents involving downed electrical wires and damaged utility poles, the danger zone should extend beyond each intact pole for a full span and to the sides for the distance that the severed wires can reach. Stay out of the danger zone until the utility company has deactivated the wires, or until trained rescuers have moved and anchored them.

Vehicle on Fire
If no other hazards are involved, such as dangerous chemicals or explosives, the ambulance should be parked no closer than 100 feet from a burning vehicle.

Hazardous Materials Threatened by Fire
When hazardous materials are either involved in or threatened by fire, the size of the danger zone is dictated by the nature of the material. Use binoculars to read the placard on the truck and refer to the *North American Emergency Response Guidebook* for a safe distance to establish your command post.

Spilled Fuel   The ambulance should be parked uphill from flowing fuel. If this is not possible, the vehicle should be parked as far from the fuel flow as possible, avoiding gutters, ditches, and gullies that may carry the spill to the parking site. Remember, your ambulance's catalytic converter is an ignition source over 1000 degrees.

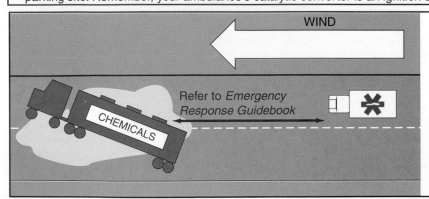

Hazardous Materials
Leaking containers of dangerous chemicals may produce a health as well as a fire hazard. When chemicals have been spilled, whether fumes are evident or not, the ambulance should be parked upwind. If the hazardous material is known, seek advice from experts through the dispatcher or CHEMTREC.

directions from the wreckage. The ambulance will be away from broken glass and other debris, and it will not impede emergency service personnel who must work in or around the wreckage. When using highway flares to protect the scene, make sure that the person igniting them has been trained in the proper technique.

- *When fuel has been spilled,* consider the danger zone to extend a minimum of 100 feet in all directions from the wreckage. In addition to parking outside the danger zone, park upwind, if possible. (Note the direction of the wind by observing flags, smoke, and so on.) Thus the ambulance will be out of the path of dense smoke if the fuel ignites. If fuel is flowing away from the wreckage, park uphill as well as upwind. If parking uphill is not possible, position the ambulance as far from the flowing fuel as possible. Avoid gutters, ditches, and gullies that can carry fuel to the ambulance. Do not use flares in areas where fuel has been spilled. Use orange traffic cones during daylight and reflective triangles at night.

- *When a collision vehicle is on fire,* consider the danger zone to extend at least 100 feet in all directions even if the fire appears small and limited to the engine compartment. If fire reaches the vehicle's fuel tank, an explosion could easily damage an ambulance parked closer than 100 feet.

- *When wires are down,* consider the danger zone as the area in which people or vehicles might be contacted by energized wires if the wires pivot around their points of attachment. Even though you may have to carry equipment and stretchers for a considerable distance, the ambulance should be parked at least one full span of wires from the poles to which broken wires are attached.

- *When a hazardous material is involved,* check the *North American Emergency Response Guidebook* (RSPA P 5800.7)—published by the U.S. Department of Transportation, Transport Canada, and the Secretariat of Communications and Transportation of Mexico—for suggestions as to where to park, or request advice from an agency such as CHEMTREC (Chemical Transportation Emergency Center, Washington, D.C., 24-hour hotline 800-424-9300 or 703-527-3887). In some cases you may be able to park 50 feet from the wreckage, as when no hazardous material has been spilled or released. In other cases, you may be warned to park 2,000 feet or more from the wreckage, as when there is the possibility that certain high explosives may detonate. In all cases, park upwind from the wreckage when you discover that a hazardous material is present at a collision site. Park uphill if a liquid is flowing, but on the same level if there are gases or fumes which may rise. Park behind some artificial or natural barrier if possible. (In Chapter 32, "Ambulance Operations," you will learn more about parking the ambulance. In Chapter 34, "Special Operations," you will learn more about hazardous materials.)

Crime Scenes and Acts of Violence

Another significant danger faced by the EMT-B is violence. Crime risks vary, but it is certain that EMT-Bs working in the field are exposed to more dangerous situations than even a few years ago. While a majority of calls go by uneventfully, the EMT-B must be conscious of dangers from many sources, including other human beings (Figure 7-1). EMT-Bs often envision violence as occurring at bar fights or on the street, but domestic violence (violence in the home) is also a cause for concern.

Protection from violence is as important as protection from the dangers at a vehicle collision. As an EMT-B, you should never enter a violent situation to provide care. Safety at a violent scene requires a careful size-up as you approach. Just as a downed wire signals danger at a collision site, there are many signals of danger from violence that you may observe as you approach the scene. These signals include:

- *Fighting or loud voices.* If you approach a scene and see or hear fighting, threatening words or actions, or the potential for fighting, there is a good

Figure 7-1 Crowds are a potential source of violence.

chance that the scene will be a danger to you.

- *Weapons visible or in use.* Any time you observe a weapon, you must use an extreme amount of caution. The weapon may actually be in the hands of an attacker (a grave danger), or simply in sight. Weapons include knives, guns, and martial arts weapons as well as any other item that may be used as a weapon.

- *Signs of alcohol or other drug use.* When alcohol or other drugs are in use, a certain unpredictability exists at any scene. It will not take long for you to observe unusual behavior from a person under the influence of one of these substances. This behavior may result in violence toward emergency personnel at the scene. Additionally, there are hazards associated with the drug culture, such as street violence and the presence of contaminated needles.

- *Unusual silence.* Emergencies are usually active events. A call that is "too quiet" should raise your suspicions. While there may be a good reason for the silence, extra care should be taken.

- *Knowledge of prior violence.* If you or a member of your crew has been to a particular location for calls involving violence in the past, extra caution must be used on subsequent calls to the same location.

Whether the call is residential or in the street, observe the scene for the signs of danger listed above and any others you may find (Figure 7-2). This brief danger assessment may be all that is required to prevent harm to you or your crew during the call.

If you observe signs of danger, there are actions that you must take to protect yourself. You learned about these actions in Chapter 2, "The Well-being of the EMT-Basic." To summarize: The specific actions you should take depend on many factors including your local protocols, the type of danger, and the help available to you. *In general, you should retreat to a position of safety, call for help, and return only after the scene has been secured by police.* Be sure to document the danger and your actions.

Body Substance Isolation (BSI) Precautions

As you perform your initial size-up of the scene, there are many important points to consider. One

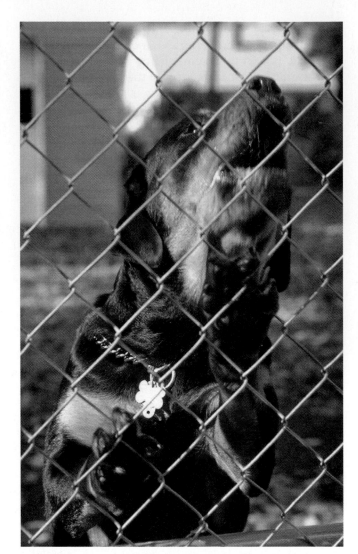

Figure 7-2   Whether the call is to a residence or to the street, a variety of hazards may be present.

very important aspect of personal protection—and one that you will need long after you have addressed any physical dangers—is body substance isolation.

You learned about BSI precautions in Chapter 2, "The Well-being of the EMT-Basic." To summarize: Body substances include blood, saliva, and any other body fluids or contents. All body substances can carry viruses and bacteria. Your patient's body substances can enter your body through cuts or other openings in your skin. They can also easily enter your body through your eyes, nose, and mouth. You are especially at risk of being infected by a patient's body substances when the patient is bleeding or coughing or sneezing or whenever you make direct contact with the patient, as in mouth-to-mouth ventilation. Infection is a two-way street, of course. Your patient can also be infected by you.

For example, at a vehicle collision that is likely to have caused severe injuries with bleeding, all personnel should wear protective gloves and eyewear. Since this potential hazard can be spotted before there is any contact with the patient, everyone should be wearing gloves before beginning patient care. If a patient requires suctioning or spits up blood, this would be another indication for protective eyewear and a mask. Whenever a patient is suspected of having tuberculosis, wear an N-95 or high efficiency particulate air (HEPA) respirator to filter out airborne particles the patient exhales or expels.

A key element of body substance isolation is always to have BSI equipment readily available, either on your person or as the first items you encounter when opening a response kit. Remember that taking proper body substance isolation (BSI) precautions early in the call will prevent needless exposure later on.

Nature of the Call

After you have assured scene safety and taken the appropriate BSI precautions, it is important to determine the nature of the call by identifying the mechanism of injury or the nature of the patient's illness.

Mechanism of Injury

The **mechanism of injury** is what causes an injury (for example, a rapid deceleration causes the knees to strike the dash of a car; a fall on ice causes a twisting force to the ankle) (Scan 7-3).

Certain injuries are considered "common" to particular situations. Injuries to bones and joints are usually associated with falls and vehicle collisions; burns are common to fires and explosions; penetrating soft-tissue injuries can be associated with gunshot wounds, and so on.

Even if you cannot determine the exact injury the patient has sustained, knowing the mechanism of injury may allow you to predict various injury patterns. For example, in many situations you will immobilize the patient's spine because the mechanism of injury, such as a forceful blow, is frequently associated with spinal injury. You do not need to know that the patient's spine is actually injured; you assume it is and treat accordingly. Knowing that the patient has fallen, should tell you to check for an injured arm or leg.

Identifying the mechanism of injury is very important when dealing with motor-vehicle collisions. For example, a collapsed or bent steering column suggests that the driver has suffered a chest-wall injury with possible rib or even lung or heart damage. A shattered, blood-spattered windshield points to the likelihood of a forehead or scalp laceration and possibly a severe blow to the head that may have caused a head or spinal injury.

The law of inertia—that a body in motion will remain in motion unless acted upon by an outside force (e.g., being stopped by striking something)—explains why there are actually three collisions involved in each motor-vehicle crash. The first collision is the vehicle striking an object. The second collision is when the body of the patient strikes the interior of the vehicle. The third collision occurs when the organs of the patient strike surfaces within the body (Figure 7-3).

A.

B.

C.

Figure 7-3 There are three collisions in a motor-vehicle crash: (A) a vehicle collision, when the vehicle strikes an object, (B) a body collision, when the person's body strikes the interior of the vehicle, and (C) an organ collision, when the person's organs strike interior surfaces of the body.

MECHANISMS OF INJURY AND AFFECTED AREAS OF THE BODY

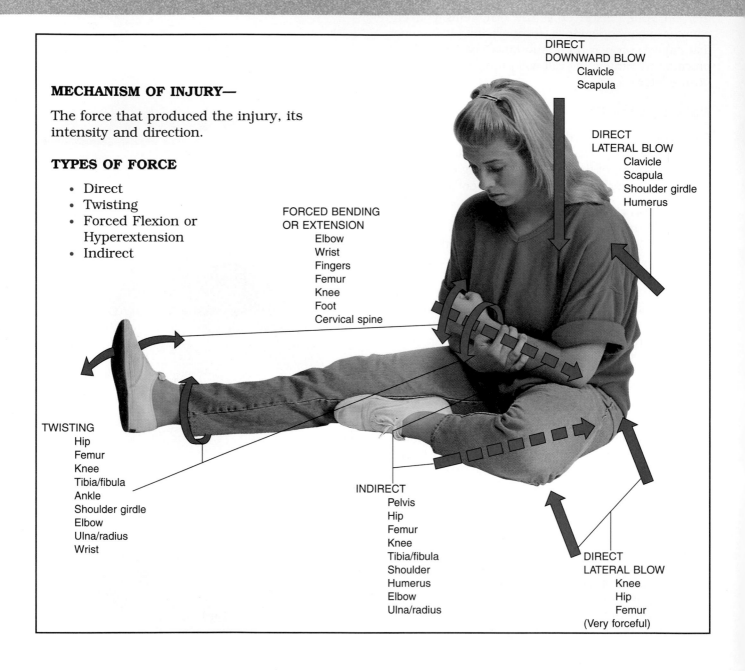

MECHANISM OF INJURY—

The force that produced the injury, its intensity and direction.

TYPES OF FORCE

- Direct
- Twisting
- Forced Flexion or Hyperextension
- Indirect

FORCED BENDING OR EXTENSION
  Elbow
  Wrist
  Fingers
  Femur
  Knee
  Foot
  Cervical spine

DIRECT DOWNWARD BLOW
  Clavicle
  Scapula

DIRECT LATERAL BLOW
  Clavicle
  Scapula
  Shoulder girdle
  Humerus

TWISTING
  Hip
  Femur
  Knee
  Tibia/fibula
  Ankle
  Shoulder girdle
  Elbow
  Ulna/radius
  Wrist

INDIRECT
  Pelvis
  Hip
  Femur
  Knee
  Tibia/fibula
  Shoulder
  Humerus
  Elbow
  Ulna/radius

DIRECT LATERAL BLOW
  Knee
  Hip
  Femur
  (Very forceful)

Figure 7-4 A head-on impact.

Identifying the type of motor-vehicle collision also provides important information on potential injury patterns:

- *Head-on collisions* have a great potential for injury to all parts of the body. Two types of injury patterns are likely: the up-and-over pattern and the down-and-under pattern. In the first pattern, the patient follows a pathway up and over the steering wheel, commonly striking his head on the windshield (especially when he was not wearing a seat belt), causing head and neck injuries. Additionally, the patient may strike his chest and abdomen on the steering wheel, causing chest injuries or breathing problems and internal organ injuries. In the second pattern, the patient's body follows a pathway down and under the steering wheel, typically striking his knees on the dash, causing knee, leg, and hip injuries (Figures 7-4 and 7-5).

- *Rear-end collisions* are common causes of neck and head injuries. The law of inertia states not only that a body in motion will remain in motion unless acted on by an outside force (as discussed earlier), but also that a body at rest will remain at rest unless acted on by an outside force (such as being pushed or jerked). This explains why neck injuries are common in a rear-end collision—the head remains still as the body is pushed violently forward by the seat back, extending the neck backward, if a headrest was not properly placed behind the head (Figures 7-6 and 7-7).

- *Side-impact collisions* (broadside, or "T-Bone") have other injury patterns. The head tends to remain still as the body is pushed laterally, causing injuries to the neck. The head, chest, abdomen,

A.

B.

Figure 7-5 In a head-on collision, an unrestrained person is likely to travel in (A) an up-and-over pathway causing head, neck, chest, and abdominal injuries or in (B) a down-and-under pathway causing hip, knee, and leg injuries.

Figure 7-6 Rear impact.

Figure 7-7 In a rear-end collision, the unrestrained person's head is jerked violently (A) backward and then (B) forward, causing neck, head, and chest injuries.

pelvis, and thighs may be struck directly, causing skeletal and internal injuries (Figures 7-8 and 7-9).

- *Rollover collisions* are potentially the most serious because of the potential for multiple impacts. Rollover collisions frequently cause ejection of anyone who is not wearing a seat belt. Expect any type of serious injury pattern (Figures 7-10 and 7-11).

- *Rotational impact collisions* involve cars that are struck, then spin. The initial impact often causes subsequent impacts (the spinning vehicle strikes another vehicle or a tree). As in a rollover collision, this can cause multiple injury patterns.

An important aspect of mechanism of injury determination is to find out where the patient was sitting in the vehicle and if he was wearing a seat belt. Note any deformities in the steering wheel, dash, pedals, or other structures within the vehicle.

You will often be able to observe important clues regarding mechanism of injury before you even exit the ambulance. At a head-on collision, for instance, you can anticipate up-and-over or down-and-under injury patterns for a driver who remains in his car and multiple injury patterns for a driver who is thrown from his car. For both patients, anticipate external injuries (from the collision of the body with auto interiors and pavement) and internal injuries (from collision of organs with the interior of the body as well as from external blunt-force or penetrating trauma). When a patient appears to have been the driver of a vehicle, look for damage to the windshield, steering wheel, dash, and pedals when you are able to do a close-up inspection. You should also observe for damage to other interior surfaces, which

Figure 7-8   Side impact.

Figure 7-9   A side-impact collision may cause head and neck injuries as well as injuries to the chest, abdomen, pelvis, and thighs.

Figure 7-10   Rollover collision.

Figure 7-11   In a rollover collision, the unrestrained person will suffer multiple impacts and possible multiple injuries.

might indicate there were additional passengers/patients.

Injuries involving motorcycles and all-terrain vehicles also have the potential to be serious. These vehicles offer the operator and passengers little protection in the event of collision. Determine whether the patient was wearing a helmet that offered some protection from head injury. Also attempt to determine whether the patient was ejected. In some cases, the operator will be thrown from the bike and strike and severely injure his hips, thighs, or legs.

Falls are another cause of injury where the extent and pattern of damage may be determined by the characteristics of the fall (Figure 7-12). Important factors to consider are the height from which the patient fell, the surface the patient fell onto, the part of the patient that hit the ground, and anything that interrupts the fall. Falls from heights of greater than 15 feet (or three times the height of the patient) are usually considered severe. Use this information to determine potential injury patterns.

Penetrating trauma, or injury caused by an object that passes through the skin or other body tissue, also has characteristics that may help in determining the extent of injury. These wounds are classified by the velocity, or speed, of the item that caused the injury. Low-velocity items are those that are propelled by hand, such as knives. Low-velocity injuries are usually limited to the area that was penetrated. Remember that there can be multiple wounds, or the blade may have been moved inside the patient, so there can be damage to multiple vital organs.

Medium-velocity wounds are usually caused by handguns and shotguns. Some forcefully propelled items such as an arrow launched from a compound bow or a ballistic knife will also cause greater velocities than the same items propelled by hand.

Bullets propelled by a high-powered or assault rifle are at a high-velocity. Medium- and high-velocity injuries can cause damage almost anywhere in the body. Bullets cause damage in two ways (Figure 7-13):

- *Damage directly from the projectile.* The bullet itself will damage anything in its path. The damage depends on the size of the bullet, its path, or whether it fragments (breaks up into smaller projectiles), the fragments taking different paths. The path of the bullet once it is inside the body is unpredictable since it may be deflected by bone or other tissue onto a totally different course.

- *Pressure-related damage, or cavitation.* This means that the velocity of the bullet as it enters the body creates a pressure wave that causes a cavity considerably greater than the size of the bullet. This cavity is temporary, but it may damage items in its path.

Blunt-force trauma is injury caused by a blow that strikes the body but does not penetrate the skin or other body tissues (for example, when one is struck by a baseball bat or thrown against a steering wheel). The energy from a blunt-force blow will travel through the body, often causing serious injury to, even rupture of, internal organs and vessels. The resulting compromise of body functions, hemorrhage, or spillage of organ contents into the body cavity may have more severe consequences for the patient than a penetrating injury. Yet signs of blunt-force trauma are often subtle and easy to overlook. The skin may appear reddened at the site of the blow, but in the prehospital setting the bluish coloration characteristic of a bruise may not have had time to appear. Your main clue that such an injury may exist will often be the presence of a mechanism of injury that *could* have caused this kind of injury.

Identifying the mechanism of injury will help you, as an EMT-B, to determine what injuries are possible and to treat these injuries accordingly, even if signs and symptoms are not present. *Never assume, based on the mechanism of injury, that there are no injuries.* Even very minor collisions may cause injuries.

Maintain a **high index of suspicion**—a keen awareness that there may be injuries—based on the mechanism of injury. Remember to maintain neck

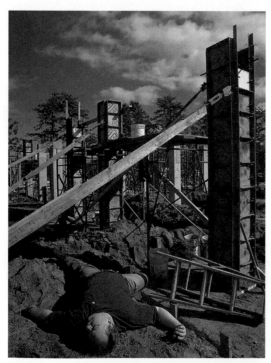

Figure 7-12 The characteristics of a fall may provide valuable clues to a patient's injuries.

A.   B.   C.

Figure 7-13 Bullets cause damage in two ways: from the bullet itself (A and C above) and from cavitation, which is the temporary cavity caused by the pressure wave (B).

and spine stabilization as patient assessment progresses.

Nature of the Illness

Identifying the **nature of the illness** for a medical patient serves the same purpose as identifying the mechanism of injury for a trauma patient: finding out what is or what may be wrong with the patient. To begin identifying the nature of a patient's illness during the scene size-up, you must scan the entire scene. Information may be obtained from many sources:

- *The patient,* when conscious and oriented, is a prime source of information about his or her condition. Your dealings with the patient will continue throughout the assessment process.
- *Family members or bystanders* can also provide important information, especially for the unconscious patient. Even when the patient is conscious and able to tell you about his condition, however, always consider the information from others who are present. Patients who are disoriented or confused may provide information that is either partially true or even untrue. Use information from all sources to piece the patient assessment "puzzle" together.

- *The scene.* While you are sizing up the scene for safety, make note of other factors that may be clues to the patient's condition. You may observe medications, which you will make a mental note to examine later. You may be struck by dangerous or unsanitary living conditions for this particular patient. This is important to note and mention to the emergency department personnel later.

Number of Patients and Adequacy of Resources

The final part of the scene size-up is determining if you have sufficient resources to handle the call. If, for example, you noted at a two-car collision that there were at least two patients—one driver still in her car and the other thrown to the pavement—you would immediately request an additional ambulance. As you approach the scene, you should actively look for clues that there may be additional patients—other passengers or pedestrians involved in the collision—and if so, you should immediately call for additional ambulances.

Sometimes you may discover a need for additional resources even in a situation that, at first,

STREET SCENES

It is the middle of the night, and you are hoping to get a few hours of sleep. You are just getting relaxed when the monitor activates. "Ambulances Bravo 5 and Delta 2 with heavy rescue to the Avenue A off-ramp for Interstate 55 to the report of a two-vehicle crash."

You are the first EMS responder to arrive, and as you approach the scene, you see both vehicles: one a passenger vehicle, the other a truck with a placard. As you do a scene size-up, you try to get the "big picture." You are concerend about where to stage your ambulance because of traffic, safety of crews, possible gasoline leaking, and not knowing what the placard on the truck identifies. You notify the dispatcher that you are on the scene and request that the Highway Pa-

trol be notified for traffic-control assistance. You find a location upwind about 100 yards from the scene. You place warning markers and flares to alert traffic and to mark the staging area for other responding units. You are putting on your turnout gear with helmet, goggles, and gloves including a reflective vest when heavy rescue arrives. You talk with the captain, and he tells you that his crew will stabilize the vehicles and handle the battery disconnects and gasoline leaks. You point out the placard that needs to be checked out.

STREET SCENE QUESTIONS

1. What other scene size-up issues are left to consider?

2. Is this scene now safe or do other precautions need to be taken?

3. What BSI precautions should be considered?

The crew from heavy rescue approaches the scene, stabilizes the vehicles, and then motions you forward. The Highway Patrol has closed off traffic

would not seem to require them. For example, you may not feel that a single-patient medical call could tax your resources, but consider the following scenarios where you may find yourself needing extra help:

• Your ambulance is called to respond to an elderly woman with chest pain. You are greeted at the door by her husband, who does not look well. He denies any complaints but is sweaty and holding his chest. Your first patient tells you that her husband has a heart condition.

• A single patient experiences back pain. This is usually not a reason for additional assistance, but this patient is immobilized on a backboard in a third-floor apartment (no elevator) and weighs 425 pounds.

• Your ambulance is called for "general weakness." Upon the arrival of you and your partner, two more persons in the same family develop the same flu-like symptoms. You appropriately suspect carbon monoxide poisoning, since they admit that they have been having furnace problems.

and the captain from heavy rescue tells you that there is no hazardous material concern. On-scene you determine that the drivers were the only occupants of the vehicles. You check one patient and, at the same time, your partner checks the other. Your patient has significant facial cuts and bruises and complains of leg pain. You realize that the gloves you are wearing will not provide the proper body substance isolation, so you put proper disposable gloves on immediately. After you try unsuccessfully to open the driver's side door next to your patient, you realize that he will require heavy rescue. The captain has already alerted his crew, and they are almost ready to use pry tools. You learn that your partner's patient is conscious and alert with no specific complaints.

STREET SCENE QUESTIONS

4. When the second ambulance arrives, where should it be located in relation to the collision scene?

5. What precautions should you take to protect the patients from any further harm while they are being extricated from the vehicle?

6. How should you plan to make sure that you can safely get the patient from the scene to the ambulance?

As heavy rescue finishes getting their tools ready, you set a protective cloth over your patient. You explain what is being done and stay next to him for reassurance. While this is going on, the second ambulance arrives, parks close to the second collision vehicle and takes over patient care. Your ambulance is relatively far away, so you ask your partner to bring it closer to prevent having to carry your patient a long distance. This makes packaging the patient for transport safer and easier. The remainder of the call is uneventful, with both patients transported safely to the hospital emergency department.

In each of these situations, what appeared to be a routine, one-patient call actually turned out to be more. An important part of scene size-up is to recognize these situations and call for help immediately. As the call progresses and you get more involved in patient care, it is less likely that you will remember to call for the additional help. It may also be too late when the help arrives if you do not call immediately.

Your response can range from simply calling for another ambulance to care for the ill husband in the first situation, or extra personnel to help move the 425-pound man in the second, to activating a multiple-casualty incident for the family with carbon monoxide poisoning. (You will learn about multiple-casualty incidents in Chapter 34, "Special Operations.") Try to anticipate the maximum numbers of patients and radio for help accordingly. Follow local protocols.

CHAPTER REVIEW

SUMMARY

Scene size-up is the first part of the patient assessment process. It is important during scene size-up to determine what, if any, threats there may be to your own safety and to the safety of others at the scene and to take appropriate body substance isolation (BSI) precautions. Next, it is important to determine the nature of the call by identifying the mechanism of injury or the nature of the patient's illness. Finally, you must take into account the number of patients and other factors at the scene to determine if you will need additional help.

KEY TERMS

blunt-force trauma injury caused by a blow that does not penetrate the skin or other body tissues.

danger zone the area around the wreckage of a vehicle collision or other incident within which special safety precautions should be taken.

index of suspicion awareness that there may be injuries.

mechanism of injury a force or forces that may have caused injury.

nature of the illness what is medically wrong with a patient.

penetrating trauma injury caused by an object that passes through the skin or other body tissues.

scene size-up steps taken by an ambulance crew when approaching the scene of an emergency call: checking scene safety, taking body substance isolation (BSI) precautions, noting the mechanism of injury or nature of the patient's illness, determining the number of patients, and deciding what, if any, additional resources to call for.

REVIEW QUESTIONS

1. For each of the following dangers, describe actions that must be taken to remain safe at a collision scene. (p. 146)
   - Leaking gasoline
   - Toxic or hazardous material spill
   - Vehicle on fire
   - Downed power lines

2. List several indicators of violence or potential violence at an emergency scene. (pp. 149–150)

3. Describe several situations where it is appropriate to wear disposable gloves. Describe situations where you would additionally wear protective eyewear and mask. Describe situations where you would wear an N95 or HEPA respirator. (pp. 150–151)

4. Describe common mechanism-of-injury-patterns. (pp. 153–154)

5. List sources of information about the nature of a patient's illness. (p. 157)

6. List several medical and trauma situations where you may require additional assistance. (pp. 157–158)

APPLICATIONS

- You are called to the scene of a shooting at a fast food restaurant. En route, you plan your scene size-up strategy. What actions do you anticipate taking on arrival?

WEB MEDIC

Visit Brady's *Emergency Care* website for direct weblinks. At **www.bradybooks.com/ emergencycare**, you will find information related to Chapter 7 topics:

- Precautions to take for specific diseases
- Accidental injury statistics
- Ice hazards

Chapter
Eight

THE INITIAL ASSESSMENT

Usually, you will take the time to do a thorough assessment (patient evaluation), transporting your patient to the hospital only after the complete assessment is finished. But if the patient has an immediately life-threatening problem—such as a blocked airway, a stoppage of breathing or heartbeat, or severe bleeding—you must provide emergency care immediately and consider the need to transport the patient without delay. One intervention for any patient with possible spine injury is to apply manual stabilization of the head and spine.

THE INITIAL ASSESSMENT

The assessment steps to discover and treat any life-threatening problems are called the **initial assessment.** It is always the first element in the total assessment of the patient. The initial assessment has six parts: forming a general impression, assessing mental status (and manually stabilizing the patient's head and neck, when appropriate—Scan 8-1), assessing airway, breathing, and circulation (and correcting any immediately life-threatening problems as soon as they were found), and determining patient priority (Scan 8-2).

Remember: If during the initial assessment, you discover any life-threatening condition, you must immediately perform the appropriate **interventions** (actions to correct those problems).

Figure 8-1 Forming a general impression includes your immediate assessment of the environment and the patient's chief complaint and appearance.

The environment can provide a great deal of information about the patient. It frequently gives clues—to the EMT-B who looks for them—about the patient's condition and history. One of the most important things it can sometimes tell you is what happened. Is there an overturned ladder, indicating that

Study Guide for the
Initial Assessment

✔ Form a general impression
✔ Assess mental status
✔ Assess airway
✔ Assess breathing
✔ Assess circulation
✔ Determine priority

Form a General Impression

Forming a general impression helps you to determine how serious the patient's condition is and to set priorities for care and transport. It is based on your immediate assessment of the environment and the patient's chief complaint and appearance (Figure 8-1).

TOPIC OVERVIEW

In this chapter, you will learn about the following topics:

- The general impression

- Manual stabilization of the spine

- Assessment of mental status using the AVPU scale

- The ABCs as part of the assessment process

- How to make a priority decision

the patient may have fallen? Has the patient been exposed to a cold outdoor environment for a long time? Or is there no apparent mechanism of injury, leading you to presume that the patient has a medical problem rather than trauma (an injury)? Although the EMT-B cannot rely completely on the patient's environment to rule out trauma, when combined with the chief complaint (e.g., the patient complaining of symptoms that sound more like a medical problem than an injury), environmental clues become extremely useful.

The **chief complaint** is the reason EMS was called, usually in the patient's own words. It may be as obvious as abdominal pain or as vague as "not feeling good." In any case, it is the patient's description of why you were called.

You form a general impression by looking, listening, and smelling. You look for the patient's age and sex—easy to determine once the patient is in sight. You look at the patient's position to see if it indicates an injury, pain, or difficulty in breathing. You listen for sounds like moaning, snoring, or gurgling respirations. You sniff the air to detect any smells like hazardous fumes, urine, feces, vomitus, or decay.

Something that is more difficult to describe than your direct observations but just as important is the feeling or sense you get when you arrive at the scene or encounter the patient. You may become anxious when you see a patient who exhibits no outward signs of illness or injury, yet "just doesn't look right" to you. Or you may feel reassured when you are dispatched to a "sick baby," but see that the infant is alert and smiling. After you gain some practice assessing and managing patients, you may develop a "sixth sense" that clues you in to the severity of a patient's condition. This is part of what is called "clinical judgment," or judgment based on experience in observing and treating patients. Some people find it easier than others to cultivate this ability, but even those who have excellent clinical judgment do not depend on it alone. A systematic approach to finding threats to life is the best way to make sure they are not missed.

HOW AND WHY?

Your AVPU determination is an important part of the initial assessment. Go to your Electronic Extras CD to find out why mental status—and changes in mental status—mean so much.

Assess Mental Status

Determining the **mental status,** or level of responsiveness, will usually be easy, since most patients are alert and responsive; that is, they are awake and will talk and answer questions sensibly. Some are not awake but will respond to verbal stimuli, such as talking or shouting. At a more depressed level, the patient will respond only to painful stimuli, such as pinching a toe or rubbing the sternum briskly. The lowest and most serious status is unresponsiveness, when the patient will not respond even to a painful stimulus. An easy way to keep these levels of responsiveness in mind is by remembering the letters **AVPU,** for *alert, verbal, painful,* and *unresponsive.*

17. Describe normal and abnormal findings when assessing skin condition. (pp. 169, 170)

18. Describe normal and abnormal findings when assessing skin capillary refill in the infant and child patient. (pp. 170, 172)

19. Explain the reason for prioritizing a patient for care and transport. (p. 169)

20. Explain the importance of forming a general impression of the patient. (pp. 163–164)

21. Explain the value of performing an initial assessment. (p. 163) (Scan 8-2, pp. 167–168)

✔ Skills

1. Demonstrate the techniques for assessing mental status.

2. Demonstrate the techniques for assessing the airway.

3. Demonstrate the techniques for assessing if the patient is breathing.

4. Demonstrate the techniques for assessing if the patient has a pulse.

5. Demonstrate the techniques for assessing the patient for external bleeding.

6. Demonstrate the techniques for assessing the patient's skin color, temperature, condition, and capillary refill (infants and children only).

7. Demonstrate the ability to prioritize patients.

For further information on these objectives . . .	See these chapters:
Objectives 4, 6, 7, 8, 9, 10, 11 (airway/breathing)	Chapter 6, "Airway Management"
Objectives 12, 13 (pulse)	Chapter 9, "Vital Signs and SAMPLE History"
Objective 14 (external bleeding)	Chapter 26, "Bleeding and Shock"
Objectives 15, 16, 17, 18 (skin/shock)	Chapter 9, "Vital Signs and SAMPLE History"; Chapter 26, "Bleeding and Shock"
Objectives 3, 4, 7, 8, 10, 11, 13, 18 (infants/children)	Chapter 13, "Pediatric, Adolescent, and Geriatric Assessment"; Chapter 31, "Infants and Children"

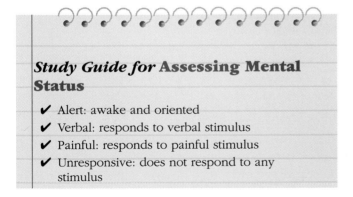

Study Guide for Assessing Mental Status

✔ Alert: awake and oriented
✔ Verbal: responds to verbal stimulus
✔ Painful: responds to painful stimulus
✔ Unresponsive: does not respond to any stimulus

A patient may be awake but confused. An awake patient's mental status can be described by specifying what he is "oriented to." Most EMS systems document orientation to person, place, and time. A patient who can speak clearly can almost always tell you his name (orientation to person). A few patients are oriented to person, but cannot tell you where they are (orientation to place). Some patients are oriented to person and place but cannot tell you the time, day, or date (orientation to time). A few EMS systems include additional questions to determine orientation.

A depressed mental status may indicate a life-threatening problem such as insufficient oxygen reaching the brain or shock (hypoperfusion). If the level of responsiveness is lower than Alert, provide high-concentration oxygen by nonrebreather mask and consider the patient a high transport priority.

MANUAL STABILIZATION OF THE HEAD AND NECK

You should apply manual stabilization on first contact with any patient who you suspect may have an injury to the spine based on mechanism of injury, or history, or signs and symptoms—that is, to virtually any trauma patient.

When you apply manual stabilization, your object is to hold the patient's head still in a neutral, in-line position. That is,

the head should be facing forward and not turned to either side nor tilted forward or backward. You must be careful not to pull or twist the patient's head but rather to hold it perfectly still and to remind the patient not to try to move it.

▲ **A.** When your patient is sitting up, position yourself just behind the patient and hold the head by spreading your fingers over the sides of the head and placing your thumbs on the back of the head.

▲ **B.** When your patient is supine, kneel behind the patient and spread your fingers and thumbs around the sides of the head to hold it steady.

If your patient is in another position, for example crumpled on his side, or is being moved by other EMS personnel, adapt the technique as practical to hold the head in a steady position in line with the spine.

PERFORMING AN INITIAL ASSESSMENT

FIRST take BSI precautions.

▲ **1** Form a **general impression** of patient and patient's environment.

▲ **2** Assess patient's **mental status.** (Intervention: high-concentration oxygen.)

▲ **3** Assess **airway.** (Intervention: Perform appropriate maneuver to open and maintain airway. If necessary, insert oro- or nasopharyngeal airway.)

▲ **4** Assess **breathing.** (Interventions: If respiratory arrest or inadequate breathing, ventilate with 100% oxygen. If breathing above 24/min, give high-concentration oxygen.)

(continued)

▲ **5** Evaluate **circulation** by taking the patient's pulse and evaluating skin temperature, color, and condition, and . . .

. . . in infants and young children also assess circulation by testing capillary refill. (Interventions: For indications of poor circulation, treat for shock. If no pulse, perform CPR.)

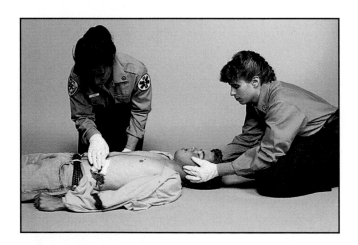

Assess for bleeding. (Intervention: Control severe bleeding.)

▲ **6** Make a decision about patient's **priority** for further assessment, interventions, or immediate transport

Assess the ABCs

You will always check the ABCs—airway, breathing, and circulation—as you look for life-threatening problems.

If the patient is alert and talking clearly or crying loudly, you know that the airway is open. If the airway is not open or is endangered (the patient is not alert, is supine, or is breathing noisily), take measures to open the airway, such as the jaw-thrust or head-tilt, chin-lift maneuver, suctioning, or insertion of an oro- or nasopharyngeal airway. If the airway is blocked, perform clearance procedures.

Once an open airway is assured, assess breathing. If the patient is in respiratory arrest, perform rescue breathing. If he is not alert and his breathing rate is slower than 8 breaths per minute, provide positive pressure ventilations with 100% oxygen. If the patient is alert and his rate is faster than 24 breaths per minute, give high-concentration oxygen by nonrebreather mask.

Once any breathing problems are corrected, assess circulation. Begin by taking the patient's pulse. If there is no pulse, perform CPR. Keep in mind, however, that cardiac arrest is not the only possible life-threatening circulation problem. Inadequate circulation and severe blood loss are also life threatening.

To evaluate circulation, assess pulse, skin, and bleeding. If the patient is light-skinned, you can check pulse and skin at the same time. As you take the radial pulse, note whether the skin at the wrist is warm, pink, and dry—indicating good circulation—or pale and clammy (cool and moist)—indicating poor circulation. If your patient is dark-skinned, you can check the color of the lips or nail beds, which should be pink.

Also check for and control severe bleeding. If even one large vessel or several smaller ones are bleeding, a patient can lose enough blood in just a minute or two to die. Quick control of severe external bleeding can be life saving. Transport decisions should take into account the potential for shock resulting from inadequate circulation and blood loss.

Determine Priority

Any life-threatening airway, breathing, or circulation problem must be treated as soon as it is discovered. Once life-threats are under control, you will decide on the patient's priority for immediate transport vs. further on-scene assessment and care.

Most patients do not need immediate transport, but a few do, and you must be able to determine which are which. If any life-threatening problem cannot be controlled or threatens to recur, or if the patient has a depressed level of responsiveness, you

Table 8-1 High-Priority Conditions
• Poor general impression
• Unresponsive
• Responsive, but not following commands
• Difficulty breathing
• Shock
• Complicated childbirth
• Chest pain with systolic blood pressure less than 100
• Uncontrolled bleeding
• Severe pain anywhere

may decide that he has an immediate priority for transport to the hospital, with assessment and care continuing en route.

There are a number of findings that indicate a high priority for transport (Table 8-1). These are conditions for which, usually, there is little or no treatment that can be given in the field that will make a difference in how well the patient does. You will learn more about these conditions in later chapters.

Initial assessment steps and interventions are summarized in Table 8-2.

PATIENT CHARACTERISTICS AND INITIAL ASSESSMENT

Patient assessment takes different forms, depending on the following characteristics of the patient:

- Whether the patient has a medical problem or trauma (injury)
- Whether the patient is responsive or unresponsive
- Whether the patient is an adult, a child, or an infant

How can the steps of initial assessment be applied to such varied types of patients? The following scenarios—plus some final paragraphs—will help to show you.

Mr. Schmidt—A Responsive Adult Medical Patient
One afternoon, you are dispatched to "an elderly man whose stomach hurts." Mrs. Schmidt greets you at the door and leads you to her husband.

Table 8-2   Initial Assessment Steps and Interventions

Medical Patient Responsive	Unresponsive	Trauma Patient Responsive	Unresponsive
1. **General Impression:** Form general impression of patient's condition.	1. **General Impression:** Form general impression of patient's condition.	1. **General Impression:** Form general impression of patient's condition. Evaluate mechanism of injury. **Intervention:** Manual stabilization of head.	1. **General Impression:** Form general impression of patient's condition. Evaluate mechanism of injury. **Intervention:** Manual stabilization of head.
2. **Mental status**—AVPU (alert)	2. **Mental status**—AVPU (responsive only to verbal or painful stimulus or not responsive). **Intervention:** High-concentration oxygen as soon as airway is open.	2. **Mental status**—AVPU (alert)	2. **Mental status**—AVPU (responsive only to verbal or painful stimulus or not responsive). **Intervention:** High-concentration oxygen as soon as airway is open.
3. **Airway** is open.	3. **Airway** is compromised. **Interventions:** Open airway with head-tilt, chin-lift; consider oro- or nasopharyngeal airway; suction as needed. For foreign body obstruction, use Heimlich maneuver or other blockage-clearing technique.	3. **Airway** is open.	3. **Airway** is compromised. **Interventions:** Open airway with jaw-thrust; consider oro- or nasopharyngeal airway; suction as needed. For foreign body obstruction, use Heimlich maneuver or other blockage-clearing technique.
4. **Breathing:** Look for rise and fall of chest, listen and feel for rate and depth of breathing. Look for work of breathing (use of accessory muscles, retractions). **Interventions:** If rate is greater than 24, high-concentration oxygen by nonrebreather mask. If breathing becomes inadequate, provide positive pressure ventilations and high-concentration oxygen. If respiratory arrest occurs, perform rescue breathing.	4. **Breathing:** Look for rise and fall of chest, listen and feel for rate and depth of breathing. Look for work of breathing (use of accessory muscles, retractions). **Interventions:** If breathing is adequate, high-concentration oxygen by nonrebreather mask. Position patient on side. If breathing is inadequate, provide positive pressure ventilations and high-concentration oxygen. If respiratory arrest, perform rescue breathing.	4. **Breathing:** Look for rise and fall of chest, listen and feel for rate and depth of breathing. Look for work of breathing (use of accessory muscles, retractions). **Interventions:** If rate is greater than 24, high-concentration oxygen by nonrebreather mask. If breathing becomes inadequate, provide positive pressure ventilations and high-concentration oxygen. If respiratory arrest occurs, perform rescue breathing.	4. **Breathing:** Look for rise and fall of chest, listen and feel for rate and depth of breathing. Look for work of breathing (use of accessory muscles, retractions). **Interventions:** If breathing is adequate, high-concentration oxygen by nonrebreather mask. Position patient on side once spinal stability is assured. If breathing is inadequate, provide positive pressure ventilations and high-concentration oxygen. If respiratory arrest, perform rescue breathing.
5. **Circulation:** Pulse, bleeding; skin color, temperature, condition (capillary refill in infants and children under 6). **Interventions:** Control bleeding. Treat for shock. If cardiac arrest, perform CPR.	5. **Circulation:** Pulse, bleeding; skin color, temperature, condition (capillary refill in infants and children under 6). **Interventions:** Control bleeding. Treat for shock. If cardiac arrest, perform CPR.	5. **Circulation:** Pulse, bleeding; skin color, temperature, condition (capillary refill in infants and children under 6). **Interventions:** Control bleeding. Treat for shock. If cardiac arrest, perform CPR.	5. **Circulation:** Pulse, bleeding; skin color, temperature, condition (capillary refill in infants and children under 6). **Interventions:** Control bleeding. Treat for shock. If cardiac arrest, perform CPR.
6. **Priority:** A responsive patient's priority depends on chief complaint, status of ABCs, and other factors.	6. **Priority:** An unresponsive patient is automatically a high priority for immediate transport.	6. **Priority:** A responsive patient's priority depends on chief complaint, status of ABCs, and other factors.	6. **Priority:** An unresponsive patient is automatically a high priority for immediate transport.

General Impression
As you approach the sofa where Mr. Schmidt is sitting, you see that he is an older male who appears ill and in pain. You see nothing around him to suggest that he has been injured. All of this suggests a medical problem rather than an injury.

Mental Status, Airway, Breathing
You introduce yourself by saying, "Hello, Mr. Schmidt. I'm Gerry Jones. I'm an emergency medical technician from the Fairfield Ambulance Service. How can I help you?" "My stomach hurts," he replies. As you ask questions, you note that Mr. Schmidt is alert and answering clearly. The fact that he is speaking in a normal way indicates that his airway is open. You can hear that his breathing is not labored. You look at his chest and note that his breathing is normal in rate and depth.

Circulation
"I'm going to take your pulse," you explain as you reach for his wrist. You quickly assess Mr. Schmidt's circulation by palpating his radial pulse, observing his skin, and looking for bleeding. His pulse is normal in rate and strength and regular in rhythm. The skin at his wrist is pink, warm, and dry. No blood is evident anywhere around him.

Priority
With the information you have gathered in just a few seconds, you conclude that Mr. Schmidt has no problems that are likely to kill him in the next few minutes. No immediate life-saving measures are required, and neither is immediate transport to the hospital. You are able, instead, to move ahead with the next steps of your assessment as Mr. Schmidt continues to rest on the sofa.

Mrs. Malone—An Unresponsive Adult Medical Patient
Your dispatcher sends you to an "unconscious" woman. Her daughter says she cannot wake her mother, Mrs. Malone, and leads you to the bedroom.

General Impression
An older woman in nightclothes is lying on her back in bed. Her eyes are closed and she is not moving.

Mental Status
You say loudly, "Mrs. Malone, can you hear me?" In response to your question, she moans a little, so you know she responds to a verbal stimulus. In your report, you will describe both the stimulus (verbal) and the response (moaning). If Mrs. Malone had not responded to verbal stimulus, you would have inflicted a painful stimulus to try to get a response from her.

Airway and Breathing
Because she is lying on her back, Mrs. Malone's airway is threatened by her tongue. Since patients with depressed responsiveness are always at risk for airway problems, you know that you need to be aggressive about opening and maintaining her airway. So even though you haven't heard any sounds indicating partial airway obstruction (like snoring or gurgling), your partner removes the pillow, tilts her head back, and lifts her chin.

Next, you evaluate her breathing by bringing your ear next to her mouth and looking for movement of her chest and abdomen as you listen and feel for the movement of air with your ear. You determine the depth of Mrs. Malone's respirations and if her breathing rate is slow or fast. If you found that her breathing was inadequate, you would ventilate Mrs. Malone with 100% oxygen.

Her respirations are in the normal range, but you will give Mrs. Malone high-concentration oxygen by nonrebreather mask anyway because her level of responsiveness is depressed. You put in a nasopharyngeal airway and move Mrs. Malone onto her side in order to help protect her airway.

Circulation
Mrs. Malone's pulse is strong, regular, and in the normal range for rate. You look for blood, but find none. The skin at her wrist is cool and dry. Because Mrs. Malone is dark-skinned, you assess for skin color at her lips and nail beds, which are pale. Although the pulse and bleeding check are normal, the pallor and coolness of her skin are slightly abnormal.

Priority
The priority of this patient is high because her mental status is depressed, her airway is at risk, and her skin indicates a circulation problem. You arrange immediate transport to the hospital, planning to continue assessment and care en route.

Clara Diller—A Responsive Child Trauma Patient
You respond to the scene where, the dispatcher says, a child has fallen.

General Impression
As you get out of the ambulance, you see a girl who is about 5 years old sitting on the sidewalk. She is crying and holding a bloody cloth on her knee. The mechanism of injury is apparent: a pair of skates indicates that she has probably taken a tumble while skating.

Mental Status, Airway, and Breathing
When you reach the patient, you kneel next to her and introduce yourself. You ask what happened. She confirms your suspicion that she fell down while trying her new skates. When you ask her, she tells you her name is Clara Diller and that her head and knee hurt. Since she is crying and answers your question easily, you determine that her mental status is alert and her airway is clear.

Because there is a mechanism of injury indicating possible trauma, you explain to her that she should not move her head and that your partner is going to hold her head to help her keep it still. Her breathing is not labored and her respiratory rate and depth are in the normal range.

Circulation
You feel Clara's radial pulse. It is slightly rapid but strong and regular. You look around her and see no blood except on the cloth and on her knee. Since it is hard to tell how much bleeding may be under the cloth, you tell Clara you want to look at her knee. You see a two-inch laceration which is oozing some blood, so you put the cloth back on and ask the neighbor who takes care of Clara to apply a little pressure to it. When you felt Clara's radial pulse, you noted that her skin is warm, pink, and dry. You also assess her capillary refill by pressing on the end of her fingernail. The color in the nail bed returns to pink in less than 2 seconds. So all indications are that Clara's circulation is good.

Priority
Based on the information you have gathered, you determine that Clara's priority for immediate transport is low. She has no significant mechanism of injury and no immediately life-threatening problems. There is no evidence that she was struck by a car or hit any object other than the sidewalk. However, since the sidewalk is a hard surface and she may have been moving fast, you maintain a high index of suspicion for possible cervical-spine injury. As soon as it is practical, you will apply a cervical collar and immobilize Clara on a backboard.

Pediatric Notes

Because Clara is a child, several other factors were different in her case than they were for your adult patients, Mr. Schmidt and Mrs. Malone.

Since children are often shy or distrustful of strangers or adults, you made a special effort to gain Clara's trust by kneeling to her level as you talked with her. Responsive children need to have some trust in the EMT-B. This may take a minute or two, but the general impression will guide you in determining how long to spend developing a rapport with the child.

Infants and children breathe faster than adults and their hearts beat faster, and you kept this in mind when you evaluated Clara's breathing and circulation.

A special part of checking circulation in infants and children is capillary refill. Nail beds are typically pink in healthy, normal people. When the end of the fingernail is gently pressed, it turns white. When the pressure is released, the nail bed turns pink again very quickly, usually in less than 2 seconds. In children, this is a good way to evaluate the circulation of blood. In an infant or small child with small nail beds, press the back of the hand or top of the foot instead. Count, "one-one thousand, two-one thousand" or say "capillary refill." If the nail or skin regains its pink color in the time it takes to say one of these, it is probably normal. Abnormal responses include prolonged and absent capillary refill (taking too long to turn pink again, or not turning pink again at all). These usually indicate problems with circulation.

Capillary refill is not a reliable sign for adults, so it is used only in infants and young children. In some adults, it is normal for capillary refill to take longer than 2 seconds, especially in the elderly. Even in infants and young children, it can be affected by factors such as the weather. Cold temperatures will prolong capillary refill. It should be used as one factor to consider in determining the priority of the young patient, but not the only one.

Like adult trauma patients, child and infant trauma patients need to have their heads immobilized in order to prevent injury to the spinal cord.

An infant has an airway that is different from an adult's, so opening an infant's or child's airway means moving the head to a neutral position, not tilting it back the way an adult's airway is opened. The mental status of unresponsive infants is typically checked by talking to the infant and flicking the feet.

You will learn about other considerations in approaching and assessing pediatric patients in Chapters 13 and 31.

Brian Sawyer—An Unresponsive Adult Trauma Patient
At the scene of a motor-vehicle collision, you go to the aid of a young man who has been thrown from his car.

General Impression
The young man appears to be approximately 25 years old. His eyes are closed and he is not moving. As you approach, you can hear snoring respirations. The mechanism of injury, the collision, and the fact that he is quite a distance from his vehicle are obvious. A police officer who has retrieved the patient's wallet tells you that his name is Brian Sawyer.

Mental Status and Airway
Your partner moves to stabilize Brian's head and the two of you position him on his back. Your partner attends to Brian's airway as you begin to check his mental status. He doesn't respond to your calling his

name, and he is unresponsive to a brisk rub of your knuckles on his sternum.

Your partner has started to treat the airway problem you both heard, snoring respirations that mean partial obstruction of the airway. Your partner manually stabilizes the head at the same time that he does a jaw thrust, which relieves the snoring sound. You listen closely and hear no other noises from his airway. If you heard gurgling or saw fluid in Brian's airway, you would suction him.

Breathing and Circulation

To evaluate breathing, you look, listen, and feel. Brian has respirations that appear normal in rate and depth. Because he is unresponsive but with adequate respirations, you decide to give Brian high-concentration oxygen by nonrebreather mask as soon as you finish checking circulation. You select an oropharyngeal airway and insert it, then apply a nonrebreather mask with 15 liters per minute of high-concentration oxygen.

You start to assess circulation by feeling the radial pulse. It is rapid and weak. There is no blood on or near the patient that you can see. His skin is pale, cool, and sweaty.

Priority

The priority you assign Brian is high. He is unresponsive to pain and his rapid, weak pulse and pale, clammy skin are signs of diminished circulation. You will spend as little time on the scene as possible. You plan to monitor his airway, place a cervical collar on him, immobilize him on a backboard, and get him to an appropriate facility quickly. Since you and your partner will both be needed to care for this patient en route to the hospital, you radio for additional personnel to drive the ambulance.

Comparing the Initial Assessments

The four patients—Mr. Schmidt, Mrs. Malone, Clara Diller, and Brian Sawyer—were very different in their characteristics. Notably:

- Mr. Schmidt and Mrs. Malone were medical patients, while Clara Diller and Brian Sawyer had suffered trauma.
- Both Mr. Schmidt and Clara Diller were responsive and neither was a priority for immediate transport.

However, both Mrs. Malone and Brian Sawyer were unresponsive and had airway and circulation problems that made them a high priority for immediate transport to the hospital.

- Clara Diller was a child, while the other three patients were adults.

There were a few obvious differences in the initial assessments of these patients. For example, both Clara Diller and Brian Sawyer, as trauma patients, required stabilization and immobilization of the head and spine, while Mr. Schmidt and Mrs. Malone, as medical patients with no evidence of any mechanism of injury, did not. For all four patients, the purpose of the initial assessment was to discover and correct any life-threatening problems. Mrs. Malone and Brian Sawyer had more problems to correct (mainly airway problems), so there were more actions to take, and the initial assessment of these two patients took a little longer than the initial assessment of Mr. Schmidt and Clara Diller.

In spite of these differences, the main thing to note is that the initial assessment steps were the same for all of them: forming a general impression; assessing mental status; checking airway, breathing, and circulation (and correcting any immediately life-threatening problems as soon as they were found); and making a priority decision regarding immediate transport vs. continued on-scene assessment and care.

These steps of the initial assessment must be followed systematically for every patient, no matter if that patient has a medical condition or trauma, is responsive or unresponsive, is an infant, child, or adult—and no matter how mild or serious that patient's condition may seem to be. If these steps are not followed consistently and systematically, it is very possible to overlook and neglect to manage a life-threatening problem.

To consider how the steps of the initial assessment are applied to responsive and unresponsive medical and trauma patients, review Table 8-2. For a summary of how the steps of the initial assessment are applied to adults, children, and infants, see Table 8-3.

TABLE 8-3   Initial Assessment of Adults, Children, and Infants

	Adults	Children 1-5 Years	Infants to 1 Year
Mental Status	AVPU: Is patient alert? responsive to verbal stimulus? responsive to painful stimulus? unresponsive? If alert, is patient oriented to person, place, and time?	As for adults	If not alert, shout as a verbal stimulus, flick feet as a painful stimulus. (Crying would be infant's response.)
Airway	Trauma: jaw-thrust Medical: head-tilt, chin-lift. Both: Consider oro- or nasopharyngeal airway, suctioning.	As for adults, but see Chapter 6 and BCLS Review for special child airway techniques. If performing head-tilt, chin-lift, do so without hyperextending (stretching) the neck.	As for children, but see Chapter 6 and BCLS Review for special infant airway techniques.
Breathing	If respiratory arrest, perform rescue breathing. If depressed mental status and inadequate breathing (slower than 8 per minute), give positive pressure ventilations with 100% oxygen. If alert and respirations are more than 24 per minute, give 100% oxygen by nonrebreather mask.	As for adults, but normal rates for children are faster than for adults (See Chapter 9 for normal child respiration rates.) Parent may have to hold oxygen mask to reduce child's fear of mask.	As for children, but normal rates for infants are faster than for children and adults. (See Chapter 9 for normal infant respiration rates.)
Circulation	Assess skin, radial pulse, bleeding. If cardiac arrest, perform CPR. See Chapter 26 on how to treat for bleeding and shock.	Assess skin, radial pulse, bleeding, capillary refill. See Chapter 9 for normal child pulse rates (faster than for adults). If cardiac arrest, perform CPR. See BCLS Review for special child techniques. See Chapter 26 on how to treat for bleeding and shock.	Assess skin, brachial pulse, bleeding, capillary refill. See Chapter 9 for normal pulse rates (faster than for infant children and adults). If cardiac arrest, perform CPR. See BCLS Review for infant techniques. See special Chapter 26 on how to treat for bleeding and shock.

STREET SCENES

Your patient is a 78-year-old unconscious male, who was shaving with his electric razor when he fell to the floor. You manually stabilize his head and neck and determine that the patient responds to painful stimuli. You then perform a jaw-thrust maneuver, assess breathing, and find that the patient has snoring respirations. So you immediately reposition the head, reassess breathing, and observe labored respirations and cyanosis around the lips. After giving the patient high-concentration oxygen by nonrebreather, circulation is assessed. In a minute or so, the patient regains consciousness and his skin color improves. He tells you his name is Danya and explains that he had suddenly felt lightheaded, sat down, and must have passed out. Later, during transport, you keep the patient on oxygen, take another set of vital signs, and gather a patient history.

STREET SCENE QUESTIONS

1. What should be done immediately upon contact with an unconscious patient who has fallen?

2. What are some considerations when opening the airway of an unconscious patient?

3. Using the AVPU scale, what is the level of responsiveness of a patient who responds to you calling out his name?

When you return to quarters, you hope to get a short break, but it's just minutes before you receive a call for a 7-year-old patient reported to be unresponsive at the Mount Hope Elementary School. Upon arrival, you are directed to the athletic field where the coach and school nurse tell you that Joey Sullivan had a seizure for the second time this month. His eyes are closed, he is not moving, and his skin color appears normal. Your partner gets

down next to the patient to assess mental status. "Hey, Joey," she calls out. He does not respond. She rubs his sternum briskly with her knuckles. There is still no response. "Unresponsive to pain," she says to you. When she tilts Joey's head back, there is a good deal of saliva visible in his mouth. Suctioning removes it without difficulty, and you administer oxygen to the patient by nonrebreather mask. You turn Joey onto his side and get a complete set of vital signs as your partner gets the stretcher. By the time you place Joey on the stretcher, he is becoming more responsive. Because of his improving mental status, you downgrade his priority and transport him with the school nurse.

STREET SCENE QUESTIONS

4. Would the cause of Joey's seizures change how you perform his initial assessment?

5. For Joey, what is the best position to prevent airway problems from occurring?

6. How did Joey's priority change during this call?

It isn't long after you leave Joey at the hospital before you are called again. "Ambulance 10, respond to the Traveler's Diner for a person having a heart attack." When you arrive, you find a woman in her mid-forties slumped in a chair. The manager tells you he thinks she is having a heart attack. You assess her airway and breathing and find she is not breathing. You are unable to ventilate her, so you perform an abdominal thrust. This results in expulsion of a piece of meat. Re-assessment reveals that she is making shallow, infrequent attempts to breathe, so you ventilate her with high-concentration oxygen. Her pulse is rapid and weak and her skin is cyanotic and sweaty. You transport her immediately as a high-priority patient.

STREET SCENE QUESTIONS

7. What is the value of following a systematic method of assessment for threats to life?

8. How much more assessment is appropriate before you transport this patient?

CHAPTER REVIEW

SUMMARY

It is essential to assess patients in a systematic way that allows for quickly finding and treating immediate threats to life. This search is called the *initial assessment*. By forming a general impression, determining mental status, evaluating airway, breathing, and circulation, and determining the patient's priority, you can find and correct the problems that could otherwise end a patient's life in just a few minutes. You will also be able to determine how urgent the patient's need to be transported is and how to conduct the rest of your assessment.

KEY TERMS

AVPU a memory aid for classifying a patient's level of responsiveness, or mental status. The letters stand for alert, verbal response, painful response, unresponsive.
chief complaint in emergency medicine, the reason EMS was called, usually in the patient's own words.
initial assessment the first element in assessment of a patient; steps taken for the purpose of discovering and dealing with any life-threatening problems. The six parts of initial assessment are: forming a general impression, assessing mental status, assessing airway, assessing breathing, assessing circulation, and determining the priority of the patient for treatment and transport to the hospital.
interventions actions taken to correct a patient's problems.
mental status level of responsiveness.

REVIEW QUESTIONS

1. List factors you will take into account in forming a general impression of a patient. (pp. 163–164)
2. Explain how to assess a patient's mental status with regard to the AVPU levels of responsiveness. (pp. 164–165)
3. Explain how to assess airway, breathing, and circulation during the initial assessment. Explain the interventions you will take for possible problems with airway, breathing, and circulation. (p. 169)
4. Explain what is meant by the term priority decision. (p. 169)
5. Explain what special interventions are required (pp. 163, 170)
   - if a patient has suffered trauma
   - if a patient is unresponsive

APPLICATIONS

You are called to respond to a "sick baby." When you arrive, you are led to a baby in its crib. Its eyes are closed. How do you conduct your initial assessment?

WEB MEDIC

Visit Brady's *Emergency Care* website for direct weblinks. At **www.bradybooks.com/ emergencycare**, you will find information related to the following Chapter 8 topics:

- Trauma
- Lung sounds

Chapter
Nine

VITAL SIGNS AND SAMPLE HISTORY

Following the initial assessment and control of any immediate life threats, you will begin a more thorough assessment of your patient. Two essential elements of this assessment will be measuring vital signs and taking a medical history. Vital signs are measurable things like pulse, blood pressure, and respirations. Because they reflect the patient's condition—and changes in the patient's condition—you will take them early and repeat them often. The medical history includes information about the present medical problem and facts about the patient that existed before the patient needed EMS. This information can affect the treatment you give. It is called a SAMPLE history because the letters in the word *SAMPLE* stand for elements of the history.

WHERE IN PATIENT ASSESSMENT?

When you begin to assess a patient, some things are obvious or easy to discover. For example, the most important part of patient assessment is the chief complaint, the reason the patient called for EMS. Usually, the patient will tell you what his complaint is. Other parts of assessment that are usually apparent as soon as you see and talk to the patient are age, sex, and general alertness. However, not all of your assessment is so obvious or so easy to find out. The vital signs and medical history, for example, are major components of assessment that will take a few minutes to complete.

Vital signs as well as the current and past medical history (SAMPLE history) are gathered on virtually every EMS patient. Occasionally, a patient will be so seriously injured or ill that you are not able to get this information because you are too busy treating immediate threats to life. This is the exception, however. The vast majority of patients you will encounter as an EMT-B should have an assessment that includes vital sign measurement and SAMPLE history gathering, among other things. If you do not get this information, you may remain unaware of important conditions, or trends in patient conditions, that require you to provide particular treatments in the field or prompt transport to a hospital.

Where do vital signs and SAMPLE history fit into the sequence of patient assessment? After the initial assessment to find and treat immediate life threats (which was the subject of Chapter 8), you will conduct a more thorough assessment known as the *focused history*

and physical exam (which will be the subject of Chapters 10 and 11). Vital signs and SAMPLE history will be obtained during the focused history and physical exam. This chapter serves as a preview of these two important procedures.

VITAL SIGNS

Vital signs are outward signs of what is going on inside the body. They include pulse; respiration; skin color, temperature and condition (plus capillary refill in infants and children); pupils; and blood pressure.

Evaluation of these indicators can give valuable information to the EMT-B. The first set of measurements you obtain are called the *baseline vital signs*. You can gain even more valuable information when you repeat the vital signs and compare them to the baseline measurements. This allows you and other members of the patient's health-care team to see trends in the patient's condition and to respond appropriately.

TOPIC OVERVIEW

In this chapter, you will learn about the following topics:

- How to obtain vital signs, including pulse, respirations, blood pressure, skin, and pupils.

- How to obtain an accurate SAMPLE history

- How to document vital signs on a prehospital report form

✔ **Knowledge and Attitude**

1. Identify the components of vital signs. (p. 179)

2. Describe the methods used to obtain a breathing rate. (p. 183)

3. Identify the attributes that should be obtained when assessing breathing. (pp. 183–184)

4. Differentiate between shallow, labored, and noisy breathing. (pp. 183–184)

5. Describe the methods to obtain a pulse rate. (pp. 180–181)

6. Identify the information obtained when assessing a patient's pulse. (pp. 180–182)

7. Differentiate between a strong, weak, regular, and irregular pulse. (pp. 181–182)

8. Describe the methods used to assess the skin color, temperature, and condition (capillary refill in infants and children). (pp. 184–185)

9. Identify the normal and abnormal skin colors. (p. 184)

10. Differentiate between pale, blue, red, and yellow skin color. (p. 184)

11. Identify the normal and abnormal skin temperature. (p. 185)

12. Differentiate between hot, cool, and cold skin temperature. (p. 185)

13. Identify normal and abnormal skin conditions. (p. 185)

14. Identify normal and abnormal capillary refill in infants and children. (p. 185)

15. Describe the methods used to assess the pupils. (pp. 185–186)

16. Identify normal and abnormal pupil size. (pp. 185–186)

17. Differentiate between dilated (big) and constricted (small) pupil size. (pp. 185–186)

18. Differentiate between reactive and non-reactive pupils and equal and unequal pupils. (pp. 185–186)

19. Describe the methods used to assess blood pressure. (pp. 185–186)

20. Define systolic pressure. (p. 185)

Another sign that gives important information about a patient's condition is mental status. It is not considered one of the vital signs; however, whenever you take the vital signs, you should also assess the patient's mental status. Chapter 8, "Initial Assessment," described how to evaluate mental status.

Note

It is essential that you record all vital signs as you obtain them, along with the time at which you took them.

Pulse

The pumping action of the heart is normally rhythmic, causing blood to move through the arteries in waves, not smoothly and continuously at the same pressure like water flowing through a pipe. A fingertip held over an artery where it lies close to the body's surface and crosses over a bone can easily feel the characteristic "beats" as the surging blood causes the artery to expand. What you feel is called the **pulse.** When taking a patient's pulse, you are concerned with two factors: rate and quality (Figure 9-1).

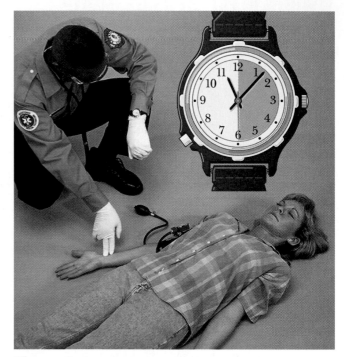

Figure 9-1   Assess pulse rate and quality. Count for 30 seconds and multiply by 2.

Pulse Rate

The **pulse rate** is the number of beats per minute. The number you get will allow you to decide if the patient's pulse rate is normal, rapid, or slow (Table 9-1).

Pulse rates vary among individuals. Factors such as age, physical condition, degree of exercise just completed, medications or other substances being taken, blood loss, stress, and body temperature all have an influence on the rate. The normal rate for an adult at rest is between 60 and 100 beats per minute. Any pulse rate above 100 beats per minute is rapid, while a rate below 60 beats per minute is slow. A rapid pulse is called **tachycardia.** A slow pulse is called **bradycardia.** An athlete may have a normal at-rest pulse rate between 40 and 50 beats per minute. This is a slow pulse rate, but it is certainly not an indication of poor health. The same pulse rate

21. Define diastolic pressure. (p. 186)

22. Explain the difference between auscultation and palpation for obtaining a blood pressure. (p. 188)

23. Identify the components of the SAMPLE history. (pp. 190–191)

24. Differentiate between a sign and a symptom. (p. 190)

25. State the importance of accurately reporting and recording the baseline vital signs. (p. 181)

26. Discuss the need to search for additional medical identification. (p. 191)

27. Explain the value of performing the baseline vital signs. (p. 181)

28. Recognize and respond to the feelings patients experience during assessment. (p. 191)

29. Defend the need for obtaining and recording an accurate set of vital signs. (p. 181)

30. Explain the rationale of recording additional sets of vital signs. (pp. 181, 189)

31. Explain the importance of obtaining a SAMPLE history. (pp. 190–191)

✔ Skills

1. Demonstrate the skills involved in assessment of breathing.

2. Demonstrate the skills associated with obtaining a pulse.

3. Demonstrate the skills associated with assessing the skin color, temperature, condition, and capillary refill in infants and children.

4. Demonstrate the skills associated with assessing the pupils.

5. Demonstrate the skills associated with obtaining blood pressure.

6. Demonstrate the skills that should be used to obtain information from the patient, family, or bystanders at the scene.

---

in a non-athletic or elderly person may indicate a serious condition. You should be concerned about the typical adult whose pulse rate stays above 100 or below 60 beats per minute.

In an emergency, it is not unusual for this rate temporarily to be between 100 and 140 beats per minute. If the pulse rate is higher than 150, or if you take a patient's pulse several times during care on scene and find him maintaining a pulse rate above 120 beats or below 50 beats per minute, consider this a sign that something may be seriously wrong with the patient and transport as soon as possible.

Table 9-1   Pulse

Normal Pulse Rates (beats per minute, at rest)

Adults	60 to 100
Infants and Children	
Adolescent 11–14 years	60 to 105
School age 6–10 years	70 to 110
Preschooler 3–5 years	80 to 120
Toddler 1–3 years	80 to 130
Infant 6–12 months	80 to 140
Infant 0–5 months	90 to 140
Newborn	120 to 160

Pulse	Significance/Possible Causes
Rapid, regular, and full	Exertion, fright, fever, high blood pressure, first stage of blood loss
Rapid, regular, and thready	Shock, later stages of blood loss
Slow	Head injury, drugs, some poisons, some heart problems, lack of oxygen in children
No pulse	Cardiac arrest (clinical death)

Infants and Children: A high pulse in an infant or child is not as great a concern as a low pulse. A low pulse may indicate imminent cardiac arrest.

Pulse Quality

Two factors determine **pulse quality:** rhythm and force. *Pulse rhythm* reflects regularity. A pulse is said to be regular when intervals between beats are constant. When the intervals are not constant, the pulse is irregular. You should report and document irregular pulse rhythms.

Pulse force refers to the pressure of the pulse wave as it expands the artery. Normally, the pulse should feel as if a strong wave has passed under your fingertips. This is a strong or full pulse. When the pulse feels weak and thin, the patient has a thready pulse.

Many disorders can be related to variations in pulse rate, rhythm, and force (Table 9-1).

Pulse rate and quality can be determined at a number of points throughout the body. During the determination of vital signs, you should initially find a **radial pulse** in patients 1 year of age and older. This is the wrist pulse, named for the radial artery found on the lateral (thumb) side of the forearm. In an infant 1 year old or less, find the **brachial pulse** in the upper arm (Figure 9-2) rather than the radial pulse. If you cannot measure the pulse on one arm, try the pulse of the other arm. When you cannot measure the radial or brachial pulse, use the **carotid pulse,** felt along the large carotid artery on either side of the neck, as you learned to do in cardiopulmonary resuscitation (CPR). Be careful when palpating a carotid pulse in a patient. Excessive pressure on the carotid artery can result in slowing of the heart, especially in older patients. If you have difficulty finding the carotid pulse on one side, try the other side, but *do not assess the carotid pulses on both sides at the same time.*

In order to measure a radial pulse, find the pulse site by placing your first three fingers on the thumb side of the patient's wrist just above the crease (to-ward the shoulder). Do not use your thumb. It has its own pulse that may cause you to measure your own pulse rate. Slide your fingertips toward the thumb side of the patient's wrist, keeping one finger over the crease. Apply moderate pressure to feel the pulse beats. A weak pulse may require applying greater pressure. But take care—if you press too hard you may press the artery shut. Remember: If you experience difficulty, try the patient's other arm.

Count the pulsations for 30 seconds and multiply by 2 to determine the beats per minute. While you are counting, judge the rhythm and force. Record the information: for example, "Pulse 72, regular and full," and the time of determination.

If the pulse rate, rhythm, or force is not normal, continue with your count and observations for a full 60 seconds.

Respiration

The act of breathing is called **respiration.** A single breath is considered to be the complete process of breathing in (called *inhalation* or *inspiration*) followed by breathing out (called *exhalation* or *expiration*). For the determination of vital signs, you are concerned with two factors: rate and quality (Figure 9-3).

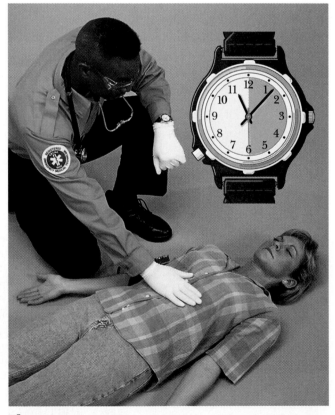

Figure 9-3 Assess respiration rate and quality. Count for 30 seconds and multiply by 2.

Figure 9-2 Palpating a brachial pulse in an infant.

Respiratory Rate

The **respiratory rate** is the number of breaths a patient takes in one minute (Table 9-2). The rate of respiration is classified as *normal, rapid,* or *slow.* The normal respiration rate for an adult at rest is between 12 and 20 breaths per minute. Keep in mind that age, sex, size, physical conditioning, and emotional state can influence breathing rates. Fear and other emotions experienced during an emergency can cause an increase in respiratory rate. However, if you have an adult patient maintaining a rate above 24 (rapid) or below 8 breaths per minute (slow), you must administer high-concentration oxygen and be prepared to assist ventilations.

Respiratory Quality

Respiratory quality, the quality of a patient's breathing, may fall into any of four categories: *normal, shallow, labored,* or *noisy.* Normal breathing means that the chest or abdomen moves an average depth with each breath and the patient is not using his accessory muscles (look for pronounced movement of the shoulder, neck, or abdominal muscles) to breathe. How can you tell if breathing is normal?

Normal depth of respiration is something you can learn to judge by watching healthy people breathe when at rest.

Shallow breathing occurs when there is only slight movement of the chest or abdomen. This is especially serious in the unconscious patient. It is important to look not only at the chest but also at the abdomen when assessing respiration. Many resting people breathe more with their diaphragm (the muscle between the chest and the abdomen) than with their chest muscles.

Labored breathing can be recognized by signs such as an increase in the work of breathing (the patient has to work hard to move air in and out), the use of accessory muscles, nasal flaring (widening of the nostrils on inhalation), and retractions (pulling in) above the collarbones or between the ribs, especially in infants and children. You may also hear stridor (a harsh, high pitched sound heard on inspiration), grunting on expiration (especially in infants), or gasping.

Noisy breathing is obstructed breathing (when something is blocking the flow of air). Sounds to be concerned about (Table 9-2) include snoring,

Table 9-2 Respirations

Normal Respiratory Rates (breaths per minute, at rest)

Adults	12 to 20
	Above 24: Serious
	Below 10: Serious
Infants and Children	
Adolescent 11–14 years	12 to 20
School age 6–10 years	15 to 30
Preschooler 3–5 years	20 to 30
Toddler 1–3 years	20 to 30
Infant 6–12 months	20 to 30
Infant 0–5 months	25 to 40
Newborn	30 to 50

Respiratory Sounds	**Possible Causes/Interventions**
Snoring	Airway blocked/ Open patient's airway; prompt transport
Wheezing	Medical problem such as asthma/ Assist patient in taking prescribed medications; prompt transport
Gurgling	Fluids in airway/ Suction airway; prompt transport
Crowing (harsh sound when inhaling)	Medical problem that cannot be treated on the scene/ Prompt transport

wheezing, gurgling, and crowing. A patient with snoring respirations needs to have his airway opened. Wheezing may respond to prescribed medication the patient has and that you may be able to assist the patient in taking. Gurgling sounds usually mean that you need to suction the patient's airway. Crowing (a noisy, harsh sound when breathing in) may not respond to any treatment you give. The patient who is crowing needs prompt transport—as do all patients with difficulty breathing.

Respiratory Rhythm

Respiratory rhythm is not important in most of the conscious patients you will see. This is because the regularity of an awake patient's breathing is affected by his speech, mood, and activity, among other things. If you observe irregular respirations in an unconscious patient, however, you should report and document it.

Start counting respirations as soon as you have determined the pulse rate. Many individuals change their breathing rate if they know someone is watching them breathe. For this reason, do not move your hand from the patient's wrist or tell the patient you are counting the respiratory rate. After you have counted pulse beats, immediately begin to watch the patient's chest and abdomen for breathing movements. Count the number of breaths taken by the patient during 30 seconds and multiply by 2 to obtain the breaths per minute. While counting, note the rate, quality, and rhythm of respiration. Record your results. For example, "Respirations are 16, normal, and regular." Record the time of the assessment.

Skin

The color, temperature, and condition of the skin can provide valuable information about your patient's circulation. There are many blood vessels in the skin. Since the skin is not as important to survival as some of the other organs (like the heart and brain), the blood vessels of the skin will receive less blood when a patient has lost a significant amount of blood or the ability to adequately circulate blood. Constriction (growing smaller) of the blood vessels causes the skin to become pale. For this reason, the skin can provide clues to blood loss as well as a variety of other conditions.

The best places to assess skin color in adults are the nail beds, the inside of the cheek, and the inside of the lower eyelids. Tiny blood vessels called capillaries are very close to the surface of the skin in all of these places, so changes in the blood are quickly reflected at these sites. They are also more accurate indicators than other sites in adults with dark complexions. In infants and children, the best places to look are the palms of the hands and the soles of the feet. In patients with dark skin you can check the lips and nail beds.

Ordinarily, the color you see (Table 9-3) in any of these places is pink. Abnormal colors include pale, cyanotic (blue-gray), flushed (red), and jaundiced (yellow). Pale skin frequently indicates poor circulation of blood. A common cause of this in the field is loss of blood. Cyanotic skin is usually a result of not enough oxygen getting to the red blood cells. Flushed skin may be caused by exposure to heat. Jaundice is a yellowish tint to the skin from liver ab-

Table 9-3 Skin Color

Skin Color	Significance/Possible Causes
Pink	Normal in light-skinned patients. Normal at inner eyelids, lips, and nail beds of dark-skinned patients.
Pale	Constricted blood vessels possibly resulting from blood loss, shock, hypotension, emotional distress
Cyanotic (blue-gray)	Lack of oxygen in blood cells and tissues resulting from inadequate breathing or heart function
Flushed (red)	Exposure to heat, emotional excitement
Jaundiced (yellow)	Abnormalities of the liver
Mottling (blotchiness)	Occasionally in patients with shock

Table 9-4   Skin Temperature and Condition

Skin Temperature/Condition	Significance/Possible Causes
Cool, clammy	Sign of shock, anxiety
Cold, moist	Body is losing heat
Cold, dry	Exposure to cold
Hot, dry	High fever, heat exposure
Hot, moist	High fever, heat exposure
"Goose pimples" accompanied by shivering, chattering teeth, blue lips, and pale skin	Chills, communicable disease, exposure to cold, pain, or fear

normalities. An uncommon skin coloration is mottling, a blotchy appearance that sometimes occurs in patients, especially children, in shock.

To determine skin temperature (Table 9-4), feel the patient's skin with the back of your hand. A good place to do this is the patient's forehead (Figure 9-4). Note if the skin feels normal (warm), hot, cool, or cold. If the patient's skin seems cold, then further assess by placing the back of your hand on the abdomen beneath the clothing. At the same time, notice condition—is the skin dry (normal), moist, or clammy (both cool and moist)? Look for "goose pimples," which are often associated with chills. Many patient problems are exhibited by changes in skin temperature and condition. Continue to be alert for major temperature differences on various parts of the body. For example, you may

note that the patient's trunk is warm but his left arm feels cold. Such a finding can reveal a problem with circulation.

 Pediatric Notes

In infants and children under 6 years of age, you should also evaluate capillary refill. Press on the nail bed—or the top of the hand or foot—and watch how long it takes for the normal pink color to return after you release it. Normally, this takes no more than 2 seconds. If it takes longer, the patient's blood is probably not circulating well. Abnormal responses include prolonged and absent capillary refill. This sign is not reliable in infants and children who have been exposed to cold temperatures.

Pupils

The **pupil** is the black center of the eye. One of the things that causes it to change size is the amount of light entering the eye. When the environment is dim, the pupil will **dilate** (get larger) to allow more light into the eye. When there is a lot of light, it will **constrict** (get smaller). So you will check a patient's pupils by shining a light into them (Figures 9-5 and 9-6). When you check pupils, you should look for three things: size, equality, and **reactivity** (reacting to light by changing size). Under ordinary conditions, pupils are neither large nor small, but midpoint. Dilated pupils are extremely large. In fact, it is usually difficult to tell what color eyes the patient has if his pupils are dilated. Both pupils are normally the same size, and when a light shines into them, they react by

Figure 9-4   Determining skin temperature.

Figure 9-5 Examining the pupils.

constricting. The rate at which they constrict should be equal. Nonreactive (fixed) pupils do not constrict in response to a bright light.

To check the patient's pupils, first note their size before you shine any light into them. Next, cover one

Constricted pupils

Dilated pupils

Unequal pupils

Figure 9-6 Constricted, dilated, and unequal pupils.

eye as you shine a penlight into the other eye. The pupil should constrict when the light is shining into it and enlarge when you remove the light. Repeat with the other eye. You should cover the eye you are not examining because light entering one eye usually affects the size of the pupils in both eyes. When you are examining a patient in direct sunlight or very bright conditions, initially cover both eyes. After a few seconds, uncover one eye and evaluate it. Cover it again and repeat with the other eye.

Pupils that are dilated, constricted to pinpoint size, unequal in size or reactivity, or nonreactive may indicate a variety of conditions (Table 9-5) including drug influence, head injury, or eye injury. Any deviations from normal should be reported and documented.

Blood Pressure

Each time the ventricle (lower chamber) of the left side of the heart contracts, it forces blood out into the circulation. The force of blood against the walls of the blood vessels is called **blood pressure.** The pressure created when the heart contracts and forces blood into the arteries is called the **systolic blood pressure.** When the left ventricle relaxes and refills, the pressure remaining in the arteries is called the **diastolic blood pressure.** These two pressures indicate the amount of pressure against the walls of the arteries and together are known as the blood pressure. When you take a patient's blood pressure, you report the systolic pressure first, the diastolic second, as "120 over 80," or "120/80."

One blood pressure reading may not be very meaningful. You will need to take several readings over a period of time while care is provided at the scene and during transport. Changes in blood pressure can be very significant. The patient's blood pressure may be normal in the early stages of some very serious problems, only to change rapidly in a matter of minutes.

Just as pulse and respiratory rates vary among individuals, so does blood pressure (Table 9-6). There is a generally accepted rule for estimating blood pressure of adults up to the age of 40. For an adult male at rest, add his age to 100 to estimate his normal systolic pressure. For an adult female at rest, add her age to 90 to estimate her normal systolic pres-

HOW AND WHY?

High blood pressure can be a very serious condition. Go to your Electronic Extras CD for tips on how to keep your own blood pressure in the safety zone.

Table 9-5 Pupils

Pupil Appearance	Significance/Possible Causes
Dilated (larger than normal)	Fright, blood loss, drugs, treatment with eye drops
Constricted (smaller than normal)	Drugs (narcotics), treatment with eye drops
Unequal	Stroke, head injury, eye injury, artificial eye
Lack of reactivity	Drugs, lack of oxygen to brain

sure. Thus, using this formula, a 36-year-old man would have an estimated normal systolic blood pressure of 136 millimeters of mercury (mmHg). (Millimeters of mercury refers to the units on the blood pressure gauge.) A 36-year-old woman would have an estimated normal systolic pressure of 126 mmHg. Normal diastolic pressures usually range from 60 to 90 mmHg.

Serious low blood pressure is generally considered to exist when the systolic pressure falls below 90 mmHg. High blood pressure exists once the systolic pressure rises above 150 or the diastolic above 90. Many individuals under stress (like that caused by

having the ambulance come to their home) will exhibit a temporary rise in blood pressure. More than one reading will be necessary to decide if a high or low reading is only temporary. If the blood pressure drops, your patient may be developing shock (however, other signs are usually more important early indicators of shock). Report any major changes in blood pressure to emergency department personnel without delay.

To measure blood pressure with a **sphygmomanometer** (the cuff and gauge), first place the stethoscope around your neck. Position yourself at the patient's side and place the blood pressure cuff

Table 9-6 Blood Pressure

Blood Pressure Normal Ranges

	Systolic	Diastolic
Adults	90 to 150	60 to 90
Infants and Children	Approx. 80 + 2 × age (yrs)	Approx. 2/3 systolic
Adolescent 11–14 years	Average 114 (88 to 140)	Average 76
School age 6–10 years	Average 105 (80 to 122)	Average 69
Preschooler 3–5 years	Average 99 (78 to 116)	Average 65

Blood Pressure	Significance/Possible Causes
High blood pressure	Medical condition, exertion, fright, emotional distress, or excitement
Low blood pressure	Athlete or other person with normally low blood pressure; blood loss; late sign of shock

Infants and children: Blood pressure is usually not taken on a child under 3 years. In cases of blood loss or shock, a child's blood pressure will remain within normal limits until near the end, then fall swiftly.

Figure 9-7 Positioning blood pressure cuff.

Figure 9-9 Measuring blood pressure by palpation.

on his arm (Figure 9-7). The cuff should cover two-thirds of the upper arm, elbow to shoulder. Be certain that there are no suspected or obvious injuries to this arm. There should be no clothing under the cuff. If you can expose the arm sufficiently by rolling the sleeve up, do so, but make sure that this roll of clothing does not become a constricting band.

Wrap the cuff around the patient's upper arm so that the lower edge of the cuff is about one inch above the crease of the elbow. The center of the bladder must be placed over the **brachial artery,** the major artery of the arm. The marker on the cuff (if provided) should indicate where you place the cuff in relation to the artery, but many cuffs do not have markers in the correct location. Tubes entering the bladder are not always in the right location, either. According to the American Heart Association, the only accurate method is to find the bladder center. Apply the cuff so it is secure but not overly tight. You are now ready to begin your determination of the patient's blood pressure.

There are two common techniques used to measure blood pressure with a sphygmomanometer: (1) **auscultation,** when a stethoscope is used to listen for characteristic sounds (Figure 9-8); and (2) **pal-**

pation, when the radial pulse or brachial pulse is palpated (felt) with the fingertips (Figure 9-9). Palpation is not as accurate as auscultation, since only an approximate systolic pressure can be determined. The technique is used when there is too much noise around a patient to allow the use of the stethoscope.

Determining Blood Pressure by Auscultation

1. *Prepare.* The patient should be seated or lying down. If the patient has not been injured, support his arm at the level of his heart.

2. *Position the cuff and the stethoscope.* Place the cuff snugly around the upper arm so that the bottom of the cuff is just above the elbow. With your fingertips, palpate the brachial artery at the crease of the elbow. Place the ear pieces of the stethoscope in your ears (the ear pieces should be pointing forward in the direction of your ear canals). Position the diaphragm of the stethoscope directly over the brachial pulse or over the medial anterior elbow (front of the elbow) if no brachial pulse can be found. Do not place the head of the stethoscope underneath the cuff, since this will give you false readings.

3. *Inflate the cuff.* With the bulb valve (thumb valve) closed, inflate the cuff. As you do so, you soon will be able to hear pulse sounds. Inflate the cuff, watching the gauge. At a certain point, you will no longer hear the brachial pulse. Continue to inflate the cuff until the gauge reads 30 mm higher than the point where the pulse sound disappeared.

4. *Obtain the systolic pressure.* Slowly release air from the cuff by opening the bulb valve, allowing the pressure to fall smoothly at the rate of approximately 5 to 10 mm per second. Listen for the start of clicking or tapping sounds. When you hear the first of these sounds, note the reading on the gauge. This is the systolic pressure.

Figure 9-8 Measuring blood pressure by auscultation.

5. *Obtain the diastolic pressure.* Continue to deflate the cuff, listening for the point at which these distinctive sounds fade. When the sounds turn to dull, muffled thuds, the reading on the gauge is the diastolic pressure. Sometimes you will not be able to hear a change in these sounds. When this happens, the point at which the sounds disappear is the diastolic pressure.

6. *Record measurements.* After obtaining the diastolic pressure, let the cuff deflate rapidly. Record the measurements and the time. For example, "BP is 140/90 at 1:10 p.m." Blood pressure is reported in even numbers. If a reading falls between two lines on the gauge, use the higher number.

If you are not certain of a reading, repeat the procedure. You should use the other arm or wait one minute before re-inflating the cuff. Otherwise, you will tend to obtain an erroneously high reading. If you are still not sure of the reading, try again or get some help. Never make up vital signs!

Note: Some patients who have high systolic blood pressures will have the pulse sounds disappear as you deflate the cuff, but reappear as you continue with deflation. When this happens, false readings may be obtained. If you determine a high diastolic reading, wait 1 to 2 minutes and take another reading. As you inflate the cuff, feel for the disappearance of the radial pulse to ensure that you are not measuring a false diastolic pressure. Listen as you deflate the cuff down into the normal range. The diastolic pressure is the reading at which the last clear sound takes place.

Determining Blood Pressure by Palpation

1. *Position the cuff, and find the radial pulse.* Apply the cuff as was described for auscultation. Then find the radial pulse on the arm to which the blood pressure cuff has been applied.

2. *Inflate the cuff.* Make certain that the adjustable valve is closed on the bulb and inflate the cuff to a point where you can no longer feel the radial pulse. Note this point on the gauge and continue to inflate the cuff 30 mm of mercury beyond this point.

3. *Obtain and record the systolic pressure.* Slowly deflate the cuff, noting the reading at which the radial pulse returns. This reading is the patient's systolic pressure. Record your findings as, for example, "blood pressure 140 by palpation" or "140/P" and the time of the determination. (You cannot determine a diastolic reading by palpation.)

Pediatric Notes

Obtain a blood pressure on every patient more than 3 years old. Blood pressures on infants and children younger than 3 are difficult to obtain with any accuracy and have little bearing on field management of the patient. You can get more useful information about the condition of an infant or very young child by observing for conditions such as a sick appearance, respiratory distress, or unconsciousness.

Vital signs are usually taken more than once. How frequently they should be repeated depends on the condition of the patient and your interventions. Stable patients need repeat vital signs at least every 15 minutes. Unstable patients need repeat vital signs at least every 5 minutes. Also repeat vital signs after every medical intervention. Record every reading of the vital signs (Figure 9-10).

Time	Pulse	Respirations	Blood Pressure
1410	88 str, reg	28	132/84

Pupils	Skin Color	Skin Temperature	Skin Condition
Equal ☑ Unequal ☐	Normal ☐	Cold ☐	Moist ☑
Reactive Ⓛ Ⓡ	Pale ☑	Cool ☑	Dry ☐
Nonreactive L R	Cyanotic ☐	Warm ☐	
Dilated ☐	Flushed ☐	Hot ☐	
Normal Size ☑	Jaundiced ☐		
Constricted ☐			

Figure 9-10 The prehospital care report (run sheet) provides spaces for recording vital signs.

OXYGEN SATURATION

Recent advances in technology now allow EMT-Bs and other health-care providers to measure the level of oxygen circulating through a patient's blood vessels. The device that does this is called a *pulse oximeter*. It sends different colors of light into the tissue at the end of a finger or on an earlobe and measures the amount of light that returns. The machine then determines the proportion of oxygen in the blood and displays the oxygen saturation percentage, also called the SpO_2.

When to Use a Pulse Oximeter

If your service has an oximeter, you should have a protocol describing when to use it. Generally, this will include all patients complaining of respiratory problems. When used properly, the device can help you to assess the effectiveness of artificial respirations, oxygen therapy, and bronchodilator (inhaler) therapy. Some services recommend its use in other patients as well. Follow your local protocols.

Interpreting Pulse Oximeter Readings

The oxygen saturation, or SpO_2, is typically 95% to 99% in a normal healthy person. A value less than 95% may sound good, but that is not really the case. A reading of 91% to 94% indicates mild hypoxia, 86% to 90% indicates moderate hypoxia, and 85% or less indicates severe hypoxia. The lower the oxygen saturation reading you get, the more aggressive your management should be. Any indication of hypoxia

is reason to administer high-concentration oxygen by nonrebreather mask. For very low readings, you will need to look at the patient's clinical condition and decide whether to ventilate the patient with high-concentration oxygen. You should try to get the SpO_2 up to at least 95%.

The reverse situation is not true; that is, a reading above 95% does NOT mean you should withhold oxygen from a patient with signs and symptoms that indicate the need for oxygen.

Cautions

• The oximeter is inaccurate with patients in shock and hypothermic patients (those whose body temperatures have been lowered by exposure to cold) because not enough blood is flowing through the capillaries for the device to get an accurate reading.

• The oximeter will produce falsely high readings in patients with carbon monoxide poisoning. This is because carbon monoxide binds with hemoglobin in the blood, producing the red color read by the device. Cigarettes produce carbon monoxide, so chronic smokers normally have 10% to 15% of their hemoglobin bound to carbon monoxide. This means their oxygen saturation readings will be higher than the actual oxygen saturation.

• Excessive movement of the patient can cause inaccurate readings. So can nail polish, if the device is attached to a finger. Carry acetone wipes to quickly remove the nail polish from a patient's fingernail before attaching the oximeter. Anemia, hypovolemia, and certain kinds of poisoning are other potential causes of falsely high oxygen saturation readings.

• The accuracy of the pulse oximeter should be checked regularly, following the manufacturer's recommendations. The batteries used to power the device must be in good condition and the probe needs to be kept clean to get accurate readings.

• Pulse oximetry is most useful in two situations: evaluating the effect of an intervention you have instituted (when you hope the SpO_2 goes up or remains high) and alerting you early to a deterioration in the patient's oxygen saturation (when the SpO_2 starts going down). Like any other device, the pulse oximeter can distract you from the patient. Keep it in its proper place. Remember, the oximeter is just another tool. Do not rely on it solely for indications of the patient's condition. *Treat the patient, not the device.*

Determining Oxygen Saturation

1. Connect the sensor lead to the monitor and clip it onto a fingertip (toe or distal foot in an infant).

2. Turn the device on. After a few seconds the device should display the SpO_2 and heart rate. Make sure the heart rate displayed on the monitor screen is the same as the patient's pulse rate (which you palpated already).

3. If you get a poor signal or "trouble" indicator, try repositioning the sensor on the finger or moving it to a different finger.

4. Once you get an accurate reading, check the oximeter reading every 5 minutes. A convenient time to do this is when you check the patient's vital signs.

SAMPLE HISTORY

An EMT-B can gain two kinds of information about the patient's present problem: signs and symptoms. A **sign** is objective—something you see, hear, feel, and smell when examining the patient. The vital signs are, of course, signs, as are sweaty skin, staggering, and vomiting, for example. A **symptom** is subjective—an indication you cannot observe but that the patient feels and tells you about. Such things as

chest pain, dizziness, and nausea are considered symptoms.

An important part of the information you should gain on all of your patients is information about the present problem (signs and symptoms) plus the past medical history—together called the **SAMPLE history** because the letters in SAMPLE stand for elements of the history: signs and symptoms, allergies, medications, pertinent past history, last oral intake, and events leading to the injury or illness. To obtain

Study Guide for SAMPLE History

✔ S — Signs and symptoms
✔ A — Allergies
✔ M — Medications
✔ P — Pertinent past history
✔ L — Last oral intake
✔ E — Events leading to the injury or illness

the SAMPLE history, ask your patient (or, if the patient is unconscious, ask the family and bystanders) these questions:

- *Signs and symptoms.* What's wrong?
- *Allergies.* Are you allergic to medications, foods, or environmentals? Is there a medical identification tag describing allergies?
- *Medications.* What medications are you currently taking (prescription, over-the-counter, or recreational)? Are you on birth control pills? Is there a medical identification tag with the names of medications on it?
- *Pertinent past history.* Have you been having any medical problems? Have you been feeling ill? Have you recently had any surgery or injuries? Have you been seeing a doctor? What is your doctor's name?
- *Last oral intake.* When did you last eat or drink? What did you eat or drink? (Food or liquids can cause symptoms or aggravate a medical condition. Also, if a patient will need to go to surgery, the hospital staff must know when he last had anything to eat or drink, since stomach contents can be vomited while a patient is under anesthesia, which is a very dangerous occurrence.)
- *Events leading to the injury or illness.* What sequence of events led up to today's problem (e.g., the patient passed out, then got into car crash versus got into car crash and then passed out)?

When conducting a patient interview:

- Position yourself close to the patient. Depending on the patient's situation, kneel or stand close to him. If possible, position yourself so that the sun or bright lights are not at your back. That way the patient will not have to squint to see you. When practical, position yourself so the patient can see your face and it is at a level close to that of the patient's face. This is especially important with children.

- Identify yourself, and reassure the patient. It is important that the patient know he is in competent hands. Maintain eye contact with the patient and state your name, that you are an Emergency Medical Technician, and the organization you represent.

- Speak in your normal voice. When you ask a question, wait for a reply. Work to gain the patient's confidence through calm conversation. Avoid inappropriate remarks like "Don't worry," and "Everything is all right." The patient knows everything is not all right.

- If you believe it to be appropriate, gently touch the patient's shoulder or rest your hand over his. A simple touch is comforting to most people.

- Learn your patient's name. Once you know it, use it in the rest of your conversations. Children will expect you to use their first names. For adults, use the appropriate Mr., Mrs., Miss, or Ms. unless they introduce themselves by their first name. If you are unsure how to address the patient, ask what he would like you to call him. You need the patient's name for completion of your forms and to give a personal touch that is often very reassuring to the patient. Having the patient's name could prove to be of great importance should he become unconscious and not be carrying any identification.

- Learn your patient's age. This will be needed for reports and communications with the medical facility.

The SAMPLE history gives valuable information about the patient's condition. This will sometimes influence the field management of the patient, but it will more often affect the patient's hospital treatment. If the patient should lose consciousness before arriving at the hospital, he will be unable to give his history. This is one of the most important reasons for the EMT to get this information.

Pediatric Notes

One of the most important factors that determines the normal range of vital signs is

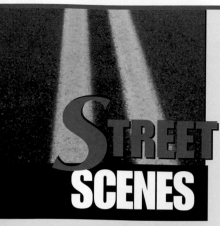

You are just sitting down to relax, when the dispatcher calls to notify you of a 73-year-old female patient with abdominal pain at 19 Oakwood Lane. Before getting to the scene, you and your partner agree that you will do the patient interview and he will assess vital signs. When you arrive, you find the patient sitting at her kitchen table. She tells you her name is Ms. Socorro Alvarez. She says she has stomach pain, "But I don't need to go to the hospital." As you look at this patient, you find that you aren't confident that this is a good decision. You start to think ABCs and realize that her airway is obviously open and clear, but her breathing seems a little rapid.

STREET SCENE QUESTIONS

1. What is your primary concern for this patient?
2. What vital signs should be taken even if a no transport decision is being considered?
3. If given the opportunity, what should the patient history include?

You tell Ms. Alvarez that if she called EMS, she must be concerned. So you ask her permission to assess her vital signs and ask her a few questions. She consents. "Tell me about the abdominal pain you had today," you ask. She explains that the pain was pretty bad and worse than the pain she had yesterday. "It is a sharp pain," she says. "It got much worse when I had a bowel movement." She tells you that her stools are black and tarry, she hasn't eaten today, and she was cleaning the kitchen when this last "attack" came on.

After your partner takes the patient's vital signs, he tells you that her pulse is 110 and thready, respirations are 28, and blood pressure is 100/70. You ask the patient if she knows her usual blood pressure, and she tells you 150/90.

STREET SCENE QUESTIONS

4. What other patient history information should be obtained?
5. Should you take another set of vital signs?
6. How might you get the patient to rethink her decision not to be transported?

You ask the patient if she is taking any medication. When she hands you two bottles from the kitchen table, you notice that her skin is pale and clammy. You write the names of the medications down and ask if she has any allergies. She tells you she is allergic to penicillin. You tell the patient that you think she really needs to go to the hospital and be seen by a doctor. You explain that her pulse is high and some of the other information she has provided needs to be evaluated. Your partner takes another set of vital signs and reports that the pulse is now 120 and thready. The other vital signs have not changed. Finally, after a bit more talk, the patient gives consent for transport.

You load the patient onto a stretcher and provide oxygen. The transport to the hospital is less than 10 minutes and uneventful. En route, your partner gives the radio report and you obtain another set of vital signs. After you transfer patient care to emergency department personnel and you are doing your paperwork, you notice a great deal of activity around her. After a while, a woman approaches and tells you that she is Mrs. Alvarez's daughter. "The doctor told me that mama is bleeding internally," she says, "and that she needed immediate medical attention. Thank you."

age. Infants and children have faster pulse and respiratory rates and lower blood pressures than adults. Compare the ranges for infants and children with those for adults in the tables in this chapter.

Another way in which infants and children under 6 differ from adults is that capillary refill can be a useful guide to the status of their circulation, which is not true of adults.

Table 9-7 Pulse, Normal Ranges

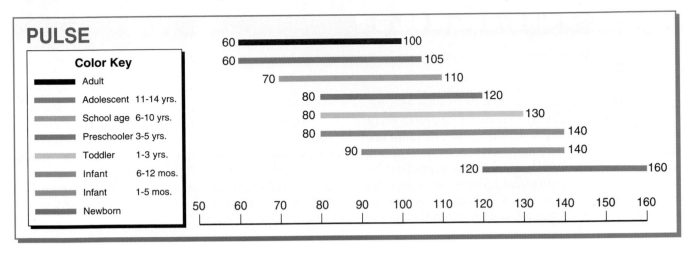

Table 9-8 Respiration, Normal Ranges

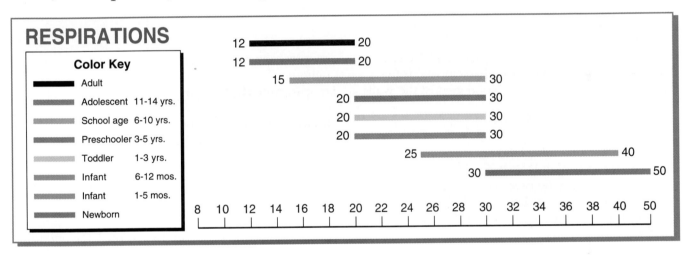

Table 9-9 Blood Pressure, Normal Ranges

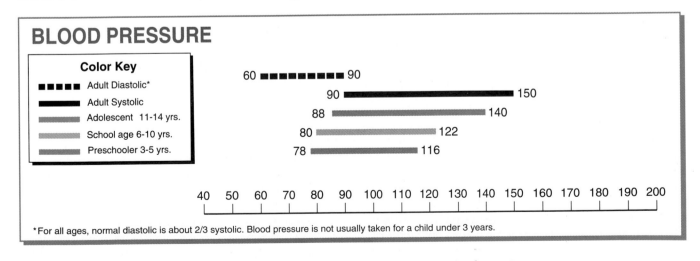

*For all ages, normal diastolic is about 2/3 systolic. Blood pressure is not usually taken for a child under 3 years.

Concept for Tables 9-7, 9-8, and 9-9 by Christine M. Yuhas, practicing EMT, State of New Jersey

CHAPTER REVIEW

Summary

As an EMT-B, you can gain a great deal of information about a patient's condition by taking a complete set of baseline vital signs. These include pulse, respirations, skin, pupils, and blood pressure. (See Tables 9-7, 9-8, and 9-9 for a summary of normal ranges for pulse, respirations, and blood pressure.) These must then be followed by repeat vital signs in order to recognize trends in the patient's condition. How often you repeat the vital signs will depend on the patient's condition.

Another source of information is the SAMPLE history. By determining the signs/symptoms, allergies, medications, pertinent past history, last oral intake, and events leading to the injury or illness, you will gain information that may affect field treatment and will be important to the definitive treatment of the patient at the hospital.

Key Terms

auscultation (os-kul-TAY-shun) listening. A stethoscope is used to auscultate for characteristic sounds.

blood pressure the force of blood against the walls of the blood vessels.

brachial (BRAY-key-al) **artery** the major artery of the arm.

brachial pulse the pulse felt in the upper arm.

bradycardia (BRAY-duh-KAR-de-uh) a slow pulse; any pulse rate below 60 beats per minute.

carotid (kah-ROT-id) **pulse** the pulse felt along the large carotid artery on either side of the neck.

constrict (kon-STRIKT) get smaller.

diastolic (di-as-TOL-ik) **blood pressure** the pressure remaining in the arteries when the left ventricle of the heart is relaxed and refilling.

dilate (DI-late) get larger.

palpation touching or feeling. A pulse or blood pressure may be palpated with the fingertips.

pulse the rhythmic beats felt as the heart pumps blood through the arteries.

pulse quality the rhythm (regular or irregular) and force (strong or weak) of the pulse.

pulse rate the number of pulse beats per minute.

pupil the black center of the eye.

radial (RAY-de-ul) **pulse** the pulse felt at the wrist.

reactivity (re-ak-TIV-uh-te) in the pupils of the eyes, reacting to light by changing size.

respiration (res-puh-RAY-shun) the act of breathing in and breathing out.

respiratory (RES-puh-ruh-tor-e) **quality** the normal or abnormal (shallow, labored, or noisy) character of breathing.

respiratory rate the number of breaths taken in one minute.

respiratory rhythm the regular or irregular spacing of breaths.

SAMPLE history the present and past medical history of a patient, so called because the elements of the history begin with the letters of the word *sample:* signs/symptoms, allergies, medications, pertinent past history, last oral intake, events leading to the injury or illness.

sign an indication of a patient's condition that is objective, or can be observed by another person; an indication that can be seen, heard, smelled, or felt by the EMT-B or others.

sphygmomanometer (SFIG-mo-mah-NOM-uh-ter) the cuff and gauge used to measure blood pressure.

symptom an indication of a patient's condition that cannot be observed by another person but rather is subjective, or felt and reported by the patient.

systolic (sis-TOL-ik) **blood pressure** the pressure created when the heart contracts and forces blood out into the arteries.

tachycardia (TAK-uh-KAR-de-uh) a rapid pulse; any pulse rate above 100 beats per minute.

vital signs outward signs of what is going on inside the body, including respiration; pulse; skin color, temperature, and condition (plus capillary refill in infants and children); pupils; and blood pressure.

REVIEW QUESTIONS

1. Name the vital signs. (p. 179)
2. Explain why vital signs should be taken more than once. (p. 179)

3. Explain the meaning of the letters S-A-M-P-L-E in patient assessment. (pp. 190–191)

APPLICATIONS

- How might the EMT-B get a SAMPLE history when a patient is unconscious?

WEB MEDIC

Visit Brady's *Emergency Care* website for direct weblinks. At **www.bradybooks.com/emergencycare**, you will find information related to the following Chapter 9 topics:

- Aging and changes in vital signs

- Breathing sounds

- Common mistakes in taking blood pressure

Chapter
Ten

ASSESSMENT OF THE TRAUMA PATIENT

Word on the Street

"We know that a patient's best chance for survival lies in our dispassionate adherence to the ABCs of survival and evaluation. Yet every time I care for someone rent by violence, I see my child, my wife, my friends, myself in his or her place for a brief moment. I look up and see the same feelings in my colleagues—physician, nurse, paramedic, EMT, even radiology tech. A flinch, and then on to work, determined that 'they ain't gonna die on my watch.' I hope that if I'm still doing this job in another 25 years, my colleagues and I will still flinch for the patient's sake."

Charles Stewart MD, FACEP

For the trauma patient—especially one whose injuries are serious—time must not be wasted at the scene. This patient needs to get to a hospital as quickly as possible. On the other hand, enough time must be spent at the scene to assess the patient adequately and give proper emergency care. How can you strike the right balance between care and speed? The key is focus. Instead of performing a time-consuming, comprehensive assessment on every patient, the EMT-B homes in on what is important for this particular patient. It is a process known as the focused history and physical exam. En route to the hospital, you may have time to do a more complete patient assessment called the detailed physical exam.

Focused History and Physical Exam for the Trauma Patient

Remember that *trauma* means "injury." Injuries can range from slight to severe, from a cut finger to a massive wound. Often you will not be able to see the injury or how serious it is, especially if it is internal. Usually, however, you will be able identify the mechanism of injury (MOI). If it is significant, you will do the focused history and physical exam differently than if the mechanism of injury is not significant.

The procedures for a trauma patient who does not have a significant mechanism of injury are discussed below. The procedures for a patient who does have a significant mechanism of injury will be discussed later in the chapter. Table 10-1 lists and contrasts the procedures for these two categories of trauma patient.

transport the patient. If the patient has no significant mechanism of injury (Table 10-2) and no immediately life-threatening injuries, you will know that you have time to assess the patient more thoroughly at the scene.

When the patient has no significant mechanism of injury, the steps of the focused history and physical exam are appropriately

How and Why?

Although pain is a good indicator of a problem, the severity of a patient's pain does not always reflect the seriousness of the injury. Some parts of the body simply have more (or less) sensory nerve endings than others. Go to your Electronic Extras CD for more information.

Study Guide for FHPE— Trauma with No Significant MOI

- ✔ Reconsider the MOI.
- ✔ Determine the chief complaint.
- ✔ Perform a focused physical exam.
- ✔ Obtain baseline vital signs.
- ✔ Take a SAMPLE history.

Trauma Patient with No Significant Mechanism of Injury

The first step of the focused history and physical exam for any trauma patient is to reconsider the mechanism of injury. The main purpose of this is to help you to determine how quickly you must

TOPIC OVERVIEW

In this chapter, you will learn about the following topics:

- The difference between a significant and non-significant mechanism of injury

- The difference between patients who need a rapid trauma assessment vs. patients who need a focused history and physical exam

- How to perform a rapid trauma assessment

- How to gather a focused history for a trauma patient

- How to perform a detailed examination for a trauma patient

✔ **Knowledge and Attitude**

1. Discuss the reasons for reconsideration concerning the mechanism of injury. (pp. 197–199, 210) (Scan 10-2, pp. 203–206)

2. State the reasons for performing a rapid trauma assessment. (pp. 211–212)

3. Recite examples and explain why patients should receive a rapid trauma assessment. (pp. 211–212)

4. Describe the areas included in the rapid trauma assessment and discuss what should be evaluated. (pp. 211–212) (Scan 10-1, p. 201; Scan 10-4, p. 214; Scan 10-5, pp. 216–218)

5. Differentiate when the rapid assessment may be altered in order to provide patient care. (pp. 211–212, 219)

6. Discuss the reason for performing a focused history and physical exam. (p. 198) (Scan 10-3, pp. 207–209)

7. Recognize and respect the feelings that patients might experience during assessment. (p. 202, 215)

8. Discuss the components of the detailed physical exam. (pp. 219–221, 225–226) (Scan 10-6, pp. 222–224)

9. State the areas of the body that are evaluated during the detailed physical exam. (p. 219)

10. Explain what additional care should be provided while performing the detailed physical exam. (pp. 219–221, 225–226)

11. Distinguish between the detailed physical exam that is performed on a trauma patient and that of the medical patient. (p. 226)

12. Explain the rationale for the feelings that these patients might be experiencing. (pp. 202, 215)

✔ **Skills**

1. Demonstrate the rapid trauma assessment that should be used to treat a patient based on mechanism of injury.

2. Demonstrate the skills involved in performing the detailed physical exam.

---

simplified. Instead of examining the patient from head to toe, you focus your assessment on just the areas that the patient tells you are painful or that you suspect may be injured because of the mechanism of injury. The assessment will include a physical exam, a set of baseline vital signs, and a SAMPLE history.

Reconsider the Mechanism of Injury

As part of scene size-up and the initial assessment, you will have already evaluated the mechanism of in-

jury. Because the mechanism of injury is so important in determining your next steps, you should now re-evaluate it. Why? When you first arrive on a scene and must take in a lot of information at once, it is easy to miss things. You are looking not only at how the patient was injured, but also for anything that might threaten you or your crew. You also have other concerns on your mind, like whether or not you need to call for help. Combine that with the stress of knowing that you may have a patient with serious injuries and it is easy to see how an EMT-B

Table 10-1 Focused History and Physical Exam—Trauma Patient	
No Significant Mechanism of Injury	**Significant Mechanism of Injury**
After scene size-up and initial assessment:	After scene size-up and initial assessment:
1. Reconsider the mechanism of injury.	1. Reconsider the mechanism of injury.
	2. Continue manual stabilization of head and neck.
	3. Consider requesting advanced life support personnel.
	4. Reconsider your transport decision.
	5. Reassess mental status.
2. Perform focused physical exam based on chief complaint and mechanism of injury.	6. Perform rapid trauma assessment.
3. Assess baseline vital signs.	7. Assess baseline vital signs.
4. Obtain a SAMPLE history.	8. Obtain a SAMPLE history.

TABLE 10-2 Significant Mechanisms of Injury

Significant Mechanisms of Injury

Ejection from vehicle

Death in same passenger compartment

Falls of more than 15 feet or 3 times patient's height

Rollover of vehicle

High-speed vehicle collision

Vehicle-pedestrian collision

Motorcycle crash

Unresponsive or altered mental status

Penetrations of the head, chest, or abdomen; e.g., stab and gunshot wounds

Additional Significant Mechanisms of Injury for a Child

Falls from more than 10 feet

Bicycle collision

Vehicle in medium speed collision

potential injuries the mechanism of injury causes you to suspect. For example, if the patient with the painful ankle suffered his injury by falling down a flight of steps, you should suspect that he may have more than just an ankle injury—including a potential spine injury that would require stabilization and, later, immobilization of the patient's head and spine.

When you assess areas of the patient's body that you suspect may be injured, you will evaluate them in two main ways: *inspecting* (looking) and *palpating* (feeling). You will look for contusions, abrasions, punctures, penetrations, burns, and lacerations. Then you will palpate for deformities, tenderness (pain on pressure), and swelling. An easy way to remember what you are trying to find is the memory aid **DCAP-BTLS** (Scan 10-1). (You can pronounce it as "Dee-cap, B-T-L-S.")

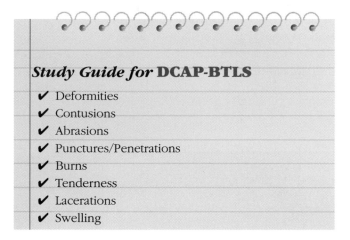

Study Guide for **DCAP-BTLS**

- ✔ Deformities
- ✔ Contusions
- ✔ Abrasions
- ✔ Punctures/Penetrations
- ✔ Burns
- ✔ Tenderness
- ✔ Lacerations
- ✔ Swelling

Deformities are just what they sound like, parts of the body that no longer have the normal shape. Common examples are broken or fractured bones that push up the skin over the bone ends. Contusions are the medical term for bruises. Abrasions, or scrapes, are some of the most common injuries you will see. Punctures and penetrations are holes in the body, frequently the result of gunshot wounds and stab wounds. When they are small, they are easy to overlook. Burns may be reddened, blistered, or charred-looking areas. *Tenderness* means that an area hurts when there is pressure on it, as when it is palpated. Pain (which is present even without any pressure) and tenderness frequently, but not always, go together. Lacerations are cuts, open wounds that sometimes cause significant blood loss. Swelling is a very common result of injured capillaries bleeding under the skin.

In order to find these signs, you will need to expose the patient. This means removing or cutting away clothing in order to see the area or areas of the body you are assessing. Be sure to tell the patient

can miss important information about the mechanism of injury.

So once the initial assessment has been completed and all life threats are under control, it is important to reconsider the mechanism of injury so you can reconsider, if necessary, the patient's priority for transport and appropriately tailor further assessment and care.

Determine the Chief Complaint

The chief complaint is what the patient tells you is the matter. For example, one patient may tell you she has cut her finger. Another may complain of pain after twisting his ankle.

Perform a Focused Physical Exam

Your decision on which areas of a patient's body to assess will depend partly on what you can see (e.g., the cut on the patient's finger) and what the patient tells you (the chief complaint, or the patient's ankle hurts). But you will not rely just on these obvious signs and symptoms. You will also pay attention to

DCAP-BTLS

▲ **D**EFORMITIES

▲ **C**ONTUSIONS

▲ **A**BRASIONS

▲ **P**UNCTURES/PENETRATIONS

▲ **B**URNS

▲ **T**ENDERNESS

▲ **L**ACERATIONS

▲ **S**WELLING

Table 10-3 Physical Exam/Trauma Assessment

Body Part	DCAP-BTLS	Plus
Head	DCAP-BTLS	Crepitation
Neck	DCAP-BTLS	Jugular vein distention Crepitation
Chest	DCAP-BTLS	Paradoxical motion Crepitation Breath sounds (present, absent, equal)
Abdomen	DCAP-BTLS	Firmness Softness Distention
Pelvis	DCAP-BTLS	Pain Tenderness Motion
Extremities	DCAP-BTLS	Distal pulse, motor function, sensation
Posterior	DCAP-BTLS	—

what you are doing and offer reassurance as necessary. Protect the patient's privacy and take steps to prevent unnecessarily long exposure to cold.

When you practice doing a physical exam, you can repeat DCAP-BTLS to yourself as you look at each body part, making sure to remember what each letter is prompting you to inspect or palpate. You will also check each part for the special signs and symptoms listed in Table 10-3 and described under "Performing the Rapid Trauma Assessment" later in this chapter.

Obtain Baseline Vital Signs and a SAMPLE History

For a trauma patient, first conduct a physical exam to assess injuries. Next, assess baseline vital signs and take a SAMPLE history (Figure 10-1).

Applying a Cervical Collar

Apply a cervical collar to any patient who you suspect may have an injury to the spine based on mechanism of injury, history, or signs and symptoms. (Remember that signs are what you observe, such as a bruise; symptoms are what the patient tells you he feels, such as pain.)

When is it appropriate to apply a cervical collar? There is a simple princi-

ple you can follow: If the mechanism of injury exerts great force on the upper body or if there is any soft-tissue damage to the head, face, or neck from trauma (such as a cut or bruise from being thrown against a dashboard), you may then assume that there is a possible cervical-spine injury. Any blow above the

Figure 10-1 Taking a SAMPLE history.

clavicles (collarbones) may damage the cervical spine. If the patient has a depressed level of responsiveness or if injury cannot be ruled out—even if the mechanism of injury is not known—suspect cervical-spine injury. When any of these conditions exists, apply a cervical collar.

There are several types of cervical-spine immobilization devices on the market. It is important when you select one that it be rigid (stiff, not easily movable) and that it be the right size. The traditional soft collar that you occasionally see someone wearing on the street has no role in immobilizing a prehospital patient's cervical spine. A soft collar provides so little restriction of neck motion that you may hear experienced EMTs refer to it as a "neck warmer."

The wrong size immobilization device may actually harm the patient by making breathing more difficult or obstructing the airway. Whatever device is used must not obstruct the airway. If the proper size collar is not available, it is better to place a rolled towel around the neck (to remind the patient not to move his head) and tape the patient's head to the backboard.

The techniques for selecting the right size cervical collar and for applying a cervical collar are presented in Scan 10-2. As you study the scan and practice applying a cervical collar, consider the following:

- Make certain that you have completed the initial assessment and that you have cared for all life-threatening problems before you apply the collar.

- Use the mechanism of injury, level of responsiveness, and location of injuries to determine the need for cervical immobilization. Apply a rigid cervical collar whenever any of these factors lead you to believe that spine injury is a possibility.

- Assess the patient's neck prior to placing the collar. Once the collar is in place, you will not be able to inspect or palpate the back of the neck.

- Reassure the patient. Having a cervical collar applied around your neck can be a constricting and frightening experience. Explain the procedure to the patient.

- Make sure the collar is the right size for the patient. The proper size rigid collar depends more on the length of the patient's neck than on the width. A large patient may not be able to wear a large collar. A small patient with a long neck may need your largest collar. The front height of the collar should fit between the point of the chin and the chest at the suprasternal (jugular) notch—the U-shaped dip where the clavicles and sternum meet. Once in place, the collar should rest on the clavicles and support the lower jaw. It should not stretch the neck (too high), it should not support the chin (too short), and it should not constrict the neck (too tight).

- Remove the patient's necklaces and large earrings before applying the collar.

- Keep the patient's hair out of the way.

- Keep the patient's head in the in-line anatomical position (a neutral position with head facing front, not tilted forward or back or turned to either side) when applying manual stabilization and the collar.

- Cervical collars alone do not provide adequate in-line immobilization. Nor is applying the collar the first step. Whenever there is the possibility of a spine injury, you must manually stabilize the patient's head and neck immediately upon first patient contact, before the collar is applied (as you learned in Chapter 8). Continue to manually stabilize the head and neck until the patient is completely immobilized and secured to a backboard. (You learned about immobilization on a backboard in Chapter 5, "Lifting and Moving," and will learn more in Chapter 29, "Injuries to the Head and Spine," and in Chapter 33, Gaining Access and Rescue Operations.)

Trauma Patient with a Significant Mechanism of Injury

When you have a patient to whom you have assigned a high priority because of problems found in the initial assessment or because of a significant mechanism of injury, you will do all of the following: reconsider the mechanism of injury, continue manual stabilization of the head and neck, consider requesting advanced life support (ALS) personnel, reconsider your transport decision, reassess the patient's mental status, and perform a rapid trauma assessment (Review Table 10-1 and see Scan 10-3).

***Study Guide for* FHPE—Trauma with a Significant MOI**

- ✔ Reconsider the MOI.
- ✔ Continue manual stabilization of the head and neck.
- ✔ Consider requesting advanced life support.
- ✔ Reconsider transport decision.
- ✔ Reassess mental status.
- ✔ Perform a rapid trauma assessment.
- ✔ Obtain baseline vital signs.
- ✔ Take a SAMPLE history.

APPLYING A CERVICAL COLLAR

▲ STIFNECK® SELECT™. (Laerdal Medical Corporation/John Hill Photography)

▲ PHILADELPHIA CERVICAL COLLAR™.

▲ PHILADELPHIA CERVICAL COLLAR™, opened.

Rigid cervical collars are applied to protect the cervical spine. DO NOT apply a soft collar.

▲ NEC-LOC™ rigid extrication collar.

▲ NEC-LOC™ rigid extrication collar, opened.

(continued)

Sizing a Cervical Collar

▲ **1.** Measure the patient's neck.

▲ **2.** Measure the collar. The chin piece should not lift the patient's chin and hyperextend the neck. Make sure the collar is not too small or tight, which would make the collar act as a constricting band.

Applying a STIFNECK® SELECT™ Collar to a Seated Patient

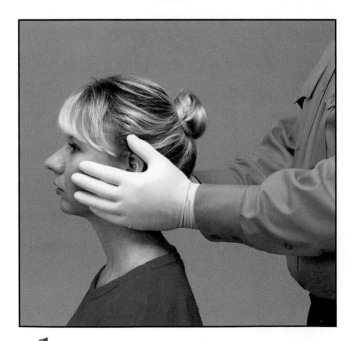

▲ **1.** Stabilize the head and neck from the rear.

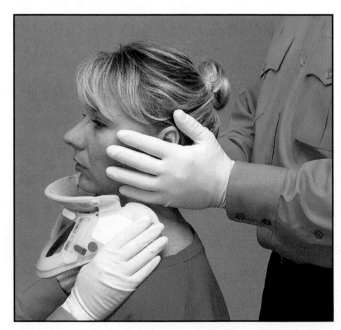

▲ **2.** Properly angle the collar for placement.

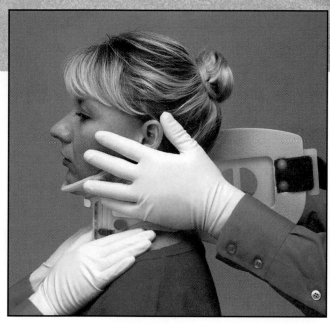

▲ **3.** Position the collar bottom.

▲ **4.** Set the collar in place around the neck.

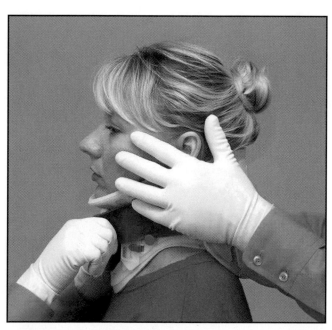

▲ **5.** Secure the collar.

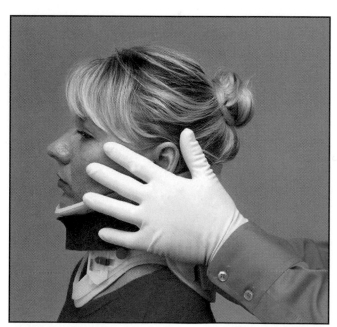

▲ **6.** Maintain manual stabilization of the head and neck.

(continued)

Applying a STIFNECK® SELECT™ Collar to a Supine Patient

▲ **1.** Kneel at the patient's head, and stabilize the head and neck.

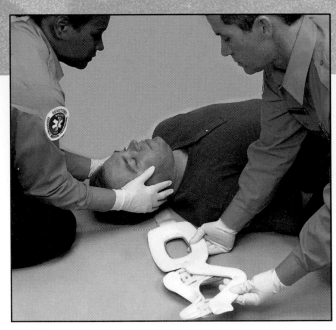

▲ **2.** Set the collar in place.

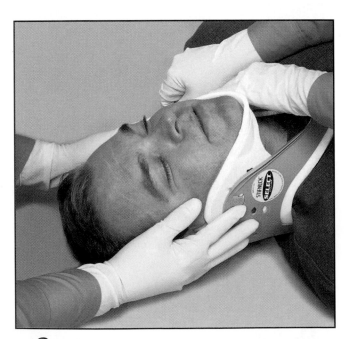

▲ **3.** Secure the collar.

▲ **4.** Continue to manually stabilize the head and neck.

FOCUSED HISTORY AND PHYSICAL EXAM- TRAUMA PATIENT

FIRST take BSI precautions.

◄ Reassess mechanism of injury (MOI). If it is not significant (e.g., patient has a cut finger), focus the physical exam (below) only on the injured part. If the MOI is significant:
- Continue manual stabilization of the head and neck.
- Consider requesting ALS personnel.
- Reconsider transport decision.
- Reassess mental status.
- Perform a rapid trauma assessment.

Rapid Trauma Assessment

Rapidly assess each part of the body for the following problems (say "Dee-cap B-T-L-S" as a memory prompt):

Deformities   **B**urns
Contusions   **T**enderness
Abrasions   **L**acerations
Punctures/Penetrations   **S**welling

▲ **HEAD:** DCAP-BTLS plus crepitation.

▲ **NECK:** DCAP-BTLS plus jugular vein distention and crepitation (then apply cervical collar).

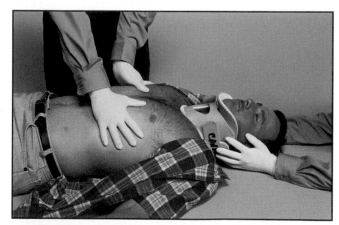

▲ **CHEST:** DCAP-BTLS plus crepitation, paradoxical motion, and breath sounds (absent, present, equal).

(continued)

▲ **ABDOMEN:** DCAP-BTLS plus firm, soft, distended.

▲ **PELVIS:** DCAP-BTLS with gentle compression for tenderness.

▲ **EXTREMITIES:** DCAP-BTLS plus distal pulse, motor function, and sensation.

▲ **POSTERIOR:** DCAP-BTLS. (To examine posterior, roll patient using spinal precautions)

Vital Signs

Assess the patient's baseline vital signs:

- Respiration
- Pulse
- Skin color, temperature, condition (capillary refill in infants and children)
- Pupils
- Blood pressure

▲ **VITAL SIGNS**

SAMPLE History

◀ Interview patient or (if patient is unresponsive), interview family and bystanders to get as much information as possible about the patient's problem. Ask about:

Signs and symptoms
Allergies
Medicines
Pertinent past history
Last oral intake
Events leading to problem

Interventions and Transport

◀ Contact on-line medical direction as needed. Perform interventions as needed.

▼ Package and transport the patient.

Note that there are several additional steps for the patient with a significant mechanism of injury as compared to the steps for the patient with no significant mechanism of injury (manual stabilization, ALS request consideration, reconsideration of transport decision, and reassessment of mental status). Also note that instead of a physical exam focused just on the area of injury, the patient with a significant mechanism of injury receives a complete, head-to-toe rapid trauma assessment.

Reconsider the Mechanism of Injury

What is a significant mechanism of injury? Simply put, it is a way of getting hurt that carries a high risk of serious injury. A patient who has been ejected from a vehicle, for example, is several times more likely to have fatal injuries than a patient who has not been ejected. A patient who is in a passenger compartment where another person died can be assumed to have sustained serious injury because of the amount of force that had to have been involved to kill the other person. Review Table 10-2, which lists a number of high-risk situations.

All of these mechanisms involve potentially large forces being exerted on a patient's body. In the case of a motor-vehicle collision, you can gain a great deal of information by walking around the vehicle and looking at all of its outside surfaces. You should also look inside the vehicle, concentrating your attention on the steering wheel, pedals, dashboard, and rear-view mirror. Look for deformities that could have been caused by a person striking the surface (Figure 10-2). Also look for intrusion of the body of the car into the passenger compartment (i.e., was the car crunched so that the inside is smaller than it used to be?). The preferred way to identify the mechanism of injury is, of course, to do it yourself. If patient care prevents this, you may ask someone else, such as a police officer at the scene, to get the information for you.

Some patients who undergo experiences like those listed in Table 10-2 will escape without serious injury, but many more will not be so lucky. For this reason, you should provide rapid assessment and treatment to any patient with a mechanism of injury listed in Table 10-2.

Although the mechanism of injury can provide a lot of information about the kinds of injuries a patient may have, there is still the possibility that patients will have "hidden injuries." These injuries are considered to be hidden because patients may have no signs or symptoms initially but later develop serious conditions that may take time to become apparent.

Seat belt injuries are a good example. There is no doubt that properly used seat belts save lives by preventing drivers and passengers from hitting hard objects inside a vehicle and by preventing them from being ejected. But seat belts can also cause injuries. When patients are in high velocity collisions, the force of being thrown forward against buckled seat belts will occasionally cause injury to the bowel and other abdominal organs. These injuries may not become apparent for several hours or even days. It is important to realize that even people who were wearing seat belts may have sustained serious injuries.

Airbags, too, may save lives but do not provide total protection from injury. Airbags prevent occupants from going through the windshield and hitting hard objects inside the vehicle. They are most effective when used in combination with seat belts. In a few instances, especially with a small driver or passenger (particularly a child) or when the front seat is pulled far forward, or when a seat belt is not in place to keep the person from being thrown forward, the expanding airbag may cause injury. Also, the driver may sustain an arm injury because of improper positioning of hands on the steering wheel or may sustain a chest injury from hitting the steering wheel after the bag deflates. When inspecting a vehicle in which an airbag has deployed, you should look at the steering wheel. Whenever you see a bent or broken steering wheel, you should treat the patient like every other patient who has a significant mechanism of injury. A good way to find this kind of damage is to remember to "lift and look" under the airbag after the patient has been removed from the vehicle (Figure 10-3).

Pediatric Notes

Infants and children are more fragile than adults. This means that a child may sustain the same injury as an adult, but from less force. For this reason, there are additional mechanisms of injury that the EMT-B needs to consider significant when children and infants are concerned (Table 10-2).

Continue Spinal Stabilization

During the initial assessment, make sure that someone is manually stabilizing the patient's head to prevent any cervical-spine injury from becoming a paralyzing spinal-cord injury. Manual stabilization must continue throughout the assessment until the patient is fully immobilized on a backboard.

Consider a Request for Advanced Life Support Personnel

Some areas of the country, particularly urban and suburban areas, have advanced life support (ALS) personnel—paramedics who respond with EMTs when they are transporting patients who might benefit from the additional interventions paramedics can provide. If this is the case where you practice as an

Figure 10-2 Deformities of the interior of a vehicle may give you clues to potential injuries in the passengers.

Figure 10-3 An airbag can prevent injuries, but once deployed, it also can conceal important information about the patient's mechanism of injury. When you see a deployed airbag, remember to "lift and look."

EMT-B, you should familiarize yourself with your local protocols. Rural EMTs do not usually have this option, but they may have other means by which to improve the patient's care before arrival at a hospital.

In some areas that are very distant from hospitals, local clinics arrange to provide advanced care to certain kinds of patients. For example, if an ambulance is an hour away from the closest hospital, but a local clinic is only 10 minutes away, the ambulance may be able to stop there with a patient in cardiac arrest. There are limits, though, on what can be done at health care centers like these. Many of them would not be able to provide additional care worth a delay in transport for awake trauma patients.

If arrangements like these exist where you work as an EMT-B, you must be familiar with the types of patients your clinic can help. The arrangements should be in writing in order to reduce confusion and prevent loss of precious time with critical patients. In any case, the patient with serious trauma must ultimately, if at all possible, be transported to a trauma center.

Reconsider Your Transport Decision

Assigning a high priority for transport is appropriate when the patient has a condition for which you can-

not provide definitive treatment—treatment that can only be provided at the hospital. As you prepare to do the rapid trauma assessment (described on the following pages), it is a good time to re-evaluate that decision. You will have had a chance to look at the mechanism of injury more closely and, if appropriate, to call for assistance from advanced life support (ALS) personnel at the scene or by intercept en route to the hospital. At this point you should take just a moment to consider again how urgently you need to transport the patient.

Reassess Mental Status

Repeat the AVPU assessment (alert, verbal response, painful response, unresponsive) as described in Chapter 8. Note whether your patient's mental status is unchanged, improved, or deteriorated. A patient who is less than fully alert or whose mental status is deteriorating is a high priority for transport.

Perform a Rapid Trauma Assessment

A patient with a significant mechanism of injury needs a rapid trauma assessment. This requires only a few moments and should be performed at the scene, before loading the patient into the ambulance, even if the patient is a high priority for transport. The care that you provide en route will be based on the results of this rapid assessment, and you will obtain valuable information to relay to the hospital staff so that they can be prepared for your patient.

During the rapid trauma assessment, you will be able to detect injuries that may later threaten life or limb. You may also find life-threatening injuries that you did not find during the initial assessment. When dealing with a responsive patient, you should ask the patient before and during the trauma assessment about any symptoms.

To perform the rapid trauma assessment, you will use your sense of sight to inspect and your sense of touch to palpate different areas of the body. You may also use your sense of hearing to detect abnormal sounds, not just from the airway but also from other areas, such as the sound of broken bones rubbing against each other. You may use your sense of smell, as well, to detect odors like gasoline, urine, feces, or vomitus.

The rapid trauma assessment emphasizes evaluation of the areas of the body where the greatest threats to the patient may be. You will evaluate the patient from head to toe, in the sequence shown below.

The signs and symptoms you will assess each area for are summarized in Table 10-3. Remember, however, that this is a quick evaluation, so you will not spend a lot of time on any one area.

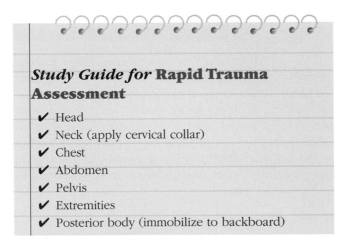

Study Guide for Rapid Trauma Assessment

- ✔ Head
- ✔ Neck (apply cervical collar)
- ✔ Chest
- ✔ Abdomen
- ✔ Pelvis
- ✔ Extremities
- ✔ Posterior body (immobilize to backboard)

Rapid Assessment of the Head. Assess the head for DCAP-BTLS and also for the sound or feel of broken bones rubbing against each other, known as **crepitation.** Run your gloved fingers through the patient's hair and palpate gently. A good way to check the back of the head in a supine patient is to start with your fingers at the top of the neck and carefully slide them upward toward the top of the patient's head. If there is blood on your gloves, there is an open wound. However, if you do not see any blood on the floor or ground, then you do not need to apply a dressing to the wound right away.

Rapid Assessment of the Neck. Assess the neck for DCAP-BTLS, crepitation, and **jugular vein distention (JVD).** Jugular vein distention is present when you can see the patient's neck veins bulging. The neck veins are usually not visible when the patient is sitting up. However, it is normal to see bulging of the neck veins when the patient is lying in a horizontal position or with his head down. Flat neck veins in a patient who is lying down may be a sign of blood loss, showing that there is not enough blood to fill them. When you see FLAT neck veins in a FLAT patient, think "blood loss."

Other things you might find when assessing the patient's anterior neck are a stoma or a tracheostomy. A **stoma** is a permanent surgical opening in the neck through which the patient breathes. A **tracheostomy** is a surgical incision held open by a metal or plastic tube. If the patient requires artificial ventilation, you may need to provide it through the stoma, as described in Chapter 6.

You may also find a medical identification medallion on a necklace when assessing the neck. Note the information on the necklace if you find one.

Application of a Cervical Collar. After you assess the head and neck, size and apply a rigid cervical spine immobilization collar. Use the principles and methods described earlier in this chapter and in Scan 10-2.

Rapid Assessment of the Chest. Next, assess the chest for DCAP-BTLS, crepitation, breath sounds, and paradoxical motion. **Paradoxical motion,** or movement of part of the chest in the opposite direction from the rest of the chest, is a sign of a serious injury. It usually occurs when a segment of ribs has broken at two ends and is "floating" free of the rest of the rib cage. (This condition is sometimes known as "flail chest.") The opposite motion of the broken section is obvious during respiration, moving inward when the lungs expand with air and outward when the lungs empty (Figure 10-4). Paradoxical motion also indicates that a great deal of force was applied to the patient's chest; in other words, there was a significant mechanism of injury.

You can check for crepitation and paradoxical motion of the chest at the same time. Start by palpating the clavicles (collarbones). Next, gently feel the sternum (breastbone). Position your hands on the sides of the chest and feel for equal expansion of both sides of the chest. During this process you may feel broken bones or floating paradoxical segments.

Palpate the entire rib cage for deformities. Use your hands to apply gentle pressure to the sides of the rib cage. If there is an injured rib and the patient is able to respond, he will tell you that it hurts. Occa-

It is important to remember that when you reach the point of examining the patient's chest in the rapid trauma assessment, you need to expose the chest if you have not already done so. However, keep the weather and the patient's privacy in mind when doing this.

Rapid Assessment of the Abdomen. When you assess the abdomen for DCAP-BTLS, also check for firmness, softness, and distention. The term **distention** is another way of saying the abdomen appears larger than normal. One of its causes can be internal bleeding. Whether the abdomen is abnormally distended or not may be a very difficult judgment to make, so do not spend a lot of time on it. You may also see a **colostomy** or **ileostomy** when you inspect the abdomen. This is a surgical opening in the wall of the abdomen with a bag in place to collect excretions from the digestive system. If you see such a bag, leave it in place and be careful not to cut it if you cut clothing away.

Palpate the abdomen by gently pressing down once on each abdominal quadrant. (Picture the abdomen divided into four segments–upper left, upper right, lower left, lower right–and press on each quadrant in turn.) If the patient tells you he has pain in a specific area of the abdomen, palpate that site last. When practical, make sure your hands are warm. Press in on the abdomen with the palm side of your fingers, depressing the surface about one inch. Many EMTs prefer to use two hands, one on top of the other at the fingertips. Normally the abdomen is soft. Firmness of the abdomen can be a sign of injury to the organs in the abdomen and internal bleeding.

Another finding you may occasionally come across when palpating a patient's abdomen is a pulsating mass. This may be an enlarged aorta. If you do feel such pulsations, do not press any farther into the abdomen. Doing so could cause further injury to a weakened blood vessel.

Rapid Assessment of the Pelvis. Next assess the pelvis for DCAP-BTLS. You may observe bleeding or **priapism,** a persistent erection of the penis that can result from spinal-cord injury or certain medical problems. If the patient is awake, ask him first if he has any pain in his pelvis. If he complains of pain, do NOT palpate the pelvis. Instead, consider the complaint of pain as reason enough to treat the patient for an injury to the pelvis. Palpating or compressing the painful pelvis of a conscious patient will not give you any more useful information, but it can produce excruciating pain and, if done too strenuously, may injure the patient.

An unconscious patient, however, cannot tell you if his pelvic area hurts. So you will gently compress the pelvis of the unconscious patient to detect

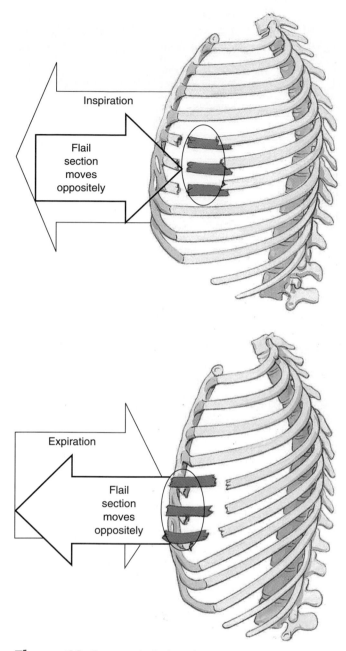

Figure 10-4 Paradoxical motion.

sionally, you may detect a crackling or crunching sensation under the skin from air that has escaped from its normal passageways.

Listen for breath sounds (Scan 10-4) just under the clavicles in the mid-clavicular line and at the bases of the lungs in the mid-axillary line. Notice whether the breath sounds are present and equal. A patient who has breath sounds that are absent or very hard to hear on one side may have a collapsed lung or other serious respiratory injury. There are many other characteristics of breath sounds, but in the trauma patient, presence and equality are the two things to look for at this time.

ASSESSING BREATH SOUNDS

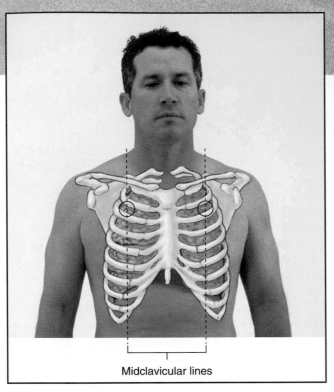

Midclavicular lines

▲ **MIDCLAVICULAR LINE**

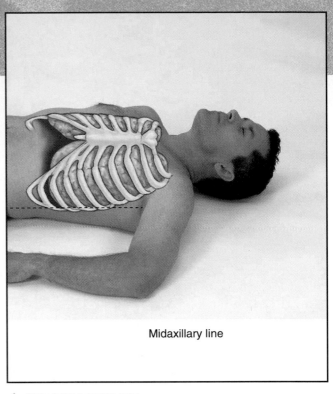

Midaxillary line

▲ **MIDAXILLARY LINE**

▲ Listen to and compare both sides of the chest. Is air entry present? Absent? Equal on both sides?

tenderness (if there is enough responsiveness to pain to cause him to flinch or groan) and motion of the bones (indicating instability or broken bones). These signs will help you determine whether you need to treat the unconscious patient for a pelvic injury.

Rapid Assessment of the Extremities. Quickly assess all four extremities for DCAP-BTLS as well as distal pulse, motor function, and sensation—that is, whether a pulse is present, the patient can move his hands and feet, and he has feeling in his hands and feet (Scan 10-5). In a conscious patient, you would touch the patient's hand or foot and ask whether he could feel your touch. If you are not sure whether the patient is telling you the truth, you can ask where on the hand or foot you are touching him. You would also test movement in the extremities of a conscious patient by asking him to squeeze your fingers in his hands and to move his feet against your hands.

If you find a deformity, diminished function, or other indication of injury to an extremity in a patient who is a high priority for transport, you will not splint the extremity at the scene but will treat it en route.

Rapid Assessment of the Posterior Body and Immobilization on a Backboard. Roll the patient onto his side as a unit (you will learn how to do a log roll maneuver in Chapter 29, "Injuries to the Head and Spine") and assess the posterior body, inspecting and palpating for DCAP-BTLS in the area of the spine and to the sides of the spine, the buttocks, and the posterior extremities. Meanwhile, have someone slide a backboard next to the patient so that, when you roll the patient back into a supine position, he is on the backboard.

If the patient has shown signs or symptoms of an injury to the pelvis, place a pneumatic anti-shock garment on the board before you roll the patient onto it. Your local protocol may direct you to place the anti-shock garment on the backboard for other kinds of trauma patients, too. (You will learn about the PASG in Chapter 26, "Bleeding and Shock.") Familiarize yourself with how local medical direction wishes you to manage these patients.

Obtain Baseline Vital Signs and a SAMPLE History. Quickly obtain a set of baseline vital signs, as discussed in Chapter 9. If the patient is unresponsive, you will not be able to get a SAMPLE history from him. If there is a friend or family member nearby, that person may be able to give you information about the patient's medical history.

In trauma situations, it is good to think of the "S" in SAMPLE as standing for not just "signs and symptoms" but also for "story," or the history of the injury. This means information like the speed of the vehicle,

whether seat belts were used, and whether the patient had a loss of consciousness. With patients who have been shot, information you should try to obtain includes the caliber of the gun, type of ammunition, and distance of the gun from the patient when the gun was discharged. When you are treating a patient who has been stabbed, try to find out the size and type of the knife.

Some General Principles

Several important principles to remember when examining a patient, mentioned throughout the chapter, are summarized below:

- Tell the patient what you are going to do. In particular, let the patient know when there may be pain or discomfort. Stress the importance of the examination and work to build the patient's confidence. Ask the patient if he understands what you are doing, and explain your actions again if needed.

- Expose any injured area before examining it, so that you can see such things as bruises and puncture wounds. Let the patient know when you must lift, rearrange, or remove any article of clothing. Do all you can to ensure the patient's privacy.

- Try to maintain eye contact. Do not turn away while you are talking or while the patient is answering your questions.

- Assume spinal injury. Unless you are sure that you are dealing with a patient who does not have a spine injury (e.g., a medical patient with no mechanism of injury or reason to suspect trauma), assume the patient has such injuries. Always assume that the unconscious trauma patient has a spine injury. Manually stabilize the head and neck on first contact with the patient, fit the patient with a properly sized cervical collar as soon as you have examined the head and neck, and fully immobilize the patient to a spine board before transport to the hospital.

- During the focused physical exam, you may stop or alter the assessment process to provide care that is necessary and appropriate for the priority of the patient. For a patient who is not a priority for rapid transport, you may pause to bandage a bleeding wound, even if the bleeding is not life threatening, or to splint an injured extremity.

- During the rapid trauma assessment, apply a cervical collar if spine injury is suspected. For a patient who is a priority for rapid transport, treatments such as controlling non-life-threatening bleeding or splinting an injured extremity may take place en route to the hospital if time and the patient's condition permit.

ASSESSING DISTAL FUNCTION

Assess all four extremities for distal pulse, motor function, and sensation. Diminished function may be a sign of injury that has compromised circulation, muscle, or nerve function. Distal function should be checked both before and after any interventions such as splinting, bandaging, and immobilization, and at intervals during transport, to be sure such interventions are not interfering with distal function. If distal function has become compromised, adjust interventions as necessary.

▲**1.** Assess distal circulation in the upper extremities by feeling for radial pulses.

▲**2.** Assess distal motor function by checking the patient's ability to move both hands.

▲**3.** Assess strength in the hands by asking the patient to squeeze your fingers.

▲ **4.** Assess distal sensation to the upper extremities by asking the patient "Which finger am I touching?" (Be sure the patient cannot see which finger.)

▲ If the patient is unresponsive, check distal sensation in the upper extremities by pinching the back of the hand. Watch and listen for a response.

▲ **5.** Check distal circulation in the lower extremities by feeling the posterior tibial pulse just behind the medial malleolus of the ankle, or . . .

▲ Feel the dorsalis pedis pulse at the top of the foot.

(continued)

▲ **6.** Assess distal motor function by checking the patient's ability to move his or her feet.

▲ **7.** Assess strength in the feet and legs by asking the patient to push against your hands.

▲ **8.** Assess distal sensation in the lower extremities by asking the patient "Which toe am I touching?" (Be sure the patient cannot see which toe.)

▲ If the patient is unresponsive, check distal sensation in the lower extremities by pinching the top of the foot. Watch and listen for a response.

Pediatric Notes

The focused history and physical exam of the pediatric (infant or child) trauma patient is very similar to the focused history and physical exam of the adult patient. One important difference is that you may need to spend more time reassuring children and explaining procedures to them. You will want to kneel or find another way to get on the same level with the child as you speak with him. Young children may be less frightened if you begin your assessment at the toes and work toward the head instead of proceeding in the usual head-to-toe direction. (Assessment of infants and children will be discussed in greater detail in Chapter 13.)

A child's airway is narrower than an adult's and more susceptible to being closed. A cervical collar that is too tight can easily constrict a child's airway. A collar that is too high can close the airway by stretching the neck. So it is especially important to choose the correct size cervical collar for a child.

DETAILED PHYSICAL EXAM

The initial assessment and the focused history and physical exam are done rapidly because of the necessity of getting the seriously injured or ill patient into the ambulance and to the hospital without delay. En route to the hospital, you may have time to do a more complete patient assessment known as the **detailed physical exam.** If you are not on a transporting unit and the ambulance has not arrived, you may do the detailed physical exam at the scene.

The purpose of the detailed physical exam is to gather additional information about the patient's injuries and conditions. Some of this information may help you to determine the proper treatment for the

Study Guide for Detailed Physical Exam

- ✔ Repeat initial assessment.
- ✔ Complete all critical interventions.
- ✔ Head
- ✔ Neck
- ✔ Chest
- ✔ Abdomen
- ✔ Pelvis
- ✔ Extremities
- ✔ Posterior
- ✔ Reassess vital signs.

patient, and some of the information you gather in the detailed physical exam will assist the emergency department staff.

The detailed physical exam is performed most often on the trauma patient with a significant mechanism of injury, less often on a trauma patient with no significant mechanism of injury, and seldom on a medical patient.

Trauma Patient with a Significant Mechanism of Injury

For a trauma patient who is not responsive or has a significant or unknown mechanism of injury, you will have assessed almost the entire body during the rapid trauma assessment—but very quickly. For this patient, a detailed physical exam may reveal signs or symptoms of injury that you missed or that have changed since the rapid trauma assessment.

Before Beginning the Detailed Physical Exam

It is important to remember that you should perform the detailed physical exam only after you have performed all critical interventions. The best way to ensure this is to repeat your initial assessment before you begin the detailed physical exam. To do this, reassess your general impression of the patient, his mental status, plus airway, breathing, and circulation.

If you are treating a severely injured patient, you may be too busy to begin or complete the detailed physical exam at all. This is not a failure on your part. Your responsibility is to give the patient the best care possible under the difficult conditions found in the field. If you do not do a complete assessment, but you keep a critical patient's airway, breathing, and circulation intact, you have helped the patient far more than if you had done the complete assessment. Performing a detailed physical exam is always a lower priority than addressing life-threatening problems. The place of the detailed physical exam among the priorities and sequence of assessment is shown in Table 10-4.

Performing the Detailed Physical Exam

If you have not already exposed the patient, you need to do so now. Since you are now in the enclosed ambulance, it is much easier to protect the patient's privacy and protect him from exposure to the environment.

The detailed physical exam will look a lot like the rapid trauma assessment that you did during the focused history and physical exam. You will look for the familiar DCAP-BTLS signs (review Scan 10-1). You will also look for certain additional signs as you examine the head, neck, chest, abdomen, pelvis, extremities, and posterior body. The only areas you will

TABLE 10-4   Detailed Physical Exam in the Sequence of Assessment Priorities

1. Scene size-up

2. Initial assessment and critical interventions for immediately life-threatening problems

3. Focused history and physical exam, plus interventions as needed

4. Repeat initial assessment for immediately life-threatening problems. Provide critical interventions as needed.

5. Detailed physical exam (time and critical-care needs permitting)

6. Ongoing assessment for life-threatening problems, plus vital signs. Provide critical interventions as needed.

Figure 10-5   Battle's sign and other signs of head injury.

assess in the detailed physical exam that you did not assess during the rapid trauma assessment portion of the focused history and physical exam will be the face, ears, eyes, nose, and mouth, as discussed below. (Also see Table 10-5 and Scan 10-6.)

Gently palpate the cranium for DCAP-BTLS and crepitation and then inspect your gloves for blood. Inspect and palpate the face for DCAP-BTLS by looking and then gently palpating the cheekbones, forehead, and lower jaw. The bones in the face are fragile and may break when subjected to significant forces.

Inspect and palpate the ears, searching for DCAP-BTLS and drainage of blood or other fluid. If found, this is an important piece of information to pass on to the emergency department staff because it may be an indication of injury to the skull. Also gently bend each ear forward to look for any bruising. (You can do this if you were careful when you applied the cervical collar to make sure you did not enclose the ears.) A bruise behind the ear of a patient is called Battle's sign (Figure 10-5) and is another important sign of skull injury to tell hospital staff about.

Next assess the eyes, inspecting for the usual DCAP-BTLS and discoloration, unequal pupils, foreign bodies, and blood in the anterior chamber (front) of the eye. Blood in the anterior chamber is not common but, when present, it is a sign that the

eye sustained significant force and is bleeding inside (Figure 10-6).

Inspect and palpate the nose for injuries or signs of injury. Look not only for DCAP-BTLS but also for drainage and bleeding.

When assessing the ears and nose, you may find blood or clear fluid draining from them. Blood may be from a laceration of that area or it may be coming from inside the skull. Clear fluid may be just from a runny nose or it may be cerebrospinal fluid (CSF). You should prevent an ear or nose that is draining blood or clear fluid from getting any dirtier than it already is. CSF surrounds the brain and spinal cord, and if it is leaking out then bacteria can get into the brain. Similarly, a wound from inside the skull that is leaking blood can also provide a route for bacteria to get in.

Open the mouth and look for DCAP-BTLS, loose or broken teeth, other objects that could cause obstruction, swelling or laceration of the tongue, unusual breath odor, and discoloration. A foreign body like a broken tooth is a potential source of airway obstruction and must be removed as soon as possible from the patient's mouth. The most common unusual breath odor is from alcoholic beverages. Other conditions besides alcohol, though, can cause similar odors.

There are only a few differences in the rest of the exam compared to what you did in the rapid trauma

TABLE 10-5 Detailed Physical Exam Compared to Rapid Trauma Assessment

Focused History and Physical Exam: Rapid Trauma Assessment		Detailed Physical Exam	
Head	DCAP-BTLS + crepitation	Head	DCAP-BTLS + crepitation
		Scalp and cranium	DCAP-BTLS + crepitation
		Face	DCAP-BTLS
		Ears	DCAP-BTLS + drainage
		Nose	DCAP-BTLS + drainage, bleeding
		Mouth	DCAP-BTLS + loose or broken teeth, objects that could cause obstruction, laceration of tongue, unusual breath odor, discoloration
Neck	DCAP-BTLS + jugular vein distention, crepitation	Neck	DCAP-BTLS + jugular vein distention, crepitation
Chest	DCAP-BTLS + paradoxical motion, crepitation, breath sounds	Chest	DCAP-BTLS + paradoxical motion, crepitation, breath sounds
Abdomen	DCAP-BTLS + firmness, softness, distention	Abdomen	DCAP-BTLS + firmness, softness, distention
Pelvis	DCAP-BTLS + pain, tenderness, motion	Pelvis	DCAP-BTLS + pain, tenderness, motion
Extremities	DCAP-BTLS + distal pulse, motor function, sensation	Extremities	DCAP-BTLS + distal pulse, motor function, sensation
Posterior	DCAP-BTLS	Posterior	DCAP-BTLS

DCAP-BTLS = deformities, contusions, abrasions, punctures/penetrations, burns, tenderness, lacerations, swelling

assessment. These differences result from either the different environment (the back of the ambulance) or from the treatment you have already given to the patient (e.g., cervical collar and immobilization on a backboard).

When you assess the neck you will be limited by the cervical collar that you placed on the patient during the focused history and physical exam (rapid trauma assessment). You will not be able to inspect or palpate the back of the neck, but you will be able to assess for DCAP-BTLS, jugular vein distention (JVD), and crepitation through the openings in the collar. You should make sure the collars you use have these openings.

Reassessing the chest can be a challenge in a moving ambulance because road noise makes breath sounds difficult to hear. Just keep in mind that you are listening for the presence and equality of breath sounds in your trauma patient, not the different kinds of abnormal sounds that are more common in medical

DETAILED PHYSICAL EXAM

The detailed physical exam is similar to the rapid trauma assessment—with some important differences:

- The head (scalp, cranium, face, ears, eyes, nose, mouth) is more thoroughly examined.
- The exam usually takes place in the ambulance, en route. Noise and motion may interfere with some procedures.
- Immobilization devices have been applied and you must work around them; for example, examining the ears through holes in the head immobilizer or below head tape, examining the neck through openings in the rigid collar, and examining only as much of the posterior as you can reach.

▲ **SCALP AND CRANIUM:** DCAP-BTLS plus crepitation.

▲ **EARS:** DCAP-BTLS plus drainage of blood and/or clear fluid.

▲ **FACE:** DCAP-BTLS.

▲ **EYES:** DCAP-BTLS plus discoloration, unequal pupils, foreign bodies, blood in anterior chamber.

▲ **NOSE:** DCAP-BTLS plus drainage of blood and/or clear fluid.

▲ **MOUTH:** DCAP-BTLS plus loose or broken teeth, objects that could cause obstruction, swelling or laceration of tongue, unusual breath odor, discoloration.

▲ **NECK:** DCAP-BTLS plus jugular vein distention, crepitation.

▲ **CHEST:** DCAP-BTLS plus paradoxical motion, crepitation.

▲ Auscultate chest for breath sounds: presence, absence, and equality.

▲ **ABDOMEN:** DCAP-BTLS plus firmness, softness, distention.

(continued)

223

▲ **PELVIS:** DCAP-BTLS plus pain, tenderness, motion.

▲ **UPPER EXTREMITIES:** DCAP-BTLS.

▲ Assess upper extremities for distal pulse, motor function, and sensation.

▲ **LOWER EXTREMITIES:** DCAP-BTLS.

▲ Assess lower extremities for distal pulse, motor function, and sensation.

▲ **POSTERIOR BODY:** DCAP-BTLS.

Figure 10-6 Blood in the anterior chamber of the eye is a sign that the eye has sustained considerable force.

patients. If you are unable to hear breath sounds because of road noise, it is generally better to continue transporting the patient to the hospital. It makes little sense to stop the ambulance and delay transport unless you can do something to treat an abnormality you find.

When it comes to reassessing the posterior body it would, of course, be inappropriate to roll the patient up off the backboard. By having the patient immobilized on a backboard, you are already treating for possible spine injury, so your primary concern at this point is to evaluate as much of the posterior body as you can reach for other injuries that may have been missed earlier. Simply reassess the flanks (sides) and as much of the spinal area as you can touch without moving the patient.

Any deformities or other indications of a musculoskeletal injury to an extremity found during the rapid trauma assessment will most likely have been temporarily immobilized by securing the patient to the spine board. It is unlikely that taking time to splint such injuries would have been appropriate at

the scene when rapid transport was a priority. En route to the hospital, if the patient's other injuries are not keeping you too busy, a good time to apply a splint to an injured extremity would be after you perform the detailed physical exam. You will learn splinting techniques in Chapter 28, "Musculoskeletal Injuries."

The rest of the detailed physical exam is essentially the same as the rapid trauma assessment, but you have more time, so you can be more thorough. This is especially true with long transports in rural or wilderness areas.

The final step of the detailed physical exam is to reassess the vital signs.

Your next priority is to make sure that the emergency department is ready for your patient. You do this by using the ambulance radio or cellular phone to notify the emergency department of the patient's condition. Depending on how far you are from the hospital and what your local protocols say, you may do this step before the detailed physical exam. If you have not yet notified the hospital, you should do it now. You will learn more about what to say to hospital personnel and how to say it in Chapter 14, "Communications."

Trauma Patient with No Significant Mechanism of Injury

When caring for a trauma patient who is responsive and has no significant mechanism of injury, you will have focused your assessment on just the areas the patient tells you hurt plus those areas that you suspect may be injured based on the mechanism of injury.

This kind of patient received all the assessment he needed while still at the scene. He does not generally need a detailed physical exam. It is important to keep a high index of suspicion, though. When in doubt, do a detailed physical exam. Be aware of the responsive trauma patient's fear and need for emotional support.

You should perform a detailed physical exam on a trauma patient who has a significant mechanism of injury and on any patient who has an unclear or unknown mechanism of injury. But the detailed physical exam is not meant for medical patients. This is because there are usually few signs an EMT-B can find in the physical exam of a medical patient that are significant or about which you can or should do anything. Most of the assessment information on medical patients comes from the history and vital signs.

Occasionally, you may come across a patient who could be either medical or trauma or both. For example, imagine you have responded to an elderly man who is found alone and unconscious, slumped over the steering wheel of his car. The car is off the road and there is no damage to it. Did the patient lose consciousness first and then drive his car off the road, or did he drive off the road and then get knocked out from a blow to the head? The safest and best thing to do for a patient like this is generally to treat him as a trauma patient who gets a rapid trauma assessment and, if there is time, a detailed physical exam—but whenever possible, also get a history from any witnesses you can find.

COMPARING ASSESSMENTS

Below are two scenarios that may help you see the difference between assessment of a trauma patient with a significant mechanism and assessment of a trauma patient with *no* significant mechanism of injury:

Clara Diller—Responsive Child with No Significant Mechanism of Injury

You have been dispatched to a 5-year-old girl, Clara, who has fallen while skating. She is crying and holding a bloody cloth to her knee. After completing the scene size-up and initial assessment, and deciding that she is not a priority for immediate transport, you begin the focused history and physical exam for a trauma patient.

Mechanism of Injury
The first step of the focused history and physical exam for a trauma patient is to reconsider the mechanism of injury. So you take a careful look around to be sure that Clara has only fallen down, not suffered a more severe incident like striking a pole or being hit by a car. There is no indication of this, and since a young child trying skates for the first time is unlikely to have been going very fast, even though a sidewalk is a hard surface to fall on, you conclude that Clara has no significant mechanism of injury. So you continue the on-scene assessment.

Chief Complaint
"Where do you hurt, Clara?" you ask her. You are not surprised when she says, "My knee hurts," because you can see that her knee is bleeding. Then she adds, "My head hurts, too." So you know that she may have struck her head. Based on the mechanism of injury—a fall to a hard surface, you suspect that she may have injured her spine as well. So you now focus your assessment according to the chief complaint and mechanism of injury. You focus not on Clara's whole body, but on her head, neck, spine, and knee.

Focused Physical Exam
You look at Clara's head and the back of her neck, searching for injuries such as contusions, abrasions, punctures or penetrations, burns, and lacerations. You find only some swelling on her forehead. Next, you gently press on her head and cervical spine, starting at the top, then moving to the back of her head and going down her neck to the large bump that indicates the lower end of the neck. You find no deformities, tenderness, or swelling. You now determine the proper cervical collar for a child Clara's size. You put it around her neck without moving her head or neck, while your partner continues to hold her head.

During the initial assessment, you controlled the bleeding from her knee. Now you tell her, "Clara, I need to lift up that cloth and look underneath. I'm going to feel around your knee, too. If it hurts, you can tell me. Okay?" Clara agrees, and you look at her knee for contusions, abrasions, punctures or penetrations, burns, or lacerations. There is only the laceration you found earlier. It is bleeding very slowly and does not appear to be deep. You palpate the area around the knee. You find no deformities or swelling, but the lateral side of the knee is tender.

Baseline Vital Signs
Next, you assess Clara's vital signs. Her pulse is 104 per minute, strong and regular. She has respirations of 24 per minute. They are normal in depth. You check her skin by looking at the palm of her hand and see

that it is pink. You feel it and determine that it is warm and dry. You squeeze the end of her fingernail and find that her capillary refill is normal. After telling Clara what you are going to do, you shine a light into her eyes and find that her pupils are equal and reactive. Again, you tell Clara what to expect before you inflate a pediatric cuff on her arm and find her blood pressure is 90/60.

History

While you are doing the focused exam, you ask Clara for more information. She is 5 years old, she tells you, and very scared because "my mommy told me not to try my new skates till later." The neighbor who takes care of Clara says, "I called Clara's mother at work when I saw her fall." You ask, "Did you see if Clara got knocked out? Even for a moment?" The neighbor tells you Clara did not lose consciousness.

Just now, Clara's mother arrives on scene. You reassure her that Clara seems to have just an injury to her knee and a slight bump on her head. You also explain that you have put a special collar on her just in case she injured her neck and that she will be placed on a spine board for the ride to the hospital.

Clara's mother is a better source of medical information than a 5-year-old, so you interview her for the SAMPLE history. You have already asked Clara what symptoms she has, so you ask her mother if Clara has any allergies or takes any medicines. You also ask about pertinent past history. She tells you that Clara has no allergies, takes no medicines, and is healthy. The neighbor tells you Clara's last food or drink was lunch a couple of hours ago. When you ask her about events leading to the injury, she tells you Clara has been feeling fine and acting normal today.

Detailed Physical Exam and Further Care

You immobilize Clara on a backboard and transport her to the emergency department. Although she has no significant mechanism of injury, there is time on the way to the hospital to do a detailed physical exam. You take special care in examining her head, since she had a bump on her forehead. You make no significant findings.

Clara's visit to the hospital is brief. Any serious head or spine injury is ruled out. She gets some ointment and a cartoon bandage for her knee. She talks excitedly about her ambulance ride all the way home.

Brian Sawyer—Unresponsive Adult with Significant Mechanism of Injury

You are caring for a young man who has been thrown to the pavement during a vehicle collision. After completing the scene size-up, you conducted an initial assessment during which you checked Brian's mental status, took steps to correct an airway problem, checked breathing and circulation, and applied high-concentration oxygen. Because your initial assessment revealed that he was unresponsive to pain and showed signs of diminished circulation (rapid, weak pulse and pale, clammy skin), you assigned Brian a high priority for rapid transport and now take just a few moments to conduct a rapid version of the focused history and physical exam for a trauma patient.

Mechanism of Injury

You have no opportunity to take a closer look at the car Brian was in because it is 20 feet away. Instead, you ask a police officer to inspect the car for any deformities that would indicate where Brian might have struck interior surfaces. The officer reports that there are no deformities in the interior of the car. However, the fact that Brian appears to have been thrown from the car is a *significant mechanism of injury*.

Manual Stabilization of the Head and Neck

Your partner started manual stabilization during the initial assessment. He continues to hold the head and neck in a neutral in-line position and keep the airway open.

Advanced Life Support Request

If you were in an area where paramedics are available to respond, this would be a good time to call them. However, in your area, you do not have this option, so you continue your focused history and physical exam.

Transport Decision

The priority you assigned Brian at the end of your initial assessment was high. After you reconsider the mechanism of injury, you confirm your decision to transport him quickly–just as soon as you complete a rapid focused history and physical exam.

Mental Status

Now you assess Brian's mental status. You determined during the initial assessment that he was unresponsive to pain. You confirm that this is still the case by pinching his shoulder muscle. There is still no response.

Rapid Trauma Assessment

The physical exam you do on Brian is different from the one you did on Clara. Clara did not have a significant mechanism of injury. She was able to tell you where she hurt, and you were able to focus your exam on just the parts identified by her complaint and mechanism of injury. You examined only her head, neck, and knee. Then you put on a cervical collar and dressed and bandaged her knee.

Brian is unresponsive to pain and cannot tell you what hurts. Even if he could, you would want to give him a more thorough exam because he had a significant mechanism of injury. Being thrown from a car during a collision is likely to produce more than just a localized cut or scrape. Yet, your examination of Brian must be speedy. You must do a more comprehensive exam than you did for Clara, but you must do it rapidly so that you can get Brian into the ambulance and en route to the hospital without delay.

So you now perform a rapid trauma assessment. As you inspect and palpate each part of his body, you look and feel for DCAP-BTLS. In addition, with particular areas of Brian's body, you also look for certain signs. You expose each part of the body as necessary. Your rapid trauma assessment of Brian goes as follows:

- *Head.* You assess Brian's head for DCAP-BTLS and crepitation (the sound or feel of broken bones rubbing against each other). You find a laceration on the back of his head that is not bleeding.

- *Neck.* You assess the neck for DCAP-BTLS, crepitation, and bulging or flat neck veins. There is no response from Brian when you palpate along his cervical spine. Brian's neck veins are flat, indicating possible blood loss, but no other abnormalities.

- *Stabilization.* You now size and apply a cervical collar. Your partner continues to hold manual stabilization as well.

- *Chest.* Next, you open Brian's shirt and assess his chest for DCAP-BTLS, crepitation, breath sounds, and paradoxical motion (movements of part of the chest in a direction that is different from the rest of the chest). You find no abnormalities.

- *Abdomen.* When you cut open Brian's trousers and assess his abdomen for DCAP-BTLS, you also check for firmness, softness, and distention. Brian's abdomen is very firm but does not look distended.

- *Pelvis.* Next, you assess Brian's pelvis for DCAP-BTLS. You find no abnormalities. Since he is not able to complain of any pain in the pelvis, you compress it gently to determine tenderness or motion. You find nothing unusual, except for confirming that his mental status is still such that he does not respond to any pain from compression.

- *Extremities.* Now you quickly assess all four extremities for DCAP-BTLS, plus distal pulse, motor function, and sensation. You find a deformity in Brian's right lower leg. You do not pause to splint the leg now but will tend to it en route to the hospital. He has weak pulses in all extremities and does not respond to a pinch there. Since he is not responsive, you cannot determine whether he has sensation or motor function.

- *Posterior and immobilization.* A firefighter has gotten a backboard from your ambulance and places it next to Brian. You and your partner roll Brian onto his side as a unit and cut away his clothing to assess his posterior body, inspecting and palpating for DCAP-BTLS. You find nothing abnormal. The firefighter places the board next to Brian and you roll him back onto the board.

You have been able to conduct the entire assessment in just a few moments. If any life-threatening problem had been discovered before or during the rapid trauma assessment, you would have altered the procedure as needed to allow for treatment of the problem.

Baseline Vital Signs
You quickly assess Brian's baseline vital signs. He has a pulse of 120, regular and weak. His respirations are 20 per minute. His skin is pale, cool, and sweaty. His left pupil is dilated and slow to react (the right pupil reacts normally to light). He has a blood pressure of 130/80.

History
No one is available to give you a SAMPLE history. You did not come across any medical identification bracelet or necklace when you assessed Brian's extremities and neck.

Detailed Physical Exam
Inside the ambulance, before conducting a detailed physical exam on Brian, you first ensure that any critical interventions are performed. You accomplish this by repeating your initial assessment. Your general impression is that he appears to have serious injuries. His mental status is still unresponsive to pain. You are now managing his airway with an oropharyngeal airway and suction. You are giving him high-concentration oxygen, but he is breathing adequately and you do not need to ventilate him. A check of his circulation shows that his radial pulse is still rapid and weak, there is no external bleeding, and his skin is pale, cool, and sweaty.

After you feel certain that Brian's ABCs are under control, you have time to undertake the detailed physical exam. You reassess his head. The main difference from the rapid trauma assessment you did at the scene is that now you pay special attention to several areas you did not evaluate in detail before: the scalp and cranium, face, ears, eyes, nose, and mouth.

You gently palpate Brian's cranium for DCAP-BTLS and crepitation. You inspect your gloves for blood and find none. You assess Brian's face for DCAP-BTLS, gently palpating his cheekbones, forehead, and lower jaw. You inspect and palpate his ears, searching for DCAP-BTLS and drainage. You see a little bit of blood in the left ear. You also gently bend each of his ears forward to look for bruising, but find none.

Next, you assess Brian's eyes, inspecting for the usual DCAP-BTLS and discoloration, unequal pupils, foreign bodies, and blood in the front of the eye. His left pupil is dilated and slow to react. You do not see any blood in the front of his eye or any other abnormalities.

Next, you assess Brian's nose, inspecting and palpating for injuries or signs of injury. In this case, you look not only for DCAP-BTLS, but also for drainage and bleeding. You do not find any.

When you assess his mouth, you open it and look for DCAP-BTLS, loose or broken teeth, other objects that could cause obstruction, swelling or laceration of the tongue, unusual breath odor, and discoloration. You do not find any of these.

STREET SCENES

It's Saturday night, and you've been assigned to one of the ambulances that covers downtown, where there is usually some kind of excitement going on. As you sit in quarters, you're listening to the scanner. The police seem to be busy with a variety of calls—disturbances, domestics, and larcenies to name a few. Then you hear on the police frequency: "Dispatch, we need an ambulance ASAP. We have a stabbing here." You don't wait for your pager to activate before you're in the ambulance bay with your partner. The pager follows shortly: "Delta 55, respond to 1512 Broadway, outside, for a stabbing. Police on the scene, and scene is secure."

Your response takes only a few minutes. When you arrive, you see a male in his 20s lying on the sidewalk. "What happened?" you ask him.

"I was mugged, hit in the face, and thrown to the ground."

At this point, you tell the patient not to move his head and that you will help by manually stabilizing it. The patient continues: "When I tried to fight them off, they stabbed me in the chest."

The patient's airway is open, but the patient is out of breath and his breathing is rapid and shallow. You check the chest and see the entrance wound. You listen for breath sounds. There is silence on the side of the wound. You put on an occlusive dressing and administer oxygen by nonrebreather. You rapidly check for external bleeding.

STREET SCENE QUESTIONS

1. What is the priority of this patient?
2. What should be done next?
3. When should vital signs be taken?

You and your partner agree that this patient needs to be rapidly transported to the trauma center. You are still holding manual stabilization of the patient's head and neck, so your partner gets a backboard and collar. A quick focused physical exam is done from head to toe. The patient has abrasions on the left cheek, the left wrist is swollen with pain on movement, and there is tenderness in both lower abdominal quadrants. A set of vital signs is taken. The SAMPLE history will be done in the ambulance. The patient is immobilized to the backboard with head immobilizer in place. During this transfer, the patient's back is checked for any wound, bleeding, and tenderness.

Once the patient is loaded in the ambulance, your partner starts toward the hospital with red light and siren. The patient is still conscious, but he is having trouble talking in complete sentences. He reports a lot of discomfort. You think there may be pressure building up in his chest because of injury to the lung.

STREET SCENE QUESTIONS

4. What should you do next?
5. What should be done for the detailed assessment, if there is time before reaching the trauma center?
6. How will DCAP-BTLS help with the assessment?

You are confident that you need to treat the patient's worsening difficulty breathing. You lift the corner of the occlusive dressing and hear some air escape. The patient starts to breathe easier almost immediately. Another set of vital signs is taken. Then the bandage over the chest wound is secured again, but only on three sides. You turn your attention to the detailed assessment, starting at the head, then chest and abdomen, and finally all four extremities. With each location, you use DCAP-BTLS to remind yourself to check for deformities, contusions, abrasions, punctures, burns, tenderness, lacerations, and swelling.

The remainder of the transport is uneventful and care is transitioned with an updated prehospital care report including the latest set of vital signs.

You go on to reassess Brian's neck, chest, abdomen, pelvis, extremities, and posterior body as you did during the rapid trauma assessment. You find no changes.

The last step in the detailed physical exam is to repeat Brian's vital signs. You obtain a pulse of 136, regular and weak; respirations of 14 per minute; skin that is still cool, pale, and sweaty; a left pupil that is still dilated and slow to react; and a blood pressure of 100/70—indicating a more rapid pulse, slower respirations, and a lower blood pressure than during the rapid trauma assessment at the scene.

You continue to care for Brian as the ambulance proceeds toward the hospital.

CHAPTER REVIEW

Summary

The focused history and physical exam of the trauma patient takes place immediately after the initial assessment. It starts with a reconsideration of the mechanism of injury. This allows you to determine which path you are going to take in assessing a patient.

The patient without a significant mechanism of injury receives a physical exam focused on areas that the patient complains about and areas that you think may be injured based on the mechanism of injury. It is important to have a high index of suspicion and evaluate any areas that you feel may have been injured. When in doubt, assess it. Next, is a set of baseline vital signs and a SAMPLE history.

The patient who has a significant mechanism of injury receives a somewhat different assessment. Assure continued manual stabilization of the head and neck, consider whether to call advanced life support personnel (if available), reconsider how urgently to transport the patient, reassess mental status, and then perform a rapid trauma assessment. In the rapid trauma assessment look for deformities, contusions, abrasions, punctures and penetrations, burns, tenderness, lacerations, and swelling, plus certain additional signs appropriate to the part being assessed (as summarized in Table 10-3). Systematically examine the head, neck, chest, abdomen, pelvis, extremities, and posterior body. After assessing the neck, apply a cervical collar. After completing the physical assessment, immobilize the patient to a spine board and get a baseline set of vital signs and a SAMPLE history.

After you have performed the appropriate critical interventions and transport has begun, the patient may receive a detailed physical exam en route to the hospital.

The detailed physical exam is every similar to the rapid trauma assessment, but it has several differences. A few more areas are assessed (scalp, cranium, face, ears, eyes, nose, and mouth). There is time to be more thorough in the assessment. And the detailed physical exam does not take place before transport unless transport is delayed.

The detailed physical exam is most appropriate for the trauma patient who is unresponsive or has a significant or unknown mechanism of injury. A responsive trauma patient with no significant mechanism of injury will seldom require a detailed physical exam. A detailed physical exam is not appropriate for most medical patients.

Key Terms

colostomy [ko-LOS-to-me] like an ileostomy, a surgical opening in the wall of the abdomen with a bag in place to collect excretions from the digestive system.

crepitation [krep-uh-TAY-shun] the grating sound or feeling of broken bones rubbing together.

DCAP-BTLS a memory aid to remember deformities, contusions, abrasions, puncture/penetrations, and symptoms of injury found by inspection or palpation during patient assessment.

detailed physical exam an assessment of the head, neck, chest, abdomen, pelvis, extremities, and posterior of the body to detect signs and symptoms of injury. It differs from the rapid trauma assessment only in that it also includes examination of the face, ears, eyes, nose, and mouth during the examination of the head, it may be done less rapidly, and it may be done en route to the hospital after earlier on-scene assessments and interventions are completed.

distention [dis-TEN-shun] a condition of being stretched, inflated, or larger than normal.

focused history and physical exam the step of patient assessment that follows the initial assessment.

ileostomy [il-e-OS-to-me] See *colostomy*.

jugular [JUG-yuh-ler] **vein distention (JVD)** bulging of the neck veins.

paradoxical [pair-uh-DOCK-si-kal] **motion** movement of a part of the chest in the opposite direction to the rest of the chest during respiration.

priapism [PRY-ah-pizm] persistent erection of the penis that may result from spinal injury and some medical problems.

rapid trauma assessment a rapid assessment of the head, neck, chest, abdomen, pelvis, extremities, and posterior of the body to detect signs and symptoms of injury.

stoma [STO-ma] a permanent surgical opening in the neck through which the patient breathes.

tracheostomy [TRAY-ke-OS-to-me] a surgical incision held open by a metal or plastic tube.

REVIEW QUESTIONS

1. Explain why it is important to reconsider the mechanism of injury at the beginning of the focused history and physical exam of a trauma patient. (pp. 197–199, 210)
2. Explain how the focused history and physical exam of a trauma patient with a significant mechanism of injury differs from that of a trauma patient with no significant mechanism of injury. (p. 226)
3. Name the signs and symptoms for which the letters DCAP-BTLS stand. (p. 199)
4. List the steps of the rapid trauma assessment and describe the kind of patient for whom the rapid trauma assessment is appropriate. (pp. 211–212)
5. What are the additional areas that you assess in the detailed physical exam that you did not evaluate in the rapid trauma assessment? (pp. 219–221, 225–226)
6. List the areas covered in the detailed physical exam. What do you look and feel for as you assess each of these areas? (pp. 219–221, 225–226)

APPLICATIONS

As an EMT-B, how would you balance the need for appropriate on-scene assessment and treatment with the need for speed in getting the patient to the hospital in each of the following situations?

- You arrive at the residence to find a patient who explains that he has accidentally cut his finger with a kitchen knife. The cut is bleeding profusely.

- You arrive at a schoolyard to find a girl who bystanders say was shot by a rival gang member. She is lying in a pool of blood but is able to speak to you.

- You are called to respond to a man who has been found unconscious on a sidewalk next to an apartment building in the middle of the night. There were no witnesses to explain what may have happened to him.

WEB MEDIC

Visit Brady's *Emergency Care* website for direct weblinks. At **www.bradybooks.com/ emergencycare**, you will find information related to the following Chapter 10 topics:

- Statistics on trauma injury
- Breath sounds

Chapter
Eleven

ASSESSMENT OF THE MEDICAL PATIENT

*W*ord on the Street

"What's the first question you should ask somebody? *What's your name?* It reminds you and everyone around you that you're not just dealing with some medical problem and, most importantly, it reminds the patient as well. Then, listen—for the appropriateness of the response, the quality of the speech, the language, and the comfort level in the voice. Look—at the symmetry of the face and the expression on it, at the eyes and pupils, at the skin color and moisture. Touch—to identify yourself as a helper and to feel the temperature. Three seconds, tops, and you know if the guy's in trouble or not."

Thom Hillson Field Supervisor

The key to moving from the initial assessment into the focused history and physical exam is reconsideration of the mechanism of injury, as well as of the patient's complaint. If there is a mechanism of injury, you will perform the focused history and physical exam for the trauma patient, which was described in Chapter 10. When the patient has a complaint that is medical in nature, and you have confirmed that there is no significant mechanism of injury, you will perform the focused history and physical exam for the medical patient—the subject of this chapter.

FOCUSED HISTORY AND PHYSICAL EXAM FOR A MEDICAL PATIENT

Responsive Medical Patient

As you learned in Chapter 8, "Initial Assessment," it makes a great deal of difference in the assessment process whether the patient is responsive or unresponsive. This is especially true of the medical patient. In trauma patients, there are often many external signs of trauma, or injury, but this is not true of a medical condition. The most important source of information about a medical patient's condition is what the patient can tell you. This is why, when the patient is awake and responsive, obtaining the patient's history comes first.

A good example of the kind of patient you will see often is awake and has a medical problem, with no immediately life-threatening problems. After you finish the initial assessment for this patient, perform a focused history and physical exam. This will tell you what you need to know in order to administer the proper treatment.

The focused history and physical exam for a medical patient has four parts: history of the present illness, SAMPLE history, focused physical exam, and baseline vital signs (Scan 11-1 and Table 11-1).

Take a History of the Present Illness

The interview you do with a patient is similar to the interview a physician conducts before a physical examination. It is a conversational information-gathering effort. Not only will you gain needed information from the interview, but you will also reduce the patient's fear and promote cooperation.

Study Guide for **FHPE—Responsive Medical Patient**

✔ History of the present illness
✔ SAMPLE history
✔ Focused physical exam
✔ Baseline vital signs

Relatives and bystanders may also serve as sources of information, but the most important source is the patient. Do not interview relatives and bystanders before you interview the patient unless the patient is unconscious or unable to communicate. You may gain information from bystanders and medical identification devices later, while you are conducting the physical examination.

TOPIC OVERVIEW

In this chapter, you will learn about the following topics:

- How to perform a focused history and physical examination for a medical patient

- The difference between patients who need a rapid physical assessment vs. patients who need a focused history and physical exam

- How to obtain a history of the present illness

- How to use the OPQRST mnemonic for history taking

DOT OBJECTIVES

✔ **Knowledge and Attitude**

1. Describe the unique needs for assessing an individual with a specific chief complaint with no known prior history. (p. 237)

2. Differentiate between the history and physical exam that is performed for responsive patients with no known prior history and responsive patients with a known prior history. (p. 234) (Scan 11-1, pp. 235–236)

3. Describe the needs for assessing an individual who is unresponsive. (pp. 238, 240–241) (Scan 11-2, p. 239)

4. Differentiate between the assessment that is performed for a patient who is unresponsive or has an altered mental status and other medical patients requiring assessment. (p. 234)

5. Attend to the feelings that these patients might be experiencing. (p. 234)

✔ **Skills**

1. Demonstrate the patient assessment skills that should be used to assist a patient who is responsive with no known history.

2. Demonstrate the patient assessment skills that should be used to assist a patient who is unresponsive or has an altered mental status.

TABLE 11-1 Focused History and Physical Exam—Medical Patient

Responsive Patient	Unresponsive Patient

1. Gather the history of the present illness: (OPQRST) from patient:
  Onset
  Provokes
  Quality
  Radiation
  Severity
  Time
	1. Conduct a rapid physical exam:
	  Head
	  Neck
	  Chest
	  Abdomen
	  Pelvis
	  Extremities
	  Posterior

2. Gather a SAMPLE history from the patient:
  Signs and symptoms
  Allergies
  Medications
  Pertinent past history
  Last oral intake
  Events leading to the illness
	2. Obtain baseline vital signs:
	  Respirations
	  Pulse
	  Skin
	  Pupils
	  Blood pressure

3. Conduct a focused physical exam (focusing on the area the patient complains about).	3. Gather the history of the present illness: (OPQRST) from family or bystanders:
	  Onset
	  Provokes
	  Quality
	  Radiation
	  Severity
	  Time

4. Obtain baseline vital signs:
  Respirations
  Pulse
  Skin
  Pupils
  Blood pressure
	4. Gather a SAMPLE history from bystanders or family:
	  Signs and symptoms
	  Allergies
	  Medications
	  Pertinent past history
	  Last oral intake
	  Events leading to the illness

Note: This table shows the general order of steps. You may alter this order in accordance with the situation and the number of EMTs available and when the patient's condition warrants immediate action due to immediate life threats.

FOCUSED HISTORY AND PHYSICAL EXAM— RESPONSIVE MEDICAL PATIENT

FIRST take BSI precautions.

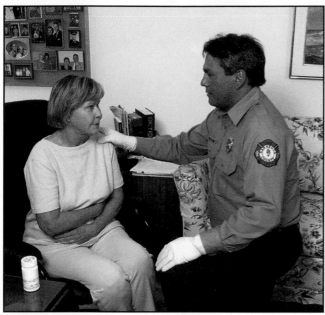

▲ **HISTORY OF PRESENT ILLNESS.** Ask the "OPQRST" questions:
Onset
Provokes
Quality
Radiation
Severity
Time

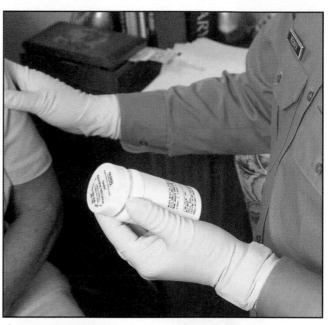

▲ **SAMPLE HISTORY.** Ask the SAMPLE questions:
Signs and symptoms
Allergies
Medications
Pertinent past history
Last oral intake
Events leading to the illness

(continued)

▲ **FOCUSED PHYSICAL EXAM.** Perform a quick assessment of affected body part or system:
Head
Neck
Chest
Abdomen
Pelvis
Extremities
Posterior

▲ **VITAL SIGNS.** Assess the patient's baseline vital signs:
Respiration
Pulse
Skin color, temperature, condition (and capillary refill in infants and children)
Pupils
Blood pressure

▲ **INTERVENTIONS AND TRANSPORT.** Perform interventions as needed, transport the patient, and contact on-line medical direction as needed.

One purpose of talking to the patient is to find out his chief complaint, the one thing that seems most seriously wrong to him. When you ask the patient what is wrong, he may tell you that several things are bothering him. If this happens, ask what is bothering him most. Find out if the patient is in pain and where he hurts. Unless the pain of one injury or medical problem masks that of another, most people will be able to tell you of painful areas.

Try to ask open-ended questions, or questions that the patient answers with responses other than "Yes" or "No." For example, do not ask "Is your chest pain dull and crushing?" Ask instead "How would you describe your pain?" In this way, you will avoid giving the patient the impression that you want a particular answer. If the patient says that he cannot describe his pain, you can try giving him several choices: "Is your pain dull, or sharp, or burning?"

An easy way to remember the questions to ask to obtain a history of the present illness is to use the letters **OPQRST**:

- *Onset.* What were you doing when it started?
- *Provokes.* Can you think of anything that might have triggered this pain?
- *Quality.* Can you describe it for me?
- *Radiation.* Where exactly is the pain? Does it seem to spread anywhere or does it stay right there?
- *Severity.* You look uncomfortable. How bad is the pain?
- *Time.* When did the pain start? Has it changed at all since it started?

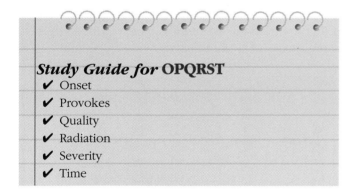

Study Guide for OPQRST
✔ Onset
✔ Provokes
✔ Quality
✔ Radiation
✔ Severity
✔ Time

Take a SAMPLE History
After finding out the patient's age, you should then get the rest of the SAMPLE history (as you learned in Chapter 9) and the name of his personal physician:

- *Signs/symptoms.* Have you had any other symptoms?
- *Allergies.* Are you allergic to anything?
- *Medications.* What medicines do you take? What do you take those for?

- *Pertinent past history.* Do you have any other medical problems? Have you ever had this kind of problem before? Who is your doctor?
- *Last oral intake.* When was the last time you ate or drank anything? What did you eat or drink?
- *Events leading to the illness.* How have you felt today? Anything out of the ordinary?

Specific Chief Complaint/No Known Prior History. Often the patient whose history you are gathering has no known prior history. For example, a patient who complains of breathing difficulty may answer "No" when you ask him if he has ever had this kind of problem before. This and other questions you ask as part of the SAMPLE history may tell you that the patient has not been under treatment for this problem and does not have any medicines on hand for the problem that you might want to assist the patient in taking. You will generally transport this patient to the hospital and provide the information to the emergency department staff.

Specific Chief Complaint/Known Prior History. Often, during the SAMPLE history interview, you will learn from your patient that he has a history relating to his chief complaint. Your patient has had this problem or something related to it before and may be under a physician's care for the problem. The patient can tell you what medical condition the current complaint probably relates to. For example, a woman with vaginal bleeding may be pregnant or have just undergone an abortion. A man who suffers a seizure may explain that he is an epileptic. Knowing this history may help you determine what interventions you can take at the scene or en route to the hospital, as well as providing information that you will give to the hospital staff. Chapters that appear later in this book will cover these and other situations and the specific prehospital interventions you can perform.

There are three situations involving a known prior history of the medical complaint that deserve special mention here. They are different from other medical emergencies because the patient may carry part of the treatment with him, and because the past medical history is essential in determining the prehospital treatment. The three situations are:

- Patient with difficulty breathing who has an inhaler prescribed by his physician
- Patient with chest pain who has nitroglycerin prescribed by his physician
- Patient with an allergic reaction who has an epinephrine auto-injector prescribed by his physician

In each of these cases, the patient has been evaluated by his physician, has been determined to have a condition that can be treated with medication the patient can carry, and has filled a prescription for that medication. You will learn more about these conditions, also, later in this book.

When a medical patient does not have a condition for which you have an intervention, you should generally transport the patient to the hospital. Similarly, when you have a patient with difficulty breathing, chest pain, or an allergic reaction, but the patient does not have his medication or has not received a prescription for a medication, you should generally transport the patient. *Note that you will generally transport the patient to the hospital even if he does have medication you can assist him in taking.* In fact, you may load the patient into the ambulance and assist him with his medication en route.

🧒 Pediatric Notes

When gathering a history from a child, be sure to kneel or find another way to get on the same level with the child. Put the OPQRST and SAMPLE questions in simple language the child can understand. Note that much of the history for a child and all of the information for an infant will need to be gathered from the parents, guardian, or other adult caretaker.

Perform a Focused Physical Exam

With responsive medical patients, the EMT-B's physical exam is usually brief. You will gather most of the important assessment information in this type of patient from the history and vital signs. The physical exam procedure will be the same as you learned for the trauma patient in Chapter 10. For each part of the body you examine, you will inspect and palpate for DCAP-BTLS (deformities, contusions, abrasions, punctures/penetrations, burns, tenderness, lacerations, swelling) plus the information that is specific to each body part. (Review Table 10-3 and Scan 10-1 in Chapter 10.) For the responsive medical patient, focus the exam on the body part that the patient has a complaint about. For example, if the patient complains of abdominal pain, you will inspect and palpate his abdomen.

How and Why?

Palpation is more than just pressing on a body part. There is a specific technique and a specific order in which to do it. Go to your Electronic Extras CD for more information on effective palpation.

Obtain Baseline Vital Signs

A complete set of baseline vital signs is essential to the assessment of a medical patient. Later assessments of the vital signs will be compared to the baseline set obtained during the focused history and physical exam to determine trends in the patient's condition.

Administer Interventions and Transport the Patient

In later chapters, you will learn when to provide treatment for specific medical conditions. The only treatment you have learned about so far that might be appropriate for a responsive patient is oxygen.

Unresponsive Medical Patient

For an unresponsive medical patient, the sequence of assessment is not the same as for a responsive medical patient. If the patient were responsive, the first step of your focused history and physical exam would be talking with the patient to obtain the history of his present illness and the SAMPLE history, followed by performing the physical exam and gathering the baseline vital signs. For an unresponsive patient, the process is done in reverse (Table 11-1 and Scan 11-2). Since you cannot obtain a history from the patient, you will begin with the physical exam and baseline vital signs. After these procedures, you will gather as much of the patient's history as you can from any bystanders or family members who may be present.

Another difference between the focused history and physical exam for both the responsive and unresponsive patients is the nature of the physical exam. For a responsive patient, you will be able to focus your exam on just the part of the body the patient complains of. Since an unresponsive patient cannot tell you where the problem is, you will need to do a rapid assessment of the entire body.

Study Guide for FHPE—Unresponsive Medical Patient

- ✔ Perform a rapid physical exam.
- ✔ Obtain baseline vital signs.
- ✔ Consider request for advanced life support.
- ✔ Take a history of the present illness and a SAMPLE history from family or bystanders.

Perform a Rapid Physical Exam

The physical exam of an unresponsive medical patient will be almost the same as the physical exam for a trauma patient. You will rapidly assess the patient's head, neck, chest, abdomen, pelvis, extremities, and

FOCUSED HISTORY AND PHYSICAL EXAM— UNRESPONSIVE MEDICAL PATIENT

FIRST take BSI precautions.

▲ **RAPID PHYSICAL EXAM.** Perform a rapid assessment of the entire body:
Head
Neck
Chest
Abdomen
Pelvis
Extremities
Posterior

▲ **VITAL SIGNS.** Assess the patient's baseline vital signs:
Respiration
Pulse
Skin color, temperature, condition (and capillary refill in infants and children)
Pupils
Blood pressure

▲ **SAMPLE HISTORY.** Interview family and bystanders to get as much information as possible about the patient's problem:
Signs and symptoms
Allergies
Medications
Pertinent past history
Last oral intake
Events leading to the illness

▲ **INTERVENTIONS AND TRANSPORT.** Contact on-line medical direction as needed, perform interventions as needed, transport the patient.

239

posterior. As you assess each area, you will look for signs of injury such as deformities, contusions, abrasions, penetrations, burns, tenderness, lacerations, and swelling (DCAP-BTLS). Other things to look for in the medical patient include:

- Neck: jugular vein distention, medical identification devices
- Chest: presence and equality of breath sounds
- Abdomen: distention, firmness or rigidity
- Pelvis: incontinence of urine or feces
- Extremities: pulse, motor function, sensation, medical identification devices

Medical ID Devices. Medical identification devices can provide important information. One of the most commonly used medical identification devices is the Medic Alert emblem shown in Figure 11-1. Over one million people wear a medical identification device in the form of a necklace or a wrist or ankle bracelet. One side of the device has a Star of Life emblem. The patient's medical problem is engraved on the reverse side, along with a telephone number to call for additional information.

When doing the physical exam, look for necklaces and bracelets or wallet cards. Never assume you know the form of every medical identification device. Check any necklace or bracelet carefully, taking care when moving the patient or any of his extremities. You should alert the emergency department staff when you arrive that the patient is wearing or carrying medical identification and tell them what is on it (diabetes or heart condition, for example).

Obtain Baseline Vital Signs

Assess the patient's pulse, respirations, skin, pupils, and blood pressure and note any abnormalities. Be sure to record your observations so later vital signs assessments can be compared with these baseline observations.

Consider a Request for ALS Personnel

In accordance with local protocols, and if advanced life support personnel are available, consider at this time if the additional services paramedics can provide would benefit your patient.

If you are serving in a rural area or other area where you do not have the option of requesting advanced life support, and if you are very distant from a hospital, there may be a closer local clinic or other health facility that has an arrangement to provide advanced care. Consider if it is worth a delay to stop at such a facility for the special care that may help stabilize your patient before you continue transporting the patient to the hospital.

If arrangements like these exist where you work as an EMT-B, you must be familiar with the types of patients this facility can help. The arrangements should be in writing in order to reduce confusion and prevent loss of precious time with critical patients.

Take a History of the Present Illness and a SAMPLE History

Since an unresponsive patient cannot talk, you will have to interview bystanders to get as much information as possible. When interviewing bystanders, determine if any are relatives or friends of the patient. They usually have more information to provide about past problems than other bystanders would have. See which of the bystanders saw what happened. When questioning bystanders, you should ask:

- *What is the patient's name?* If the patient is obviously a minor, ask if the parent or guardian is present or if he or she has been contacted.
- *What happened?* You may be told that the patient fell off a ladder, appeared to faint, fell to the ground and began seizing, was hit on the head by a falling object, or other possible clues.
- *Did the bystander see anything else?* For example, was the patient clutching his chest or head before he fell?
- *Did the patient complain of anything before this happened?* You may learn of chest pain, nausea, concern about odors where he was working, or other clues to the problem.
- *Does the patient have any known illnesses or problems?* This may provide you with information about heart problems, alcohol abuse, allergies, or other problems that could cause a change in the patient's condition.

Figure 11-1 A medical identification device.

- *Is the patient taking any medications?* Be sure to use the word "medications" or "medicines." If you say "drugs" or some other term, bystanders may not answer you, thinking that you are asking questions as part of a criminal investigation. In rare cases, you may feel that the bystanders are holding back information because the patient was abusing drugs. Remind them that you are an EMT-B and you need all the information they can give you so proper care can begin.

While gathering the patient's history, you should also see if there is a "Vial of Life" or similar type of sticker on the main outside door, closest window to the main door, or the refrigerator door. If so, patient information and medications can usually be found in the refrigerator. (The Vial of Life is not used in all regions.)

Administer Interventions and Transport the Patient

There is not usually much information gained from the focused history and physical examination of an unresponsive medical patient that will change treatment in the field. The most important thing to look for is mechanism of injury or signs of injury that would make you suspect a spine injury. Either of these would mean that you need to immobilize the patient's spine. Most of the time, the information you gather in your assessment of unresponsive medical patients will be particularly helpful to the staff in the emergency department. Emergency physicians and nurses depend on EMT-Bs to evaluate the scene carefully and to gather as much useful information as possible that they cannot get in the hospital.

COMPARING ASSESSMENTS

Below are two scenarios that may help you see the difference between assessment of a responsive medical patient and assessment of an unresponsive medical patient.

Mr. Schmidt—Responsive Adult Medical Patient

You have been dispatched to an older man who is complaining of stomach pain. After completing the scene size-up, you conduct the initial assessment. You determine that Mr. Schmidt is alert and that his airway, breathing, and circulation are not compromised. You decide that he is a medical patient with no immediately life-threatening problems and you proceed to the focused history and physical exam for a medical patient.

History
You tell Mr. Schmidt that you need to get some information about his condition. You start by asking him questions that will give you the history of the present illness:

You: When did the pain start, Mr. Schmidt?
Mr. Schmidt: About two hours ago.

You: Can you describe it for me?
Mr. Schmidt: It's kind of a burning pain.

You: Has it changed at all since it started?
Mr. Schmidt: It's gotten worse, especially in the last hour.

You: Where exactly is the pain?
Mr. Schmidt: (points to his upper abdomen) Right here.

You: Does it seem to spread anywhere or does it stay right there?
Mr. Schmidt: It just stays right here.

You: What were you doing when it started?
Mr. Schmidt: I was talking with my wife.

You: Can you think of anything that might have triggered this pain?
Mr. Schmidt: No, not really.

You: You look uncomfortable. How bad is the pain?
Mr. Schmidt: Pretty bad. I've never had a pain this bad.

Now that you have the history of the present illness, you can find out the patient's age and proceed with the rest of the SAMPLE history:

You: How old are you, Mr. Schmidt?
Mr. Schmidt: I'm 68.

You: Have you had any other symptoms?
Mr. Schmidt: Well, I've been sick to my stomach.

You: Do you have any pain in your chest, arms, neck, or shoulders?
Mr. Schmidt: No.

You: Have you vomited?
Mr. Schmidt: No.

You: Have you had any diarrhea?
Mr. Schmidt: No.

You: Are you allergic to anything?
Mr. Schmidt: Just cats.

You: What medicines do you take?
Mr. Schmidt: Ibuprofen and Minipress.

You: What do you take those for?
Mr. Schmidt: I have arthritis and high blood pressure.

You: Do you have any other medical problems?
Mr. Schmidt: No.

You: Have you ever had this kind of problem before?
Mr. Schmidt: No.

You: Who is your doctor?
Mr. Schmidt: Dr. Anderson.

You: When was the last time you ate or drank anything?
Mr. Schmidt: I had dinner about three hours ago.

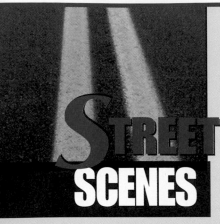

Just as we sat down to eat lunch, our ambulance was dispatched to a local health club for a 50-year-old female having an asthma attack. Upon arrival, we found the scene to be safe. Taking BSI precautions, we were directed to the women's locker room where we found our patient sitting on a workout bench.

"Hello. How can we help you today?" I asked. My general impression was of an alert middle-aged woman in moderate respiratory distress.

"Oh, I'm having an asthma attack," she said. I could see her airway was open, but breathing was rapid and moderately labored. I observed no bleeding, found her skin to be normal, and her radial pulse to be slightly rapid but strong and regular.

STREET SCENE QUESTIONS

1. What priority is this patient?
2. What are the next steps in the management of this patient?

Satisfied there were no life threats for which I had to provide immediate intervention, I determined this patient's priority to be medium in severity with the potential to get worse.

"What's your name?" I asked. She told me her name was Andrea.

"What were you doing when the difficulty breathing started?" I asked. It turned out she had been exercising on the treadmill. I noted she spoke in complete sentences and did not have to stop every few words to catch her breath. I asked Juan, my partner, to begin administering oxygen by way of a nonrebreather mask. While Juan was doing that, I continued my examination.

You: How have you felt today? Anything out of the ordinary?

Mr. Schmidt: No, it was a pretty normal day.

Focused Physical Exam

The next step in assessment is a focused physical exam. Since Mr. Schmidt is complaining of abdominal pain, you unbutton his shirt to expose his abdomen so you can inspect and palpate it. His abdomen does not appear distended, but there is some tenderness in the upper half.

Vital Signs

Next, you assess Mr. Schmidt's baseline vital signs. His pulse is 92, regular and full. Respirations are 20 and unlabored. Skin is normal (warm, pink, and dry). Blood pressure is 140/86. Because his complaint is of abdominal pain, which has no relationship to the brain, you do not need to check his pupils.

Together, the initial assessment, history, physical exam, and vital signs did not give you any reason to believe that Mr. Schmidt needed oxygen. (If your protocols had told you to, however, or if you wished, you could have given Mr. Schmidt oxygen. It would not harm him.) Throughout the exam you reassured Mr. Schmidt and tried to calm his fears. Now you move Mr. Schmidt to your stretcher and put him in the position in which he is most comfortable: sitting. You and your partner move him to the ambulance and begin the trip to the hospital.

Mrs. Malone—Unresponsive Adult Medical Patient

You arrive at the home of an older woman whose daughter has reported that she cannot waken her mother. After completing the scene size-up, you conduct the initial assessment. You find that Mrs. Malone only responds to verbal stimulus by moaning. Her airway is endangered because of her depressed level of responsiveness and the fact that she is supine. Your partner performs a head-tilt, chin-lift to open and protect the airway and you provide high-concentration oxygen by nonrebreather mask. Her circulation is normal. Because of her depressed level of responsiveness and threatened airway, you determine that Mrs. Malone is a high priority for transport to the hospital—but before loading her into the ambulance you will quickly conduct the focused history and physical exam for a medical patient.

Rapid Physical Exam

Because Mrs. Malone is unresponsive, you have no way of knowing what part of her body to focus on. So you do a rapid assessment of her head, neck, chest, abdomen, pelvis, extremities, and posterior in just the same way as you would for an unresponsive trauma patient. As you assess each area of her body, you remove enough clothing to be able to inspect and palpate it, then quickly replace the clothing. You find no abnormalities.

3. What part of the focused history and physical exam should follow next?

4. What signs or symptoms would you look for to determine if the patient was getting better or worse?

"What do you think caused your shortness of breath?" I asked. She told me that she's had a mild case of asthma for about 10 years and that it was exercise induced. I asked how long she had been having trouble breathing with this episode. "About 10 minutes," she said.

I knew that many asthmatics carry their own medication for asthma, so I asked what medications she was taking. "I have an inhaler, but I left it at home. I think it's called Al Butterball or something like that." I asked her if it was "albuterol" and she nodded her head.

Meanwhile, Juan had placed the oxygen mask on Andrea's face. I asked if she was allergic to anything and she shook her head no. While I listened to lung sounds, Juan obtained baseline vitals. I noted that the lung sounds were equal but noisy, like a whistling sound. Juan informed me that her pulse was 120 and regular; skin was warm and dry; respirations were 24 and slightly labored; and her blood pressure was 130/70.

Andrea accepted our offer to transport her to the emergency department, so we put her on the stretcher in her position of comfort, sitting up. During the short trip to the hospital, I used the radio to inform the emergency department of our patient's condition and treatment, took another set of vital signs, and re-assessed the patient. She appeared to be a little better, but her breathing was still slightly labored and a little noisy. She did not have any of the signs that would have made me think she was getting worse, things like retractions above the clavicles and between the ribs, the ability to speak only a few words at a time, and cyanosis, particularly of the lips and nailbeds. After we transferred Andrea to the care of the emergency department staff, we returned to service.

Vital Signs

Your partner finds that Mrs. Malone has a pulse of 92, strong and regular. Her respirations are 20, full and non-labored. Skin is cool and dry. Pupils are equal and reactive. Blood pressure is 160/90. Everything is in the normal range except for her high blood pressure. You note this, but it does not require any action on your part.

You have placed Mrs. Malone in the recovery position, and you now check her airway again. Since you turned her on her side, you have not heard any abnormal sounds from her airway like snoring or gurgling. This, and the fact that she is breathing adequately, means that her airway is open. You check the oxygen and confirm that you are administering oxygen at 12 to 15 liters per minute by nonrebreather mask.

History

Because Mrs. Malone has a decreased level of responsiveness and you could not get a history by interviewing her, you need to depend on others to provide as much of this information as possible. The family member who met you at the door is Mrs. Malone's daughter, Florence. You question her to find out what happened and what medical history her mother has.

You: What happened?
Florence: I think she had a convulsion.

You: What happened to make you say that?
Florence: Well, I heard some choking sounds from the room next door, and when I came in her arms and legs were moving around.

You: Was it both arms and both legs?
Florence: Yes, I think so.

You: Was anyone with her when this started?
Florence: No, no one else was home.

You: When did this happen?
Florence: About 10 minutes ago, just before I called 9-1-1.

You: How long did you see her arms and legs moving?
Florence: I think it was only about a minute, but it felt like a lot longer when it was happening.

You: Has she ever had anything like this happen before?
Florence: I don't think so, but my mother lives alone, so I'm not sure.

You: How old is your mother?
Florence: She's 60.

You: Is she allergic to anything?
Florence: Not that I know of.

You: Does she take any medicines?
Florence: No, I don't think so.

You: Is she generally healthy?
Florence: Yes, although sometimes she gets migraines.

You: Does she take any medicine for her migraines?
Florence: No, she used to, but she had to stop taking it because it made her feel so tired.

You: When did she stop taking the medicine?
Florence: Oh, that was months ago.

You: Do you know when she last ate?
Florence: We had lunch about four hours ago—just a cheese sandwich and some tomato soup. I was starting to make dinner when this happened.

You: Can you think of anything unusual that happened today that might explain what happened to your mother?
Florence: No, it seemed like a normal day until just a little while ago.

You: I think you were right when you said she had a convulsion, or seizure. What you described sounds a lot like a seizure. We're going to take her to the

hospital to be checked by a doctor in the emergency department.
Florence: Thank you. Should I come with you or drive to the hospital myself?

You: You're welcome to come with us, but it might be easier for you to get home if you drive.
Florence: OK. I'll meet you there.

You: Don't follow the ambulance too closely. Take your time and be careful.

Having completed the focused history and physical exam, you move Mrs. Malone to your stretcher and take her to the ambulance for transport to the hospital. You will not do a detailed physical exam en route because there is no reason to suspect injuries of the kind that a detailed physical exam would assess. Since Mrs. Malone is unresponsive, however, you maintain a high index of suspicion and remain ready to do a more detailed exam en route if anything about her condition should change so as to cause you to suspect that she may have been injured.

Mrs. Malone's condition is potentially very serious. At the hospital, she will be scheduled for a series of tests and referred to a specialist.

CHAPTER REVIEW

SUMMARY

The focused history and physical exam of the medical patient takes two forms. You assess the responsive patient by getting a history of the present illness (a fuller description of the chief complaint), and a SAMPLE history, then performing a physical exam of affected parts of the body before getting baseline vital signs. The primary purpose of gathering this information is to determine the proper treatment of the patient.

In unresponsive medical patients, since they cannot communicate, history gathering will not provide

as much useful information. In these patients, it is appropriate to start the assessment with a rapid physical exam. This exam looks almost the same as the trauma patient's rapid assessment. Baseline vital signs come next, and then you interview bystanders, family, and friends to get any history that can be obtained. You may not change any field treatment as a result of the information gathered here, but the results of the assessment may be very important to the emergency department staff.

KEY TERMS

OPQRST a memory device for the questions asked to get a description of the present illness: Onset, Provokes, Quality, Radiation, Severity, Time.

Review Questions

1. Explain how and why the focused history and physical exam for a medical patient differs from the focused history and physical exam for a trauma patient. (p. 233)

2. Explain how and why the focused history and physical exam for a responsive medical patient differs from the focused history and physical exam for an unresponsive medical patient. (p. 234)

Applications

As an EMT-B, how would you deal with the following situations?

• What questions would you ask to get a history of the present illness from a patient with a chief complaint of chest pain?

• You are trying to get information from the very upset son of an unresponsive man. He is the only available family member. He is so upset that he is having difficulty talking to you. How can you quickly get him to calm down and give you his father's medical history?

• You are interviewing a very pleasant older man. Unfortunately, your assessment is taking a long time because he does not answer your questions and instead starts talking about other things. He lives alone and appears to be lonely. How should you handle this?

Web Medic

Visit Brady's *Emergency Care* website for direct weblinks. At **www.bradybooks.com/ emergencycare**, you will find information related to the following Chapter 11 topics:

• Breathing sounds

• Heart sounds

• Common mistakes in taking blood pressure

Chapter
Twelve

ONGOING ASSESSMENT

*W*ord on the Street

"Taking vital signs may seem like a mundane chore destined to have you fill out blocks on the prehospital care report, but if one vital sign is an observation, two are a comparison, and at least three sets will provide you with a trend. In an instance of impending shock, this attention to detail should give you an early jump on assessing circulatory compromise. Ongoing assessment may not seem glamorous, but finding a potential life threat is pretty satisfying."

Jeff Grunow, MSN, NREMT-P
Director, Prehospital Education,
Carolinas Medical Center

An appropriate assessment at the scene and en route to the hospital allows you to detect and treat injuries and illnesses. Your job does not stop there, though. The patient's condition can change, either gradually or suddenly. You will be able to detect these changes by performing a series of steps called the ongoing assessment.

ONGOING ASSESSMENT

It is important to observe and re-observe your patient, not only to determine his condition when you first see him, but also to detect any changes. The patient may exhibit an obvious change like loss of consciousness or more subtle differences such as restlessness, anxiety, or sweating. These may indicate a change in blood circulation. Some patients may take a turn for the worse before they reach the hospital, although this is uncommon, or you may see patient improvement, possibly in response to interventions you perform.

You will perform the ongoing assessment on every patient after you have finished performing life-saving interventions and, often, after you have done the detailed physical exam. Sometimes you may skip doing a detailed physical exam because you are too busy taking care of life-threatening problems, or for a medical or non-critical trauma patient for whom the detailed physical exam would not yield useful information. The ongoing assessment, however, must never be skipped except when life-saving interventions prevent doing it. Even in the latter situation, one partner can often perform the ongoing assessment while the other continues life-saving care.

Throughout the assessment procedures that take place on the way to the hospital, remember to explain to a conscious patient what you are doing, to talk in a reassuring tone, and to consider the patient's feelings, such as anxiety or embarrassment.

Pediatric Notes

Remember to keep eye contact with a conscious child, staying as much as possible on the child's level, and explaining what you are doing in a quiet and reassuring voice.

Components of the Ongoing Assessment

During the **ongoing assessment,** you will repeat key elements of assessment procedures you have already performed. You will repeat the initial assessment (to check for life-threatening problems), reassess vital signs, repeat the focused assessment related to the patient's specific complaint or injuries, and check any interventions you have performed (see Scan 12-1).

***Study Guide for* Ongoing Assessment**

✔ Repeat the initial assessment.
✔ Reassess vital signs.
✔ Repeat the focused assessment related to specific complaint or injuries.
✔ Check interventions.

Repeat the Initial Assessment

Begin the ongoing assessment by repeating the initial assessment to recheck for life-threatening problems:

- Reassess mental status.
- Maintain an open airway.

TOPIC OVERVIEW

In this chapter, you will learn about the following topics:

- How to perform an ongoing assessment
- The significance of changes in vital signs over time
- The difference in ongoing assessments for stable vs. unstable patients

DOT OBJECTIVES

✔ **Knowledge and Attitude**

1. Discuss the reasons for repeating the initial assessment as part of the ongoing assessment. (pp. 247–248)

2. Describe the components of the ongoing assessment. (pp. 247–248) (Scan 12-1, p. 249)

3. Describe trending of assessment components. (pp. 248, 250)

4. Explain the value of performing an ongoing assessment. (p. 247)

5. Recognize and respect the feelings that patients might experience during assessment. (p. 247)

6. Explain the value of trending assessment components to other health professionals who assume care of the patient. (p. 250)

✔ **Skills**

1. Demonstrate the skills involved in performing the ongoing assessment.

- Monitor breathing for rate and quality.
- Reassess the pulse for rate and quality.
- Monitor skin color and temperature.
- Reestablish patient priorities.

Remember, life-threatening problems that were not present or were brought under control during the initial assessment may develop or redevelop before the patient reaches the hospital. For example, the mental status of the patient who was responsive and alert may begin to deteriorate—a significant trend and worrisome sign. The airway that was open may become occluded, the patient who was breathing adequately on his own may now require respiratory support, other signs such as a rapid pulse, cool skin, and pallor may indicate the onset of shock. Life threats must be watched for continually and managed immediately when discovered.

Pediatric Notes

The mental status of an unresponsive child or infant can be checked by shouting (verbal stimulus) or flicking the feet (painful stimulus). An expected response would be crying.

When reassessing the circulation of a young child or infant, do not forget to check capillary refill. Remember that when you press on a nail bed and then release the pressure, the pink color should return in less than two seconds. Counting "one-one thousand, two-one thousand" or saying "capillary refill" takes about two seconds, so the pink color should return before you finish saying either of these. In small children who have very small nail beds, press on the top of a hand or foot to check capillary refill.

Reassess and Record Vital Signs

During the focused history and physical exam you took and recorded a set of baseline vital signs: pulse, respiration, skin, pupils, and blood pressure. During the ongoing assessment, you will reassess and record the vital signs, comparing the results with the baseline measurements and any other vital signs mea-

surements you may have taken, for example during the detailed physical exam, if you conducted one.

It is especially important to record each vital sign measurement as soon as you obtain it. In this way, you will not need to worry about remembering the different numbers you get for pulse rate, blood pressure, and respiratory rate. When you have more than one set of vital signs, it becomes even easier to forget them if you have not written them down. Another reason to document your ongoing assessment is so that you can see trends in the patient's condition, which we will discuss later in this chapter.

Repeat the Focused Assessment

You may find many changes as you repeat the physical exam. For example, a chest injury may become apparent as muscles get tired and you see paradoxical motion that was not present when you first assessed the patient (paradoxical motion is present when a part of the chest goes in as the patient inhales and goes out as the patient exhales, opposite to the motion of the rest of the chest). The abdomen may become distended, a sign that you are especially likely to see if you have a long transport. As you learn more about specific injuries and illnesses in later chapters, you will learn more signs to look for in your ongoing assessment.

Check Interventions

Whenever you check the interventions that you have performed for a patient, try to take a fresh look at the patient. Attempt to see the patient as though you had never seen him before. This may help you to evaluate the adequacy of your interventions more objectively and to adjust them as necessary. Always do the following:

- Assure adequacy of oxygen delivery and artificial ventilation.
- Assure management of bleeding.
- Assure adequacy of other interventions.

The fact that you put the patient on oxygen initially does not prevent the tank from running out

ONGOING ASSESSMENT

▲ **1.** Repeat the initial assessment.

▲ **2.** Reassess and record vital signs.

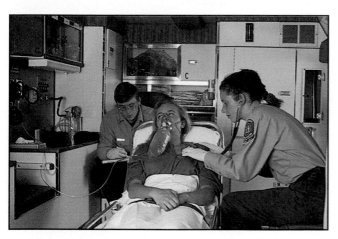

▲ **3.** Repeat the focused assessment.

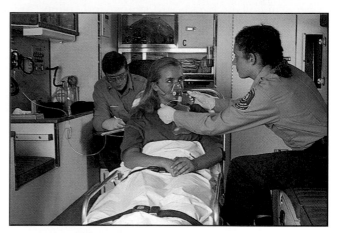

▲ **4.** Check interventions.

later, or the tubing from becoming disconnected. A good habit to develop is to check the entire path of the oxygen from the tank to the patient. This means looking at the regulator on the tank and confirming that it has sufficient oxygen and that the flowmeter is set to the proper flow. Make sure that the tube is firmly connected to the regulator. Follow the tubing and make sure there are no kinks that would prevent the flow of oxygen. Look at the mask. Make sure the tubing is connected to it, and that it is the proper mask, a nonrebreather (sometimes simple or rebreather masks are accidentally stocked in an ambulance). Confirm that the mask is snug on the patient's face and that the nonrebreather bag does not completely deflate when the patient inhales. Increase the flow rate if it does. With practice, this sequence of steps will take just a few seconds.

Wounds that stopped bleeding can start bleeding again, so it is important to check them as part of the ongoing assessment. Check any bandage you have applied and make sure it is dry with no blood seeping through. When an unbandaged wound is in a location where you cannot see it, gently palpate it with gloved hands and check your gloves for blood.

Also be sure to check other interventions, such as cervical collars, backboard straps, and splints. Any of these can slip and need adjustment.

Observing Trends

Because ongoing assessment is a means of determining **trending** (changes over time) in the patient's condition, you will need to repeat the ongoing assessment steps frequently. Be sure to record your findings and compare them to earlier findings. It is important to notice and document any changes or trends. In later chapters, you will learn about specific trends to look for in patients' vital signs. For example, when you reach Chapter 26, "Bleeding and Shock," you will learn about trends in the pulse rate and blood pressure as signs of shock.

Based on your findings, you may need to institute new treatments or adjust treatments you have already started. Your findings, in particular any trends you have noted, will also be important information for the hospital staff and will let them know if the patient's condition is improving or deteriorating.

Ongoing Assessment for Stable and Unstable Patients

The patient's condition, as well as the length of time you spend with the patient, will determine just how often you will conduct the ongoing assessment. The more serious the patient's condition, the more often

you will do it. The recommended intervals are as follows:

- *Every 15 minutes for a stable patient,* such as a patient who is alert, has vital signs in the normal range, and has no serious injury
- *Every 5 minutes for an unstable patient,* such as a patient who has an altered mental status, difficulty with airway, breathing, or circulation, including severe blood loss, or a significant mechanism of injury

Whenever you believe there may have been a change in the patient's condition, repeat at least the initial assessment. In this way, you will detect signs of life-threatening conditions as soon as possible.

When in doubt, repeat the ongoing assessment every 5 minutes or as frequently as possible.

COMPARING ASSESSMENTS

Below are two scenarios that may help you see the difference between an ongoing assessment of a responsive medical patient and assessment of an unresponsive medical patient.

Mr. Schmidt—Responsive Adult Medical Patient
You have been dispatched to an older man who is complaining of stomach pain. You complete the scene size-up and initial assessment. You determine that there is no mechanism of injury, that Mr. Schmidt is alert, and that his airway, breathing, and circulation are not compromised. Since he is alert and has no immediate life threats, he is not a priority for immediate transport. You conduct the focused history and physical exam, discovering that Mr. Schmidt is suffering a burning pain localized to his upper abdomen that started about two hours ago and is getting worse. He reports no history of any similar disorder. The physical exam reveals some tenderness in the upper quadrants but no distention. His vital signs are normal. You load him into the ambulance for transport to the hospital, placing him in a position he finds comfortable, sitting up. Deciding that a detailed physical exam will not be useful, you proceed with ongoing assessment en route.

Ongoing Assessment—Stable Medical Patient
To begin the ongoing assessment, you repeat the initial assessment to check for any immediately life-threatening problems. You get a general impression of an older man who is in discomfort. By talking to him, you confirm that his mental status is alert and his airway and breathing are adequate. You check circulation by feeling his radial pulse and looking for external bleeding. His radial pulse is normal in rate and strength and regular in rhythm. The skin at his

wrist is warm, pink, and dry. You do not see any blood around him. You conclude that Mr. Schmidt's condition has not changed and he is still not a high priority patient.

Next, you repeat and record the vital signs. Mr. Schmidt has a pulse of 88, regular and full, respirations 20 and unlabored, skin normal (warm, pink, and dry), and blood pressure 134/88. His pulse and blood pressure are somewhat lower than when you assessed them during the focused history and physical exam, but well within normal ranges, probably indicating that he is somewhat calmer than before. You record your new findings.

Now you repeat the focused history and physical exam. When you ask Mr. Schmidt about his abdominal pain, he tells you there has been no change. He is still a little nauseated, but does not feel as though he will vomit. Nevertheless, you anticipate that he may vomit, so you keep a basin nearby. You very gently palpate his abdomen again. He reports no change in the amount of tenderness present, and you find no firmness or distention.

Next, you check interventions you have performed. In Mr. Schmidt's case, the only intervention that was appropriate was positioning. You ask Mr. Schmidt whether you can make him more comfortable, but he says he is fine sitting up.

The trip to the hospital takes about 20 minutes, so 15 minutes after you leave the scene, you repeat the ongoing assessment and find no changes in Mr. Schmidt's condition.

At the hospital, Mr. Schmidt is diagnosed with an ulcer, given a prescription for medication, and advised to consult with Dr. Anderson, his regular physician.

Brian Sawyer—Unresponsive Adult Trauma Patient
You have witnessed a collision in which Brian, the driver, was thrown from his car. You complete the scene size-up and initial assessment, determining that there is a significant mechanism of injury and that Brian is unresponsive with a compromised airway. Your partner stabilizes Brian's spine and performs a jaw-thrust. You insert an oral airway and administer high-concentration oxygen. You assign Brian a high priority for transport and quickly complete the rapid trauma assessment, finding a head laceration, flat neck veins, and a deformity to his right leg. You apply a cervical collar during the rapid trauma assessment. As soon as the assessment is finished, you immobilize Brian to a backboard, load him into the ambulance, and conduct a detailed physical exam en route, making no further significant findings. You then proceed immediately to the ongoing assessment.

Ongoing Assessment—Unstable Trauma Patient
You and your partner both need to be with this critically injured patient on the way to the hospital. Fortunately during your initial assessment, when you

realized how seriously injured Brian might be, you asked dispatch to send another qualified driver so the two of you could continue to work on Brian en route to the hospital. In accordance with your local protocol, you told the driver to drive to the closest hospital able to provide quality trauma care.

You start the ongoing assessment by repeating the initial assessment to check for life-threatening problems. First you reassess Brian's mental status. When he does not respond to your shouting his name, you pinch his shoulder. There is no response. You re-evaluate his airway by putting your ear next to his mouth and listening for abnormal sounds like snoring, gurgling, or stridor. There is a little bit of gurgling, so you suction his mouth. When you listen again, you hear no more abnormal sounds. You also look in Brian's mouth. You see nothing that could cause his airway to become obstructed. Next, you look at Brian's breathing. It is now slow (approximately 8 per minute) and shallow, so you get the flow-restricted, oxygen-powered ventilation device for your partner, who starts to ventilate Brian at a rate of 12 per minute. Brian's pulse is rapid and weak. His skin is still pale, cool, and sweaty. You reconfirm that Brian is a high-priority patient. In fact, his condition is even more serious than before, because you now need to assist his ventilations.

The next step in the ongoing assessment is to repeat and record vital signs. Brian has a pulse of 132, regular and weak, respirations of 8 and shallow, and a blood pressure of 100 by palpation. As you record these findings, you note that his pulse and blood pressure have not changed from your earlier readings, but—as you noted when repeating the initial assessment of respiration—his breathing has now slowed to a dangerous level that requires assisted ventilations.

Next you repeat the rapid trauma assessment. You palpate the laceration on the back of Brian's head and check your gloves but find no fresh blood. The deformity to his right leg is temporarily stabilized by his immobilization on the backboard. You find no additional injuries.

Finally, you check the interventions you performed for Brian. You confirm that oxygen is running into the flow-restricted, oxygen-powered ventilation device and that Brian's chest is rising with each ventilation. There is no bleeding to control. Now you check the other interventions: the cervical collar, straps, and long backboard. The collar is the right size and is in the right place (sometimes cervical collars can slip). The straps are snug, and Brian has not moved on the board. You find time now to splint his injured leg.

During the ride to the hospital, you repeat your ongoing assessment every 5 minutes (performing any needed interventions), recording your findings and noting any trends in his condition.

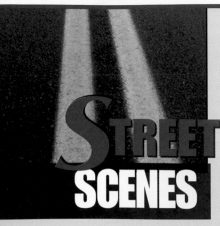

We received a call for an elderly woman with a possible stroke. After taking the appropriate BSI precautions, we assured scene safety and entered the house. An older man, identifying himself as the patient's husband, met us at the door. As he led us to the kitchen, he explained that he came home after being out for a while and found his wife unable to stand up. When we reached the kitchen, we found Althea Stokes sitting in a chair.

My general impression was of an elderly woman who appeared awake, but was slumped onto her left side. As I introduced myself, I noticed the patient's eyes were open and she appeared awake, but her speech was slow and slurred. She did not appear to be in pain. A small amount of saliva was drooling onto her blouse. Her airway was open (at least for the moment); breathing appeared normal and unlabored; there was no sign of bleeding; and her radial pulse was strong, slightly rapid, and very irregular. I assigned Mrs. Stokes a medium priority as a medical patient. In our BLS system, calling for advanced life support is not an option.

STREET SCENE QUESTIONS

1. How does the patient's mental status affect the way you maintain the patient's airway?

2. What questions should you ask the patient and her husband?

We wiped the saliva away from the patient's mouth and considered how to maintain her airway. If she should lose consciousness, we should be prepared to suction. In the meantime, we made a mental note to keep an eye on further potential threats to her airway.

Since the patient was having difficulty speaking, I got most of the focused history from Mr. Stokes. His 82-year-old wife is usually alert and very active, he informed us. She was fine when he left about four hours ago, but when he came home, she was slumped over in the chair and couldn't seem to move her left arm and leg. When I asked Mrs. Stokes if she was having any pain or difficulty breathing, she slowly responded with slurred speech, "No, I'm not." As my partner gathered vital signs, I looked at the patient more carefully. The right side of her face seemed to be drooping, especially her cheek and upper eyelid. When I asked her to hold her arms out in front of her, she picked up her right arm, but could barely move her left one. When I asked her to smile, only the left side of her face moved. Her pupils were equal and reactive to light. Her vital signs were pulse 92 and irregular, BP 180/96, respirations 20 and unlabored.

According to Mr. Stokes, the only medical problem his wife had was high blood pressure, for which she takes just one medication, Vasotec. She had no allergies to medications. She was a patient of Dr. Newman and had not been hospitalized recently.

Because her brain might not be getting enough oxygen, we gave her 10 liters per minute by nonre-

The importance of the ongoing assessment became clear in Brian's case. Unlike Mr. Schmidt, the medical patient whose condition improved somewhat during the trip to the hospital, Brian took a turn for the worse. Because you closely re-evaluated his airway, you discovered that he had some fluid in his pharynx (which caused the gurgling sound), and so you suctioned him. His respiratory rate had decreased to the point where his breathing was inadequate, and so your partner began to assist his ventilations with a flow-restricted, oxygen-powered ventilation device.

The value of looking at trends also became apparent. If you look at Brian's vital signs (Table 12-1), you can see that his respiratory rate was decreasing, a bad sign in an unresponsive patient. During the course of Brian's recovery, you check with hospital personnel from time to time to see how he's doing. You are told that the quick work you and your partner did in opening Brian's airway and assisting his ventilations have prevented any brain damage that might have occurred. Brian is transferred to the rehabilitation institute and, after several months, returns to work.

breather mask. We took special care to put Mrs. Stokes on her left side on the stretcher so she would be able to still move her right arm and saliva would not obstruct her airway.

STREET SCENE QUESTIONS

3. How should you perform an ongoing assessment on this patient?

En route, we contacted the receiving hospital and reported on Mrs. Stokes's condition and treatment. I repeated the patient's vital signs and this time got a pulse of 88 and irregular, BP 170 by palpation, and respirations of 22 and unlabored. When I asked the patient how she felt now, she replied in a clear voice, "Why, much better, young man." Surprised at this sudden improvement, I proceeded to assess her again. She could now hold both arms up in front of her with her eyes closed. When she smiled, there was no longer any sign of a deficit. Cheered up by this turn of events, I confirmed that her husband's version of events was accurate. I also learned that Mrs. Stokes had led an interesting life, having been a history teacher for 40 years.

About 5 minutes after this improvement, I noticed that the patient seemed to be having trouble speaking again. When I asked her to hold her arms out in front of her, she was able to pick both of them up, but her left arm drifted off and fell down. Her smile barely showed her teeth. When I asked her to repeat the phrase, "The sky is blue in Cincinnati," she could get only the first few words out and only with great difficulty. Concerned about these changes in the patient's condition, I called the hospital again and advised them of the developments.

When we arrived at the emergency department a few minutes later, Mrs. Stokes's condition had not changed again. The nurse undressed her and the emergency physician assessed her as we prepared the ambulance for the next call and completed our patient care report. Just as I was finishing the report, the doctor came out of the patient's room. "Well, I'm glad you brought this patient here," he said. "She's not a candidate for clot-busting drugs, but since this is a teaching hospital, we can offer Mrs. Stokes the opportunity to participate in a research project evaluating a new experimental treatment for stroke."

"Do you think she's really having a stroke? Her condition kept changing, getting better and then getting worse again," I asked.

"We often see changes in the condition of stroke patients in the first few hours of the episode. It can make assessment a real challenge. I'm glad you were able to detect the changes and let us know about them."

With a new appreciation for the value of an ongoing assessment, we returned to our service area ready for another call.

TABLE 12-1 Vital Sign Trends for Brian Sawyer

Assessment Step	Pulse	Respirations	Blood Pressure
Focused history/physical exam	120, regular and weak	20 and normal	130/80
Detailed physical exam	136, regular and weak	14 and normal	100/70
Ongoing assessment	132, regular and weak	8 and shallow	100/P (by palpation)

CHAPTER REVIEW

Summary

The ongoing assessment is the last step in your assessment of a patient. You will repeat it every 15 minutes for a stable patient and at least every 5 minutes for an unstable patient. This means repeating the initial assessment, vital signs, focused assessment, and checking the interventions you performed for the patient. Interventions you need to check include oxygen, bleeding, spine immobilization, and splints.

Key Terms

ongoing assessment a procedure for detecting changes in a patient's condition. It involves four steps: repeating the initial assessment, repeating and recording vital signs, repeating the focused assessment, and checking interventions.

trending changes in a patient's condition over time, such as slowing respirations or rising pulse rate, that may show improvement or deterioration, and that can be shown by documenting repeated assessments.

Review Questions

1. Name the four steps of the ongoing assessment and list what assessments you will make during each step. (pp. 247–248)

2. Explain the value of recording, or documenting, your assessment findings, and explain the meaning of the term *trending*. (p. 250)

Applications

What do you need to do if your ongoing assessment turns up one of these findings?

- Gurgling respirations

- Bag on nonrebreather mask collapses completely when the patient inhales
- Snoring respirations

WEB MEDIC

Visit Brady's *Emergency Care* website for direct weblinks. At **www.bradybooks.com/ emergencycare**, you will find information related to the following Chapter 12 topics:

- Aging and vital signs

Chapter
Thirteen

PEDIATRIC, ADOLESCENT, AND GERIATRIC ASSESSMENT

You learned how to assess a patient in Chapters 8 through 12. The principles you learned pertain to all patients. However, when your patient is at one of the extremes of age, you will need to make some adjustments in how you proceed. This is especially true with regard to communication.

PEDIATRIC PATIENT

Just as a 6-year-old child is different from a 35-year-old adult, so is a 4-week-old infant different from a 12-year-old child. Children are constantly growing and learning and hence changing. In an ideal world, we might be able to tell exactly how a 4-year-old will behave. In reality, we have to put children into broad categories according to how children of their age group behave on the average. No system of categorizing children is perfect, but each has advantages for particular uses.

For basic life support (rescue breathing and CPR), the American Heart Association defines an infant as birth to 1 year, a child as 1 to 8 years, and an adult as anyone over 8. These age ranges do not always apply to the care of children in other medical or trauma cases. In general emergency care, the following age categories are more useful to keep in mind:

- Newborns and infants: birth to 1 year
- Toddlers: 1 to 3 years
- Preschool: 3 to 6 years
- School age: 6 to 12 years
- Adolescent: 12 to 18 years

There will be calls when it will not be possible to find out the age of the patient and you will have to guess at the age, based on the child's physical size and emotional reactions.

Psychological and Personality Characteristics

Each age group has its own general characteristics of psychology and personality that will affect the way you assess and care for the patient. These are outlined in Table 13-1.

Anatomical and Physiological Differences

Infants and children differ from adults not only in psychology but also in anatomy and physiology. (Review the special characteristics of infants and children in Chapter 4, "The Human Body.") Understanding some of these differences will help you do a better job of assessing and caring for young patients. Key differences have to do with the head, airway and respiratory system, chest and abdomen, body surface, and blood volume.

Head

A child's head is proportionately larger and heavier than an adult's until about the age of 4. The implication for emergency care is that you should suspect head injury whenever there is a serious mechanism of injury because a child is likely to be propelled forward head first.

Infants up to about one year or 18 months of age will have a "soft spot," or anterior fontanelle, which is flat and soft while the child is quiet. The fontanelle is just anterior to the center of the skull. A sunken fontanelle may indicate dehydration. A bulging fontanelle may indicate elevated intracranial pressure. The fontanelle also normally bulges when the infant is crying.

Airway and Respiratory System

The infant and child's neck muscles are immature and the airway structures are narrower and less rigid

TOPIC OVERVIEW

In this chapter, you will learn about the following topics:

- Anatomical and physiological differences of infants, children, and adults
- Patient assessment techniques for pediatric patients
- Patient assessment techniques for geriatric patients
- Communication techniques for different age groups

DOT OBJECTIVES

✔ **Knowledge and Attitude**

1. Identify the developmental considerations for the following age groups: (pp. 258–259)

—infants   —school age

—toddlers   —adolescent

—preschool

2. Describe differences in anatomy and physiology of the infant, child, and adult patient. (pp. 252–261)

3. Differentiate the response of the ill or injured infant or child (age specific) from that of an adult. (pp. 258–259)

✔ **Skills**

1. Demonstrate the assessment of the infant and child.

Note: There are no objectives in the national standard curriculum on geriatric patients.

than an adult's. There are several more special characteristics you should be aware of (Figure 13-1):

- The mouth and nose are smaller and more easily obstructed than in adults.
- The tongue takes up more space proportionately in the mouth than in adults.
- Newborns and infants are obligate nose breathers. This means they will not know to open their mouths to breathe when the nose becomes obstructed.
- The trachea (windpipe) is softer and more flexible in infants and children.
- The trachea is narrower and is easily obstructed by swelling or foreign objects.
- The chest wall is softer, and infants and children tend to depend more on their diaphragms for breathing.

Table 13-1   Developmental Characteristics of Infants and Children

Age Group	Characteristics	Assessment and Care Strategies
Newborns and infants—birth to 1 year 	• Infants do not like to be separated from their parents. • There is minimal stranger anxiety. • Infants are used to being undressed but like to feel warm, physically and emotionally. • The younger infant follows movement with his eyes. • The older infant is more active, developing a personality. • They do not want to be "suffocated" by an oxygen mask.	• Have the parent hold the infant while you examine him. • Be sure to keep him warm— warm your hands and stethoscope before touching the infant. • It may be best to observe breathing from a distance, noting the rise and fall of the chest, the level of activity, and skin color. • Examine the heart and lungs first and the head last. This is perceived as less threatening to the infant and therefore less likely to start him crying. • A pediatric nonrebreather mask may be held near the face to provide "blow-by" oxygen.
Toddlers—1 to 3 years 	• Toddlers do not like to be touched or separated from their parents. • Toddlers may believe that their illness is a punishment for being bad. • Unlike infants, they do not like having their clothing removed. • They frighten easily, overreact, have a fear of needles, pain. • Toddlers may understand more than they communicate. • They begin to assert their independence. • They do not want to be "suffocated" by an oxygen mask	• Have a parent hold the child while you examine him. • Assure the child that he was not bad. • Remove an article of clothing, examine, and then replace the clothing. • Examine in a trunk-to-head approach to build confidence. (Touching the head first may be frightening.) • Explain what you are going to do in terms the toddler can understand (taking the blood pressure becomes a squeeze or a hug on the arm).

Table 13-1   continued

Age Group	Characteristics	Assessment and Care Strategies
Preschool—3 to 6 years	• Preschoolers do not like to be touched or separated from their parents. • They are modest and do not like their clothing removed. • Preschoolers may believe that their illness is a punishment for being bad. • Preschoolers have a fear of blood, pain, and permanent injury. • They are curious, communicative, and can be cooperative. • They do not want to be "suffocated" by an oxygen mask.	• Have a parent hold the child while you examine him. • Respect the child's modesty. Remove an article of clothing, examine, and then replace the clothing. • Have a calm, confident, reassuring, respectful manner. • Be sure to offer explanations about what you are doing. • Allow the child the responsibility of giving the history. • Explain as you examine. • A pediatric nonrebreather mask may be held near the face to provide "blow-by" oxygen.
School age—6 to 12 years	• This age group cooperates but likes their opinions heard. • They fear blood, pain, disfigurement, and permanent injury. • School age children are modest and do not like their bodies exposed.	• Allow the child the responsibility of giving the history. • Explain as you examine. • Present a confident, calm, respectful manner. • Respect the child's modesty.
Adolescent—12 to 18 years	• Adolescents want to be treated as adults. • Adolescents generally feel that they are indestructible but may have fears of permanent injury and disfigurement. • Adolescents vary in their emotional and physical development and may not be comfortable with their changing bodies.	• Although they wish to be treated as adults, they may need as much support as children. • Present a confident, calm, respectful manner. • Be sure to explain what you are doing. • Respect modesty. You may consider assessing them away from their parents. Have the physical exam done by an EMT-B of the same sex as the patient if possible.

These differences in respiratory anatomy pose several implications for the emergency treatment you provide to an infant or a child:

• Because infants are obligate nose breathers, be sure to suction secretions from the nose as needed to help the patient breathe.

• Hyperextension or flexion of the neck (tipping the head too far back or letting it fall forward) may result in airway obstruction. A folded towel under the shoulders of a supine infant or young child will help to keep the airway in a neutral in-line position (Figure 13-2).

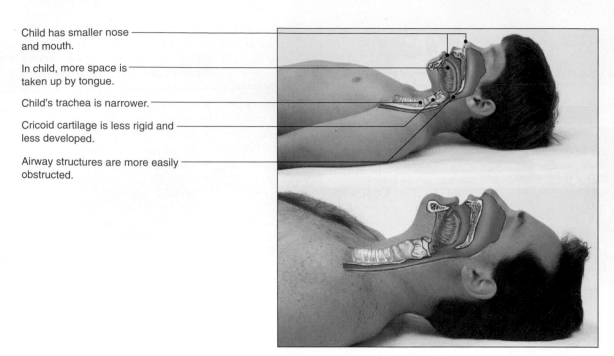

Child has smaller nose and mouth.

In child, more space is taken up by tongue.

Child's trachea is narrower.

Cricoid cartilage is less rigid and less developed.

Airway structures are more easily obstructed.

Figure 13-1 Comparison of child and adult respiratory passages.

A

B

Figure 13-2 (A) When an infant or young child is supine, the head will tip forward, obstructing the airway. (B) To keep the airway aligned, place a folded towel under the shoulders.

- "Blind" finger sweeps are not performed when trying to clear an airway obstruction in an infant or child because your finger might force the obstruction back and wedge it in the narrow trachea.

Chest and Abdomen

The less developed and more elastic chest structures of an infant or child make labored or distressed breathing obvious from a distance. The muscles above the sternum and between the ribs, and the ribs themselves, will pull inward when breathing is labored. Infants and young children are abdominal breathers, using their diaphragms for breathing more than adults. Watch the abdomen as well as the chest to evaluate breathing.

In addition, the fact that musculoskeletal structures of the chest and abdomen are less well developed means that the vital organs are not as well protected from injury as are those of adults.

Body Surface

A child's body surface area is larger in proportion to the body mass, making the child more prone to heat loss through the skin. This makes infants and children more vulnerable to hypothermia, an abnormally low body temperature. (See Chapter 22, "Environmental Emergencies.") They must be kept covered and warm.

With regard to burns, because an infant's or child's head, body, and extremities are proportioned differently from an adult's (the head being larger, for example), the extent of a burn is estimated differently for a child, using a special formula that will be described in Chapter 27, "Soft-Tissue Injuries."

Blood Volume

As you would expect, the blood volume of a pediatric patient is less than the blood volume of an adult. A newborn does not have enough blood to fill a 12-ounce soda can, and an 8-year-old has only about 2 liters of blood. Therefore, a blood loss that might be considered moderate in an adult can be life threatening for a child.

Interacting with the Pediatric Patient

You will not be able to interview infants, and most toddlers are poor communicators. However, the parents or the care providers who called for help can usually provide a history of a small child's illness or injury.

Preschoolers can usually be interviewed if you take your time and keep your language simple. School-age children will be able to describe more clearly how they feel and what happened. They will talk with you honestly but may feel that the injury or illness is a punishment for something they did. They must be reassured and told it is all right to feel sick or hurt or to cry.

If parents, teachers, or care providers are at the scene, talk with them but do not exclude the child. Seeing that familiar adults are being included gains the child's confidence if you follow up by talking directly to the child. If the parents are injured, you may not be able to get information from them, and the child needs to know that someone is caring for his or her parent as well.

All patients have some degree of fear at the emergency scene. Infants and children are usually more fearful than adults because they lack experience with illness and injury. In addition to this, children are easily frightened by the unknown. Since so many details of the emergency scene are unknowns, it is easy to see why emergencies can be scary for children. The elements associated with the emergency (pain, noise, bright lights, cold) can set off a panic reaction in infants.

At an emergency, if the child does not understand you, or believes that you do not understand in return, fear will increase. If the child is to communicate, he must remain calm. Putting the child at ease is a very important part of the care you must provide. Some children, when stressed, will act like a younger child. This is called *regression*.

Any problems faced by the child will be intensified if the parents are not at the scene. Children find security by being with their parents when facing new problems or emergencies. Asking for mom or dad may be the child's first priority, even above that of having your help.

When dealing with pediatric patients you should:

1. Identify yourself simply by saying "Hi, I'm Pat. What's your name?"

2. Let the child know that someone will call his or her parents.

3. Determine if there are life-threatening problems and treat them immediately. If there are no problems of this nature, continue at a relaxed pace. Fearful children cannot take the pressure of a rapidly paced assessment and confusing questions fired at them by a stranger.

4. Let the child have any nearby toy that he may want.

5. Kneel or sit at the child's eye level (Figure 13-3). Assure that bright light is not directly behind you and shining into the child's eyes.

6. SMILE. This is a familiar sign from adults that reassures children.

7. Touch the child or hold his hand or foot. Very young children sometimes like to have their toes played with. A child who does not wish to be touched will let you know. Do not force the issue; smile and provide comfort through your conversation.

8. Do not use any equipment on the child without explaining what you will do with it. Many children fear the medical items that are so familiar to the

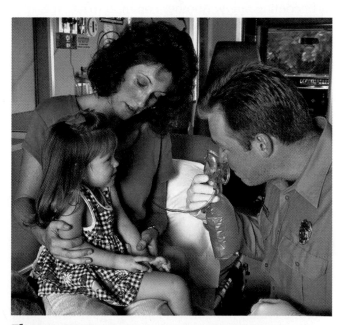

Figure 13-3 Kneel or sit at the child's eye level.

EMT-B, thinking they will cause pain. Always tell the child what you are going to do as you take vital signs and do a physical exam. Do not try to explain the entire procedure at once. Instead, explain each step as you do it. Use simple language and remember that children tend to take things literally. If you tell a young child "I'm going to take your pulse," he may think you are going to take something away from him. Instead say, "I'm going to hold your wrist for a minute." If the child is older, explain why.

9. Let the child see your face, and make eye contact without staring at the child. (Staring makes children uncomfortable.) Speak directly to the child, making a special effort to speak clearly and slowly in words he can understand. Be sure the child can hear you.

10. Stop occasionally to find out if the child understands. Never assume the child understood you, but find out by asking questions if the child is old enough to respond.

11. NEVER LIE TO THE CHILD. Tell him when the examination may hurt. If the child asks if he is sick or hurt, be honest, but be sure to add that you are there to help and will not leave. Let the child know that other people also will be helping.

Supporting the Parents or Other Care Providers

Parents may react in one of several ways when their child suffers a sudden life-threatening injury or illness. Their first reaction may be one of denial or shock. Some parents will react by crying, screaming, or becoming angry. Another common reaction is self-blame and guilt. In all of these instances, be calm, reassuring, and supportive. Use simple language to explain what has happened and what is being done to and for their child.

In some cases, an upset parent may interfere with your care of the child. This is a natural reaction to protect the child from further harm. Usually, you can persuade the parent to assist you by asking him to hold the child's hand, give you a medical history, or comfort the child. If the parent is out of control, however, and cannot or will not cooperate, have a friend or relative of the parent remove him from the scene.

At this point, it should be noted that not all children live with two parents in a traditional nuclear family. The child may have a single parent or may be living with a grandparent or other relative or even with someone who is not related to the child. Whoever the child's full-time caretaker or guardian is, that person is likely to have the same emotional re-

sponses in an emergency as any parent. The EMT-B should be sensitive to the fact that the child may or may not call this person "Mommy" or "Daddy" and may be upset if asked where his mother or father is. Tact is often required to find out who is responsible for the child and what the child calls that person. Though "parent" or "mom and dad" appear in this chapter, keep in mind that the terms are being used to stand for any person or persons who act as parents, guardians, or principal caretakers to the child.

You need to gain confidence and calm the emotions of all the people around the scene in order to be able to treat the child effectively. Your interactions with the child will show everyone present your concern, and the manner in which you provide care will show your professionalism.

In general, involving the parent in the care of the child helps both the child and the parent. The most effective method may be to have the parent hold the child in a position of comfort on his lap, if appropriate, during assessment and treatment procedures. Offer as much emotional support as possible to the parent. *However, never forget that the child (not the parent) is your patient. Do not allow communication with the parent to distract you from care of the child.*

Assessing the Pediatric Patient

The steps of assessment are the same for the pediatric patient as they are for the adult patient. Below, certain special concerns for assessment of the pediatric patient are discussed.

Scene Size-up and Safety—Pediatric
When entering the area where there is a pediatric patient, enter slowly and make some important observations. The first is to determine if the scene is safe. Even though it is a rare occurrence, sometimes there may be a risk from violence or abusive behavior, possibly directed toward the child. Look around carefully for any mechanism of injury.

BSI precautions must be taken for the usual reasons. Additionally, be aware that ordinary childhood diseases can be devastating when contracted by an adult.

Initial Assessment—Pediatric

Forming a General Impression. A great deal of information can and should be gathered from the doorway, before you approach and possibly upset the patient. From across the room, you can gain a general impression of the child. First decide: Is the child well or sick? The child's general appearance and behavior will usually provide the answer.

A child who is alertly watching your approach, squirming and able to talk with you, or vigorously crying obviously has an open airway, is breathing, and has a pulse and blood pressure. If the child is silent, appears to be sleeping deeply, or is unresponsive, the child's airway, breathing, and circulation must be assessed immediately.

As you approach and form your general impression, make the following observations:

- *Mental status.* The well child is alert. The sick child may be drowsy, inattentive, or sleeping.
- *Effort of breathing.* The well child's breathing should be unlabored. The sick child will be making a visible effort to breathe, including flared nostrils and retractions or pulling in of the tissues between the ribs.
- *Skin color.* A sick child may be pale, cyanotic, or flushed.
- *Quality of cry or speech.* In general, a strong cry or normal speech indicate a well child with good air exchange. The child who can speak only in short sentences or grunts has significant respiratory distress.
- *Interaction with the environment or others.* The healthy child exhibits normal behavior for his age. He moves around, plays, is attentive, establishes eye contact, and interacts with his parents. The sick child may be silent, listless, or unconscious.
- *Emotional state.* The well child's emotional state is appropriate to the situation. Crying may be his normal response to pain or fear. A withdrawn child or one who is emotionally flat is probably a sick child.
- *Response to you.* A well child may be interested in you or afraid of you. A sick child will give little attention to a stranger.
- *Tone and body position.* A sick child may be limp with poor muscle tone. Pediatric patients with respiratory distress often assume characteristic positions that seem to help them breathe (e.g., leaning forward with hands on knees).

Assessing Mental Status. Use the AVPU method of assessing mental status, taking the child's age and development into account. You may need to shout to elicit a response to verbal stimulus. Tap or pinch the patient to test for response to painful stimulus. Never shake an infant or child.

Assessing the Airway. Consider not only whether the airway is open but whether it is endangered. A depressed mental status, secretions, blood, vomitus, foreign bodies, face or neck trauma, and lower respiratory infections may all compromise the airway. *Be careful not to hyperextend the child's neck.*

Assessing Breathing. First assess if the patient is breathing or not. If the patient is not breathing or is breathing inadequately, provide artificial ventilations with supplemental oxygen. If the patient is experiencing respiratory distress, provide high-concentration oxygen by pediatric nonrebreather mask. (See Chapter 17, "Respiratory Emergencies," and Chapter 31, "Infants and Children.")

To assess breathing, observe the following:

- *Chest expansion.* There should be equal movement on both sides of the chest.
- *Effort of breathing.* Watch for nasal flaring when the patient inhales, and retractions or "pulling in" of the sternum and ribs with inhalation.
- *Sounds of breathing.* Listen for stridor, crowing, or other noisy respirations. Breath sounds should be present and equal on both sides of the chest. Note the presence of grunting at the end of expiration, a worrisome sign.
- *Breathing rate.* Normal respiratory rates for infants and children are 12 to 20 per minute in an adolescent, 15 to 30 per minute in a child, 25 to 50 per minute in an infant. Breathing that is either faster or slower than normal is inadequate and requires artificial ventilation as well as oxygen.
- *Color.* Cyanosis (blue color) indicates that the patient is not getting enough oxygen.

Assessing Circulation. As with an adult, check for normal warm, pink, and dry skin and normal pulse as indications of adequate circulation and perfusion. For assessment, check the radial pulse in a child, the brachial pulse in an infant. For basic life support, check the carotid pulse in a child, the brachial or femoral pulse in an infant (Figure 13-4). In infants and children 5 years old or younger, also check capillary refill. When you press on the nail bed or press the top of a hand or foot, the area will turn white. If circulation is adequate, the normal pink color will return in less than 2 seconds, or in less time than it takes to say "capillary refill." Check for and control any blood loss.

Identifying Priority Patients. A patient who is a high priority for immediate transport is one who:

- Gives a poor general impression
- Is unresponsive or listless
- Has a compromised airway
- Is in respiratory arrest or has inadequate breathing or respiratory distress
- Has a possibility of shock
- Has uncontrolled bleeding

A

B

Figure 13-4 For basic life support, check the (A) brachial pulse or (B) femoral pulse in an infant.

Focused History and Physical Exam—Pediatric

At times, the child may be the only source of a history. He may be at school or another place where medical records are not kept or where adults who know his medical history are not present. Get as much history as you can from the child by asking simple questions that cannot be answered with a yes or no. A child who cannot tell you where it hurts can usually point to the area.

Perform a focused physical exam for a medical patient and a rapid trauma exam for a trauma patient, as you would for an adult. Explain to the awake child what you are doing, and do the exam in trunk-to-head order to avoid frightening the child.

Take and record vital signs, assessing blood pressure only in children older than 3, using an appropriately-sized cuff (Figure 13-5). See Table 13-2 for normal ranges of pediatric vital signs.

Detailed Physical Exam—Pediatric

The EMT-B normally performs the physical examination or body assessment in head-to-toe order; but on alert infants and small children this is reversed. Starting with the toes or trunk and working your way toward the head will let the child get used to you and your touch before you, who after all are a stranger, attempt to touch him around the head and face. Playing with infants' feet often puts them at ease.

Unless there are possible injuries that indicate the child should not be moved, a young child should be held on the parent's lap during the physical exam. Many EMS teams carry clean toys that can be given to a child during the physical exam. The toys can provide comfort to the child and allow you to explain the examination by using the toy as model. Point to

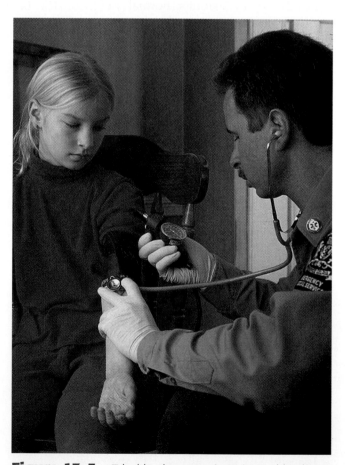

Figure 13-5 Take blood pressure in patients older than 3 years.

Table 13-2 Normal Vital Sign Ranges: Infants and Children

Normal Pulse Rate (beats per minute, at rest)

Newborn	120–160
Infant 0–5 months	90 to 140
Infant 6–12 months	80 to 140
Toddler 1–3 years	80 to 130
Preschooler 3–5 years	80 to 120
School age 6–10 years	70 to 110
Adolescent 11–14 years	60 to 105

Normal Respiration Rate (breaths per minute, at rest)

Newborn	30 to 50
Infant 0–5 months	25 to 40
Infant 6–12 months	20 to 30
Toddler 1–3 years	20 to 30
Preschooler 3–5 years	20 to 30
School age 6–10 years	15 to 30
Adolescent 11–14 years	12 to 20

Blood Pressure Normal Ranges

	Systolic	Diastolic
	Approx. 80 plus 2 × age	Approx. 2/3 Systolic
Preschooler 3–5 years	average 99 (78 to 116)	average 65
School age 6–10 years	average 105 (80 to 122)	average 69
Adolescent 11–14 years	average 114 (88–140)	average 76

Note: A high pulse in an infant or child is not as great a concern as a low pulse. A low pulse may indicate imminent cardiac arrest. Blood pressure is usually not taken in a child under 3 years. In cases of blood loss or shock, a child's blood pressure will remain within normal limits until near the end, then fall swiftly.

an area on the toy to show the child where you must touch and where you will bandage when you need to provide emergency care. This type of one-to-one communication also helps build parent and bystander confidence, letting them know that a professional, compassionate EMT-B is caring for the child. (If you use a toy, then give it to the child to keep.)

Most very young children will suffer no embarrassment when clothing is removed or repositioned during the exam. Nonetheless, protect the child from the stares of onlookers. Many children around the age of 5 to 8 go through a stage of intense modesty. You may have to keep explaining why you must remove certain articles of clothing. Many parents, teachers, and day care personnel teach children that strangers should not remove their clothing or touch them. The children that you examine may not understand your intentions and may resist. Some children may become upset because they feel you are taking something away from them. Take your time and do not rush children into accepting all that is happening. Remember that children lose body heat rapidly, so if you expose them, quickly cover them with a blanket.

The assessment of an infant or child is done to look for the same signs of injury and illness as in the case of the adult patient. However, you should take special care with components of the exam as discussed below (Figure 13-6).

Head. Do not apply pressure to the "soft spots" (fontanelles) of an infant. The skin over the anterior fontanelle is normally level with the skull, or slightly sunken, and may bulge naturally when the infant cries or be abnormally sunken if the infant is dehydrated. Meningitis and head trauma cause the fontanelle to bulge due to increased intracranial pressure. Accidents involving infants and children can often produce head injuries.

Nose and Ears. Look for blood and clear fluids from the nose and ears. Suspect skull fractures if present. Children are nose breathers and mucus or blood clot obstructions will make it hard for them to breathe.

Neck. Children are vulnerable to spinal-cord injuries because the head is proportionately larger and heavier. It also has less support because muscles and bone structures are less developed. In medical emergencies, the neck may be sore, stiff, or swollen.

Airway. Keep the infant's head in the neutral position and the child's head in the neutral-plus or sniffing position (chin thrust forward to maintain an open airway). If there is no suspicion of spinal injury, place a flat, folded towel under the patient's shoulders to get the appropriate airway opening. Children's airways are more pliable and smaller than an adult's. Hyperextension or hyperflexion may close off the airway. For medical respiratory problems, the child will probably want to sit up.

Chest. Listen closely for even air entry and the sounds of breathing on both sides of the chest. Be alert for wheezes and other noises. Check for symmetry, bruising, paradoxical movement, and retraction of the sternum or the muscles between the ribs. Remember that a child's soft ribs may not break, but there may be underlying injuries to the organs within the chest.

Abdomen. Note any rigid or tender areas and distention. Because a child's abdominal organs (especially the spleen and liver) are large in relation to the size of the abdominal cavity, and because there is little protection offered by the still-undeveloped abdominal muscles, these organs are more susceptible to trauma than an adult's. Any injury that impedes the movement of the diaphragm will compromise a young child's breathing, as most children 8 years of age or younger are abdominal breathers.

Pelvis. In trauma, check for stability of the pelvic girdle.

Extremities. Perform a neurological assessment with capillary refill and distal pulse, motor function, and sensation check. With an infant or young child, you do

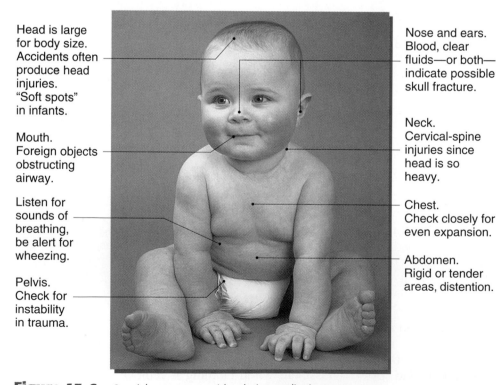

Head is large for body size. Accidents often produce head injuries. "Soft spots" in infants.

Mouth. Foreign objects obstructing airway.

Listen for sounds of breathing, be alert for wheezing.

Pelvis. Check for instability in trauma.

Nose and ears. Blood, clear fluids—or both— indicate possible skull fracture.

Neck. Cervical-spine injuries since head is so heavy.

Chest. Check closely for even expansion.

Abdomen. Rigid or tender areas, distention.

Figure 13-6 Special areas to consider during pediatric assessment.

not have to press on a nail bed. You can quickly check capillary refill by squeezing a hand or foot, forearm or lower leg. Check for painful, swollen, and deformed injury sites. (The bones of an infant or child are more pliable so they bend, splinter, and buckle before they fracture.)

Ongoing Assessment—Pediatric

Pediatric patients are dynamic—constantly changing. Continual assessment is essential to good patient care. A rule of thumb for infants and children is: *Don't take your eyes off them for a minute!*

As time permits, the following should be done. In some cases where the patient is seriously ill or traumatized, maintaining the airway and supporting ventilations will keep the EMT-B from performing a detailed physical exam and a complete history.

1. Reassess mental status
2. Maintain open airway
3. Monitor breathing
4. Reassess pulse
5. Monitor skin color, temperature, and moisture
6. Reassess vital signs
   — every 5 minutes in unstable patients
   — every 15 minutes in stable patients
7. Assure that all appropriate care and treatment are being given.

Figure 13-7   Treat the adolescent with respect.

How and Why?

It is important for you to recognize the signs of child abuse so that you can be one more safeguard against it. Go to your Electronic Extras CD to learn more.

Child Abuse and Neglect

Abuse and neglect of children is a serious and all-too-common problem. Be aware of any signs that the pediatric patient's illness or injury is the result of abuse or neglect and report these signs according to your state laws and local protocols. Child abuse and neglect will be discussed in detail in Chapter 31, "Infants and Children."

ADOLESCENT PATIENT

In many ways, adolescent patients are almost like adult patients. Certainly they like to be treated as adults and are very sensitive to violations of their dignity or a manner they believe is patronizing. On the other hand, when ill or injured or frightened, they often need as much emotional support as younger children (Figure 13-7).

Adolescents should be able to tell you exactly what happened and how they feel. However, in the presence of parents or peers, an adolescent patient may not be completely communicative or cooperative. He may be embarrassed, intimidated by the attention, trying to hide the fact that he was doing something wrong, or feel pressure to show bravado. Tact may be required to get information from the adolescent patient, and assessment may be more productive if this patient can be taken aside or into a private area.

The young adolescent is often embarrassed or worried about the changes occurring to his or her body and uncertain if these changes are "normal." Handling the clothing of a teenager of the opposite sex can be awkward for the EMT-B as well as for the patient. In most cases, a simple preliminary description of the examination will set the patient at ease. However, you should make sure that both the adolescent and the parents understand what you are going to do and why it must be done. When possible, have the exam conducted by or in the presence of an EMT-B of the same sex as the patient.

However, do not delay patient evaluation and care because you or the patient may be embarrassed. As a professional, you must put such feelings aside and act in a manner that will allow the patient to relax and understand that there is no need for embarrassment.

Most people living in the United States today can remember visiting their grandparents when they were growing up. This was not always the case. The average age has increased significantly over the last two centuries. Today, one out of every eight persons in the U.S. is 65 years or older. By the year 2040, one of every five persons will be at least 65. Fortunately, with longer lives we are also seeing healthier lives. Those over 85 are the fastest growing age group.

Among those over 65 years, certain medical conditions are common: almost half have arthritis, about a third have high blood pressure and heart disease, more than a quarter have some kind of hearing impairment, and about one tenth have diabetes or some kind of visual impairment. Despite these medical problems, more than half of those 85 years or older live alone or with just a spouse. In the 65–74 age group, even more live independently.

Contrary to popular opinion, only about 5% of the older population resides in nursing homes.

Some medical authorities believe that starting at about age 30, our organ systems lose about 1% of their function each year (the "1% rule"), which can make it difficult to distinguish between the normal effects of aging and the effects of disease. This is one reason why it is important to find out early what a patient's normal or baseline condition is. One way to do this is to ask how the patient is different compared to a week ago. This

Table 13-3 Physiological Effects of Aging and Implications for Assessment

Change	Result	Implications for Assessment
Depositing of cholesterol on arterial walls that have become thicker	Increased risk of heart attack and stroke, hypertension	Heart attack and stroke more likely
Decreased cardiac output	Diminished activity and tolerance of physical stress	More prone to falls
Decreased elasticity of lungs and decreased activity of cilia	Decreased ability to clear foreign substances from lungs	Higher risk of pneumonia and other respiratory infections
Fewer taste buds, less saliva; less acid production and slower movement in digestive system	Difficulty chewing and swallowing; less enjoyment of eating; difficulty digesting and absorbing food; constipation; early feeling of fullness when eating	Weight loss; abdominal pain common
Diminished liver and kidney function	Increased toxicity from alcohol and medications; diminished ability of blood to clot	Need for reduced doses of medication; bleeding tendencies
Diminished function of thyroid	Decreased energy and tolerance of heat and cold	Increased risk of hypothermia and hyperthermia
Decreased muscle mass, loss of minerals from bones	Decreased strength	Falls more likely; minor falls more likely to cause fractures
Multiple medical conditions	Many different medications, sometimes prescribed by different physicians	Increased risk of medication error; potentially harmful medication interactions common
Death of friends and family	Depression; loss of social support	Increased risk of suicide
Loss of skin elasticity, shrinking of sweat glands	Thin, dry, wrinkled skin	Increased risk of injury (The EMT-B must handle the patient gently to avoid injuring skin and subcutaneous tissues.)

information can be very helpful in distinguishing a chronic condition from a new problem.

Just as children change as they get older, so do adults, though not always in ways that are apparent. The function of many body systems diminishes as a person ages. Table 13-3 describes some of these changes and their implications for assessment by the EMT-B.

Older patients make up a much higher proportion of patients transported by EMS than would be expected from their numbers in society. In fact, older patients are at least twice as likely to use EMS. They also are more likely than younger patients to have a medical problem, rather than an injury.

The most common reasons for EMS to be called to an older person include cardiac and respiratory problems, neurological problems like stroke, and injuries from a fall. The elderly are less likely than the younger population to be involved in a motor-vehicle collision and sustain injuries in that way.

Communicating with the Geriatric Patient

Although most elderly people are healthy and able to live on their own, a sizable number of them have conditions that can hamper communication, such as hearing loss or deterioration of vision. Many also wear dentures that, if not fitted properly, can make speech difficult or even painful. Table 13-4 lists some of the physiological effects of aging that may affect communication and EMT-B actions that can help to offset these problems.

A few of the elderly have a significant deterioration of memory and overall intellectual ability from Alzheimer's disease (a chronic organic disorder resulting in dementia) or other conditions. However, do not assume that confusion in your elderly patient is "normal," or the result of long-term mental deterioration. Unless someone who knows the patient can confirm that this is a chronic condition, suspect that an altered mental status may be the result of the present illness or injury.

When you are speaking to any patient, it is important that the patient see and hear you. This is especially true in the elderly patient who has a hearing impairment or poor peripheral vision. Keep in mind that speaking loudly to a patient does not mean speaking down to a patient. Treat the patient with respect and dignity (Figure 13-8). Begin by calling the patient by his last name. Ask the patient how he would like to be addressed before assuming that you may use his first name. Whenever possible, speak to the patient at the same level, crouching, or even kneeling down if you need to.

Assessing the Geriatric Patient

The steps of assessment for geriatric patients are the same as those for other patients. Some particular things to be aware of and to look for include the following.

Scene Size-up and Safety— Geriatric

When you approach an elderly person's residence, look both outside and inside for clues as to the patient's physical and mental abilities. Is the outside of the house conscientiously cared for, or is the paint on the house peeling and the garden untended? When you enter the home, besides looking for potential dangers to you and your crew, look at the general condition of the residence. Is half-eaten food sitting in the living room? Is something unrecognizable drying up in a pan on the stove? Is the house dirty? Are items left out in the open where someone can trip on them?

A very important question to ask is what is the temperature? Like infants, older people cannot regulate their body temperatures very well. They need an environment that frequently feels uncomfortably warm to younger people. Even at such temperatures, some older people still wear several layers of clothing to retain sufficient heat. This can become a problem when a heat wave occurs and the older person fails to feel the temperature rising. A life-threatening rise in body temperature can result. (See Chapter 22, "Environmental Emergencies.")

Initial Assessment—Geriatric

Forming a General Impression. Now that you have looked at the patient's surroundings, look at the patient. What is the level of his distress? Is he leaning forward with hands on knees gasping for

Table 13-4 Effects of Aging with Implications for Communication

Change	Result	EMT-B Communication Strategies
Clouding and thickening of lens in eye	Cataracts; poor vision, especially peripheral vision	Position yourself in front of patient where you can be seen; put hand on arm of blind patient to let patient know where you are.
Shrinkage of structures in ear	Decreased hearing, especially ability to hear high frequency sounds; diminished sense of balance	Speak clearly; check hearing aids as necessary.
Deterioration of teeth and gums	Patient needs dentures, but they may inflict pain on sensitive gums, so patient doesn't always wear them	If patient's speech is unintelligible, ask patient to put his dentures in.

Figure 13-8 Position yourself at the patient's level, make good eye contact, and speak slowly and clearly.

breath? Is he lying on a hospital bed apparently unresponsive and breathing through an open mouth? Is he sitting in a chair in no acute distress?

Assessing Mental Status. This can be very challenging, because some older people have an abnormal mental status as part of their baseline condition. If family members or caregivers are available, it is important you find out from them what normal is for this patient.

Assessing the Airway. Evaluating the airway of an older patient is very similar to evaluating the airway of other patients with two major exceptions. You may find it difficult to extend the head and flex the neck of an older patient because of arthritic changes in the bones of the neck. The best thing to do in this case is not to try to force the head back, but instead to thrust the jaw forward to pull the tongue out of the airway.

The other difficulty you may come across is dentures. If a patient's dentures are secure, there is usually no reason to remove them. If, however, they are loose or ill-fitting, it is best to remove them from the mouth of an unresponsive patient to prevent them from becoming an airway obstruction.

Assessing Breathing. Older patients are at higher risk of foreign body airway obstruction. Two major risk factors are large, poorly chewed pieces of food and dentures. If you are unable to ventilate an older patient, reposition the head and try to ventilate again. If this does not work, initiate the sequence of steps to relieve a foreign body airway obstruction.

Assessing Circulation. Finding a radial pulse in an older patient is usually no different from finding a pulse in other patients. What you may notice in these patients, though, is that the pulse is often irregularly irregular, i.e., completely without any kind of cycle or regularity. This is the result of a very common arrhythmia (abnormal heart rhythm) in older people. The irregularity is not a reason for concern in itself.

Identifying Priority Patients. Older patients are less likely to show severe symptoms in certain conditions, so it can be difficult to determine a patient's priority. For example, most people having a heart attack experience significant chest pain. An older person is more likely to have just the sudden onset of weakness with no chest pain. Keep a high index of suspicion for serious conditions in elderly patients, even if symptoms are seemingly mild or vague.

Focused History and Physical Exam—Geriatric

History. Obtaining a history of the present illness can be challenging when the patient is elderly. He may answer questions very slowly or even inappropriately. It may be difficult to understand his speech, or he may have difficulty understanding your questions. Regardless of the particular circumstances, you must gather as much information as you can from the patient and from other sources.

When interviewing the patient, be sure to introduce yourself, speak slowly and clearly, and position yourself where he can easily see you. If he is answering your questions slowly and your initial assessment did not reveal any immediate threats to life, give him additional time. Be sure to ask just one question at a time. Similarly, if the patient's speech is slurred but still understandable, do not rush him. Doing so could easily fluster him, delaying responses even more, and destroy any rapport you have established. If the patient's speech is difficult to understand because his dentures are not in place, ask him to put them in if appropriate.

Sometimes a patient will answer questions very slowly because he is *clinically depressed,* or so sad or blue that his eating and sleeping habits are altered, he feels fatigued, his memory or concentration is impaired, his self-confidence is low, and he may even have thoughts of suicide. About one tenth of older people have clinical depression. However, do not be fooled into thinking that a patient who is depressed has no other problems. Depression can both mimic and mask other serious medical problems.

Another possibility you may find when interviewing a patient is that the family tells you he was wrong in some of his responses. This is sometimes a result of a neurological condition, but it can also be caused by medications the patient is taking, especially if there are many of them (Figure 13-9) or the dose is too high for some.

A variation of this is the patient who gives you a story of having gone out to the movies last night but who, according to family members, has not left the house in years. This is called *confabulation*. The patient is replacing lost circumstances with imaginary ones. These made-up experiences are usually quite believable and the patient is typically very pleasant to talk to. Nonetheless, the experiences are not real and may very well change if you ask the same question a few minutes later. Confabulation can be caused by a number of neurological conditions.

This points out the importance of gathering information from family members and others who are familiar with the patient's condition. If the patient lives with a spouse or other family members, they can frequently be an excellent source of information about his medications, SAMPLE history, and even the history of the present illness. Similarly, visiting nurses can provide a great deal of this information.

Figure 13-9 Older patients often take multiple medications.

Physical Exam. When performing a physical exam on an older person, keep the patient's dignity in mind. Explain what you are going to do before you do it and replace as soon as possible any clothing you remove. Many older people have a high threshold for pain. An extremity that is obviously fractured may cause very little discomfort to some patients. On the other hand, some of these patients have a very low threshold for pain. You will need to judge this for yourself when doing a physical exam.

Baseline Vital Signs. Vital signs of the elderly are similar to those of other adults, with only a few exceptions. As people age, the systolic blood pressure has a tendency to increase. It usually does not require treatment. Many older patients you meet will be on medication for hypertension, usually defined as a diastolic pressure over about 90 mmHg. These medications can have significant side effects, including weakness and dizziness, especially on standing up quickly from a sitting or supine position.

The skin loses much of its elasticity as it ages, leading to dry skin that is thin and fragile. Applying pressure that is too heavy, even with just your fingertips, can be enough to cause the skin to tear in some patients. Be careful when pulling or lifting a patient to be as gentle as possible.

The pupils are not round and reactive to light in some older patients. Eye sur-

gery or pre-existing conditions may have given the pupil an abnormal shape or the inability to react to light normally. Certain eye drops can also prevent normal reactions to light. When you find this condition, inquire as to whether it is normal before assuming the patient has a serious condition based on this sign.

Detailed Physical Exam—Geriatric

The detailed physical exam for older patients is the same as for other adults. You may come across some unusual findings because of the patient's age or condition, though.

Head and Neck. When evaluating the head, be especially attentive. Injuries to the head and face are very common in older patients who have sustained a fall or been involved in a motor-vehicle collision (Figure 13-10). In fact, falls and motor-vehicle collisions account for the overwhelming majority of injuries in patients over 65 years.

The neck may be stiff and the head may be far forward of where it normally is because of changes in the spine. This can be a challenge to deal with when you suspect a neck injury and must immobilize the patient. Use folded towels or other materials to keep the head in its normal position, prevent hyperextension, and make the patient more comfortable.

Chest and Abdomen. The chest and abdomen are not commonly injured, but keep in mind the decreased sensitivity to pain that many older people have. Serious abdominal problems that would cause a younger person agony may produce only slight discomfort for older patients.

Pelvis and Extremities. The hip or proximal femur is commonly fractured in a fall, especially in women. This is partly because more women than men survive to be old, but even more so because women are very prone to loss of calcium from bone. This leads to so much weakening of the bone that a fracture is sometimes the cause of a fall rather than a result. Other areas on the extremities are also injured sometimes because of this weakening of the bone.

Spine. The back is sometimes injured in a fall, but it is very commonly injured in motor-vehicle collisions. Again, because of abnormal curvature that sometimes accompanies aging, immobilizing these patients can be very challenging. Do your best to keep the vertebrae in alignment

Figure 13-10 Extrication of an elderly patient from a motor-vehicle collision.

and to reduce the patient's discomfort as much as possible.

Ongoing Assessment—Geriatric

Children who deteriorate are likely to experience sudden changes in condition. Although that can happen in elderly patients, it is more common for them to show a slow, steady decline in condition. This can be deceiving because the patient does not suddenly tell you or show sudden signs that his condition is going downhill. Instead, you may be lulled into a false sense of security because there is little or no appreciable change from one minute to the next. Guard against this by performing an ongoing assessment at regular intervals and comparing your findings to those you recorded previously. Look for trends that indicate trouble.

Keep in mind the elements of the ongoing assessment:

1. Reassess mental status
2. Maintain open airway
3. Monitor breathing
4. Reassess pulse
5. Monitor skin color, temperature, and moisture

6. Reassess vital signs
   —every 5 minutes in unstable patients
   —every 15 minutes in stable patients

7. Assure that all appropriate care and treatment are being given.

Additional Concerns

Falls. The significance of a fall for an older person should not be underestimated. Of older patients seen in an emergency department for a fall, one quarter will die within a year. Death may not be a direct result of the fall, but instead may be a result of complications from the fall. For example, while recuperating from bruised ribs sustained in a fall, a 74-year-old woman may not breathe as deeply as normal because of the pain associated with inhalation. As a result of not coughing and other changes in the lung associated with aging, if this patient comes down with pneumonia, she is more likely to die from complications of the disease.

Often, a fall is just an indication of a more serious problem. A number of older people fall because of abnormal heart rhythms. Others fall because of a stroke or internal bleeding from an ulcer. Whenever

possible and when time allows, assess the patient not only for injuries that may have resulted from the fall, but also for a cause of the fall.

EMT-Bs can help prevent falls. When you enter an older person's home, look for potential hazards. Table 13-5 lists a number of hazards and what you or the patient's family or friends can do to correct them.

Elder Abuse and Neglect. Elder abuse and neglect have occurred for many years but have only recently received the attention they deserve. There are essentially three ways in which elders can be abused or neglected: physically, psychologically, and financially. Physical abuse and neglect includes pushing, shoving, hitting, shaking, or improperly feeding an older person. It occasionally includes sexual abuse. Psychological abuse and neglect includes threats, insults, or ignoring an older person ("the silent treatment"). Financial abuse and neglect is the exploitation or misuse of an older person's belongings or money.

Detecting elder abuse and neglect can be difficult. Even though falls are

Table 13-5   Making a Home Safer for the Elderly

Hazard	Intervention	Reason
Torn or slippery rugs	Repair or replace.	To prevent tripping and slipping
Chair without armrests	Install armrests.	To provide leverage in getting out of chair
Chair with low back	Replace with a chair with high back.	To support neck; prevent falling backward for patients who must rock to get out of chair
Chair with wheels	Replace with a chair with sturdy legs.	To prevent chair from sliding when elder is getting into or out of it
Temperature too low	Maintain temperature at 72°F in winter.	To prevent hypothermia
Obstructing furniture	Move items so that clutter is minimized and pathways are clear.	To help those with poor mobility and poor peripheral vision
Slippery bathtub	Install skid-resistant strips or mat.	To provide more stable footing
Missing handrails on stairways	Install handrail.	To allow elder to grab onto support

common in the elderly, evaluate any injury in this age group with an eye toward recognizing signs of abuse or neglect. Many states have laws that require the reporting of such suspicions. Be aware of the laws in your state and local protocols and take whatever actions you are permitted to take to help the victim of abuse.

Loss of Independence. It is hard for younger adults to understand how disruptive a serious injury or illness can be to an older person. Years of independence can vanish in an instant, leaving the patient in the care of strangers. Even worse, he goes to a hospital where many friends and perhaps a spouse have gone, never to return. The EMT-B can ease this transition by treating the patient in a respectful, dignified manner. Do not minimize the patient's fears and concerns. Instead, acknowledge them and try to put them in perspective.

Ask the patient if he would like you to lock up before you leave the house. Inquire about the care of any pets and whether there is a trusted neighbor who can take care of them for awhile. If you can honestly say it, reassure the patient that most patients you have seen with this particular problem do well and return home in good condition. A friendly hand on the forearm, if you feel the patient will accept it, can be very reassuring. Asking the patient during transport about what he has done over the course of a lifetime can be not only therapeutic for the patient, but enlightening for you as well. Above all, treat the patient in a respectful, empathetic manner.

COMPARING ASSESSMENTS

The scenario below may help you see the special considerations involved in assessing pediatric and geriatric patients.

Dispatch

Two ambulance crews, including you and three other EMT-Bs, have been dispatched to care for four victims of carbon monoxide inhalation: 71-year-old Dolores McAuliffe and her grandchildren, Andrea (16 years old), Megan (10 years old), and Eddie (11 months old). You find the patients inside a neighbor's home, Mrs. McAuliffe and Megan supine on the floor, Andrea standing nearby with Eddie crying in her arms.

Assessment of 71-Year-Old Woman

Initial Assessment

Your general impression is of an unresponsive older woman. When you assess Mrs. McAuliffe's mental status, you find that she moans in response to a painful stimulus. The firefighter has already opened her airway. He reports that he performed a jaw-thrust with no head tilt because her neck seems somewhat arthritic and stiff. You confirm that her airway is open and note that her breathing is adequate in both rate and depth. You assess her circulation by palpating a strong, rapid radial pulse. Her skin is pale and slightly sweaty. You find no external bleeding. You assign her a high priority because of her altered mental status and her threatened airway. You administer oxygen by nonrebreather mask at 12 liters per minute.

Focused History and Physical Exam—Medical

Since Mrs. McAuliffe cannot communicate, you delay the history to perform a rapid physical exam. You find no injuries or other abnormalities. You obtain baseline vital signs of pulse 112 and irregular, BP 180/90, respirations 24 and regular, pupils equal and reactive. The history has to be gathered from others at the scene. Firefighters inform you that the alarm that went off was a carbon-monoxide alarm. On arrival, the firefighters found Mrs. McAuliffe in the cellar between the clothes dryer and the furnace and immediately evacuated her. The neighbors know that Mrs. McAuliffe often babysits for her grandchildren but don't know much about her medical history. They think she may have a heart problem. A firefighter is sent to recover Mrs. McAuliffe's purse, which contains some prescribed medications you will bring with her to the hospital.

Assessment of 10-Year-Old Girl

Initial Assessment

Your partner's general impression is of a moaning 10-year-old girl. Megan's mental status is awake and crying. Her airway is open and her breathing is adequate in both rate and depth. Your partner's assessment of circulation reveals a strong, rapid radial pulse. Skin is flushed and dry. There is no apparent external bleeding. Megan's priority is high because of the nature of the illness: carbon monoxide poisoning. Your partner calms the child as she begins administering oxygen by pediatric nonrebreather mask at 12 liters per minute and continues with her assessment.

Focused History and Physical Exam—Medical

At first, like many sick children, Megan is withdrawn and not interested in communicating with your partner, who is a stranger to her. However, by treating Megan in a calm and friendly manner, your partner is able to gain her attention and confidence. The history your partner can gather is scant, however. The firefighter says Megan was found lying on the living room floor, very drowsy, and was quickly carried out of the house. Megan confides that the whole family started feeling sick at the same time and that right now her head hurts. A rapid physical exam reveals no injuries or other abnormalities. Baseline vital signs are pulse 140, regular and strong, BP 100/70, and respirations of 28 and regular.

"Unit 10, respond to the senior citizen housing center on Martin Luther King, Jr. Avenue for a patient having difficulty breathing." When you arrive, you stop for a moment at the doorway and notice that the apartment is messy. The patient is a 67-year-old male sitting upright in a chair with rapid respirations and wheezing. You ask why he has called EMS, and he responds in short sentences, telling you that he is having trouble catching his breath and may be having an asthma attack. Your partner tells the patient she wants to give him oxygen. While a nonrebreather is set up, you perform an initial assessment.

STREET SCENE QUESTIONS

1. What is your initial priority for providing care to this patient?

2. After the initial assessment is completed, what assessment information should be obtained next?

3. Why is the condition of the apartment significant?

The patient's airway is open and his respirations are 24 per minute with wheezing upon exhalation. Your partner continues to obtain additional vitals, and you get a SAMPLE history. When you ask the patient if he is taking any medications, he asks if you could speak up because he doesn't hear well. You reposition yourself in front of the patient and speak clearly, without shouting, at a greater volume. He responds by pointing to a shoe box full of pill bottles and two inhalers. You ask if he has been taking his medications and, appearing confused, he says he doesn't remember which ones he took today. When asked if someone knows about his medication schedule, he states that he lives alone. Your partner reports the following vital signs: respirations are 28, pulse is 110, blood pressure is 160/100, skin is moist, and pupils equal and reactive. You and your partner tell the patient that you want to take him to the hospital. He agrees, and you package and move him to the ambulance.

Assessment of 11-Month-Old Infant

Initial Assessment
The general impression formed by the EMT-B from the other ambulance is of an infant who appears in no acute distress. Eddie's mental status is awake and calm. He is moving energetically in Andrea's arms and looking around curiously at all the activity in the room. His airway is open and his breathing is adequate in both rate and depth. The assessment of circulation reveals a strong, rapid brachial pulse. Skin is warm, pink, and dry. There is no apparent external bleeding. Although Eddie does not appear to be in distress, his priority is high because of the nature of the illness, carbon monoxide poisoning. The EMT-B starts to administer high-concentration oxygen. Eddie fights the mask, but he tolerates "blow-by" administration with his big sister holding the mask near his face.

Focused History and Physical Exam—Medical
Eddie's history—provided by Andrea—includes the fact that his sister had placed him upstairs in a crib when the family started feeling ill, so he was relatively far from the malfunctioning furnace. The EMT-B who is assessing Eddie gets him giggling happily by playing with his toes, then conducts a rapid physical exam in toe-to-head sequence. The exam reveals no injuries or other abnormalities. Baseline vital signs are pulse 128, regular and strong, respirations of 30 and regular.

Assessment of 16-Year-Old Girl

Initial Assessment
The general impression is of a teenage girl who appears in no acute distress. Andrea's mental status is awake and oriented, although she is quite anxious about her grandmother, sister, and brother. Her airway, breathing, and circulation are all normal. Although she appears to be well, her priority is high because she has been exposed to carbon monoxide. The EMT-B gives her high-concentration oxygen, but first thinks to enlist Andrea's help in showing the mask to Eddie, smiling, and saying "Look what I get to put on!" so Eddie won't be frightened by the mask on his sister's face.

4. Based on the assessment, would you expect this patient's condition to worsen? How should you be prepared if it does?

5. What additional assessment should be done en route to the hospital? How often should the vital signs be taken?

6. What information about the patient's living situation seems significant enough to provide to the hospital staff?

You briefly discuss the patient situation with your partner and you decide that a transport with red lights and siren seems appropriate as the patient's breathing rate is increasing and you may need to assist ventilations with a bag-valve mask. You also decide, based on the patient's confused state and inability to breathe deeply, not to assist him with one of his inhalers. As you proceed to the hospital, with your partner driving, you reassess vital signs and find the patient's respiratory rate has returned to 24 and the patient is starting to talk in longer sentences. You ask some additional medical history questions about previous asthma attacks and the patient seems more lucid. You are communicating well with the patient, and he is hearing you. In fact, he provides the name of his daughter and gives you a telephone number. The patient seems less anxious and, about 5 minutes before arrival at the hospital, he has a respiratory rate of 20 with wheezing still present. You contact the hospital by radio, provide patient information, and give an ETA.

While completing your prehospital care report, you remember the condition of the apartment and that this patient lives alone. Before leaving, you share this information with the charge nurse and suggest that if this patient is sent home, he may need living assistance as well as help with his care, such as medications. The nurse thanks you and tells you that she will ask a case manager to follow up.

Focused History and Physical Exam—Medical
Andrea's history includes the fact that she had been upstairs with her baby brother and, like him, farther from the furnace than her sister and grandmother. The female EMT-B has gained Andrea's confidence by treating her with professionalism and respect. Andrea admits that she is afraid she has done herself some permanent injury by breathing carbon monoxide and also feels guilty that she didn't do more to help her grandmother and siblings. The EMT-B is able to comfort and reassure her. She explains to Andrea the elements of the rapid physical exam before she conducts it. She is careful to protect Andrea's privacy during the exam, which reveals no injuries or other abnormalities. Baseline vital signs are pulse 70, regular and strong, BP 94/60, respirations of 18 and regular.

Back-up drivers have been sent to the scene so both members of each ambulance crew can attend to their patients en route. You continue administering oxygen to Mrs. McAuliffe and Megan. Mrs. McAuliffe begins to become more awake, and by the time you arrive at the emergency department, she is alert and complaining of a terrible headache and nausea. Her vital signs return to the normal range and you turn over her care to emergency department staff. Megan's head still hurts, but she is far less drowsy. By the time your ambulance arrives at the emergency department, both of your patients are looking and feeling better. In the other ambulance, Andrea and Eddie both continue to receive oxygen and seem quite well when they arrive at the emergency department.

At the hospital, blood tests on the patients confirm that they all were exposed to carbon monoxide, Mrs. McAuliffe receiving the most exposure, Megan a moderate exposure, and Andrea and Eddie only a minor exposure. All four are expected to make a good recovery.

CHAPTER REVIEW

SUMMARY

People are most dependent on others for help, especially when illness or injury strikes, at the extremes of age. By taking into account a child's age and developmental characteristics, you will be able to perform a more thorough assessment that will lead to less commotion and disturbance for the child's family. Similarly, by considering an older person's physical and emotional condition, you will be able to gather needed medical information in a way that preserves the dignity of our elders.

REVIEW QUESTIONS

1. Describe key differences in the anatomy and physiology of infants and children with regard to (pp. 258–261):
   —head
   —airway and respiratory system
   —chest
   —abdomen
   —body surface
   —blood volume
2. Describe how each of the differences you named for question 1, above, will affect your assessment of the infant or child patient. (pp. 262–267)
3. Describe ways of calming and interacting effectively with the infant or child patient with the parent or caregiver. (p. 262)

4. Explain some of the elements of a general impression of the infant or child patient that you can obtain "from the doorway"—before you approach the patient. (pp. 262–263)
5. Describe how to approach an elderly patient who has vision and hearing impairments. (p. 269)
6. What question should you ask to determine if an elderly patient's condition is normal or a change from baseline? (p. 270)
7. Name some of the most common medical conditions that cause EMS to be called for elderly patients. Name the most common mechanism of injury to elderly patients. (pp. 268–269)

APPLICATIONS

You respond to an elderly woman who has fallen and injured her hip. When you arrive, you find a 90-year-old woman lying on the kitchen floor, alert and oriented, complaining of hip pain. She is somewhat hard of hearing. Her 91-year-old husband is very upset over what happened and blaming himself for her fall. How should you approach your assessment of the patient? How should you deal with her husband?

Visit Brady's *Emergency Care* website for direct weblinks. At **www.bradybooks.com/ emergencycare**, you will find information related to the following Chapter 13 topics:

- Child abuse
- Elder abuse

Chapter
Fourteen

COMMUNICATIONS

There are three types of communication that you will learn about in this chapter: radio communication, the verbal report at the hospital, and interpersonal communication. As the name implies, radio communication is conducted by radio. Technology has allowed the use of cellular phones and other equipment to be used where radio transmissions were previously the only choice. The verbal report is your chance to convey information about your patient directly to the hospital personnel who will be taking over his care. Interpersonal communications are important in dealing with other EMT-Bs, the patient, family and bystanders, medical direction, and other members of the EMS system.

COMMUNICATIONS SYSTEMS AND RADIO COMMUNICATION

Radio equipment is often taken for granted since it is now so common (Figure 14-1). However, the development of radio links between dispatchers, mobile units, and hospitals has been one of the key contributors to improvement in EMS over the years. Imagine if you had to call the dispatcher by phone every few minutes to see if there is a call! And without radio transmissions from ambulances, hospitals would be unable to prepare for the arrival of patients, as they do now.

Communications Systems

There are a number of components to any radio or communications system: **base stations, mobile radios, portable radios, repeaters, cellular phones,** and other devices.

- *Base stations* are two-way radios that are at a fixed site such as a hospital or dispatch center.
- *Mobile radios* are two-way radios that are used or affixed in a vehicle. Most are actually mounted inside the vehicle. These devices have lower transmitting power than base stations. The unit used to measure output power of radios is the **watt.** The output of a mobile radio is generally 20–50 watts with a range of 10–15 miles.
- *Portable radios* are hand-held two-way radios with an output of 1–5 watts. This type of radio is important because it will allow you to be in touch with the dispatcher, medical direction, and other members of the EMS system while you are away from the ambulance.
- *Repeaters* are devices that are used when transmissions must be carried over a long distance. Repeaters may be in ambulances or placed in various areas around an EMS system. The repeater picks up signals from lower-power units, such as mobile and portable radios, and re-transmits them at a higher power. The re-transmission is done on another frequency (Figure 14-2).
- *Cellular phones* are phones that transmit through the air instead of over wires so that the phones can be transported and used over a wide area. These devices are becoming more widely available and popular around the country. In many areas where the distances or expense is too great to set up a conventional EMS radio system, cellular phones allow EMS communications through an already established commercial system.

TOPIC OVERVIEW

In this chapter, you will learn about the following topics:

- Communication skills used when interacting with the patient
- Radio procedures used at various stages of the EMS call
- Delivery and format of a radio report to the hospital
- Delivery and format of a verbal hand-off report

DOT OBJECTIVES

New technology is developing almost constantly. Microwave radio transmissions are used in some areas. In others, radio communications are carried via phone lines for part of the signal's journey from one point to another. Digital radio equipment permits transmission of some standard messages, such as ambulance identification or arrival at the scene, by punching a key. The messages are transmitted in a condensed form that helps keep busy frequencies less crowded.

Since radios are so important to EMS today, many systems have back-up radios. This means that in the event of power failure or malfunction, another option is available. If the base station fails, there may

be a back-up radio or alternative power supply available. If the mobile radio in your ambulance malfunctions, portable radios or phones may be used in its place.

Note that radio systems require preventive maintenance and repair, just as the ambulance and your EMS equipment do. Radio equipment must be treated with care on a daily basis and not mishandled.

Radio Communication

EMS is just one of many public services that use radio communication. To maintain order on the airwaves, the Federal Communications Commission (FCC) assigns and licenses radio frequencies. This is to prevent two or more agencies from trying to use the same frequency and interfering with each other's communications. There are also strict rules about interfering with emergency radio traffic and prohibiting profanities or offensive language.

Some general rules for radio transmissions should always be followed. These rules prevent delays and allow all persons to use the frequencies. There may be some minor variations within your EMS system, but always keep in mind the principles shown in Table 14-1.

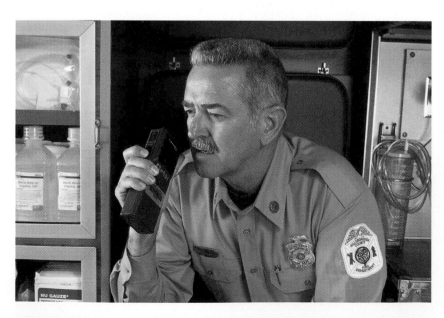

Figure 14-1 Communication from the ambulance can be by radio or cellular phone.

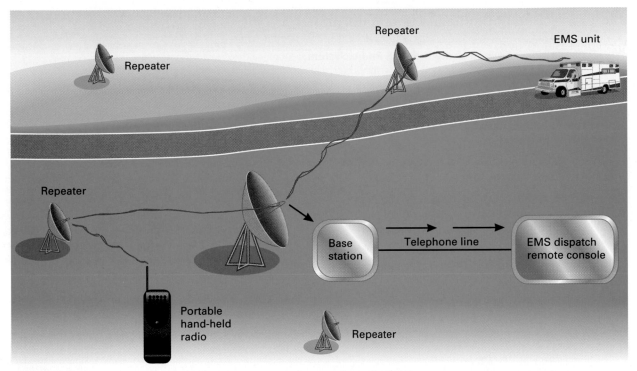

Figure 14-2 Example of an EMS communication system using repeaters.

Radio Transmissions Throughout the Call

When the Emergency Medical Dispatcher (EMD) receives the initial call for help, the call most often comes via telephone but may also be radioed from another agency, such as the police. After proper information is obtained, the units are dispatched. The following is a sample flow of information between the dispatcher and units in the field. You are the EMT-B on ambulance number 6:

Dispatcher: Ambulance 6 . . .
You: Ambulance 6. Go ahead.
Dispatcher: Ambulance 6, respond to 1243 Magnolia Boulevard—that's one-two-four-three Magnolia Boulevard—for an assault. The police are en route. Stand by at the corner of Magnolia and Third until the police report the scene secure.
You: Ambulance 6 received that. Will stand by at Magnolia and Third.

Without a prompt and efficient receipt and dispatch of information, the ambulance could easily be sent to the wrong location. In this situation, the dispatcher also relayed important safety information. Since the call was for an assault, the dispatcher "staged" the ambulance, or ordered it to stand by, until the scene is safe.

You respond to the assigned location, reporting your arrival to the dispatcher:

You: Dispatcher, Ambulance 6 is arriving at the staging area.

Dispatcher: Message received, Ambulance 6. I will advise you when the scene is secure.

Most scenes are safe. However, in this case the dispatcher has decided, from the nature of the call and other information she was able to obtain, that it is not. Police arrive at the scene and separate the parties involved in the assault. The police radio the dispatcher and advise that the scene is secure. The next transmission is to your ambulance:

Dispatcher: Ambulance 6, the police report that the scene is secure. Respond in.
You: Message received by Ambulance 6. (You drive two blocks to the scene and report to the dispatcher.) Dispatcher, Ambulance 6 is at the scene.
Dispatcher: Ambulance 6 at the scene (gives the time on the 24-hour clock) at 1310 hours.

The dispatcher records all the times from the time of the original call, the time dispatched, at the staging area, and finally at the scene. Should this case go to court, the records of the dispatch center, your care report, and the dispatch audio tape of the call may be subpoenaed. Unless there is a need for medical direction or assistance from the scene, the next call will be when you are en route to the hospital:

You: Dispatcher, Ambulance 6 is en route to Mercy Hospital with one patient.
Dispatcher: Ambulance 6 en route to Mercy Hospital at 1323 hours.

Table 14-1   Principles of Radio Communication

Follow These Principles When Using the EMS Radio System:

- Make sure that your radio is on and the volume is adjusted properly.

- Reduce background noise by closing the vehicle window when possible.

- Listen to the frequency and ensure that it is clear before beginning a transmission.

- Press the "press to talk" (PTT) button on the radio, then wait one second before speaking. This prevents cutting off the first few words of your transmission.

- Speak with your lips about 2 to 3 inches from the microphone.

- When calling another unit or base station, use their unit number or name, followed by yours. "Dispatcher, this is Ambulance 2."

- The unit being called will signal that the transmission should start by saying "go ahead" ("Ambulance 2, this is the dispatcher. Go ahead") or another regionally accepted term. If the unit you are calling tells you to "stand by," wait until they tell you they are ready to take your transmission.

- Speak slowly and clearly.

- Keep the transmissions brief. If it takes longer than 30 seconds, stop at that point and pause for a few seconds so that emergency traffic can use the frequency if necessary.

- Use plain English. Avoid codes.

- Do not use phrases like "be advised." These are implied and serve no purpose.

- Courtesy is assumed, so there is no need to say "please," "thank you," and "you're welcome."

- When transmitting a number that might be unclear (15 may sound like 16 or 50), give the number, then repeat the individual digits. Say "15, one-five."

- Anything said over the radio can be heard by the public on a scanner. Do not use the patient's name over the radio. For the same reason, do not use profanities or statements that tend to slander any person. Use objective, impartial statements.

- Use "we" instead of "I." As an EMT-B, you will rarely be acting alone.

- "Affirmative" and "negative" are preferred over "yes" and "no" because the latter are difficult to hear.

- Give assessment information about your patient, but avoid offering a diagnosis of the patient's problem. For example, say "Patient complains of chest pain," but not "Probably having a heart attack."

- After transmitting, say "Over." Wait for acknowledgment that the person to whom you were speaking heard your message.

- Avoid slang or abbreviations that are not authorized.

- Use EMS frequencies only for authorized EMS communication.

You will call the hospital via radio or phone to advise them of the status of your patient and the estimated time of arrival (ETA). When arriving at the hospital, you again advise the dispatcher:

You: Ambulance 6 is arriving at Mercy Hospital.
Dispatcher: Ambulance 6 at Mercy at 1334 hours.

You will note that the dispatcher gives the time after most transmissions. This will allow you to record times if they are required on your patient care record. The dispatcher also usually acknowledges by briefly repeating the message to assure that she has acknowledged the right unit. If two units happened to transmit at exactly the same time and the dispatcher simply acknowledged a transmission, both units would think that the dispatcher heard them when, actually, only one unit was able to get through.

After turning the patient over to the hospital staff and preparing the ambulance for the next run, you will advise the dispatcher that you are leaving the hospital. You may also find it part of your local procedure to advise the dispatcher when you are back in your district or area and when you are back in quarters (the station or ambulance garage).

A majority of these transmissions were made between the mobile radio within the ambulance and the dispatcher at a base station. Remember, when you have one available, bring your portable radio with you whenever you leave the ambulance. You may need to call for assistance during scene size-up if hazards or multiple patients are found, and the portable radio allows you to do it without running back to the ambulance to make the call on the fixed unit.

Medical Radio Reports

Reports must be made to medical personnel as part of almost every call. These reports may be by radio, verbal (in person), or in writing. The radio report is specifically structured to present pertinent facts about the patient without telling more detail than necessary. Too much detail ties up the radio frequency and takes up the time of hospital personnel.

Experienced EMT-Bs often try to "paint a picture" of the patient in words. This requires knowledge of radio procedure and practice. If you have a critical patient, your radio report should make that clear. This can be done by describing the chief complaint, injuries, vital signs, treatments, and mechanism of injury. Even with critical patients you must keep a clear, steady tone to your voice. Resist the urge to talk fast or appear excited as it will prevent effective communication.

A medical radio report has twelve parts (Table 14-2). Below is an example, broken into its individual parts, of a report you might make to the hospital:

1. **Unit identification and level of provider**
   Memorial Hospital, this is Community BLS Ambulance 6 en route to your location . . .

2. **Estimated time of arrival**
   . . . with a 15-minute ETA.

3. **Patient's age and sex**
   We are transporting a 68-year-old male patient . . .

4. **Chief complaint**
   . . . who complains of pain in his abdomen.

5. **Brief, pertinent history of the present illness**
   Onset of pain was 2 hours ago and is accompanied by slight nausea.

6. **Major past illnesses**
   The patient has a history of high blood pressure and arthritis

7. **Mental status**
   He is alert and oriented, never lost consciousness.

8. **Baseline vital signs**
   His vital signs are pulse 88 regular and full, respirations 20 and unlabored, skin normal, and blood pressure 134 over 88.

9. **Pertinent findings of the physical exam**
   Our exam revealed tenderness in both upper abdominal quadrants. They did not appear rigid.

10. **Emergency medical care given**
    For care, we have placed him in a position of comfort.

11. **Response to emergency medical care**
    The level of pain has not changed during our care. Mental status has remained unchanged. Vital signs are basically unchanged.

12. **If your system requires contacting medical direction, or if you have questions**
    Does medical direction have any orders?

After giving this information, you will continue with ongoing assessment of the patient en route to the hospital. Additional vital signs will be taken, there may be changes in the patient's condition, or you may discover new information about the patient, particularly on long transports. In some systems, you should radio this additional information to the hospital in a follow-up radio call while en route (follow local protocols).

When medical direction is contacted, orders may be given to the EMT-B. The on-line physician may order you to assist in administering the patient's own medication, or order the administration of a medication you carry on the ambulance, or give other orders. In any case, the communication between you and medical direction must be clear and concise to avoid misinterpretations that can inadvertently harm the patient. For example, a patient may have a medication for chest pain called nitroglycerin. This medication, as you will learn in Chapter 16, "General Pharmacology," is one that you may assist the patient in taking (according to local protocols). The medication should be given only if the patient's blood

---

Table 14-2   Radio Medical Report

Twelve Parts of a Radio Medical Report

1. Unit identification and level of provider
2. Estimated time of arrival
3. Patient's age and sex
4. Chief complaint
5. Brief, pertinent history of the present illness
6. Major past illnesses
7. Mental status
8. Baseline vital signs
9. Pertinent findings of the physical exam
10. Emergency medical care given
11. Response to emergency medical care
12. Contact medical direction if required or if you have questions

pressure is above a certain level. If there is a misunderstanding between you and the physician and this medication is ordered improperly, harm may come to the patient.

To avoid misunderstanding and miscommunication, use the following guidelines when communicating with medical direction:

- Give the information to medical direction clearly and accurately. Speak slowly and clearly. The orders of the physician will be based on what you report.
- After receiving an order for a medication or procedure, repeat the order word for word. You may also ask to do a procedure or give a medication and be denied by medical direction. Repeat this also.
- If an order is unclear, ask the physician to repeat it. After you have a clear understanding of the order, repeat it back to the physician.
- If an order appears to be inappropriate, question the physician. There may have been a misunderstanding. Your questioning may prevent the inappropriate administration of a medication. If the physician verifies the order, he may explain to you why he has given you that particular order.

THE VERBAL REPORT

At the hospital, you will give a written report on your patient to hospital personnel. (See Chapter 15, "Documentation.") However, it will take some time to complete your written report, so the first information you give to hospital personnel will be your verbal report.

As you transfer your patient to the care of the hospital staff, introduce the patient by name. Then summarize the same kind of information you gave over the radio, pointing out any information that is updated or different from your last radio report. Include the following in your verbal report:

- Chief complaint
- History that was not given previously
- Additional treatment given en route
- Additional vital signs taken en route

INTERPERSONAL COMMUNICATION

While communication between two or more human beings is a skill that you have learned over the years, many people still do not communicate as well as they could. Communicating with patients and others who are in crisis is even more difficult. While interpersonal communication could be presented as a course in itself, the following guidelines will help when dealing with patients, families, friends, and bystanders:

- *Use eye contact.* Make frequent eye contact with your patient. It shows that you are interested in your patient and that you are attentive. Failure to make eye contact signals that you feel uneasy around the patient. (If your patient is avoiding eye contact, consider that in some cultures eye contact is considered rude. You may want to match your behavior to the patient's in this situation.)
- *Be aware of your position and body language.* Your positioning in respect to the patient is important. If you are higher than the patient, you may appear intimidating. If possible, position yourself at or below the patient's eye level (Figure 14-3). This will be less threatening to the patient. Body language is also important. Standing with your arms crossed or not directly facing the patient (a closed stance) sends a signal to the patient that you are not interested. Use a more open stance (arms down, facing the patient), when it can be done safely, to communicate a warmer attitude.

A closed or more serious stance may sometimes be beneficial, however, when you need to

HOW AND WHY?

Sometimes a failure to communicate is caused by a lack of privacy. Go to your Electronic Extras CD for tips on building trust and rapport.

Figure 14-3 Position yourself at or below the patient's eye level to be less intimidating and to aid communication.

calm or direct bystanders at the scene. Standing above a patient may convey authority and can be done to gain control when necessary.

Watch the patient's body language to see how your communication with him is going. If the patient uses a closed stance, your communication efforts may not be working.

- *Use language the patient can understand.* Speak slowly and clearly. Do not use medical or other terms that the patient will not understand. Explain procedures before they are performed, to prevent anxiety.

- *Be honest.* Honesty is important. You will frequently be asked questions that you will not have the answer to: "Is my leg broken?" "Am I having a heart attack?" At other times you will know the answer to the question, but it is not pleasant: "Will it hurt when you put that splint on?" If the answer is yes, tell the truth. Explain that you will do it as gently as possible to reduce pain, but some pain may be experienced. It is much worse to lie to the patient and have them find out that you were not being truthful. This will erode the patient's confidence in you as well as in other EMT-Bs and medical personnel the patient may meet later on.

- *Use the patient's proper name.* Especially with senior citizens and other adults, do not assume familiarity. As a general rule, call patients as they introduce themselves to you. If a person many years older than you introduces himself as William Harris, it might be best to call him Mr. Harris as a sign of respect. Immediately calling him "Bill" when he clearly stated his name was "William" would be disrespectful. If, after you call him "Mr. Harris," he says "Please call me Bill," you have shown respect and can then use the less formal name. If in doubt, ask what the patient would like to be called.

- *Listen.* If you ask the patient a question, get an answer, then have to ask again, it will show the patient that you were not listening. If you are not listening, the patient will feel that you are not interested in what he has to say, or that you just don't care. If you ask a question, wait for the answer. Then write it down so you will not forget.

If a person has a mental disability or is hard of hearing, speak slowly and clearly. Do not talk down to the patient. If the patient has a hearing disability, he may read lips or, in any case, seeing your lips may help him understand what you are saying. So be sure that a deaf or hearing-impaired person can see your mouth when you talk.

Remember that a person who is blind or has a visual deficit can usually hear, so do not give in to the temptation to speak to him loudly or unnaturally. For the visually impaired person, you will want to take extra effort to explain anything that is happening that he cannot see.

You may also find people who do not speak the same language as you. In this case, use an interpreter (for example, a family member or friend who speaks both languages) or a manual that provides translations. You may also find that your communications center or medical direction has someone available who speaks the patient's language.

The elderly are a rapidly growing segment of the population who often need EMS care. These older patients may have medical problems simply because of their age. They may also be more prone to falls and serious injury from trauma due to the condition of their bones and body systems.

Many elderly patients are well oriented and physically able. Others, however, may have problems with hearing, sight, or orientation that have come on with age. These patients may seem confused or simply find it difficult to communicate. In spite of their sensory limitations, of course, these patients still have needs and feelings. They deserve patience, kindness, and understanding—along with proper emergency care (Figure 14-4).

Pediatric Notes

Since children sometimes can be difficult to assess and communicate with, it is often best to involve the parents of the child when

Figure 14-4 Be considerate of the elderly patient.

You are just about to leave the hospital emergency department after your last run, when the dispatcher calls on the portable radio. You answer: "Go ahead, dispatch. This is Ambulance 40." Unfortunately, your radio will not transmit out of the hospital, so you call the communications center by telephone. The dispatcher informs you of a 9-1-1 call from a cell phone reporting someone trapped in a vehicle on the side of the road near mile marker 21 on Route 15. The sheriff and a fire department First Response unit with extrication equipment have been dispatched. Your response time is approximately 15 minutes.

While en route, you receive a transmission from the dispatcher that the deputy sheriff reports only one patient who is trapped and unresponsive. You are now 10 minutes from the scene and the next transmission that you hear is the First Response unit arriving on scene.

STREET SCENE QUESTIONS

1. What type of scene safety information do you want to know from the sheriff's deputy?

2. Should you contact the First Responders or wait until they contact you?

3. What patient information would be helpful to know?

You radio the dispatcher and request that he contact the deputy sheriff on the scene to find out what the best access is and where you can stage the ambulance. As you finish this transmission, you hear: "Ambulance 40, this is Fire Rescue 8 at the scene." You acknowledge, and they provide you with the following information: "Patient is unconscious with an open airway, breathing is 24 and labored, pulse is 120, pale and diaphoretic, with possible head and chest trauma. He was wearing a seatbelt but no air bag deployment. He needs to be extricated which should take about 10 minutes. Consider rapid extrication to a backboard. A cervical collar is already in place."

You are now 4 minutes from the scene and the dispatcher notifies you that you should approach using the northbound lane, which has been blocked off. In addition, Fire Rescue 8 has identified a safe

---

communicating. Two rules of adult communication are critically important to children:

- Always come down to the child's level (Figure 14-5). Never stand above a child. You literally tower over the child and appear very intimidating. Crouching down reduces the size difference and greatly improves communication. If the child is not critically ill, you might even take the time to sit on the floor and get slightly below the child in the beginning.

- Children often sense lies even faster than adults. It is important to tell the truth to children. Remember, you may be the first contact from the EMS system that the child has ever had. Work to make it positive.

Figure 14-5 Stay at a child's eye level or lower.

location to stage the ambulance close to the crash site. As you approach the scene, you are advised that a helicopter has been requested for transport to the trauma center.

STREET SCENE QUESTIONS

4. What information should be provided to the incident commander upon arrival?

5. What type of coordinated effort between Ambulance 40 and Fire Rescue 8 should be done to ensure the best care?

6. What information about both the patient's condition and the landing zone need to be relayed to the helicopter?

As you pull up to the scene, you are directed to an area about 30 feet from the crashed vehicle. The extrication is underway. You approach the incident commander who tells you that the helicopter is 15 minutes from the scene and he is having a landing zone prepared. You are advised to work with Fire Rescue 8 to provide patient care and oversee rapid extrication to a backboard when freed.

You identify yourself to the fire captain and ask what equipment is needed. He tells you that the pa-tient will be out in a matter of minutes and he thinks that rapid extrication would be most appropriate. He has two firefighters available to help with boarding the patient. He asks if you think the plan will work and for any suggestions. You tell him the plan sounds good.

While your partner is getting the needed equipment, you get additional patient information and ask what is the best way to access the patient. You reassess the patient and convey the information to the helicopter, which is making its landing approach.

You agree with your partner and the crew from Fire Rescue 8 on who will do what to stabilize the patient's head and neck and to rotate the patient onto the backboard. The procedure goes quickly and smoothly. You reassess the patient and obtain a new set of vital signs. The flight medics are now next to the patient, and you update them on patient status. You assist with care and loading onto the helicopter. As the helicopter lifts off, you think how well this call went and realize that communication among all the emergency providers made a significant difference.

CHAPTER REVIEW

SUMMARY

Communication is not as tangible a skill as putting on a splint or taking a pulse, but it is a very important part of every call. Communication may be face to face with people—hospital personnel, other EMT-Bs, patients, family, bystanders, and others. Radio communication is important as your link to the dispatcher and medical direction. Use communication by any means or method carefully and accurately.

KEY TERMS

base station a two-way radio at a fixed site such as a hospital or dispatch center.

cellular phone a phone that transmits through the air instead of over wires so that the phone can be transported and used over a wide area.

mobile radio a two-way radio that is used or affixed in a vehicle.

portable radio a hand-held two-way radio.

repeater a device that picks up signals from lower-power radio units, such as mobile and portable radios, and re-transmits them at a higher power. It allows low-power radio signals to be transmitted over longer distances.

watt the unit of measurement of the output power of a radio.

REVIEW QUESTIONS

1. List several guidelines for proper use of the EMS radio system. (p. 282)
2. List the steps of a medical radio report and describe the communication that may be necessary during each part. (p. 283)
3. List several guidelines for effective interpersonal communication with patients. (pp. 284–286)

APPLICATIONS

The following information, describing a patient, is in random order. Organize the information and present a medical radio report as if you were radioing the hospital.

Chest pain radiating to the shoulder
56 years old
Oxygen applied at 15 liters per minute via nonrebreather
Alert and oriented
Female

Came on 20 minutes ago while mowing the lawn
History of high blood pressure and diabetes
ETA 20 minutes
Pulse 86, respirations 22, skin cool and moist, blood pressure 110/66
Oxygen relieved the pain slightly
Denies difficulty breathing
You are requesting orders from medical direction
You are on Community BLS Ambulance 4
Lungs sounds equal on both sides
Placed in a position of comfort

Visit Brady's *Emergency Care* website for direct weblinks. At **www.bradybooks.com/emergencycare**, you will find information related to the following Chapter 14 topics:

- Cellular 9-1-1
- The 9-1-1 system

Chapter
Fifteen

DOCUMENTATION

Documentation is an important part of the patient care process and lasts long after the call. The report you write will become a part of the patient's permanent hospital record. As records of your agency, your reports and those written by other EMT-Bs become a valuable source for research on trends in emergency medical care and a guide for continuing education and quality improvement. A report you have written may be used as evidence in a legal case. Documentation has short-term benefits as well. Noting vital signs and patient history will help you remember important facts about the patient during the course of the call.

PREHOSPITAL CARE REPORT

The record that you produce during a call is called a *prehospital care report* or, informally, a PCR. Your region or service may use a different name for the same kind of document, such as trip sheet, run report, or another name.

Prehospital care reports vary from system to system and state to state. While the information that is required to complete each is relatively similar, the method used to record the data may be somewhat different. *Written reports* are those that have portions with narrative areas, areas to record vital signs in written number form, and check boxes (Figure 15-1). *Computerized reports* are those that are completed by shading boxes to record data and then scanned for easy data storage and evaluation. In order to be scanned correctly, each box must be filled in completely with no stray marks (Figure 15-2).

A recent development in prehospital care reports is the *electronic clipboard*. This device is a computer in a clipboard format. The computer is able to recognize handwriting and convert it to computer text. The data are stored and eventually downloaded to a larger

computer. The computers, also called *pen-based computers*, may be attached to printers at receiving hospitals to print out a hard copy of the report for the emergency department staff (Figure 15-3).

Functions of the Prehospital Care Report

The prehospital care report has many functions. It is the record of patient care, serves as a legal document, provides information for administrative functions, aids education and research, and contributes to quality improvement. These functions are discussed in the following paragraphs.

Patient Care Record

The prehospital care report conveys important information about the patient to members of the EMS system and beyond. Although you provide a verbal report to the hospital staff before you leave the patient, your written record allows emergency department personnel to see the status of the patient when you arrived on scene, the care you gave, and how the patient's status may have changed during your care. An example of this would be the emergency department

TOPIC OVERVIEW

In this chapter, you will learn about the following topics:

● Components and procedures for the written run report

● Legal aspects and benefits of documentation

● Documentation concerns in patient refusal

✔ **Knowledge and Attitude**

1. Explain the components of the written report and list the information that should be included in the written report. (pp. 292, 295–298)

2. Identify the various sections of the written report. (pp. 292, 295–298)

3. Describe what information is required in each section of the prehospital care report and how it should be entered. (pp. 292, 295–298)

4. Define the special considerations concerning patient refusal. (pp. 298, 300–301)

5. Describe the legal implications associated with the written report. (pp. 298, 300–301)

6. Discuss all state and/or local record and reporting requirements. (pp. 302, 305)

7. Explain the rationale for patient care documentation. (p. 292)

8. Explain the rationale for the EMS system gathering data. (p. 292)

9. Explain the rationale for using medical terminology correctly. (p. 298)

10. Explain the rationale for using an accurate and synchronous clock so that information can be used in trending. (p. 295)

✔ **Skills**

1. Complete a prehospital care report.

staff looking back at your original set of vital signs to compare the current condition of the patient with the condition of the patient when he was first found at the scene.

The prehospital care report becomes part of the patient's permanent hospital record.

Legal Document

The prehospital care report also serves as a legal document, which may be called for at any legal proceeding resulting from the call. The person who wrote the report will ordinarily go to court with the form. If the patient was the victim or perpetrator of a crime, the report and the writer may be called into court to testify about the call during criminal proceedings. Civil law proceedings for negligence in injuries (e.g., a patient falls in a shopping mall and sues) are another reason that your report may be examined.

Unfortunately, there may be a time when the report is being examined because you are the subject of a lawsuit. Fortunately, this is rare and usually preventable, but in this case too, the report in which you documented the circumstances and the care you gave will be very important.

Administrative Purposes

Depending on the service you belong to, you may have to obtain insurance and billing information from the patient or patient's family. This may be recorded on your prehospital care report, or on a separate form, or both.

Education and Research

Your report may be examined later as part of a research project. Analysis of statistics compiled from prehospital care reports can reveal patterns and trends in EMS management and care. For example, analysts may see instances in which response time could be improved or ways of scheduling and deploying units to prepare for busy areas and times.

Statistics also may justify a request for additional resources.

Prehospital care reports can help management keep track of each EMT-B's experience and skills. Extra practice may be scheduled during continuing education sessions for skills that the reports reveal are underutilized, for instance. When an unusual or uncommon type of call has taken place, the prehospital care report may be used for demonstration of how to document such a case.

Quality Improvement

Most organizations have a Quality Improvement (QI)—or Quality Assurance (QA) or Total Quality Management (TQM)—system in place by which calls are routinely reviewed for conformity to current medical and organizational standards. Examination of prehospital care reports is one major way of conducting this review. At times, QI evaluations reveal excellent care by an EMT-B team that deserves special recognition and a "pat on the back."

Elements of the Prehospital Care Report

Data Elements

Each individual box in the prehospital care report is called a *data element*. While some elements may seem insignificant, each is actually an important part of the report and the description of the patient and response. These elements are necessary for research as well as for documenting the call.

To aid in research across many states and regions, the U. S. Department of Transportation has developed a *minimum data set*. These are the minimum elements recommended to be included in all prehospital care reports nationwide. There is also a standardized definition of what each element means. Over a period of time, it is hoped, the minimum data set will be widely adopted. The minimum data set is briefly summarized in Table 15-1.

Figure 15-1 Example of a prehospital care report with fill-in boxes and a narrative space.

Figure 15-2 Example of a prehospital care report that is scannable by computer.

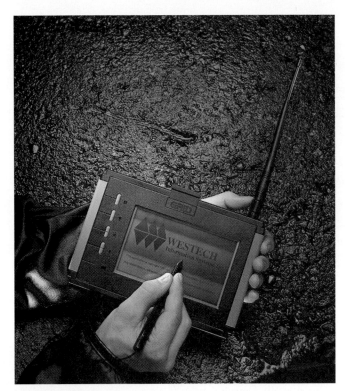

Figure 15-3 A pen-based computer can read handwriting and convert it to computer text.

The prehospital care report can be broken down into several sections, each containing different types of information. The sections include run data, patient data, check boxes, and the narrative section.

Run Data

This section includes the agency name, unit number, date, times, run or call number, and crew members' names, certification levels, and numbers (Figure 15-4). Times recorded must be accurate and synchronous (by clocks or watches that show the same time). Be sure to use the time as given by the dispatcher when noting times on your report. Unless your watch or the ambulance clock displays exactly the same time as the dispatch center, the times on your report will not match. There may be a difference of several minutes between the time displayed on your watch and the dispatch center's official time.

This time difference may seem insignificant but is actually very important in such areas as determining how long a patient has been in cardiac arrest, trends in patient condition, or measurement of system efficiency in response times.

Patient Data

This section contains information about the patient, the patient's condition throughout the call, and the care given to the patient (Figure 15-5). This is the major portion of your report. Specifically, it contains:

- Patient's name, address, date of birth, age, sex
- Billing and insurance information (in many jurisdictions)
- Nature of the call
- Mechanism of injury
- Location where the patient was found
- Treatment administered before arrival of the EMT-B (by bystanders, First Responders)
- Signs and symptoms, baseline and subsequent vital signs
- SAMPLE history
- Care administered and the effect that the care had on the patient (e.g., improved, no change)
- Changes in condition throughout the call

Check Boxes

Many prehospital care reports have check boxes for many data elements. This can be an efficient way to document parts of the call. In some cases, you will write a number or a few words into a short blank (Figure 15-6).

Table 15-1   Minimum Data Set

Patient Information

Gathered at the time of the EMT-B's initial contact with patient upon arrival at scene, following all interventions, and upon arrival at medical facility:

- Chief complaint
- Level of responsiveness (AVPU)—mental status
- Systolic blood pressure for patients greater than 3 years old
- Skin perfusion (capillary refill) for patients less than 6 years old
- Skin color and temperature
- Pulse rate
- Respiratory rate and effort

Administrative Information

- Time of incident report
- Time unit notified
- Time of arrival at patient
- Time unit left scene
- Time of arrival at destination
- Time of transfer of care

Prehospital Care Report

Agency Name	ARLINGTON RESCUE		MILEAGE			USE MILITARY TIMES	
			END	2 4 4 9 6	CALL REC'D	0 7 0 5
Dispatch Information	CARDIAC		BEGIN	2 4 4 7 6	ENROUTE	0 7 0 7
Call Location	124 CYPRUS ST 2nd FLOOR		TOTAL	0 0 0 2 0	ARRIVED AT SCENE	0 7 1 9

CHECK ONE ☒ Residence ☐ Health Facility ☐ Farm ☐ Indus. Facility ☐ Other Work Loc. ☐ Roadway ☐ Recreational ☐ Other

LOCATION CODE 0 1 2 4

FROM SCENE 0 7 3 8

CALL TYPE AS REC'D	MECHANISM OF INJURY		
☒ Emergency	☐ MVA (✓ seat belt used) N/A	☐ Knife	AT DESTIN 0 7 5 4
☐ Non-Emergency	☐ Fall of ___ feet N/A	☐ Machinery	IN SERVICE 0 8 1 0
☐ Stand-by	☐ Unarmed assault	☐ ___	IN QUARTERS 0 8 3 2
	☐ GSW		

Figure 15-4 One section of a prehospital care report contains run data.

Narrative

The narrative section of a prehospital care report is less structured than the fill-in blanks and check-box sections. It provides space to write information about the patient that cannot fit into fill-in blanks or check-off boxes (Figure 15-7).

Experienced EMT-Bs consider a good prehospital care report as one that "paints a picture" of their patient. The report, as mentioned previously, is read by many people and is a vital part of the patient's record. When hospital personnel or your quality improvement team reads your report, it should tell the patient's story fully and appropriately.

Remember, you were there throughout the call and are familiar with the patient, his chief complaint, and the care you gave. The people who read your report will have no prior knowledge of the call or the patient. It is imperative that you provide complete, accurate, and pertinent information about your patient and present the information in a logical order. The following guidelines will help you prepare narrative portions of your prehospital care reports:

- *Include both objective and pertinent subjective information.* Objective statements are those that are observable, measurable, or verifiable, such as "The patient has a swollen, deformed extremity." This is backed up by your visual observation. Or an objective statement might be "The patient's blood pressure was 110/80," based on a measurement you took. Or it might be "Patient uses a prescribed inhaler," a verifiable fact provided by the patient.

Subjective information is information from an individual point of view. It may be provided by the patient as a symptom ("I feel dizzy"). It also

CHIEF COMPLAINT		TIME	RESP	PULSE	B.P.	LEVEL OF CONSCIOUSNESS	R PUPILS L	SKIN
"MY CHEST HURTS"	V I T A L	0724	Rate: 18 ☒ Regular ☐ Shallow ☐ Labored	Rate: 88 ☐ Regular ☒ Irregular	148/88	☒ Alert ☐ Voice ☐ Pain ☐ Unresp.	☒ Normal ☒ — ☐ Dilated ☐ ☐ Constricted ☐ ☐ Sluggish ☐ ☐ No-Reaction ☐	☐ Unremarkable ☒ Cool ☒ Pale ☐ Warm ☐ Cyanotic ☐ Moist ☐ Flushed ☐ Dry ☐ Jaundiced
PAST MEDICAL HISTORY ☐ None ☒ Allergy to ASPIRIN ☐ Hypertension ☐ Stroke ☐ Seizures ☐ Diabetes ☐ COPD ☒ Cardiac ☐ Other (List) ☐ Asthma	S I G	0730	Rate: 18 ☒ Regular ☐ Shallow ☐ Labored	Rate: 84 ☐ Regular ☒ Irregular	144/86	☒ Alert ☐ Voice ☐ Pain ☐ Unresp.	☒ Normal ☒ — ☐ Dilated ☐ ☐ Constricted ☐ ☐ Sluggish ☐ ☐ No-Reaction ☐	☐ Unremarkable ☒ Cool ☒ Pale ☐ Warm ☐ Cyanotic ☐ Moist ☐ Flushed ☐ Dry ☐ Jaundiced
Current Medications (List) CARDIZEM	N S	0745	Rate: 20 ☒ Regular ☐ Shallow ☐ Labored	Rate: 88 ☐ Regular ☒ Irregular	144/86	☒ Alert ☐ Voice ☐ Pain ☐ Unresp.	☒ Normal ☒ — ☐ Dilated ☐ ☐ Constricted ☐ ☐ Sluggish ☐ ☐ No-Reaction ☐	☐ Unremarkable ☒ Cool ☒ Pale ☐ Warm ☐ Cyanotic ☐ Moist ☐ Flushed ☐ Dry ☐ Jaundiced

Figure 15-5 One section of a prehospital care report is devoted to patient data.

TREATMENT GIVEN

☑ Moved to ambulance on stretcher/backboard
☐ Moved to ambulance on stair chair
☐ Walked to ambulance
☐ Airway Cleared
☐ Oral/Nasal Airway
☐ Esophageal Obturator Airway/Esophageal Gastric Tube Airway (EOA/EGTA)
☐ Endotracheal Tube (E/T)
☑ Oxygen Administered @ [1][5] L.P.M., Method **NON-REBREATHER MASK**
☐ Suction Used
☐ Artificial Ventilation Method _____
☐ C.P.R. in progress on arrival by: ☐ Citizen   ☐ PD/FD/Other First Responder   ☐ Other
☐ C.P.R. Started @ Time ▶ [ ][ ][ ][ ]   Time from Arrest Until C.P.R. ▶ [ ][ ][ ] Minutes

☐ Bleeding/Hemorrhage Controlled (Method Used: _____)
☐ Spinal Immobilization Neck and Back
☐ Limb Immobilized by   ☐ Fixation   ☐ Traction
☐ (Heat) or (Cold) Applied
☐ Restraints Applied, Type _____
☐ Baby Delivered @ Time _____ In County _____
   ☐ Alive   ☐ Stillborn   ☐ Male   ☐ Female
☐ Transported in Trendelenburg position
☐ Transported in left lateral recumbent position
☑ Transported with head elevated
☐ Other _____

Figure 15-6   Most prehospital care reports have check boxes for some data elements.

may be provided by the EMT-B, such as your general impression of the patient ("Patient appears to have difficulty breathing") or your evaluation of the patient's behavior or emotional state ("Patient appears agitated and hostile"). Avoid subjective statements that are merely opinions, beyond your level of training or scope of practice ("I do not believe that the leg is broken" or "Patient is probably having a heart attack"), or are irrelevant ("Patient's daughter was rude").

Prehospital care reports are designed to be factual documents. Use objective statements whenever possible and only pertinent subjective statements. If you record something you did not observe yourself, put it in quotation marks (e.g., A bystander stated that "the patient passed out at the wheel before crashing"). Placing a statement in quotation marks and identifying the source lets readers of the report know where the information came from.

The chief complaint is another piece of information that is usually given in quotes. If a patient is conscious and oriented, he will usually tell you why he or someone else called you ("My chest hurts"). If the patient is not conscious or oriented, the person who called EMS may provide the chief complaint (He said he "felt faint and then passed out"). Since the chief complaint is in someone else's words, it should be placed in quotes.

In documenting your assessment procedures, remember to document important observations about the scene, such as suicide notes, weapons, and any other facts that would be important for patient care but not available to the emergency department personnel.

- *Pertinent negatives* are examination findings that are negative (things that are not true), but are important to note. For example, if a patient has chest pain, you will ask that patient if he has difficulty breathing. If the patient says he does not have difficulty in breathing, that is an important piece of negative information. On your prehospital care report, you would note "the patient denies difficulty breathing." Negative information often applies to trauma patients. For example, if the mechanism of injury indicates that there may be an injury to the arm but the patient says he feels no pain, you would note "the patient denies pain in right arm." Documenting pertinent negatives lets other medical professionals know that you thought to examine these areas and that the findings were negative. Not documenting them might leave the reader wondering if this area was explored at all.

  Note: The simple fact that there is no pain or complaint of difficulty does not mean that the patient should not be treated. If the patient's medical condition or if the mechanism of injury so

NARRATIVE

THE PATIENT DEVELOPED A SUDDEN ONSET OF CHEST PAIN WHILE WATCHING TV. THE PAIN IS SUBSTERNAL, CRUSHING, AND RADIATES TO THE LEFT SHOULDER AND ARM. THE PATIENT STATES THAT THIS PAIN IS "EXACTLY THE SAME AS WHEN I HAD A HEART ATTACK 2 YEARS AGO." HE DENIES LOSS OF CONSCIOUSNESS OR DIFFICULTY BREATHING....

Figure 15-7   The narrative portion of a prehospital care report provides space to write information that will not fit into check-off boxes or fill-in blanks.

indicates, treat the patient despite absence of pain or other symptoms.

- *Avoid radio codes and non-standard abbreviations.* Codes you may use on the radio may not be familiar to hospital personnel, so do not use them in written documentation. Abbreviations, when used properly, make writing efficient and accurate, but non-standard abbreviations will cause confusion and possibly lead to errors in patient care.

- *Write legibly and use correct spelling.* A prehospital care report will have absolutely no value if it cannot be read, so take the time to make your handwriting readable. Unclear writing, misread by others, may cause errors that could harm the patient. Additionally, your QI team will be unable to read the report for review, and it will have no value for research or training. Spelling is also important. If you cannot properly spell a word, look it up (many ambulances and emergency departments have medical dictionaries) or use another word.

- *Use medical terminology correctly.* Be sure that any medical terms you use are used correctly. If you are not sure of the meaning of a term, look it up in a medical dictionary or use everyday language to describe the condition instead. Careless use of medical terms could make your report unclear or cause a misunderstanding that might result in harm to the patient.

- *If it's not written down, you didn't do it.* This is a statement that you will most likely hear from your instructor and experienced EMT-Bs in the field. It explains an important concept of EMS documentation. Make sure that you document all your interventions thoroughly. If you did not document them, it will appear as if they were never performed when the call is later reviewed.

The most important function of the prehospital care report is to present an accurate representation of the patient's condition throughout the call, the patient's history and vital signs, treatments performed, and changes or lack of changes in the patient's condition following treatments.

SPECIAL DOCUMENTATION ISSUES

Legal Issues

There are several legal issues pertaining to prehospital care reports and other documents you may be asked to complete. These include issues of confidentiality, patient refusals, falsification, and error correction.

Confidentiality

The prehospital care report itself and the information it contains are strictly confidential. The information must not be discussed with or distributed to unauthorized persons. State or local regulations will indicate to whom the information may be distributed. Obviously, the receiving hospital must receive patient care information so they can treat the patient properly. Most reports have a copy that will be left at the hospital. Confidentiality has been discussed in Chapter 3, "Medical/Legal and Ethical Issues."

Patient Refusals

In Chapter 3, the issue of liability when patients refuse treatment was discussed. It is one of the foremost causes of liability for EMT-Bs and their EMS systems. Several suggestions were presented in Chapter 3 on what to do when a patient refuses care or transportation.

All actions you have taken to persuade the patient to go to the hospital must be documented. Additionally, you will have to make notes on the patient's competency, or his ability to make an informed, rational decision on his medical needs. If the patient was not capable of making this determination for any reason—including age, intoxication (alcohol and/or other drugs), mental competency, or as a result of the patient's medical condition—actions you took to protect the patient must also be documented. The patient must be informed of the potential results of not going to the hospital or of refusing your care.

The fact that a patient refuses transport to a hospital does not mean that you should not perform an assessment. If the patient greets you with a statement such as "I don't know why my daughter called, because I'm not going anywhere," you may still be able to persuade the patient to get "checked out." Perform as much of a physical exam as possible, including vital signs. Document all of your findings and emergency care given on the prehospital care report. This information will be important to give to medical direction when you talk to them. Be sure to consult medical direction, according to your local protocols, whenever there is a patient refusal.

Most EMS agencies have a refusal-of-care form to use in the event that you have done your best to persuade the patient to accept care or transport and the patient still refuses. This form may be part of either the prehospital care report or a separate document. You should make sure the patient reads and signs this form (Figure 15-8). It is rare that a patient will refuse to sign the form, but if he does, be sure to document this, as well, and note the names of witnesses to the refusal. If possible, when a patient refuses to

REFUSAL INFORMATION SHEET

PLEASE READ AND KEEP THIS FORM!

This form has been given to you because you have refused treatment and/or transport by Emergency Medical Services (EMS). Your health and safety are our primary concern, so even though you have decided not to accept our advice, please remember the following:

1) The evaluation and/or treatment provided to you by the EMS providers is not a substitute for medical evaluation and treatment by a doctor. We advise you to get medical evaluation and treatment.

2) Your condition may not seem as bad to you as it actually is. Without treatment, your condition or problem could become worse. If you are planning to get medical treatment, a decision to refuse treatment or transport by EMS may result in a delay which could make your condition or problem worse.

3) Medical evaluation and/or treatment may be obtained by calling your doctor, if you have one, or by going to any hospital Emergency Department in this area, all of which are staffed 24 hours a day by Emergency Physicians. You may be seen at these Emergency Departments without an appointment.

4) If you change your mind or your condition becomes worse and you decide to accept treatment and transport by Emergency Medical Services, please do not hesitate to call us back. We will do our best to help you.

5) DON'T WAIT! When medical treatment is needed, it is usually better to get it right away.

I have received a copy of this information sheet.

PATIENT SIGNATURE: _____ DATE: _____

WITNESS SIGNATURE: _____ DATE: _____

AGENCY INCIDENT #: _____ AGENCY CODE: _____

NAME OF PERSON FILLING OUT FORM: _____

G 11A

Figure 15-8 Example of a refusal information sheet.

The 49 year old female patient, according to her daughter, "passed out" suddenly. She was in that condition for about 3-5 minutes. The daughter stated that the patient "came to" gradually. Upon our arrival she was fully conscious and oriented. The daughter denies observing any seizure activity. She states that the patient passed out in a chair and did not fall or injure herself as a result of the incident. The patient denies any problems such as chest pain or difficulty breathing. She denies allergies. Her last oral intake was about 2 hours ago (sandwich and coffee). The patient denies any past medical history or current medications.

Vital signs noted above show no abnormalities between two sets taken at a 15 minute interval. The patient refuses transportation to the hospital and has signed the refusal form attached to this report. Her daughter is present with her at her residence and witnessed the refusal. The patient appears competent and oriented. She was advised to call back at any time should she need our assistance or transportation to the hospital of her choice. She was also advised that her failure to go to the hospital may result in a return or worsening of the previous symptoms which, depending on the underlying cause, could result in a serious medical problem or even death.

The patient's daughter will stay with her for several hours and then provide follow-up calls throughout the evening to make sure the patient is all right. The patient was encouraged to contact her family physician for follow-up care as soon as possible. Since the patient did not have one, a sticker listing our phone number was placed on her phone. We contacted medical direction about the situation and spoke to Dr. Baker at Mercy Hospital. She had no further suggestions.

Figure 15-9 Document a patient refusal of care thoroughly in the narrative portion of the prehospital care report.

sign a refusal form, get the witnesses to sign a statement confirming that the patient has refused care or transport.

You should also include information about the patient refusal in the narrative section of the prehospital care report. A sample documentation of a patient refusal that might go into the narrative portion of the prehospital care report is shown in Figure 15-9.

You will note that the narrative shown in Figure 15-9 contains many points of information, including pertinent negatives. The report states that the patient "denies" chest pain or difficulty in breathing. Statements from the patient's daughter are noted as to the source: "according to her daughter . . ." and "The daughter denies seeing any seizure activity."

Before you leave the patient who has refused care or transport, be sure to make alternative care suggestions, such as encouraging him to seek care from a doctor, and document them. Try to be sure that a responsible family member or friend remains with the patient. Make sure that person also understands that the patient should seek care. Never convey the impression that you are annoyed about being called to the scene "for nothing." Make certain the patient understands that if his condition worsens or if he changes his mind, he can call EMS and you or another EMT-B team will gladly come back.

Falsification

Prehospital care reports document the information obtained and the care rendered during the call. False entries or misrepresentations on a report are usually intended to cover up serious flaws in assessment or in care. However, falsification may actually make the problem look worse when it is uncovered.

There are two types of errors that may be committed during a call: omission and commission. Errors of omission are those in which an important part of the assessment or care was left out. An example is oxygen. If a patient is experiencing chest pain, oxygen is an appropriate treatment. If it is overlooked for any reason, never write that oxygen was administered when it was not.

Occasionally, because of events during transport to a hospital, an EMT may only be able to get one set of vital signs. Never be tempted to write down an extra set of vital signs when none were taken. Just don't do it! Document only the vital signs that were taken. If there is a reason why you have only taken one set, document the reason (e.g., "The patient became combative and disoriented en route, preventing a second set of vital signs.").

Errors of commission are actions performed on the patient that are wrong or improper. An example of this is incorrect administration of medication. There are certain medications that you will be able to administer or assist the patient in administering to himself. This is a great responsibility. If a medication was administered when it was not indicated, it is important to tell medical direction and document the incident on the prehospital care report. Failure to document exactly what happened may have a negative effect on the patient's care. The hospital may think that the patient's condition is due to some other cause. In other situations, the hospital may re-administer the medication, not realizing that it had already been given.

Document the situation surrounding any error of omission or commission and explain exactly what happened. Document what was done to correct the situation, including advising medical direction and verbally notifying hospital personnel.

Falsification or misrepresentation on a prehospital care report leads to poor patient care because the facts were not documented, and hospital personnel may be misled about the patient's condition and the care he received. Falsification or misrepresentation may also lead to the suspension or revocation of your certification or license as an EMT-B.

You will avoid falsifications if you follow this rule: Write everything important that did happen and nothing that didn't.

Correction of Errors

Prehospital care reports are not always written in ideal circumstances. You may even find yourself being dispatched to another call before you finish writing up your last one. In situations such as this, you may inadvertently write incorrect information on the report.

Any time there is incorrect information on the report, it must be corrected. If the report is still intact (all copies attached and not yet distributed), draw a single horizontal line through the error, initial it, then write the correct information beside it (Figure 15-10). Do not completely cross out the error or obliterate it. This may be looked on by others as an attempt to cover up a mistake in patient care.

If the error is discovered at a later date, after the report has been submitted, draw a single line through the error, mark the area with your initials and the date, and add the correct information to the end of the report or on a separate note. This should be done in a different color ink when possible so the change will be obvious. Copies of the report may have already been distributed to other agencies, your quality improvement committee, insurance companies, or attorneys, and a corrected copy may need to be sent. Make sure that you place the date on the changes so the most recent copy is identifiable. If information has been omitted and you wish to add it, be sure also to date this information and place your initials by the added information.

| COMMENTS | PATIENT COMPLAINS OF PAIN IN HIS ~~RIGHT~~ [DL] LEFT SHOULDER THAT RADIATES TO THE LEFT ARM. |

Figure 15-10 Cross out an error with a single line and initial the change.

Special Situations

Multiple-Casualty Incidents

An incident in which there are many patients or injuries—such as a multiple-vehicle collision, a major fire, or a plane crash—causes many logistical problems for an EMS system. Documentation of information for each individual patient may be difficult. A patient in a multiple-casualty incident (MCI) will probably be moved from one treatment area to another at the scene and then receive transport to a hospital. Possibly patients will be transported to several different hospitals. It is very important to keep the information with the patient as he moves through the system. This is often done through the use of a triage tag (Figure 15-11). This tag is affixed to the patient and used to record chief complaint and injuries, vital signs, and treatments given. At a point later in the emergency, the tag will be used to complete a traditional prehospital care report.

When completing a prehospital care report for a patient involved in a multiple-casualty incident, it will not be possible to provide the detail that you would normally provide for a single-patient call. This is an understandable consequence of the MCI. Your region or agency will have requirements for what information must be completed on the report during an MCI.

Special Situation Reports

Many states use a supplemental form for advanced life support (ALS) calls or additional documentation for calls that were complex or involved (Figure 15-12).

Your activities as an EMT-B may also take you to some unusual situations that will require documentation on a form other than a prehospital care report. Such forms are usually specific to a local agency rather than mandated statewide (Figure 15-13). Some examples of situations that might require this kind of special report include:

- Exposure to infectious disease
- Injury to yourself or another EMT-B
- Hazardous or unsafe scenes to which other crews should be alerted

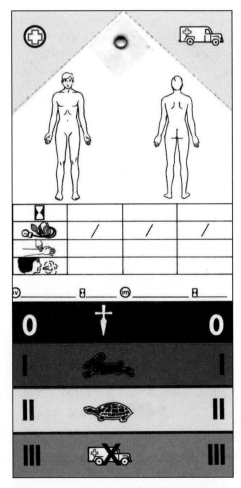

Figure 15-11 During a multiple-casualty incident, triage tags are used to document information for each patient.

USE BALL POINT PEN ONLY.

CONTINUATION FORM
for the
Prehospital Care Report

Press Down Firmly. You're Making 4 Copies.

M D Y
DATE   RUN NO.

AGENCY CODE   VEH. ID

Name

Agency Name

Enter PCR ID# (Top Center of PCR)

ADDITIONAL HISTORY & PHYSICAL EXAM FINDINGS

Weight in Kilograms

R BREATH SOUNDS L	NECK VEINS	EDEMA	ABDOMEN
☐ Normal ☐	☐ Normal	☐ Pedal	☐ Normal
☐ Decreased ☐	☐ Distended	☐ Sacral	☐ Tender
☐ Absent ☐	**TRACHEAL SHIFT**	☐ Ascites	☐ Rigid
☐ Rales ☐		☐ Other	☐ Distended
☐ Rhonchi ☐	R L		☐ Other
☐ Wheezes ☐	☐ ☐		

SERIAL VITAL SIGNS, EKG, RHYTHMS, MEDICATIONS AND TREATMENT

TIME	RESP.	PULSE	B.P.	LEVEL OF CONSCIOUSNESS	EKG RHYTHMS	DEFIBRILLATION CARDIOVERSION	MEDICATIONS			DOSE	ROUTE
	Rate: ☐ Regular ☐ Shallow ☐ Labored	Rate: ☐ Regular ☐ Irregular		☐ Alert ☐ Voice ☐ Pain ☐ Unresp.	☐ NSR ☐ Brady ☐ Asystole ☐ IVR ☐ V. Fib. ☐ V. Tach. ☐ PVC ☐ SVT ☐ Other___		☐ Epinephrine ☐ Atropine ☐ Dextrose ☐ Lidocaine ☐ Lasix	☐ Dopamine ☐ Sodium Bicarb. ☐ Isoproterenol ☐ Other___	☐ Naloxone ☐ Bretylium ☐ Nitroglycerin		☐ IV ☐ ET ☐ IM ☐ SL ☐ SQ ☐ PO ☐ Nebulizer
	Rate: ☐ Regular ☐ Shallow ☐ Labored	Rate: ☐ Regular ☐ Irregular		☐ Alert ☐ Voice ☐ Pain ☐ Unresp.	☐ NSR ☐ Brady ☐ Asystole ☐ IVR ☐ V. Fib. ☐ V. Tach. ☐ PVC ☐ SVT ☐ Other___		☐ Epinephrine ☐ Atropine ☐ Dextrose ☐ Lidocaine ☐ Lasix	☐ Dopamine ☐ Sodium Bicarb. ☐ Isoproterenol ☐ Other___	☐ Naloxone ☐ Bretylium ☐ Nitroglycerin		☐ IV ☐ ET ☐ IM ☐ SL ☐ SQ ☐ PO ☐ Nebulizer
	Rate: ☐ Regular ☐ Shallow ☐ Labored	Rate: ☐ Regular ☐ Irregular		☐ Alert ☐ Voice ☐ Pain ☐ Unresp.	☐ NSR ☐ Brady ☐ Asystole ☐ IVR ☐ V. Fib. ☐ V. Tach. ☐ PVC ☐ SVT ☐ Other___		☐ Epinephrine ☐ Atropine ☐ Dextrose ☐ Lidocaine ☐ Lasix	☐ Dopamine ☐ Sodium Bicarb. ☐ Isoproterenol ☐ Other___	☐ Naloxone ☐ Bretylium ☐ Nitroglycerin		☐ IV ☐ ET ☐ IM ☐ SL ☐ SQ ☐ PO ☐ Nebulizer
	Rate: ☐ Regular ☐ Shallow ☐ Labored	Rate: ☐ Regular ☐ Irregular		☐ Alert ☐ Voice ☐ Pain ☐ Unresp.	☐ NSR ☐ Brady ☐ Asystole ☐ IVR ☐ V. Fib. ☐ V. Tach. ☐ PVC ☐ SVT ☐ Other___		☐ Epinephrine ☐ Atropine ☐ Dextrose ☐ Lidocaine ☐ Lasix	☐ Dopamine ☐ Sodium Bicarb. ☐ Isoproterenol ☐ Other___	☐ Naloxone ☐ Bretylium ☐ Nitroglycerin		☐ IV ☐ ET ☐ IM ☐ SL ☐ SQ ☐ PO ☐ Nebulizer
	Rate: ☐ Regular ☐ Shallow ☐ Labored	Rate: ☐ Regular ☐ Irregular		☐ Alert ☐ Voice ☐ Pain ☐ Unresp.	☐ NSR ☐ Brady ☐ Asystole ☐ IVR ☐ V. Fib. ☐ V. Tach. ☐ PVC ☐ SVT ☐ Other___		☐ Epinephrine ☐ Atropine ☐ Dextrose ☐ Lidocaine ☐ Lasix	☐ Dopamine ☐ Sodium Bicarb. ☐ Isoproterenol ☐ Other___	☐ Naloxone ☐ Bretylium ☐ Nitroglycerin		☐ IV ☐ ET ☐ IM ☐ SL ☐ SQ ☐ PO ☐ Nebulizer
	Rate: ☐ Regular ☐ Shallow ☐ Labored	Rate: ☐ Regular ☐ Irregular		☐ Alert ☐ Voice ☐ Pain ☐ Unresp.	☐ NSR ☐ Brady ☐ Asystole ☐ IVR ☐ V. Fib. ☐ V. Tach. ☐ PVC ☐ SVT ☐ Other___		☐ Epinephrine ☐ Atropine ☐ Dextrose ☐ Lidocaine ☐ Lasix	☐ Dopamine ☐ Sodium Bicarb. ☐ Isoproterenol ☐ Other___	☐ Naloxone ☐ Bretylium ☐ Nitroglycerin		☐ IV ☐ ET ☐ IM ☐ SL ☐ SQ ☐ PO ☐ Nebulizer
	Rate: ☐ Regular ☐ Shallow ☐ Labored	Rate: ☐ Regular ☐ Irregular		☐ Alert ☐ Voice ☐ Pain ☐ Unresp.	☐ NSR ☐ Brady ☐ Asystole ☐ IVR ☐ V. Fib. ☐ V. Tach. ☐ PVC ☐ SVT ☐ Other___		☐ Epinephrine ☐ Atropine ☐ Dextrose ☐ Lidocaine ☐ Lasix	☐ Dopamine ☐ Sodium Bicarb. ☐ Isoproterenol ☐ Other___	☐ Naloxone ☐ Bretylium ☐ Nitroglycerin		☐ IV ☐ ET ☐ IM ☐ SL ☐ SQ ☐ PO ☐ Nebulizer

COMMENTS:

MEDICAL FACILITY CONTACTED

C R E W	ADDITIONAL NAME — CREW ☐ EMS-FR ☐ EMT ☐ AEMT #	ADDITIONAL NAME — CREW ☐ EMS-FR ☐ EMT ☐ AEMT #	ADDITIONAL NAME — CREW ☐ EMS-FR ☐ EMT ☐ AEMT #	ADDITIONAL NAME — CREW ☐ EMS-FR ☐ EMT ☐ AFMT #

© COPYRIGHT 1986 NEW YORK STATE DEPARTMENT OF HEALTH

EMS 100A (11/86) provided by NYS-EMS PROGRAM

AGENCY COPY/**WHITE**   HOSPITAL PATIENT RECORD COPY/**PINK**   RESEARCH COPY/**BLUE**   EXTRA SERVICE COPY/**GREEN**

PAGE _____ OF _____

Figure 15-12 Example of a supplemental form.

Special Incident Report

Town of Colonie
Department of Emergency Medical Services ⎯⎯⎯⎯⎯⎯⎯⎯

Date of Incident: _____   Time: _____   REMO #: _____

Town Run #: _____   Reported by: _____   Zone: _____

Type of Incident: ☐ MCI   ☐ Rescue   ☐ Personnel Matter   ☐ Injury   ☐ Accident with an EMS vehicle
☐ Infectious Disease Exposure   ☐ Scene Conflict   ☐ Other _____

Total # of Patients: ☐ #P-1: _____   ☐ #P-2: _____   ☐ #P-3: _____   ☐ #P-0: _____
Elapsed Scene Time: *(First unit arrival to last unit to hospital)* _____
Total Time of Incident: _____

Describe the Incident Below:
Attach any additional documentation such as news clipppings and the pre-hospital care report.
Attach additional sheets if necessary.

_____
_____
_____
_____
_____
_____
_____
_____
_____
_____
_____
_____
_____
_____
_____
_____
_____
_____
_____

Signature: _____   Date: _____

- -

Office Use Only
This incident relates to: ☐ Day Operation: TOT   ☐ Night Operations: TOT: ☐ Administration: TOT:
_____   _____   _____

Disposition: _____
_____
                                                                    Date: _____

Notifications/Copies: ☐ Director   ☐ Deputy Director   ☐ Supervisors
                        ☐ Deputy Supervisors   ☐ Senior Medics   ☐ Zone Coordinator(s)
                        ☐ Other _____   Zone: ☐ 2 ☐ 3 ☐ 4

Figure 15-13   Example of a special incident report.

STREET SCENES

You and your partner have just finished a call involving a motor-vehicle crash involving two vehicles. It was the first call of the day, just after you had checked out the ambulance but before you had time for breakfast. It is now 9:30 a.m. and you are sitting at a desk in the emergency department doing the prehospital care report. Although the patient didn't seem to be hurt badly, he had been complaining of lower back pain. Based on the patient complaint and the patient assessment, you decide to do a full immobilization.

STREET SCENE QUESTIONS

1. What information is important to include in the prehospital care report?

Although your partner is hurrying you, you write a very complete and thorough prehospital care report. You detail the patient's pulses, motor function, and sensation in all extremities before and after immobilization, including the fact that you observed the patient had difficulty moving his left foot and that it felt numb. The patient also told you that he was wearing only a lap-style seatbelt at the time of the crash, and that he had a considerable amount of pain. He had not moved from the vehicle prior to the arrival of EMS.

STREET SCENE QUESTIONS

2. What is the importance of doing an accurate and thorough prehospital care report?

3. Should you have your partner read and comment on the prehospital care report before considering it complete?

4. What are the ramifications of having a prehospital care report in the hospital record that is different from the original copy on file with your EMS agency?

After writing your prehospital care report, your partner reviews it and a copy is left at the hospital for inclusion in the hospital chart. You manage to make it to breakfast, and you put this call behind you.

A few months later the director of your ambulance service stops you and asks if you remember this call. You think for a moment but only have a vague recollection. He informs you that the patient has started a lawsuit and claims that he sustained damage as the result of prehospital care. The prehospital care report has been reviewed by the ambulance service's lawyer, who believes that it will be a very good defense and the case will probably be dismissed. The director hands you a copy of the prehospital care report, and as you read it, you start to remember the call. You had forgotten about the patient's complaint of pain and other symptoms.

As he walks away, the director tells you that good documentation will make all the difference in how this case gets decided. This is very different from a case he had a few years ago when an EMT-B changed the service's copy of the PCR after he left a copy at the hospital. The lawyer for the plaintiff noticed the discrepancies and made things very difficult for the service.

- Referrals to social service agencies for elderly or other patients in need of home care
- Mandatory reports for child or elderly abuse

This list is not all-inclusive. If there is any situation that requires extra documentation, the special report form may be the place to note it. It is important to remain accurate and objective when filling out this type of report, especially in an unusual or emotional situation. Follow local guidelines for the documentation of confidential information in these reports and for distribution of copies to appropriate agencies or persons.

CHAPTER REVIEW

SUMMARY

Documentation is an important skill. A properly completed prehospital care report, or PCR, provides important patient care and medical information about your patient. This form will become a permanent record in the patient's hospital chart as well as in the files of your agency. It may be used to help determine future treatments or as a legal document in a court proceeding. Your report will also be vital in charting trends, research, and quality improvement. Your report should "paint a picture" of your patient and his condition, accurately describing your contact with the patient throughout the call.

REVIEW QUESTIONS

1. Explain the term "minimum data set" and why it is important. (p. 292)
2. Explain what is meant by "objective" and "subjective" information in the narrative portion of the prehospital care report. Explain what is meant by "a pertinent negative." (pp. 296–297)
3. Explain how spelling and the use of codes, abbreviations, and medical terms relate to writing a clear and accurate narrative report. (p. 298)
4. List some important steps to take and information to include when documenting a patient refusal. (pp. 298, 300–301)
5. Describe some possible consequences of falsifying information on a prehospital care report. (p. 301)
6. Describe how to properly correct an error in a prehospital care report. (p. 301)

• Write a narrative report for a call you have been on. If you have not yet been on an ambulance, write one that describes an injury or illness that has happened to you or a family member. If a prehospital care report form is available, complete the whole form, including the check-off or fill-in boxes as well as the narrative portion.

WEB MEDIC

Visit Brady's *Emergency Care* website for direct weblinks. At **www.bradybooks.com/emergencycare**, you will find information related to the following Chapter 15 topics:

• Dispatch and confidentiality

Chapter
Sixteen

GENERAL PHARMACOLOGY

*W*ord on the Street

"Very few patients can deteriorate so rapidly as one experiencing anaphylaxis or a severe allergic reaction. Wheezing, airway swelling, rash, and cardiovascular collapse seemed to happen in moments. Previously, all EMTs could do was maintain the airway, hope for ALS backup, and put the pedal to the metal! Today the EMT-Basic is trained to assist the patient in taking an epinephrine self-injector—a life-saving skill that both you and your patient will be thankful for. So, although these calls are infrequent, pay close attention to your instructor when this material is covered—it can save a life!"

Bob Elling, MPA, REMT-P Faculty,
American College of Prehospital Medicine

The study of drugs—their sources, characteristics, and effects—is called **pharmacology.** Note that although EMS personnel use the terms *medications* and *drugs* interchangeably, the public often associates the word *drugs* with illegal or abused substances. So when dealing with the public, use the terms *medicines* or *medications.*

This chapter introduces the medications carried by EMT-B on the ambulance, as well as prescribed medications the EMT-B may assist the patient in taking with approval from medical direction. You will learn the forms of medications your patients may be taking, as well as the names for common types of medications and why they are used.

MEDICATIONS EMT-BASICS CAN ADMINISTER

There are six medications that you will be able to administer or assist with in the field. They are activated charcoal, oral glucose, oxygen, prescribed inhalers, nitroglycerin, and epinephrine auto-injectors. The information that follows is a brief introduction to each of these drugs.

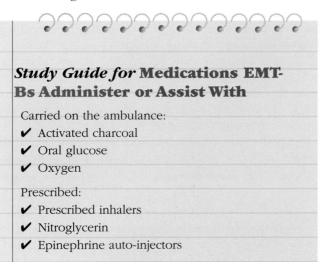

Study Guide for Medications EMT-Bs Administer or Assist With

Carried on the ambulance:
- ✔ Activated charcoal
- ✔ Oral glucose
- ✔ Oxygen

Prescribed:
- ✔ Prescribed inhalers
- ✔ Nitroglycerin
- ✔ Epinephrine auto-injectors

Medications on the Ambulance

As an EMT-B, you will carry activated charcoal, oral glucose, and oxygen on the ambulance. Under specific circumstances that will be described later, you will be able to administer these medications to patients.

Activated Charcoal
Activated charcoal is a powder prepared from charred wood, usually premixed with water to form a slurry for use in the field (Figure 16-1). It is used to treat a poisoning or overdose when a substance is swallowed and is in the patient's digestive tract. Activated charcoal will adsorb some poisons (bind them to the surfaces of the charcoal) and help prevent them from being absorbed by the body. The procedure for administering activated charcoal will be found in Chapter 21, "Poisoning and Overdose Emergencies."

Oral Glucose
Glucose is a kind of sugar. **Oral glucose** is a form of glucose that can be taken by mouth as a treatment for a conscious patient (able to swallow) with an altered mental status and a history of diabetes. The brain is very sensitive to low levels of sugar, which can be caused by poorly managed diabetes, and this can be a cause of the altered mental status. Oral glucose usually comes as a tube of gel (Figure 16-2) that you can apply to a tongue depressor and place between the patient's cheek and gum or under the tongue. This allows the patient to swallow the glucose so it can be easily absorbed into the digestive tract and bloodstream, which carries it to the brain. This may begin to reverse the patient's potentially

TOPIC OVERVIEW

In this chapter, you will learn about the following topics:

- Which medications may be carried by the EMT-B and which the EMT-B may assist patients with

- What to consider when administering any medication

- The role of medical direction in medication administration

✔ **Knowledge and Attitude**

1. Identify which medications will be carried on the unit. (p. 309)

2. State the medications carried on the unit by the generic name. (p. 309)

3. Identify the medications which the EMT-Basic may assist the patient with administering. (pp. 309–312)

4. State the medications the EMT-Basic can assist the patient with by the generic name. (pp. 309–312)

5. Discuss the forms in which the medications may be found. (p. 313)

6. Explain the rationale for the administration of medications. (pp. 309–312)

✔ **Skills**

1. Demonstrate general steps for assisting patient with self-administration of medications.

2. Read the labels and inspect each type of medication.

life-threatening condition. The procedure for administering oral glucose will be found in Chapter 19, "Diabetic Emergencies and Altered Mental Status."

Oxygen

Oxygen is a gas commonly found in the atmosphere. Pure oxygen is used as a drug to treat any patient whose medical or traumatic condition causes him to be hypoxic (low in oxygen) or in danger of becoming hypoxic (Figure 16-3). Throughout this text, you have learned and will learn many situations in which a patient should be given oxygen. Specific methods of administering oxygen may be found in Chapter 6, "Airway Management."

Prescribed Medications

The three medications described next—prescribed inhaler, nitroglycerin, and epinephrine auto-injector—are drugs that, as an EMT-B, you may assist the patient in taking if they have been prescribed for the patient by a physician.

Prescribed Inhalers

There are various medications that patients carry to help them through a period of difficulty breathing. Most often patients with diseases like asthma, emphysema, or chronic bronchitis carry a "bronchodilator," a medication designed to enlarge constricted bronchial tubes, making breathing easier. Many of these medications can be carried in an **inhaler**, which contains an aerosol form of a medication the patient can spray directly into his airway (Figure 16-4). Examples of these medications include: albuterol, Ventolin, Proventil, and Volmax.

Since many bronchodilators also have an effect on the heart, an increased heart rate and patient jitteriness are common side effects of treatment.

Figure 16-1 Activated charcoal is often used in poisoning cases.

Figure 16-2 Oral glucose may help a patient with diabetes.

Figure 16-3 Oxygen is a powerful drug.

Figure 16-4 A prescribed inhaler may help a patient who has respiratory problems.

You may need to have permission from medical direction to help a patient self-administer a prescribed inhaler. Be sure to determine that the inhaler is actually the patient's and not that of a family member or bystander. You may need to seek permission from medical direction by phone or radio, or there may be a standing medical order that permits you to assist a patient with this kind of medication. *Always comply with the protocols of your EMS system.* More details on the use of a prescribed inhaler will be found in Chapter 17, "Respiratory Emergencies."

Nitroglycerin

Many patients with problems such as recurrent chest pain, or a history of heart attack, carry **nitroglycerin** pills or spray. Nitroglycerin (Figure 16-5) is a drug that helps to dilate the coronary vessels which supply the heart muscle with blood. It is often called just "nitro." A common trade name is Nitrostat.

This drug is taken by the patient when he begins to have chest pain he believes to be cardiac in origin. It is not uncommon for EMT-Bs to treat patients who have already taken a nitroglycerin pill or who are carrying a bottle of nitroglycerin tablets and have not thought to try one. (Many patients are instructed by their physician to take up to three nitroglycerin pills for their chest pain and, if the chest pain persists, to call EMS.)

Be sure to determine that the nitroglycerin is actually the patient's and not that of a family member or bystander.

Since nitro causes a dilation of blood vessels, a drop in the patient's blood pressure is always a potential side effect of administration. If this should occur, you may also need to lay the patient down and raise the legs as you re-contact medical direction for advice.

You may need to seek permission from medical direction by phone or radio, or there may be a standing medical order that permits you to assist a patient with nitroglycerin administration. *Always comply with the protocols of your EMS system.* More information on assisting a patient in taking nitroglycerin will be found in Chapter 18, "Cardiac Emergencies."

Figure 16-5 Nitroglycerin is often prescribed for chest pain.

HOW **AND** **W**HY?

Sometimes drugs can interact. Go to your Electronic Extras CD to learn why it is necessary to ask patients if they are taking Viagra before assisting them in taking nitroglycerin.

Epinephrine Auto-Injectors

When a patient is highly allergic to something like shellfish, penicillin, or a bee sting, he may have a very severe reaction. This reaction may cause life-threatening changes in the airway and circulation. The reaction can be reversed by using **epinephrine.** Epinephrine is a medication that will help to constrict the blood vessels and relax airway passages.

Because severe allergic reactions may reach a life-threatening stage in a very short time, epinephrine must be administered quickly. Many patients who are prone to severe allergic reactions carry an epinephrine auto-injector (Figure 16-6). This is a syringe with a spring-loaded needle that will release and inject epinephrine into the muscle when the auto-injector is pushed against the thigh. Epi-Pen® is the trade name of a commonly carried epinephrine auto-injector. If you need to assist a patient with the use of an epinephrine auto-injector, be sure to determine that the auto-injector is actually the patient's and not that of a family member or bystander.

Since epinephrine has a potent effect on the heart and vascular system, increased heart rate and blood pressure commonly occur after its administration to the patient.

You may need to seek permission from medical direction by phone or radio, or there may be a standing medical order that permits you to assist a patient with an epinephrine auto-injector. Always comply with the protocols of your EMS system. More information on assisting a patient in using an epinephrine auto-injector is included in Chapter 20, "Allergic Reactions."

GENERAL INFORMATION ABOUT MEDICATIONS

Drug Names

Every drug or medication is listed in the *U.S. Pharmacopoeia* (USP), which is a comprehensive government publication. Each drug is listed by its generic name (a general name that is not the brand name of any manufacturer), but, in fact, each drug actually has at least three names: the chemical name, the generic name, and one or more trade (brand) names given the drug by various manufacturers. For example, *epinephrine* is a generic drug name. Its chemical name is B- (e, 4 dihydroxyphenyl) -a-methylamino-ethanol. (Chemical names are technical formulas used only by scientists or manufacturers.) As mentioned earlier, Epi-Pen® is the trade name of an epinephrine auto-injector.

HOW **AND** **WHY?**

Some medications are available over the counter, others are by prescription only. Still others are controlled. Go to your Electronic Extras CD for more information on how medications are classified.

What You Need To Know When Giving a Medication

Every drug has **indications,** or specific signs, symptoms, or circumstances under which it is appropriate to administer the drug to a patient. For example, nitroglycerin is indicated when a patient has chest pain or squeezing, dull pressure. Each drug also has **contraindications,** or specific signs, symptoms, or circumstances under which it is not appropriate, and may be harmful, to administer the drug to the patient. For example, nitroglycerin is contraindicated (should not be given) if the patient has low blood pressure, because nitroglycerin, in dilating the arteries, causes a slight drop in the systolic blood pressure.

A **side effect** is any action of a drug other than the desired actions. Some side effects are predictable, like the drop in blood pressure from nitroglycerin. If you were not aware of the side effect of a drop in blood pressure and gave the drug to a patient who

Figure 16-6 An epinephrine auto-injector can reverse a severe allergic reaction.

started out with low blood pressure, the results could be devastating. The patient's blood pressure might "bottom out"—definitely not a desirable effect for a cardiac patient.

Medications come in many different forms. A few examples are:

- Compressed powders or tablets, such as nitroglycerin pills
- Liquids for injection, such as the epinephrine in an auto-injector
- Gels, such as the paste in a tube of oral glucose
- Suspensions, such as the thick slurry of activated charcoal in water
- Fine powder for inhalation, such as that in a prescribed inhaler
- Gases for inhalation, such as oxygen
- Sub-lingual (under-the-tongue) sprays such as a nitroglycerin spray
- Liquid that is vaporized, such as a fixed-dose nebulizer

Before administering a drug to any patient, confirm the order and write it down. Then check the "four rights" by asking yourself the following questions as you select the medication and confirm that it is not expired:

- Do I have the *right patient?*
- Is this the *right medication?*
- Is this the *right dose?* Generally, a dose is given in milligrams.

- Am I giving this medication by the *right route* of administration?

The route by which the drug is administered affects the rate that the medication enters the bloodstream and arrives at its target organ to achieve its desired effect. Routes of administration include:

- Oral, or swallowed
- Sublingual, or dissolved under the tongue
- Inhaled, or breathed into the lungs, usually in tiny aerosol particles as from an inhaler or as a gas such as oxygen
- Intravenous, or injected into a vein
- Intramuscular, or injected into a muscle
- Subcutaneous, or injected under the skin
- Endotracheal, or sprayed directly into a tube inserted into the trachea

After any medication is given to a patient, it is important that you reassess the patient to see how the drug has affected him. Obtain another set of vital signs and compare them to the vital signs that you took before administering the medication. The ongoing assessment of the patient should include an evaluation of the changes in the patient's condition and vital signs after administration of medication. Be sure to document the response of the patient to each drug intervention. For example, "The patient's respiratory distress decreased after 5 minutes of high-concentration oxygen by nonrebreather mask."

MEDICATIONS PATIENTS OFTEN TAKE

It would be impossible to learn and carry around in your head all the types of medications you might discover your patients are taking. However, the medications a patient is taking may be a clue to a preexisting medical condition or, if improperly used, a cause of the patient's current problem. For example, a patient who is taking antihypertensives and antidiabetics might also be taking or misusing other medications that can contribute to an altered mental status—perhaps Dilantin to control seizures, codeine for pain, or Inderal for a heart rhythm disorder.

It is a good idea to have a resource from which you can find out additional information about a patient's medications en route to the hospital. Many ambulances carry a *Physician's Desk Reference,* or *PDR,* for this purpose. Most EMT-Bs carry, or have available to them, a pocket guide that contains useful information such as commonly used abbreviations. These pocket guides usually list the most commonly prescribed medications along with the general category of that medication to help you understand what the medication may be used for. However, remember that *your main purpose in finding out what medications the patient is taking is not to make a diagnosis but to report this information to medical direction and hospital personnel.*

Table 16-1 lists the seven most common categories of medications you will find in the field that are relevant to patient care, with a few examples of medications in each category. There are many other drugs and drug categories in addition to those listed in the table.

Table 16-1   Medications Patients Often Take

Analgesics
Drugs prescribed for pain relief

- propoxyphene (Darvon)
- nalbuphine (Nubain)
- morphine (Astramorph PF, Duramorph, MS Contin, Roxanol)
- acetaminophen (Anacin-3, Panadol, Tempra, Tylenol)
- ibuprofen (Actiprofen, Advil, Excedrin IS, Motrin, Novoprofen, Nuprin)
- aspirin (Ecotrin, Emprin)
- codeine

Antiarrhythmics
Drugs prescribed for heart rhythm disorders

- digoxin (Lanoxin)
- propranolol (Inderal)
- verapamil (Calan, Calan SR, Isoptin, Isoptin SR, Verclan)
- procainamide (Procan SR, Promine, Pronestyl)

Anticonvulsants
Drugs prescribed for prevention and control of seizures

- carbamazepine (Epitol, Tegretol)
- phenytoin (Dilantin)
- primidone (Mysoline)
- phenobarbital (Phenobarbital, Phenobarbital Sodium, Solfoton)
- valproic acid (Depakene)

Antihypertensives
Drugs prescribed to reduce high blood pressure

- captopril (Capoten)
- clonidine (Catapres)
- guanabenz (Wytensin)
- hydralazine (Apresoline, Hydralazine HCL)
- hydrochlorothiazide (Esidrix, HydroDiuril, Oretic)
- methyldopa (Aldomet)
- nifedipine (Adalat, Adalat CC, Procardia)

Bronchodilators
Drugs that relax the smooth muscles of the bronchial tubes. These medications provide relief of bronchial asthma and allergies affecting the respiratory system.

- albuterol (Proventil, Ventolin, Volmax)
- aminophylline
- isoetharine (Bronkometer, Bronkosol)
- metaproterenol (Alupent, Metaproterenol Sulfate, Metaprel)
- terbutaline (Brethaire, Brethine, Bricanyl)
- theophylline (Theo-Dur, T-Phyl, Uniphyl)

Antidiabetic agents
Drugs prescribed to diabetic patients to control hyperglycemia (high blood sugar)

- chlorpropamide (Diabinese)
- glipizide (Glucotrol)
- glyburide (DiaBeta, Glynase Prestab, Micronase)
- insulin (Humulin, Novolin, NPH, Humalog)
- metformin (Glucophage)

Antidepressant agents
Drugs prescribed to help regulate the emotional activity of the patient to minimize the peaks and valleys in their psychological and emotional state

- amitriptyline (Elavil)
- amoxapine (Asendin)
- bupropion (Wellbutrin)
- clomipramine (Anafranil)
- desipramine (Desipramine HCl, Norpramin)
- doxepin (Adapin, Sinequan, Sinequan Concentrate)
- fluoxetine (Prozac)
- imipramine (Tofranil, Tripamine)
- nefazodone (Serzone)
- nortriptyline (Aventyl, Pamelor)
- paroxetine (Paxil)
- protriptyline (Vivactil)
- sertraline (Zoloft)
- trimipramine (Surmontil)

Note: Generic names are lowercase. Trade names are capitalized.

STREET
SCENES

It is winter and cold, so you are not too surprised when the dispatcher tells you to respond to the mall for a 62-year-old male patient with chest pain. During winter, many cardiac patients walk for exercise in the mall, and this is not the first cardiac call you have had there. When you arrive, you find the patient sitting in a chair. You introduce yourself and your partner, ask the patient his name, and then say, "Well, Mr. Edwards, why was EMS called?"

"I was doing my usual morning walk," he explains, "when I started to get chest pain. I thought it might go away but it didn't. I got concerned and asked the security guard to call 9-1-1."

As your partner administers oxygen by nonrebreather and takes a set of vital signs, you ask the patient: "On a scale of 1 to 10, with 10 being the worst pain you've ever had, how would you rate the chest pain you're having now?" He tells you that it is a 7. You ask him to describe the pain and to point to where it is located. He says that it feels like a dull pain and points to the center of his chest. He also says the pain does not radiate. The patient seems pale, and his skin is dry. After a bit more questioning, he tells you the last time this happened he took nitro for relief.

STREET SCENE QUESTIONS

1. What additional patient history should you obtain?

2. Should you let the patient take nitroglycerin? Why, or why not?

3. Are vital signs important if nitroglycerin is going to be taken by the patient?

You ask Mr. Edwards if he has nitroglycerin with him now. He says his wife has it, but she went to a store in another part of the mall and should be back shortly. You then ask about other medications, and the patient tells you he is on propranolol and a diuretic. Next, you ask if he has ever had a heart attack. The patient tells you that he had one about a year and a half ago with an angioplasty. Vital signs are: pulse 90, blood pressure 120/90, and respirations of 24 and labored. When his wife shows up, she attempts to administer a pill, but you ask her to wait.

STREET SCENE QUESTIONS

4. What information do you want to know about the nitroglycerin?

5. How should the nitroglycerin be administered?

3. When should vital signs be taken again?

At your request, the patient's wife gives you the nitroglycerin bottle so you can check the expiration date. At the same time, you check to make sure that it is the patient's specific prescription. It all checks. According to standing orders in your system, with these signs and symptoms including a systolic blood pressure over 100, a nitro may be given without radio contact with medical direction. You tell the patient that you are going to put the pill under his tongue and he should let it dissolve. You specifically tell Mr. Edwards not to swallow.

About a minute after the patient is given the pill, he complains of a slight headache. You tell him this is a possible side effect of taking nitro and not to be concerned. After another minute goes by, you ask the patient to rate the chest pain on a scale of 1 to

PATIENT NAME: Francis Edwards						PATIENT AGE: 62		

CHIEF COMPLAINT

"Chest pain"

PAST MEDICAL HISTORY

- [ ] None
- [ ] Allergy to _____
- [ ] Hypertension   [ ] Stroke
- [ ] Seizures   [ ] Diabetes
- [ ] COPD   [ ] Cardiac
- [ ] Other (List)   [ ] Asthma

Previous MI, angioplasty

Current Medications (List)
nitroglycerin, propranolol, lasix

VITAL SIGNS

TIME	RESP	PULSE	B.P.	MENTAL STATUS	R PUPILS L	SKIN
1000	Rate: 24 [ ] Regular [ ] Shallow [X] Labored	Rate: 90 [X] Regular [ ] Irregular	120 / 90	[✓] Alert [ ] Voice [ ] Pain [ ] Unresp.	[✓] Normal [✓] [ ] Dilated [ ] [ ] Constricted [ ] [ ] Sluggish [ ] [ ] No-Reaction [ ]	[ ] Unremarkable [ ] Cool [✓] Pale [✓] Warm [ ] Cyanotic [ ] Moist [ ] Flushed [✓] Dry [ ] Jaundiced
1015	Rate: 20 [X] Regular [ ] Shallow [ ] Labored	Rate: 90 [X] Regular [ ] Irregular	120 / 90	[✓] Alert [ ] Voice [ ] Pain [ ] Unresp.	[✓] Normal [✓] [ ] Dilated [ ] [ ] Constricted [ ] [ ] Sluggish [ ] [ ] No-Reaction [ ]	[ ] Unremarkable [ ] Cool [✓] Pale [✓] Warm [ ] Cyanotic [ ] Moist [ ] Flushed [✓] Dry [ ] Jaundiced
1030	Rate: 18 [X] Regular [ ] Shallow [ ] Labored	Rate: 80 [X] Regular [ ] Irregular	110 / pal-pation	[✓] Alert [ ] Voice [ ] Pain [ ] Unresp.	[✓] Normal [✓] [ ] Dilated [ ] [ ] Constricted [ ] [ ] Sluggish [ ] [ ] No-Reaction [ ]	[ ] Unremarkable [ ] Cool [✓] Pale [✓] Warm [ ] Cyanotic [ ] Moist [ ] Flushed [✓] Dry [ ] Jaundiced

NARRATIVE

On arrival we were met by a conscious, alert, somewhat anxious 62-year-old male with a chief complaint of a sudden onset of substernal chest pressure while walking. He is sitting upright in a chair, somewhat ashen. Upon questioning, patient states that the pain is similar to previous cardiac-related chest discomfort and is 7 on the 10 scale. He denies any radiation down his arm or toward his jaw. He also denies any relief with the brief wait while sitting. Our treatment begins with O_2 at 10 LPM via nonrebreather. While assessing the patient, his wife arrived with his nitroglycerin prescription. Administered one of patient's 0.4 mg nitro sublingually per BLS protocol. Patient states significant relief with the nitro and O_2 prior to transport.

10 again. About a 2 he replies. "In fact, the pain is almost gone," he tells you. Your partner takes another set of vital signs because blood pressure can drop with nitro, but there is no change. You package the patient for transport and move to the ambulance, making sure you keep the AED close by. You give Mrs. Edwards a short update and explain to her that you will take the nitroglycerin bottle with the patient. The transport to the hospital is uneventful with another set of vital signs taken en route.

CHAPTER REVIEW

SUMMARY

The following are medications carried on the ambulance that the EMT-B may administer to a patient under specific conditions: activated charcoal, oral glucose, and oxygen. The following medications are those that, if prescribed for the patient, the EMT-B may assist the patient in taking: prescribed inhalers, nitroglycerin, and epinephrine in auto-injectors. You may need to have permission from medical direction to administer or assist the patient with a medication. Follow local protocols.

There is a wide variety of medications that a patient may be taking. You will try to find out what medications a patient is taking when you take the SAMPLE history. These drugs may be identified by a variety of generic and trade names. Your main purpose in finding out what medications the patient is taking is to report this information to your medical director or hospital personnel.

KEY TERMS

activated charcoal a powder, usually pre-mixed with water, that will adsorb some poisons and help prevent them from being absorbed by the body.

contraindications (KON-truh-in-duh-KAY-shunz) specific signs or circumstances under which it is not appropriate and may be harmful to administer a drug to a patient.

epinephrine (ep-uh-NEF-rin) a drug that helps to constrict the blood vessels and relax passages of the airway. It may be used to counter a severe allergic reaction.

indications specific signs or circumstances under which it is appropriate to administer a drug to a patient.

inhaler a spray device with a mouthpiece that contains an aerosol form of a medication that a patient can spray into his airway.

nitroglycerin (NYE-tro-GLIS-uh-rin) a drug that helps to dilate the coronary vessels that supply the heart muscle with blood.

oral glucose (GLU-kos) a form of glucose (a kind of sugar) given by mouth to treat an awake patient (who is able to swallow) with an altered mental status and a history of diabetes.

oxygen a gas commonly found in the atmosphere. Pure oxygen is used as a drug to treat any patient whose medical or traumatic condition may cause them to be hypoxic, or low in oxygen.

pharmacology (FARM-uh-KOL-uh-je) the study of drugs, their sources, characteristics, and effects.

side effect any action of a drug other than the desired action.

REVIEW QUESTIONS

1. Name the drugs that are carried on the ambulance and may be administered by the EMT-B under certain circumstances. (p. 309)
2. Name the drugs that the EMT-B may assist the patient in taking if they have been prescribed for him and with approval by medical direction. (p. 310)
3. Medications may take the form of tablets. Name several other forms that medications may have. (p. 313)
4. Name the four "rights" you must check before administering a medication. (p. 313)
5. Name several routes by which medications may be administered. (p. 313)

APPLICATIONS

- A patient is complaining of chest pain. "Here's some nitroglycerin," says a family member. "Give him that." What do you do?

WEB MEDIC

Visit Brady's *Emergency Care* website for direct weblinks. At **www.bradybooks.com/ emergencycare**, you will find information related to the following Chapter 16 topics:

- Metered dose inhalers
- Nitroglycerin

Chapter
Seventeen

RESPIRATORY EMERGENCIES

As an EMT-B, you will encounter some patients who are having breathing difficulty but who nevertheless are breathing adequately. You will provide oxygen by nonrebreather mask to these patients and complete an on-scene assessment before transporting them to the hospital. At other times, you will encounter patients whose respiratory problems are more severe. They may be having such extreme difficulty moving air in and out of their lungs that their breathing is no longer adequate to support life. These patients will require much more rapid care, which will probably include artificial respiration.

The difference between adequate and inadequate breathing is one of the most important concepts in this chapter.

RESPIRATION

Respiratory Anatomy and Physiology

You learned about the respiratory system in Chapter 4, "The Human Body," and in Chapter 6, "Airway Management." In preparation for this chapter, you should review in those chapters the following structures of the respiratory system: nose, mouth, oropharynx, nasopharynx, epiglottis, trachea, cricoid cartilage, larynx, bronchi, lungs, alveoli, and diaphragm.

The diaphragm is a muscular structure that divides the chest cavity from the abdominal cavity. During a normal respiratory cycle, the diaphragm and other parts of the body work together to allow the body to inhale (breathe in) and exhale (breathe out) air. The respiratory cycle progresses as follows (Figure 17-1):

- *Inspiration.* The active process that uses the contraction of several muscles to increase the size of the chest cavity is called **inspiration.** The intercostal (rib) muscles and the diaphragm contract. The diaphragm lowers and the ribs move upward and outward. The expanding size of the chest cavity causes air to flow into the lungs. Another term for inspiration is **inhalation.**
- *Expiration.* A passive process, **expiration** involves the relaxation of the rib muscles and diaphragm. The ribs move downward and inward, while the diaphragm rises. This movement causes the chest cavity to decrease in

size and causes air to flow out of the lungs. Another term for expiration is **exhalation.**

Review in Chapter 4 how oxygen and carbon dioxide are exchanged through the alveoli and capillaries of the lungs, and through the capillaries and cells throughout the body. The exchange of oxygen and carbon dioxide, both in the lungs and in the body's cells, is critical to support life. There are many things that can go wrong within the body that will alter this vital exchange. Primarily, these problems are with the respiratory system or the circulatory system. This chapter will discuss the respiratory system, problems with breathing, and their effects on the body. Problems with the circulatory system will be discussed in Chapter 18, "Cardiac Emergencies."

TOPIC OVERVIEW

In this chapter, you will learn about the following topics:

- The difference between adequate and inadequate air exchange
- How to identify and treat a patient with breathing difficulty
- Use of a prescribed inhaler and how to assist a patient with one
- How to document findings and care of a patient with breathing difficulty

DOT OBJECTIVES

✔ **Knowledge and Attitude**

1. List the structure and function of the respiratory system. (p. 321)

2. State the signs and symptoms of a patient with breathing difficulty. (pp. 323–324, 325–326)

3. Describe the emergency medical care of the patient with breathing difficulty. (pp. 324, 327)

4. Recognize the need for medical direction to assist in the emergency medical care of the patient with breathing difficulty. (pp. 327, 329)

5. Describe the emergency medical care of the patient with breathing distress. (pp. 324, 327)

6. Establish the relationship between airway management and the patient with breathing difficulty. (pp. 324, 325, 327)

7. List signs of adequate air exchange. (pp. 322–323)

8. State the generic name, medication forms, dose, administration, action, indications, and contraindications for the prescribed inhaler. (p. 329) (Scan 17-1, p. 330; Scan 17-2, p. 331))

9. Distinguish between the emergency medical care of the infant, child, and adult patient with breathing difficulty. (pp. 324, 325)

10. Differentiate between upper airway obstruction and lower airway disease in the infant and child patient. (p. 325)

11. Defend EMT-Basic treatment regimens for various respiratory emergencies. (pp. 324, 327)

12. Explain the rationale for administering an inhaler. (p. 329)

✔ **Skills**

1. Demonstrate the emergency medical care for breathing difficulty.

2. Perform the steps in facilitating the use of an inhaler.

Adequate Breathing

It is easy to take breathing for granted. Fortunately, we do not consciously have to tell ourselves to inhale and exhale. The brain does that automatically.

As you learned in Chapter 6, "Airway Management," breathing may be classified as adequate or inadequate. Simply stated, adequate breathing is breathing that is sufficient to support life. Inadequate breathing is not. Your assessment of the adequacy of a patient's breathing may be vital to his survival.

Adequate breathing falls within certain ranges that are considered "normal." The patient will not appear to be in distress. He will be able to speak full sentences without having to catch his breath. His color, mental status, and orientation will be normal. Normal breathing may be determined by observing for rate, rhythm, and quality:

- *Rate.* Rates of breathing that are considered normal vary by age. For an adult, a normal rate is 12–20 breaths per minute. For a child, it is 15–30 breaths per minute. For an infant, it is 25–50 breaths per minute.

- *Rhythm.* Normal breathing rhythm will usually be regular. Breaths will be taken at regular intervals and will last for about the same length of time. Remember that talking and other factors can make normal breathing slightly irregular.

INSPIRATIONS AND EXPIRATIONS

RELAXED

CONTRACTION
Inspiration begins

INSPIRATION

RELAXED
Passive expiration begins

Figure 17-1 The process of respiration.

Table 17-1 Adequate and Inadequate Breathing

	Adequate Breathing	Inadequate Breathing
Rate	Adult: 12–20/minute Child: 15–30/minute Infant: 25–50/minute	Above or below normal rates for the patient's age group
Rhythm	Regular	May be irregular

Quality
    Breath Sounds
    Chest Expansion
    Effort of Breathing
	Present and equal
	Adequate and equal
	Unlabored, normal respiratory effort
		Diminished, unequal, or absent
		Inadequate or unequal
		Labored: increased respiratory effort; use of accessory muscles (may be pronounced in infants and children and involve nasal flaring, seesaw breathing, grunting, and retractions between the ribs and above the clavicles and sternum)

- *Quality.* Breath sounds, when auscultated with a stethoscope, will normally be present and equal when the lungs are compared to each other. When observing the chest cavity, both sides should move equally and adequately to indicate a proper air exchange. The depth of the respirations must be adequate.

Inadequate Breathing

Inadequate breathing is breathing that is not sufficient to support life. If left untreated, this condition will surely lead to death. It is one of your most important tasks as an EMT-B to identify and treat patients with inadequate breathing. Assessment and treatment are begun early in the call and must be continued throughout your time with the patient. Patients who are breathing adequately at first may deteriorate into inadequate breathing later on (Table 17-1).

● Patient ASSESSMENT

Inadequate Breathing

If the patient is not breathing adequately to support life, you may see any of the following conditions:

- *Rate.* The patient with inadequate breathing will have a breathing rate that is out of the normal ranges. Very slow breaths and very rapid breaths may not allow enough air to enter the lungs, re-

sulting in not enough oxygen being distributed throughout the body.

Agonal respirations (also called dying respirations) are sporadic, irregular breaths that are usually seen just before respiratory arrest. They are shallow and gasping with only a few breaths per minute. This breathing pattern is clearly a sign of inadequate breathing.

- *Rhythm.* The rhythm of inadequate breathing may be irregular. However, rhythm is not an absolute indicator of adequate or inadequate breathing. Remember that someone who is talking or is aware that you are observing his respirations may have slight irregularities, even though his breathing is adequate. On the other hand, a patient may have a regular rate, even when his breathing is inadequate.

- *Quality.* When breathing is inadequate, breath sounds may be diminished or absent. The depth of respirations (tidal volume) will be inadequate or shallow. Chest expansion may be inadequate or unequal and respiratory effort increased. You may note the use of accessory muscles (muscles other than the diaphragm and the intercostal muscles, such as the muscles of the neck and abdomen) in breathing. Since oxygenation of the body's tissues is reduced, the skin may be pale or cyanotic (blue) and feel cool and clammy to the touch.

In patients who have a diminished level of responsiveness or who are totally unresponsive, sounds such as snoring and gurgling also indicate a serious airway problem that requires immediate intervention.

Pediatric Notes

Respiratory problems can be very serious in infants and children. Since children rarely have heart attacks or other problems of adulthood, respiratory conditions, statistically, are a leading killer of infants and children. With this in mind, you must begin respiratory treatment of infants and children with a thorough and accurate assessment and prompt, proper care.

The structure of infants' and children's airways differs somewhat from that of adults:

- *Airway.* All airway structures are smaller in an infant or child than in an adult and therefore are more easily obstructed.
- *Tongue.* Infants' and children's tongues are proportionately larger and therefore take up more space in the mouth than an adult's tongue.
- *Trachea.* The trachea is smaller, softer, and more flexible in infants and children, which may lead to obstruction from swelling or trauma more easily than in adults. The cricoid cartilage is less developed and less rigid.
- *Diaphragm.* Infants and children depend more heavily on the diaphragm for respiration since the chest wall is softer. This is why infants and small children in respiratory distress exhibit "seesaw breathing" in which the movement of the diaphragm causes the chest and abdomen to move in opposite directions.

Be aware that some signs of inadequate breathing are unique to or more prominent in infants and children. So, be on the lookout for these signs:

- Nasal flaring (widening of the nostrils)
- Grunting
- Seesaw breathing
- Retractions (pulling in of the muscles) between the ribs (intercostal), above the clavicles (supraclavicular), and above the sternum (suprasternal).

Patient *CARE*

Inadequate Breathing

There is a wide range of function between adequate respirations and complete stoppage of breathing (respiratory arrest). You must pay careful attention to the patient's breathing throughout the call. It is not enough to simply make sure he is breathing. The patient must be breathing adequately! If at any time you find that he is not breathing adequately, the treatment of this condition is your first patient-care priority.

When you determine, by the signs discussed under Patient Assessment, above, that a patient's breathing is inadequate, you will provide artificial ventilation with supplemental oxygen. In order of preference, the means of providing artificial ventilation are:

1. Pocket face mask with supplemental oxygen

2. Two-rescuer bag-valve mask with supplemental oxygen

3. Flow-restricted, oxygen-powered ventilation device

4. One-rescuer bag-valve mask with supplemental oxygen

The means of providing artificial ventilation were discussed in Chapter 6, "Airway Management." Make sure that you are properly trained with the device that you are using for ventilation. If supplemental oxygen is not immediately available, begin artificial respirations without supplemental oxygen and attach the oxygen supply to the mask as soon as it is available.

If you are uncertain about whether a patient's breathing is inadequate and requires artificial ventilation, provide artificial ventilation. In the rare circumstance when a patient with inadequate breathing is conscious enough to fight artificial ventilation, transport immediately and consult medical direction.

Adequate and Inadequate Artificial Ventilation

Like breathing, artificial ventilation can be adequate or inadequate. When you are performing artificial ventilation adequately, the chest will rise and fall with each artificial ventilation. The adequate rate for artificial ventilation is 12 breaths per minute for adults, and 20 per minute for infants and children.

When you are providing artificial ventilation without chest compressions (patient has a pulse), monitor the pulse carefully. With adequate artificial ventilation, the pulse rate should return to normal. Since the pulse in adults will rise from a lack of oxygen, a pulse that remains the same or increases may indicate inadequate artificial ventilation. Naturally, if the pulse disappears this indicates that the patient is in cardiac arrest, and you will need to begin chest compressions (CPR).

Pediatric Notes

Pediatric patients differ from adults in many ways. There are few differences that are more important in emergency care than those within the respiratory system. When adult patients experience a decrease in oxygen in the bloodstream (hypoxia), their pulse increases.

In infants and children with respiratory difficulties, you may observe a slight increase in pulse early, but soon the pulse will drop significantly. *A low (or brady-cardic) pulse in infants and small children in the setting of a respiratory emergency usually means trouble!* This is a sharp contrast from adults where it is a good sign when their pulse lowers to a more normal level.

If you observe a pulse below the expected rates for infants and children, evaluate your ventilations or oxygen therapy thoroughly. In ventilations, make sure that you have an open airway and that the chest rises with each breath. *Nothing is more important for infants and children than adequate airway care!* In any situation make sure that the oxygen tank has not run out and that the tubing has not kinked or slipped off the delivery device or oxygen cylinder.

For any patient—adult, child, or infant—if the chest does not rise and fall with each artificial ventilation, or the pulse does not return to normal, increase the force of ventilations. If the chest still does not rise, check that you are maintaining an open airway by the head-tilt, chin-lift maneuver (if there is no suspected spine injury) or by the jaw-thrust maneuver (if spine injury is possible). Insert an oropharyngeal or nasopharyngeal airway as needed to prevent the tongue from blocking the airway. Suction fluids and foreign matter from the airway as necessary, or perform the Heimlich maneuver and finger sweeps as needed to clear large airway obstructions. (Deliver alternating series of back blows and chest thrusts to clear airway obstructions in infants. Do not perform blind finger sweeps—remove only visible objects—in infants and children.) If you are using supplemental oxygen, check that all connections are secure and that the tubing has not kinked.

Review the techniques of airway maintenance and artificial ventilation in Chapter 6, "Airway Management," and in "Basic Cardiac Life Support Review" in the back of this book.

In infants and children, it is especially important to distinguish between an upper airway obstruction and a lower airway disease if there appears to be a blockage of the airway. If the airway is blocked by the tongue, blood, secretions, or debris, consider suctioning, performing finger sweeps, or inserting an oropharyngeal or nasopharyngeal adjunct to help maintain an open airway.

However, infants and children are also subject to lower respiratory diseases or infections that may result in swelling of the airway passages. With some of these diseases, it is dangerous to probe or place anything in the patient's mouth or pharynx because this may set off spasms along the airway.

Refrain from placing anything in the patient's mouth and transport as quickly as possible if you see the following signs of a lower respiratory problem:

- Wheezing
- Increased breathing effort on exhalation
- Rapid breathing without stridor (a harsh, high-pitched sound)

For more about assessing and treating respiratory conditions in infants and children, see Chapter 13, "Pediatric, Adolescent, and Geriatric Assessment" and Chapter 31, "Infants and Children."

BREATHING DIFFICULTY

Breathing difficulty is a frequent chief complaint, representing a patient's feeling of labored, or difficult, breathing. Although there are objective signs associated with breathing difficulty (listed on the next page), the "difficulty" that is reported to you by the patient is a subjective perception of the patient. The amount of distress the patient feels may or may not reflect the actual severity of his condition. His breathing may be more adequate or less adequate than he feels it is. You should not rely entirely on the patient's report to decide how serious the condition really is. You will need to perform an assessment to help you make that determination.

It is important to remember that a patient with breathing difficulty may have either adequate or inadequate breathing. You may encounter two patients, at different times, who tell you that they are having difficulty breathing ("I can't catch my breath" or a similar complaint). One patient may be having minor difficulty due to a preexisting respiratory condition but still have adequate breathing. His condition is not life threatening. The other patient, who has offered exactly the same complaint, may be having a problem such as an allergic reaction and severe difficulty breathing. Your examination of this patient may reveal inadequate breathing that requires immediate artificial ventilation.

Difficulty in breathing may have many causes ranging from ongoing medical conditions to illnesses such as pneumonia and other infections, to cardiac problems that cause disturbances in the respiratory system.

Breathing Difficulty

Symptoms of breathing difficulty include a feeling of shortness of breath or tightness in the chest and restlessness or anxiety. Signs of breathing difficulty are as follows (Figure 17-2):

- Increased pulse rate
- Decreased pulse rate (especially in infants and children)
- Changes in the breathing rate (above or below normal levels)
- Changes in breathing rhythm
- Pale, cyanotic, or flushed skin
- Noisy breathing which may be described as
  —Audible wheezing (heard without stethoscope)
  —Gurgling
  —Snoring
  —Crowing
  —Stridor (harsh, high-pitched sound during breathing, usually due to upper airway obstruction)
- Inability to speak full sentences (or at all) due to breathing difficulty
- Use of accessory muscles to breathe
- Retractions
- Altered mental status

- Coughing
- Flared nostrils, pursed lips
- Patient positioning
  —Tripod position (patient leaning forward with hands on knees or another surface)
  —Sitting with feet dangling, leaning forward
- Unusual anatomy (barrel chest)

The focused history and physical exam for patients with respiratory emergencies involves an appropriate interview and an examination of the chest and respiratory structures. Use the letters OPQRST to remember which questions to ask about the respiratory difficulty:

O—*Onset.* When did it begin?

P— *Provocation.* What were you doing when this came on?

Q—*Quality.* Can you describe the feeling you have?

R—*Radiation.* Does the feeling seem to spread to any other part of your body? Do you have pain or discomfort anywhere else in your body?

S—*Severity.* On a scale of 1 to 10, how bad is your breathing trouble? (10 is worst, 1 best)

T—*Time.* How long have you had this feeling?

Ask if the patient has taken any prescribed medications or done anything else to help relieve his condition. This may affect the treatment provided by you and the treatment provided later at the hospital.

Figure 17-2   Signs and symptoms of breathing difficulty.

Figure 17-3   A patient with chronic obstructive pulmonary disease (COPD).

Patient *CARE*

Breathing Difficulty

When a patient is suffering from breathing difficulty, provide the following care:

- *Assessment.* Assess the airway during the initial assessment and then frequently throughout the call. Assist respiration with artificial ventilations and supplemental oxygen whenever the patient has or develops inadequate breathing.

- *Oxygen.* Oxygen is the main treatment for any patient in respiratory difficulty. If the patient is breathing adequately, use a nonrebreather mask at 12 to 15 liters per minute to provide oxygen. Use a nasal cannula only in cases where the patient will not tolerate a mask. If the patient has inadequate breathing, provide supplemental oxygen while performing artificial ventilations.

- *Positioning.* If the patient is experiencing breathing difficulty but is breathing adequately, place him in a position of comfort. Most patients with breathing difficulty feel they can breathe better sitting up. This is not possible if the patient has inadequate breathing, since the patient would need to be supine to receive assisted ventilations.

- *Prescribed inhaler.* If the patient has a prescribed inhaler, you may be able to assist the patient in taking this medication. This would be done after consultation with medical direction, often during transportation to the hospital. (More information will be provided on prescribed inhalers later in this chapter.)

You may hear from other EMT-Bs that oxygen must be administered to some patients with caution—or not at all. This is because of a condition sometimes called the *hypoxic drive.* (You read about hypoxic drive in Chapter 6.) This occurs in a few patients who have lung diseases such as emphysema or chronic bronchitis. For many years it was recommended that oxygen not be given, or be given cautiously, to such patients for fear that oxygen would destroy their "drive to breathe." It is now widely believed that more harm is done by withholding oxygen than could be done by administering oxygen. Even with patients who have these diseases, never withhold oxygen from a patient in respiratory distress.

Oxygen is a drug. Like all drugs, it must be administered responsibly and with careful monitoring of the patient. If breathing becomes inadequate or stops during oxygen administration, provide artificial ventilation. This kind of adverse response to oxygen, however, would rarely have time to develop during the short duration of prehospital care and is almost unheard of during EMS calls. More likely, the patient's worsening condition is due to a respiratory emergency, not to the application of oxygen.

HOW AND WHY?

Not all inhalers are designed to help respiratory distress. Some inhalers are prescribed steroids or other medications, which will not help the patient in respiratory distress right away. Go to your Electronic Extras CD for more information.

RESPIRATORY DISEASES

It is not necessary to diagnose a patient's condition to provide effective treatment as an EMT-B. In fact, the care for all respiratory conditions is essentially the same, as described earlier in this chapter. The information that follows on chronic obstructive pulmonary diseases (Figure 17-3) and asthma is provided to enrich your knowledge of respiratory diseases.

Chronic Obstructive Pulmonary Disease (COPD)

Emphysema—as well as chronic bronchitis, black lung, and many undetermined respiratory illnesses that cause the patient problems like those seen in emphysema—are all classified as chronic obstructive pulmonary disease (COPD).

COPD is mainly a problem of middle-aged or older patients. This is because these disorders take time to develop as tissues in the respiratory tract react to irritants. Cigarette smoking causes the overwhelming majority of cases of COPD. Occasionally other irritants such as chemicals, air pollutants, or repeated infections cause this condition.

Chronic bronchitis and emphysema are compared in Figure 17-4. In chronic bronchitis, the bronchiole lining is inflamed. Excess mucus is formed. The cells in the bronchioles that normally clear away accumulations of mucus are not able to do so. The sweeping apparatus on these cells, the cilia, have been damaged or destroyed.

In emphysema, the walls of the alveoli break down, greatly reducing the surface area for respiratory exchange. The lungs begin to lose elasticity. These factors combine to allow stale air laden with carbon dioxide to be trapped in the lungs, reducing the effectiveness of normal breathing efforts.

Many COPD patients will exhibit characteristics of both emphysema and chronic bronchitis. Usually the reason a COPD patient calls the ambulance is that a recent upper respiratory infection has caused an acute worsening of the disease.

A very few COPD patients develop a hypoxic drive to trigger respirations. In patients without COPD, the brain determines when to breathe based on increased levels of carbon dioxide in the blood. Since COPD patients develop a tolerance to their body's high levels of carbon dioxide, the brain learns to rely, instead, on low oxygen levels as the trigger to breathe. The higher oxygen levels that result from oxygen administration may, in rare cases, signal the COPD patient to reduce breathing or even to stop breathing (develop respiratory arrest).

In most cases, however, the hypoxic drive will not be a problem in the prehospital setting. The patient's need for oxygen will outweigh the risk involved with administration. If the patient has a possible heart attack or stroke, is developing shock, or has respiratory distress, a higher concentration of oxygen will be required in spite of the potential problems. *If oxygen is required by the COPD patient, do not withhold it.*

Constantly monitor the patient. If the patient's breathing becomes inadequate or stops, be prepared to assist respirations through artificial ventilation, and contact medical direction.

Asthma

Seen in young and old patients alike, asthma is an episodic disease (a disease that only affects the patient at irregular intervals). This is far different from chronic bronchitis and emphysema, both of which afflict the patient continually. Asthma also differs from chronic bronchitis and emphysema in that it does not produce a hypoxic drive. Although the disease is episodic, an asthma attack can be life threatening. Between episodes, the asthmatic patient can lead a normal life.

An asthma attack may be triggered by an allergic reaction to something inhaled, swallowed, or injected into the body. Attacks can be precipitated by insect stings, air pollutants, infection, strenuous exercise, or emotional stress. When an asthma attack occurs, the small bronchioles that lead to the air sacs of the lungs become narrowed because of contractions of the muscles that make up the air-

Normal   Chronic Bronchitis   Emphysema

Mucus plugs and inflammation

Decreased surface area

Figure 17-4 Chronic bronchitis and emphysema are chronic obstructive pulmonary diseases.

way. To complicate matters, there is an overproduction of thick mucus. The combined effects of the contractions and the mucus cause the small passages to practically close down, severely restricting air flow.

The air flow is mainly restricted in one direction. When the patient inhales, the expanding lungs exert an outward pull, increasing the diameter of the airway and allowing air to flow into the lungs. During exhalation, however, the opposite occurs and the stale air becomes trapped in the lungs. This requires the patient to exhale the air forcefully, producing the characteristic wheezing sounds associated with asthma.

THE PRESCRIBED INHALER

HOW AND WHY?

Prescribed inhalers can help patients in respiratory distress. The proper delivery of these medications is not an easy task—especially when a patient is not calm! Go to your Electronic Extras CD for more information.

A patient with a respiratory problem may have an inhaler prescribed by a physician. You will need to get permission from medical direction to help the patient use the inhaler. Remember to find out if the patient has already used the inhaler before your arrival. Keep in mind that a patient may overuse the inhaler prior to your arrival, so it is important to determine exactly when and how many times the inhaler has been used. Be sure to give this information to medical direction.

The metered-dose inhaler gets its name from the fact that each activation of the inhaler provides a metered, or exactly measured, dose of medication. Most patients simply refer to the device as their "inhaler" or "puffer." The inhaler is prescribed for patients with respiratory problems that cause **bronchoconstriction** (constriction, or blockage, of the bronchi that lead from the trachea to the lungs) or other types of lung obstructions. The inhalers contain a drug that dilates, or enlarges, the air passages, making breathing easier.

When patients use an inhaler, they often are excited or nervous because they are short of breath. Many do not use their inhaler properly. Some people have never had proper instruction in use of their inhaler. Make sure to calm the patient the best you can and coach him to use the inhaler properly, as follows:

1. As with any medication, assure that you have the right patient, the right medication, the right dose, and the right route. Check the expiration date. Make sure the inhaler is at room temperature or warmer. Shake the inhaler vigorously several times.

2. Make sure that the patient is alert enough to use the inhaler properly.

3. Make sure the patient first exhales deeply.

4. Have the patient put his lips around the opening and press the inhaler to activate the spray as he inhales deeply.

5. After the patient inhales, make sure he holds his breath as long as possible so the medication can be absorbed. This may be difficult with a patient who is anxious, but unless the medication is held in the lungs, it will have minimal or no value.

Your role will involve more coaching than actually administering the medication. The proper sequence for administration of a prescribed inhaler is shown in Scan 17-1. Inhalers are described in detail in Scan 17-2. Follow local protocols and consult medical direction, if required, before assisting a patient with an inhaler.

Documentation Tips— Respiratory Emergencies

Difficulty in breathing can mean different things to different people. When documenting a respiratory complaint, attempt to get the patient to describe the difficulty in his own words and note them in the narrative portion of your prehospital care report. Put the patient's exact words in quotation marks. The patient's description may be anything from "I can't catch my breath" to "It hurts when I try to breathe deeply." The way the patient describes the complaint is valuable information.

You may also use the "1 to 10" scale (10 being the worst) to help the patient describe difficulty in breathing. This may be especially helpful when documenting the effects of an inhaler. A patient may describe her breathing difficulty as "9" before using the inhaler. After using the inhaler, she may say her difficulty was reduced to "3 or 4." You may find that the inhaler makes no difference or that it relieves the distress totally. In any case, having the patient assign a numerical value lets you, medical direction, and hospital personnel know more exactly how your patient feels.

PRESCRIBED INHALER—PATIENT ASSESSMENT AND MANAGEMENT

▲ 1. The patient has the indications for use of an inhaler: signs and symptoms of breathing difficulty and an inhaler prescribed by a physician.

▲ 2. Contact medical direction and obtain an order to assist the patient with the prescribed inhaler.

3. Assure the four "rights" for administration of a medication:
- Right patient
- Right medication
- Right dose
- Right route

Check expiration date, shake inhaler, make sure inhaler is room temperature or warmer, and make sure patient is alert.

▲ 4. Coach the patient in the use of inhaler. Tell him he should exhale deeply, inhaler to activate spray, inhale, and in so medication can be ab-

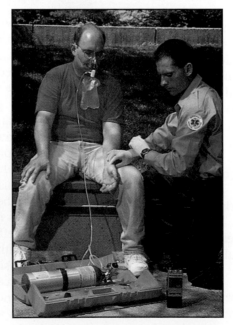

▲ 5. After use of inhaler, reassess the patient: take vital signs, perform a focused exam, and determine if breathing is adequate.

A "spacer" device between inhaler and patient allows more effective use of medication. If the patient has a spacer, it should be attached to the inhaler before use. The patient should then follow the manufacturer's instructions. It is important to note two things about using a spacer: (1) timing is not as critical as long as the patient presses the inhaler *before* inhaling, and (2) the patient should inhale deeply but *slowly*.

PRESCRIBED INHALER

Medication Name

1. Generic: albuterol, isoetharine, metaproterenol
2. Trade: Proventil, Ventolin, Bronkosol, Bronkometer, Alupent, Metaprel

Indications
Meets all of the following criteria:

1. Patient exhibits signs and symptoms of respiratory emergency.
2. Patient has physician-prescribed hand-held inhaler.
3. Medical direction gives specific authorization to use.

Contraindications

1. Patient is unable to use device (e.g., not alert).
2. Inhaler is not prescribed for patient.
3. No permission has been given by medical direction.
4. Patient has already taken maximum prescribed dose prior to EMT-B's arrival.

Medication Form
Hand-held metered-dose inhaler

Dosage
Number of inhalations based on medical direction's order or physician's order

Administration

1. Obtain order from medical direction, either on-line or off-line.
2. Assure right patient, right medication, right dose, right route, and patient alert enough to use inhaler.
3. Check expiration date of inhaler.
4. Check if patient has already taken any doses.
5. Assure inhaler is at room temperature or warmer.
6. Shake inhaler vigorously several times.
7. Have patient exhale deeply.
8. Have patient put her lips around the opening of the inhaler.
9. Have patient depress the hand-held inhaler as she begins to inhale deeply.
10. Instruct patient to hold her breath for as long as she comfortably can so medication can be absorbed.
11. Put oxygen back on patient.
12. Allow patient to breathe a few times and repeat second dose if so ordered by medical direction.
13. If patient has a spacer device for use with her inhaler (device for attachment between inhaler and patient to allow for more effective use of medication), it should be used.

Actions
Beta agonist bronchodilator dilates bronchioles, reducing airway resistance.

Side Effects

1. Increased pulse rate
2. Tremors
3. Nervousness

Reassessment Strategies

1. Gather vital signs.
2. Perform focused reassessment of chest and respiratory function.
3. Observe for deterioration of patient; if breathing becomes inadequate, provide artificial respirations.

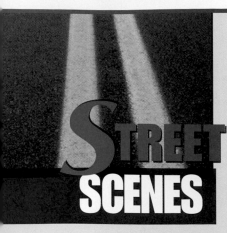

STREET SCENES

Carmela Bartolone has been diagnosed with emphysema. She spends many days housebound on a home oxygen unit. But on this particular spring day, she felt that she should work in her flower garden. As she starts to pull weeds, she doesn't realize how much her rate of breathing is picking up. She soon finds that she is unable to catch her breath and unable to get back to the house. A neighbor sees Carmela having a problem breathing and asks if she needs anything. Carmela's response is "Get help!"

Your pager is activated, and the only information the dispatcher provides is "a female patient with difficulty breathing." The dispatcher also advises you that the ALS response unit is unavailable. Upon arrival, you find Mrs. Bartolone in a lawn chair with her husband and neighbor standing next to her, trying to get her to slow her breathing. You ask some quick medical questions and realize that the neighbor saw what happened, the husband has the medical history, and the patient can't talk in full sentences because of severe dyspnea.

STREET SCENE QUESTIONS

1. What is the first thing you should do for this patient?

2. What questions should you ask the husband? The neighbor?

After you perform an initial assessment, you decide to get patient information from the husband. He states that Mrs. Bartolone has emphysema from many years of smoking two packs of cigarettes a day. He says this same type of attack happened once before about 6 months ago. At that time, she was taken to the hospital and needed to be intubated and placed on a ventilator. She is on a number of medications, which he needs to get from inside the house. He reports no known allergies or other medical history.

STREET SCENE QUESTIONS

3. What is the significance of the medical history provided by the husband?

4. How much oxygen should the patient receive?

The fact that Mrs. Bartolone had to be put on a ventilator makes you realize that this patient is at risk of deteriorating very quickly. As you evaluate her breathing again, you note her respiration rate is still rapid. Your partner counts it at 36. You notice the patient's lips are bluish, her nostrils are flaring, and she is pushing herself up in the chair to make it easier to breathe. Your partner informs you that the patient is using the muscles of the chest and stomach to help her breathe. Mrs. Bartolone is becoming less restless because she is getting drowsy, a sign that action is needed. Your partner recommends that you assist respirations with a bag-valve mask and you concur. As you start to hook up the oxygen reservoir, the husband returns with the patient's inhalers and tells you the patient only gets 2 liters per minute on her home unit. He also tells you that the doctor stressed she should not get more than that.

STREET SCENE QUESTIONS

5. Is the patient a good candidate for use of an inhaler?

6. Should this patient be considered a high priority with red light and siren for transport to the hospital?

You and your partner agree that this patient needs ventilations assisted with a high concentration of oxygen and transport without delay. Her normal 2 liters per minute of oxygen are not enough to oxygenate her in this condition. You transport while assisting ventilations. You would like to help her use her inhaler but your protocol requires the patient to be alert and you know you are doing the patient a lot of good by ventilating her with high-concentration oxygen.

While en route, your partner notifies the hospital by radio of the patient's condition, treatment being provided, and an ETA of 10 minutes. You are able to ventilate the patient well by yourself, but that also means you are unable to get repeat vital

PATIENT NAME: *Carmela Bartolone* **PATIENT AGE:** *74*

CHIEF COMPLAINT

Dyspnea

PAST MEDICAL HISTORY

- [ ] None
- [ ] Allergy to _____
- [ ] Hypertension   [ ] Stroke
- [ ] Seizures   [ ] Diabetes
- [ ] COPD   [ ] Cardiac
- [x] Other (List)   [ ] Asthma

Emphysema

Current Medications (List)

2 LPM O$_2$ by NC, ipratropium & albuterol inhalers

	TIME	RESP	PULSE	B.P.	MENTAL STATUS	R PUPILS L	SKIN
V I T A L S I G N S	1 0 2 8	Rate: **36** [ ] Regular [ ] Shallow [x] Labored	Rate: **110** [x] Regular [ ] Irregular	**160** / **90**	[x] Alert [ ] Voice [ ] Pain [ ] Unresp.	[ ] Normal [ ] Dilated [ ] Constricted [ ] Sluggish [ ] No-Reaction	[ ] Unremarkable [x] Cool [ ] Pale [ ] Warm [x] Cyanotic [ ] Moist [ ] Flushed [x] Dry [ ] Jaundiced
	1 0 4 0	Rate: **12** *Assisted* [ ] Regular [ ] Shallow [ ] Labored	Rate: *Approx.* **100** [ ] Regular [x] Irregular		[ ] Alert [x] Voice [ ] Pain [ ] Unresp.	[ ] Normal [ ] Dilated [ ] Constricted [ ] Sluggish [ ] No-Reaction	[ ] Unremarkable [x] Cool [ ] Pale [ ] Warm [x] Cyanotic [ ] Moist [ ] Flushed [x] Dry [ ] Jaundiced
	1 0 5 5	Rate: **12** *Assisted* [ ] Regular [ ] Shallow [ ] Labored	Rate: *Approx.* **110** [x] Regular [ ] Irregular		[ ] Alert [x] Voice [ ] Pain [ ] Unresp.	[ ] Normal [ ] Dilated [ ] Constricted [ ] Sluggish [ ] No-Reaction	[ ] Unremarkable [x] Cool [x] Pale [ ] Warm [ ] Cyanotic [ ] Moist [ ] Flushed [x] Dry [ ] Jaundiced

NARRATIVE

74-year-old female patient found in her yard complaining of severe difficulty in breathing which

began while working in the garden. Patient was unable to speak in full sentences. She was using accessory muscles

to breathe, displayed nasal flaring, and had cyanosis about the lips. Shortly after our arrival the patient became

drowsy. We provided assisted ventilations via BVM with supplemental oxygen.

Patient has history of smoking and emphysema. An episode similar to this about 6 months ago resulted in the

patient being intubated and placed on a ventilator. Patient did not experience relief from rest. She denies chest pain

or other complaints. She is on oxygen via cannula at home. Patient transported to the hospital. BVM assisted

ventilations continued en route. Patient's condition improved slightly with assisted ventilations (increased level of

consciousness). Unable to obtain second set of vital signs due to insufficient personnel and assisting ventilations.

signs. Keeping your priorities in mind, you continue ventilating and estimate her pulse rate by checking it quickly and frequently between ventilations. The patient seems more alert as you arrive at the emergency department. There you provide a prehospital care report to the waiting physician, which includes the patient history you obtained from the husband. As you start to leave the patient area, the doctor thanks you for being aggressive by assisting ventilations.

CHAPTER REVIEW

SUMMARY

Respiratory emergencies are common calls that require diligent assessment, care, and emotional support. It is very important to evaluate your patient for adequate breathing throughout the call. If at any time you find breathing inadequate, you must assist ventilations. Providing artificial ventilation to a patient promptly may prevent him from slipping into respiratory arrest—and death!

For a patient who is experiencing difficulty breathing but whose breathing is adequate, administration of high-concentration oxygen by nonrebreather mask, coaching the patient in the use of a prescribed inhaler if the patient has one, placing the patient in a position of comfort, and providing reassurance are the key treatments the EMT-B can provide.

KEY TERMS

bronchoconstriction constriction, or blockage, of the bronchi that lead from the trachea to the lungs.

exhalation (EX-huh-LAY-shun) another term for expiration.

expiration (EK-spuh-RAY-shun) a passive process in which the intercostal (rib) muscles and the diaphragm relax, causing the chest cavity to decrease in size and forcing air from the lungs.

inhalation (IN-huh-LAY-shun) another term for inspiration.

inspiration (IN-spuh-RAY-shun) an active process in which the intercostal (rib) muscles and the diaphragm contract, expanding the size of the chest cavity and causing air to flow into the lungs.

REVIEW QUESTIONS

1. List the normal rates of breathing for adults, children, and infants. List the other signs of adequate breathing. (pp. 322, 323)
2. List the signs of inadequate breathing. (pp. 323–324)
3. Explain the treatment you will give, as an EMT-B, when a patient's breathing is inadequate. (pp. 324, 325)
4. List the signs and symptoms of breathing difficulty. (p. 326)
5. Explain the treatments you may give, as an EMT-B, for breathing difficulty when breathing is adequate. (p. 327)
6. Explain the steps to follow before, during, and after helping a patient to use a prescribed inhaler. (pp. 329–331)
7. List some differences between adult and infant/child respiratory systems. (p. 324)
8. List some special considerations in the assessment and treatment of infants and children with respiratory problems. (pp. 324, 325)

APPLICATIONS

For each of the following patients, state whether the patient's breathing seems adequate or inadequate-and explain your reasoning:

• A 45-year-old male patient experiencing severe difficulty in breathing. His respirations are 36/minute and very shallow. He has minimal chest expansion and can barely speak.

• A 65-year-old female who tells you that she has trouble breathing. Her respirations are 20/minute and slightly labored. Her respirations are regular and there appears to be good chest expansion.

• A 3-year-old patient who has had a respiratory infection recently. Her parents called because she is having difficulty breathing. You observe retractions of the muscles between the ribs and above the collarbones as well as nasal flaring. The child seems drowsy. Respirations are 40/minute.

WEB MEDIC

Visit Brady's *Emergency Care* website for direct weblinks. At **www.bradybooks.com/ emergencycare**, you will find information related to the following Chapter 17 topics:

• COPD

• Emphysema

• Chronic bronchitis

• Asthma

• Pneumonia

Chapter
Eighteen

CARDIAC EMERGENCIES

*W*ord on the Street

"My first medical director gave a lecture that was so good I memorized it. Twenty-one years later I can still quote all of it: 'Air is good.' Short and cute, but it drove home the message: the simple things are the most important. Cardiac arrests in the field give us our assessment at its most basic—the ABCs, we don't have to go any further. As my EMS education progressed, they gave me more toys for my jump kit—some neat stuff, and getting neater—but I try to remember what I learned from that lecture. Finish this sentence: Air is _____."

James B. Allen, BS, NREMT-P
Past President, NAEMT
Captain, Clinton (MS) Fire & Rescue

As an EMT-B, you may often encounter a patient who complains of chest discomfort. Sometimes this discomfort will be the result of a cardiac (heart) problem—possibly a heart attack, possibly some other cardiac disorder. You will be able to provide these patients with oxygen, which is the most important drug in the treatment of heart problems. You may also be able to assist patients with taking nitroglycerin. Most patients with chest pain will not be having heart attacks. In fact, they may not have a heart problem at all. Keep in mind that oxygen will not harm patients who are not having heart problems and may be of great benefit to those who are.

Occasionally, you will encounter a patient who is in cardiac arrest—whose normal heartbeat and circulation of blood have completely stopped. CPR can help postpone death for a short time, but defibrillation must be performed as quickly as possible. Defibrillation, which will be covered in the second part of this chapter, is the application of an electrical shock to the chest in order to restart the normal action of the heart. Cardiac arrest is one of the few situations in which you may actually be able to save someone's life by acting quickly and efficiently.

CARDIAC ANATOMY AND PHYSIOLOGY

You learned about the cardiovascular system (made up of the heart and the blood vessels) and circulation of the blood in Chapter 4, "The Human Body." Before continuing through this chapter on cardiac emergencies, you should review that material. In particular, you should review:

- Flow of blood through the chambers of the heart (the atria and ventricles), and the cardiac conductive system (the electrical impulses and specialized muscles that cause the heart to contract)
- Composition of the blood (red and white blood cells, platelets, and plasma)
- Flow of blood through the arteries, veins, arterioles, venules, and capillaries, and the names and positions of major blood vessels
- Circulation of blood between the heart and the lungs and between the heart and the rest of the body
- How heart function and the circulation of blood relate to pulse (review the peripheral and central pulses) and blood pressure (review systolic and diastolic pressure; also review Chapter 9, "Vital Signs and SAMPLE History")
- Shock (hypoperfusion)

You may also wish to review the diagrams of the heart, the cardiovascular system, the cardiac conductive system, and the circulatory system in Chapter 4, and the diagram of the cardiovascular system in the "Anatomy and Physiology Plates" at the end of this book.

CARDIAC COMPROMISE

Cardiac compromise is a blanket term that refers to any kind of problem with the heart. There are many different ways in which patients' hearts show that

TOPIC OVERVIEW

In this chapter, you will learn about the following topics:

● How to identify a patient with chest discomfort/pain

● Treatment for a patient with chest discomfort/pain

● Your role in the administration of prescribed nitroglycerin

● How to use an AED on a patient in cardiac arrest

● How to document findings and care of patients with cardiac emergencies

DOT OBJECTIVES

---

they are in trouble. One reason for this is that there are many different kinds of problems the heart can experience. A coronary artery may become narrowed or blocked, a one-way valve may stop working properly, or the specialized tissue that carries electrical impulses may function abnormally.

Just as there are many different problems the heart can experience, there is a very wide variety of signs and symptoms associated with these problems. Most of these signs and symptoms can also result from problems that have nothing to do with the heart. Many patients with heart trouble will complain of pain in the center of the chest. Others may have only mild chest discomfort or no pain at all. Some may experience difficulty breathing, while still others have only the sudden onset of sweating, nausea, and vomiting.

Since the signs and symptoms of a heart problem can vary so greatly, it is much safer for the EMT-B to treat all patients with certain signs and symptoms as though they are having a heart problem—cardiac compromise—instead of trying to decide whether or not the patient has a heart problem or what kind of heart problem it might be. (Some common cardiovascular disorders will be discussed later in this chapter as background information, but you do not need this information to recognize and treat the symptoms associated with such disorders. Definitive diagnosis and care will be provided at the hospital.)

The best known symptom of a heart problem is chest pain. Typically, a patient describes this pain as crushing, dull, heavy, or squeezing. Sometimes the patient will vehemently deny having pain, but may

How and Why?

Although the heart attack rate of women under age 70 is lower than that of men, the mortality rate for women is actually higher. Go to your Electronic Extras CD for more.

28. Discuss the special considerations for rhythm monitoring. (pp. 351, 362)

29. List the steps in the operation of the automated external defibrillator. (pp. 352, 357–358) (Scan 18-3, pp. 354–356)

30. Discuss the standard of care that should be used to provide care to a patient with persistent ventricular fibrillation and no available ACLS. (pp. 353, 358)

31. Discuss the standard of care that should be used to provide care to a patient with recurrent ventricular fibrillation and no available ACLS. (p. 358)

32. Differentiate between single rescuer and multi-rescuer care with an automated external defibrillator. (p. 359)

33. Explain the reason for pulses not being checked between shocks with an automated external defibrillator. (p. 358)

34. Discuss the importance of coordinating ACLS trained providers with personnel using automated external defibrillators. (p. 358)

35. Discuss the importance of post-resuscitation care. (pp. 358–359)

36. List the components of post-resuscitation care. (pp. 358–359)

37. Explain the importance of frequent practice with the automated external defibrillator. (pp. 365–366)

38. Discuss the need to complete the Automated Defibrillator: Operator's Shift Checklist. (pp. 364–365)

39. Discuss the role of the American Heart Association (AHA) in the use of automated external defibrillation. (pp. 348–349)

40. Explain the role medical direction plays in the use of automated external defibrillation. (p. 366)

41. State the reasons why a case review should be completed following the use of the automated external defibrillator. (pp. 365–366)

42. Discuss the components that should be included in a case review. (pp. 365–366)

43. Discuss the goal of quality improvement in automated external defibrillation. (pp. 365–366)

44. Define the function of all controls on an automated external defibrillator, and describe event documentation and battery defibrillator maintenance. (pp. 361–362)

45. Defend the reasons for obtaining initial training in automated external defibrillation and the importance of continuing education. (p. 366)

46. Defend the reason for maintenance of automated external defibrillators. (pp. 364–365)

✔ Skills

1. Demonstrate the assessment and emergency medical care of a patient experiencing chest pain or discomfort.

2. Perform the steps in facilitating the use of nitroglycerin for chest pain or discomfort.

3. Demonstrate the assessment and documentation of patient response to nitroglycerin.

4. Demonstrate the application and operation of the automated with external defibrillator.

5. Demonstrate the maintenance of an automated external defibrillator.

6. Demonstrate the assessment and documentation of patient response to the automated external defibrillator.

7. Demonstrate the skills necessary to complete the Automated Defibrillator: Operator's Shift Checklist.

8. Practice completing a prehospital care report for patients cardiac emergencies.

---

admit to some pressure. Some patients will describe this sensation as just a discomfort. This is a good example of why you should have a patient describe in his own words how he is feeling. If you ask some of these patients whether they are having chest pain, they will tell you they are not because to them it is not pain. When a patient is having difficulty describing the sensation, try suggesting several choices, as you learned in Chapter 11, "Assessment of the Medical Patient."

The pain, pressure, or discomfort associated with cardiac compromise commonly radiates along the arms, down to the upper abdomen, or up to the jaw. Patients complain of radiation to the left arm more than the right, but either (or both) is possible.

Another frequent complaint (and sometimes the only complaint in a patient with cardiac compromise) is difficulty breathing, called **dyspnea.** If the patient does not complain of difficulty breathing, specifically ask the patient about it. Sometimes the pain is so intense that patients focus their atten-

tion on that and do not mention other important symptoms.

A patient with cardiac compromise is often anxious. In some patients, this takes the form of a feeling of impending doom, which the patient may express to you or others. Occasionally, you will see a patient whose anxiety displays itself through irritability and a short temper.

Other common symptoms in patients with cardiac compromise are nausea and pain or discomfort in the upper abdomen (epigastric pain). Some of these patients also vomit. A less common finding is loss of consciousness. This may result from the heart beating too fast or too slow to adequately supply the brain with oxygenated blood. Usually, the patient regains consciousness quickly.

There are also several signs you will see in some of these patients. These include the sudden onset of sweating and an abnormal pulse or blood pressure. Many patients who have sudden onset of sweating think they are coming down with the flu, but this may result from the denial that is common in these patients. They refuse to acknowledge, at least consciously, that they may be having heart problems. The pulse may be abnormally slow (slower than 60 beats per minute, called **bradycardia**) or abnormally fast (faster than 100 beats per minute, called **tachycardia**) and will frequently be irregular. Some patients complain of palpitations, which are irregular or rapid heartbeats they feel as a fluttering sensation in the chest. A few patients are hypotensive (systolic blood pressure less than 90), while others are hypertensive (systolic greater than 150 or diastolic greater than 90).

Patients with cardiac compromise can have many different presentations. Some complain of pressure or pain in the chest with difficulty breathing and a history of heart problems. Others may have just mild discomfort that they ignore for several hours or that goes away and returns. Between 10% and 20% of patients who are having heart attacks have no chest discomfort at all. Because of these many possibilities and because of the potentially severe complications of heart problems, it is important to have a high index of suspicion and treat patients with any of these signs and symptoms for cardiac compromise. The treatment will not hurt them and may help them.

Management of Cardiac Compromise

The management of a patient with cardiac compromise is detailed below and in Scan 18-1.

Patient ASSESSMENT

Cardiac Compromise

After performing your initial assessment, perform a focused history and physical exam. Get a history of the present illness by asking the OPQRST questions (inquire about onset, provocation, quality, radiation, severity, and time). Also get a SAMPLE history (signs/symptoms, allergies, medications the patient may be taking, pertinent past history, last oral intake, events leading to the present emergency). Then take baseline vital signs.

The following signs and symptoms are often associated with cardiac compromise:

- Pain, pressure, or discomfort in the chest or upper abdomen (epigastrium)
- Difficulty breathing
- Palpitations
- Sudden onset of sweating and nausea or vomiting
- Anxiety (feeling of impending doom, irritability)
- Abnormal pulse
- Abnormal blood pressure

Patient CARE

Cardiac Compromise

Follow these steps for the emergency care of a patient with suspected cardiac compromise:

How **AND** **W**HY?

Many treatments are available for heart-attack patients. Go to your Electronic Extras CD to learn more about the most up-to-date care.

1. Place the patient in a position of comfort, typically sitting up. This is especially true of patients with difficulty breathing. Patients who are hypotensive (systolic blood pressure less than 90) will usually feel better lying down. This position allows more blood to flow to the brain. Occasionally, you will see a patient who has both difficulty breathing and hypotension. It may be very difficult to find a good position in this case. The best way to determine the proper position is to ask the patient what position will relieve his breathing difficulty without making him weak or lightheaded.

2. Apply high-concentration oxygen through a nonrebreather mask if not already done. If the patient has or develops an altered mental status, you will need to open and maintain the patient's airway. If the patient is not breathing adequately, you will also need to ventilate him. Always be prepared for the patient to go into cardiac arrest. (Procedures for cardiac arrest will be discussed later in this chapter.)

3. Transport immediately if the patient has any one of the following:

- No history of cardiac problems
- History of cardiac problems, but does not have nitroglycerin
- Systolic blood pressure of less than 100

4. Give the patient (or help the patient take) nitroglycerin (Scan 18-2) if *all* of the following conditions are met:

- Patient complains of chest pain
- Patient has a history of cardiac problems
- Patient's physician has prescribed nitroglycerin (NTG)
- Patient has the nitroglycerin with him
- Systolic blood pressure is greater than 100 systolic
- Medical direction authorizes administration of the medication

MANAGING CHEST PAIN

FIRST take BSI precautions.

▲ **1.** Perform the initial assessment.

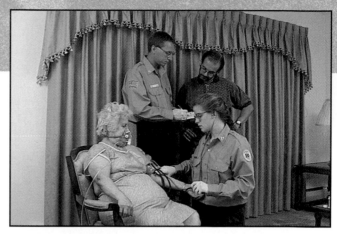

▲ **2.** Provide high-concentration oxygen by nonrebreather mask. Perform the focused history and physical exam for a medical patient. Document findings.

▲ **3.** If the patient meets nitroglycerin criteria and has prescribed nitroglycerin, ask her about the last dose taken. Consult medical direction before assisting the patient with taking medication.

▲ **4.** Check the four rights: right patient, right drug, right dose, right route. Check the expiration date.

(continued)

▲ **5.** Remove the oxygen mask. Ask patient to open her mouth and lift her tongue.

▲ **6.** Place the nitroglycerin tablet under the tongue, or . . .

If the nitroglycerin is in spray form, spray the medication under her tongue according to label directions.

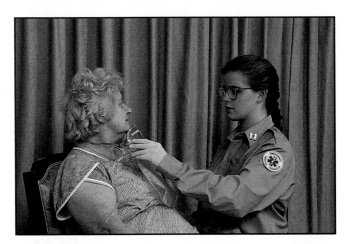

▲ **7.** Have the patient close her mouth and hold the nitroglycerin under her tongue, where the medication will be quickly absorbed.

◄ **8.** Replace the oxygen mask, reassess the patient, and document findings.

NITROGLYCERIN

Medication Name
1. Generic: nitroglycerin
2. Trade: Nitrostat™, Nitrolingual®

Indications
All of the following conditions must be met:

1. Patient complains of chest pain.
2. Patient has a history of cardiac problems.
3. Patient's physician has prescribed nitroglycerin (NTG).
4. Systolic blood pressure is greater than 100 systolic.
5. Medical direction authorizes administration of the medication.

Contraindications
Patient has hypotension, or a systolic blood pressure below 100.

1. Patient has a head injury.
2. Patient is an infant or child.
3. Patient has already taken the maximum prescribed dose.

Medication Form
Tablet, sublingual (under-the-tongue) spray

Dosage
One dose. Repeat in 5 minutes, if no relief, systolic blood pressure remains above 100, and if authorized by medical direction, up to a maximum of three doses.

Administration
1. Perform focused assessment for cardiac patient.
2. Take blood pressure. (Systolic pressure must be above 100.)
3. Contact medical direction, if no standing orders.
4. Assure right medication, right patient, right dose, right route. Check expiration date.

5. Assure patient is alert.
6. Question patient on last dose taken and effects. Assure understanding of route of administration.
7. Ask patient to lift tongue, and place tablet or spray dose under tongue (while wearing gloves) or have patient place tablet or spray under tongue.
8. Have patient keep mouth closed with tablet under tongue (without swallowing) until dissolved and absorbed.
9. Recheck blood pressure within 2 minutes.
10. Record administration, route, and time.
11. Perform reassessment.

Actions
1. Relaxes blood vessels
2. Decreases workload of heart

Side Effects
1. Hypotension (lowers blood pressure)
2. Headache
3. Pulse rate changes

Reassessment Strategies
1. Monitor blood pressure.
2. Ask patient about effect on pain relief.
3. Seek medical direction before readministering.
4. Record assessments.

5. After giving one dose of the nitroglycerin, repeat another dose in 5 minutes if *all* of the following conditions are met:

- Patient experiences no relief
- Systolic blood pressure remains greater than 100 systolic
- Medical direction authorizes another dose of the medication

Administer a maximum of three doses of nitroglycerin, reassessing vital signs and chest pain after each dose. If the blood pressure falls below 100 systolic, treat the patient for shock (hypoperfusion). Transport promptly.

Note

Transportation of a patient with a heart condition must be carried out in a thoughtful, calm, and careful fashion. A rough ride with sudden starts, stops, and turns and siren wailing is likely to increase the patient's fear and apprehension, placing additional stress on the heart. Speed is important; the patient must reach the hospital quickly. However, the judicious use of siren or horn must be balanced against the possibility of worsening the patient's condition.

Documentation Tip— Nitroglycerin Administration

Be sure to document the patient's vital signs, especially blood pressure, before the first dose of nitroglycerin is administered and after each dose. Make sure to find out how many doses of nitroglycerin the patient took before you arrived. Ask the patient about the effect of the medication on the chest pain or discomfort, and record the patient's responses. It is vital information for hospital personnel to know if and how the patient has responded to nitroglycerin, since response or lack of response are important clues to the cause of the patient's difficulty.

Pediatric Notes

Children usually have very healthy hearts, so it is rare for an EMT-B to see a pediatric patient with a cardiac problem. Most such problems are congenital; that is, the child is born with them, so they are discovered before the newborn leaves the nursery. You may see a child who has had cardiac surgery or has learned to live with his problem through changes in lifestyle or medication. In cases like these, parents are frequently very well informed and can be of great assistance.

CARDIOVASCULAR DISORDERS

Cardiac compromise and its associated signs and symptoms can be caused by a number of disorders that affect the condition and function of the blood vessels and the heart. (Keep in mind that, as an EMT-B you do not need to know that your patient's signs and symptoms are caused by a cardiovascular problem, much less be able to diagnose the specific disorder. The information about cardiovascular disorders given here is intended to serve only as general background.)

The majority of cardiovascular emergencies are caused, directly or indirectly, by changes in the inner walls of arteries. These arteries can be part of the systemic (total body), pulmonary (lung), or coronary (heart) circulatory systems. Problems with the heart's electrical and mechanical functions also cause cardiovascular emergencies.

Coronary Artery Disease

The heart is a muscle—a very active muscle. Like all other muscles, it needs oxygen to contract. The blood that is pumped through the chambers of the heart does not provide oxygen to the heart itself. Instead, the heart muscle is supplied with oxygenated blood by special blood vessels: the coronary arteries.

When the coronary arteries are narrowed or blocked, blood flow is reduced, thereby reducing the amount of oxygen delivered to the heart. This might not be noticed when the body is at rest or at a low activity level. However, when the body is subject to stress or exertion, the heart rate (beats per minute) increases. With the increased heart rate comes an increased need for oxygen. Arteries that are narrowed or blocked cannot supply enough blood to meet the demands of the heart.

Two conditions, atherosclerosis and arteriosclerosis, commonly cause the narrowing or blockage of arteries. **Atherosclerosis** is a build-up of fatty deposits on the inner walls of arteries (Figure 18-1). This build-up causes a narrowing of the inner vessel diameter, restricting the flow of blood. Fats and other particles combine to form this deposit, known as *plaque*. As time passes, calcium can be deposited at the site of the plaque, causing the area to harden.

Arteriosclerosis is a stiffening or hardening of the artery wall resulting from

Figure 18-1 Atherosclerosis, the process of plaque formation on the interior wall of an artery.

calcium deposits. Often called "hardening of the arteries," this condition causes the vessel to lose its elasticity, changing blood flow and increasing blood pressure.

In both atherosclerosis and arteriosclerosis, the amount of blood passing through the artery is restricted. The rough surface formed inside the artery can facilitate formation of blood clots, which narrow the artery even more. The clot and debris from the plaque form a **thrombus.** A thrombus can reach a size where it causes an **occlusion** (cutting off) of blood flow, or it may break loose to become an **embolism** and move to occlude the flow of blood somewhere downstream in a smaller artery. In cases of partial or complete blockage, the tissues beyond the point of blockage will be starved of oxygen and may die. If this blockage involves a large area of the heart (as in a heart attack) or the brain (causing one kind of stroke), the results may be quickly fatal.

When such diseases affect the arteries of the heart, they are commonly called **coronary artery disease (CAD).** Coronary artery disease is a serious health problem that results in hundreds of thousands of deaths yearly in the United States.

There are factors that put a person at risk of developing CAD. Some of these risk factors, such as heredity (a close relative who has CAD) and age, cannot be changed. However, there are also many risk factors that can be modified to reduce the risk of coronary artery disease. These include hypertension (high blood pressure), obesity, lack of exercise, elevated blood levels of cholesterol and triglycerides, and cigarette smoking.

Many patients have more than one of these risk factors. Fortunately, the damage caused by the second group of risk factors may be reversed or slowed by changing behavior. Smokers can return to the risk level of a non-smoker soon after quitting. Medication and weight loss can lower high blood pressure. Improved diet and exercise can help the other controllable factors.

In the majority of cardiac-related medical emergencies, it is the reduced blood supply to the myocardium (heart muscle) that causes the emergency. The most common symptom of this reduced blood supply is chest pain. Patients may have symptoms that range anywhere from mild chest pain to cardiac arrest. Angina pectoris (chest pain), acute myocardial infarction (heart attack), and congestive heart failure—all conditions that can be related to CAD—are discussed later in this chapter.

Aneurysm

Another cause of cardiovascular system disorder stems from weakened sections in the arterial walls. Each weak spot that begins to dilate (balloon) is known as an **aneurysm.** This weakening can be related to other arterial diseases, or it can exist independently. When a weakened section of an artery bursts, there can be rapid, life-threatening internal bleeding (Figure 18-2). Tissues beyond the rupture can be damaged because the oxygenated blood they need is escaping and not reaching them. If a major artery ruptures, death from shock can occur very quickly. When an artery in the brain ruptures, a severe form of stroke occurs. The severity is

A   **B**

Figure 18-2   (A) A weakened area in the wall of an artery will tend to balloon out, forming a sac-like aneurysm, which may eventually burst. (B) A ruptured aneurysm.

dependent on the site of the stroke and the amount of blood loss.

Electrical Malfunctions of the Heart

Electrical impulses generated within the heart are responsible for the rhythmic beating of the heart that pumps blood throughout the body. A malfunction of the heart's electrical system will generally result in an **arrhythmia,** an irregular, or absent, heart rhythm. Arrhythmias include bradycardia (abnormally slow, less than 60 beats per minute), tachycardia (abnormally fast, greater than 100 beats per minute), as well as rhythms that may be present when there is no pulse (in cardiac arrest) including ventricular fibrillation, ventricular tachycardia, pulseless electrical activity, and asystole (described later in this chapter).

Mechanical Malfunctions of the Heart

Another complication sometimes seen with a myocardial infarction, or heart attack, is mechanical pump failure. A lack of oxygen has caused the death of a portion of the myocardium. The dead area can no longer pump and contract. If a large enough area of the heart dies, the pumping action of the whole heart will be affected. This can lead to cardiac arrest, shock, pulmonary edema (fluids "backing up" in the lungs), or congestive heart failure (discussed later in this chapter). A few heart attack patients suffer cardiac rupture as the dead tissue area of the heart muscle bursts open. This occurs days after a heart attack.

Deterioration or malfunction of the valves of the heart is also a common component of cardiovascular disorders such as congestive heart failure.

Angina Pectoris

Angina pectoris means, literally, a pain in the chest. Coronary artery disease has narrowed the arteries that supply the heart. During times of exertion or stress, the heart works harder. The portion of the myocardium supplied by the narrowed artery becomes starved for oxygen. When the myocardium is deprived of oxygen, chest pain—angina pectoris—is the most frequent result (Figure 18-3). This pain is sometimes called an angina attack.

Since the pain of angina pectoris comes on after stress or exertion, the pain will frequently diminish when the patient stops the exertion. As the oxygen demand of the heart returns to normal, the pain subsides. Seldom does this painful attack last longer than 3 to 5 minutes.

Another indication that the patient has a history of this condition is if the patient has the medication **nitroglycerin.** Nitroglycerin is a medication that dilates the blood vessels. This results in more blood staying in the veins of the body, so there is less blood coming back to the heart. With less blood to pump out, the heart does not have to work as hard. Nitroglycerin is available in tablets that are placed under the patient's tongue to dissolve, and also in sprays and patches. The patches have adhesive that keeps them on the skin. They gradually release nitroglycerin throughout the day.

Most angina patients are advised by their doctors to take nitroglycerin for their chest pain. Patients are usually told to rest and are allowed to take three nitroglycerin doses over a 10-minute period. If there is no relief of symptoms after that time, they are instructed to call for help.

Acute Myocardial Infarction

The condition in which a portion of the myocardium (heart muscle) dies as a result of oxygen starvation is known as **acute myocardial infarction (AMI)** (Figure 18-4). Often called a heart attack by lay persons, AMI is brought on by the narrowing or occlusion of the coronary artery that supplies the region with blood. Rarely, the interruption of blood flow to the myocardium may be due to the rupturing of a coronary artery (aneurysm).

The American Heart Association reports over a million cases of AMI in the United States each year. Hundreds of thousands of deaths annually are the result of cardiovascular disease. A major portion of these are cases of **sudden death,** a cardiac arrest that occurs within 2 hours of the onset of symptoms. In most cases, sudden death occurs outside of hospitals. The patient may have no prior symptoms of coronary artery disease. Nearly 25% of these individuals have no previous history of cardiac problems.

A variety of factors can cause an AMI. Coronary artery disease is usually the underlying reason for the incident. However, for some patients, factors often regarded as harmless may trigger an AMI. These factors include chronic respiratory problems, unusual exertion, or severe emotional stress.

The treatment of AMI has changed radically over recent years. Previously, patients were admitted to coronary care units where they were observed and, when emergencies occurred, treated with varying degrees of success. Now, some patients receive treatment with medications called **thrombolytics** to dissolve the clot that is blocking the coronary artery. To be most effective, these medications must be administered early. With each hour that passes before they are administered, they become less and less likely to dissolve the clot. Many patients with myocardial infarctions are not candidates for

Figure 18-3   Angina pectoris, or chest pain, results when a coronary artery is blocked, depriving an area of the myocardium of oxygen.

Labels: Coronary arteries · Partial block producing chest pain · Area of decreased blood supply

Figure 18-4 (A) Cross-section of a myocardial infarction, and (B) a heart with normal and infarcted tissue.

this treatment, but those who are must reach the hospital quickly.

Congestive Heart Failure

Congestive heart failure (CHF) is a condition of excessive fluid build-up in the lungs and/or other organs and body parts because of the inadequate pumping of the heart. The fluid build-up causes **edema,** or swelling. The disorder is termed congestive because the fluids congest, or clog, the organs. It is termed heart failure because the congestion both results from and also aggravates failure of the heart to function properly. The congestion may also result from and aggravate failure of the lungs to function properly.

Congestive heart failure may be brought on by diseased heart valves, hypertension, or some form of obstructive pulmonary disease such as emphysema. CHF is often a complication of AMI. Congestive heart failure often progresses as follows:

1. A patient sustains an AMI. Myocardium in the area of the left ventricle dies. (Recall the function of the heart: the left is the side of the heart that receives oxygenated blood from the lungs and

pulmonary circulation and pumps it to the rest of the body.)

2. Because of the damage to the left ventricle, blood backs up into the pulmonary circulation and then the lungs. Fluid accumulation in the lungs is called **pulmonary edema.** This edema causes a poor exchange of oxygen between the lungs and the bloodstream, and the patient experiences shortness of breath, or dyspnea. Listening to this patient's lungs with a stethoscope may reveal crackling or bubbly lung sounds called *rales.* Some patients cough up blood-tinged sputum from their lungs.

3. Left heart failure, if untreated, commonly causes right heart failure. The right side of the heart (which receives blood from the body and pumps it to the lungs) becomes congested because the clogged lungs cannot receive more blood. In turn, fluids may accumulate in the dependent (lower) extremities, the liver, and the abdomen. Accumulation of fluid in the feet or ankles is known as **pedal edema.** The abdomen may become noticeably distended. In a bedridden patient, fluid collects in the sacral area of the spine.

The signs and symptoms of CHF may include:

- Tachycardia (rapid pulse, 100 beats per minute or more)
- Dyspnea (shortness of breath)
- Normal or elevated blood pressure
- Cyanosis
- Diaphoresis (profuse sweating), or cool and clammy skin
- Pulmonary edema, sometimes coughing up of frothy white or pink sputum
- Anxiety or confusion due to hypoxia (inadequate supply of oxygen to the brain and other tissues) caused by poor oxygen/carbon dioxide exchange
- Pedal edema
- Engorged, pulsating neck veins (late sign)
- Enlarged liver and spleen, with abdominal distention (late sign)

The CHF patient may be on medications for this condition. Often patients will tell you that they take a water pill for fluid build-up. This refers to a *diuretic,* a medication that helps remove fluid from the circulatory system. Other medications may increase the strength of the cardiac contraction to counteract the heart failure.

CARDIAC ARREST

In a typical ambulance service, only 1% to 2% of emergency calls are cardiac arrests. Most patients with heart problems do not go into cardiac arrest while they are under your care. Nonetheless, EMS systems exert a great deal of time and energy on attempts to resuscitate these patients. The odds of bringing a cardiac-arrest patient back to life have increased considerably over the last 10 or 15 years. As the problem of cardiac arrest has received more attention, EMS researchers, physicians, administrators, and providers have learned more about what is effective and what is not.

Chain of Survival

The American Heart Association has summarized the most important factors that affect survival of cardiac arrest patients in its chain of survival concept. The chain (Figure 18-5) has four elements: (1) early access, (2) early CPR, (3) early defibrillation, and (4) early advanced care. An EMS system where each of these links is strong is much more likely to bring back a patient from cardiac arrest than a system with weaknesses in the chain. This has been shown in systems that tried to strengthen just one link (early defibrillation) without strengthening the other links.

Early Access

Early access means that the person who sees someone collapse or finds someone unresponsive calls a dispatcher who quickly gets EMS responding to the emergency. Unfortunately, this is easier said than done. The lay public, unlike EMS providers, are not used to recognizing emergencies. It takes longer for them to realize that an emergency exists and that they should call for help right away. Even when a layperson does decide to make the call for help, there may still be obstacles.

Many areas still do not have 9-1-1. This means that emergency services have seven-digit telephone numbers that laypeople cannot be expected to remember. Even though many phone companies list emergency numbers on the inside cover of their directories, this adds an extra step to the process and delays even further the call for help. Many EMS agencies in this position have public information programs that include the distribution of telephone stickers with emergency numbers on them. Since Americans change residence frequently (and buy new telephones more often than that), emergency services must make these stickers available frequently and easily.

Early CPR

Early CPR can increase survival significantly. About the only time it does not help is when defibrillation reaches the patient within approximately 2 minutes. Since this is rarely the case in real life, this means EMS agencies need to address this factor. There are at least three ways in which CPR can be delivered earlier: get CPR-trained professionals to the patient faster, train laypeople in CPR, and train dispatchers to instruct callers in how to perform CPR.

An efficient way to get CPR to patients faster in many areas is to send CPR-trained professionals to the scene. This may mean police, firefighters, secu-

| EARLY | EARLY | EARLY | EARLY |
| ACCESS | CPR | DEFIBRILLATION | ADVANCED CARE |

ᵣe 18-5 The chain of survival (American Heart Association).

rity officers, or lifeguards. Whoever it is needs to receive notification of the possible need for CPR as soon as possible. They also need to be in the right place in order to be able to respond quickly to where they are needed.

Some EMS agencies have CPR courses for the lay public as part of their public information and education programs, but too many do not. It is especially important to train the right laypeople. Teaching CPR to elementary and high school students is good, especially in the long run, but they are not usually present when someone goes into cardiac arrest. The typical cardiac arrest patient is a male in his 60s, so it is not surprising to learn that the typical witness of a cardiac arrest is a woman in her 60s. Middle-aged and older people need CPR courses at least as much as children and adolescents.

A surprisingly effective way to get a layperson to perform CPR is for a dispatcher to instruct the caller over the phone. This has been done in a number of areas and has produced significant increases in the survival rate from cardiac arrest. The quality of CPR done by untrained laypeople instructed by dispatchers is comparable to CPR done by laypeople who were trained in CPR previously. Emergency Medical Dispatchers (EMDs) are trained to give such instructions. Pre-arrival dispatch instructions to guide other dispatchers in this step are available.

Early Defibrillation

Early defibrillation has received a great deal of attention the last few years. This is because it is the single most important factor in determining survival from cardiac arrest.

Although a lot of emphasis has been put on defibrillation, frequently there has not been enough attention paid to early defibrillation. With a few thousand dollars, an agency can purchase an automated defibrillator. The hard part is getting it to the patient in cardiac arrest early enough to be effective. If the response time of the defibrillator (time from call received to arrival of the defibrillator) is longer than 8 minutes, virtually no one survives cardiac arrest. This is true even with early CPR. Although 8 minutes is really the maximum response time for effective defibrillation, the sooner the defibrillator arrives, the more likely it is that a patient will survive cardiac arrest. This is one time when it is literally true that every minute counts.

One way to get around long ambulance response times is to provide defibrillators to other emergency services providers. Some EMS systems have used innovative ways to make sure that a defibrillator arrives in time. In urban and suburban areas, police officers and firefighters have sometimes been equipped with the machines since they may arrive before the ambu-

lance. In rural areas, some EMTs and First Responders carry defibrillators in their personal vehicles so that the patient who needs a defibrillator gets it in time.

Early Advanced Care

Early advanced care is second only to defibrillation in the drama and excitement it stirs in laypeople. Putting a breathing tube into someone's throat (endotracheal intubation), putting a needle into someone's arm (starting an intravenous line), and administering medications into an IV line are all activities that laypeople may not understand, but they are actions that the public has come to expect. They are also apparently responsible for a higher survival rate.

The most common way for patients to get advanced cardiac life support (ACLS) is through EMT-Paramedics who either respond to the scene or rendezvous with a basic life support unit en route to the hospital. In some areas, there are EMTs who have more training than EMT-Bs, but less than EMT-Paramedics. Their level of practice is frequently called EMT-Cardiac, EMT-Critical Care, or EMT-Intermediate. They may be able to perform interventions that can improve survival of these patients. Another method that is not quite as fast is for EMT-Bs to transport patients not to a hospital, but to a clinic or other medical facility that is closer. Any such arrangements need to be made before they are actually needed and should be in writing in the form of protocols. These protocols should be approved by your medical director.

EMS systems that have early access, early CPR, early defibrillation, and early advanced care have survival rates from cardiac arrest that are much higher than systems with one or more weak links in the chain of survival.

Management of Cardiac Arrest

As an EMT-B, you can provide two links in the chain of survival: early CPR and early defibrillation. You studied CPR in your basic life support course, which was required as a prerequisite to your EMT-Basic course. You can review CPR in Basic Cardiac Life Support Review at the end of this book.

The rest of this chapter will emphasize the role of defibrillation in treating cardiac arrest patients. Managing a patient in cardiac arrest means you need to be able to:

- Perform one- and two-rescuer CPR (Ordinarily, you will do two-rescuer CPR when you are on duty, but you must be able to perform one-rescuer CPR while your partner is preparing equipment or while you are en route to a medical facility.)
- Use an automated external defibrillator
- Request advanced life support (when available) to continue the chain of survival

- Use a bag-valve-mask device with oxygen
- Use a flow-restricted, oxygen-powered ventilation device
- Lift and move patients
- Suction a patient's airway
- Use airway adjuncts (oropharyngeal and naso-pharyngeal airways)
- Take BSI precautions to protect yourself (and patients)
- Interview bystanders and family members to obtain facts related to the arrest

Most of the patients you see with chest pain or difficulty breathing will remain alert and in good condition while you are assessing or treating them, but a few will go into cardiac arrest before you arrive at the hospital. For this reason, you must be prepared for cardiac arrest whenever you have a patient with chest discomfort or difficulty breathing. This means bringing the defibrillator to the scene when you are dispatched to one of these calls and having the defibrillator nearby while you are transporting.

Automated External Defibrillator (AED)

Types of AEDs

There are two ways someone can defibrillate. The traditional method (manual defibrillation) is for the operator to look at the patient's heart rhythm on a screen, decide the rhythm is shockable, lubricate and charge two paddles, and deliver a shock to the patient's chest. An automated defibrillator, on the other hand, contains a computer that analyzes the patient's heart rhythm after the operator applies two monitoring-defibrillation pads to the patient's chest (Figure 18-6).

There are two types of automated external defibrillators: semiautomatic and fully automatic. Semiautomatic defibrillators, the more common type, advise the EMT-B to press a button that will cause the machine to deliver a shock through the pads. Semiautomatic defibrillators are sometimes called "shock advisory defibrillators." Fully automated defibrillators do not advise the EMT-B to take any action. They deliver the ~hock automatically once enough en-

ergy has been accumulated. All the EMT-B has to do to use a fully automatic defibrillator is assess the patient, turn on the power, and put the pads on the patient's chest. The information below about how to operate an AED applies principally to a semiautomatic AED.

How AEDs Work

Like all muscles, the heart produces electrical impulses. By putting two monitoring electrodes on the chest, it is possible to "see" the electrical activity of the heart. An AED can analyze this cardiac rhythm and determine whether or not it is a rhythm for which a shock is indicated. The microprocessors and the computer programs used to do this have been tested extensively and have been very accurate, both in the laboratory and in the field.

Figure 18-6   Automated external defibrillators (AEDs).

Today's AEDs are very reliable in distinguishing between rhythms that need shocks and rhythms that do not need shocks.

When AEDs deliver shocks inappropriately, it is almost always the result of human error. This occurs because the operator did not assess the patient properly (AEDs are designed only for use on patients in cardiac arrest), did not use the AED properly, or did not maintain the machine. The chance of mechanical error is always present, but it is small. Maintaining the AED in good operating order; attaching an AED only to unresponsive, pulseless, nonbreathing patients; practicing frequently; and following your local protocols are the best ways to avoid making an error that could affect a patient.

Often, a cardiac event such as a spasm or blockage of a coronary artery (myocardial infarction or heart attack) is associated with a disturbance of the heart's electrical, or conduction, system, which must function normally if the heart is to continue to beat with a regular rhythm. The most common conditions that result in cardiac arrest are *shockable* rhythms:

- Ventricular fibrillation
- Ventricular tachycardia

The primary electrical disturbance resulting in cardiac arrest is **ventricular fibrillation (VF).** Up to 50% of all cardiac arrest victims will be in VF if EMS personnel arrive in the first 8 minutes or so. The heart in VF may have plenty of electrical energy, but it is totally disorganized. Chaotic electrical activity originating from many sites in the heart prevents the heart muscle from contracting normally and pumping blood. If you could see a heart in VF, it would appear to be quivering like a bag of worms. VF is considered a "shockable rhythm;" that is, VF is a rhythm for which defibrillation is effective.

Automated external defibrillators are also designed to shock a rhythm known as **ventricular tachycardia (V-tach),** if it is very fast. In ventricular tachycardia (a very unusual cardiac arrest rhythm observed in less than 10% of all out-of-hospital cases), the heart rhythm is organized, but it is usually quite rapid. The faster the heart rate, the more likely it is that ventricular tachycardia will not allow the heart's chambers to fill with enough blood between beats to produce blood flow sufficient to meet the body's needs, especially that of the brain. Pulseless V-Tach is considered a shockable rhythm.

Some patients with ventricular tachycardia are awake, even with very fast heart rates. If an AED was attached to one of these patients, it would charge up and advise a shock. Since the patient has a pulse and is awake, this would be inappropriate. This is one of the reasons the AED should be attached only to patients in cardiac arrest.

Nonshockable rhythms include:

- Pulseless electrical activity (PEA)
- Asystole

In 15% to 20% of cardiac arrest victims, the rhythm is called **pulseless electrical activity (PEA);** that is, the heart muscle itself fails even though the electrical rhythm remains relatively normal. This condition of relatively normal electrical activity but no pumping action means that the heart muscle is severely and almost always terminally sick. Or it may mean that the patient has lost too much blood. The heart could pump if it had something to pump, but there is no fluid in the system. Defibrillation cannot help these people because their heart's electrical rhythm is already organized and slow (unlike ventricular tachycardia, where the rhythm is organized but very fast). PEA is not considered a shockable rhythm.

In the remaining 20% to 50% of cardiac arrest victims, the heart has ceased generating electrical impulses altogether. This is a condition called **asystole.** When this happens, there is no electrical stimulus to cause the heart muscle to contract, and so it does not. As a result, there is no blood flow, and the patient has no pulse or respirations and is unconscious. (This condition is commonly called "flatline," because the wavy line displayed on an ECG when there is electrical activity goes flat with asystole.) This condition can be the result of untreated ventricular fibrillation, a sick heart, a terminal illness, or severe blood loss. Asystole is not considered a shockable rhythm.

By adding up the numbers, you can see that automated defibrillators will shock at most only about 6 or 7 of every 10 cardiac arrest patients to whom they are attached: those suffering from the disturbed rhythms of ventricular fibrillation and ventricular tachycardia. For patients suffering from pulseless electrical activity (heart muscle failure) or asystole (complete lack of electrical activity), defibrillation will not be effective.

Note

As an EMT-B, you cannot diagnose heart ailments or causes of cardiac arrest. You must initiate CPR and defibrillation as rapidly as possible and, if defibrillation is not successful in restoring heart function, continue CPR to prevent biological death until the patient's care can be taken over at a medical facility or by those with advanced skills.

Coordinating CPR and AED for a Patient in Cardiac Arrest

During your course in cardiopulmonary resuscitation, you learned to interrupt CPR only when necessary and for as short a period as possible. Since you will be using a defibrillator on patients in cardiac arrest, you need to understand some additional circumstances when you should interrupt CPR.

If you are touching the patient when the AED is analyzing the rhythm, there can be interference from the electrical impulses of your heart and from movement of the patient's muscles. This can fool the computer in the AED into believing there is a shockable rhythm when there really isn't one or vice versa. It is also true that if a shock is delivered when you are touching the patient, the shock can be transmitted to you. Although it is not likely to cause you serious harm, you could be injured.

For these reasons, no one should ventilate, do chest compressions, or in any way touch the patient when the rhythm is being analyzed or a shock is being delivered.

Defibrillation is more effective than CPR in restoring a patient's pulse, so stopping CPR to allow for rhythm analysis and defibrillation is actually better for the patient. You may stop CPR for up to 90 seconds in order to give three shocks. You should resume CPR only after you deliver the first three shocks or you get a no-shock-indicated message (Figure 18-7 and Scan 18-3).

⬤ Patient *ASSESSMENT*

Cardiac Arrest

As with all calls, you should protect yourself from infectious diseases by using BSI equipment and taking BSI precautions. This is especially important in the case of a cardiac arrest where blood and other body fluids are commonly found. Patient assessment includes the following:

- Perform the initial assessment. If a bystander is doing CPR when you arrive, have the bystander stop. Verify pulselessness (no carotid pulse) and **apnea** (no breathing). Look for external blood loss.
- After CPR has been resumed, perform a focused history and physical exam. Inquire about onset, trauma, and signs and symptoms that were present before the patient collapsed. Get a SAMPLE history if you can. Do not let history gathering interfere with or slow down defibrillation.

⬤ Patient *CARE*

Cardiac Arrest

Emergency care of a patient in cardiac arrest includes the following:

1. Begin or resume CPR.

2. Determine whether the patient is a candidate for the AED:

- If the patient is an adult (at least 8 years old for the purpose of defibrillation) who has not sustained trauma, proceed with the AED.
- If the patient is less than 8 years old OR the patient has sustained trauma before collapse, do not attach the AED unless you are ordered to do so by medical direction. Continue CPR and transport.

3. Turn on the defibrillator power.

4. Begin the narrative if the AED has a voice recorder. You should describe who you are, what the situation is, and what you are doing as you do it. Do not delay your actions in order to describe them.

5. Attach the monitoring-defibrillation pads to the cables if pads are not pre-attached.

6. Bare the patient's chest (if not already done). Place the pads so that the one attached to the white cable is in the angle between the sternum and the right clavicle and the one attached to the red cable is over the lower left ribs ("white to right, red to ribs"). (This will be the patient's left and right, not your left and right.) Press the pads firmly on the chest to ensure good contact. Once in a while, you may have a male patient whose chest is so hairy that the pads do not make good contact. Use a hospital razor to quickly shave some of the hair away, and use a new pair of pads.

7. Stop CPR and clear the patient (make sure no one is touching the patient).

✋ Note

As stated earlier, about half of all patients in cardiac arrest have nonshockable heart rhythms. If this is the case, when you press the "analyze" button, the AED will give a "No shock" message. In other cases, the AED may give you a "Deliver shock" message and then, after one or more shocks are delivered, will give a "No shock" message on a subsequent try. (When the AED gives a "No shock" message, it may be very bad news—

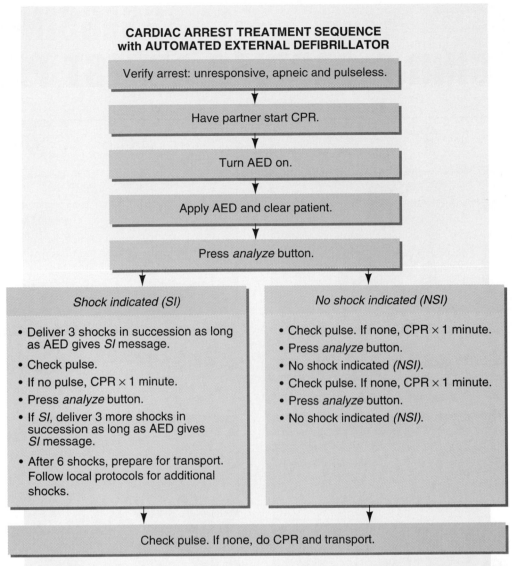

CARDIAC ARREST TREATMENT SEQUENCE with AUTOMATED EXTERNAL DEFIBRILLATOR

Verify arrest: unresponsive, apneic and pulseless.

↓

Have partner start CPR.

↓

Turn AED on.

↓

Apply AED and clear patient.

↓

Press *analyze* button.

Shock indicated (SI)

- Deliver 3 shocks in succession as long as AED gives *SI* message.
- Check pulse.
- If no pulse, CPR × 1 minute.
- Press *analyze* button.
- If *SI*, deliver 3 more shocks in succession as long as AED gives *SI* message.
- After 6 shocks, prepare for transport. Follow local protocols for additional shocks.

No shock indicated (NSI)

- Check pulse. If none, CPR × 1 minute.
- Press *analyze* button.
- No shock indicated (*NSI*).
- Check pulse. If none, CPR × 1 minute.
- Press *analyze* button.
- No shock indicated (*NSI*).

Check pulse. If none, do CPR and transport.

Notes:

Whenever a *no shock indicated (NSI)* message appears, check for a pulse.

If the patient regains a pulse, check breathing. Ventilate with high-concentration oxygen, or give oxygen by nonrebreather mask as needed.

If you initially shock the patient and then receive an *NSI* message before giving six shocks, follow the steps in the above right-hand column.

If you initially receive an *NSI* message and then on a subsequent analysis receive a *shock indicated (SI)* message, follow the steps in the above left-hand column.

Occasionally you may need to shift back and forth between the two columns. If this happens, follow the steps until one of the indications for transport (described below) occurs.

Transport as soon as one of the following occurs:

• You have administered six shocks.

• You have received three consecutive *NSI* messages (separated by one minute of CPR).

• The patient regains a pulse.

If you shock the patient out of cardiac arrest and he arrests again, start the sequence of shocks from the beginning.

Figure 18-7 AED cardiac arrest treatment sequence.

ASSESSING AND MANAGING A CARDIAC ARREST PATIENT

▲ **1.** On arrival, briefly question those present about arrest events. (If a rescuer already on scene is performing CPR, direct him to stop.)

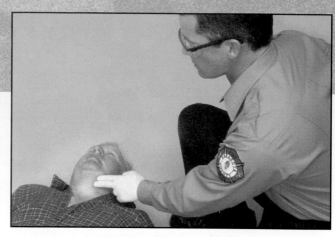

▲ **2.** Verify absence of spontaneous pulse.

▲ **3.** One EMT-B provides CPR; the other sets up AED.

▲ **4.** Turn on the AED power.

NOTE: At earliest opportunity, call for ALS intercept.

◄ **5.** Connect two defibrillator pads to cables, following color code. Remove backing. Place one pad on upper right chest, one on lower left ribs.

▲ **6.** Say "Clear!" Ensure that all individuals are clear of patient.

▲ **7.** After everyone is clear, press the "analyze" button and wait for the AED to analyze the rhythm.

▲ **8.** If advised by the AED, press button to deliver a shock. Repeat analysis and shock delivery until three shocks have been delivered.

▲ **9.** Verify presence or absence of a spontaneous carotid pulse.

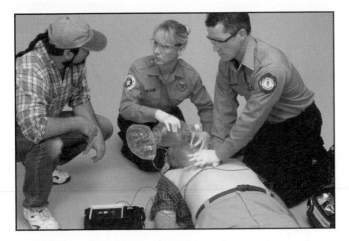

▲ **10.** If pulse is absent, direct resumption of CPR. Gather additional information on arrest events.

▲ **11.** Check patient's pulse during CPR to confirm effectiveness of compressions.

(continued)

▲ **12.** Direct insertion of airway adjunct.

▲ **13.** Direct ventilation of patient with high-concentration oxygen.

▲ **14.** After 1 minute of CPR, have all individuals stand clear and repeat sequence of three analyses and shocks by AED.

▲ **15.** Check patient's carotid pulse.

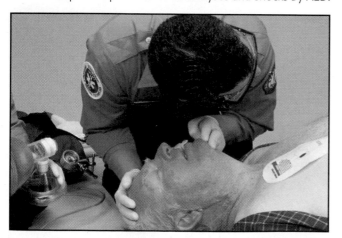

▲ **16.** If there is a spontaneous pulse, check patient's breathing. Note that in many cases, even when a pulse has ___ed, the patient will require ventilatory assistance.

▲ **17.** If breathing is adequate, provide high-concentration oxygen by nonrebreather mask. If breathing is inadequate, ventilate patient with high-concentration oxygen. Transport without delay.

the patient has a nonshockable heart rhythm and cannot be helped by the defibrillator. Or it may be very good news—the electrical rhythm of the patient's heart has responded successfully to earlier shocks. In the latter case, even though the heart's electrical activity has recovered, another stint of CPR may be required to get enough oxygen into the muscle cells of the heart to start it beating again.)

If a "Deliver shock" message is received each time the "analyze" button is pressed, proceed as follows:

8. When you get a "Deliver shock" message:

- Deliver the first shock.
- If necessary, press the "analyze" button to re-analyze the rhythm (get a "Deliver shock" message), and deliver a second shock.
- If necessary, press the "analyze" button to re-analyze the rhythm (get a "Deliver shock" message), and deliver a third shock.

The set of shocks you have just delivered is called a "set of three stacked shocks"—"stacked" because they are delivered with no pause for a pulse check or CPR after the first two shocks.

9. After the first set of three stacked shocks, check the carotid pulse. If the patient has a pulse, check breathing. Then:

- If the patient is breathing adequately, give high-concentration oxygen by nonrebreather mask and transport.
- If the patient is not breathing adequately, provide artificial ventilations with high-concentration oxygen and transport.

10. If the patient does not have a pulse, resume CPR for 1 minute. (Do not waste time checking the pulse again after the 1 minute of CPR. If there is a pulse, the AED will give you a "No shock" message.)

11. Repeat a cycle of three stacked shocks just as you did in step 8. This will complete the second set of three stacked shocks.

12. Assuming there is no on-scene ACLS (such as EMT-Paramedics), you should transport the patient when *any one* of the following occurs:

- Patient regains a pulse (determined during the pulse check before CPR or after the AED gives a "No shock" message).
- Six shocks have been delivered (two sets of three stacked shocks).
- The machine gives three consecutive messages (separated by 1 minute of CPR) that no shock is advised.

If a "No shock" message is received when "analyze" button is pressed, proceed as follows:

13. When the machine advises "No shock," check the patient's pulse.

a. If the patient has a pulse, check breathing.

- If the patient is breathing adequately, give high-concentration oxygen by nonrebreather mask and transport.
- If the patient is not breathing adequately, artificially ventilate with high-concentration oxygen and transport.

b. If the patient has *no* pulse, resume CPR for 1 minute, then:

- Analyze the rhythm a second time. When you get a "No shock" message, check the pulse. If the patient has a pulse, follow the steps described above. If there is no pulse, resume CPR for 1 minute.
- Analyze the rhythm a third time. When you get a "No shock" message again, if there is a pulse, follow step 13a and transport. If there is no pulse, resume CPR and transport. Do not request any further analyses with the AED.

In a few cardiac arrest patients, the heart rhythm may be shockable one minute and not shockable the next. This can lead to potentially confusing messages. *If confusing "Deliver shock" and "No shock" messages are received, proceed as follows:*

14. After any rhythm analysis, if the machine advises "No shock" check the pulse. Then:

a. If the patient has a pulse, check breathing.

- If the patient is breathing adequately, give high-concentration oxygen by nonrebreather mask and transport.
- If the patient is not breathing adequately, artificially ventilate with high-concentration oxygen and transport.

b. If the patient has *no* pulse and you have *not* already delivered six shocks or gotten three consecutive "No shock" messages, resume CPR for 1 minute, then analyze the rhythm again. If the AED gives a "Deliver shock" message, deliver up to two sets of three stacked shocks (a total of six shocks), with 1 minute of CPR separating the two sets. (Do not deliver more than a total of six shocks including those you gave before receiving the "No shock" message.)

Continue analyzing the rhythm, checking for a pulse as appropriate, doing CPR, and delivering shocks as described above until any one of the following occurs:

- The patient regains a pulse.
- Six shocks have been delivered.
- The machine gives three consecutive messages (separated by 1 minute of CPR) that no shock is advised.

Remember

If at any time you get a "No shock" message and determine that the patient has a pulse, check the patient's breathing. If breathing is adequate, provide high-concentration oxygen by nonrebreather mask and transport. If breathing is inadequate, provide artificial ventilations with high-concentration oxygen and transport.

Special Considerations for AED Use

General Principles

- One EMT-B operates the defibrillator, one does CPR. This prevents the EMT-B who is operating the defibrillator from being distracted.
- Defibrillation comes first. Do not hook up oxygen or do anything that delays analysis of the rhythm or defibrillation.
- You must be familiar with the particular model of AED used in your area.
- All contact with the patient must be avoided during analysis of the rhythm.
- State "Clear!" and be sure everyone is clear of the patient before delivering every shock.
- No defibrillator is capable of working without properly functioning batteries. Check the batteries at the beginning of your shift and carry an extra.
- If you have delivered six shocks (a rare occurrence) and you have no ALS back-up, prepare the patient for transport. You may deliver additional shocks at the scene or en route if local medical direction approves.
- An AED cannot analyze a rhythm accurately in a moving emergency vehicle. You must completely stop the vehicle in order to analyze the rhythm if more shocks are ordered.
- It is not safe to defibrillate in a moving ambulance.
- Pulse checks should not occur during rhythm analysis. Typically, there will be no pulse check after shocks 1 and 2 and shocks 4 and 5. Checking a pulse at these times would slow down defibrilla-

tion and is not necessary. If the AED makes a mistake, it is much more likely to fail to give a shock than it is to give an inappropriate shock.

- There is some evidence suggesting that patients may benefit from a brief stint of CPR before defibrillation when response has been delayed for more than 4 minutes. Follow your local protocols.

Coordination with ALS Personnel

You do not need to have an advanced life support (ALS) team at the scene in order to use an AED, but the sooner the patient receives advanced cardiac life support (ACLS), the greater the patient's chance of survival. If you have an ALS team available, notify them of the arrest as soon as possible (preferably before you even arrive on scene). Whether you postpone transport and wait for the ALS team at the scene or start transport and rendezvous with them should be in local protocols approved by your medical director. Your actions may depend on the location of the arrest and the estimated time of arrival of the ALS team.

If the ALS team arrives before you have finished the first cycle of stacked shocks, they should allow you to complete a cycle of three shocks. They should then institute the advanced care that they can give. They may allow you to defibrillate later, but that will be their decision. Since they are the most highly trained providers at the scene, they are responsible for the overall care of the patient.

Coordination with Others Who Defibrillate Before You Arrive

First Responders, police officers, security officers, and others may defibrillate the patient before you arrive. If this happens, you should let the operator of the AED complete a cycle of three stacked shocks before you take over care of the patient. After three shocks are delivered, or a "No shock" message is received, work with the operator to bring about an orderly transfer of care.

In some areas, you may need to take the first AED to the hospital with the patient so that data can be retrieved from the machine. Your protocols should address this. They also should tell you whether or not to switch from the first AED to your own.

Post Resuscitation Care

After you have run through the automated external defibrillation protocol, the patient will be in one of three conditions: (1) The patient has a pulse. In this case, you will need to keep a close eye on his airway and be aggressive in keeping it open. Keep the defibrillator on the patient during transportation in case the patient goes back into arrest. En route, perform a focused assessment based on what the patient tells you is bothering him, and perform an ongoing assessment every 5 minutes. (2) If the patient has no pulse, the AED will have given you a "No shock indicated" message, or (3) the AED may be prompting you to analyze the rhythm because it "thinks" there is a shockable rhythm. In either case, you will need to resume CPR. (You will not perform further defibrillation once you have completed the six shocks of the AED protocol unless the patient has recovered a pulse and then, later, goes back into cardiac arrest.)

For all of these patients, you will need to use the techniques of lifting and moving that you learned in Chapter 5. You will also need to consider how and where to meet ALS personnel (if available).

Patients Who Go Back into Cardiac Arrest

A patient who has been resuscitated from cardiac arrest is at high risk of going back into arrest. This change may be difficult to detect since most patients who have just been resuscitated are unconscious and many of them will need assisted ventilation. Since you are breathing for the patient, you may not notice that he no longer has a pulse. This is why, on unconscious patients who have recovered a pulse, you should check the pulse frequently (approximately every 30 seconds). The AED may alert you that it "thinks" the patient has a shockable rhythm. If you get such a prompt from the defibrillator, check for a pulse immediately. If you find that there is no pulse, then:

1. If you are en route, stop the vehicle.
2. Have someone else start CPR, if the AED is not immediately ready.
3. Analyze the rhythm.
4. Deliver a shock if indicated.
5. Continue with two sets of three stacked shocks separated by 1 minute of CPR or as your local protocol directs.

Witnessed Arrests in the Ambulance

Occasionally, you will be transporting a conscious patient with chest pain who becomes unconscious, pulseless, and apneic (not breathing). Although there are no guarantees, you have a very good chance of getting this patient back because you can defibrillate very shortly after the patient goes into a shockable rhythm. If this happens, stop the vehicle and treat him like any other patient in cardiac arrest.

Single Rescuer with an AED

Some EMT-Bs will be alone or have no one else nearby who can do CPR when they reach the patient. If this happens, the sequence of steps to take changes slightly. Since CPR is a way of supporting the body's organs until defibrillation is available, it makes little sense to start CPR instead of using the AED. In this situation, you should:

1. Perform the initial assessment.
2. Assure pulselessness and apnea. Attempt ventilation, preferably with a pocket face mask. Determine pulselessness but do not start chest compressions. In this way, you can be sure that the patient's arrest is not caused by a foreign body airway obstruction.
3. Turn on the AED and begin the narrative if the machine has a voice recorder.
4. Attach the device in the usual way.
5. Initiate analysis of the rhythm.
6. Deliver up to three shocks as advised by the AED.
7. Call for additional help, start CPR, and follow your protocol. Call for additional EMS help only after you get a "No shock" message, the patient regains a pulse, or you have delivered three shocks.

Contraindications

The only contraindications to using a defibrillator are for patients under 8 years of age and/or less than 55 lbs (25 kg.). Any other patient in cardiac arrest will receive defibrillation.

There are patients for whose condition defibrillation will not be the best or the only remedy. An example is trauma. If a patient has a serious traumatic injury and is in cardiac arrest, this is most likely caused by severe blood loss or damage to one or more vital organs. Even if the patient were defibrillated, success would be highly unlikely. It is also important to note that as an EMT you are to spend as little time as possible at the scene of a serious traumatic injury, since the patient requires immediate transport to a facility where surgery can be performed to correct these injuries. Spending extra time performing repeated defibrillation will increase transport time. You will learn more about this in Chapter 26, Bleeding and Shock.

Another case where defibrillation may not always be effective is hypothermia (very low body temperature). Patients who are severely hypothermic are usually warmed in a controlled setting before defibrillation is performed. Some systems recommend three shocks (one series) in the event of cardiac arrest. If this does not work, the patient should be transported immediately.

Ask your instructor or refer to your local protocols for guidelines for defibrillating patients who have experienced trauma or are severely hypothermic. In addition, national standards established for the use of AEDs are sometimes revised as new technology and information becomes available. Your EMS system will keep you advised of these updates and may alter future protocols for AED use based on the most current information.

Safety Note

When you defibrillate a patient, you are delivering electrical current through a patient's chest. That current can be carried or conducted to you under certain conditions. Although it is unlikely to put you into cardiac arrest, this electricity can harm you. You can prevent this and other potentially harmful effects from occurring by following a few basic principles (Figure 18-8).

Do not defibrillate a soaking wet patient. Water is a very good conductor of electricity, so either dry the patient's chest or move him out of the wet environment (bring him inside, away from the rain, for example).

Do not defibrillate the patient if he is touching anything metallic that other people are touching. Metal is also a very good conductor of electricity. This means that you must be careful if the patient is on a metal floor or deck, and you must make sure no one is touching the stretcher when you deliver a shock. It is a good idea to make sure no one is touching anything, including a bag-valve mask, that is in contact with the patient.

If you see a nitroglycerin patch on the patient's chest, remove it carefully before defibrillating. The plastic in the patch (not the nitroglycerin) may explode from the rapid melting that a defibrillatory shock can cause. This problem has been reported only when the patch is on the chest. Be sure to wear gloves when you remove the patch. It is designed to release nitroglycerin through the skin, and it will not discriminate between the patient's skin and yours. The last thing you need at a cardiac arrest is a headache from nitroglycerin.

Be absolutely sure that before every shock you say "Clear!" and look from the patient's head to his toes to ensure no one is touching the patient or any conductive material that the patient is touching.

Operating a Fully Automatic Defibrillator

A fully automatic defibrillator will assess the patient's rhythm and determine whether a shock is needed. If it senses that a shock is needed, a fully automatic defibrillator will automatically charge to a preset energy level and deliver the shock, all without any further action by the rescuer. Some models of fully automatic defibrillators have only two controls: an "On" button

DO NOT defibrillate if...

...anyone is touching patient. (Be sure everyone is clear.)

...Patient is wearing nitroglycerin patch. (Remove patch.)

...patient is touching metal. (Move away from metal.)

...patient is wet or patient is lying in water. (Dry the patient.)

Figure 18-8　Be alert to safety hazards when using an AED. Do not defibrillate a patient who is wet or in contact with metal. Before defibrillation, remove a nitroglycerin patch that is on the chest. Do not defibrillate until everyone is clear of the patient.

and an "Off" button. Fully automatic defibrillators also make use of voice synthesizers to verbally announce instructions and warnings such as "Stop CPR" and "Stand Back" and "Check breathing and pulse."

Operating a fully automatic defibrillator is very similar to operating a semiautomatic defibrillator. You start with the initial assessment, begin CPR, turn on the machine, and attach it to the patient. The defibrillator will announce "Stop CPR" and begin analyzing the patient's rhythm. If a shock is indicated, the fully automatic defibrillator will repeatedly announce "Stand back," charge to 200 joules of energy, and deliver the shock. Do not touch or move the patient when you hear the warning "Stand back."

Remain clear of the patient. Immediately following delivery of the first shock, the fully automatic defibrillator will again analyze the rhythm. If the patient still has a rhythm for which a shock is indicated, the defibrillator will once again warn "Stand back" and charge to 200–300 joules of energy. The second shock will be delivered as soon as the charging process is complete.

Continue to remain clear of the patient. The process continues automatically until the third shock of 360 joules has been delivered or until the patient has a rhythm for which a shock is not indicated.

IMPLANTS AND SURGERIES

With the rapidly expanding medical technology available, the EMT-B may be presented with patients who have undergone surgeries or had special electronic devices implanted in the body. The ABCs, including CPR and appropriate oxygen delivery, will not change because of prior surgery or conditions. Defibrillation can be performed on such a patient, although the positioning of defibrillation pads on the patient's chest may need to be adjusted to avoid contact with an implanted device.

Some of the devices and surgeries you may observe in the field include the following:

• *Cardiac pacemaker* (Figure 18-9). When the heart's natural pacemaker does not function properly, an artificial pacemaker can be surgically implanted to perform the same function. This pacemaker helps the heart beat in a normal, coordinated fashion. It is often placed below one of the clavicles, is visible as a small lump, and can be palpated. If you notice a lump under a clavicle, do not put a defibrillation pad over it. Try to put the pad at least several inches away while staying in the general area where you want the pad.

Occasionally pacemakers malfunction. Although this situation is rare, it is possible. A malfunctioning pacemaker usually results in a slow or irregular pulse. The patient may have signs of shock due to the fact the heart is not beating properly. Pacemaker failure can be life threatening. Remember that care for patients with implanted pacemakers and signs of a cardiac emergency are the same as for those without a pacemaker. You should arrange for an ALS intercept and transport the patient immediately.

• *Implanted defibrillator.* These implanted devices are not yet as common as pacemakers but may be observed in the field. Cardiologists are sometimes able to identify patients who are at high risk of going into ventricular fibrillation. They sometimes receive a miniature defibrillator surgically implanted in the chest. When the patient develops a lethal cardiac rhythm, the implanted defibrillator detects it and shocks the patient. Since the implanted defibrillator is directly attached to the heart, low energy levels are needed for each shock. The presence of the implanted defibrillator should not pose a threat to the EMT-B. Emergency care, CPR, and defibrillation for this patient are the same as for other cardiac patients.

• *Cardiac bypass surgery.* The coronary artery bypass has become a relatively common procedure in cardiac surgery. A blood vessel from another part of the body is surgically implanted to bypass an occluded coronary artery. This helps restore blood flow to a section of the myocardium. Should a patient with a suspected myocardial infarction tell you that he has had bypass surgery, or if you observe a midline surgical scar on the chest of an unconscious patient, provide the same emergency care, including CPR and defibrillation, as for any other patient.

Figure 18-9 An implanted pacemaker is visible in this patient's right chest.

After three shocks have been delivered or the patient has a rhythm that should not be shocked, the defibrillator will announce "Check breathing and pulse" and then enter an inactive monitoring mode. At this point, check for a spontaneous pulse and breathing.

If a pulse is present, immediately prepare the patient for transportation to a hospital. Leave the defibrillator connected to the patient. Continue life-support measures as necessary, including the administration of oxygen and assisted ventilations.

If there is no pulse, leave the defibrillator connected and resume CPR. After 60 seconds the fully automatic defibrillator will prompt you to "Stop CPR," following which it will again analyze the patient's rhythm. If a shock is indicated, the defibrillator will warn you to "Stand back" and then deliver up to three more shocks.

If a shock is not indicated or after the three additional shocks have been delivered, the fully automatic defibrillator will prompt you to "Check breathing and pulse," following which it will enter a perpetual monitoring mode. If there is no pulse, perform CPR. If the patient has a pulse, continue preparations for transportation.

During the perpetual monitoring mode, the fully automatic defibrillator will continually assess the patient's heart rhythm, although it will not be able to deliver additional shocks without further action on your part, even if a rhythm develops for which a shock is indicated. If this should happen, you will hear a beep followed by the prompt "Check breathing and pulse." Stop immediately if you are performing CPR and carefully check for a spontaneous pulse and regular respirations. If there is no pulse, clear the area, press the "On" button, and repeat the steps outlined above.

Remember

Not all models of fully automatic defibrillators function in exactly the same manner as described here. Consult the user's manual for the defibrillator you will be using for accurate and detailed instructions.

Advantages of Automated External Defibrillation

Only 15 years ago, it was unthinkable for EMT-Bs to defibrillate patients in cardiac arrest. Now, EMT-Bs are expected to be trained and equipped to perform this potentially life-saving intervention. Probably the biggest reason this situation has changed is the improvement in technology that allows defibrillators to determine whether a patient's rhythm is shockable quickly and accurately.

This means that initial training and continuing education are much easier and simpler than that required for manual defibrillation in which the operator has to be able to read and analyze the heart rhythms that the AED does automatically. This is especially true in areas where EMT-Bs see few cardiac arrests, such as in rural areas. Automated defibrillation is actually easier to learn and remember than CPR. This does not mean that EMT-Bs are "well programmed robots." You still must carefully perform an initial assessment to assure that the patient is in cardiac arrest, you must memorize the treatment sequence, and you must always act with the safety of the patient and others in mind.

Another advantage of automated defibrillation is the speed of the procedure. An EMT-B can deliver the first shock within 1 minute of arrival at the patient's side. This is difficult to do with manual defibrillation.

Automation also requires that the operator defibrillate through adhesive pads instead of paddles. This is safer and allows for more accurate and consistent electrode placement. Since the operator does not have to hold paddles on the patient's chest, there is almost no chance of "arcing," the passage of electrical current outside the chest from too little paddle pressure. Certainly, the level of anxiety of the EMT-B is lower when he can push a button to deliver a shock instead of holding charged paddles on a patient's chest.

Some AEDs may allow for monitoring of the rhythm of patients who are not in cardiac arrest. This can be confusing for the EMT-B, since he is not trained in rhythm recognition and cannot treat nonshockable rhythms. A rhythm screen can be very distracting and take attention away from the patient. If you monitor patients with chest pain or difficulty breathing, make sure that this is allowed by your medical director.

Importance of Speed

Recall that a major factor in the survival of a person who is in cardiac arrest is the amount of time that elapses from the moment of collapse until the start of defibrillation. This time period has four phases:

1. EMS access time
2. Dispatch time
3. Ambulance response time
4. Assessment and shock time

For EMS to be effective, each of these time segments must be as short as possible (Table 18-1).

EMS Access Time. This is the time that passes from the time a person collapses in cardiac arrest until someone notifies the EMS system. A person who collapses in front of another person (a witnessed arrest)

Table 18-1   Minimizing the Time from Collapse to Defibrillation

Time Component	Objective	Goal	Method
EMS access time	To minimize the time from collapse until someone places a call for help	1.0 min	An increased community awareness of the need for calling for an ambulance quickly; more public CPR programs
Dispatch time	To minimize the time it takes for an EMS dispatcher to elicit information from a caller and get a defibrillator-equipped unit on the road	0.5 min	Better dispatcher training; improved call-handling procedures
Response time	To minimize the time it takes to get a trained defibrillator team to the patient	3.0 min	Strategic placement of AEDs with first-response personnel
Shock time	To minimize the time it takes to deliver the first shock	1.5 min	Use AEDs; continually practice to maintain peak efficiency

should have a far greater chance of survival than a person who collapses in an isolated place away from other people; the person seeing the collapse can call for an ambulance. Someone seeing a person collapse in cardiac arrest is no guarantee that an ambulance will be called immediately, however. In fact, most witnesses to a collapse delay calling for an ambulance for 2 minutes or more, and many delay calling for 4 to 6 minutes and longer.

Obviously, members of the public should be trained in CPR. But the public should also be trained to call for an ambulance immediately upon seeing someone collapse, even though they know CPR. Any delay in activating the community EMS system results in delayed defibrillation.

Dispatch Time. The second phase of a defibrillation effort begins with receipt of the call for help by a dispatcher and ends with the alert of an ambulance crew. This time segment should be kept as short as possible. The dispatcher rapidly determines whether the call is for a cardiac problem (by asking the caller about difficult breathing, unconsciousness, and the like). Then the dispatcher immediately sends out an EMS unit with a defibrillator. Once this is done, the dispatcher acquires additional information from the caller.

Ambulance Response Time. The third phase of the collapse-to-defibrillation period is the time from dispatch until the ambulance arrives at the location of the stricken person. Ambulance response time varies

considerably from community to community, as well as from one area to another within large communities. Response times are often long in large cities where congested streets are a problem and in small communities where volunteers must respond to the ambulance garage from homes and places of business. The fastest ambulance response times are generally in towns and small cities that are large enough to have an ambulance service staffed around the clock by in-station crews, but small enough so traffic and response distances are not problems.

One way to shorten the time from dispatch to the arrival of a defibrillator in communities that do not have in-station crews is to station and equip a trained EMT in the community with an AED 24 hours a day. Thus, when a call for a potential cardiac problem is received, that trained individual can respond directly to the scene with the defibrillator while other EMTs respond to the station to get the ambulance. This approach works. In one group of small communities, the time it took to get a defibrillator on the road was reduced from 7.5 minutes to 2.5 minutes. Placing with First Responders in large cities has proved equally effective in reducing the response time of a trained individual with a defibrillator.

Assessment and Shock Time. The final phase of a defibrillation period is the time that elapses from the moment a rescuer arrives at the side of the stricken person to the moment the first shock is delivered. As with each of the other phases of the collapse-to-

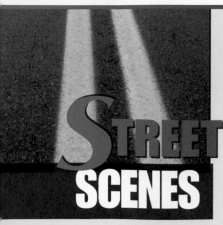

STREET SCENES

Mary Anderson is an active 70-year-old who lives by herself in an apartment. She just returned home from shopping and is sitting down eating lunch, when she feels some chest discomfort that she believes is indigestion. She thinks it will go away, but it doesn't. She stops eating and goes into the living room to sit on the couch, which makes her feel out of breath. She thinks about calling her doctor but doesn't want to be a bother. Unfortunately, the discomfort is now turning into pain and she feels numbness in her left arm. So, she finally calls her doctor and asks what to do. After hearing the symptoms, her doctor calls 9-1-1 to have an ambulance take her to the hospital. Almost 2 hours have passed since Mary started having signs and symptoms.

You are having a late lunch, which you have only half finished, when a tone comes over your radio. "Ambulance 32, respond to a 70-year-old cardiac at the Maple Tree Apartments, #2-D, a third-party call from a physician's office."

When you arrive on scene, your partner says he knows a stair chair will be needed to get the patient from the second floor. He gets the stair chair, and you get the first-in bag.

STREET SCENE QUESTIONS

1. What type of emergency equipment needs to be taken to the side of every potential cardiac patient?

You proceed to the patient's apartment. As you enter, you notice the patient sitting on the couch looking pale and anxious. You ask her why EMS was called. She responds by telling you about her discomfort and her trouble breathing. She also mentions that the pain has become worse. You ask the patient on a scale of 1 to 10 (with 10 being the worst pain she ever had) what the pain was initially and what is it now. She answers, "3 in the beginning, but now it is 8." Your partner comes through the door with the AED and you give him a quick overview. You both agree that the ALS unit needs to be requested. You radio the dispatcher, who gives you an ETA of 5 minutes.

STREET SCENE QUESTIONS

2. What are the treatment priorities for this patient?
3. What assessment information do you need to obtain next?

Your partner gets a set of vital signs, and you place the patient on a nonrebreather at 10 liters per minute. You do a SAMPLE history, with the most significant additional information being high blood pressure, for which she takes medication and has been compliant. Your partner has just finished taking vital signs, when the patient gasps and appears to go unconscious.

STREET SCENE QUESTIONS

4. What should you do next?

The patient is found to be unresponsive and not breathing. As your partner ventilates the patient, you attach the AED and hit the "analyze" button. The AED indicates the need to shock. You and your partner stand clear. The AED discharges. The device tells you to "check pulse." You check the pulse and find it to be slow. You check respirations and continue assisting ventilations. As you start to check the blood pressure, the EMT-Paramedic arrives.

defibrillation period, this time segment must be kept as short as possible if life-saving efforts are to be effective: ideally 1 minute or less.

The shorter the collapse-to-defibrillation time, the greater the chance for survival. A person who can be shocked in 4 to 6 minutes or less after collapse has a good chance of surviving. A person who cannot be shocked within 8 minutes of the moment of collapse has only a slim chance of surviving.

Because the ambulance response time alone approaches 8 minutes in many communities, the importance of implementing creative approaches to shortening the time from collapse to shock cannot be overemphasized. The goals listed in Table 18-1, if achieved, should result in a witnessed VF survival rate of 25% or higher.

Defibrillator Maintenance

Because human error is so common, the U. S. Food and Drug Administration convened a panel of experts to review reports of defibrillator malfunctions. The experts drafted a checklist of actions that the de-

PATIENT NAME: Mary Anderson **PATIENT AGE:** 70

CHIEF COMPLAINT

Chest pain, witnessed cardiac arrest

PAST MEDICAL HISTORY

- [ ] None
- [ ] Allergy to _____
- [x] Hypertension
- [ ] Seizures
- [ ] COPD
- [ ] Other (List)
- [ ] Stroke
- [ ] Diabetes
- [ ] Cardiac
- [ ] Asthma

Current Medications (List)
  Unknown antihypertensive

VITAL SIGNS

TIME	RESP	PULSE	B.P.	MENTAL STATUS	R PUPILS L	SKIN
1215	Rate: 32 / [ ] Regular / [x] Shallow / [ ] Labored	Rate: 120 / [x] Regular / [ ] Irregular	140/84	[x] Alert / [ ] Voice / [ ] Pain / [ ] Unresp.	[✓] Normal [✓] / [ ] Dilated / [ ] Constricted / [ ] Sluggish / [ ] No-Reaction	[ ] Unremarkable / [✓] Cool [✓] Pale / [ ] Warm [ ] Cyanotic / [✓] Moist [ ] Flushed / [ ] Dry [ ] Jaundiced
1222	Rate: 0 / [ ] Regular / [ ] Shallow / [ ] Labored	Rate: 0 / [ ] Regular / [ ] Irregular	0/0	[ ] Alert / [ ] Voice / [ ] Pain / [✓] Unresp.	[✓] Normal [✓] / [ ] Dilated / [ ] Constricted / [ ] Sluggish / [ ] No-Reaction	[ ] Unremarkable / [✓] Cool [✓] Pale / [ ] Warm [ ] Cyanotic / [✓] Moist [ ] Flushed / [ ] Dry [ ] Jaundiced
1240	Rate: 28 / [ ] Regular / [x] Shallow / [ ] Labored	Rate: 110 / [x] Regular / [ ] Irregular	130/80	[ ] Alert / [✓] Voice / [ ] Pain / [ ] Unresp.	[✓] Normal [✓] / [ ] Dilated / [ ] Constricted / [ ] Sluggish / [ ] No-Reaction	[ ] Unremarkable / [ ] Cool [ ] Pale / [✓] Warm [ ] Cyanotic / [ ] Moist [ ] Flushed / [✓] Dry [ ] Jaundiced

NARRATIVE

On arrival, we met a conscious, alert, 70-year-old female who states a sudden onset of indigestion-like chest discomfort, which worsened with rest and began to radiate down her left arm. She appears somewhat anxious. She states the onset occurred after shopping and while eating her lunch. The chest discomfort quickly resulted in shortness of breath and 8 on 10 chest pain. She has been suffering from worsening pain for about 2 hours. We placed the patient on 100% O$_2$ via nonrebreather mask. While assessing the patient, she suddenly became unresponsive and was noted to be pulseless and apneic. AED was applied, and one shock was administered. Pulse returned but respirations were initially absent. Patient ventilated via two-rescuer BVM. Paramedics arrived on scene and provided ALS care. Patient began breathing adequately en route to hospital. O$_2$ was continued at 10 LPM via NRB. She was verbally responsive by arrival at hospital.

The paramedic starts an intravenous line and administers medication. The patient starts to breathe on her own. You prepare for transport and 20 minutes later you arrive in the emergency department with a conscious patient. A few weeks later you hear that Mrs. Anderson has recovered fully and is expected to return to an active life style.

fibrillator operator should complete on each shift (Figure 18-10). One of the most common problems with AEDs has been battery failure. It is especially important that you make sure the battery is charged and that you have a spare with the defibrillator. A defibrillator with a dead battery helps no one.

You should use the checklist at the beginning of every shift in order to be sure that you have all the supplies you will need and that the AED is functioning properly. The time to discover a problem is before you need the defibrillator, not when you are at the scene of a cardiac arrest.

Quality Improvement

There are many ways you can evaluate and improve your ability to resuscitate patients in cardiac arrest. These methods should be part of your service's quality improvement (QI) program. The defibrillation part of your QI program involves a number of things, including medical direction, initial training, maintenance of skills, case review, trend analysis, and strengthening the links in the chain of survival. Every participant in the EMS system has a role to play in QI, whether it is the patient who comes back to thank you, the physician who praises you for a job

Figure 18-10 Make sure the AED battery is charged and that you have a spare battery.

AED, and solid-state memory modules and magnetic tape recordings stored in the machine. The report should evaluate the timeliness of the EMT-B's actions, the accuracy of the machine, and any other factors that affect survival. The EMT-B should receive a copy of the medical director's report or other feedback each time he uses an AED.

Most EMT-Bs will not use an AED very often. It becomes very easy, then, for them to forget what they learned about defibrillation. This is one of the reasons continuing education and skill maintenance are so important. These sessions should occur at least every 90 days and should include review of past cases, descriptions of changes in the program, and demonstration of cardiac-arrest management and defibrillation. The American Heart Association publishes a variety of guidelines and additional information on automated external defibrillation.

An important part of a QI program is looking at patient outcomes. Since cardiac arrests are uncommon events, few services will have enough arrest cases over a reasonable period of time to be able to conclude how well they are doing. Data collection over large regions, or even states, will give a better idea of how well things are going and where improvements need to occur. All of this depends on EMS agencies collecting and submitting the right data to the right place. This means that the information EMT-Bs collect and document has far-reaching consequences.

well done, the nurse who follows up on the patient's in-hospital course, or the EMT-B who uses the defibrillator and then documents the call.

Medical direction is an essential component of any defibrillation program. The medical director needs to be involved with all aspects of the program. This includes equipment selection (such as whether or not to get an AED with a voice recorder), initial training and evaluation, case review, continuing education, and skill maintenance. The EMT-B defibrillates under the medical director's license to practice medicine, so the medical director has a strong motivation to be involved.

An EMT-B who completes AED training in an EMT-Basic course is allowed to defibrillate only under certain conditions. He must meet the requirements of state laws and regulations and the medical director.

One of the best ways to improve your performance is by looking at how you performed when you actually managed an arrest. Every time an EMT-B uses an AED, the medical director or his designated representative must review the case. This can be done through several means, including the written report, voice ECG tape recorders in certain models of

Pediatric Notes

Since children usually have healthy hearts, cardiac arrest in children is rarely the result of heart problems. Instead, it usually is caused by respiratory problems like foreign body airway obstruction or drowning. For this reason, airway management and artificial ventilation are the best way to resuscitate these patients. Children rarely go into shockable rhythms, so automated external defibrillation is not appropriate for cardiac arrest in children under 8 years of age or approximately 55 pounds. It will almost always result in delays to definitive in-hospital care and rarely help the patient.

Documentation Tip—Cardiac Arrests

Cardiac arrests are stressful, strenuous calls, but after you catch your breath, remember to document what you did and the patient's response to it. For example, it is a good idea to write that the patient's chest rose with ventilations and that a carotid pulse was palpable with chest compressions (assuming that was the case).

CHAPTER REVIEW

SUMMARY

Patients with cardiac compromise can have many different presentations. Some complain of pressure or pain in the chest with difficulty breathing and a history of heart problems. Others may have just mild discomfort that they ignore for several hours or that goes away and returns. Between 10% and 20% of patients having heart attacks have no chest discomfort at all. Because of these many possibilities and because of the potentially severe complications of heart problems, it is important to have a high index of suspicion and treat patients with these symptoms for cardiac compromise. The treatment will not hurt them and may help them. These patients need high-concentration oxygen and prompt, safe transportation to definitive care. You may be able to assist patients who have their own nitroglycerin in taking it, thereby relieving pain and anxiety.

Every EMS system should strive to strengthen the links in the chain of survival. It is not enough just to provide AEDs and train people how to use them. Only if there is early access, early CPR, early defibrillation, and early advanced care will EMS systems be able to save as many patients as possible from cardiac arrest. All of these things must be integrated with a quality improvement system that provides superb initial training, strong medical direction, individual case review, and encouragement to provide excellent care.

KEY TERMS

acute myocardial infarction (AMI) (ah-KUTE MY-o-KARD-e-ul in-FARK-shun) the condition in which a portion of the myocardium dies as a result of oxygen starvation; often called a heart attack by lay persons.

aneurysm (AN-u-rizm) the dilation, or ballooning, of a weakened section of the wall of an artery.

angina pectoris (AN-ji-nah [or an-JI-nah] PEK-to-ris) pain in the chest, occurring when blood supply to the heart is reduced and a portion of the heart muscle is not receiving enough oxygen.

apnea (ap-ne-ah) no breathing.

arrhythmia (ah-RITH-me-ah) a disturbance in heart rate and rhythm.

arteriosclerosis (ar-TE-re-o-skle-RO-sis) a condition in which artery walls become hard and stiff due to calcium deposits.

asystole (ay-SIS-to-le) a condition in which the heart has ceased generating electrical impulses.

atherosclerosis (ATH-er-o-skle-RO-sis) a build-up of fatty deposits on the inner walls of arteries.

bradycardia (bray-di-KAR-de-ah) when the heart rate is slow, usually below 60 beats per minute.

cardiac compromise a blanket term for any heart problem.

cardiovascular system the heart and the blood vessels.

congestive heart failure (CHF) the failure of the heart to pump efficiently, leading to excessive blood or fluids in the lungs, the body, or both.

coronary artery disease (CAD) diseases that affect the arteries of the heart.

dyspnea (DISP-ne-ah) shortness of breath; labored or difficult breathing.

edema (eh-DEEM-uh) swelling resulting from a buildup of fluid in the tissues.

embolism (EM-bo-lizm) a thrombus, or clot of blood and plaque, that has broken loose from the wall of an artery.

Nitroglycerin (NTG) a medication that dilates the blood vessels.

occlusion (uh-KLU-zhun) blockage, as of an artery by fatty deposits.

pedal edema accumulation of fluid in the feet or ankles.

pulmonary edema accumulation of fluid in the lungs.

pulseless electrical activity (PEA) a condition in which the heart's electrical rhythm remains relatively normal, yet the mechanical pumping activity fails to follow the electrical activity, causing cardiac arrest.

sudden death a cardiac arrest that occurs within two hours of the onset of symptoms. The patient may have no prior symptoms of coronary artery disease.

tachycardia (tak-e-KAR-de-ah) when the heart rate is fast, above 100 beats per minute.

thrombus (THROM-bus) a clot formed of blood and plaque attached to the inner wall of an artery.

ventricular fibrillation (VF) (ven-TRIK-u-ler fib-ri-LAY-shun) a condition in which the heart's electrical impulses are disorganized, preventing the heart muscle from contracting normally.

ventricular tachycardia (V-Tach) (ven-TRIK-u-ler tak-i-KAR-de-uh) a condition in which the heartbeat is quite rapid; if rapid enough, ventricular tachycardia will not allow the heart's chambers to fill with enough blood between beats to produce blood flow sufficient to meet the body's needs.

REVIEW QUESTIONS

1. What position is best for a patient with (p. 340):
   a. Difficulty breathing and a blood pressure of 110/70?
   b. Chest pain and a blood pressure of 180/90?
2. What is the best way to transfer down a flight of stairs a patient with difficulty breathing, chest pressure, and a blood pressure of 160/100? (Chapter 5)
3. Describe how to "clear" a patient before administering a shock. (p. 352)
4. List three safety measures to keep in mind when using an AED. (p. 360)
5. List the steps in the application of an AED. (pp. 352, 357–358)

APPLICATIONS

• Evaluate the system you work or live in with respect to the chain of survival. Which links are strong and which need work? How successful is your system in resuscitating patients from cardiac arrest?

Visit Brady's *Emergency Care* website for direct weblinks. At **www.bradybooks.com/emergencycare**, you will find information related to the following Chapter 18 topics:

- Early defibrillation
- Cardiac compromise

Some of the material in this chapter on defibrillation and the AED has been adapted from material written by Kenneth R. Stults, M.S., former Director of The University of Iowa Hospitals and Clinics, Emergency Medical Services Learning Resources Center.

Chapter
Nineteen

DIABETIC EMERGENCIES AND ALTERED MENTAL STATUS

When you are called to the scene of a diabetic emergency, your task will not be to diagnose or treat diabetes but rather to recognize and treat a condition that diabetes, or the poor management of diabetes, has caused. The first indication that the patient is diabetic may be an altered mental status. There will often be other clues, such as a medical identification necklace, insulin or other diabetic medication in the refrigerator or purse, or information provided by family members, friends, or coworkers.

To do your job, you do not have to understand all the complications of diabetes, but you must be ready to administer glucose if your assessment turns up a history of diabetes, an altered mental status, and assurance that the patient can swallow. However, the following information about diabetes may provide some perspective.

DIABETES

Glucose, a form of sugar, is the body's basic source of energy. The sugars that a person eats are converted into glucose, which is then absorbed into the bloodstream. However, this blood sugar cannot simply pass from the bloodstream into the body's cells. To enter the cells, **insulin,** a hormone produced by the pancreas, must be present. Without insulin, the cells can be surrounded by glucose but still starve for this sugar. The insulin/glucose relationship has been described as a "lock and key" mechanism. Consider insulin the key. Without the insulin "key," glucose cannot enter the locked cells (Figure 19-1).

When sugar intake and insulin production are balanced, the body can effectively use sugar as an energy source. If, for some reason, insulin production decreases, glucose cannot be used by the cells. This glucose remains in circulation, increasing in concentration as more sugars are digested by the person. The level of blood sugar climbs, eventually to be spilled over into the urine. High sugar leads to increased urine output, which in turn makes the patient abnormally thirsty.

Diabetes mellitus, often called "sugar diabetes" or just "diabetes," is brought about by decreased insulin production or, more commonly in older patients, by the inability of the body's cells to use insulin properly, resulting in high blood sugar. The person suffering from this condition is a diabetic.

Hypoglycemia

The most common medical emergency for the diabetic is a condition called **hypoglycemia,** or low blood sugar. (*Hypo* means "less than normal" or "deficient." *Glyc* means "sugar.") Hypoglycemia is caused when the diabetic does any one of the following:

- Takes too much insulin, (or, less commonly, oral medication used to treat diabetes), thereby putting too much sugar into the cells and leaving too little sugar in the blood
- Reduces sugar intake by not eating
- Overexercises or overexerts himself, thus using sugars faster than normal
- Vomits a meal, emptying the stomach of sugar as well as other food

TOPIC OVERVIEW

In this chapter, you will learn about the following topics:

- Various levels of altered mental status
- Treatment of a patient with altered mental status
- How to identify patients who should receive oral glucose and how to administer glucose
- How to document findings and care of patients with altered mental status

✔ Knowledge and Attitude

1. Identify the patient taking diabetic medications with altered mental status and the implications of a diabetes history. (pp. 373, 376)

2. State the steps in the emergency medical care of the patient taking diabetic medicine with an altered mental status and a history of diabetes. (p. 376) (Scan 19-1, pp. 374–375)

3. Establish the relationship between airway management and the patient with altered mental status. (pp. 372, 376, 379, 380)

4. State the generic and trade names, medication forms, dose, administration, action, and contraindications for oral glucose. (pp. 373, 376) (Scan 19-2, p. 377)

5. Evaluate the need for medical direction in the emergency medical care of the diabetic patient. (p. 376)

6. Explain the rationale for administering oral glucose. (pp. 372, 376)

✔ Skills

1. Demonstrate the steps in the emergency medical care for the patient taking diabetic medicine with an altered mental status and a history of diabetes.

2. Demonstrate the steps in the administration of oral glucose.

3. Demonstrate the assessment and documentation of patient response to oral glucose.

4. Demonstrate how to complete a prehospital care report for patients with diabetic emergencies.

When blood sugar is thus reduced, an altered mental status, possibly unconsciousness, even permanent brain damage can occur quickly if the sugar is not replenished.

Rapid onset, abnormal behavior, and very sweaty skin are all typical of a sudden drop in blood sugar level. Quick administration of glucose, when it can be done without threatening the airway (that is, if the patient is conscious and can swallow), is critical to this patient's outcome. Glucose must be given promptly, before the patient becomes unconscious.

Blood Glucose Meters

One of the many advances in managing diabetes in the last few years has been the development of portable, reliable blood glucose meters (Figure 19-2). People with diabetes now routinely test the level of glucose in their blood at least once a day, sometimes as often as five or six times a day. By determining the amount of glucose in their blood, they can determine

very precisely how much insulin they should take. Keeping blood glucose levels as close to normal as possible leads to significantly fewer diabetes-related complications (heart disease, blindness, and kidney failure, to name a few), so a person with diabetes has a strong motivation to keep his blood glucose level within the normal range.

A patient uses a blood glucose meter by pricking a finger and placing a drop of blood on a test strip. The glucose meter evaluates the change in chemical composition of the material on the strip and displays a number. In the United States, this number usually shows the amount of glucose in milligrams per deciliter (100 ml) of blood, also called *milligrams percent*. Outside of the U.S., the meter may use a different system of measuring glucose to report results.

The EMT-B may encounter a blood glucose meter in one of two ways: the patient owns a glucose meter or the EMS agency carries one on the ambulance. If the patient has a glucose meter, the patient or a family member can use it to determine the pa-

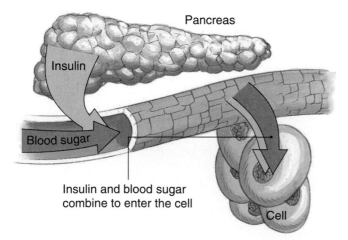

Figure 19-1 Insulin is needed to help the cells take in glucose.

Figure 19-2 Many diabetics use home glucometers to test their blood glucose levels.

tient's blood glucose level. Generally, EMT-Bs should not use a patient's glucose meter. There are many different types of these devices on the market, each with its own instructions for use, which may be very different from device to device. Additionally, there is no way for the EMT-B to know whether the test strips have been stored properly or when the device was last calibrated. These facts are very important, if the reading is to be accurate.

Some EMS agencies carry blood glucose meters and allow EMT-Bs to use them. If this is the case in your area, your service will instruct you in the details of how to use the device. The steps generally include preparing the meter and test strip, cleaning the patient's finger, pricking it with a sterile lancet, placing a drop of blood on the strip, and waiting for the machine to display a reading.

A value less than 80 mg percent in a symptomatic diabetic is typical of hypoglycemia and indicates the need for prompt administration of glucose. A reading over 120 or 140 (depending on the manufacturer's instructions) indicates *hyperglycemia*, a condition which requires treatment in a health-care setting more advanced than an ambulance.

A reading inconsistent with the patient's symptoms (such as 25 mg percent in a patient who is alert and oriented) should make the EMT-B question the result. There are many potential causes of inaccurate results, including insufficient blood on the test strip, a strip past its expiration date or not stored properly, or a meter that needs calibration. Although many people use blood glucose meters appropriately and accurately, it is quite common to get an inaccurate reading, especially when the device is not used properly. It is critical for any health-care provider, who is using a blood glucose meter to test a patient's blood, to have the proper training in use of the device and be thoroughly familiar with its care and maintenance. Calibration and testing on a regularly scheduled basis are essential if the device is to give accurate results.

Most EMS agencies do not let EMT-Bs use blood glucose meters, primarily because it should not change the EMT-B's management of a patient. *Follow your local protocol.* The steps described below will guide you in providing appropriate care to a patient who has diabetes and an altered mental status.

Diabetic Emergencies

Prehospital treatment of the diabetic depends on rapid identification of the patient with an altered mental status and a history of diabetes. (See Scan 19-1.) To assess the patient:

1. Perform an initial assessment. Identify altered mental status.

2. Perform a focused history and physical exam. Gather the history from the patient or bystanders.

- Gather a history of the present episode. Ask about how the episode occurred, time of onset, duration, associated symptoms, any mechanism of injury or other evidence of trauma, whether there have been any interruptions to the episode, seizures, or a fever.

- During the SAMPLE history, determine if the patient has a history of diabetes. Question the patient or bystanders about such a history. Look for a medical identification bracelet, wallet card, or other identification of a diabetic condition. Look in the refrigerator or elsewhere at the scene for medications such as insulin, or a medication with a trade name for insulin (Humulin, Lente), or an oral medication used to treat diabetes (Glucotrol, Micronase) (Figure 19-3). Also ask about the patient's last meal, last medication dose, and any related illnesses.

3. Determine if the patient is alert enough to be able to swallow.

Insulin in refrigerator
Wallet card
Oral medication
Medical ID bracelet or necklace

Figure 19-3 Look for indications that the patient may have a history of diabetes.

MANAGEMENT OF A DIABETIC EMERGENCY

▲ **1.** Perform an initial assessment. Determine if the patient's mental status is altered.

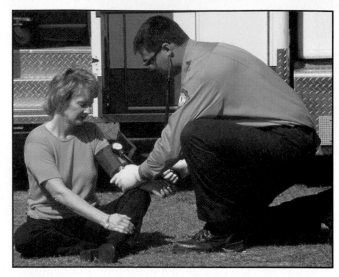

▲ **2.** Perform a focused history and physical exam and take the patient's vital signs. Be sure to find out if she has a history of diabetes. Observe for a medical identification device.

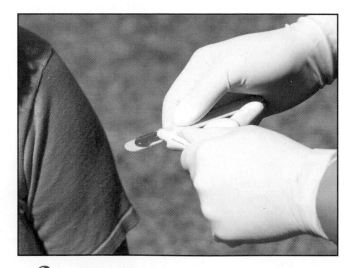

▲ **3.** If the patient has a history of diabetes, has an altered mental status, and is alert enough to swallow, prepare to administer oral glucose by squeezing it onto a tongue depressor.

▲ **4.** Then insert the tongue depressor and oral glucose into the patient's mouth between the cheek and gum. Or, if appropriate, allow the patient to squeeze the oral glucose directly into her own mouth.

▲ **5.** The patient should then remove the tongue depressor from her own mouth. If the patient has lost consciousness, remove it yourself.

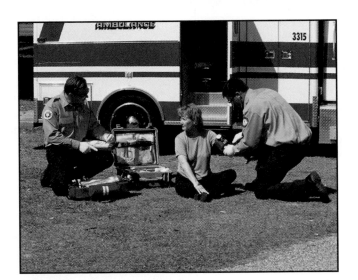

▲ **6.** Reassess the patient. If she does not improve, be prepared to provide basic life support. Consult medical direction to see if you should administer more glucose.

4. Take baseline vital signs. (In some jurisdictions, oral glucose will be administered before the vital signs are taken.)

The following signs and symptoms are associated with a diabetic emergency:

- Rapid onset of altered mental status
  - after missing a meal on a day the patient took prescribed insulin
  - after vomiting a meal on a day the patient took prescribed insulin
  - after an unusual amount of physical exercise or work
  - may occur with no identifiable predisposing factor
- Intoxicated appearance, staggering, slurred speech, to unconsciousness
- Cold, clammy skin
- Elevated heart rate
- Hunger
- Uncharacteristic behavior
- Anxiety
- Combativeness
- Seizures

Patient *CARE*

Diabetic Emergencies

Emergency care of a patient with a diabetic emergency includes the following (see Scans 19-1 and 19-2):

1. Determine if all of the following criteria for administration of oral glucose are present: The patient has a history of diabetes, an altered mental status, and is awake enough to swallow.

2. If the patient meets the criteria for administration of oral glucose, it may be given by applying it to a tongue depressor and placing it in the patient's mouth between cheek and gum. Alternatively, if he is able, let the patient squeeze the glucose from the tube directly into his mouth.

3. Reassess the patient. If the patient's condition does not improve after administration of oral glucose, consult medical direction about whether to administer more. If at any time the patient loses consciousness, remove the tongue depressor from his mouth and take steps to assure an open airway.

If the patient is not awake enough to swallow, treat him like any other patient with an altered mental status. That is, secure the airway, provide artificial ventilations if necessary, and be prepared to perform CPR if needed. Position the patient appropriately. If the patient does not need to be ventilated, place him in the recovery position (on his side) so that he is less likely to choke on or to aspirate fluids or vomitus into his lungs. Request an ALS intercept if available.

Pediatric Notes

Diabetic children are more at risk for medical emergencies than diabetic adults. Children are more active and may exhaust blood sugar levels by playing hard—especially if they have taken their prescribed insulin. Children are also less likely to be disciplined about eating correctly and on time. As a consequence, children are more at risk of hypoglycemia.

Documentation Tips— Diabetic Emergencies

With diabetic emergencies, note the nature of the onset of altered mental status (rapid or gradual) according to the patient, friends, family, or bystanders. But also remember to document the patient's mental status throughout the call. A change in mental status may indicate an alteration in the patient's blood sugar level. Document mental status on the AVPU scale (alert, verbal stimulus, painful stimulus, unresponsive). If alert, check for orientation to person, place, and time. The patient may be responsive but confused.

Administration of glucose may dramatically improve your patient's mental status. Make sure to document the patient's vital signs, as well as mental status, both before and after administration of this or any medication.

OTHER CAUSES OF ALTERED MENTAL STATUS

In addition to diabetic emergencies, there are many causes of altered mental status in which the patient is confused or disoriented. Examples include alcohol use, overdose of other drugs, metabolic abnormalities, head trauma, brain tumor, infectious diseases such as meningitis, and hypoxia. In all cases, gather a careful history, calm the patient, maintain an open airway, provide high-concentration oxygen, and transport to the hospital.

The following sections provide additional information on two other causes of altered mental status: seizure disorders and stroke.

ORAL GLUCOSE

Medication Name
1. Generic: Glucose, oral
2. Trade: Glutose, Insta-glucose

Indications
Patients with altered mental status and a known history of diabetes mellitus

Contraindications
1. Unconsciousness
2. Known diabetic who has not taken insulin for days
3. Unable to swallow

Medication Form
Gel, in toothpaste-type tubes

Dosage: One tube

Administration
1. Assure signs and symptoms of altered mental status with a known history of diabetes.
2. Assure patient is conscious.
3. Administer glucose.
   a. Place on tongue depressor between cheek and gum.
   b. Self-administered between cheek and gum
4. Perform ongoing assessment.

Actions: Increases blood sugar

Side Effects
None when given properly. May be aspirated by the patient without a gag reflex.

Reassessment Strategies
If patient loses consciousness or seizes, remove tongue depressor from mouth.

Additional information on diabetes

Types of Diabetes

There are two major classifications of diabetes mellitus: Type I and Type II. Type I, or insulin-dependent, diabetes occurs in individuals with little or no ability to produce insulin. It has been called "juvenile diabetes," since it tends to begin in childhood. The Type I diabetic must inject doses of supplemental insulin at least once a day.

Type II, or non-insulin-dependent, diabetes occurs in individuals who can produce insulin but in insufficient amounts and/or whose body cells cannot use the insulin properly. This disorder usually develops in adults and has been called "maturity-onset diabetes." Diabetes in adulthood is usually associated with obesity and is seen more often in older than in younger people. Type II diabetes can often be controlled without supplemental insulin through supervised diets and oral medications.

The danger of undetected and untreated diabetes is severe. As the condition develops, the diabetic can become weak and lose weight even with increased sugar and fat intake. Advanced diabetes is often associated with such complications as heart disease, kidney disease, and blindness.

Hyperglycemia

Although hypoglycemia, or low blood sugar (discussed at the beginning of this chapter) is the most common cause of diabetic emergency, another possible problem is overly high blood sugar, or **hyperglycemia.** (*Hyper* means "more than normal" or "excessive." *Glyc* means "sugar.") Like hypoglycemia, hyperglycemia can be life threatening.

Hyperglycemia occurs because the diabetic does not produce enough natural insulin to take sugar out of the blood and into the cells, and because of any one of the following:

• He has not taken enough insulin to make up for this deficiency.

• He has forgotten to take his insulin.

• He has overeaten.

• He has an infection that has upset his insulin/glucose balance.

With hyperglycemia, not only is there too much sugar in the blood, there is too little sugar in the cells. The body attempts to overcome the lack of sugar in the cells by using other foods for energy, particularly stored fats. However, fats are not an efficient alternative to glucose, and the waste products of fat utilization, ketones (compounds that are in the same class as those used to make fingernail polish remover) begin to concentrate in the blood, turning the blood acidic. The person will drink large quantities of water to offset the loss of fluids through excess urination, caused by the body's attempt to get rid of extra sugar. If untreated, the acidity of the blood and the loss of fluids eventually lead to a condition known as diabetic *ketoacidosis*, which can lead to death.

Hypoglycemia and Hyperglycemia Compared

Many students find that they confuse hypoglycemia and hyperglycemia. Fortunately, it is not necessary to distinguish between the two conditions in order to give the proper treatment. There are three typical differences between hypoglycemia and hyperglycemia:

• *Onset.* Hyperglycemia usually has a slower onset, while hypoglycemia tends to come on suddenly. This is because some sugar still reaches the brain in hyperglycemic (high blood sugar) states. With hypoglycemia (low blood sugar), it is possible that no sugar is reaching the brain. Seizures may occur.

• *Skin.* Hyperglycemic patients often have warm, red, dry skin. Hypoglycemic patients have cold, pale, moist, or "clammy" skin.

• *Breath.* The hyperglycemic patient often has acetone breath (like nail polish remover), while the hypoglycemic patient does not.

Also, patients who are hyperglycemic frequently breathe very deeply and rapidly, as though they have just run a race. Dry mouth, intense thirst, abdominal pain, and vomiting are all common signs and symptoms of this condition. The proper treatment is given under close medical supervision in a hospital.

There appear to be clear-cut differences between the signs and symptoms of hyperglycemia and hypoglycemia, but distinguishing between them in the field can be difficult and is not necessary. Giving glucose will help the hypoglycemic patient by getting needed sugar into the bloodstream and to the brain. Although the hyperglycemic patient already has too much sugar in his blood, the extra dose of glucose will not have time to cause damage in the short time before he reaches the hospital and can be diagnosed and treated. This is why "sugar (glucose) for everyone" is the rule of thumb for diabetic emergencies, whether the patient is hypo- or hyperglycemic, and why you do not need to distinguish between the two conditions.

Note: Some hyperglycemic and hypoglycemic patients will appear to be intoxicated. Always suspect a diabetic problem in cases that seem to involve no more than intoxication. Remember that the patient intoxicated on alcohol may also be a diabetic, with the alcohol breath covering the acetone odor of diabetic ketoacidosis. The alcoholic diabetic is a good candidate for a diabetic emergency, because he tends to neglect eating and taking insulin during prolonged drinking and usually has a low blood sugar level.

Seizure Disorders

If the normal functions of the brain are upset by injury, infection, or disease, the electrical activity of the brain can become irregular. This irregularity can bring about a sudden change in sensation, behavior, or movement, called a **seizure** (also called a fit, spell, or attack by nonmedical people). Some seizures involve uncontrolled muscular movements called *convulsions*.

A seizure is not a disease in itself, but rather a sign of some underlying defect, injury, or disease. The most common cause of seizures in adults is failure to take anti-seizure medication. The most common cause of seizures in infants and children 6 months to 3 years of age is high fever (febrile seizures). Other categories of seizures include:

- *Toxic.* Drug or alcohol use, abuse, or withdrawal can cause seizures. (Toxic means "poisonous"—the drug or alcohol has worked as a poison.)
- *Brain tumor.* A brain tumor may occasionally cause seizures.
- *Congenital brain defects.* Seizures due to congenital defects of the brain (defects one is born with) are most often seen in infants and young children.
- *Infection.* Swelling or inflammation of the brain caused by an infection can cause seizures.
- *Metabolic.* Seizures can be caused by irregularities in the patient's body chemistry (metabolism).
- *Trauma.* Head injuries can cause seizures. So can scars formed at the site of previous brain injuries.
- *Idiopathic.* These occur spontaneously, with an unknown cause. This is often the case with seizures that start in childhood.

In addition, convulsive seizures may be seen with:

- Epilepsy
- Stroke
- Measles, mumps, and other childhood diseases
- Hypoglycemia
- Eclampsia (a severe complication of pregnancy)
- Hypoxia (lack of oxygen)
- Heat stroke (resulting from exposure to high temperatures)

Epilepsy is perhaps the best-known of the conditions that result in seizures. Some people are born with epilepsy, while others develop epilepsy after a head injury or surgery. Conscientious use of medications allows most epileptics to live normal lives without seizures of any type. Remember that, while a patient with seizures may be an epileptic, epilepsy is only one condition that causes seizures.

Not all seizures are alike. The type of seizure most people associate with epilepsy and other seizure disorders is the generalized tonic-clonic seizure—a seizure in which the person falls to the floor and has severe convulsions. This is the kind of seizure for which EMS will most likely be called. (Types of seizures are discussed later in the chapter.)

Patient ASSESSMENT

Seizure Disorders

As an EMT-B, it is not your job to diagnose the cause of a seizure. However, it is very important to be able to describe the seizure to emergency department personnel. If you have not observed the seizure (usually EMS is called after the seizure has taken place), always try to find out what the seizure was like by asking the following questions of bystanders. Be sure to record and report your findings.

- What was the person doing before the seizure started?
- Exactly what did the person do during the seizure—movement by movement—especially at the beginning? Was there loss of bladder or bowel control?
- How long did the seizure last?
- What did the person do after the seizure? Was he asleep (and for how long)? Was he awake? Was he able to answer questions? (If you are present during the seizure, use the AVPU scale to assess mental status.)

Patient CARE

Seizure Disorders

Emergency care of a patient with a seizure disorder includes the following:

If you are present when a convulsive seizure occurs
- Place the patient on the floor or ground. If there is no possibility that spine injury has occurred, position the patient on his side for drainage from the mouth.
- Loosen restrictive clothing.
- Remove objects that may harm the patient.
- Protect the patient from injury, but do not try to hold the patient still during convulsions (Figure 19-4).

After convulsions have ended
- Protect the airway. A patient who has just had a generalized seizure will sometimes drool and will usually be very drowsy for a little while, so you may need to suction the airway. If there is no possibility of spine injury, position the patient on his side for drainage from the mouth.
- If the patient is cyanotic (blue), assure an open airway and provide artificial ventilations with supplemental oxygen.

Figure 19-4 Protect the seizure patient from injury.

- Treat any injuries the patient may have sustained during the convulsions, or rule out trauma. Head injury can cause seizures, or the patient may have injured himself during the seizure. Immobilize the neck and spine if trauma is suspected.
- Transport to a medical facility, monitoring vital signs and respirations closely.

Note: Never place anything in the mouth of a seizing patient. Many objects can be broken and obstruct the patient's airway.

The epileptic is often knowledgeable about his condition, medications, and history. Since seizures may be common for the patient, he may refuse

transportation. The patient should be encouraged to accept transportation to a hospital for examination. Should the patient continue to refuse, he should not be left alone after the seizure, and he must not drive. A competent person must remain with the patient.

Warning

Seizures usually last no more than 1 to 3 minutes. When the patient has two or more convulsive seizures without regaining full consciousness and lasting 5 to 10 minutes or more, it is known as **status epilepticus.** Some systems consider all patients who are still seizing when EMS arrives on the scene to be in status epilepticus. This is a high-priority emergency requiring immediate transport to the hospital and possible ALS intercept (having an advanced life support team meet your ambulance en route). The airway must be opened and suctioned and a high concentration of oxygen should be administered at the scene and while en route.

Pediatric Notes

Remember that seizures caused by high fevers and idiopathic seizures (with no known cause) are common in children. Seizures in children who frequently have them are rarely life threatening. However, as an EMT-B, you should treat any seizure in an infant or child as if it is life threatening.

TYPES OF SEIZURES

Just as it is not your job to diagnose the cause of a seizure, it is not your job to identify the type of seizure. Your job as an EMT-B is to gather a history and provide other normal assessment and care as described above. However, some background information about types of seizures can provide perspective.

The generalized tonic-clonic seizure in which the person falls to the floor and has severe convulsions, described earlier, is only one of four common types of seizures in two classifications: partial seizures and generalized seizures.

Partial Seizures

In a simple partial seizure (also called focal motor, focal sensory, or Jacksonian) there is tingling, stiffening, or jerking in just one part of the body. There may also be an aura, which is a sensation such as a smell, bright lights, a burst of colors, or a rising sensation in the stomach. There is no loss of consciousness. However in some cases the jerking may spread and develop into a tonic-clonic seizure.

A complex partial seizure (also called psychomotor or temporal lobe) is often preceded by an aura. This type of seizure is characterized by abnormal behavior that varies widely from person to person. It may involve confusion, a glassy stare, aimless moving about, lip smacking or

chewing, or fidgeting with clothing. The person may appear to be drunk or on drugs. He is not violent but may struggle or fight if restrained. Very rarely, such extreme behavior as screaming, running, disrobing, or showing great fear may occur. There is no loss of consciousness, but there may be confusion and no memory of the episode afterward. In some cases, the seizure may develop into a tonic-clonic seizure.

Generalized Seizures

In a tonic-clonic (also called grand mal) seizure, there is often no aura or other warning. The person may cry out before falling to the floor. This type of seizure is characterized by unconsciousness and major motor activity. The patient will thrash about wildly, using his entire body. The convulsion usually lasts only a few minutes and has three distinct phases:

- *Tonic phase.* The body becomes rigid, stiffening for no more than 30 seconds. Breathing may stop, the patient may bite his tongue (rare), and bowel and bladder control could be lost.
- *Clonic phase.* The body jerks about violently, usually for no more than 1 or 2 minutes (some can last 5 minutes). The patient may foam at the mouth and drool. His face and lips often become cyanotic.

- *Postictal phase.* This begins when convulsions stop. The patient may regain consciousness immediately and enter a state of drowsiness and confusion, or he may remain unconscious for several hours. Headache is common.

An absence seizure (also called petit mal) is brief, usually only 1 to 10 seconds. There is no dramatic motor activity and the person usually does not slump or fall. Instead there is a temporary loss of concentration or awareness. An absence seizure may go unnoticed by everyone except the person and knowledgeable members of his family. A child may suffer

several hundred absence seizures a day, severely interfering with his ability to pay attention and do well in school. Absence seizures often stop before adulthood but sometimes worsen and become tonic-clonic seizures.

Patient care for the generalized tonic-clonic seizure was described earlier. For a simple or complex partial seizure, do not restrain the person; simply remove objects from his path and gently guide him away from danger. For an absence seizure, if you are aware that it has occurred, simply provide the patient with any information he may have missed.

STROKE

One of the many causes of altered mental status may be a **stroke.** Also called a **cerebral vascular accident (CVA),** a stroke refers to the death or injury of brain tissue that is deprived of oxygen. This can be caused by blockage of an artery that supplies blood to part of the brain or bleeding from a ruptured blood vessel in the brain. A stroke caused by a blockage is called an *ischemic stroke.* It can occur when a clot or embolism occludes an artery or as the result of atherosclerosis. This mechanism is responsible for most strokes.

A stroke caused by bleeding into the brain is called a *hemorrhagic stroke.* It frequently is the result of longstanding hypertension. It also can occur because of a weak area of an artery (an aneurysm) that bulges out and eventually ruptures, forcing the brain into a smaller than usual space within the skull.

Different patients experiencing a stroke may have very different signs and symptoms, depending on the size and location of the arteries involved. One of the most common signs is one-sided weakness (hemiparesis). Because the left side of the brain controls movement on the right side of the body (and vice versa), someone with right-sided weakness from

a stroke actually has a problem on the left side of his brain. However, the nerves that control the face muscles do not necessarily cross over in the same way, so sagging or drooping on one side of the face is not a reliable sign of injury to the opposite side.

A less common, but very important, sign of stroke is a headache caused by bleeding from a ruptured vessel. If you find in gathering a history that the patient cried out in pain, clutched his head and collapsed, this is very important information to relay to the hospital staff. This patient may have had a particular kind of bleeding from an artery under the arachnoid layer of the meninges (the meninges are several layers of tissue that surround the brain and spinal cord). This is called a *subarachnoid hemorrhage.* Fortunately, most stroke patients are not hemorrhaging and do not experience headaches.

In many cases, you will find it difficult to communicate with the stroke patient. The damage to the brain sometimes causes a partial or complete loss of the ability to use words. The patient may be able to understand you but will not be able to talk or will have great difficulty with speech. Sometimes, the patient will understand you and know what he wants to say, but he will say the wrong words. This difficulty in using words is known as *expressive aphasia.* Aphasia is a general term that refers to difficulty in communication. Another form of it is *receptive*

aphasia. In this case, the patient can speak clearly, but cannot understand what you are saying, so he will clearly say things that do not make much sense or are inappropriate for the situation.

Patient ASSESSMENT

Stroke

A very good way to evaluate conscious patients for stroke is to evaluate three items that constitute the Cincinnati Stroke Scale (Scan 19-3):

- Ask the patient to grimace or smile. (Demonstrate to the patient what you want him to do, making sure that you show your teeth. This allows you to test control of the facial muscles.) A normal response is for the patient to move both sides of his face equally and to show you his teeth. An abnormal response is unequal movement or no movement at all.
- Ask the patient to close his eyes and extend his arms straight out in front of him for 10 seconds. A normal response is for the patient to move both arms at the same time. An abnormal response is for one arm to drift down or not move at all.
- Ask the patient to say something like "The sky is blue in Cincinnati." An uninjured person's speech is usually clear. A

stroke patient is more likely to show an abnormal response to the test, like slurred speech, the wrong words, or no speech at all.

Other signs and symptoms of stroke include:

- Confusion
- Dizziness
- Numbness, weakness or paralysis (usually on one side of the body)
- Loss of bowel or bladder control
- Impaired vision
- High blood pressure
- Difficult respiration or snoring
- Nausea or vomiting
- Seizures
- Unequal pupils
- Headache
- Loss of vision in one eye
- Unconsciousness (uncommon)

Patient CARE

Stroke

It is not necessary to determine that a stroke has taken place, although you may suspect it. There are many problems that can mimic strokes, including tumor or in-fection in the brain, head injury, and hypo-glycemia. Treat the patient as you would any patient with similar symptoms:

- For a conscious patient who can maintain his airway, calm and reassure him, monitor the airway, and administer high-concentration oxygen. Transport the patient in a semi-sitting position.

- For an unconscious patient, or a patient who cannot maintain his airway, maintain an open airway, provide high-concentration oxygen, and transport with the patient lying on the affected side.

Note: A common occurrence is for an EMT-B to respond to a patient described as being confused, weak on one side, and having difficulty speaking. The EMT-B arrives, only to find an elderly patient who is alert, oriented, and perfectly normal. This patient may have had a *transient ischemic attack* or *TIA,* sometimes called a mini-stroke by laypeople. When this condition occurs, a patient looks as though he is having a stroke because he has the typical signs and symptoms of the condition. However, unlike stroke, a patient with a TIA has complete resolution of his symptoms without treatment within 24 hours (usually much sooner).

With TIA, small clots may be temporarily blocking circulation to part of the brain. When the clot breaks up, the pa-tient's symptoms resolve because the affected brain tissue had only a short period of hypoxia and did not sustain permanent damage. This patient is at significant risk of having a full-blown stroke. If the patient wishes to refuse transport, you have a responsibility to attempt to persuade the patient to be evaluated as soon as possible so that a stroke can be prevented.

Because of recent research into the treatment of stroke, you may have special protocols for management and transport of patients with signs and symptoms of stroke. New treatments are being used and tried in many hospitals, but time is of the essence if any of these treatments is to be effective. There appears to be a very narrow window within which assessment must be completed and treatment must be started. Most stroke patients are not good candidates for some of the newest treatments, but this is a decision that will be made in the hospital, not in the field. Become familiar with these protocols if they are used in your area.

Until recently, in-hospital management of stroke was mostly a matter of watching, waiting, and hoping. With new treatments on the horizon and more attention being paid to traditional treatments like rehabilitation, there is more reason to hope than ever before that a patient with a stroke will recover.

CINCINNATI PREHOSPITAL STROKE SCALE

▲ **1.** Assess for facial droop.

▲ **2.** Assess for arm drift.

▲ **3.** Assess for speech difficulties.

STREET SCENES

While on your day off, you receive a telephone call about working a shift at the county fair. It sounds like fun, so you agree. That Friday night, you and your partner are on stand-by with an ambulance at the first-aid tent. It is 10 p.m. and the evening has been quiet. Just when you think that it will also be uneventful, you receive a call on the radio that security has an intoxicated person they want you to examine on the midway. Upon arrival, you find a male patient in his 20s, sitting and talking in slurred speech to a deputy sheriff. A security guard tells you that the patient was wandering down the midway and talking incoherently. "I'm sure he's drunk," he tells you, "but the rules say you have to take a look before we transport to the security office."

STREET SCENE QUESTIONS

1. Does this patient need a thorough assessment?
2. What is the first concern when starting to assess this patient?
3. What types of underlying medical problems might make a patient appear to be drunk?

As your partner approaches the patient, he is met with what appears to be an angry patient, who says, "That's all I need—another cop." The patient then pushes the deputy sheriff away, and he turns to you. "This guy is just another drunk," your partner says, "and we are out of here." You almost buy into your partner's hasty evaluation, but you notice a bracelet on the patient's wrist. You approach, introduce yourself, and ask the patient if you can check him out. He reluctantly agrees, and as you take a pulse, which is rapid, you see that his bracelet indicates he has diabetes.

STREET SCENE QUESTIONS

4. Does your assessment plan change at this point?
5. How will you get a SAMPLE history if the patient is alone?
6. What is the priority level of this patient? Is there a need to call for ALS assistance?

After initial and focused assessments, you find the patient's airway is open with no mucus or other secretions noted, his breathing is at 24 breaths per minute, and his pulse rate is 110.

Just as you finish taking vital signs, a person approaches who says he is a friend. He confirms that your patient is a diabetic and that he took his insulin before they left for the fair. "He expected to eat here," the friend tells you, "but he was trying to win at the midway games and must have forgotten." You and your partner agree that he could tolerate oral glucose. You explain to your patient what you are doing and apply some to the inside of his cheek. In a few minutes he starts to become more alert, and soon he says he feels fine.

The ALS unit is now on the scene and has checked his sugar level. It is in a normal range. The patient does not want to be transported and, after you talk to medical direction, he is allowed to leave with his friend who promises to take him directly to a diner for something to eat. You call back in service and, as you walk to the ambulance, you remind your partner that you can never assume anything. Every patient needs an assessment.

SAMPLE DOCUMENTATION

| PATIENT NAME: | John Poitier | | | | PATIENT AGE: | 26 | |

CHIEF COMPLAINT

Altered mental status

PAST MEDICAL HISTORY

- [ ] None
- [ ] Allergy to _____
- [ ] Hypertension [ ] Stroke
- [ ] Seizures [x] Diabetes
- [ ] COPD [ ] Cardiac
- [ ] Other (List) [ ] Asthma

Current Medications (List)

Insulin

VITAL SIGNS

TIME	RESP	PULSE	B.P.	MENTAL STATUS	R PUPILS L	SKIN
2005	Rate: 24 [x] Regular [ ] Shallow [ ] Labored	Rate: 110 [x] Regular [ ] Irregular	130/80	[ ] Alert [x] Voice [ ] Pain [ ] Unresp.	[x] Normal [x] [ ] Dilated [ ] [ ] Constricted [ ] [ ] Sluggish [ ] [ ] No-Reaction [ ]	[ ] Unremarkable [ ] Cool [ ] Pale [ ] Warm [ ] Cyanotic [x] Moist [ ] Flushed [ ] Dry [ ] Jaundiced
2012	Rate: 28 [x] Regular [ ] Shallow [ ] Labored	Rate: 120 [x] Regular [ ] Irregular	120/78	[ ] Alert [x] Voice [ ] Pain [ ] Unresp.	[x] Normal [x] [ ] Dilated [ ] [ ] Constricted [ ] [ ] Sluggish [ ] [ ] No-Reaction [ ]	[ ] Unremarkable [ ] Cool [ ] Pale [x] Warm [ ] Cyanotic [x] Moist [ ] Flushed [ ] Dry [ ] Jaundiced
2020	Rate: 24 [x] Regular [ ] Shallow [ ] Labored	Rate: 100 [x] Regular [ ] Irregular	126/84	[x] Alert [ ] Voice [ ] Pain [ ] Unresp.	[x] Normal [x] [ ] Dilated [ ] [ ] Constricted [ ] [ ] Sluggish [ ] [ ] No-Reaction [ ]	[ ] Unremarkable [ ] Cool [ ] Pale [x] Warm [ ] Cyanotic [ ] Moist [ ] Flushed [x] Dry [ ] Jaundiced

NARRATIVE EMS called to the scene of what appears to be an intoxicated male patient. According to a deputy sheriff and a security guard, patient was found wandering down the midway of a fair, talking incoherently. Patient initially presents as agitated and mildly combative but eventually consents to medical evaluation. Patient is noted to be a diabetic via his medical identification bracelet. This is confirmed by a companion on scene. The patient took insulin but did not eat. The patient is verbally responsive, able to follow instructions, and able to protect his airway. We administered oral gulcose on standing order. A tongue blade with the glucose was placed into patient's mouth along cheek. After administration of glucose, patient became fully alert. He refused transportation to hospital. We contacted Dr. Stiglmeier at medical direction, who agreed with the refusal as long as patient agreed to eat and stay with a friend. Patient was advised of the potential dangers in refusal of care and signed a release witnessed by the deputy sheriff. Patient and his companion were advised of signs of diabetic problems and were advised to call again if he had problems.

CHAPTER REVIEW

SUMMARY

Diabetic emergencies are usually caused by poor management of the patient's diabetes. Often this involves a condition brought about by hypoglycemia, or low blood sugar. The chief sign of this condition is altered mental status. Whenever a patient has an altered mental status and a history of diabetes and can swallow, the treatment to be administered by the EMT-B is oral glucose.

Seizures are sometimes experienced by diabetic patients but also have a number of other causes. When a patient experiences a seizure, assess and treat for possible spinal injury, protect the patient's airway, and provide oxygen as needed. Gather information about the seizure to give to hospital personnel.

A stroke, or cerebrovascular accident (CVA), is caused when an artery in the brain is blocked or ruptures. Signs and symptoms commonly include an altered mental status, numbness or paralysis on one side, and difficulty with speech, among others. Assure an open airway and provide high-concentration oxygen. Transport promptly.

KEY TERMS

cerebrovascular (suh-RE-bro VAS-ku-ler) **accident** (CVA) See *stroke*.

diabetes mellitus (di-ah-BEE-tez MEL-i-tus) also called "sugar diabetes" or just "diabetes," the condition brought about by decreased insulin production. The person with this condition is a diabetic.

epilepsy (EP-uh-lep-see) a medical condition that causes seizures. With proper medication, many epileptic patients will no longer have seizures.

glucose (GLU-kos) a form of sugar, the body's basic source of energy.

hyperglycemia (HI-per-gli-SEE-me-ah) high blood sugar.

hypoglycemia (HI-po-gli-SEE-me-ah) low blood sugar.

insulin (IN-suh-lin) a hormone produced by the pancreas or taken as a medication by many diabetics.

seizure (SEE-zher) a sudden change in sensation, behavior, or movement. The most severe form of seizure produces violent muscle contractions called *convulsions*.

status epilepticus (STAY-tus or STAT-us ep-i-LEP-ti-kus) a prolonged seizure or when a person suffers two or more convulsive seizures without regaining full consciousness.

stroke a condition of altered function caused when an artery in the brain is blocked or ruptured, disrupting the supply of oxygenated blood or causing bleeding into the brain. Also called a *cerebrovascular accident (CVA)*.

REVIEW QUESTIONS

1. List the chief signs and symptoms of a patient who is having a diabetic emergency. (pp. 373, 376)
2. Explain how you can determine a medical history of diabetes. (p. 373)
3. Explain what treatment may be given by an EMT-B for a diabetic emergency and the criteria for giving it. (p. 376)
4. Tell whether treatment for a diabetic emergency should be given before or after baseline vital signs are taken. (Answer according to your local protocol.)
5. Explain the care an EMT-B will ordinarily give for a patient who has had a seizure. (pp. 379–380)
6. Explain the care that should be given to a conscious and to an unconscious patient with suspected stroke. (p. 382)

APPLICATIONS

• You are dispatched to a "man behaving oddly" at a train station. When you arrive, you find that the man is unconscious. "He's drunk," a bystander tells you. "He was staggering and slurring his words." As you assess the patient, you find a medical identification bracelet that tells you he is a diabetic. Do you administer oral glucose? How do you proceed?

WEB MEDIC

Visit Brady's *Emergency Care* website for direct weblinks. At **www.bradybooks.com/emergencycare**, you will find information related to the following Chapter 19 topics:

• Diabetes and insulin

• Stroke

• Seizures and epilepsy

Chapter
Twenty

ALLERGIC REACTIONS

Allergic reactions can be mild or extremely severe. A mild allergic reaction can develop into a severe reaction rapidly. A severe allergic reaction can quickly become life threatening. For these reasons, prompt recognition and appropriate assessment and treatment of allergic reactions can be critical.

ALLERGIC REACTIONS

HOW AND WHY?

Some substances cause allergic reactions in large groups of the population, while others affect only a small number of people. Go to your Electronic Extras CD to learn more about the process of allergic reactions.

A natural response of the human body's immune system is to react to any foreign substance—to defend the body by neutralizing or getting rid of the foreign material. Sometimes the immune response is exaggerated, and this exaggerated reaction is called an **allergic reaction.** Almost any of a wide variety of substances can be an **allergen,** something that causes an allergic reaction. For example, cat dander can be an allergen. A person who is allergic to cat dander will itch and sneeze whenever a cat is nearby. The reaction is unpleasant but harmless.

In some people, however, contact with certain foreign substances triggers an immune response that gets out of hand. Consider bee stings. Most people have no reaction to a bee sting other than pain and some swelling at the sting site. A few people have very severe, life-threatening reactions to bee stings. This kind of severe allergic reaction is called **anaphylaxis,** or *anaphylactic shock.* In anaphylaxis, exposure to the allergen will cause blood vessels to dilate rapidly and cause a drop in blood pressure (hypotension). Many tissues may swell, including those that line the respiratory system. This swelling can obstruct the airway, leading to respiratory failure.

Something that all allergic reactions share is that people do not have them the first time they are exposed to an allergen. This is because the body's immune system has not "learned" to recognize the allergen yet. The first time someone is exposed to an allergen, the immune system forms antibodies in response. These antibodies are an attempt by the body to "attack" the foreign substances. A particular antibody will combine with only the allergen it was formed in response to (or another allergen very similar to the original one). The second time the person is exposed to the allergen, the antibodies already exist in the person's body. This time, the allergen combines with the antibody and results in dilation of the blood vessels, swelling, and difficulty breathing.

Causes of allergic reactions (in some individuals) include (Figure 20-1):

- *Insects.* The stings of bees, yellow jackets, wasps, and hornets can cause rapid and severe reactions.
- *Foods.* Foods such as nuts, eggs, milk, and shellfish can cause reactions. In most cases, the effect is slower than that seen with insect stings. An exception is peanuts. Peanut allergies are frequently very severe and very rapid in onset. Many people with allergies to one food will have allergies to

TOPIC OVERVIEW

In this chapter, you will learn about the following topics:

- How to identify a patient experiencing an allergic reaction

- Differences between a mild allergic reaction and anaphylaxis

- How to treat a patient experiencing an allergic reaction

- Who should be assisted with an epinephrine auto-injector

- How to document findings and care of patients with allergic reactions

1. Recognize the patient experiencing an allergic reaction. (p. 392)

2. Describe the emergency medical care of the patient with an allergic reaction. (p. 393) (Scan 20-1, pp. 394–395)

3. Establish the relationship between the patient with an allergic reaction and airway management. (pp. 389, 391–392)

4. Describe the mechanisms of allergic response and the implications for airway management. (pp. 389–390, 391–392)

5. State the generic and trade names, medication forms, dose, administration, action, and contraindications for the epinephrine auto-injector. (p. 393) (Scan 20-2, p. 396)

6. Evaluate the need for medical direction in the emergency medical care of the patient with an allergic reaction. (p. 393)

7. Differentiate between the general category of those patients having an allergic reaction and those patients having an allergic reaction and requiring immediate medical care, including immediate use of epinephrine auto-injector. (pp. 389, 393)

8. Explain the rationale for administering epinephrine using an auto-injector. (p. 393)

✔ Skills

1. Demonstrate the emergency medical care of the patient experiencing an allergic reaction.

2. Demonstrate the use of epinephrine auto-injector.

3. Demonstrate the assessment and documentation of patient response to an epinephrine injection.

4. Demonstrate proper disposal of equipment.

5. Demonstrate completing a prehospital care report for patients with allergic emergencies.

related foods (for example, someone who is allergic to almonds is more likely to be allergic to walnuts). Again, peanuts are an exception. People who are allergic to peanuts do not necessarily have any other allergies, including nuts (in part because peanuts are legumes, not nuts).

- *Plants.* Contact with certain plants such as poison ivy, poison sumac, and poison oak can cause a rash that is sometimes severe. (See Figure 20-2.) The rash associated with poison ivy is actually an allergic reaction. Approximately two-thirds of the population is allergic to the oil on poison ivy leaves. Plant pollen also causes allergic reactions in many people, but rarely anaphylaxis.

- *Medications.* Antitoxins and drugs, especially antibiotics such as penicillin, may cause severe reactions. Just as with foods, people who are allergic to one kind of antibiotic can be allergic to related antibiotics. In the course of evaluating patients, you will hear many of them say they are allergic to penicillin or other antibiotics.

- *Others.* Dust, chemicals, soaps, make-up, and a variety of other substances can cause allergic reactions, occasionally severe, in some people.

One particular product EMT-Bs should be aware of as a possible allergen is latex. Only in the last few years have health-care providers recognized allergic reactions to latex for what they are. Two groups of people are especially likely to be allergic to latex. One of these groups is patients with conditions that require multiple surgeries. The repeated exposure to the latex in doctors' and nurses' gloves is probably the reason many such patients develop a severe allergy to latex. This is very important to understand,

Insect stings

Plants

Food

Medications

Figure 20-1 Substances that may cause allergic reactions.

Figure 20-2   (A) Poison ivy, (B) poison sumac, and (C) poison oak.

because if you wear latex gloves when treating a patient with a latex allergy, you may actually cause an allergic or anaphylactic reaction in the patient.

The other group that is becoming more sensitive to latex is health-care professionals, including EMT-Bs. Again, this is probably because of more frequent exposure to latex as a result of practicing BSI precautions. Fortunately, there are ways to avoid latex. Manufacturers of medical equipment are generally happy to provide information about which of their products contain latex and to suggest vinyl or other latex-free substitutes.

Safety Note

If you notice that your hands seem to be red and itchy after a call, you may be developing an allergy to latex. If you are allergic to latex, it is very important that you protect yourself from further exposure to this allergen. If you do not, the signs will get worse as you continue to wear latex gloves. Some people become extremely sensitive to latex, so it is important that you tell this to any health-care provider who is caring for you as a patient. Also discuss this with your own physician so that you become as informed as possible about this topic and learn how to protect yourself.

There is no way to predict the exact course of allergic reaction. Severe reactions most often take place immediately, but they are occasionally delayed 30 minutes or more. A mild allergic reaction may turn into more serious anaphylactic shock in a matter of minutes. When you have a patient with an exposure to a known allergen but who is displaying only minor signs and symptoms, you must closely monitor the patient for signs of the condition becoming more serious. This

HOW AND WHY?

Itching can be very unpleasant. Some say it can be more unpleasant than pain. Individuals with extreme itching will continue to scratch even when pain is the result. Go to your Electronic Extras CD for more information.

patient's airway may swell and close off in just a few minutes. Be prepared to manage the airway and to administer epinephrine if so advised by medical direction.

The signs and symptoms of allergic reaction or anaphylactic shock can include:

Skin
- Itching
- **Hives** (red, itchy, possibly raised blotches on the skin—Figure 20-3), especially around an insect sting
- Flushing (red skin)
- Swelling of face (especially the eyes and lips), neck, hands, feet, or tongue
- Warm, tingling feeling in the face, mouth, chest, feet, and hands

Respiratory
- Patient may report a feeling of tightness in his throat or chest
- Cough
- Rapid breathing
- Labored, noisy breathing
- Hoarseness, muffled voice, or loss of voice entirely
- Stridor (harsh, high-pitched sound during inspiration)
- Wheezing (audible without a stethoscope)

Cardiac
- Increased heart rate
- Decreased blood pressure

Generalized findings
- Itchy, watery eyes
- Headache
- Runny nose
- Patient expresses a sense of impending doom

Figure 20-3 Hives are red, itchy blotches, sometimes raised, that often accompany an allergic reaction.

Signs and symptoms of shock
- Altered mental status
- Flushed, dry skin or pale, cool, clammy skin
- Nausea or vomiting
- Changes in vital signs: increased pulse, increased respirations, decreased blood pressure

Distinguishing Anaphylaxis from Mild Allergic Reaction

Any of the signs and symptoms discussed above can be associated with an allergic reaction. To be considered a severe allergic reaction, or anaphylaxis, the patient must have either respiratory distress or signs and symptoms of shock.

● Patient ASSESSMENT

Allergic Reaction or Anaphylaxis

Conduct the usual assessment sequence, as follows:

1. Perform the initial assessment and care for any immediately life-threatening problems with the airway, breathing, or circulation.

2. Perform a focused history and physical exam. Inquire about

- History of allergies
- What patient was exposed to
- How patient was exposed (contact, ingestion, etc.)
- What signs and symptoms the patient is having
- Progression (What happened first, next? How rapidly?)
- Interventions (Has any care been provided? Has the patient taken any medication?)

3. Assess baseline vital signs and get the remainder of the SAMPLE history.

Suspect an allergic reaction whenever the patient has come in contact with a substance that has caused an allergic reaction in the past, and whenever the patient complains of itching, hives, or difficulty breathing (respiratory distress), or shows signs or symptoms of shock (hypoperfusion).

Remember

When the above signs and symptoms of allergic reaction include either respiratory distress or signs and symptoms of shock (hypoperfusion), assume that it is a severe allergic reaction (anaphylaxis).

Allergic Reaction or Anaphylaxis

1. *Manage the patient's airway and breathing.* Apply high-concentration oxygen through a nonrebreather mask, if you have not already done so during the initial assessment. If the patient has or develops an altered mental status, open and maintain the patient's airway. If the patient is not breathing adequately, provide artificial ventilations.

2. You may be able to assist the patient in administering an epinephrine auto-injector. To find out if it is appropriate, consider each of the following:

- IF the patient has come in contact with a substance that caused an allergic reaction in the past, AND IF the patient has respiratory distress or exhibits signs and symptoms of shock, AND IF the patient has a prescribed epinephrine auto-injector, then *contact medical direction and, if so ordered, assist the patient with the auto-injector* (Scan 20-1). Record the administration of the epinephrine auto-injector. Transport. Reassess 2 minutes after epinephrine administration and record reassessment findings.

- IF the patient has come in contact with a substance that caused an allergic reaction in the past, AND IF the patient complains of respiratory distress or exhibits signs and symptoms of shock, AND IF the patient does not have a prescribed epinephrine auto-injector available or has never had one prescribed, then *care for shock and transport immediately.*

- IF assessment findings show that the patient has come in contact with a substance that caused an allergic reaction in the past, BUT the patient is NOT wheezing or showing signs of respiratory distress or shock (hypoperfusion), then continue with the focused assessment. Consult medical direction and, only if the patient has an epinephrine auto-injector and if medical direction so orders, administer epinephrine. If the patient does not have an epinephrine auto-injector, consider requesting an ALS intercept. Paramedics carry and can administer epinephrine.

You probably will not see many patients with allergic reactions, but most of them will be able to give you a history of allergies. Once in a while, you will see a patient who has no history and is having his first allergic reaction. In this case, the patient will not be carrying an epinephrine auto-injector because his physician has not prescribed one. Treat the patient for shock and transport immediately.

Remember

A patient with an allergic reaction may have a compromised airway or respiratory function, or these conditions may develop as the allergic reaction progresses. Carefully monitor the patient's airway and breathing throughout care and transport.

In your ongoing assessment, you will frequently find that the patient's condition improves, but sometimes it will deteriorate. You may need to give additional doses of epinephrine in this case. You will be able to do this only if the patient has one or more extra auto-injectors AND you have remembered to ask the patient to bring them in the ambulance. Auto-injectors on the market today can give only one dose of epinephrine. If a patient has an extra epinephrine auto-injector, bring it along.

SELF-ADMINISTERED EPINEPHRINE

For years, physicians have prescribed **epinephrine** in the form of bee sting kits, AnaKits®, or EpiPens® for patients who are susceptible to severe allergic reactions. Epinephrine is a hormone produced by the body. When administered as a medication, it will constrict blood vessels (helping to raise the blood pressure and improve perfusion) and will dilate the bronchioles (helping to open the airway and improve respiration).

Many people who are subject to severe allergic reactions are prescribed an epinephrine auto-injector by their physician to carry with them and use when such a reaction occurs. The reason it is important for such a patient to carry an epinephrine auto-injector is that an allergic reaction can become life threatening so quickly that there is not enough time to transport the patient to a hospital to receive the medication. An auto-injector is a spring-loaded needle and syringe with a single dose of epinephrine that will automatically release and inject the medication.

When authorized by medical direction, you may administer or help the patient administer a dose of epinephrine from an auto-injector that has been prescribed for the patient by a physician. After you make sure that the auto-injector is prescribed for the patient and that the liquid is clear (if you can see it), remove the cap and press the injector firmly against the patient's thigh. Hold it there until the entire dose is injected. (Injection on the outside of the thigh midway between waist and knee is recommended.) On reassessment 2 minutes after the epinephrine is administered, in addition to some relief of symptoms, expect the patient's pulse to have increased.

The procedure for administering an epinephrine auto-injector is shown in Scan 20-1. Information about epinephrine auto-injectors is summarized in Scan 20-2.

ASSESSING AND MANAGING AN ALLERGIC REACTION

FIRST take BSI precautions.

▲ Patient suffers severe allergic reaction.

▲ **1.** Perform an initial assessment. Provide high-concentration oxygen by nonrebreather mask.

▲ **2.** Perform a focused history and physical exam. Obtain a SAMPLE history.

▲ **3.** Take the patient's vital signs.

▲ **4.** Find out if the patient has a prescribed epinephrine auto-injector and if it is prescribed for this patient. Then check expiration date and for cloudiness or discoloration if liquid is visible. Contact medical direction.

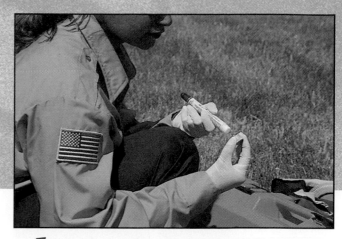

▲ **5.** If medical direction orders use of the epinephrine auto-injector, prepare it for use by removing the safety cap.

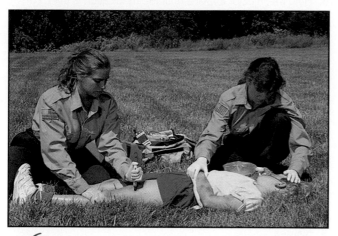

▲ **6.** Then press the injector against the patient's thigh to trigger release of the spring-loaded needle and inject the dose of epinephrine into the patient.

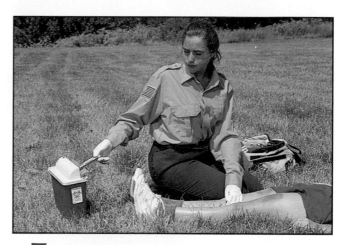

▲ **7.** Dispose of the used injector in a portable biohazard container.

▲ **8.** Document the patient's response to the medication.

▲ **9.** Perform an ongoing assessment, paying special attention to the patient's ABCs and vital signs en route to the hospital.

EPINEPHRINE AUTO-INJECTOR

Medication Name
1. Generic: epinephrine
2. Trade: Adrenalin™
3. Delivery system: EpiPen® or EpiPen® Jr.

Indications
Must meet the following three criteria:
1. Patient exhibits signs of a severe allergic reaction, including either respiratory distress or shock (hypoperfusion).
2. Medication is prescribed for this patient by a physician.
3. Medical direction authorizes use for this patient.

Contraindications
No contraindications when used in a life-threatening situation

Medication Form
Liquid administered by an auto-injector—an automatically injectable needle-and-syringe system

Dosage
Adult: one adult auto-injector (0.3 mg)
Infant and child: one infant/child auto-injector (0.15 mg)

Administration
1. Obtain patient's prescribed auto-injector. Ensure:
   a. Prescription is written for the patient who is experiencing the severe allergic reaction.
   b. Medication is not discolored (if visible).
2. Obtain order from medical direction, either on-line or off-line.
3. Remove cap from auto-injector.

4. Place tip of auto-injector against patient's thigh.
   a. Lateral portion of the thigh
   b. Midway between waist and knee
5. Push the injector firmly against the thigh until the injector activates.
6. Hold the injector in place until the medication is injected (at least 10 seconds).
7. Record activity and time.
8. Dispose of injector in biohazard container.

Actions
1. Dilates the bronchioles
2. Constricts blood vessels

Side Effects
1. Increased heart rate
2. Pallor
3. Dizziness
4. Chest pain
5. Headache
6. Nausea
7. Vomiting
8. Excitability, anxiety

Reassessment Strategies
1. Transport
2. Continue focused assessment of airway, breathing, and circulatory status.

If patient's condition continues to worsen (decreasing mental status, increasing breathing difficulty, decreasing blood pressure):

a. Obtain medical direction for an additional dose of epinephrine
b. Treat for shock (hypoperfusion)
c. Prepare to initiate basic life support procedures (CPR, AED)

If patient's condition improves, provide supportive care:

a. Continue oxygen
b. Treat for shock (hypoperfusion)

Epinephrine is a very powerful medication. It not only saves lives, it can also occasionally take lives. One of the good things epinephrine does for patients is make the heart beat more strongly. This is beneficial when the patient is hypoperfusing (that is, when the patient is in shock), because one reason for the hypoperfusion is that the patient's blood vessels are dilated and blood is not returning to the heart as quickly. Unfortunately, once you give a drug, you cannot take it back. If the dose of epinephrine in the auto-injector is more than the patient needs, the patient's heart will be working harder than it needs to. This can be dangerous in a patient with a heart condition or who is hypertensive (has high blood pressure).

This is one of the reasons why EMT-Basics are taught to *give epinephrine only to patients who have been prescribed auto-injectors by their physicians.* They have been evaluated by physicians who have considered the patient's history and physical condition, were satisfied that a patient is a good candidate for epinephrine, and wrote a prescription.

Some patients receive instruction from their physicians in how to use the auto-injector, but others will be uncomfortable or afraid to use one because of unfamiliarity with the device and will prefer to have you help them with it. Ordinarily, when a health-care provider gives an injection, the clothing over the injection site is rolled up or down and the area is cleansed with an alcohol pad. These steps are not necessary with an epinephrine auto-injector. The risk of giving a patient an infection because you did not take those steps is so small, in fact, that the manufacturer's instructions for auto-injectors do not advise patients to take those steps. Your protocols may direct you to act differently. Follow your local protocols.

One of the most difficult things you may have to do is distinguish between the patient with a (localized) allergic reaction, who should not receive epinephrine, and the patient with a (generalized) anaphylactic reaction, who should be given epi-

nephrine. Patients can and do present in many different ways. One patient in anaphylaxis may have severe difficulty breathing with no hives or decreased blood pressure, while another patient may have a rapid heartbeat and decreased blood pressure with no difficulty breathing. The important thing to recognize in any patient is the presence of EITHER RESPIRATORY DISTRESS OR SIGNS AND SYMPTOMS OF SHOCK (HYPOPERFUSION). One of these needs to be present for the patient to be in anaphylaxis.

Pediatric Notes

Epinephrine auto-injectors come in two different sizes. The adult size contains an adult dose of 0.3 mg. The child size (for a child weighing less than 66 pounds) has 0.15 mg. Infants rarely experience anaphylactic reactions because their immune systems have not matured enough to develop the kinds of antibodies that cause anaphylactic reactions. Allergic reactions are common in older children, though. Fortunately, many children "grow out" of their allergies as they mature. Parents frequently will have a great deal of useful information about the child's medical history.

Documentation Tip—Allergic Reactions

The administration of epinephrine, like all medications, needs to be documented carefully. This is especially true with a medication this strong. Epinephrine can be life saving, but it can occasionally be fatal. Epinephrine has powerful effects on the heart and will increase the workload of the heart significantly. It is very important that anyone caring for the patient, after you hand the patient over to more advanced providers, know how much epinephrine the patient has received and when and what effects the medication had on the patient, both good and bad. This will allow for better care of the patient after you are gone.

As you are responding to a remote neighborhood in your district for an unknown problem, your dispatcher gives you further information about the call. She states that an elderly male has been stung several times by hornets but has not developed difficulty breathing. The dispatcher also tells you there is an ALS unit responding from the other side of town.

As you arrive on scene, you see an older woman coming out to greet you. She appears upset as she tells you that her 78-year-old husband was doing some work in their storage shed. "I was working in the kitchen when I heard him yelling my name. As I ran outside, I could see him waving his arms around, trying to scare away the hornets."

You find Mr. Meeker sitting forward on a lawn chair at the rear of the house. You notice immediately he is using accessory muscles to breathe and that his face and neck appear flushed. He attempts to explain what has happened but is unable to speak in complete sentences.

STREET SCENE QUESTIONS

1. What is your impression of Mr. Meeker's condition?
2. What do you think might be happening to him?

As you apply a nonrebreather mask to the patient, Mrs. Meeker tells you that he has an allergy to hornet stings and the last time he was stung was shortly after he returned from the South Pacific during WWII. You ask, "Does your husband carry an Epi-Pen?" She tells you no. He has no other allergies, he takes an aspirin daily, and had a heart attack nine years ago.

You suspect the patient might be experiencing an allergic reaction to the insect stings and that this could be a life-threatening reaction.

As you place Mr. Meeker in the ambulance, your partner reassures the patient's wife and advises her to be careful as she follows the ambulance to the hospital. En route, you assess vital signs and find that the patient's pulse is 136 and thready, his respirations are 28 and shallow, oxygen saturation (his SAO_2) is 93% on 15 liters per minute O_2, and he has a blood pressure of 92/60. You notice the patient's respiratory count is falling and that he has become extremely fatigued by breathing.

STREET SCENE QUESTIONS

3. What do you suspect is beginning to happen to your patient?
4. What further treatment should you render?

When you reassess the patient's breathing more closely, you notice his respiratory rate has dropped significantly to about 12. Although that number is in the normal range for an adult, you realize that the depth of the patient's respirations is so shallow that he is not breathing adequately. You connect the bag-valve mask to the oxygen tank and ventilate Mr. Meeker about 12 times a minute, making sure you ventilate him deeply enough to make his chest rise. After a few breaths, you are able to match your ventilations to the patient's so that he is not fighting against the BVM.

As you arrive at the hospital, you advise the emergency department staff that you have a 78-year-old male who has been stung by several hornets and you suspect a severe allergic reaction. The staff relieves you of patient care and thanks you for the report.

PATIENT NAME: Joshua Meeker   **PATIENT AGE:** 78

CHIEF COMPLAINT		TIME	RESP	PULSE	B.P.	MENTAL STATUS	R PUPILS L	SKIN
Hornet sting. Possible allergic reaction.	V I T A L S I G N S	1 1 4 7	Rate: 28 ☐ Regular ☒ Shallow ☐ Labored	Rate: 136 ☐ Regular ☐ Irregular	92 / 60	☒ Alert ☐ Voice ☐ Pain ☐ Unresp.	☒ Normal ☒ ☐ Dilated ☐ Constricted ☐ Sluggish ☒ No-Reaction	☐ Unremarkable ☐ Cool ☐ Pale ☒ Warm ☐ Cyanotic ☐ Moist ☒ Flushed ☒ Dry ☐ Jaundiced
PAST MEDICAL HISTORY ☐ None ☒ Allergy to _Hornet stings. NKMA_ ☐ Hypertension ☐ Stroke ☐ Seizures ☐ Diabetes ☐ COPD ☐ Cardiac ☐ Other (List) ☐ Asthma			Rate: ☐ Regular ☐ Shallow ☐ Labored	Rate: ☐ Regular ☐ Irregular	/	☐ Alert ☐ Voice ☐ Pain ☐ Unresp.	☐ Normal ☐ ☐ Dilated ☐ Constricted ☐ Sluggish ☐ No-Reaction	☐ Unremarkable ☐ Cool ☐ Pale ☐ Warm ☐ Cyanotic ☐ Moist ☐ Flushed ☐ Dry ☐ Jaundiced
Heart attack 9 yrs ago Current Medications (List) _Aspirin_			Rate: ☐ Regular ☐ Shallow ☐ Labored	Rate: ☐ Regular ☐ Irregular	/	☐ Alert ☐ Voice ☐ Pain ☐ Unresp.	☐ Normal ☐ ☐ Dilated ☐ Constricted ☐ Sluggish ☐ No-Reaction	☐ Unremarkable ☐ Cool ☐ Pale ☐ Warm ☐ Cyanotic ☐ Moist ☐ Flushed ☐ Dry ☐ Jaundiced

NARRATIVE Dispatched for possible allergic reaction. Upon arrival, found 78 y/o male sitting upright leaning forward outside on lawn chair. Per patient and wife, patient stung several times (unknown exact number) by hornets while working in storage shed. Patient unable to ambulate back to house and alert his wife. Initial assessment showed patient oriented x 3. Patient in obvious respiratory distress; using accessory muscles to breathe. Flushed and blotchy skin noted to patient's neck and face. Immediately administered 15 LPM O_2 via NRB and placed patient into unit and transported. En route, patient became too exhausted to breathe and BVM used to assist respirations. Vitals en route are stated above. Upon arrival to Med-Valley General, updated that staff on patient's condition and transferred patient and care. No changes at the time.

CHAPTER REVIEW

SUMMARY

Allergic reactions are common. Anaphylaxis, a true life-threatening allergic reaction, is rare. The most common symptom in all of these cases is itching. Patients with anaphylaxis, though, will also display life-threatening difficulty breathing and/or signs and symptoms of shock (hypoperfusion). These patients will also be extremely anxious. Their bodies are in trouble and are letting them know it.

Fortunately, most of these patients know about their condition and manage to avoid exposure to the allergens they are sensitive to. Their physicians have often prescribed epinephrine auto-injectors for them for the times when they are exposed.

By quickly recognizing the condition, consulting medical direction, and administering the appropriate treatment, you can literally make the difference between life and death for these patients.

KEY TERMS

allergen something that causes an allergic reaction.
allergic reaction an exaggerated immune response.
anaphylaxis (an-ah-fi-LAK-sis) a severe or life-threatening allergic reaction in which the blood vessels dilate, causing a drop in blood pressure, and the tissues lining the respiratory system swell, interfering with the airway. Also called *anaphylactic shock*.
auto-injector a syringe pre-loaded with medication that has a spring-loaded device which pushes the

needle through the skin when the tip of the device is pressed firmly against the body.
epinephrine (EP-uh-NEF-rin) a hormone produced by the body. As a medication, it constricts blood vessels and dilates respiratory passages and is used to relieve severe allergic reactions.
hives red, itchy, possibly raised blotches on the skin that often result from allergic reactions.

REVIEW QUESTIONS

1. What are the indications for administration of an epinephrine auto-injector? (p. 396)
2. List some of the more common causes of allergic reactions. (pp. 389–390)

3. List signs or symptoms of an anaphylactic reaction associated with each of the following: (p. 392)
   — skin
   — respiratory system
   — cardiovascular system

APPLICATIONS

- You are treating an alert 5-year-old boy who has many environmental allergies and who now has hives on his neck, chest, and arms after playing inside the home of neighbors who own a cat. One of his many allergies is to cats. He has a pulse of 100, BP of 90/60, and respirations of 20 and unlabored. Capillary refill is normal. He has no other signs or symptoms. Do you think the physician in the emergency department will order the use of a child-size EpiPen®? If yes, why? If no, why not?

WEB MEDIC

Visit Brady's *Emergency Care* website for direct weblinks. At **www.bradybooks.com/emergencycare**, you will find information related to the following Chapter 20 topics:

- Stinging insects
- Food allergies
- Anaphylaxis

Chapter
Twenty-One

POISONING AND OVERDOSE EMERGENCIES

*W*ord on the Street

"Early in my career, I answered a phone call to our fire station from a very sad woman. She said she wanted to die. I spoke with her for a few minutes while we tried to trace her call. The whole time she sounded as if she was eating peanut M&Ms. After building enough trust with her, I got her to tell me her address and to accept some help. Then I asked her what she had been eating since it sounded so delicious. 'My antidepressant pills,' she answered."

David Page Emergency Health Services, Inver Hills Community College, St. Paul, MN

How can you know that the patient you encounter at the scene of an emergency call has been poisoned? Family members or bystanders may, of course, report this fact when they call for help. There may be clues at the scene, such as empty pill bottles or containers of toxic substances, and the patient's signs and symptoms may indicate poisoning or overdose. After you identify and treat immediately life-threatening problems, such as airway or breathing difficulties, your main assessment task will be to gather information for medical direction, who will guide your care and management of the poisoning or overdose patient.

POISONING

A **poison** is any substance that can harm the body, sometimes seriously enough to create a medical emergency. In the United States, there are more than a million cases of poisoning annually. Although some of these result from murder or suicide attempts, most are accidental and involve young children. These accidents usually involve common substances such as medications, petroleum products, cosmetics, and pesticides. In fact, a surprisingly large percentage of chemicals in everyday use contain substances that are poisonous if misused.

We usually think of a poison as some kind of liquid or solid chemical that has been ingested by the poisoning victim. This is often the case, but many living organisms are capable of producing a **toxin,** a substance that is poisonous to humans. For example, some mushrooms and other common plants can be poisonous if eaten. These include some varieties of house plants, including the rubber plant and certain parts of holiday plants such as mistletoe and holly berries. Bacterial contaminants in food may produce toxins, some of which can cause deadly diseases (such as botulism).

A great number of substances can be considered poisons, with different people reacting differently to various poisons (Table 21-1). As odd as it may seem, what may be a dangerous poison for one person may have little effect on another person. For most poisonous substances, the reaction is far more serious in the ill and the elderly.

Once on or in the body, poisons can do damage in a variety of ways. A poison may act as a corrosive or irritant, destroying skin and other body tissues. A poisonous gas can act as a suffocating agent, displacing oxygen in the air. Some poisons are systemic poisons, causing harm to the entire body or to an entire body system. These poisons can critically depress or overstimulate the central nervous system, cause vomiting and diarrhea, prevent red blood cells from carrying oxygen, or interfere with the normal biochemical processes in the body. The actual effect and extent of damage is dependent on the nature of the poison, on its concentration, and sometimes on how it enters the body. These factors vary in importance depending on the patient's age, weight, and general health.

TOPIC OVERVIEW

In this chapter, you will learn about the following topics:

- Different types of poisons and how they enter the body

- How to identify patients who have overdosed or who have had contact with poisons

- Which overdose/poisoning patients should receive activated charcoal

- Role of medical control in poisoning and overdose cases

- How to document findings and care of patients with a poisoning/overdose emergency

DOT OBJECTIVES

✔ Knowledge and Attitude

1. List various ways that poisons enter the body. (p. 405)

2. List signs and symptoms associated with poisoning. (pp. 403, 404, 405–406, 412)

3. Discuss the emergency medical care for the patient with possible overdose. (pp. 419–420, 422)

4. Describe the steps in the emergency medical care for the patient with suspected poisoning. (pp. 409, 410, 413, 422) (Scan 21-1, p. 407; Scan 21-3, p. 411; Scan 21-4, p. 415)

5. Establish the relationship between the patient suffering from poisoning or overdose and airway management. (pp. 410, 417, 419)

6. State the generic and trade names, indications, contraindications, medication form, dose, administration, actions, side effects, and reassessment strategies for activated charcoal. (pp. 406, 409) (Scan 21-2, p. 408)

7. Recognize the need for medical direction in caring for patient with poisoning or overdose. (pp. 405–406, 409, 413, 419)

8. Explain the rationale for administering activated charcoal. (pp. 406, 409)

9. Explain the rationale for contacting medical direction early in the prehospital management of the poisoning or overdose patient. (pp. 405, 409)

✔ Skills

1. Demonstrate the steps in the emergency medical care for the patient with possible overdose.

2. Demonstrate the steps in the emergency medical care for the patient with suspected poisoning.

3. Perform the necessary steps required to provide a patient with activated charcoal.

4. Demonstrate the assessment and documentation of patient response.

5. Demonstrate proper disposal of equipment for the administration of activated charcoal.

6. Demonstrate completing a prehospital care report for patients with a poisoning or overdose emergency.

Table 21-1   Common Ingested Poisons

Substance	Signs and Symptoms
acetaminophen	Nausea and vomiting. There may be no signs or symptoms.
acids and alkalis	Burns on or around the lips. Burning in mouth, throat, and abdomen. Vomiting.
antihistamines and cough or cold preparations	Hyperactivity or drowsiness. Rapid pulse, flushed skin, dilated pupils.
aspirin	Delayed signs and symptoms, including ringing in the ears, deep and rapid breathing, bruising.
food poisoning	Different types of food poisoning have different signs and symptoms of varying onset. Most include abdominal pain, nausea, vomiting, and diarrhea, sometimes with fever.
insecticides	Slow pulse, excessive salivation and sweating, nausea, vomiting, diarrhea, difficulty breathing, constricted pupils.
petroleum products	Characteristic odor of breath, clothing, vomitus. If aspiration has occurred, coughing and difficulty breathing.
plants	Wide range of signs and symptoms, ranging from none to nausea and vomiting to cardiac arrest.

INHALATION

Sprays

Cleaning fluid

INJECTION

Drugs

INGESTION

Lye

Rat poison

Drain cleaners

ABSORPTION

Household cleaners

Insecticides

Figure 21-1 Poisons enter the body by way of ingestion, inhalation, absorption, and injection.

Poisons can be classified into four types, according to how they enter the body: **ingested, inhaled, absorbed,** and **injected** (Figure 21-1):

- *Ingested poisons* (poisons that are swallowed) can include many common household and industrial chemicals, medications, improperly prepared foods, plant materials, petroleum products, and agricultural products made specifically to control rodents, weeds, insects, and crop diseases.

- *Inhaled poisons* (poisons that are breathed in) take the form of gases, vapors, and sprays. Again, many of these substances are in common use in the home, industry, and agriculture. Such poisons include carbon monoxide (from car exhaust, wood-burning stoves, and furnaces), ammonia, chlorine, insect sprays, and the gases produced from volatile liquid chemicals (*volatile* means "able to change very easily from a liquid into a gas;" many industrial solvents are volatile).

- *Absorbed poisons* (poisons taken into the body through unbroken skin) may or may not damage

the skin. Many are corrosives or irritants that will injure the skin and then be slowly absorbed into body tissues and the bloodstream, possibly causing widespread damage. Others are absorbed into the bloodstream without injuring the skin. Examples of these poisons include insecticides and agricultural chemicals. Contact with a variety of plant materials and certain forms of marine life can lead to skin damage and possible absorption into tissues under the skin.

- *Injected poisons* (poisons inserted through the skin). The most common injected poisons include illicit drugs injected with a needle and venoms injected by snake fangs or insect stingers. These will be discussed under "Substance Abuse," later in this chapter, and in Chapter 22, "Environmental Emergencies."

Ingested Poisons

Ingested poisons are those that have been swallowed. An ingested poison is often a toxic substance that a curious child has eaten or drunk. In adults, an ingested poison is often a medication on which the patient has accidentally or deliberately overdosed.

Safety Note

Sometimes patients who have ingested poisons will require assisted ventilations. Direct mouth-to-mouth ventilation in such a case is dangerous, not only because of the danger of contracting an infectious disease but also because of possible contact with poisonous substances remaining on the patient's lips, in the airway, or in his vomitus. Use a pocket face mask with a one-way valve, a bag-valve-mask unit with supplemental oxygen, or positive-pressure ventilation when providing ventilations to a patient who is suspected of ingesting a poison.

If intentional poisoning or attempted suicide is suspected, approach the scene with caution and have police back up if indicated.

Patient *ASSESSMENT*

Ingested Poisons

You must gather information quickly in cases of possible ingested poisoning. In order to determine if activated charcoal is appropriate, on-line medical direction will need certain information:

- *What substance was involved?* Many products have similar names. It is important to get the exact spelling of the substance. If it is possible and safe, bring the container to the hospital with the patient.

- *When did the exposure occur?* Some poisons act very quickly and will require immediate treatment. Others may take longer to affect the body, which may allow for other treatments to be used. It is important for emergency department personnel to know as closely as possible the time of ingestion so that appropriate testing and treatment can be done.

    It is sometimes difficult to determine the time of the exposure from family members or witnesses. If you cannot get an exact time, determine when the earliest and latest possible times of exposure were.

- *How much was ingested?* This may be as easy as counting the number of tablets left in a brand new prescription or as difficult as estimating the amount of gasoline spilled on a garage floor. When the amount cannot be estimated reliably, determine the maximum amount that might have been ingested.

- *Over how long a period did the ingestion occur?* Someone who takes certain medication chronically and then overdoses on it may require very different hospital treatment from the patient who has the same overdose but has never taken that medication before.

- *What interventions have the patient, family, or well-meaning bystanders taken?* Many traditional home remedies for medical problems are harmful, particularly when someone has been exposed to enough of a substance to suffer ill effects. Product labels have been improved over the last few years, but some still contain inaccurate or even dangerous instructions for management of potentially toxic exposures.

- *What is the patient's estimated weight?* This, in combination with the amount of substance ingested, may be critical in determining the appropriate treatment.

- *What effects is the patient experiencing from the ingestion?* Nausea and vomiting are two of the most common results of poison ingestion, but you may also find altered mental status, abdominal pain, diarrhea, chemical burns around the mouth, and unusual breath odors.

Activated Charcoal

To provide the proper emergency care for ingested poisons (Scan 21-1), follow the instructions given to you by medical direction or your regional poison control center. In some cases of ingested poisoning, medical direction will order administration of activated charcoal (Scan 21-2).

Activated charcoal works through *adsorption,* the process of one substance becoming attached to the surface of another. Ordinary charcoal adsorbs some substances, but activated charcoal is different because it has been manufactured to have many cracks and crevices. As a result, activated charcoal has an increased amount of surface available for poisons to bind to (similar to corrugated cardboard which, if you cut it open, has many more surfaces than you would expect by looking at the smooth outer surface). Activated charcoal is not an antidote, but through the adsorption or binding process, in many cases it will prevent or reduce the amount of poison available for the body to absorb.

Many poisons are adsorbed by activated charcoal, but not all. Since there are millions of potential poisons available and the number is always increasing, it makes little sense to memorize lists of poisons where activated charcoal should not be used. Instead, medical direction (possibly in consultation with a poison control center) will determine whether the use of activated charcoal is appropriate.

There are, however, a few instances you should know about where the use of activated charcoal is contraindicated:

- Patient who cannot swallow obviously cannot swallow activated charcoal.
- Patient with altered mental status might choke on activated charcoal and aspirate it into the lungs.
- Patient who has ingested acids or alkalis should not take activated charcoal because the caustic material may have severely damaged the mouth, throat, and esophagus. Activated charcoal cannot help the damage that has already been done, and swallowing it may cause further damage. Examples of such caustic substances are oven cleaners, drain cleaners, toilet bowl cleaners, and lye.
- Patient who has accidentally swallowed while siphoning gasoline should not be given activated charcoal. This patient will be coughing violently and possibly aspirating the gasoline. This patient will be unable to swallow activated charcoal.

Many brands of activated charcoal are on the market, but some have greater surface area than others. Medical direction can guide you in the selection of an appropriate brand.

Some patients, especially those who have taken an intentional overdose, may refuse to take activated charcoal. Never attempt to force a patient to swallow activated charcoal. If the patient refuses, notify medical direction and continue ongoing assessment and care.

Some EMS systems may direct EMT-Bs to administer an activated charcoal mixture that includes sorbitol, a cathartic, or rapid-acting laxative. Hospital

INGESTED POISONS

FIRST take BSI precautions.

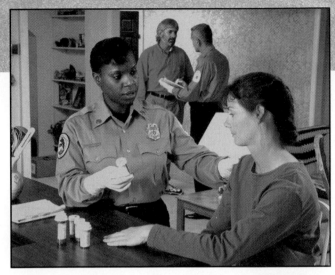

▲ **1.** Quickly gather information.

▲ **2.** Call medical direction on the scene or en route.

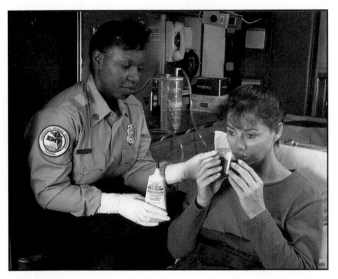

▲ **3.** If directed, administer activated charcoal. You may wish to administer the medication in an opaque cup that has a lid with a hole for a straw.

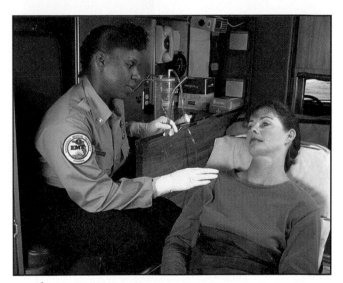

▲ **4.** Position patient for vomiting and save all vomitus. Have suction equipment ready.

SAFETY NOTE When a patient has ingested a poison, it provides another reason to avoid mouth-to-mouth contact. Provide ventilations through a pocket face mask or other barrier device.

407

ACTIVATED CHARCOAL

Medication Name

1. Generic: activated charcoal
2. Trade: SuperChar, InstaChar, Actidose, Liqui-Char, and others

Indications

1. Poisoning by mouth

Contraindications

1. Altered mental status
2. Ingestion of acids or alkalis
3. Inability to swallow

Medication Form

1. Pre-mixed in water, frequently available in plastic bottle containing 12.5 grams of activated charcoal
2. Powder—should be avoided in field

Dosage

1. Adults and children: 1 gram activated charcoal/kg of body weight
2. Usual adult dose: 25–50 grams
3. Usual pediatric dose: 12.5–25 grams

Administration

1. Consult medical direction.
2. Shake container thoroughly.

3. Since medication looks like mud, patient may need to be persuaded to drink it. Providing a covered container and a straw will prevent patient from seeing the medication and so may improve patient compliance.
4. If patient does not drink the medication right away, the charcoal will settle. Shake or stir it again before administering.
5. Record the name, dose, route, and time of administration of the medication.

Actions

1. Activated charcoal adsorbs (binds) certain poisons and prevents them from being absorbed into the body.
2. Not all brands of activated charcoal are the same; some adsorb much more than others, so consult medical direction about the brand to use.

Side Effects

1. Black stools
2. Some patients may vomit, particularly those who have ingested poisons that cause nausea. If patient vomits, repeat the dose once.

Reassessment Strategies

1. Be prepared for the patient to vomit or further deteriorate.

ACTIVATED CHARCOAL VS. SYRUP OF IPECAC

A traditional treatment for poisoning used to be syrup of ipecac. This orally administered drug causes vomiting in most people with just one dose. During recent years, however, it has been used less and less as the use of activated charcoal has increased. Ipecac stimulates both the stomach and the vomiting center in the brain, but it typically takes 15 to 20 minutes to work. If the first dose had not caused vomiting within 20 to 30 minutes, a second dose was typically given (almost everyone vomits after two doses of ipecac). When vomiting does occur, it results, on the average, in removal of less than a third of the stomach contents. Combine the slowness and relative ineffectiveness of syrup of ipecac with the potential for the patient to become drowsy or unconscious in 20 minutes, thus chancing aspiration of vomitus by a non-alert patient, and the disadvantages of ipecac become clear.

Although poison control centers frequently instruct parents of young children in the proper use of syrup of ipecac, activated charcoal is the medication of first choice for healthcare providers in most poisoning and overdose cases. This is why the national standard EMT-B curriculum now includes the use of activated charcoal and not syrup of ipecac.

staff frequently administer sorbitol in order to enhance activated charcoal's ability to prevent absorption of poisons by speeding their passage through the gastrointestinal tract. Because it acts so quickly, sorbitol is not used in most EMS systems, especially those with long transport times.

Dilution. Occasionally, medical direction will give an order for dilution of a poisonous substance. This means an adult patient should drink one to two glasses of water or milk, whichever is ordered. A child should typically be given half to one glass. Dilution with water may slow absorption slightly. Milk may soothe stomach upset. This treatment is frequently advised for patients who, medical direction or poison control determines, do not need transport to a hospital.

Patient *CARE*

Ingested Poison

Emergency care of a patient who has ingested poison includes the following:

1. Detect and treat immediately life-threatening problems in the initial assessment. Evaluate the need for prompt transport for critical patients.

2. Perform a focused history and physical exam, including SAMPLE history. Use gloved hands to carefully remove any pills, tablets, or fragments from the patient's mouth.

3. Assess baseline vital signs.

4. Consult medical direction. As directed, administer activated charcoal to adsorb the poison, or water or milk to dilute it. This can usually be done en route.

5. Transport the patient with all containers, bottles, and labels from the substance.

6. Perform ongoing assessment en route.

Pediatric Notes

It is the nature of infants and children to explore their world—and to get into and often taste whatever they find. Children will swallow substances adults cannot imagine swallowing, including horrible-tasting poisonous substances like bleach or lye. The natural curiosity of children makes them the most frequent victims of accidental poisoning.

It is important to find out an infant's or child's weight, which—in combination with the estimated amount of the poisonous substance that was ingested—will help medical direction determine appropriate treatment.

As an EMT-B, always assume that the infant or child has ingested a lethal amount of the poison. Because it is usually extremely difficult or impossible to be sure exactly how much the child has taken in, always treat for the worst. Call medical direction, administer the recommended treatments, and transport the child to the hospital.

ANTIDOTES

Many lay people think that every poison has an antidote, a substance that will neutralize the poison or its effects. The opposite is true. There are only a few genuine antidotes, and they can be used only with a very small number of poisons. Modern treatment of poisonings and overdoses consists primarily of prevention of absorption when possible (such as by administration of activated charcoal) and good supportive treatment (such as airway maintenance, administration of oxygen, treatment for shock). In a small number of poisonings, advanced treatments are administered in a hospital (administration of antidotes and dialysis).

Inhaled Poisons

Inhaled poisons are those that are present in the atmosphere and that you, as well as the patient, are at risk of breathing in. Carbon monoxide poisoning is a common problem. Other possible inhaled poisons include chlorine gas (often from swimming pool chemicals), ammonia (often released from household cleaners), sprayed agricultural chemicals and pesticides, and carbon dioxide (from industrial sources).

Safety Note

If you suspect that a patient has inhaled a poison, approach the scene with care. Some EMS systems provide training in the use of protective clothing and self-contained breathing apparatus to be used in a hostile environment (such as chlorine gas, ammonia, or smoke). Remember that many inhaled poisons can also be absorbed through the skin. Go only where your protective equipment and clothing will allow you to go safely to perform your mission, and only after you have been trained in the use of this equipment. *Do only what you have been trained to do and go only where your protective equipment will allow you to go safely. If you are underequipped or undertrained, get someone there who is properly equipped and trained.*

Patient ASSESSMENT

Inhaled Poisons

Gather the following information as quickly as possible:

- *What substance was involved?* Get its exact name.
- *When did the exposure occur?* Estimate as well as you can when the patient was exposed to the poisonous gas by finding out the earliest and latest possible times of exposure.
- *Over how long a period did the exposure occur?* The longer someone is exposed to a poisonous gas, the more poison will probably be absorbed.
- *What interventions has anyone taken?* Did someone remove the patient or ventilate the area right away? When did this happen?
- *What effects is the patient experiencing from the exposure?* Nausea and vomiting are very common in poisoning of all types. With inhaled poisons, find out if the patient is having difficulty breathing, chest pain, coughing, hoarseness, dizziness, headache, confusion, seizures, or altered mental status.

Patient CARE

Inhaled Poisons

The principal prehospital treatment of inhaled poisoning consists of maintaining the airway and supporting respiration (Scan 21-3). In the case of inhaled poisoning, oxygen is a very important drug. Some inhaled poisons prevent the blood from transporting oxygen in the normal manner. Some prevent oxygen from getting into the bloodstream in the first place. In either case, your ability to keep the airway open, ventilate as needed, and give high-concentration oxygen may make the difference in the survival and quality of life of the patient who has inhaled a poison.

Emergency care steps include the following:

1. If the patient is in an unsafe environment, have trained rescuers remove the patient to a safe area. Detect and treat immediately life-threatening problems in the initial assessment. Evaluate the need for prompt transport for critical patients.

2. Perform a focused history and physical exam, including SAMPLE history and vital signs.

3. Administer high-concentration oxygen. This is the single most important treatment for inhaled poisoning after the patient's airway is opened.

4. Transport the patient with all containers, bottles, and labels from the substance.

5. Perform ongoing assessment en route.

Carbon Monoxide

Carbon monoxide is one of the most common inhaled poisons, usually associated with motor-vehicle exhaust and fire suppression. The number of cases has increased recently because of the carbon monoxide that can accumulate from the use of improperly vented wood-burning stoves and the use of charcoal for heating and indoor cooking in areas without adequate ventilation. Malfunctioning oil, gas, and coal-burning furnaces and stoves can also be sources of carbon monoxide.

Since carbon monoxide is an odorless, colorless, and tasteless gas, you will not be able to directly detect its presence without special equipment. Look for indications of possible carbon monoxide poisoning like wood-burning stoves, doors that lead to a garage, or bedrooms above a garage where motor repair work is in progress, and evidence that suggests the patient has spent a long period of time sitting in an idling motor vehicle. When inhaled, carbon monoxide prevents the normal carrying of

INHALED POISONS

SAFETY NOTE In the presence of hazardous fumes or gases, wear protective clothing and self-contained breathing apparatus or wait for those who are properly trained and equipped to enter the scene and bring the patient out.

▲ **1.** Remove patient from source of the poison.

▲ **2.** Establish an open airway.

▲ **3.** Insert an oropharyngeal airway and administer high-concentration oxygen by nonrebreather mask.

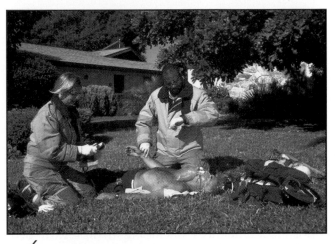

▲ **4.** Gather the patient's history, take baseline vital signs, and expose the chest for auscultation.

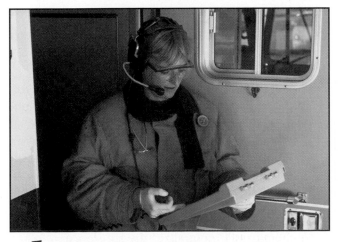

▲ **5.** Contact medical direction.

▲ **6.** Transport the patient.

411

oxygen by the red blood cells. Long exposure, even to low levels of the gas, can cause dramatic effects. Death may occur as hypoxia becomes more severe.

The signs and symptoms of carbon monoxide poisoning are deceptive, because they can resemble those of the flu. Specifically, you may see:

- Headache, especially "a band around the head"
- Dizziness
- Breathing difficulty
- Nausea
- Cyanosis
- Altered mental status; in severe cases, unconsciousness may result

Note

There is a commonly accepted idea that a carbon monoxide victim will have cherry red lips. In fact, cherry red skin is NOT typically seen in patients with carbon monoxide poisoning.

You should suspect carbon monoxide poisoning whenever you are treating a patient with vague, flu-like symptoms who has been in an enclosed area. This is especially true when a group of people in the same area have similar symptoms. A patient with carbon monoxide poisoning may begin to feel better shortly after being removed from the dangerous environment. It is still very important to continue to administer oxygen and to transport these patients to a hospital. Oxygen is an antidote for carbon monoxide poisoning, but it takes time to "wash out" the carbon monoxide from the patient's bloodstream. These patients need medical evaluation because they can have serious consequences, including neurological deficits, from their exposure.

Absorbed Poisons

Absorbed poisons frequently irritate or damage the skin. Some poisons can be absorbed with little or no damage to the skin.

Safety Note

Just as poisonous substances can be absorbed by patients, they can also be absorbed by EMT-Bs. It is critical that the EMT-B take protective measures to prevent exposure to these substances. It may be necessary for firefighters to decontaminate a patient before the EMT-B touches him.

SMOKE INHALATION

Smoke inhalation is a serious problem associated with the scenes of thermal and chemical burns. The smoke from any fire source contains many poisonous substances. Modern building materials and furnishings often contain plastics and other synthetics that release toxic fumes when they burn or are overheated. It is possible for the substances found in smoke to burn the skin, irritate the eyes, injure the airway, cause respiratory arrest, and, in some cases, cause cardiac arrest.

As an EMT-B, you will most likely find irritated (reddened, watering) eyes and, of far greater concern, injury to the airway associated with smoke.

Signs of an airway injured by smoke inhalation include:

- Difficulty breathing
- Coughing
- Breath that has a "smoky" smell or the odor of chemicals involved at the scene
- Black (carbon) residue in the patient's mouth and nose
- Black residue in any sputum coughed up by the patient
- Nose hairs singed from super-heated air

Move the patient to a safe area and provide the same care you would provide for any inhaled poison: Assess the patient, administer high-concentration oxygen, and transport.

Note: The body's reaction to toxic gases and foreign matter in the airway can often be delayed. Convince all smoke inhalation patients that they must be seen by a physician, even if they are not yet feeling serious effects.

Patient ASSESSMENT

Absorbed Poisons

Gather the following information as quickly as possible:

- *What substance was involved?* Get its exact name.
- *When did the exposure occur?*
- *How much of the substance was the patient exposed to?* How large an area of skin was the substance on?
- *Over how long a period did the exposure occur?* The longer someone's skin is exposed to a poison, the more likely it is to be well absorbed.
- *What interventions has anyone taken?* Did someone attempt to wash the substance off the patient? If so, with what? Did anyone attempt to use a chemical to "neutralize" the substance?

- *What effects is the patient experiencing from the exposure?* Common signs and symptoms include a liquid or powder on the patient's skin, burns, itching, irritation, and redness.

Patient CARE

Absorbed Poisons

Emergency care of a patient with absorbed poisons includes the following:

1. Detect and treat immediately life-threatening problems in the initial assessment. Evaluate the need for prompt transport of critical patients.

2. Perform a focused history and physical exam, including SAMPLE history and vital signs. This includes removing contaminated clothing while protecting oneself from contamination.

3. Remove the poison by doing one of the following:

- *Powders:* Brush powder off the patient, then continue as for other absorbed poisons.
- *Liquids:* Irrigate with clean water for at least 20 minutes and continue en route if possible.
- *Eyes:* Irrigate with clean water for at least 20 minutes and continue en route if possible.

4. Transport the patient with all containers, bottles, and labels from the substance.

5. Perform ongoing assessment en route.

The most important part of the treatment of a patient with an absorbed poison is to get the poison off the skin or out of the eye (Scan 21-4). The best way to do this is by irrigating the skin or the eye with large amounts of clean water. A garden hose or fire hose can be used to irrigate the patient's skin, but care must be taken not to injure the skin further with high pressure.

"Neutralizing" acids or alkalis with solutions such as dilute vinegar or baking soda in water should NOT be done. When incidents like these occur, such substances are almost never readily available. Even if they were, they would not be appropriate. They have never been shown to help, and there is good reason to believe they would make matters worse. When an acid is mixed with an alkali, it is true that the two may be neutralized. It is also true, though, that this reaction produces heat. Skin that has been injured already by an acid or alkali may be further damaged by attempts to neutralize the chemical.

FOOD POISONING

Another way someone can be poisoned is through food that has been handled or cooked improperly. Food poisoning can be caused by several different bacteria that grow when exposed to the right conditions. This frequently happens when raw meat, poultry, or fish is left at room temperature before being cooked or the food does not reach a high enough temperature to kill the bacteria. Signs and symptoms vary somewhat, depending on the bacteria involved, but frequently include nausea, vomiting, abdominal cramps, diarrhea, and fever.

You can prevent food poisoning at home and at the station by washing hands, utensils, cutting boards, and any surface the food touches before and especially after any contact with raw meat, fish, or poultry (the bacteria can easily be spread to other foods from hands or surfaces); by storing and cooking foods at appropriate temperatures; and by not leaving raw or cooked foods at room temperature for long periods of time.

Injected Poisons

As mentioned earlier, the most common injected poisons are illicit drugs injected with a needle and the venom of snakes and insects.

Documentation Tips—Poisoning

With any kind of poisoning, be sure to gather and document the following kinds of information that medical direction and hospital personnel will need:

- *Route of poisoning.* Note whether the poison was ingested, inhaled, absorbed, or injected.
- *Substance.* Write down the exact name and spelling of the substance.
- *Amount.* Estimate how much of the substance the patient took in or was exposed to. If the exact amount is unknown, note any clues ("The 1-liter bottle was half empty," for example). Put witnesses' exact words in quotation marks ("There was this funny smell, like nail polish remover").
- *Time.* Document when the ingestion or exposure took place and over how long a period of time.
- *Interventions.* Write down any actions the patient, family members, or bystanders took before you arrived, such as having the patient swallow something or inducing vomiting.

POISON CONTROL CENTERS

Emergency care in poisoning cases presents special problems for the EMT-B. Signs and symptoms can vary greatly. Some poisons produce a characteristic set of signs and symptoms very quickly, while others are subtle and slow to appear. Poisons that act almost immediately usually produce obvious signs, and the particular poison or its container is often still nearby. Slow-acting poisons can produce effects that mimic an infectious disease or some other medical emergency.

There will be times when you will not know the substance that caused the poisoning. In some of these cases, an expert may be able to tell, based on the combination of signs and symptoms. Even when you know the source of the poison, correct emergency care procedures may still be in question. Ideas about proper care keep changing as more research is done on poisoning. This constant change makes it impossible to print guides and charts for poison control and care that will be up to date when you use them. Although manufacturers have improved the instructions on many container labels, many still have inaccurate or even dangerous advice.

Fortunately, a network of poison control centers exists to provide information and advice to both lay people and health-care providers. In most localities, a poison control center can be reached 24 hours a day.

An EMT-B should consult a poison control center only when directed by local protocol. In most cases, EMT-Bs get medical direction from physicians or nurses who are in hospital emergency departments. Unless special arrangements have been made, the poison control center staff does not have the authority to provide on-line medical direction. If the poison control center staff does have the authority to do so, they can tell you what should be done for most cases of poisoning.

If you are permitted to communicate directly with the poison control center in your area, do so by telephone. Even if you have radio contact with your local poison control center, the telephone is the preferred way to communicate. The staff member may need to talk to you for several minutes, far too long a period to monopolize the air waves. The telephone will also allow you to maintain patient confidentiality. Make certain you have memorized the number and/or carry the poison control center number with you into the residence—perhaps pasted inside your kit—so that you do not have to return to the rig to get it.

To help the poison control center staff, gather all of the information you need before you call.

Many people have the impression that the poison control center should be called only for cases of ingested poisonings. The center's staff can provide valuable care information for all types of poisoning.

Your community may have special poisoning problems. Not every community is exposed to rattlesnakes, jellyfish, or powerful agricultural chemicals. Many EMS systems have compiled lists of poisoning problems specific for their areas. Check to see if this has been done for the area in which you will be an EMT-B.

- *Patient's weight.* If the poison was ingested, note the patient's body weight. If no one knows, write down your best estimate.
- *Effects of poisoning.* Document any effects of the poisoning the patient has experienced (such as nausea or vomiting, dizziness, difficulty breathing, altered mental status, itching, burning).
- *Effects of treatment.* Document the patient's response to treatments you or others have given.

PREVENTION

Preventing poisoning is, of course, preferable to having to treat it. The EMT-B's own home and the squad building should be "childproofed" against poisoning by keeping medications and other dangerous substances out of children's reach. The EMT-B can also share poisoning prevention information with members of the public during school visits and community outreach activities.

ALCOHOL AND SUBSTANCE ABUSE

As an EMT-B, you will see many patients whose conditions are caused either directly or indirectly by alcohol or substance abuse. Although these are often thought of as urban problems, the abuse of alcohol and other drugs crosses all geographic and economic boundaries.

Alcohol Abuse

Many persons consume alcohol without any problems. Others occasionally or chronically abuse alcohol. Although alcohol is legal (for adults), it must not be forgotten that alcohol is a drug and has a potent effect on the central nervous system. Emergencies arising from the use of alcohol may be due to the effect of alcohol that has just been con-

HOW AND WHY?

Alcoholism, or chronic alcohol abuse, affects more than 10 million people in the U.S. Approximately 200,000 deaths annually are due to alcohol-related medical conditions. Go to your Electronic Extras CD to learn more.

ABSORBED POISONS

SAFETY NOTE Take care to protect your skin from contact with poisonous substances. Wear protective clothing. If necessary, have firefighters or others who are properly protected hose off the patient before you touch him.

FIRST take BSI precautions.

▲ **1.** Remove patient from the source or the source from patient. Avoid contaminating yourself with the poison.

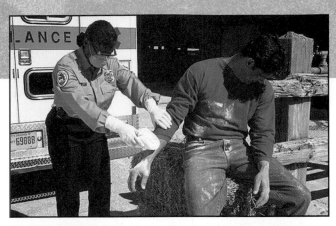

▲ **2.** Brush powders from the patient. Be careful not to abrade the patient's skin.

▲ **3.** Remove contaminated clothing and other articles.

▲ **4.** Irrigate with clean water for at least 20 minutes. Catch contaminated run-off and dispose of it safely.

▲ **5.** Contact medical direction.

▲ **6.** Transport the patient.

sumed, or it may be the result of the cumulative effects of years of alcohol abuse.

EMT-Bs often do not take alcohol abuse patients seriously. This may be partially due to the belligerent or unusual behavior they often exhibit. In addition, frequent calls for intoxicated persons may cause the EMT-B to become callous toward them. The hygiene of many of these patients on the street leaves much to be desired. Nevertheless, provide care for the patient suffering from alcohol abuse the same as you would for any other patient. Patients who appear intoxicated must be treated with the same respect and dignity as those who are "sober."

Above all, you must not neglect your duty to provide medical care. Not only do alcohol-abuse patients often have injuries from accidents and falls, but they are also candidates for many medical emergencies. Chronic drinkers often have derangements in blood sugar levels, poor nutrition, the potential for considerable gastrointestinal bleeding, and other problems. A person can be both intoxicated and having a heart attack or hypoglycemia. If the patient has ingested alcohol and other drugs, this can produce a serious medical emergency. When alcohol is combined with other depressants such as antihistamines and tranquilizers, the effects of alcohol can be more pronounced and, in some cases, can be lethal.

Since EMT-B safety is a critical part of all calls, do not hesitate to ask for police assistance with any patient who appears intoxicated or irrational or exhibits potentially dangerous behavior. The nature of intoxication is such that a passive person may suddenly become aggressive. Always be prepared for this event. (See Chapter 23, "Behavioral Emergencies.")

Patient ASSESSMENT

Alcohol Abuse

Keep in mind that, while alcohol may be the patient's only problem, there may be another problem present. Conduct a complete assessment to identify any medical emergencies. Remember that diabetes, epilepsy, head injuries, high fevers, hypoxia, and other medical problems may make the patient appear to be intoxicated when he is not. Also look for injuries. Do not allow the presence of alcohol or the signs and symptoms of alcohol abuse override your suspicions of other medical problems or injuries.

Since getting a SAMPLE history from any patient who appears intoxicated will be difficult and perhaps unreliable, your powers of observation and resourcefulness will be tested. Family members and bystanders may provide important information.

The signs and symptoms of alcohol abuse include those listed below:

- Odor of alcohol on the patient's breath or clothing. By itself, this is not enough to conclude alcohol abuse. Be certain that the odor is not "acetone breath," as with some diabetic emergencies.
- Swaying and unsteadiness of movement
- Slurred speech, rambling thought patterns, incoherent words or phrases
- A flushed appearance to the face, often with the patient sweating and complaining of being warm
- Nausea or vomiting
- Poor coordination
- Slowed reaction time
- Blurred vision
- Confusion
- Hallucinations, visual or auditory ("seeing things" or "hearing things")
- Lack of memory (blackout)
- Altered mental status

The alcoholic patient may not be under the influence of alcohol but, instead, may be suffering from alcohol **withdrawal.** This can be a severe reaction occurring when the patient cannot obtain alcohol, is too sick to drink alcohol, or has decided to quit drinking suddenly. The alcohol-withdrawal patient may experience seizures or **delirium tremens (DTs),** a condition characterized by sweating, trembling, anxiety, and hallucinations. In some cases, alcohol withdrawal can be fatal.

Signs of alcohol withdrawal include the following:

- Confusion and restlessness
- Unusual behavior, to the point of demonstrating "insane" behavior
- Hallucinations
- Gross tremor (obvious shaking) of the hands
- Profuse sweating
- Seizures (common and often very serious)

NOTE THAT ALL PATIENTS WITH SEIZURES OR DTs MUST BE TRANSPORTED TO A MEDICAL FACILITY AS SOON AS POSSIBLE.

Warning

Be on the alert for signs—such as depressed vital signs—that the patient has mixed alcohol and drugs. Also, when interviewing the intoxicated patient or the patient suffering from alcohol withdrawal, do not begin by asking the patient if he is taking drugs. He may react to this question as if you are gathering evidence of a crime. Ask if any medications have been taken while drinking. If necessary, when you are certain that the patient knows you are concerned about his well-being, you can repeat the question using the word "drugs."

Patient *CARE*

Alcohol Abuse

Since these patients often vomit, take BSI precautions, including gloves, mask, and protective eyewear as necessary. To provide basic care for the intoxicated patient and the patient suffering alcohol withdrawal, follow these steps:

1. Stay alert for airway and respiratory problems. Be prepared to perform airway maintenance, suctioning, and positioning of the patient should the patient lose consciousness, seize, or vomit. Help the patient during vomiting so that vomitus will not be aspirated. Have a rigid-tip suction device ready. Provide oxygen and assist respirations as needed.

2. Be alert for changes in mental status as alcohol is absorbed into the bloodstream. Talk to the patient in an effort to keep him as alert as possible.

3. Monitor vital signs.

4. Treat for shock.

5. Protect the patient from self-injury. Use restraint as authorized by your EMS system. Request assistance from law enforcement if needed. Protect yourself and your crew.

6. Stay alert for seizures.

7. Transport the patient to a medical facility if indicated.

Note: In some systems, patients under the influence of alcohol who are not suffering from a medical emergency or apparent injury are not transported. They are given over to the police. This may not be wise since some patients having an alcohol-related emergency may die unless they receive additional care. In addition, EMS personnel may have missed a medical problem or injury. Remember that the patient's condition may worsen as the alcohol continues to be absorbed by his system. Be especially careful of patients with even minor head injuries, since subdural hematoma (see Chapter 29, "Injuries to the Head and Spine") is common in alcoholics.

Also note that A PATIENT UNDER THE INFLU-ENCE OF ALCOHOL CANNOT MAKE AN IN-FORMED REFUSAL OF TREATMENT OR TRANS-PORT. If the patient refuses treatment or transport, you should nevertheless treat and arrange for transport of the patient as necessary on the basis of implied consent. Document this in your prehospital care report.

Substance Abuse

Substance abuse is a term that indicates a chemical substance is being taken for other than therapeutic (medical) reasons. Many substances have legitimate purposes when used properly. When these same substances are abused, the results can be devastating.

Individuals who abuse drugs and other chemical substances should be considered to have an illness. They have the right to the same professional emergency care as any other patient.

The most common drugs and chemical substances that are abused, and lead to problems requiring an EMS response, can be classified as **uppers, downers, narcotics, hallucinogens,** and **volatile chemicals.**

- *Uppers* are stimulants that affect the nervous system and excite the user. Many abusers use these drugs in an attempt to relieve fatigue or to create feelings of well-being. Examples are caffeine, amphetamines, and cocaine. Cocaine may be "snorted," smoked, or injected. Other stimulants are frequently in pill form.

- *Downers* have a depressant effect on the central nervous system. This type of drug may be used as a relaxing agent, sleeping pill, or tranquilizer. Barbiturates are an example, usually in pill or capsule form.

- *Narcotics* are drugs capable of producing stupor or sleep. They are often used to relieve pain and to quiet coughing. Many drugs legitimately used for these purposes (such as codeine) are also abused, affecting the nervous system and changing many of the normal activities of the body, often producing an intense state of relaxation or feeling of well-being. Illegal narcotics such as heroin are commonly abused. Heroin is usually injected into a vein. Other narcotics are in pill form.

- *Hallucinogens* such as LSD and PCP are mind-affecting drugs that act on the nervous system to produce an intense state of excitement or a distortion of the user's perceptions. This class of drugs has few legal uses. They are often eaten or dissolved in the mouth and absorbed through the mucous membranes.

- *Volatile chemicals* can give an initial "rush" and then act as a depressant on the central nervous system. Cleaning fluid, glue, model cement, and solutions used to correct typing mistakes are commonly abused volatile chemicals.

Substance Abuse

As an EMT-B, you will not need to know the names of the very many abused drugs or their specific reactions. It is far more important for you to be able to detect possible drug abuse at the overdose level and to relate certain signs to certain types of drugs and drug withdrawal. Table 21-2 provides some of the names of commonly abused drugs. Do not worry about memorizing this list. Read it through so that you can place some of the more familiar drugs into categories in terms of drug type.

Table 21-2   Commonly Abused Drugs

Uppers	Downers	Narcotics	Mind-Altering Drugs	Volatile Chemicals
AMPHETAMINE (Benzedrine, bennies, pep pills, ups, uppers, cartwheels)	AMOBARBITAL (blue devils, downers barbs, Amytal)	CODEINE (often in cough syrup)	*Hallucinogenic*	AMYL NITRATE (snappers, poppers)
BIPHETAMINE (bam)	BARBITURATES (downers, dolls, barbs, rainbows)	DEMEROL	DMT	BUTYL NITRATE (locker room, rush)
COCAINE (coke, snow, crack)	CHLORAL HYDRATE (knockout drops, Noctec)	DILAUDID	LSD (acid, sunshine)	CLEANING FLUID (carbon tetrachloride)
DESOXYN (black beauties)	ETHCHLORVYNOL (Placidyl)	FENTANYL (Sublimaze)	MESCALINE (peyote, mesc)	FURNITURE POLISH
DEXTROAMPHETAMINE (dexies, Dexedrine)	GLUTETHIMIDE (Doriden, goofers)	HEROIN ("H," horse, junk, smack, stuff)	MORNING GLORY SEEDS	GASOLINE
METHAMPHETAMINE (speed, crank, meth, crystal, diet pills, Methedrine)	METHAQUALONE (Quaalude, ludes, Sopor, sopors)	METHADONE (dolly)	PCP (angel dust, hog, peace pills)	GLUE
METHYLPHENIDATE (Ritalin)	NONBARBITURATE SEDATIVES (various tranquilizers and sleeping pills: Valium or diazepam, Miltown, Equanil, meprobamate, Thorazine, Compazine, Librium or chlordiazepoxide, reserpine, Tranxene or chlorazepate and other benzodiazepines)	MORPHINE	PSILOCYBIN (magic mushrooms)	HAIR SPRAY
PRELUDIN		OPIUM (op, poppy)	STP (serenity, tranquillity, peace)	NAIL POLISH REMOVER
		MEPERIDINE (Demerol)	*Nonhallucinogenic*	PAINT THINNER
	PARALDEHYDE	PAREGORIC (contains opium)	HASH	TYPEWRITING CORRECTION FLUIDS
	PENTOBARBITAL (yellow jackets, barbs, Nembutal)	TYLENOL WITH CODEINE (1, 2, 3, 4)	MARIJUANA (grass, pot, tea, wood, dope)	
	PHENOBARBITAL (goofballs, phennies, barbs)		THC	
	SECOBARBITAL (red devils, barbs, Seconal)			

The signs and symptoms of substance abuse, dependency, and overdose can vary from patient to patient, even for the same drug or chemical. The problem is made more complex by the fact that many substance abusers take more than one drug or chemical at a time. Often, you will have to carefully combine the information gained from the signs and symptoms, the scene, the bystanders, and the patient in order to determine that you may be dealing with substance abuse. In many cases, you will not be able to identify the substance involved.

When questioning the patient and bystanders, you will get better results if you begin by asking if the patient has been taking any medications. Then, if necessary, ask if the patient has been taking drugs.

Some significant signs and symptoms related to specific types of drugs include those listed below. These are offered for your information in helping you to recognize possible drug abuse in general. Your patient care will not change as a result of this knowledge, but information you can gather about what kind of drug the patient may have been taking will be useful to hospital personnel.

Signs and symptoms of drug abuse include:

- *Uppers*. Excitement, increased pulse and breathing rates, rapid speech, dry mouth, dilated pupils, sweating, and the complaint of having gone without sleep for long periods. Repeated high doses can produce a "speed run." The patient will be restless, hyperactive, and usually very apprehensive and uncooperative.
- *Downers*. Sluggish, sleepy patient lacking typical coordination of body and speech. Pulse and breathing rates are low, often to the point of a true emergency.
- *Hallucinogens*. Fast pulse rate, dilated pupils, and a flushed face. The patient often "sees" or "hears" things, has little concept of real time, and may not be aware of the true environment. Often what he says makes no sense to the listener. The user may become aggressive or be very timid.
- *Narcotics*. Reduced rate of pulse and rate and depth of breathing, often seen with a lowering of skin temperature. The pupils are constricted, often pinpoint in size. The muscles are relaxed and sweating is profuse. The patient is very sleepy and does not wish to do anything. In overdoses, coma is common. Respiratory arrest or cardiac arrest may develop rapidly.
- *Volatile chemicals*. Dazed or showing temporary loss of contact with reality. The patient may develop coma. The linings of the nose and mouth may show swollen membranes. The patient may complain of a "funny numb feeling" or "tingling"

inside the head. Changes in heart rhythm can occur. This can lead to death.

Warning

When reading the above list, you will have noticed that many of the indications of drug abuse are similar to those for quite a few medical emergencies. As an EMT-B, you must never assume drug abuse occurring by itself. You must be on the alert for medical emergencies, injuries, and combinations of drug abuse problems and other emergencies.

In addition to the effects of long-term drug use and overdose, you may encounter cases of severe drug withdrawal. Withdrawal occurs when the long-term user of certain drugs such as narcotics suddenly stops taking the drug. As in reactions to the use of various drugs, withdrawal varies from patient to patient and from drug to drug.

In most cases of drug withdrawal, you may see:

- Shaking
- Anxiety
- Nausea
- Confusion and irritability
- Hallucinations (both visual and auditory—"seeing things" or "hearing things")
- Profuse sweating
- Increased pulse and breathing rates

Patient *CARE*

Substance Abuse

Your care for the drug-abuse patient will be basically the same for all drugs and will not change unless you are so ordered by medical direction. *When providing care for substance-abuse patients, make certain that you are safe and identify yourself as an EMT-B to the patient and bystanders. Since these patients often vomit, take BSI precautions, including gloves, mask, and protective eyewear as necessary.*
Emergency care includes the following:

1. Perform an initial assessment. Provide basic life support measures if required.

2. Be alert for airway problems and inadequate respirations or respiratory arrest. Provide oxygen and assist ventilations if needed.

3. Treat for shock.

4. Talk to the patient to gain his confidence and to help maintain his level of responsiveness. Use his

You and your partner are assigned to the night shift when you are dispatched out for a "possible poisoning." You arrive on scene within 4 minutes to find a 20-year-old female sitting on the couch with a small child in her arms. The female, Anna Prince, states that she is the child's mother and she believes the child has ingested some lamp oil. The child's name is Maria, and she is 8 months old. Anna states, "I was doing the dishes when I turned around and saw Maria with the oil candle in her hands. I don't know how much she drank or how much she spilled." Maria is crying and coughing excessively, but she is alert and responds to her mother. Her skin is warm, dry, and pink. You also notice that there is some lamp oil on the front of Maria's shirt.

STREET SCENE QUESTIONS

1. What questions would you ask the patient's mother next?

2. What signs or symptoms should you inquire about?

You continue to gather information about the situation and discover that the time of exposure occurred approximately 3–4 minutes before 9-1-1 was activated. Anna also reports that she neither has the original container that the lamp oil was purchased in, nor does she remember how much oil was left in the candle. You estimate the total container size to be 100 cc and determine that half of the oil is missing. Anna also reports that she gave Maria some water, but Maria vomited after drinking a small amount.

As you continue with your assessment, you find that Maria has a clear upper airway. Her mucous membranes are pink and moist, and her pupils are equal and reactive to light. Anna states that Maria has been sick lately and that she weighed 20 pounds at her last doctor's visit. Maria is currently taking Children's Tylenol for fever reduction, has no known medical allergies, and the only medical history that her mother reports is a recent fever and mild cough. Maria's current vital signs include a strong pulse of 140 and regular; respirations are 36 with crying and coughing; and an oxygen saturation of 97%.

STREET SCENE QUESTIONS

3. What treatments would you initate?

4. Should you contact someone for advice? If yes, then who?

You provide the patient with blow-by oxygen from a mask attached to a teddy bear and set the flow rate at 10 liters per minute. You place the child in a car seat that is securely anchored to the ambulance stretcher for transport. The mother also is secured in a seat inside the ambulance. You take the lamp oil candle with you.

You contact poison control, and they advise you that the main concern for Maria is related to aspiration of the oil into the lungs. They advise you that the oil may be a petroleum product with a hydrocarbon base and that activated charcoal and syrup of ipecac are contraindicated. You also contact medical direction; they agree with the recommendations from poison control and order only supportive care.

During transport, you continually monitor your patient's airway and ventilatory status. When you repeat vital signs, respirations are 32 and slightly labored and pulse is 128, regular, and strong. As you arrive at the emergency department, Maria has stopped crying but continues to cough. No other changes occur during the transport.

name often, maintain eye contact, and speak directly to the patient.

5. Perform a rapid trauma exam or detailed physical exam to assess for signs of injury to all parts of the body. Assess carefully for signs of head injury.

6. Look for gross soft-tissue damage on the extremities resulting from the injection of drugs ("tracks"). Tracks usually appear as darkened or red areas of scar tissue or scabs over veins.

7. Protect the patient from self-injury and attempting to hurt others. Use restraint as authorized by your EMS system. Request assistance from law enforcement if needed.

8. Transport the patient as soon as possible.

9. Contact medical direction according to local protocols.

10. Perform ongoing assessment with monitoring of vital signs. Stay alert for seizures, and be on guard for vomiting that could obstruct the airway.

11. Continue to reassure the patient throughout all phases of care.

PATIENT NAME: Maria Prince

PATIENT AGE: 8 months

CHIEF COMPLAINT
Coughing, possible ingested poisoning

PAST MEDICAL HISTORY
- ☒ None
- ☐ Allergy to _____
- ☐ Hypertension ☐ Stroke
- ☐ Seizures ☐ Diabetes
- ☐ COPD ☐ Cardiac
- ☐ Other (List) ☐ Asthma

Recent fever with mild cough

Current Medications (List)
Children's Tylenol

VITAL SIGNS

TIME	RESP	PULSE	B.P.	MENTAL STATUS	R PUPILS L	SKIN
2051	Rate: **36** ☐ Regular ☐ Shallow ☒ Labored	Rate: **140** ☒ Regular ☐ Irregular		☒ Alert ☐ Voice ☐ Pain ☐ Unresp.	☒ Normal ☒ ☐ Dilated ☐ ☐ Constricted ☐ ☐ Sluggish ☐ ☐ No-Reaction ☐	☐ Unremarkable ☐ Cool ☐ Pale ☒ Warm ☐ Cyanotic ☐ Moist ☐ Flushed ☒ Dry ☐ Jaundiced
2056	Rate: **32** ☐ Regular ☐ Shallow ☒ Labored	Rate: **128** ☒ Regular ☐ Irregular		☒ Alert ☐ Voice ☐ Pain ☐ Unresp.	☒ Normal ☒ ☐ Dilated ☐ ☐ Constricted ☐ ☐ Sluggish ☐ ☐ No-Reaction ☐	☐ Unremarkable ☐ Cool ☐ Pale ☒ Warm ☐ Cyanotic ☐ Moist ☐ Flushed ☒ Dry ☐ Jaundiced
	Rate: ☐ Regular ☐ Shallow ☐ Labored	Rate: ☐ Regular ☐ Irregular		☐ Alert ☐ Voice ☐ Pain ☐ Unresp.	☐ Normal ☐ Dilated ☐ Constricted ☐ Sluggish ☐ No-Reaction	☐ Unremarkable ☐ Cool ☐ Pale ☐ Warm ☐ Cyanotic ☐ Moist ☐ Flushed ☐ Dry ☐ Jaundiced

NARRATIVE

Responded to a possible poisoning. Upon arrival, we found an 8-month-old female in the arms of her mother. Mother stated that she "was doing the dishes when I turned around and saw Maria with an oil candle in her hands. I do not know how much she drank or how much she spilled." Mother reports child's weight as 20 pounds. Time of exposure was approximately 3-4 minutes before 9-1-1 activation. Patient received some water, which she vomited back up, prior to our arrival. Approximate amount of lamp oil ingested may have been as much as 50 cc.

Assessment revealed a crying and coughing infant, who appeared alert and responding to her mother. Upper airway was clear. Skin was warm and dry. Mucous membranes were moist and pink. Pupils were equal and reactive to light. Vitals above.

Treatment consisted of blow-by O$_2$ at 10 liters per minute. During transport, patient was kept with her mother to reduce anxiety. Lamp oil also transported for identification purposes. Poison control and medical direction contacted; both recommended only airway support and continued assessment. Upon arrival at ED, patient ceased her crying, but her cough was still present. No other changes during transport.

Safety Note

Many drug abusers may appear calm at first and then become violent as time passes. Always be on the alert and ready to protect yourself. If the patient creates an unsafe scene and you are not a trained law enforcement officer, GET OUT and find a safe place until the police arrive.

When dealing with drug abuse, you must also protect yourself from the substance itself. Many hallucinogens can be absorbed through the skin and mucous membranes. Intravenous drug users may possess hypodermic syringes, which pose a hazard of infectious disease transmission through accidental punctures. Take BSI precautions and follow all infection exposure control procedures. Never touch or taste any suspected illicit substance.

CHAPTER REVIEW

Summary

Poisonings and overdoses are frequent causes of medical emergencies. When responding to a poisoning or possible poisoning:

1. Perform initial assessment and immediately treat life-threatening problems. Assure an open airway. Administer high-concentration oxygen if the poison was inhaled or injected.

2. Perform a focused history and physical exam, including baseline vital signs. Find out if the poison was ingested, inhaled, absorbed or injected, what substance was involved, how much poison was taken in, when and over how long a period exposure took place, what interventions others have already done, and what effects the patient experienced.

3. Consult medical direction. As directed, administer activated charcoal or water or milk for ingested poisons. Remove the patient who has inhaled a poison from the environment and administer high-concentration oxygen; remove poisons from the skin by brushing off or diluting.

4. Transport the patient with all containers, bottles, and labels from the substance.

5. Perform ongoing assessment en route.

6. Carefully document all information about the poisoning, interventions, and the patient's responses.

Key Terms

absorbed poisons poisons that are taken into the body through unbroken skin.

activated charcoal a substance that adsorbs many poisons and prevents them from being absorbed by the body.

antidote a substance that will neutralize the poison or its effects.

delirium tremens (duh-LEER-e-um TREM-uns) **(DTs)** a severe reaction that can be part of alcohol withdrawal, characterized by sweating, trembling, anxiety, and hallucinations. Severe alcohol withdrawal with the DTs can lead to death if untreated.

dilution (di-LU-shun) thinning down or weakening by mixing with something else. Ingested poisons are sometimes diluted by drinking water or milk.

downers depressants, such as barbiturates, that depress the central nervous system, often used to bring on a more relaxed state of mind.

hallucinogens (huh-LOO-sin-uh-jens) mind-affecting or mind-altering drugs that act on the central nervous system to produce excitement and distortion of perceptions.

ingested poisons poisons that are swallowed.

inhaled poisons poisons that are breathed in.

injected poisons poisons that are inserted through the skin, for example by needle, snake fangs, or insect stinger.

narcotics a class of drugs that affect the nervous system and change many normal body activities. Their legal use is for the relief of pain. Illicit use is to produce an intense state of relaxation.

poison any substance that can harm the body by altering cell structure or functions.

toxin a poisonous substance secreted by bacteria, plants, or animals.

uppers stimulants such as amphetamines that affect the central nervous system to excite the user.

volatile chemicals vaporizing compounds, such as cleaning fluid, that are breathed in by the abuser to produce a "high."

withdrawal referring to alcohol or drug withdrawal in which the patient's body reacts severely when deprived of the abused substance.

REVIEW QUESTIONS

1. What are four ways in which a poison can be taken into the body? (p. 405)
2. What is the sequence of assessment steps in cases of poisoning? (pp. 405–406, 410, 412–413, 422)
3. What information must you gather in a case of poisoning before contacting medical direction? (pp. 405–406, 410, 412–413)
4. What are the emergency care steps for ingested poisoning? (p. 409)
5. What are the emergency care steps for inhaled poisoning? For absorbed poisoning? (pp. 410, 413)

APPLICATIONS

A local farmer calls 9-1-1, concerned because one of his farm hands has tried to clean up some spilled pesticide powder with his hands. On arrival, you find that the patient insists he has brushed all the powder off, feels fine, and doesn't need to go to the hospital.

As he talks, he continues to make brushing motions at his jeans on which you can see the marks of a powdery residue. How do you manage the situation?

WEB MEDIC

Visit Brady's *Emergency Care* website for direct weblinks. At **www.bradybooks.com/ emergencycare**, you will find information related to the following Chapter 21 topics:

- Poisoning
- Poisoning prevention

Chapter
Twenty-Two

ENVIRONMENTAL EMERGENCIES

Environmental emergencies can occur in any setting—wilderness, rural, suburban, and urban areas. They include exposure to both heat and cold, near-drownings and other water-related injuries, and bites and stings from insects, spiders, snakes, and marine life. The keys to effective management are recognizing the patient's signs and symptoms and providing prompt and proper emergency care. However, as an EMT-Basic, you also must recognize that exposure may not be the only danger to the patient. Environmental emergencies can involve preexisting or cause additional medical problems and injury.

EXPOSURE TO COLD

How the Body Loses Heat

If the environment is too cold, body heat can be lost faster than it can be generated. The body attempts to adjust by reducing perspiration and circulation to the skin—shutting down avenues by which the body usually gets rid of excess heat. Muscular activity in the form of shivering and the rate at which fuel (food) is burned within the body both increase to produce more heat. At a certain point, however, not enough heat is generated to be available to all parts of the body. This may result in damage to exposed tissues and a general reduction or cessation of body functions.

To be able to prevent or compensate for heat loss, the EMT-B must be aware of the ways in which a body loses heat:

- *Conduction.* The direct transfer of heat from one material to another through direct contact is called **conduction.** Heat will flow from a warmer material to a cooler one. Body heat transferred directly into cool air is a problem, but when the body or clothing gets wet, **water chill** is an even greater problem because water conducts heat away from the body 25 times faster than still air. Heat loss through conduction can be a major problem when a person is lying on a cold floor or another cold surface. A person who is standing or walking around in cold weather will lose less heat than a person who is lying on the cold ground.
- *Convection.* When currents of air or water pass over the body, carrying away heat, **convection** occurs. The effects of a cold environment are worsened when moving water or air surround the body. **Wind chill** is a frequent problem. The more wind, the greater the heat loss. For example, if it is 10°F with no wind, the body will lose heat, but if there is a 20 mph wind, the amount of heat lost by the body is much greater—the same as if it were minus 25°F.
- *Radiation.* In conduction and convection, heat is "picked up" by the surrounding (still or moving) air or water. In **radiation,** the body's atoms and molecules send out rays of heat as they move and change. If you were in the vacuum of outer space with no air or water around to pick up heat, you would still lose heat by radiating it out into space. Most radiant heat loss occurs from a person's head and neck.

TOPIC OVERVIEW

In this chapter, you will learn about the following topics:

- Effects of heat and cold on the body
- Treatment of conditions caused by heat and cold
- Personal safety concerns in water emergencies
- Signs, symptoms, and treatment of near-drowning patients
- Signs, symptoms, and treatment of patients who have experienced bites or stings
- How to document findings and care of patients with environmental emergencies

DOT OBJECTIVES

✔ **Knowledge and Attitude**

1. Describe the various ways that the body loses heat. (pp. 425–426)

2. List the signs and symptoms of exposure to cold. (pp. 427–430)

3. Explain the steps in providing emergency medical care to a patient exposed to cold. (pp. 428–433)

4. List the signs and symptoms of exposure to heat. (pp. 432, 433)

5. Explain the steps in providing emergency care to a patient exposed to heat. (pp. 432, 433)

6. Recognize the signs and symptoms of water-related emergencies. (pp. 433–434)

7. Describe the complications of near drowning. (p. 434) (Scan 22-1, pp. 436–438)

8. Discuss the emergency medical care of bites and stings. (pp. 443, 445–447)

✔ **Skills**

1. Demonstrate the assessment and emergency medical care of a patient with exposure to cold.

2. Demonstrate the assessment and emergency medical care of a patient with exposure to heat.

3. Demonstrate the assessment and emergency medical care of a near-drowning patient.

4. Demonstrate completing a prehospital care report for patients with environmental emergencies.

- *Evaporation.* **Evaporation** occurs when the body perspires or gets wet. As perspiration or water on the skin or clothing vaporizes, the body experiences a generalized cooling effect.

- *Respiration.* **Respiration** causes loss of body heat as a result of exhaled warm air. The amount of heat loss depends on the outside air temperature as well as the rate and depth of respirations.

Generalized Hypothermia

When cooling affects the entire body, a problem known as **hypothermia,** or general cooling, develops. Exposure to cold reduces body heat. With time, the body is unable to maintain its proper core (internal) temperature. If allowed to continue, hypothermia leads to death. (See Table 22-1 for a description of the stages of hypothermia.)

Note

Be aware that hypothermia can develop in temperatures well above freezing.

Predisposing Factors

Patients with injuries, chronic illness, or certain other conditions will show the effects of cold much sooner than healthy persons. These conditions include

---

Table 22-1   Stages of Hypothermia

Core Body Temperature		Symptoms
99°F—96°F	37.0°C—35.5°C	Shivering.
95°F—91°F	35.5°C—32.7°C	Intense shivering, difficulty speaking.
90°F—86°F	32.0°C—30.0°C	Shivering decreases and is replaced by strong muscular rigidity. Muscle coordination is affected and erratic or jerky movements are produced. Thinking is less clear, general comprehension is dulled, possible total amnesia. Patient generally is able to maintain the appearance of psychological contact with surroundings.
85°F—81°F	29.4°C—27.2°C	Patient becomes irrational, loses contact with environment, and drifts into stuporous state. Muscular rigidity continues. Pulse and respirations are slow and cardiac arrhythmias may develop.
80°F—78°F	26.6°C—20.5°C	Patient loses consciousness and does not respond to spoken words. Most reflexes cease to function. Heartbeat slows further before cardiac arrest occurs.

shock (hypoperfusion), burns, head and spinal-cord injuries, generalized infection, and diabetes with hypoglycemia. Those under the influence of alcohol or other drugs also tend to be affected more rapidly and more severely than others. The unconscious patient lying on the cold ground or other cold surface is especially prone to rapid heat loss through conduction and will tend to have greater cold-related problems than one who is conscious and able to walk around.

Geriatric Notes

Hypothermia is often an especially serious problem for the aged. The effects of cold temperatures on the elderly are more immediate. During the winter months, many older citizens on small fixed incomes live in unheated rooms or rooms that are kept too cool. Failing body systems, chronic illnesses, poor diets, certain medications, and a lack of exercise may combine with the cold environment to bring about hypothermia.

Pediatric Notes

Since infants and young children are small with large skin surface areas in relation to their total body mass and little body fat, they are especially prone to hypothermia. Because of their small muscle mass, infants and children do not shiver very much or at all—another reason for the susceptibility of the very young to the cold.

Obvious and Subtle Exposure

At times, it is obvious that a patient has been exposed to cold and is probably suffering from hypothermia. With other patients, however, exposure is subtle—that is, not so obvious, not the first thing you may think of. Consider, for example, the elderly patient who has fallen during the night and is not discovered until morning. A broken hip or other injuries may claim your attention, but if your patient has been on the cold floor all night, he is probably also suffering from hypothermia. The patient trapped in a wrecked auto is probably suffering a variety of injuries, but if the weather is cool and extrication from the vehicle takes a while, the patient can easily develop hypothermia as well.

Consider the possibility of hypothermia in the following situations when another condition or injury may be more obvious:

- *Ethanol (alcohol) ingestion.* Has the intoxicated patient passed out on a cold floor or been wandering around outdoors in cool or cold weather?
- *Underlying illness.* Does the patient have a circulatory disorder or other condition that makes him especially susceptible to cold?

- *Overdose or poisoning.* Has the patient been lying in a cold garage or on a cold floor? Is he sweating heavily in a cool environment with evaporation causing excessive heat loss?
- *Major trauma.* Has the patient been lying on the ground or trapped in wreckage during cold weather? Is shock (hypoperfusion, or inadequate circulation of the blood) preventing parts of the body from being warmed by circulating blood?
- *Outdoor resuscitation.* Is your patient getting too cold? If your patient is a near-drowning victim who has been in the water, has exposure to cool water caused hypothermia?
- *Decreased ambient temperature* (for example, room temperature). Is your patient living in a home or apartment that is too cold?

Geriatric Notes

Remember that older patients require an ambient temperature that would feel too warm to a younger person. If that patient's environment is slightly cool, even a temperature that might feel quite comfortable to you, consider hypothermia.

Remember that the injured patient is more susceptible to the effects of cold. Protect the patient who is entrapped or for any other reason must remain in a cool or cold environment for a period of time. The major course of action is to prevent additional body heat loss. It may be neither practical nor possible to replace wet clothing, but you can at least create a barrier to the cold with blankets, a salvage cover, an aluminized blanket, a survival blanket, or even articles of clothing. A plastic trash bag can serve as protection from wind and water. Keep in mind that the greatest area of heat loss may be the head. Provide some sort of head covering for the patient.

When the patient's injuries allow, place a blanket between his body and the cold ground. Rotate warm blankets from the heated ambulance to the patient. If the patient will remain trapped for a period of time, plug holes in the wreckage with blankets.

Patient *ASSESSMENT*

Hypothermia

Consider the impact of the following factors: air temperature, wind chill and/or water chill, the patient's age, the patient's clothing, health of the patient including underlying illness and existing injuries, how active the patient was during exposure, and possible alcohol or drug use.

The signs and symptoms of hypothermia include the following. Note that decreasing mental status and decreasing motor function both correlate with the degree of hypothermia.

- Shivering in early stages when core body temperature is above 90°F. In severe cases shivering decreases or is absent.
- Numbness, or reduced-to-lost sense of touch
- Stiff or rigid posture in prolonged cases
- Drowsiness and/or unwillingness or inability to do even the simplest activities. In prolonged cases, the patient may become irrational, drift into a stuporous state, or actually remove clothing.
- Rapid breathing and rapid pulse in early stages. Slow to absent breathing and pulse in prolonged cases. Blood pressure may be low to absent.
- Loss of motor coordination, such as staggering or inability to hold things
- Joint/muscle stiffness, or muscular rigidity
- Decreased level of consciousness, or unconsciousness. In extreme cases, the patient has a "glassy stare."
- Cool abdominal skin temperature. (Place the back of your hand inside the clothing and against the patient's abdomen.)
- Skin may appear red in early stages. In prolonged cases, skin is pale to cyanotic. In most extreme cases, some body parts are stiff and hard (frozen).

During initial assessment, be sure to check an awake patient's orientation to person, place, and time. (Can he tell you his name? Where he is? What day it is?) Perform a focused history and physical exam to help you estimate the extent of hypothermia. Assume severe hypothermia if shivering is absent.

Passive and Active Rewarming

Passive rewarming allows the body to rewarm itself. It involves simply covering the patient and taking other steps, including removal of wet clothing, to prevent further heat loss, allowing the body to rewarm itself. **Active rewarming** includes application of an external heat source to the body. All EMS systems permit passive rewarming. Some allow the active rewarming of a hypothermic patient who is alert and responding appropriately. Many do not. Follow local protocols.

Active rewarming can prove to be a dangerous process if the patient's condition is more serious than believed. If you are allowed to rewarm a patient with hypothermia who is alert and responding appropriately, do not delay transport. Rewarm the patient while en route. *The emergency care steps listed below and on the next page assume a protocol that permits active rewarming of a patient who is alert and responding appropriately. Follow your local protocols.*

● Patient *CARE*

Hypothermic Patient Alert and Responding Appropriately

For the hypothermic patient who is alert and responding appropriately, proceed with active rewarming:

1. Remove all of the patient's wet clothing. Keep the patient dry, dress the patient in dry clothing, or wrap in dry warm blankets. Keep the patient still and handle very gently. Do not allow the patient to walk or exert himself. Do not massage extremities.

2. During transport, actively rewarm the patient. Gently apply heat to the patient's body in the form of heat packs, hot water bottles, electric heating pads, warm air, radiated heat, and even your own body heat. *Do not warm the patient too quickly.* Rapid warming will circulate peripherally stagnated cold blood and rapidly cool the vital central areas of the body, possibly causing cardiac arrest. If transport is delayed, move the patient to a warm environment if at all possible.

3. Provide care for shock. Provide oxygen, warmed and humidified if possible.

4. Give the alert patient warm liquids slowly. When warm fluids are given too quickly, circulation patterns change, sending blood away from the core to the skin and extremities. Do not allow the patient to eat or drink stimulants.

5. Except in the mildest of cases (shivering), transport the patient. Continue to provide high-concentration oxygen and monitor vital signs. *Never allow a patient to remain in, or return to, a cold environment.*

Take the following precautions when actively rewarming a patient:

- Rewarm the patient slowly. Handle the patient with great care, just as if there were unstabilized cervical-spine injuries.
- Use **central rewarming.** Heat should be applied to the lateral chest, neck, armpits, and groin. You must avoid rewarming the limbs. If they are warmed first, blood will collect in the extremities due to vasodilation (dilation of blood vessels) and cause a fatal form of shock (see

Chapter 26, "Bleeding and Shock"). If you rewarm the trunk and leave the lower extremities exposed, you can control the rewarming process and help prevent most of the problems associated with the procedure.

- If transport must be delayed, a warm bath is very helpful, but keep the patient alert enough so that he does not drown. Do not warm the patient too quickly.
- Keep the patient at rest. Do not allow the patient to walk, and avoid rough handling. Such activity may set off severe heart problems, including ventricular fibrillation. Since the blood is coldest in the extremities, exercise or unnecessary movement could quickly circulate the cold blood and lower the core body temperature.

Patient *CARE*

Hypothermic Patient Unresponsive or not Responding Appropriately

A patient who is unresponsive or not responding appropriately has severe hypothermia. For this patient, provide passive rewarming. Do not try to actively rewarm the patient with severe hypothermia. Remove the patient from the environment and protect him from further heat loss. Active rewarming may cause the patient to develop ventricular fibrillation.

For the patient with severe hypothermia, you should:

1. Assure an open airway.

2. Provide high-concentration oxygen that has been passed through a warm-water humidifier. If necessary, the oxygen that has been kept warm in the ambulance passenger compartment can be used. If there is no other choice, oxygen from a cold cylinder may be used.

3. Wrap the patient in blankets. If available, use insulating blankets. Handle the patient as gently as possible. Rough handling may cause ventricular fibrillation. Do not allow the patient to eat or drink stimulants. Do not massage extremities.

4. Transport immediately.

Extreme Hypothermia

In extreme cases of hypothermia, you will find the patient unconscious with no discernible vital signs. The heart rate can slow to less than 10 beats per minute, and the patient will feel very cold to your touch (core body temperature may be below 80°F). Even so, it is possible that the patient is still alive! Provide emergency care as follows:

- Assess the carotid pulse for 30–45 seconds. If there is no pulse, start CPR immediately and prepare to apply the AED.
- If there is a pulse, follow the care steps for a patient who is unresponsive or not responding appropriately as listed above.

Because the hypothermic patient may not reach biological death for over 30 minutes, the hospital staff will not pronounce a patient dead until after he is rewarmed and resuscitative measures applied. This means you cannot assume that a severe hypothermia patient is dead on the basis of body temperature and lack of vital signs. As medical personnel point out, "You're not dead until you're warm and dead!"

Localized Cold Injuries

Cold-related emergencies also can result from **local cooling.** Local cooling injuries are those affecting particular (local) parts of the body. Localized cold injuries are classified as early or superficial, and late or deep.

Local cooling most commonly affects the ears, nose, face, hands, and the feet and toes. When a part of the body is exposed to intense cold, blood flow to that part is limited by the constriction of blood vessels. When this happens, tissues freeze. Ice crystals can form in the skin, and in the most severe cases, gangrene (localized tissue death) can set in and ultimately lead to the loss of the body part.

As you read the following pages, notice how the signs and symptoms of early or superficial cold injuries are progressive. First, the exposed skin reddens in light-skinned individuals, or in dark-skinned individuals the skin color lightens and approaches a blanched (reduced-color or whitened) condition. As exposure continues, the skin takes on a gray or white blotchy appearance. Exposed skin becomes numb because of reduced circulation. If the freezing process continues, all sensation is lost and the skin becomes dead white.

Patient *ASSESSMENT*

Early or Superficial Local Cold Injury

Early or superficial local cold injuries (sometimes called frostnip) are brought about by direct contact with a cold object or exposure to cold air. Wind chill and water chill also can be major factors. Tissue damage is minor and response to care is good. The tip of the nose, tips of the ears, upper cheeks, and fingers (all areas that are usually exposed) are most susceptible to early or superficial local cold injuries. The injury, as its name suggests, is localized with clear demarcation of its limits. Patients are often unaware of the onset of an early local cold injury until someone indicates that there is something unusual about the person's skin color. Signs and symptoms include:

- Affected area in patients with light skin reddens; dark skin lightens. Both then blanch (whiten). Once blanching begins, the color change can take place very quickly.
- Affected area feels numb to the patient.

Figure 22-1 Local cold injuries.

Patient CARE

Early or Superficial Local Cold Injury

Emergency care for early local cold injury is as follows:

1. Get the patient out of the cold environment.

2. Warm the affected area.

3. If the injury is to an extremity, splint and cover it. Do not rub or massage, and do not re-expose to the cold.

Usually, the patient can apply warmth from his own bare hands, blow warm air on the site, or if the fingers are involved, hold them in the armpits. During recovery from an early local cold injury, the patient may complain about tingling or burning sensations, which is normal. If the condition does not respond to this simple care, begin to treat for a late or deep local cold injury.

Patient ASSESSMENT

Late or Deep Local Cold Injury

Late or deep local cold injury (also known as *frostbite*) develops if an early or superficial local cold injury goes untreated. In late or deep local cold injury, the skin and subcutaneous layers of the body part are affected. Muscles, bones, deep blood vessels, and organ membranes can become frozen. Signs and symptoms include:

- Affected skin appears white and waxy. When the condition progresses to actual freezing, the skin turns mottled or blotchy, the color turns from white to grayish yellow and finally to grayish blue. Swelling and blistering may occur (Figure 22-1).
- Affected area feels frozen, but only on the surface. The tissue below the surface is still soft and has its normal resilience, or "bounce." With freezing, the tissues are not resilient and feel frozen to the touch. (**Note:** Do not squeeze or poke the tissue. The condition of the deeper tissues can be determined by feeling gently. Do the assessment as if the affected area had a fractured bone.)

Patient CARE

Late or Deep Local Cold Injury

Initial emergency care for late or deep local cold injury—frostbite and freezing—is as follows:

1. Administer high-concentration oxygen.

2. Transport to a medical facility without delay, protecting the frostbitten or frozen area by covering it and handling it as gently as possible.

3. If transport must be delayed, get the patient indoors and keep him warm. Do not allow the patient to drink alcohol or smoke, because constriction of blood vessels and decreased circulation to the injured tissues may result. Rewarm the frozen part as per local protocol, or request instructions from medical direction.

Note

Never listen to myths and folktales about the care of frostbite. Never rub a frostbitten or frozen area. Never rub snow on a frostbitten or frozen area. There are ice crystals at the capillary level; rubbing the injury site may cause them to seriously damage the already injured tissues. Do not break blisters or massage the injured area. Do not allow the patient to walk on an affected extremity. *Do not thaw a frozen limb if there is any chance it will be refrozen.*

Active Rapid Rewarming of Frozen Parts

Active rewarming of frozen parts is seldom recommended. The chance of permanently injuring frozen tissues with active rewarming is too great. Consider it only if local protocols recommend it, if you are instructed to do so by medical direction, or if transport will be severely delayed and you cannot reach medical direction for instructions. If you are in a situation where you must attempt rewarming without instructions from a physician, follow the procedure described here.

You will need warm water and a container in which you can immerse the entire site of injury without the limb touching the sides or bottom of the container. If you cannot find a suitable container, fashion one from a plastic bag supported by a cardboard box or wooden crate (Figure 22-2). Proceed as follows:

1. Heat water to between 100°F and 105°F. You should be able to put your finger into the water without experiencing discomfort.

2. Fill the container with the heated water and prepare the injured part by removing clothing, jewelry, bands, or straps.

3. Fully immerse the injured part. Do not allow the injured area to touch the sides or bottom of the

container. Do not place any pressure on the affected part. Continuously stir the water. When the water cools below 100°F, remove the affected part and add more warm water. The patient may complain of moderate pain as the affected area rewarms or he may experience intense pain. Pain is usually a good indicator of successful rewarming.

4. If you complete rewarming of the part (it no longer feels frozen and is turning red or blue), gently dry the affected area and apply a dry sterile dressing. Place dry sterile dressings between fingers and toes before dressing hands and feet. Next, cover the site with blankets or whatever is available to keep the area warm. Do not allow these coverings to come in direct contact with the injured area or to put pressure on the site. First try to build some sort of framework on which the coverings can be placed.

5. Keep the patient at rest. Do not allow the patient to walk if a lower extremity has been frostbitten or frozen.

6. Make certain that you keep the entire patient as warm as possible without overheating. Cover the patient's head with a towel or small blanket to reduce heat loss. Leave the patient's face exposed.

7. Continue to monitor the patient.

8. Assist circulation according to local protocol (some systems recommend rhythmically and carefully raising and lowering the affected limb).

9. Do not allow the limb to refreeze.

10. Transport as soon as possible with the affected limb slightly elevated.

EXPOSURE TO HEAT

Effects of Heat on the Body

The body generates heat as a result of its constant internal chemical processes. A certain amount of this heat is required to maintain normal body temperature. Any heat that is not needed for temperature maintenance must be lost from the body. If it is not, **hyperthermia,** an abnormally high body temperature, will be the result. Left unchecked, it will lead to death. Heat and humidity are often associated with hyperthermia.

As you learned earlier, heat is lost through the lungs or the skin. Mechanisms of heat loss include conduction, convection, radiation, evaporation, and respiration. Consider what can happen to the body in a hot environment. Air being inhaled is warm, possibly warmer than the air being exhaled. The skin may absorb more heat than it loses. When high humidity is added, the evaporation of perspiration slows. To

Figure 22-2   Rewarming the frozen part.

make things even more difficult, consider all this in an environment that lacks circulating air or a breeze, which would increase convection and evaporative heat loss.

Since evaporative heat loss is reduced in a humid environment, moist heat can produce dramatic body changes in a short time. Moist heat usually tires people quickly, frequently stopping them from harming themselves through overexertion. Dry heat, on the other hand, often deceives people. They continue to work or remain exposed to excess heat far beyond what their bodies can tolerate. This is why you may see problems caused by dry heat exposure more often than those seen in moist heat exposure.

The same rules of care apply to heat emergencies as to any other emergency. You will need to perform the appropriate steps of assessment, remaining alert for problems other than those related to heat. Collapse due to heat exposure, for example, may result in a fall that can fracture bones. Pre-existing conditions such as dehydration, diabetes, fever, fatigue, high blood pressure, heart disease, lung problems, or obesity may hasten or intensify the effects of heat exposure, as will ingestion of alcohol and other drugs.

Age, diseases, and existing injuries all must be considered. The elderly may be affected by poor thermoregulation, prescription medications, and lack of mobility. Newborns and infants also may have poor thermoregulation. Always consider the problem to be greater if the patient is a child or elderly, injured or living with a chronic disease.

Patient with Moist, Pale, Normal-to-Cool Skin

Prolonged exposure to excessive heat can create an emergency in which the patient presents with moist pale skin that may feel normal or cool to the touch. The individual perspires heavily, often drinking large quantities of water. As sweating continues, salts are lost, bringing on painful muscle cramps (sometimes called *heat cramps*). A person who is actively exercising can lose more than a liter of perspiration per hour.

Healthy individuals who have been exposed to excessive heat while working or exercising may experience a form of shock brought about by fluid and salt loss. It is often seen among firefighters, construction workers, dock workers, and those employed in poorly ventilated warehouses. It is a particular problem during prolonged heat waves. This condition is sometimes known as *heat exhaustion*.

Patient ASSESSMENT

Heat Emergency Patient with Moist, Pale, Normal-to-Cool Skin

Signs and symptoms of a heat emergency patient with moist, pale, and normal-to-cool skin include:

- Muscular cramps, usually in the legs and abdomen
- Weakness or exhaustion, sometimes dizziness or periods of faintness
- Rapid, shallow breathing
- Weak pulse
- Heavy perspiration
- Loss of consciousness is possible

Patient CARE

Heat Emergency Patient with Moist, Pale, Normal-to-Cool Skin

Emergency care of a heat emergency patient with moist, pale, and normal-to-cool skin includes the following:

1. Remove the patient from the hot environment and place in a cool environment (such as in shade or an air-conditioned ambulance).

2. Administer oxygen by nonrebreather mask at 15 liters per minute.

3. Loosen or remove clothing to cool the patient by fanning without chilling him. Watch for shivering.

4. Put patient in a supine position with legs elevated. Keep him at rest.

5. If the patient is responsive and not nauseated, have him drink water. If the patient is unresponsive or vomiting, transport to the hospital with patient on his left side.

6. If patient experiences muscular cramps, apply moist towels over cramped muscles.

7. Transport.

Patient with Hot, Dry or Moist Skin

When a person's temperature-regulating mechanisms fail and the body cannot rid itself of excessive heat, you will see a patient with hot, dry, or possibly moist skin. When the skin is hot—whether dry or moist—this is a true emergency. It is a condition that is sometimes known as heat stroke. The problem is compounded when, in response to loss of fluid and salt, the patient stops sweating, which prevents heat loss through evaporation. Athletes, laborers, and others who exercise or work in hot environments commonly develop this condition. So do the elderly who live in poorly ventilated apartments without air conditioning, and children left in cars with the windows rolled up. More cases of patients with hot, dry skin are reported on hot, humid days. However, many cases occur from exposure to dry heat.

Patient ASSESSMENT

Heat Emergency Patient with Hot, Dry or Moist Skin

Signs and symptoms of a heat emergency patient with hot and dry or hot and moist skin include:

- Rapid, shallow breathing
- Full and rapid pulse
- Generalized weakness
- Little or no perspiration
- Loss of consciousness or altered mental status
- Dilated pupils
- Seizures may be seen; no muscle cramps

Patient CARE

Heat Emergency Patient with Hot, Dry or Moist Skin

Emergency care of a heat emergency patient with hot and dry or hot and moist skin is as follows (Figure 22-3):

1. Remove the patient from the hot environment and place in a cool environment (in the ambulance with air conditioner running on high).

2. Remove clothing. Apply cool packs to neck, groin, and armpits. Keep the skin wet by applying water by sponge or wet towels. Fan aggressively.

3. Administer oxygen by nonrebreather mask at 15 liters per minute.

4. Transport immediately. Should transport be delayed, find a tub or container, immerse the patient up to the neck in cooled water, and monitor vital signs throughout process.

Pediatric Notes

For infants or young children, cooling is started using tepid (lukewarm) water. This

Figure 22-3 In heat-emergency cases where the patient's skin is hot (and either dry or moist), cool aggressively.

water can then be replaced with cooler water at the recommendation of medical direction.

Beware of what you are told by some patients. They may not believe heat emergencies are serious. Many simply want to return to work. Nevertheless, conduct a thorough initial assessment plus a focused history and physical exam. If you have any doubts, tell the patient why he should be transported and seek his permission to do so. You may have to spend a little time with some patients to gain their confidence.

WATER-RELATED EMERGENCIES

Water-Related Accidents

Drowning or near-drowning is the first thing people think of in connection with water-related accidents. However, there are many types of injuries resulting from many types of accidents that can occur on or in the water. Boating, water-skiing, wind surfing, jet-skiing, diving, and scuba-diving accidents can produce fractured bones, bleeding, soft-tissue injuries, and airway obstruction. Even auto collisions can send vehicles or passengers into the water, resulting in any of the injuries usually associated with motor vehicle collisions as well as the complications caused by the presence of water.

Medical problems such as heart attacks can also cause or be caused by water accidents or can simply take place in, on, or near the water. Remember, too, that some water accidents happen far away from pools, lakes, or beaches. Bathtub drownings do occur. Adults, as well as children, can drown in only a few inches of water.

Safety Note

Do not attempt a rescue in which you must enter deep water or swim, unless you have been trained to do so and are a very good swimmer. Except for shallow pools and open shallow waters with uniform bottoms, the problems faced in water rescue are too great and too dangerous for the poor swimmer or untrained person. If this bothers you— having to stand by, not being able to help—then take a course in water safety and rescue. Otherwise, if you attempt a deep water or swimming rescue, you will probably become a victim yourself.

Patient ASSESSMENT

Water-Related Accidents

Learn to look for the following problems in water-related-accident patients:

- *Airway obstruction.* This may be from water in the lungs, foreign matter in the airway, or swollen airway tissues (common if the neck is injured in a dive). Spasms along the airway may be present in cases of near-drowning.
- *Cardiac arrest.* This is often related to respiratory arrest or occurs before the near-drowning.
- *Signs of heart attack.* Some untrained rescuers too quickly conclude that chest pains are due to muscle cramps as a result of swimming.
- *Injuries to the head and neck.* These are expected to be found in boating, water-skiing, and diving accidents, but they are also very common in swimming accidents.
- *Internal injuries.* While doing the focused physical exam, stay on the alert for musculoskeletal injuries, soft-tissue injuries, and internal bleeding.
- *Generalized cooling, or hypothermia.* The water does not have to be very cold and the length of stay in the water does not have to be very long for hypothermia to occur.
- *Substance abuse.* Alcohol and drug use are closely associated with adolescent and adult drownings. Elevated blood alcohol levels have been found in over 30% of drowning victims. The screening for drug use has not been as extensive as that done for alcohol, but research indicates that other drugs are a contributory factor in many water-related accidents.

- *Drowning or near-drowning.* The patient may be discovered under or face down in the water. He may be unconscious and without discernible vital signs or may be conscious, breathing, and coughing up water.

Provide assessment and care for any of the above problems as you have learned in relevant chapters of this text. Drowning and near-drowning are discussed in detail, below.

Drowning and Near-Drowning

The process of drowning begins as a person struggles to keep afloat in the water. He gulps in large breaths of air as he thrashes about. When he can no longer keep afloat and starts to submerge, he tries to take and hold one more deep breath. As he does, water may enter the airway. There is a series of coughing and swallowing actions, and the victim involuntarily inhales and swallows more water. As water flows past the epiglottis, it triggers a reflex spasm of the larynx. This spasm seals the airway so effectively that no more than a small amount of water reaches the lungs. Unconsciousness soon results from hypoxia (oxygen starvation).

About 10% of the people who drown die just from the lack of air. In the remaining victims, the person attempts a final respiratory effort and draws water into the lungs, or the spasms subside with the onset of unconsciousness and water freely enters the lungs.

As an EMT-B, you should start using the term **near-drowning.** Obviously, if the patient is breathing and coughing up water, he has not drowned but has nearly drowned. This is only part of what we mean by near-drowning. If a patient has "drowned" in lay person's terms, he is not necessarily biologically dead. Resuscitation efforts may keep the patient biologically alive long enough for more advanced measures to save the patient's life.

Only when sufficient time has passed to render resuscitation useless has **drowning** truly taken place. Some patients in cold water can be resuscitated after 30 minutes or more in cardiac arrest. Once the water temperature falls below 70°F, biological death may be delayed. The colder the water, the better are the patient's chances for survival, unless generalized hypothermia produces lethal complications.

Rescue Breathing In or Out of the Water
Transport for the near-drowning patient should not be delayed. You may initiate care when the patient is out of the water (already out when you arrive or in the water when you arrive but rescued by others before you initiate care). At other times you may need to be able to initiate care while the patient is still in

the water—especially rescue breathing and immobilization for possible spine injuries. Chest compressions will be effective only after the patient is out of the water.

If needed, rescue breathing should begin without delay. If you can reach the nonbreathing patient in the water, provide ventilations as you support him in a semi-supine position. Continue providing ventilations while the patient is being immobilized and removed from the water. If the patient is already out of the water, begin rescue breathing or CPR on the land.

You may find resistance as you ventilate the near-drowning patient. You will probably have to ventilate more forcefully than you would other patients. Remember, you must provide air to the patient's lungs as soon as possible.

A patient with water in the lungs usually has water in the stomach, which will add resistance to your efforts to provide rescue breathing or CPR ventilations. Since the patient may have spasms along the airway, or swollen tissues in the larynx or trachea, you may find that some of the air you provide will go into the patient's stomach. Remember, the same problem will occur if you do not properly open the airway or if your ventilations are too forceful.

If gastric distention interferes with artificial ventilation, place the patient on his left side. With suction immediately available, the EMT-B should place his hand over the epigastric area of the abdomen and apply firm pressure to relieve the distention. This procedure should be done only if the gastric distention interferes with the EMT-B's efforts to artificially ventilate the patient effectively.

Safety Note

Unless you are a very good swimmer and trained in water rescue, do not go into the water to save someone. Such training is available from the American Red Cross and the YMCA in the form of water safety and rescue courses.

Care for Possible Spinal Injuries in the Water

Injuries to the cervical spine are seen with many water-related accidents. Most often, these injuries are received during a dive or when the patient is struck by a boat, skier or ski, surfer or surfboard. Even though cervical-spine injuries are the most common of the spine injuries seen in water-related accidents, there can be injury anywhere along the spine.

In water-related accidents, assume that the unconscious patient has neck and spinal injuries. Should the patient have head injuries, also assume that there are neck and spinal injuries. Keep in mind that a patient found in respiratory or cardiac arrest will need resuscitation started before you can immobilize the neck and spine. Also, realize that you may not be able to carry out a complete assessment for spinal injuries while the patient is in the water. Take care to avoid aggravating spinal injuries, but do not delay basic life support. Do not delay removing the patient from the water if the scene presents an immediate danger. When possible, keep the patient's neck rigid and in a straight line with the body's midline (Scan 22-1). Use the jaw-thrust maneuver to open the airway.

If the patient with possible spinal injuries is still in the water, you are a good swimmer, and you are able to aid in the rescue, secure the patient to a long spine board before removing him from the water. This will help prevent permanent neurological damage or paralysis. This type of rescue requires special training in the use of the spine board while in the water. This rigid device can "pop up" very easily from below the water surface. Make certain that you know how to control the board and how to work in the water.

● Patient *CARE*

Water-Related Accidents

In all cases of water-related accidents, assume that the unconscious patient has neck and spinal injuries. If the patient is rescued by others while you wait on shore, or if the patient is out of the water when you arrive, you should:

1. Do an initial assessment, protecting the spine as much as possible.

2. Provide rescue breathing. If there is no pulse, begin CPR and prepare to apply the AED. Protect yourself by using a pocket face mask with a one-way valve or bag-valve-mask unit.

3. Look for and control profuse bleeding. Since the patient's heart rate may have slowed down, take a pulse for 60 seconds in all cold-water rescue situations before concluding that the patient is in cardiac arrest.

4. Provide care for shock (as described in Chapter 26), administer a high concentration of oxygen, and transport the patient as soon as possible.

5. Continue resuscitative measures throughout transport. Initial and periodic suctioning may be needed.

The near-drowning patient receiving rescue breathing or CPR should be transported as soon as possible. If resuscitation and immediate transport are not required, cover the patient to conserve body heat and complete a focused history and physical exam.

WATER RESCUE
WITH POSSIBLE SPINAL INJURY

SAFETY NOTE Unless you are a very good swimmer and trained in water rescue, do not go into the water to save someone.

HEAD-CHIN SUPPORT

TWO RESCUERS IN SHALLOW WATER

▲ When there are two rescuers present, perform the head-chin support technique to provide in-line stabilization of a patient in shallow water.

HEAD-SPLINT SUPPORT

ONE RESCUER IN SHALLOW WATER

▲ **1.** When you find a patient face down in shallow water, position yourself alongside the patient.

▲ **2.** Extend the patient's arms straight up alongside his or her head to create a splint.

▲ **3.** Begin to rotate the torso toward you.

▲ **4.** As you rotate the patient, lower yourself into the water.

▲ **5.** Maintain manual stabilization by holding the patient's head between his arms.

(continued)

HEAD-CHIN SUPPORT TECHNIQUE

ONE RESCUER IN DEEP WATER

▲ **1.** When you find a patient face down in deep water, position yourself beside him. Support his head with one hand and his mandible with the other.

▲ **2.** Then rotate the patient by ducking under him.

▲ **3.** Continue to rotate until the patient is face up.

▲ **4.** Maintain in-line stabilization until a backboard is used to immobilize the patient's spine.

Uncover only those areas of the patient's body involved with the stage of the assessment. Care for any problems or injuries detected during the assessment in the order of their priority.

If spinal injury is not suspected, place the patient on his left side to allow water, vomit, and other secretions to drain from the upper airway. Suction as needed. When transport is delayed and you believe that the patient can be moved to a warmer place, do so without aggravating any existing injuries. Do not allow the near-drowning patient to walk. Transport the patient.

Information supplied to the dispatcher or to the hospital from the scene and during transport is critical in cases of near-drowning. The hospital emergency department staff needs to know if this is a fresh- or salt-water drowning, if it took place in cold or warm water, and if it is related to a diving accident. You may be asked to transport the patient to a special facility or to a center having a hyperbaric chamber when decompression therapy is needed.

Diving Accidents

Water-related accidents often involve injuries that occur when individuals attempt dives or enter the water from diving boards. In the majority of these accidents, the patient is a teenager. Basically the same types of injuries are seen in dives taken from diving boards, poolsides, docks, boats, and the shore. The injury may be due to the diver striking the board or some object on or under the water. From great heights, injury may result from impact with the water.

Most diving accidents involve the head and neck, but you will also find injuries to the spine, hands, feet, and ribs in many cases. Any part of the body can be injured depending on the position that the diver is in when he strikes the water or an object. This means that you must perform an initial assessment. You must also perform a focused history and physical exam on all diving accident patients. Do not overlook the fact that a medical emergency may have led to the diving accident.

Emergency care for diving accident patients is the same as for any accident patient, if they are out of the water. Care provided in the water and during removal from the water is the same as for any patient who may have neck and spine injuries. Remember, assume that any unconscious or unresponsive patient has neck and spinal injuries.

SCUBA DIVING ACCIDENTS

Scuba (self-contained underwater breathing apparatus) diving accidents have increased with the popularity of the sport, especially since many untrained and inexperienced persons are attempting dives. Today, there are more than 2 million people who scuba dive for sport or as part of their industrial or military job. Added to this are a large number who decide to "try it one time," without the benefits of lessons or supervision. Well-trained divers seldom have problems. Those with inadequate training place themselves at great risk.

Scuba diving accidents include all types of body injuries and near-drownings. In many cases, the scuba diving accident was brought about by medical problems that existed prior to the dive. There are two special problems seen in scuba diving accidents. They are air emboli in the diver's blood and decompression sickness.

An **air embolism**—more accurately called arterial gas embolism (AGE)—is the result of gases leaving a damaged lung and entering the bloodstream. Severe damage may lead to a collapsed lung. Air emboli (gas bubbles in the blood) are most often associated with divers who hold their breath because of inadequate training, equipment failure, underwater emergency, or when trying to conserve air during a dive. However, a diver may develop an air embolism in very shallow water (as little as 4 feet). An automobile-collision victim also may suffer an air embolism if, when trapped below water, he takes gulps of air from air pockets held inside the vehicle. When freed, the patient may develop air emboli the same as a scuba diver.

Decompression sickness is usually caused when a diver comes up too quickly from a deep, prolonged dive. The quick ascent causes nitrogen gas to be trapped in the body tissues and then in the bloodstream. Decompression sickness in scuba divers takes from 1 to 48 hours to appear, with about 90% of cases occurring within 3 hours of the dive. Divers increase the risk of decompression sickness if they fly within 12 hours of a dive. Because of this delay, carefully consider all information gathered from the patient interview and reports from the patient's family and friends. This information may provide the only clues relating the patient's problems to a scuba dive.

The signs and symptoms of scuba diving problems may include the following:

Air Embolism (rapid onset of signs and symptoms)
- Blurred vision
- Chest pains
- Numbness and tingling sensations in the extremities

- Generalized or specific weakness, possible paralysis
- Frothy blood in mouth or nose
- Convulsions
- Rapid lapse into unconsciousness
- Respiratory arrest and cardiac arrest

Decompression Sickness
- Personality changes
- Fatigue
- Deep pain to the muscles and joints (the "bends")
- Itchy blotches or mottling of the skin
- Numbness or paralysis
- Choking
- Coughing
- Labored breathing
- Behavior similar to intoxication (such as staggering)
- Chest pains
- Collapse leading to unconsciousness
- Skin rashes that keep changing in appearance (in some cases)

For a patient with signs and symptoms of either air embolism or decompression sickness, follow the same emergency care steps:

1. Maintain an open airway.

2. Administer the highest possible concentration of oxygen by nonrebreather mask.

Figure 22-4   Proper positioning of a scuba diving accident patient.

3. Rapidly transport all patients with possible air emboli or decompression sickness.

4. Contact medical direction for specific instructions concerning where to take the patient. You may be sent directly to a hyperbaric trauma care center.

5. Keep the patient warm.

6. Position the patient either supine or on either side (Figure 22-4). Continue to monitor the patient. You may have to reposition the patient to ensure an open airway.

The Diver Alert Network (DAN) was formed to assist rescuers with the care of underwater diving accident patients. The staff, which is available on a 24-hour basis, can be reached by phoning (919) 684-8111. Collect calls will be accepted for actual emergencies. DAN can give you or your dispatcher information on assessment and care and how to transfer the patient to a hyperbaric trauma care center. (A hyperbaric trauma care center is one that has a special pressure chamber for treatment of such conditions.) For nonemergencies, call (919) 684-2948.

Note: The well-trained scuba diver makes use of a preplanned dive chart. The dive chart, if it is available, may provide you with useful information concerning the nature and duration of the dive. This chart must be transported with the patient.

WATER RESCUES

The following is the order of procedures for a water rescue (Figure 22-5), most of which can be performed short of going into the water: *reach, throw and tow, row, go.*

- *Reach.* When the patient is responsive and close to shore or poolside, try to reach him by holding out an object for him to grab. Then pull him from the water. Make sure your position is secure. Line (rope) is considered the best choice. If no line is available, use a branch, fishing rod, oar, stick, or other such object, even a towel, blanket, or article of clothing. If no object is available or you have only one opportunity to grab the person (e.g., in strong currents), position yourself flat on your stomach and extend your hand or leg to the patient (not recommended for the nonswimmer). Again, make certain that you are working from a secure position.

- *Throw and tow.* Should the person be conscious and alert but too far away for you to reach and pull from the water, throw an object that will float (Figure 22-6). A personal flotation device (PFD or lifejacket) or ring buoy (life preserver) works best. Other buoyant objects include foam cushions, logs, plastic picnic containers, surf boards, flat boards, large beach balls, and plastic toys. Two empty, capped, plastic milk jugs can keep an adult afloat for hours. Inflatable splints can be used if there is nothing at the scene that will float.

Once the conscious patient has a flotation device, try to find a way to tow him to shore. From a safe position, throw the patient a line or another flotation device attached to a line. If you are a good swimmer and you know how to judge the water, wade out no deeper than waist high, wear a personal flotation device, and have a safety line that is secured on shore.

- *Row.* When the patient is too far from shore to allow for throwing and towing, or is unresponsive, you may be able to row a boat to the patient. Do not attempt to row to the patient if you cannot swim. Even if you are a good swimmer, wearing a per-

Reach

Throw and Tow

Row

Figure 22-5 First try to *reach* and pull the patient from the water. If that fails, *throw* him anything that will float and *tow* him from the water. If that fails, *row* to the patient.

sonal flotation device while in the boat is required.

If the patient is conscious, tell him to grab an oar or the stern (rear end) of the boat. You must exercise great care when helping the patient into the boat. This is even trickier when you are in a canoe. Should the canoe tip over, stay with it and hold onto its bottom and side. Most canoes will stay afloat.

• *Go.* As a last resort, when all other means have failed, you can go into the water and swim to the patient. You must be a good swimmer, trained in water rescue and lifesaving. Untrained rescuers can become victims themselves.

ICE RESCUES

Every winter people fall through ice while skating or attempting to cross an ice-covered body of water. Often, the scene becomes a multiple-rescue problem as individuals try to reach the victim and also fall

Figure 22-6 Throw the patient any object that will float.

through the ice. The number-one rule in ice rescue is to protect yourself. Formal ice rescue training is available. A cold-water submersion suit and personal flotation device should be worn during any ice rescue attempt (Figure 22-7).

There are several ways in which you can reach a patient who has fallen through ice:

• Flotation devices can be thrown to the patient.

• A rope in which a loop has been formed can be tossed to the patient. He can put the loop around his body so that he can be pulled onto the ice and away from the danger area.

• A small, flat-bottomed aluminum boat is probably the best device for an ice rescue. It can be pushed stern (rear end) first by other rescuers and pulled to safety by a rope secured to the bow (front end). The primary rescuer will remain dry and safe should the ice break. The patient can be pulled from the water or allowed to

Figure 22-7 Safe ice rescues require proper equipment.

grasp the side of the boat, although he may be unable to grasp or to hold on for long.

• A ladder is an effective tool often used in ice rescue. It can be laid flat and pushed to the patient, then pulled back by an attached rope. The ladder also can serve as a surface on which a rescuer can spread out his weight if he must go onto the ice to reach the patient. The ladder should have a line that can be secured by a rescuer in a safe position. Any rescuer on the ladder should have a safety line.

Remember that the patient may not be able to do much to help in the rescue process. Hypothermia may interfere with his mental and physical capabilities in a matter of minutes.

Whenever possible, do not work alone when trying to perform an ice rescue. If you must work alone, do not walk out onto the ice. Never go onto ice that is rapidly breaking. Never enter the water through a hole in the ice in order to find the victim. Your best course of action will be to work with others, from a safe ice

surface or the shore. When there is no other choice, you and your fellow rescuers can elect to form a human chain to reach the patient. However, this is not the safest method to employ, even when all the rescuers are wearing personal flotation devices and using safety lines.

Expect to find injuries to most patients who have fallen through the ice. Treat for hypothermia according to local protocols and treat for any injuries. Transport all patients who have fallen through ice.

BITES AND STINGS

Insect Bites and Stings

Insect stings, spider bites, and scorpion stings are typical sources of injected poisons, or toxins—substances produced by animals or plants that are poisonous to humans. (**Venom** is a term for a toxin produced by some animals such as snakes, spiders, and certain marine life forms.) Commonly seen insect stings are those of wasps, hornets, bees, and ants. Insect stings and bites are rarely dangerous. However, 5% of the population of the U. S. will have an allergic reaction, which may result in shock. Those who are hypersensitive develop severe anaphylactic shock that is quickly life threatening (see Chapter 20, "Allergic Reactions").

All spiders are poisonous, but most species cannot get their fangs through human skin. The black widow spider and the brown recluse, or fiddleback, spider (Figure 22-8) are two that can, and their bites can produce medical emergencies. Almost all brown recluse bites are painless, and patients seldom recall being bitten. The characteristic lesion appears in only 10% of cases, and then only after up to 12 hours (Figure 22-9). EMT-Bs are seldom called to respond to a brown recluse bite. Black widow bites cause a more immediate reaction.

Scorpion stings are common in the Southwest U.S. They do not ordinarily cause deaths, but one rare species (*centroroides exilcauda*) is dangerous to humans and can cause serious medical problems in children, including respiratory failure.

Note: Bites and stings belong in the class of injected poisons discussed in Chapter 21, "Poisoning and Overdose Emergencies."

A

B

Figure 22-8   (A) Black widow spider, and (B) a brown recluse spider.

Figure 22-9 Brown recluse spider bite.

Patient ASSESSMENT

Insect Bites and Stings

Gather information from the patient, bystanders, and the scene. Find out whatever you can about the insect or other possible source of the poisoning. The signs and symptoms of injected poisoning can include those listed below:

- Altered states of awareness
- Noticeable stings or bites on the skin
- Puncture marks (especially note the fingers, forearms, toes, and legs)
- Blotchy skin (mottled skin)
- Localized pain or itching
- Numbness in a limb or body part
- Burning sensations at the site followed by pain spreading throughout the limb
- Redness
- Swelling or blistering at the site
- Weakness or collapse
- Difficult breathing and abnormal pulse rate
- Headache and dizziness
- Chills
- Fever
- Nausea and vomiting
- Muscle cramps, chest tightening, joint pains
- Excessive saliva formation, profuse sweating
- Anaphylaxis

Patient CARE

Insect Bites and Stings

As an EMT-B, you are not expected to be able to identify insects and spiders. Proper identification of these organisms is best left to experts. If the problem has been caused by a creature that is known locally and is not normally dangerous (such as a bee, wasp, or puss caterpillar), the major concern will be anaphylactic shock. If anaphylactic shock does not develop, care is usually simple.

If the cause of the bite or sting is unknown, or the organism is unknown, the patient should be seen by a physician. Call medical direction or take the patient to a medical facility and let experts decide on the proper treatment for the patient. If possible, transport the stinging object or organism in a sealed container, taking care not to handle it without proper protection, even if it is dead. If you can accomplish this safely, you may save precious minutes needed to identify the toxin.

To provide emergency care for injected toxins:

1. Treat for shock, even if the patient does not present any of the signs of shock.

2. Call medical direction. Skip this only if the organism is known and your EMS system has a specific protocol for care.

3. To remove the stinger or venom sac, the traditional advice is to scrape the site with a blade or a card and to avoid pulling with tweezers which, it was thought, might squeeze more venom into the wound. However, recent research indicates that how you remove the stinger or venom sac is far less important than doing so quickly.

4. Remove jewelry from affected limbs in case the limb swells, which would make removal more difficult later.

5. If local protocol permits and if the wound is on an extremity (not a joint), place constricting bands above and below the sting or bite site. This is done to slow the spread of venom in the lymphatic vessels and superficial veins. The band should be made of ¾-inch to 1½-inch-wide soft rubber or other wide soft material. It should be placed about 2 inches from the wound. The band must be loose enough to slide a finger under it. It should not cut off circulation.

6. Keep the limb immobilized and the patient still to prevent distribution of the poison to other parts of the body. (Note: Some EMS systems recommend placing a cold compress on the wound. Most EMS systems do not use cold for any injected toxin. Follow local protocol.)

A

B

Figure 22-10 The pit vipers include (A) water moccasin, (B) rattlesnake, and (C) copperhead. The coral snake (D) is also poisonous.

Snakebites

Snakebites require special care but are usually not life threatening. Nearly 50,000 people in the U. S. are bitten by snakes each year. Over 8,000 of these cases involve poisonous snakes, but on the average fewer than 10 deaths are reported annually. (In the U. S., more people die each year from bee and wasp stings than from snakebites.) The signs and symptoms of snakebite poisoning may take several hours to appear. If death does result, it is usually not a rapidly occurring event unless anaphylactic shock develops. Most victims who die survive at least one to two days.

In the U. S. there are two types of native poisonous snakes—pit vipers (including rattlesnakes, copperheads, and water moccasins) and coral snakes (Figure 22-10). Up to 25% of pit viper bites and 50% of coral bites are "dry bites" without venom injection, but the venomous bite from a diamondback rattler or coral snake is considered very serious. Since each person reacts differently to snakebite, you should consider the bite from any known poisonous snake or any unidentified snake to be a serious emergency. Staying calm and keeping the patient calm and at rest is critical. Since reaction time is slow, there is time to transport the patient without haste.

Patient ASSESSMENT

Snakebite

Unless you are dealing with a known species of snake that is not considered poisonous, consider all snakebites to be from poisonous snakes. The patient

C

D

Figure 22-10 continued

or bystanders may say that the snake was not poisonous, but they could be mistaken. The signs and symptoms of snakebite may include the following:

- Noticeable bite on the skin. This may appear as nothing more than a discoloration.
- Pain and swelling in the area of the bite. This may be slow to develop, taking from 30 minutes to several hours.
- Rapid pulse and labored breathing
- Progressive general weakness
- Vision problems (dim or blurred)
- Nausea and vomiting
- Seizures
- Drowsiness or unconsciousness

If the dead or captured snake is at the scene, your role as an EMT-B is not to identify the snake but to transport it in a sealed container along with the patient. Arrange for separate transport of a live specimen. Do not transport a live snake in the ambulance.

Should you see the live, uncaptured snake, take great care or you may be its next victim. When possible, note its size and coloration. Getting close enough to look for details of the eyes or for a pit between the eye and mouth is foolish. How you classify a snake, whether it is dead or alive, will probably have little to do with subsequent care. The medical center staff will arrange to have an expert classify a captured or dead specimen, and they have protocols to determine care if the snake has not been captured. Unless you are an expert in capturing snakes, do not try to catch the snake. Never delay care and transport in order to capture the snake.

Patient *CARE*

Snakebite

Emergency care of a patient with snakebite includes:

1. Call medical direction.

2. Treat for shock and conserve body heat. Keep the patient calm.

3. Locate the fang marks and clean the site with soap and water. There may be only one fang mark.

4. Remove any rings, bracelets, or other constricting items on the bitten extremity.

5. Keep any bitten extremities immobilized—the application of a splint will help. Try to keep the bite at the level of the heart or, when this is not possible, below the level of the heart.

6. Apply light constricting bands above and below the wound if ordered by medical direction. (See more information on constricting bands below.)

7. Transport the patient, carefully monitoring vital signs.

Warning

Do not place an ice bag or cold pack on the bite unless you are directed to do so by a physician or local protocol. Do not cut into the bite and suction or squeeze unless you are directed

It's very cold out and it's been snowing for hours. Shortly after sundown, you get dispatched to a downtown area for an "unknown man down" call. En route you say to your partner, "Do you think this will be one of our regulars?" As you pull up to the scene, you are met by a police officer who tells you that the man sitting by the heater grate in the sidewalk was going to be taken to the shelter "but something didn't seem right." You get the first-in bag and approach the patient. You ask his name and he says "Frank." You ask for a last name but he doesn't respond.

"Well, Frank, what's going on?" He just stares. "Do you have any pain?" Again no response. He just sits with his arms folded over his chest and appears to be shivering. "Frank, we think you need to go to the hospital to get checked out."

"What?" he whispers. You ask the patient if he can stand up but his response is unintelligible. You get the cot and load for transport. The police officer asks you what's wrong and you tell him that you think the patient might be hypothermic.

STREET SCENE QUESTIONS

1. What concerns might you have for this patient?
2. What assessment needs to be performed?
3. Should you rewarm this patient? If so, when should you start?

When you get into the ambulance, you repeat your initial assessment, checking breathing closely and looking for any external bleeding. Again, you ask the patient if he knows where he is but he responds only with groans. You notice that his clothing is wet, so you turn up the heat in the patient compartment, take off his wet jacket and shirt, and wrap him in more blankets. He is still shivering. You take a set of vital signs and determine the BP is 90/60, pulse is 120, respiration rate is 28 and shallow, and the skin is flushed. When you feel the abdomen with the back of your hand, it feels cool. You do not smell any alcohol on the patient and when you check distal pulses, motor function, and sensation, you find that he can move all extremities but it is difficult and almost seems painful. His pupils respond to light but appear sluggish. You decide to administer oxygen by nonrebreather. You also decide not to actively rewarm the patient, but keep him wrapped in blankets, covering his head and keeping the heater turned up.

STREET SCENE QUESTIONS

4. How often should you take vital signs?
5. When moving the patient out of the ambulance and onto the hospital stretcher, what precautions should be taken?

You decide to take another set of vital signs after 5 minutes because you think that this patient could be at risk for respiratory arrest or sudden cardiac death. You make sure the AED and the respiratory equipment are close at hand. Vital signs are about the same. You call the hospital, give your report, and advise an ETA of about 5 minutes. When you get there, you remind your partner that this patient

to do so by a physician. Never suck the venom from the wound using your mouth. Instead, use a suction cup. Suctioning is seldom done.

Apply constricting bands above and below the fang marks. Each band should be about two inches from the wound, but never place the bands on both sides of a joint, such as above and below the knee. Since the typical coral snakebite is to a finger or a toe, due to its small mouth, just a single band may be placed above a coral snakebite. If the bite is to a finger, the band can be applied to the wrist.

The purpose of the constricting bands is to restrict the flow of lymph, not of blood. They should be made of ¾-inch to 1½-inch-wide soft rubber. If only one band is available, place it above the wound (between the wound and the heart). If no bands are available, use a handkerchief or other wide soft material. The bands should be snug but not tight enough to cut off circulation. Monitor for a pulse at the wrist or ankle, depending on the extremity involved. Check to be certain that tissue swelling does not cause the constricting bands to become too tight.

Poisoning from Marine Life

Poisoning from marine life forms can occur in a variety of ways—from eating improperly prepared

PATIENT NAME: *Frank*								PATIENT AGE: *Unknown*	

CHIEF COMPLAINT

Altered mental status

PAST MEDICAL HISTORY

- [ ] None
- [ ] Allergy to _____
- [ ] Hypertension
- [ ] Stroke
- [ ] Seizures
- [ ] Diabetes
- [ ] COPD
- [ ] Cardiac
- [ ] Other (List)
- [ ] Asthma

Unknown

Current Medications (List)

Unknown

VITAL SIGNS

TIME	RESP	PULSE	B.P.	MENTAL STATUS	R PUPILS L	SKIN
2130	Rate: *28* [ ] Regular [x] Shallow [ ] Labored	Rate: *120* [x] Regular [ ] Irregular	*90* / *60*	[ ] Alert [x] Voice [ ] Pain [ ] Unresp.	Normal [ ] Dilated [ ] Constricted [ ] [x] Sluggish [x] No-Reaction [ ]	[ ] Unremarkable [x] Cool [ ] Pale [ ] Warm [ ] Cyanotic [ ] Moist [x] Flushed [ ] Dry [ ] Jaundiced
2135	Rate: *28* [ ] Regular [x] Shallow [ ] Labored	Rate: *120* [x] Regular [ ] Irregular	*90* / *60*	[ ] Alert [x] Voice [ ] Pain [ ] Unresp.	Normal [ ] Dilated [ ] Constricted [ ] [x] Sluggish [x] No-Reaction [ ]	[ ] Unremarkable [x] Cool [ ] Pale [ ] Warm [ ] Cyanotic [ ] Moist [x] Flushed [ ] Dry [ ] Jaundiced
	Rate: [ ] Regular [ ] Shallow [ ] Labored	Rate: [ ] Regular [ ] Irregular	/	[ ] Alert [ ] Voice [ ] Pain [ ] Unresp.	Normal [ ] Dilated [ ] Constricted [ ] Sluggish [ ] No-Reaction [ ]	[ ] Unremarkable [ ] Cool [ ] Pale [ ] Warm [ ] Cyanotic [ ] Moist [ ] Flushed [ ] Dry [ ] Jaundiced

NARRATIVE *EMS requested to the scene by local police, who state they found the patient sitting on a heater grate alongside the sidewalk in soaking wet clothing. They state that the patient did not appear alert, so EMS was requested. On our arrival, patient responds to loud verbal stimuli with occasional inappropriate responses. Patient is obviously shivering and initially appears to be hypothermic. Once patient is loaded in the ambulance via the cot, the heat is turned up. We removed patient's wet clothing and gently dried him prior to wrapping him in warm, dry blankets. Oxygen therapy is initiated prior to transporting the patient with as gentle a ride as possible. The patient is turned over to the hospital slightly more alert and oriented.*

needs to be handled gently. You also get another blanket from the emergency department before you make the move. The patient seems to be warming up and you don't want to put him at any additional risk. When you get into the emergency department, you smoothly move the patient to the stretcher and give the prehospital care report. As you are leaving, Frank looks at you and says: "Thanks, you're nice."

seafood or poisonous organisms to stings and punctures. Patients who have ingested spoiled, contaminated, or infested seafood may develop a condition that resembles anaphylactic shock. They should receive the same care as any patient in anaphylactic shock. During care, you must be prepared for vomiting. Most patients will show the signs of food poisoning. The care for seafood poisoning is the same as for all other food poisonings.

It is extremely rare for someone in the U.S. to eat a poisonous variety of marine life. Creatures such as puffer fish and paralytic shellfish are not readily available. For all cases of suspected poisoning due to ingestion, call your on-line medical direction or the poison control center as local protocol directs you. Be prepared for vomiting, convulsions, and respiratory arrest.

Venomous marine life forms producing sting injuries include the jellyfish, the sea nettle, the Portuguese man-of-war, coral, the sea anemone, and the hydra. For most victims, the sting produces pain with few complications. Some patients may show allergic reactions and possibly develop anaphylactic shock. These cases require the same care as rendered for any case of anaphylactic shock. Stings to the face, especially those near or on the lip or eye, require a physician's attention. Rinsing the affected area with vinegar or rubbing alcohol will reduce the pain of the sting. Be careful not to let vinegar or, especially, rubbing alcohol get into the patient's mouth or eyes.

Puncture wounds occur when someone steps on or grabs a stingray, sea urchin, spiny catfish, or other form of spiny marine animal. Although it is true that soaking the wound in non-scalding hot water for 30 minutes will break down the venom, you should not delay transport. Puncture wounds must be treated by a physician and the patient may need a tetanus inoculation. Remember, the patient could react to the venom by developing anaphylactic shock.

Documentation Tips— Environmental Emergencies

In addition to routine observations and measurements related to the patient's signs and symptoms, include the following:

- If the injury is related to exposure to heat, cold, water, or ice, briefly describe environmental conditions. If possible, provide good estimates of measurements, such as temperature and factors relating to wind chill and water chill.
- Ask the patient what caused the emergency. He or she might forget to tell you that the near-drowning was caused by "sudden chest pain" or that the exposure to cold was due to trauma from a fall.
- If the injury is caused by a bite or sting, record the patient's or a bystander's description of the insect or animal. Include size and color if possible.
- Ask the patient or witnesses if the patient lost consciousness. Document all changes in mental status.
- Record vital signs early. Take several sets and record the intervals so hospital personnel can note the rate of change.

CHAPTER REVIEW

SUMMARY

Patients suffering from exposure to heat or cold must be removed from the harmful environment as quickly and as safely as possible. Rewarming or cooling procedures approved by local protocol should be performed as needed. Immediate resuscitation of the water-related emergency patient may require quick and persistent intervention. For injection or ingestion of the poisons of insects, spiders, snakes, and marine life, call medical direction and follow local protocol.

KEY TERMS

active rewarming application of an external heat source to rewarm the body of a hypothermic patient.
air embolism gas bubble in the bloodstream. The plural is *air emboli*. The more accurate term is *arterial gas embolism (AGE)*.
central rewarming application of heat to the lateral chest, neck, armpits, and groin of a hypothermic patient.
conduction the direct transfer of heat from one material to another through direct contact.

convection carrying away of heat by currents of air or water or other gases or liquids.
decompression sickness a condition resulting from nitrogen trapped in the body's tissues caused by coming up too quickly from a deep, prolonged dive. A symptom of decompression sickness is "the bends," or deep pain in the muscles and joints.
drowning death caused by changes in the lungs resulting from immersion in water.

evaporation the change from liquid to gas. When the body perspires or gets wet, evaporation of the perspiration or other liquid into the air has a cooling effect on the body.

hyperthermia (HI-per-THURM-e-ah) an increase in body temperature above normal, life-threatening in its extreme.

hypothermia (HI-po-THURM-e-ah) generalized cooling that reduces body temperature below normal, life-threatening in its extreme.

local cooling cooling or freezing of particular (local) parts of the body.

near-drowning the condition of having begun to drown but still able to be resuscitated.

passive rewarming covering a hypothermic patient and taking other steps to prevent further heat loss and help the body rewarm itself.

radiation sending out energy, such as heat, in waves into space.

respiration breathing. During respiration, body heat is lost as warm air is exhaled from the body.

toxins substances produced by animals or plants that are poisonous to humans.

venom a toxin (poison) produced by certain animals such as snakes, spiders, and some marine life forms.

water chill chilling caused by conduction of heat from the body when the body or clothing is wet.

wind chill chilling caused by convection of heat from the body in the presence of air currents.

REVIEW QUESTIONS

1. Describe when it is appropriate to treat a cold emergency with active rewarming and when you should perform passive rewarming. (pp. 428–431)
2. List five situations in which a patient may be suffering from hypothermia along with another, more obvious medical condition or injury. (p. 427)
3. Name the signs and symptoms of a late or deep localized cold injury. (p. 430)

4. Describe the management of a patient suffering from heat emergency who has moist, pale, and cool skin. (p. 432)
5. Describe the management of a patient suffering from a heat emergency who has hot, dry skin. (p. 433)
6. Describe the proper care for a patient suffering from snakebite. (pp. 445–446)

APPLICATIONS

• You are called to respond to an elderly woman who has fallen while walking in the park on a cool fall day. How should you manage assessment and care of this patient?

WEB MEDIC

Visit Brady's *Emergency Care* website for direct weblinks. At **www.bradybooks.com/ emergencycare**, you will find information related to the following Chapter 22 topics:

• Heat and cold emergencies
• Aquatic safety and water rescue

Chapter
Twenty-Three

BEHAVIORAL EMERGENCIES

*W*ord on the Street

"Experience will help you develop the street smarts it takes to handle unusual calls. Though even with years under my belt, I can still be surprised. Like the time we responded to a diabetic patient, who ended up pulling a knife, or when we picked up the same patient for 'transport to the hospital for detox' three times in the same day, or when we had to handle a suicidal patient. Like every other call, you have to respond in a professional, caring, competent manner. The things to keep foremost in mind are your personal safety, the safety of your crew, and the safety of the patient."

Dawson Blackmore, Jr.
EMT-I and EMS Instructor

As an EMT-Basic, you will respond to many emergencies in which the patient is behaving in unexpected and sometimes dangerous ways. The unusual behavior may be the result of stress, physical trauma or illness, drug or alcohol abuse, or mental illness. Whatever the apparent cause, do not hesitate to request police assistance whenever you feel it is necessary. Local protocol may even require it. Once the scene is secure, you will be able to provide appropriate emergency care.

BEHAVIORAL EMERGENCIES

What Is a Behavioral Emergency?

We all exhibit behavior. **Behavior** is defined as the manner in which a person acts or performs. Behavior involves any or all activities of a person, including physical and mental activity. Of course, behavior differs from person to person and from situation to situation.

A **behavioral emergency** exists when a person exhibits abnormal behavior—that is, behavior within a given situation that is unacceptable or intolerable to the patient, the family, or the community.

A key part of that definition is "within a given situation." You may have observed, in your own life or in that of friends or family, that behavior varies, depending on the situation at hand. For example, if a person is notified unexpectedly of the death of a loved one, a common reaction is screaming, crying, throwing things, or other emotional outbursts. In the context of the situation, this behavior would not be unusual. If the same behaviors were exhibited for no apparent reason in the middle of a shopping center, they might indicate a behavioral emergency.

Remember that you will be exposed to persons from other cultures and with different lifestyles. Some behaviors may seem unusual to you but might be quite normal to the person performing them. Behavioral conditions require patient assessment, just like any other emergency. Remain objective. Do not judge patients hastily or solely on the way they look or act.

Physical Causes of Altered Behavior

There are many medical and traumatic conditions that are likely to alter a patient's behavior. These problems may include:

- *Low blood sugar,* which may be the cause of rapid onset of erratic or hostile behavior (similar to alcohol intoxication), dizziness and headache, fainting, seizures, sometimes coma, profuse perspiration, hunger, drooling, and rapid pulse but normal blood pressure. (See Chapter 19, "Diabetes and Altered Mental Status.")
- *Lack of oxygen,* which may cause restlessness and confusion, cyanosis (blue or gray skin), and altered mental status.

TOPIC OVERVIEW

In this chapter, you will learn about the following topics:

- How to identify patients who are experiencing a behavioral emergency

- How to recognize potentially dangerous patients and act with safety in mind

- Methods of calming and interacting with patients experiencing behavioral emergencies

- How to restrain a patient safely and effectively

- How to document findings and care of patients with behavioral emergencies

DOT OBJECTIVES

✔ **Knowledge and Attitude**

1. Define behavioral emergencies. (p. 451)

2. Discuss the general factors that may cause an alteration in a patient's behavior. (pp. 451–452)

3. State the various reasons for psychological crises. (pp. 452–453)

4. Discuss the characteristics of an individual's behavior which suggest that the patient is at risk for suicide. (p. 454)

5. Discuss special medical/legal considerations for managing behavioral emergencies. (pp. 456, 458–459) (Scan 23-1, p. 457)

6. Discuss the special considerations for assessing a patient with behavioral problems. (pp. 453, 454, 455)

7. Discuss the general principles of an individual's behavior which suggest that he is at risk for violence. (p. 455)

8. Discuss methods to calm behavioral emergency patients. (pp. 452–453, 454–455)

9. Explain the rationale for learning how to modify your behavior toward the patient with a behavioral emergency. (pp. 452–453, 454–455)

✔ **Skills**

1. Demonstrate the assessment and emergency medical care of the patient experiencing a behavioral emergency.

2. Demonstrate various techniques to safely restrain a patient with a behavioral problem.

- *Inadequate blood to the brain or stroke,* which may cause confusion or dizziness, impaired speech, headache, loss of function or paralysis of extremities on one side of body, nausea and vomiting, and rapid full pulse.

- *Head trauma,* which can cause personality changes ranging from irritability to irrational behavior, altered mental status, amnesia or confusion, irregular respirations, elevated blood pressure, and decreasing pulse.

- *Mind-altering substances,* which can cause highly variable signs and symptoms depending on the substance ingested. (See Chapter 21, "Poisoning and Overdose Emergencies.")

- *Excessive cold,* which may cause shivering, feelings of numbness, altered mental status, drowsiness, staggering walk, slow breathing, and slow pulse.

- *Excessive heat,* which may cause decreased or complete loss of consciousness. (See Chapter 22, "Environmental Emergencies.")

When dealing with someone who appears to be having a behavioral emergency, always consider the possibility that his unusual behavior is caused by something other than a psychological problem (Figure 23-1).

Situational Stress Reactions

When faced with severe, unexpected stress, most patients will display emotions such as fear, grief, and anger. These are typical stress reactions at the accident scene and common reactions to serious illness and death. In the vast majority of cases, as you begin to take control of the situation and treat the patient as an individual, personal interaction will inspire confidence in your ability to help. The patient will begin to calm down and may even begin to feel able to cope with the emergency.

Be as unhurried as you can. If you rush your patient assessment and interview, the patient may feel as if the situation is out of control. The patient also may believe that you are concerned about the problem and not about him. Let the patient know that you are there to help.

Whenever you care for a patient who is displaying typical stress reactions, act in a calm manner, giving the patient time to gain control of his emotions.

Figure 23-1   There are many reasons why a patient may experience an altered mental status.

Quietly and carefully evaluate the situation, keeping your own emotions under control. Let the patient know that you are listening to what he is saying, and explain things to the patient honestly. Stay alert for sudden changes in behavior.

By acting in this manner, you are applying crisis management techniques to help the patient deal with stress. If the patient does not begin to interact with you or calm down, and if there are no apparent physical causes for the behavior, you must assume that there is a problem of a more serious nature, such as a psychiatric problem. Proceed according to the recommendations in the following segments of this chapter.

EMERGENCY CARE FOR BEHAVIORAL EMERGENCIES

Psychiatric Emergencies

There is a wide range of psychiatric problems. One patient with a psychiatric condition may be withdrawn and not wish to communicate while another may be agitated, talkative, or exhibiting bizarre or threatening behavior. Some patients may act as if they wish to harm themselves or others.

Follow these general rules to deal with a patient who is experiencing a behavioral or psychiatric emergency:

HOW AND WHY?

Many psychiatric patients have been prescribed powerful medications to control their conditions. However, abuse of those same medications can be fatal. Go to your Electronic Extras CD to learn more about common medications and their side effects.

- Identify yourself and your role.
- Speak slowly and clearly. Use a calm and reassuring tone.
- Listen to the patient. You can show you are listening by repeating part of what the patient says back to him.
- Do not be judgmental. Show compassion, not pity.
- Use positive body language. Avoid crossing your arms or looking uninterested.
- Acknowledge the patient's feelings.
- Do not enter the patient's personal space. Stay at least 3 feet from the patient. Making the patient feel closed in can cause an emotional outburst.
- Be alert for changes in the patient's emotional status. Watch for increasingly aggressive behavior and take appropriate safety precautions.

● Patient *ASSESSMENT*

Behavioral or Psychiatric Emergency

To assess a patient who appears to be suffering a behavioral or psychiatric emergency:

- Perform a careful scene size-up.
- Identify yourself and your role. It may not be obvious to the patient who you are and what you intend to do.
- Complete an initial assessment, including assessment of the patient's mental status (level of responsiveness; orientation to person, place, and time).
- Perform as much of the focused and detailed examinations as possible. Be alert for medical and traumatic conditions that could be causing the patient's behavior.
- Gather a thorough patient history. This will alert you to past psychiatric problems, psychiatric medications the patient may be taking (or not taking—causing the outburst). This may also alert you to conditions such as diabetes that can closely mimic a psychiatric condition.

Common presentations, or signs and symptoms, of patients experiencing psychiatric emergencies include:

- Panic or anxiety
- Unusual appearance, disordered clothing, poor hygiene
- Agitated or unusual activity, such as repetitive motions, threatening movements, or withdrawn stance
- Unusual speech patterns, such as too rapid or pressured-sounding speech (as if being forced out), or inability to carry on a coherent conversation
- Bizarre behavior or thought patterns
- Suicidal or self-destructive behavior
- Violent or aggressive behavior with threats or intent to harm others

● Patient *CARE*

Behavioral or Psychiatric Emergency

Emergency care of a patient having a behavioral or psychiatric emergency includes:

- Be alert for personal or scene safety problems throughout the call.
- Treat any life-threatening problems during the initial assessment.

- Be alert for medical or traumatic conditions that could mimic a behavioral emergency.

- Be prepared to spend time talking to the patient. Use the skills listed earlier in dealing with the patient. Remember to talk in a calm, reassuring voice. Use positive body language and good eye contact. Avoid unnecessary physical contact and quick movements.

- Encourage the patient to discuss what is troubling him.

- Never play along with any visual or auditory hallucinations that a patient may be experiencing. Do not lie to the patient.

- If it appears it will help, involve family members or friends in the conversation. Evaluate the response of the patient to the presence of others. If it agitates the patient, ask the others to leave.

Suicide

Each year in this country, thousands of people commit suicide. Many more suffer both physical and emotional injuries in suicide attempts. Anyone may become suicidal if emotional distress is severe, regardless of gender, age, or ethnic, social, or economic background.

HOW AND WHY?

Suicide and suicide attempts are all too common. Did you know that some single-occupant motor-vehicle collisions may actually be suicide attempts? Go to your Electronic Extras CD to find out more about suicide.

People attempt suicide for many reasons, including depression caused by chemical imbalance, the death of a loved one, financial problems, the end to a love affair, poor health, loss of esteem, divorce, fear of failure, and alcohol and drug abuse. People attempt to end their lives by any one of a variety of methods. You may observe suicides or attempted suicides by drug overdose, hanging, jumping from high places, ingesting poisons, inhaling gas, wrist-cutting, self-mutilation, stabbing, or shooting.

Safety Note

Whenever you are called to care for a patient who has attempted or may be about to attempt suicide, your first concern must be your own safety. Not all patients will wish to harm you, but the mechanism used to attempt suicide will be capable of causing death. It could intentionally or accidentally be turned on you.

Potential or Attempted Suicide

Factors often associated with a risk for suicide are listed below. Although some or even all of them may be present in a patient, it is not possible to use these characteristics to predict who will or who will not commit suicide.

- *Depression.* Take seriously a patient's feelings and expressions of despair or suicidal thoughts.

- *High current or recent stress levels.* If so, take the threat of suicide seriously.

- *Recent emotional trauma,* such as job loss, loss of a significant relationship, serious illness, arrest, imprisonment.

- *Age.* High suicide rates occur at ages 15–25 and over age 40. The elderly are a population where suicide rates are increasing.

- *Alcohol and drug abuse.*

- *Threats of suicide.* The patient may have told others that he is considering suicide. Take all threats of suicide seriously.

- *Suicide plan.* A patient who has a detailed suicide plan is more likely to commit suicide. Look for a plan that includes a method to carry out the suicide, notes, giving away personal possessions, or getting affairs in order.

- *Previous attempts or suicide threats,* including a history of self-destructive behavior. Often patients who have attempted suicide are considered to be "looking for attention" and are not taken seriously. However, statistics reveal that a person who has attempted suicide in the past is more likely to commit suicide than one who has not.

- *Sudden improvement from depression.* A patient who has made the decision to commit suicide may actually appear to be coming out of a depression. The fact that the decision has been made and an end is in sight can cause this apparent "improvement." You may find family members and friends of suicidal patients who will report that the patient had seemed "better" in the past few days.

Potential or Attempted Suicide

Patients who are in an emotional, psychiatric, or attempted-suicide emergency are cared for in similar ways. In all cases, your personal interaction with the patient is key. Try to establish visual and verbal contact as soon as possible. Avoid arguing. Make no threats, and show no indication of using force.

Remember that you are the first professional to begin both the physical and mental health care of the patient. The more reassurance you can provide for the patient, the easier it will be for the hospital emergency department staff to continue care.

Emergency care includes the following:

1. Treatment must begin with scene size-up. Make sure it is safe to approach the patient. If the scene is not safe, request assistance from the police and wait until they have secured the scene. Do not leave the patient alone unless you are at risk of physical harm. Try to talk with the patient from a safe distance until the police arrive. Take BSI precautions.

2. When the scene is secure, look for and treat life-threatening problems to the extent that the patient will permit it. Seek police assistance in restraining the patient if necessary for care of life-threatening problems.

3. As possible, perform a focused history and physical exam and provide emergency care.

4. Perform a detailed physical exam only if it is safe and you suspect the patient may have an injury.

5. Perform ongoing assessment. Watch for sudden changes in the patient's behavior and physical condition.

6. Contact the receiving hospital and report on current mental status and other essential information.

Note that a physical exam may be difficult with the emotional or psychiatric patient. You may not be able to proceed beyond the initial assessment.

Throughout your interaction with the patient speak slowly, and patiently await answers to your questions. As you gain the patient's confidence, explain what questions must be answered and what must be done as part of the physical exam and taking vital signs. Let the patient know that you think it would be best if he goes to the hospital and that you need his cooperation and help. Back off if necessary. If the patient's fear or aggression increases, do not push the issues of the examination or transport. Instead, try to reestablish the conversation and give the patient more time before you again say that going to the hospital is a good idea.

Transport all suicidal patients. Seek police assistance if necessary. Report any attempted suicide or expression of suicidal thoughts to the medical facility, police, or government agency designated by your state law and local protocols.

Aggressive or Hostile Patients

Aggressive or disruptive behavior may be caused by trauma to the brain and nervous system, metabolic disorders, stress, alcohol, other drugs, or psychological disorders. Sometimes you will know that your patient is aggressive from the information you receive from dispatch. Other times the scene may provide quick clues (such as drugs, yelling, unclean conditions, broken furniture). Neighbors, family members, or bystanders may tell you that the patient is dangerous or angry or has a history of aggression or combativeness. The patient's stance (tense muscles, fists clenched, or quick irregular movements, for example) or his position in the room may give you an early warning of possible violence. On rare occasions, you may start with an apparently calm patient who suddenly turns aggressive.

Safety Note

When a patient acts as if he may hurt himself or others, *your first concern must be your own safety.* Take the following precautions:

- Do not isolate yourself from your partner or other sources of help. Make certain that you have an escape route. Do not let the patient come between you and the door. Should a patient become violent, retreat and wait for police assistance.
- Do not take any action that may be considered threatening by the patient. To do so may bring about hostile behavior directed against you or others.
- Always be on the watch for weapons. Stay out of kitchens. They are filled with dangerous weapons. Stay in a safe area until the police can control the scene.
- Be alert for sudden changes in the patient's behavior.

Patient *ASSESSMENT*

Aggressive or Hostile Patient

Your assessment of the aggressive or hostile patient may never go beyond the initial assessment phase. Most of your time may be spent trying to calm the patient and ensuring everyone's safety. An aggressive or hostile patient:

- Responds to people inappropriately
- Tries to hurt himself or others
- May have a rapid pulse and breathing
- Usually displays rapid speech and rapid physical movements
- May appear anxious, nervous, "panicky"

Aggressive or Hostile Patient

Follow these steps for the emergency care of an aggressive or hostile patient:

1. Treatment begins with scene size-up. Make sure it is safe to approach the patient. Request assistance from law enforcement before approaching if necessary. Practice BSI precautions.

2. Seek advice from medical direction if the patient's behavior prevents normal assessment and care procedures.

3. As part of ongoing assessment, watch for sudden changes in the patient's behavior.

4. Seek assistance from law enforcement, as well as from medical direction, if restraint seems necessary.

Reasonable Force and Restraint

Reasonable force is the force necessary to keep a patient from injuring himself or others. Reasonableness is determined by looking at all circumstances involved, including the patient's strength and size, type of abnormal behavior, mental status, and available methods of restraint. Understand that you may protect yourself from attack, but otherwise you must avoid actions that can cause injury to the patient.

In addition, in most localities an EMT-B cannot legally restrain a patient, move a patient against his will, or force a patient to accept emergency care—even at the family's request. The restraint and forcible moving of patients is usually within the jurisdiction of law enforcement. The police (and in some areas a physician) can order you to restrain and transport a patient to the appropriate medical facility. However, the physician is not empowered to order you to take action that could place you in danger. If police order restraint and transport, they must assist with these procedures as necessary. Remember to follow local protocol.

Never try to assist in restraining a patient unless there are sufficient personnel to do the job. You must be able to ensure your safety and the safety of the patient. If you help the police or a physician to restrain a patient, make certain that the restraints are humane. Handcuffs and plastic "throwaway" criminal restraints should not be used because of the soft-tissue damage they can inflict. Initially, the police may have to use such restraints. However, in some states they can be replaced with soft restraints such as leather cuffs and belts. If authorized in your state and by local protocol, an ambulance should carry leather cuffs, a waist-size belt, and at least three short belts. Restraints for the wrists and ankles can be made from gauze roller bandages.

Do not remove police restraints until you and the police are certain that soft restraints will hold the patient. To ensure everyone's safety once they are on, remember not to remove soft restraints, even if the patient appears to be acting rationally.

Follow these guidelines when a patient must be restrained (Scan 23-1):

- Be sure to have adequate help.
- Plan your activities.
- Estimate the range of motion of the patient's arms and legs and stay beyond range until ready.
- Once the decision to restrain the patient has been reached, act quickly.
- Have one EMT-B talk to and reassure the patient throughout the restraining procedure.
- Approach with four persons, one assigned to each limb, all to act at the same time.
- Secure all four limbs with restraints approved by medical direction.
- Position the patient face up or face down. The position will be dictated by what the restraining process itself permits, the patient's condition (e.g., injuries, breathing problems), and local protocols. Monitor the patient's airway. Never "hog tie" the patient or restrain the patient in any manner that will impair breathing. Patients who have been improperly restrained have died as a result of a condition called **positional asphyxia.** Monitor all restrained patients carefully.
- Use multiple straps or other restraints to ensure that the patient is adequately secured. Anticipate that the patient's behavior may turn more violent and be sure that restraint is adequate for this possibility.
- If the patient is spitting on rescuers, place a surgical mask on the patient if he has no breathing difficulty or likelihood of vomiting and if local protocols permit, or have rescuers wear protective masks, eye wear, and clothing.
- Reassess the patient's distal circulation frequently and adjust restraints as safe and necessary if distal circulation is diminished.
- Use sufficient force, but avoid unnecessary force.
- Document the reasons why the patient was restrained and the technique of restraint.

Documentation Tips— Behavioral Emergencies

It is important to document your observations and actions when writing your report of a

RESTRAINING A PATIENT

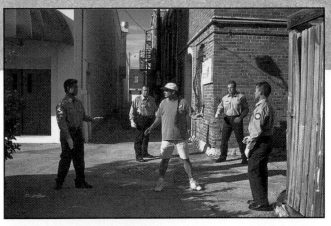

▲ **1.** Plan your approach to the patient in advance and remain outside the range of his arms and legs until you are ready to act.

▲ **2.** Assign one EMT to each limb, and approach the patient at the same time.

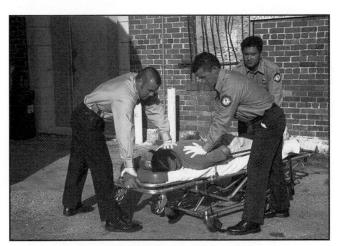

▲ **3.** Place the patient on the stretcher as his condition and local protocols indicate. Do not let go until he is properly secured.

▲ **4.** Use multiple straps or other soft restraints to secure the patient to the stretcher.

◀ **5.** When the patient is secure, assess his distal circulation and monitor his airway and breathing continually.

It's a sunny summer afternoon and relatively quiet, when you are dispatched to a small manufacturing company for an individual "acting in a bizarre manner." The dispatcher is trying to get additional information, but it is difficult. Your response time is 5 minutes, and you are met outside by the manager. He tells you that about 15 minutes ago a worker kicked a table and disrupted some of the equipment. When he was approached by coworkers, he said "Stay away, or I *will* hurt myself." The manager says the patient has a knife, but no one has seen it.

STREET SCENE QUESTIONS

1. What is your first and most important concern?
2. How should you handle the matter of scene safety?
3. When should you approach the patient?

You contact the dispatcher who informs you that two police officers are responding and should be on scene in three minutes. You make sure that your crew and bystanders are in a safe position in the event the patient exits the building. When the officers pull up, you tell them what you know. The police tell you to wait outside. They enter the building and find the patient still very agitated. While you wait outside, a coworker of the patient approaches and says that she might have some information that could help. Supposedly, the patient is on antidepressant drugs and his wife recently left him. She believes that he could hurt himself but she doubts he will hurt anyone else. At this point, one of the police officers tells you that the patient is calm and they have frisked him.

STREET SCENE QUESTIONS

4. How should the patient be approached?
5. What are the safety concerns when working with an agitated patient?
6. Does this patient need a medical assessment?

You decide that only you should approach the patient so as not to overwhelm him. There is already a police officer standing next to him. As you approach, you introduce yourself and tell the patient that you need to ask some questions and get some medical information. You listen to him and, during the medical history, you ask if he has taken more medication than he should. He says that he took his morning dose but that is all. You take a set of vital signs and continue to listen. After a few minutes, the patient agrees to go to the hospital with you.

You ask your partner to move the ambulance to a back door so the patient doesn't have to pass coworkers on the way out. You have discussed the situation with the police officers and you feel confident that there is no longer a safety issue and that they won't be

behavioral emergency call. Document your observations of the patient objectively and professionally. Do not interject opinions or unprofessional comments (e.g., "The patient was acting like he was nuts"). Describe behavior in exact terms (e.g., "The patient was pacing with clenched fists. He was shouting all words. He referred to himself as 'god' and referred to the police as 'devils'").

Document the scene thoroughly. If a patient demolished his own apartment and possessed a knife, document this in your report. Hospital and mental-health personnel will not have been able to see the scene, making your accurate documentation essential for continuing care.

When documenting, include statements that support your belief that the patient might have harmed himself or others had you not provided care. If you suspect use of alcohol or other drugs by the patient, this too should be documented. If injury or illness are suspected as causes of the behavioral emergency, document facts that support this possibility as well.

Be sure to include in your report the names of law enforcement or other witnesses.

Transport to an Appropriate Facility

Your medical protocols or procedures should direct you to the most appropriate medical facility within your service area. Not all hospitals are prepared to treat behavioral emergencies.

Medical/Legal Considerations

A patient who refuses emergency care or transport is a significant medical/legal risk for EMS agencies and

PATIENT NAME: Robert Lanctot					PATIENT AGE: 38		

CHIEF COMPLAINT

Threatening to injure self

PAST MEDICAL HISTORY

- [ ] None
- [ ] Allergy to _____
- [ ] Hypertension
- [ ] Seizures
- [ ] COPD
- [x] Other (List)
- [ ] Stroke
- [ ] Diabetes
- [ ] Cardiac
- [ ] Asthma

Depression, marital problems

Current Medications (List)

Unknown antidepressant

VITAL SIGNS

TIME	RESP	PULSE	B.P.	MENTAL STATUS	R PUPILS L	SKIN
1015	Rate: 20 [x] Regular [ ] Shallow [ ] Labored	Rate: 90 [x] Regular [ ] Irregular	120/80	[x] Alert [ ] Voice [ ] Pain [ ] Unresp.	[x] Normal [ ] Dilated [ ] Constricted [ ] Sluggish [ ] No-Reaction	[x] Unremarkable [ ] Cool [ ] Pale [ ] Warm [ ] Cyanotic [ ] Moist [ ] Flushed [ ] Dry [ ] Jaundiced
	Rate: [ ] Regular [ ] Shallow [ ] Labored	Rate: [ ] Regular [ ] Irregular		[ ] Alert [ ] Voice [ ] Pain [ ] Unresp.	[ ] Normal [ ] Dilated [ ] Constricted [ ] Sluggish [ ] No-Reaction	[ ] Unremarkable [ ] Cool [ ] Pale [ ] Warm [ ] Cyanotic [ ] Moist [ ] Flushed [ ] Dry [ ] Jaundiced
	Rate: [ ] Regular [ ] Shallow [ ] Labored	Rate: [ ] Regular [ ] Irregular		[ ] Alert [ ] Voice [ ] Pain [ ] Unresp.	[ ] Normal [ ] Dilated [ ] Constricted [ ] Sluggish [ ] No-Reaction	[ ] Unremarkable [ ] Cool [ ] Pale [ ] Warm [ ] Cyanotic [ ] Moist [ ] Flushed [ ] Dry [ ] Jaundiced

NARRATIVE *EMS requested to the scene by manager, who states the patient had a very sudden onset of disruptive behavior and threatened to injure himself with a knife. The patient appears very agitated when approached by police officers. According to a coworker, patient is on an unknown antidepressant and had a recent break up with his wife. After being calmed by police, patient consents to transportation for evaluation. Patient is cooperative and denies taking an overdose of his medication or any other injury.*

needed for the transport. The police searched the patient for weapons and found none. The patient is placed on the stretcher with all safety straps applied. You listen to the patient all the way to the hospital, being compassionate and acknowledging the patient's feelings as well as you can. Your partner calls the hospital on the radio and gives an ETA of 5 minutes.

Later, as you walk away from the patient in the emergency department, he smiles and thanks you for listening.

EMT-Bs. What should you do when a behavioral emergency patient refuses or resists your efforts to provide care?

Most states have a provision in law that will allow a patient to be transported against his will if he is a danger to himself or others. This is an exception to the rule that patients must provide consent for their care and transportation. Know your state laws on treating patients without consent. Many states give this authority to law enforcement personnel. It will always be beneficial to have the police present if the patient must be restrained as a matter of safety.

You may also be required to contact medical direction about the psychiatric patient who refuses care. Many communities have mental health teams that will respond to the scene to help with the care of a patient with behavioral problems. This team will also help evaluate the need for transporting the patient against his will.

Emotionally disturbed patients sometimes accuse EMS personnel of sexual misconduct. If possible, EMT-Bs of the same sex as the patient should attend to emergency care of disturbed patients. For the aggressive or violent patient, make sure law enforcement officers accompany you to the hospital to protect you and the patient. In the event of a legal problem, they can serve as third-party witnesses.

For more information on this topic, review Chapter 3, "Medical/Legal and Ethical Issues."

CHAPTER REVIEW

SUMMARY

As an EMT-Basic, you will respond to many behavioral emergencies. Because the treatment for these patients usually requires long-term management, little medical intervention can be done in the acute situation. However, how you interact with the patient during the emergency can make a difference—to the patient and to the medical professionals who take over. On these calls remember that you must assure your own safety, consider the legal ramifications of your actions, document the circumstances, and transport the patient in a safe and effective manner to an appropriate facility. Know your local protocols.

KEY TERMS

behavior the manner in which a person acts.
behavioral emergency when a patient's behavior is not typical for the situation; when the patient's behavior is unacceptable or intolerable to the patient, his family, or the community, or when the patient may harm himself or others.
positional asphyxia death of a person due to a body position that restricts breathing for a prolonged time.

REVIEW QUESTIONS

1. Name several conditions that can alter a person's mental status and behavior. (pp. 451–452)
2. List several methods that can help calm the patient suffering a behavioral or psychiatric emergency. (pp. 453, 456)
3. Describe the signs and symptoms of a behavioral or psychiatric emergency. (p. 453)
4. Describe what you can do when scene-size up reveals that it is too dangerous to approach the patient. (p. 455)
5. List several factors that can help you assess the patient's risk for suicide. (p. 454)
6. List several methods that can help calm the psychiatric emergency patient. (pp. 452–453, 454–455)
7. Research your state law. Then describe the circumstances that must exist for you to treat and transport a behavioral emergency patient without consent.

APPLICATIONS

- You are called to respond to an intoxicated minor who is physically aggressive, threatens suicide, and whose parents permit you to treat but not transport. How would you manage this patient?

Visit Brady's *Emergency Care* website for direct weblinks. At **www.bradybooks.com/ emergencycare**, you will find information related to the following Chapter 23 topics:

- Suicide
- Mental illness
- Violence

Chapter
Twenty-Four

OBSTETRICS AND GYNECOLOGICAL EMERGENCIES

*W*ord on the Street

"Childbirth is a natural process that has gone on for many years before the 'invention' of medical professionals. In fact, I have responded to many calls where a surprised dad had delivered a baby before we arrived and things went just fine. Remember three things: you are there to calm, support, and assist; in the very rare instance of a complication, you must be prepared; and always appreciate the joy and wonder a birth will bring you."

Daniel Limmer EMT-P, Textbook Author

Childbirth is a natural process that existed long before there were EMTs. During your career as an EMT-Basic, you may be called upon to assist with an out-of-hospital delivery. One of your main responsibilities in this situation will be to help calm the patient and family members through your unruffled professional manner. However, because childbirth is not a common occurrence in the prehospital setting, it might be easy to get flustered and seem uncertain about the procedures you are performing. So it is important that you learn about childbirth and practice the procedures required to assist with delivery. If you are ever called upon to assist in a delivery, your skills will contribute to decreased stress and better care of the mother and baby.

ANATOMY AND PHYSIOLOGY OF CHILDBIRTH

Pregnancy and Delivery

The developing baby is called a **fetus** (Figure 24-1). During pregnancy, the fetus grows in the mother's **uterus,** a muscular organ also called the *womb* (Figure 24-2). When the mother is in labor, the muscles of the uterus contract at ever-shortening intervals and push the baby through the neck of the uterus, known as the **cervix.** The cervix must dilate some 4 inches (10 cm) during labor to allow the baby's head to pass into the **vagina,** or birth canal, so that delivery can take place.

More than just the fetus develops within the uterus during pregnancy. Attached to the wall of the uterus is a special organ called the **placenta.** Composed of both maternal and fetal tissues, the placenta serves as an exchange area between mother and fetus. Oxygen and nutrients (and drugs, nicotine, and alcohol) from the mother's bloodstream are carried across the placenta to the fetus. Carbon dioxide and certain other wastes cross from fetal circulation to maternal circulation. Since the placenta is an organ of pregnancy, it is expelled after the baby is born.

The mother's blood does not flow through the body of the fetus. The fetus has a circulatory system. Blood from the fetus is sent through blood vessels in the **umbilical cord** to the placenta where the blood picks up nourishment from the mother, then returns through the umbilical cord to the fetus's body. The umbilical cord, about 1 inch wide and 22 inches long at birth, is fully expelled with the birth of the baby and the delivery of the placenta.

While developing in the uterus, the fetus is enclosed and protected within a thin, membranous "bag of waters" known as the **amniotic sac.** This sac contains 1 to 2 quarts of liquid, called amniotic fluid. It allows the fetus to float during development, acts as a cushion between the fetus and minor injury, and helps maintain a constant fetal body temperature. In the vast majority of cases, the amniotic sac breaks during labor and the fluid gushes from the birth canal. This is a normal condition of childbirth that also provides a natural lubrication to ease the infant's progress through the birth canal.

TOPIC OVERVIEW

In this chapter, you will learn about the following topics:

- How to identify a patient at risk of immediate childbirth

- Care of the mother before, during, and after delivery

- Care of the baby during and after delivery (including potential complications)

- Neonatal resuscitation procedures

- How to document findings and care of patients with obstetric and gynecological emergencies

✔ **Knowledge and Attitude**

1. Identify the following structures: uterus, vagina, fetus, placenta, umbilical cord, amniotic sac, perineum. (pp. 463, 476)

2. Identify and explain the use of the contents of an obstetrics kit. (pp. 466–467)

3. Identify predelivery emergencies. (pp. 468, 481–484)

4. State indications of an imminent delivery. (pp. 466, 467–468)

5. Differentiate the emergency medical care provided to a patient with predelivery

emergencies from a normal delivery. (pp. 481–484)

6. State the steps in the predelivery preparation of the mother. (p. 469)

7. Establish the relationship between body substance isolation and childbirth. (p. 469)

8. State the steps to assist in the delivery. (pp. 469–470) (Scan 24-1, p. 471)

9. Describe care of the baby as the head appears. (p. 470)

10. Describe how and when to cut the umbilical cord. (pp. 473–474)

11. Discuss the steps in the delivery of the placenta. (p. 475)

12. List the steps in the emergency medical care of the mother post-delivery. (pp. 475–476)

13. Summarize neonatal resuscitation procedures. (pp. 472–473)

14. Describe the procedures for the following abnormal deliveries: breech birth, prolapsed cord, limb presentation. (pp. 476–479)

15. Differentiate the special considerations for multiple births. (pp. 479–480)

16. Describe special considerations of meconium. (p. 481)

The 9 months of pregnancy are divided into three 3-month periods, or *trimesters*. During the first trimester, the fetus is being formed. As the fetus remains quite small, there is little uterine growth during this period. After the third month, the uterus grows rapidly, reaching the umbilicus (navel) by the fifth month and the epigastrium (upper abdomen) by the seventh month. Other changes in a woman's body during this time include increased blood volume, increased cardiac output, and increased heart rate. The blood pressure is usually decreased slightly, and there is slowed digestion. One very important change is a massive increase in vascularity (presence of blood and blood vessels) of the uterus and related structures.

Crowning occurs when the presenting part of the baby first bulges from the vaginal opening. The *presenting part* is defined as the part of the infant that is first to appear at the vaginal opening during labor. Usually, the presenting part of the baby is the head. The normal head-first birth is called a **cephalic presentation.** If the buttocks or both feet of the baby deliver first, the birth is called a **breech presentation** or breech birth.

Labor

Labor is the entire process of delivery. There are three stages of labor (Figure 24-3):

- *First stage* starts with regular contractions and the thinning and gradual dilation of the cervix and ends when the cervix is fully dilated.
- *Second stage* is the time from when the baby enters the birth canal until he is born.
- *Third stage* begins after the baby is born and lasts until the **afterbirth** (placenta, umbilical cord, and some tissues from the amniotic sac and the lining of the uterus) is delivered.

The first stage of labor is also called the *dilation period*. Picture the uterus as a long-neck bottle. In order to expel the contents, the neck of the bottle must be stretched to the size of a wide-mouth jar. Before the cervix can fully dilate, the long neck of the cervix must be shortened and thinned (this process is called *effacement*) to the wide-mouth-jar shape.

Sometimes several days before the onset of actual labor, uterine muscles begin mild contractions and slight dilation occurs as the cervix begins to thin. When actual labor begins, the contractions of the uterus that occur during the first stage continue the thinning and dilation process, and the infant's head begins to move downward. The cervix gradually shortens and thins enough (wide-mouth-jar shape) to become flush with the vagina or fully open to the birth canal.

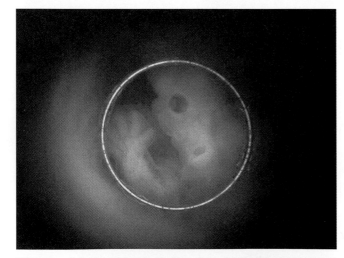

Figure 24-1 Endoscopic photograph of a five-week-old live fetus in the uterus. A hand and eye are clearly visible.

17. Describe the special considerations of a premature baby. (pp. 480–481)

18. Discuss the emergency medical care of a patient with a gynecological emergency. (p. 485)

19. Explain the rationale for understanding the implications of treating two patients (mother and baby). (pp. 475, 476)

✔ **Skills**

1. Demonstrate the steps to assist in the normal cephalic delivery.

2. Demonstrate necessary care procedures of the fetus as the head appears.

3. Demonstrate infant neonatal procedures.

4. Demonstrate post-delivery care of the infant.

5. Demonstrate how and when to cut the umbilical cord.

6. Attend to the steps in the delivery of the placenta.

7. Demonstrate the post-delivery care of the mother.

8. Demonstrate the procedures for the following abnormal deliveries: vaginal

bleeding, breech birth, prolapsed cord, limb presentation.

9. Demonstrate the steps in the emergency medical care of the mother with excessive bleeding.

10. Demonstrate completing a prehospital care report for patients with obstetrical/gynecological emergencies.

The cycle of contractions starts far apart and becomes shorter as birth approaches. Typically, these contractions range from every 30 minutes down to 3 minutes apart, or less. Labor pains accompany the contractions.

As the fetus moves downward and the cervix dilates, the amniotic sac usually breaks. Normally, the amniotic fluid is clear. Fluid that is greenish or brownish-yellow in color may be an indication of maternal or fetal distress during labor and is called **meconium staining.** The full dilation of the cervix signals the end of the first stage of labor. Women giving birth for the first time will remain in this first stage for an average of 16 hours. However, some

women may remain in this stage for no more than 4 hours, especially if this is not the first child.

There may be a watery, bloody discharge of mucus (not bleeding) associated with the first stage of labor. Part of this initial discharge will be from a mucus plug that was in the cervix. This is usually mixed with blood and is called the *bloody show*. It is not necessary to wipe it away. Watery, bloody fluids discharging from the vagina are typical for all three stages of labor.

The second stage of labor begins after the full dilation of the cervix. During this time, contractions become increasingly frequent. Labor pains will become more severe. In the second stage of labor, the

Amniotic sac

Umbilical cord

Placenta

Uterus

Cervix

Rectum

Bladder

Pubic bone

Vagina

Figure 24-2   Structures of pregnancy.

First stage:
beginning of contractions to full cervical dilation

Second stage:
baby enters birth canal and is born

Third stage:
delivery of the placenta

Figure 24-3 Three stages of labor.

cramping and abdominal pains associated with the first stage of labor still may be present, but most women report a major new discomfort, that of feeling they have to move their bowels. This is caused as the baby's body moves and places pressure on the rectum. The moment of birth is nearing, and the EMT-B will have to decide whether to transport or to keep the mother where she is and prepare to assist with delivery.

The third stage of labor begins shortly after the baby is born. Contractions will resume and continue until the placenta is delivered. The contractions and labor pains may be as painful and severe as the second stage. The third stage usually lasts 10 to 20 minutes.

Labor Pains

The contractions of the uterus produce normal labor pains. Most women report the start of labor pains as an ache in the lower back. As labor progresses, the pain becomes most noticeable in the lower abdomen, with the intensity of pain increasing. The pains come at regular intervals, lasting from 30 seconds to 1 minute and occur at 2- to 3-minute intervals. When the uterus starts to contract, the pain begins. As the muscles relax, there is relief from the pain. Labor pains may start, stop for a while, then start up again.

As an EMT-B, you should time the following characteristics of labor pains:

- *Contraction time, or duration.* The time from the beginning of contraction to when the uterus relaxes (from start to end).
- *Contraction interval, or frequency.* The time from the start of one contraction to the beginning of the next (from start to start).

When contractions last 30 seconds to 1 minute and are 2 to 3 minutes apart, delivery of the baby may be imminent.

NORMAL CHILDBIRTH

Role of the EMT-Basic

Your primary role will be to determine whether the delivery will occur on scene and, if so, to assist the mother as she delivers her child.

 Remember

EMT-Bs do not deliver babies; mothers do!

Assisting the mother and providing care is much easier if a few basic items are kept as part of the ambulance supplies. You will need a sterile obstetric kit that contains the items required for preparation of the mother, delivery, and initial care of the newborn (Figure 24-4). This kit should include

- Several pairs of sterile surgical gloves to protect from infection

Figure 24-4 Contents of an OB (obstetric) kit.

- Towels or sheets for draping the mother
- 1 dozen 2 × 2 (or 4 × 4) gauze pads (sponges) for wiping and drying the baby
- 1 rubber bulb syringe (3 oz.) to suction the baby's mouth and nostrils
- Cord clamps or hemostats to clamp the umbilical cord (plus extra clamps in case of a multiple birth)
- Umbilical cord tape to tie the cord
- 1 pair of surgical scissors to cut the cord
- 1 baby blanket to wrap the baby and keep him warm
- Several individually wrapped sanitary napkins to absorb blood and other fluids
- Plastic bag

Occasionally, in an off-duty situation, you may need to assist in the delivery of a baby without using a sterile delivery pack. A few simple supplies can be used to assist the mother:

- Clean sheets and towels to drape the mother and wrap the newborn
- Heavy flat twine or new shoelaces to tie the cord (do not use thread, wire, or light string since these may cut through the cord)
- A towel or plastic bag to wrap the placenta after its delivery
- Clean, unused rubber gloves and eyewear. The lack of gloves and eyewear will mean possible exposure to infectious diseases.

Normal Delivery

Evaluating the Mother

A simple series of questions, an examination for crowning, and determination of vital signs will allow you make the decision for transport. However, do not let the "urgency" of this decision upset the mother. Your patient needs emotional support at this time. Your calm, professional actions will help her feel more at ease and assure her that the required care will be provided for both her and the unborn child.

✋ Remember

It is best to transport an expecting mother unless, based on your evaluation, you expect delivery within a few minutes.

To begin to evaluate the mother:

1. Ask her name, age, and expected due date.

2. Ask if this is her first pregnancy. The average time of labor for a woman having her first baby is about 16 to 17 hours. The time in labor is typically shorter for subsequent births, unless the mother has given birth to more than four or five babies already. In some women with numerous deliveries, the uterus will continue to act like a well-toned muscle; in others, it will be less effective and delivery will take longer.

3. Ask her how long she has been having labor pains, how often she is having pains, and if her "bag of waters" has broken. Ask "Have you had any bleeding or bloody show?" At this point, with a woman having her first delivery, you may think that you can make a decision about transport. However, you should continue with the evaluation procedure. Also, begin to time the frequency and length of the contractions.

4. Ask her if she is straining or if she feels as though she needs to move her bowels. If she says yes, this usually means that the baby has moved into the birth canal and is pressing the vaginal wall against the rectum. Do not allow the mother to go to the bathroom as she may deliver the infant into the toilet. Birth will probably occur very soon. The mother may tell you that she can feel the baby trying to move out through her vaginal opening. In such cases, birth is probably very near.

5. Examine the mother for crowning (Figure 24-5). This is a visual inspection to see if there is bulging

Figure 24-5 Crowning of the infant's head.

at the vaginal opening or if the presenting part of the baby is visible. If part of the baby's head or presenting part is visible with each contraction, then birth is imminent.

6. Feel for uterine contractions. You may have to delay this procedure until the patient tells you she is having labor pains. Tell her what you are going to do, then place the palm of your gloved hand on her abdomen, above the navel. This can be done over the top of the patient's clothing. You should be able to feel her uterus and its contraction. All contractions should be timed. Keep track of the duration and frequency of the contractions. The uterus and the tissues between this organ and the skin will feel more rigid as the delivery of the baby nears.

7. Take vital signs at this time if you do not have a partner to do it. Alert the medical facility staff if the mother's vital signs are abnormal.

Examining for crowning may be embarrassing to the mother, the father, and any required bystanders. For this reason, it is important that you fully explain what you are doing and why. Be certain that you protect the mother from the stares of bystanders. In a polite but firm manner, ask everyone who does not belong at the scene to leave. Carefully help the patient remove enough clothing to allow you an unobstructed view of the vaginal opening.

Remember

A professional appearance coupled with a professional manner instills confidence in patients and bystanders alike.

If this is the woman's first delivery, she is not straining, and there is no crowning, there is little reason why she cannot be transported to a medical facility for delivery. On the other hand, if this is not her first delivery, and she is straining, crying out, and complaining about having to go to the bathroom, birth will probably occur too soon for transport. If the mother is having labor pains from contractions that are about 2 minutes apart, birth is very near. If you determine that delivery is imminent based on the presence of crowning or other signs, local protocol may require you to contact medical direction for the decision to commit to delivery on the site. If delivery does not occur in 10 minutes, contact medical direction for permission to initiate transport of the mother.

You may find a patient who is afraid of transport because she believes that birth will occur along the way. Assure her that you believe there is enough time before delivery. Let her know that you are trained to assist with the delivery and that the ambulance is well equipped to handle her needs and care for the newborn should she deliver en route. If crowning occurs during transport, stop the ambulance and prepare for delivery.

If your evaluation of the patient leads you to believe that birth is too near at hand for transport, you and your partner should prepare to assist the mother with delivery. Remember, as part of the preparation, the patient will need emotional support.

Remember

Do not allow the mother to go to the bathroom, even though she says that she has to move her bowels. Birth is probably only a few minutes away. Do not allow the mother to hold her legs together or use any other method to attempt to delay the delivery.

Supine Hypotensive Syndrome

Near the time of birth, the weight of the uterus, coupled with the infant's weight, placenta, and amniotic fluid, approximates 20–24 pounds. When the mother is in a supine position, this heavy mass will tend to compress the inferior vena cava, a major blood vessel, reducing return of blood to the heart, reducing cardiac output and resulting in a low blood pressure. This causes dizziness and a drop in blood pressure, a set of signs and symptoms known as **supine hypotensive syndrome.** This syndrome is also referred to as *vena cava compression syndrome.* The body begins to compensate, when it senses the drop in blood pressure, by contracting the uterine arteries and redirecting blood to the major organs. This can affect the fetus severely.

The drop in blood pressure signals shock, but the method of treating for shock (hypoperfusion) by elevating the legs is not effective in this instance because it does not relieve pressure on the vena cava.

To counteract or avoid the possible drop in blood pressure, all third-trimester patients should be transported on their left side. A pillow or rolled blanket should be placed behind the back to maintain proper positioning.

Preparing the Mother for Delivery

When your evaluation leads you to believe birth is imminent, you must immediately prepare the mother for delivery. To do so, you should:

1. Control the scene so that the mother will have privacy. (Her birthing coach may remain.) If you are not in a private room and transfer to the ambulance is not practical (crowning is present), ask bystanders to leave.

2. In addition to surgical gloves, you and your partner should put on gowns, caps, face masks, and eye protection since there is a high probability of splashing blood and other body fluids during delivery.

3. Place the mother on a bed, floor, or the ambulance stretcher. Elevate the buttocks with blankets or a pillow. Have the mother lie with knees drawn up and spread apart. You will need about 2 feet of work space below the woman's buttocks to place and initially care for the newborn. Having the patient positioned on the stretcher may speed transport if complications arise.

4. Remove any of the patient's clothing or underclothing that obstructs your view of the vaginal opening. Use sterile sheets or sterile towels to cover the mother as shown in Figure 24-6. Clean sheets, clean cloths, towels, or materials such as tablecloths can be used if you do not have an obstetric kit.

5. Position your assistant—your partner, the father, or someone the mother agrees to have assist you—at the mother's head. This person should stay alert to help turn the mother's head should she vomit. As well, this person should provide emotional support to the mother, soothing and encouraging her.

6. Position the obstetric kit near the patient. All items must be within easy reach.

Note: If delivery is to take place in an automobile, position the mother flat on the seat. Arrange her legs so that she has one foot resting on the seat and the other foot resting on the floor.

Figure 24-6   Preparing the mother for delivery.

Delivering the Baby

Position yourself in such a way that you have a constant view of the vaginal opening. Be prepared for the baby to come at any moment.

Be prepared for the patient to experience discomfort. Delivering a child is a natural process, but it will be accompanied by pain. Your patient may also have intense feelings of nausea. If this is her first child, she may be very frightened. All these factors may cause your patient to be uncooperative at times. You must remember that the patient is in pain and she may feel ill. She will need emotional support.

During delivery, talk to the mother. Encourage her to relax between contractions. Continue to time her contractions from the beginning of one contraction to the beginning of the next. Encourage her not to strain unless she feels she must. Remind her that her feeling of a pending bowel movement is usually just pressure caused by the baby moving into her birth canal. Encourage her to breathe deeply through her mouth. She may feel better if she pants, although she should be discouraged from breathing rapidly and deeply enough to bring on hyperventilation. If her "bag of waters" breaks, remind her that this is normal.

Note

Unless there are signs of complications, consider the delivery to be normal if there is a cephalic presentation. Observe any unusual color in the amniotic fluid.

To assist the mother with a normal delivery:

1. Continue to keep someone at the mother's head to provide support, monitor vital signs, and be alert for vomiting. If no one is on hand to help, be alert for vomiting and check vital signs between contractions.

2. Position your gloved hands at the mother's vaginal opening when the baby's head starts to appear. Do not touch the area around the vagina except to assist with the delivery. For legal reasons, it is always preferable for both your protection and the patient's to have your partner present at all times when you are touching a woman's vaginal area.

3. Place one hand below the baby's head as it delivers (Figure 24-7 and Scan 24-1). Spread your fingers evenly, remembering that the skull contains "soft spots" or *fontanelles.* Support the baby's head, but avoid pressure to these soft areas at the top and sides of the skull. A slight, well-distributed pressure may help prevent an explosive delivery. Keeping one hand on the baby's head and using the other hand to hold a sterile towel to support the tissue between the mother's vagina and anus can help prevent tearing of this tissue during delivery of the head. DO NOT PULL ON THE BABY!

4. If the amniotic sac has not broken by the time the baby's head is delivered, use your finger to puncture the membrane. Pull the membranes away from the baby's mouth and nose. The amniotic fluid should be clear. Examine the amniotic fluid for meconium staining, which will appear to be a dark green-black color. Meconium-stained amniotic fluid is caused by fetal feces (wastes) released during labor, usually because of maternal or fetal stress. If meconium is present, prepare to suction the infant immediately. If the meconium is aspirated (breathed in) by the fetus, the baby can develop pneumonia or other infections.

5. Once the head delivers, check to see if the umbilical cord is wrapped around the baby's neck. Tell the mother not to push while you check. If she can "pant," or take short quick breaths for just a moment, it may help relieve the urge to push while you check. Then gently loosen the cord if necessary. Even though the umbilical cord is very tough, rough handling may cause it to tear. If the cord is wrapped around the baby's neck, try to place two fingers under the cord at the back of the baby's neck. Bring the cord forward, over the baby's upper shoulder and head.

If you cannot loosen or slip the cord over the baby's head, the baby cannot be delivered. So immediately clamp the cord in two places using the clamps provided in the obstetric kit. Be very careful not to injure the baby. With extreme care, cut the cord between the two clamps. Gently unwrap the ends of the cord from around the baby's neck, and then proceed with the delivery.

6. Check the baby's airway. Most babies are born face down and then rotate to the right or left. Support the baby's head so that it does not touch the mother's anal area. When the entire head of the baby is visible, continue to support the head with one hand and, with the other hand, wipe the mouth and nose with sterile gauze pads. Use the rubber bulb syringe to suction the baby's mouth, then the nose.

Compress the syringe BEFORE placing it in the baby's mouth. Suction the mouth first, then the nostrils. Carefully insert the tip of the syringe about 1 to 1½ inches into the baby's mouth and release the bulb to allow fluids to be drawn into the syringe. Control the release with your fingers. Withdraw the tip and discharge the syringe's contents onto a towel. Repeat this procedure two or three times in the baby's mouth and once or twice in each nostril. The tip of the syringe should not be inserted more than ½ inch into the baby's nostril.

7. Help deliver the shoulders. The upper shoulder (usually with some delay) will deliver next, followed quickly by the lower shoulder. You must support the baby throughout this entire process. Gently guide the baby's head downward, to assist the mother in delivering the baby's upper shoulder. After the upper shoulder has delivered, if the lower shoulder is slow to deliver, assist the mother by gently guiding the baby's head upward.

8. Support the baby throughout the entire birth process. Remember that newborns are very slippery. As the feet are born, grasp them to assure a good

Figure 24-7 Delivering the infant's head.

ASSISTING IN A NORMAL DELIVERY

FIRST take BSI precautions.

Note: Assist the mother by supporting the baby throughout the birth process.

▲ **1.** Support the infant's head.

▲ **2.** Suction the infant's mouth and nose.

▲ **3.** Aid in the birth of the upper shoulder.

▲ **4.** Support the trunk.

▲ **5.** Support the feet.

▲ **6.** Keep the infant level with the vagina until the umbilical cord stops pulsating.

471

hold on the baby. Never pick up a baby by the feet as they are very slippery and you could drop the child. Once the feet are delivered, lay the baby on his side with his head slightly lower than his body. This is done to allow blood, fluids, and mucus to drain from the mouth and nose. Suction the mouth and nose again with the bulb syringe. Keep the baby at the same level as the mother's vagina until the umbilical cord stops pulsating. Wrap the infant in a warm, dry blanket.

9. Note the exact time of birth.

Caution

Some deliveries are explosive. Do not squeeze the baby, but do provide adequate support. You can prevent an explosive delivery by using one hand to maintain slight pressure on the baby's head, avoiding direct pressure to the infant's soft spot on the skull.

The Newborn

Assessing the Newborn

The vigor of an infant should be assessed as soon as he is born. If you arrive after the birth, it is still your responsibility to make the assessments based on your first observations. Remember, however, that care for the infant and the mother should not be delayed. *The assessment is meant to take place while these other activities are being performed.*

Your EMS system may call for a general or a specific evaluation protocol. A general evaluation usually calls for noting ease of breathing, the heart rate, crying, movement, and skin color. A normal newborn should have a pulse greater than 100/min, be breathing easily, crying (vigorous crying is a good sign), moving his extremities (the more active, the better), and show blue coloration at the hands and feet only. Five minutes later, these signs should still be apparent, with breathing becoming more relaxed. The blue coloration may or may not disappear, but it should not spread to other parts of the body.

Caring for the Newborn

Even with a normal delivery, each step in the care of the baby is essential for his survival. To care for the newborn, you should first place the baby on a sterile sheet on the bed or padded table surface, keeping the baby close to the level of the mother's vagina so that the infant's blood does not transfuse back into the placenta. Do not place the infant on the mother's abdomen at this time (not until after the cord is clamped and cut—see later in this chapter).

During the birth process, the infant is passive. Once the baby is born, he very quickly becomes ac-

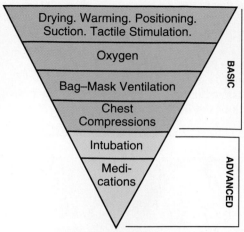

Figure 24-8 Inverted pyramid of neonatal resuscitation.

tive. Exposure to the air is usually enough to stimulate the infant to breathe. As you suction, dry, and warm the baby, he is stimulated even more. If the newborn does not breathe on his own after suctioning, drying, and warming for 30 seconds, begin resuscitation measures.

Resuscitation of the Newborn

Neonatal resuscitation follows an inverted pyramid. As Figure 24-8 shows, most newborns with abnormal assessment findings respond to relatively simple maneuvers. Few require CPR or advanced life support measures.

Follow these steps for initial care of the newborn:

1. Clear the baby's airway. Use a bulb syringe, suctioning the mouth first and then the nostrils. Squeeze the bulb before inserting the syringe into the baby's mouth. Release the bulb to create suction. It may be necessary to use a sterile gauze pad to clear mucus and blood from around the baby's nose and mouth.

Note

When the nostrils are suctioned, the baby may gasp or begin breathing and aspirate any meconium, blood, fluids, or mucus from his mouth into his lungs. That is why it is imperative to suction the mouth before the nostrils.

2. Keep the baby on his side and again suction the mouth, then the nose with a rubber bulb syringe (Figure 24-9). If necessary, you can cradle the baby in your arms. However, it is best to keep the baby on the cot or table surface.

3. Establish that the baby is breathing. Usually the baby will be breathing on his own by the time you

Figure 24-9 Suction the mouth and then the nose of the newborn.

clear the airway. A newborn should begin breathing within 30 seconds. If he does not, then you must "encourage" the baby to breathe (Figure 24-10). Usually, a gentle but vigorous rubbing of the baby's back will promote spontaneous respiration. Should this method fail, snap one of your index fingers against the sole of the baby's foot. Do not hold the baby up by his feet and slap his bottom! Do not become alarmed if the hands and feet of a breathing newborn appear slightly blue. It is not uncommon for this blue color to remain for the first few minutes.

If assessment of the infant's breathing reveals shallow, slow, or absent respirations, provide artificial ventilations at a rate of 40 to 60 per minute.

Remember: Provide only small puffs of air to the neonate if using mouth to mask, and small squeezes on the bag if using an infant-size bag-valve-mask device. Reassess the infant's respiratory efforts after 30 seconds. If there is no change in the effort of breathing, continue with ventilations and reassessment.

4. Assess the infant's heart rate. If the heart rate is less than 100 beats per minute, then provide artificial ventilations at a rate of 40 to 60 per minute. Reassess the heart rate after 30 seconds. If the heart rate is between 60 and 80 per minute and rising, continue to provide artificial ventilations and reassess again in 30 seconds. If the heart rate on reassessment is less than 60 per minute, or between 60 and 80 per minute and not rising, continue ventilations and initiate chest compressions, as shown in Figure 24-11. Chest compressions in the neonate should be delivered at a rate of 120 compressions per minute, midsternum with two thumbs, fingers supporting the back. Depth of compression is ½ to ¾ inch. The ratio of compressions to breaths is 3 compressions to 1 breath.

5. If the child has adequate respirations and a pulse rate greater than 100 per minute, but exhibits cyanosis of the face and/or torso, provide supplemental oxygen. Oxygen is best delivered at 10–15 liters per minute using oxygen tubing placed close to, but not directly into, the infant's face.

Cutting the Umbilical Cord

In a normal birth, the infant must be breathing on his own before you clamp and cut the cord. Before clamping and cutting the cord, palpate the cord with your fingers to make sure it is no longer pulsating. The general procedure for umbilical cord care is as follows:

1. Keep the infant warm. Dry off the baby and wrap him in a baby blanket or infant swaddler, clean towel, or sheet prior to clamping the cord (Figure 24-12). Do not wash the infant. Sometimes the mother may request you to do so, but it is best to leave the protective coating (called the *vernix*) on the infant until he reaches the medical facility.

2. Use the sterile clamps or umbilical tape found in the obstetric kit. Use extreme care with any tying done to the cord, forming the knot slowly to avoid cutting the cord. Ties should be made using a square knot (right over left, then left over right).

3. Apply one clamp or tie to the cord about 10 inches from the baby. This leaves enough cord for intravenous lines to be used by paramedics or the staff at the hospital if they are needed.

4. Place a second clamp or tie about 7 inches from the baby. The proximal clamp should be about the width of 4 fingers from the neonate.

5. Cut the cord between the clamps or knots using sterile surgical scissors (Figure 24-13). Use caution and protect your eyes when cutting the cord as a spurt of blood is very common. Never untie or unclamp a cord once it

Figure 24-10 It may be necessary to stimulate the newborn to breathe.

Figure 24-11 Deliver chest compressions at 120 per minute, midsternum with two thumbs, at a depth of ½ to ¾ inches. For a very small infant (inset), the thumbs may be overlapped.

is cut. The placental end of the cord should be placed on the drape over the mother's legs to avoid contact with expelled blood, feces, and fluids. Examine the fetal end of the cord for bleeding. Do not attempt to adjust the clamp or retie the knot. Should bleeding continue, apply another tie or clamp as close to the original as possible.

6. Be careful when moving the baby so that no trauma is brought to the clamped cord. If the cord does not remain closed off completely, the baby may bleed to death from seemingly little blood loss. In most cases, the cord vessels will collapse and seal themselves.

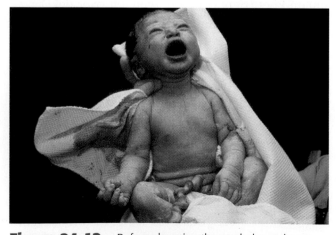

Figure 24-12 Before clamping the cord, dry and wrap the infant to keep him warm.

Figure 24-13 Cutting the umbilical cord.

Warning

Do not tie, clamp, or cut the cord of a baby who is not breathing on his own unless you have to do so to remove the cord from around the baby's neck during birth, or unless you have to perform CPR on the infant. Do not cut or clamp a cord that is still pulsating.

Keeping the Baby Warm

It is critical that the baby be kept warm. Wrap the newborn in an infant swaddler and a warmed blanket or towel and let the mother hold the infant on her abdomen (Figure 24-14). Bubble wrap can also be used. It provides padded protection, warmth (prewarm it), and allows visual monitoring of the infant. Be sure to cover the infant's head (but not the face). During the delivery of the placenta, have your partner hold the baby unless the mother insists otherwise. Keep the ambulance warm.

Assisting at a Birth When Off Duty

If you are assisting at a birth when off duty, you will probably be able to find all the items you need to tie and cut the cord. If no clamps or tying devices are on hand, use clean shoelaces or similar soft, clean ties. You may delay clamping and tying the cord if the infant will receive this care within 30 minutes. If you tie the cord, you believe it will be some time before transport and transfer, and you do *not* have sterile

Figure 24-14 Place the baby on the mother's abdomen. Write the mother's last name and time of delivery on a tape, fold it so the adhesive does not touch the baby's skin, and place it around the baby's wrist.

scissors, soak scissors in alcohol for several minutes and use them to cut the cord. If the baby is still attached to the placenta when the organ is delivered, wrap the placenta in a towel and transport infant and placenta as a unit. The placenta should be placed at the same level as the baby, or slightly higher. Careful monitoring of the baby must be maintained.

Caring for the Mother

Remember that you have two patients to care for: the infant and the mother. Care for the mother includes helping her deliver the placenta, controlling vaginal bleeding, and making her as comfortable as possible.

Delivering the Placenta

The third stage of labor is the delivery of the placenta with its umbilical cord section, membranes of the amniotic sac, and some of the tissues lining the uterus (Figure 24-15). (All of these together are known as the afterbirth.) Placental delivery begins with a brief return of the labor pains that stopped when the baby was born. You will notice a lengthening of the cord, which indicates the placenta has separated from the uterus. In most cases, the placenta will be expelled within a few minutes after the baby is born.

Although the process may take 30 minutes or longer, avoid the urge to put pressure on the abdomen over the uterus to hasten delivery of the placenta. If mother and baby are doing well, and there are no respiratory problems or significant uncontrolled bleeding, transportation to the hospital can be delayed up to 20 minutes while awaiting delivery of the placenta.

Save all afterbirth tissues. The attending physician will want to examine the placenta and other tissues for completeness since any afterbirth tissues remaining in the uterus pose a serious threat of

Figure 24-15 Delivery of the placenta.

infection and prolonged bleeding to the mother. Try to catch the afterbirth in a container. Place the container in a plastic bag, or wrap it in a towel, paper, or plastic. If no container is available, catch the afterbirth in a towel, paper, or a plastic bag. Label this material "placenta" and include the name of the mother and the time the tissues were expelled.

Remember: If the placenta does not deliver within 20 minutes of the baby's birth, transport the mother and baby to a medical facility without delay.

Note

Some EMS systems recommend transport without waiting for delivery of the placenta. There may be a condition in which the placenta does not separate from the uterine wall, and it is important for mother and baby to get to the hospital. You can always stop the ambulance to deliver the placenta if it crowns en route.

Controlling Vaginal Bleeding After Birth

Delivery of the baby and placenta is ALWAYS accompanied by some bleeding from the vagina. Although the blood loss is usually no more than 500 cc, it may be profuse. To control vaginal bleeding after delivery of the baby and placenta, you should:

1. Place a sanitary napkin over the mother's vaginal opening. Do not place anything in the vagina.

2. Have the mother lower her legs and keep them together. Tell her that she does not have to "squeeze" her legs together. Elevate her feet.

3. Massaging the uterus will help it contract (Figure 24-16). This will help control bleeding. Feel the mother's abdomen until you note a "grapefruit-sized" object. This is her uterus. Rub this area lightly with a circular motion. It should contract and become firm, and bleeding should diminish.

4. The mother may want to nurse the baby. This will aid in the contraction of the uterus. Some pediatricians recommend the baby not nurse until a doctor has examined it.

The skin between the vagina and the anus is known as the **perineum.** A tearing of tissue can occur in the perineum at the vaginal opening during the birth process. The mother may feel the discomfort from this torn tissue. Let her know that this is normal and that the problem will be quickly cared for at the medical facility. Treat the torn perineum as a wound. Dress by applying a sanitary napkin and applying some pressure.

Providing Comfort to the Mother

Keep contact with the mother throughout the entire birth process and after she has delivered. Your care for the mother does not end when you have completed your duties with the placenta and vaginal bleeding. Take her vital signs frequently. Be aware that she has just undergone a tremendous emotional experience and small acts of kindness will be appreciated and remembered. Childbirth is a rigorous task, and a woman is physically exhausted at the conclu-

sion of delivery. Wiping her face and hands with a damp washcloth and then drying them with a towel will do wonders to refresh her and prepare her for the trip to the hospital. Replace blood-soaked sheets and blankets. Make sure that both she and the baby are warm.

When delivery occurs at home, ask a member of the family or a trusted neighbor to help you clean up. You should clean up whatever disorder EMS care has caused in the house; however, you should not delay transport in order to complete these activities. In some areas, local protocol may have you return to the house after transport in order to complete the clean-up process. If you do, you will have to be accompanied by a member of the family. Be sure to properly dispose of items that have been in contact with blood and other body fluids in a biohazard container.

Remember

Birth is an exciting and joyous event. Talking to the mother and paying attention to her new baby are part of total patient care. A good rule to follow is to treat your patient as you would wish a member of your family to be treated.

CHILDBIRTH COMPLICATIONS

Complications of Delivery

Although most babies are born without difficulty, complications may occur during and after delivery. We have already considered three such complications: the cord around the neck, an unbroken amniotic sac, and infants who need encouragement to breathe. These problems can be handled by simple procedures. However, there are other complications that can threaten the life of both mother and newborn and for which definitive treatment is beyond the EMT-B's level of training. For emergencies such as breech presentation, prolapsed umbilical cord, and limb presentation, you will provide high-concentration oxygen and rapid transport to the hospital.

Breech Presentation

Breech presentation is the most common abnormal delivery. It involves a buttocks-first or both-legs-first delivery (Figure 24-17). The risk of birth trauma to the baby is high in breech deliveries. In addition there is an increased risk of prolapsed cord (see the next section). In addition, meconium staining often occurs with breech presentations.

Control Bleeding

Figure 24-16 After delivery of the placenta, massage the uterus to help control vaginal bleeding.

Figure 24-17 Breech delivery.

Patient ASSESSMENT

Breech Presentation

If you evaluate a woman in labor and find the baby's buttocks or both legs presenting, rather than the head presenting, this is a breech presentation. Although breech presentations can spontaneously deliver successfully, the complication rate is high.

Patient CARE

Breech Presentation

Emergency care of a patient with a breech presentation includes the following:

1. Initiate rapid transport upon recognition of a breech presentation.

2. Never attempt to deliver the baby by pulling on his legs.

3. Provide high-concentration oxygen.

4. Place the mother in a head-down position with the pelvis elevated.

5. If the body delivers, support him and prevent an explosive delivery of the head.

6. After delivery, care for the baby, cord, mother, and placenta as in a cephalic delivery.

Prolapsed Umbilical Cord

Sometimes during delivery, the umbilical cord presents first (this is most common in breech births) and the cord is squeezed between the vaginal wall and the head of the baby. The cord is pinched, and oxygen supply to the baby may be totally interrupted. This occurrence is known as a **prolapsed umbilical cord.**

Patient ASSESSMENT

Prolapsed Umbilical Cord

If, upon viewing the vaginal area, you see the umbilical cord presenting, the cord is prolapsed.

Patient CARE

Prolapsed Umbilical Cord

Follow the steps below when the umbilical cord is prolapsed (Figure 24-18):

1. Position the mother with her head down and buttocks raised with a blanket or pillow, using gravity to lessen pressure on the birth canal.

2. Provide the mother with a high concentration of oxygen by way of a nonrebreather mask to

- Elevate hips, administer oxygen, and keep mother warm
- Keep baby's head away from cord
- Do not attempt to push cord back
- Wrap cord in sterile moist towel
- Transport mother to hospital, continuing pressure on baby's head

Figure 24-18 Prolapsed umbilical cord.

increase the concentration carried over to the infant.

3. Check the cord for pulses and wrap the exposed cord, using a sterile towel from the obstetric kit. The cord must be kept warm.

4. Insert several fingers of your gloved hand into the mother's vagina so that you can gently push up on the baby's head or buttocks to keep pressure off of the cord. You will be pushing up through the cervix. This may be the only chance that the baby has for survival, so continue to push up on the baby until a physician relieves you. You may feel the cord pulsating when pressure is released.

5. Keeping mother, child, and EMT-B as a unit, transport immediately to a medical facility. Be prepared to stay in this position until you reach the hospital.

6. All patients with prolapsed cords require rapid transport. Have your partner obtain vital signs while en route to the hospital if possible.

Limb Presentation

A **limb presentation** occurs when a limb of an infant protrudes from the vagina. The presenting limb is commonly a foot when the baby is in the breech position. Limb presentations cannot be delivered in the prehospital setting. Rapid transport is essential to the baby's survival.

● Patient ASSESSMENT

Limb Presentation

When checking for crowning, you may see an arm, a single leg, or an arm and leg together, or a shoulder and an arm (Figure 24-19). If one or more limbs present, there is often a prolapsed umbilical cord as well.

● Patient CARE

Limb Presentation

When you discover a limb presentation, take these emergency care steps:

1. If there is a prolapsed cord, follow the same procedures as you would for any delivery involving a prolapsed cord. Remember, you have to keep pushing up on the baby until relieved by a physician. The baby must be kept off of the cord if he is to survive.

2. Transport the mother immediately to a medical facility.

3. Place the mother in a head down position with the pelvis elevated.

4. Administer a high concentration of oxygen with a nonrebreather mask.

Figure 24-19   Limb presentation.

Remember

For a limb presentation, do not try to pull on the limb or replace the limb into the vagina. Do not place your gloved hand into the vagina, unless there is a prolapsed cord.

Multiple Birth

When more than one baby is born during a single delivery, it is called a **multiple birth.** A multiple birth, usually twins, is not considered a complication, provided that the deliveries are normal. Twins are generally delivered in the same manner as a single delivery, one birth following the other. However, if a multiple birth is encountered, you should have enough personnel and equipment to be prepared for multiple resuscitations. Call for assistance if needed.

When delivering twins, identify the infants as to order of birth (one and two, or A and B).

Patient ASSESSMENT

Multiple Birth

If the mother is under a physician's care, she will probably be aware that she is carrying twins. Without this information, you should consider a multiple birth to be a possibility if the mother's abdomen appears unusually large before delivery, or it remains very large after delivery of one baby. If the birth is multiple, labor contractions will continue and the second baby will be delivered shortly after the first. The second baby may present in a breech position, usually within minutes of the first birth. The placenta(s) are delivered normally (Figure 24-20).

Separate placentas

One placenta

Figure 24-20   Multiple births.

Multiple Birth

When assisting in the delivery of twins, follow these steps:

1. Clamp or tie the cord of the first baby before the second baby is born.

2. The second baby may be born either before or after the placenta is delivered. Assist the mother with the delivery of the second baby.

3. Provide care for the babies, umbilical cords, placenta(s), and the mother as you would in a single-baby delivery.

4. The babies will probably be smaller than in a single birth, so special care should be taken to keep them warm during transport.

Premature Birth

By definition, a **premature infant** is one who weighs less than 5½ pounds at birth, or one who is born before the 37th week of pregnancy.

Premature Birth

Since you probably will not be able to weigh the baby, make a determination as to whether the baby is full-term or premature based on the mother's information and the baby's appearance. By comparison with a normal full-term baby, the head of a premature infant is much larger in proportion to the small, thin, red body (Figure 24-21).

Premature Birth

Premature babies need special care from the moment of birth. The smaller the baby, the more important is the initial care. You should take the following steps when providing care for the premature infant:

1. Keep the baby warm. Premature infants are at great risk of developing hypothermia. Once breathing, the baby should be dried and wrapped snugly in a warm blanket. Additional protection can be provided by an outer wrap of plastic bubble wrap (keep away from the face) or a small reflective blanket. Premature babies lack fat deposits that

A

B

Figure 24-21 (A) Full-term newborn and (B) a premature newborn after 24 weeks of gestation.

would normally keep them warm. Some EMS systems in cold regions are using a plastic or bubble wrap or bag for the infant, covered by a blanket. This helps maintain warmth and allows for easier visual inspection of the clamped cord to check for bleeding. A stockinet cap should be placed on the baby's head to help reduce heat loss.

2. Keep the airway clear. Continue to suction fluids from the nose and mouth using a rubber bulb syringe. Keep checking to see if additional suctioning is required.

3. Provide ventilations and/or chest compressions as outlined earlier based upon the baby's pulse and respiratory effort. In some cases, resuscitation may not be possible if the baby is extremely premature.

4. Watch the umbilical cord for bleeding. Examine the cut end of the cord carefully. If there is any sign of bleeding, even the slightest, apply another clamp or tie closer to the baby's body.

5. Provide oxygen. Do not blow a stream of oxygen directly on the baby's face, but arrange for oxygen to flow past the baby's face. If available, use a humidified source of oxygen.

6. Avoid contamination. The premature infant is susceptible to infection. Keep him away from other people. Do not breathe on his face.

7. Transport the infant in a warm ambulance. The desired temperature is between 90°F and 100°F. Use the ambulance heater to warm the patient compartment prior to transport. In the summer months, the air conditioning should be turned off and all compartment windows should be closed or adjusted to keep the desired temperature.

8. Call ahead to the emergency department.

Meconium

As noted earlier, meconium is a result of the fetus defecating (putting out wastes). It is a sign of fetal or maternal distress.

Patient ASSESSMENT

Meconium

Meconium stains amniotic fluid greenish or brownish-yellow in color. Infants born with meconium are at increased risk for respiratory problems, especially if aspiration of the meconium occurs at birth.

Patient CARE

Meconium

If you see meconium staining in the amniotic fluid, follow these steps:

1. To reduce the risk of aspiration, do not stimulate the infant before suctioning the oropharynx.

2. Suction the mouth and then the nose.

3. Maintain an open airway.

4. Provide artificial ventilations and/or chest compression as indicated by effort of breathing and heart rate.

5. Transport as soon as possible.

Emergencies in Pregnancy

There are a number of predelivery emergencies that can arise in the pregnant patient prior to labor or childbirth.

Excessive Prebirth Bleeding

A number of conditions can cause excessive prebirth bleeding late in pregnancy. Whether the vaginal bleeding is associated with abdominal pain or not, the risk to both the mother and the unborn child is great.

One such condition is **placenta previa,** a condition in which the placenta is formed in an abnormal location (low in the uterus and close to or over the cervical opening) that will not allow for a normal delivery of the fetus. As the cervix dilates, the placenta tears. Another such condition is **abruptio placentae,** a condition in which the placenta separates from the uterine wall. This can be a partial or a complete abruption. Either placenta previa or abruptio placenta may occur in the third trimester. Both are potentially life threatening to the mother and fetus.

A pregnant woman does not have to be in labor to have excessive bleeding from the vagina. Bleeding in early pregnancy may be due to a miscarriage. If the bleeding occurs late in pregnancy, it may be due to problems involving the placenta.

Patient ASSESSMENT

Excessive Prebirth Bleeding

Signs and symptoms of excessive prebirth bleeding include the following:

- Main sign is usually profuse bleeding from the vagina.

- Mother may or may not experience associated abdominal pain.
- During initial assessment, look for signs of shock.
- Obtain baseline vital signs. A rapid heartbeat may indicate significant blood loss.

Patient *CARE*

Excessive Prebirth Bleeding

- Treatment is based on signs and symptoms. If signs of shock exist, treat with high-concentration oxygen and rapid transportation.
- Place a sanitary napkin over the vaginal opening. Note the time of napkin placement. DO NOT PLACE ANYTHING IN THE VAGINA. Replace pads as they become soaked, but save all pads for use in evaluating blood loss.
- Save all tissue that is passed.

Ectopic Pregnancy

In normal pregnancy, the fertilized egg will begin to divide in the oviduct (fallopian tube) and eventually implant in the wall of the uterus. In an **ectopic pregnancy,** implantation may take place in an oviduct, the cervix of the uterus, or in the abdominopelvic cavity. These areas or organs cannot contain or support the developing fetus.

Patient *ASSESSMENT*

Ectopic Pregnancy

The problems related to this condition are seen early in pregnancy. Women may have signs and symptoms including those indicating shock due to internal bleeding. This condition can be life threatening and, as the saying goes, "Any woman of child bearing age with abdominal pain is to be considered an ectopic pregnancy until proven otherwise by the physician in the emergency department."

Be alert to recognize the following signs and symptoms as they develop:

- Acute abdominal pain, often beginning on one side or the other
- Vaginal bleeding
- Rapid and weak pulse (a later sign)
- Low blood pressure (a very late sign)

Patient *CARE*

Ectopic Pregnancy

Emergency care includes the following:

1. Consider the need for immediate transport.

2. Position the patient for shock.

3. Care for shock.

4. Provide high-concentration oxygen by nonrebreather mask.

5. Do not give the patient anything by mouth.

Seizures in Pregnancy

Seizures in pregnancy, sometimes caused by conditions called **eclampsia,** tend to occur late in pregnancy. The seizures are usually associated with high blood pressure and **preeclampsia,** or swelling of the extremities. Seizures in pregnancy pose a serious threat to both the mother and unborn baby.

Patient *ASSESSMENT*

Seizures in Pregnancy

A seizure may be associated with any of the following:

- Elevated blood pressure, which increases the risk of abruptio placentae
- Excessive weight gain
- Extreme swelling of face, hands, ankles, and feet
- Headache

Patient *CARE*

Seizures in Pregnancy

Emergency care of a pregnant patient with seizures includes the following:

1. Ensure and maintain an open airway.

2. Administer high-concentration oxygen by nonrebreather mask.

3. Transport the patient positioned on her left side.

4. Handle her gently at all times. Rough handling may induce more seizures.

5. Keep her warm, but do not overheat.

6. Have suction ready.

7. Have a delivery kit ready.

Miscarriage and Abortion

For a number of reasons, the fetus and placenta may deliver before the 28th week of pregnancy—generally before the baby can live on his own. This occurrence is an **abortion.** When it happens on its own, it is called a **spontaneous abortion,** more commonly known as a **miscarriage.** An **induced abortion** is an abortion that results from deliberate actions taken to stop the pregnancy.

Patient ASSESSMENT

Miscarriage and Abortion

Women having a miscarriage that requires them to seek emergency care generally have the following signs and symptoms:

- Cramping abdominal pains not unlike those associated with the first stage of labor
- Bleeding ranging from moderate to severe
- A noticeable discharge of tissue and blood from the vagina

Ask the patient about the starting date of her last menstrual period. If it has been more than 24 weeks, be prepared with a delivery pack. Premature infants may survive if they receive rapid neonatal intensive care.

Patient CARE

Miscarriage and Abortion

1. Obtain baseline vital signs.

2. If signs of shock are present, provide a high concentration of oxygen by a nonrebreather mask. Treatment should be based on signs and symptoms.

3. Help absorb vaginal bleeding by placing a sanitary napkin over the vaginal opening. Do not pack the vagina.

4. Transport as soon as possible.

5. Replace and save all blood-soaked pads.

6. Save all tissues that are expelled. Do not attempt to replace or pull out any tissues that are being expelled through the vagina.

7. Provide emotional support to the mother. Emotional support is very important. When speaking to the patient, her family, or where bystanders may hear you, ALWAYS use the term *miscarriage* instead of spontaneous abortion. Most people associate the word *abortion* with an induced abortion, not a miscarriage. It is essential to talk with the patient to gain her confidence and to allow you to provide emotional support.

Trauma in Pregnancy

Obviously the pregnant patient, as any other accident victim, can sustain injury. However, especially during the last two trimesters, the uterus and fetus are also subject to injuries when the mother is injured. Injuries to the uterus may be blunt or penetrating. In both cases, the greatest danger to mother and baby is hemorrhage (bleeding) and shock.

The most common cause of blunt trauma is automobile collisions, but falls or beatings also account for many injuries. The uterus is well designed to protect the baby. The fetus is inside the uterus, a muscular chamber filled with fluid. The uterus acts as an efficient shock absorber. Thus most minor trauma to the abdomen, such as a blow or fall, does not harm the fetus.

Automobile collisions are a different story. The magnitude of forces is great. Because of its size and location, the uterus is frequently injured. Sudden blunt trauma to the abdomen during the later months of pregnancy may cause uterine rupture or premature separation of the placenta (abruptio placentae). Other blunt trauma injuries, such as a ruptured spleen or liver, may also occur. Rupture of the diaphragm may occur with blunt trauma during later pregnancy. Multiple trauma with fractures of the pelvis can cause laceration or tearing of the vessels in the pelvis with massive hemorrhage. The common problem with most blunt injuries to the pregnant abdomen or pelvis is massive bleeding and shock.

If a pregnant woman is injured in an accident, such as a motor-vehicle collision or a fall, perform a patient assessment and treat her injuries as you would those of any other trauma patient.

Patient ASSESSMENT

Trauma in Pregnancy

Follow these patient assessment steps:

- During initial assessment and assessment of vital signs, remember the following about the physiology of pregnant women:
  - The pregnant patient has a pulse that is 10–15 beats per minute faster than the nonpregnant female. Vital signs may be interpreted as being suggestive of shock when they are normal for the pregnant female.
  - A woman in later pregnancy may have a blood volume that is up to 48% higher than her nonpregnant state. With hemorrhage, 30%–35% blood loss may occur before otherwise healthy pregnant females exhibit signs or symptoms.
  - Although shock is more difficult to assess in the pregnant patient, it is the most likely cause of prehospital death from injury to the uterus.
- Question the conscious patient to determine if she has received any blows to the abdomen, pelvis, or back.

- Ask the patient if she has had bleeding or rupture of the bag of waters. When in doubt, examine the vaginal area for bleeding, being certain to provide privacy.
- Examine the unconscious patient for abdominal injuries, remembering to consider the mechanism of injury.

Patient *CARE*

Trauma in Pregnancy

Remember that maintenance of respiration and circulation and the control of bleeding are vital not only to the mother but also to the fetus. A developing fetus is critically dependent on the uninterrupted oxygenated blood supply that enters the placenta. What is good for the mother is good for the baby. Since the mother-to-be may have undetected internal bleeding or the fetus may be injured, provide the following care to the injured mother:

1. Provide resuscitation if necessary.

2. Provide a high concentration of oxygen by using a nonrebreather mask. (Oxygen requirements of the woman in later pregnancy are 10%–20% greater than normal. If in doubt, give oxygen.)

3. Because of slowed digestion and delayed gastric emptying, there is a greater risk the patient will vomit and aspirate. Be ready with suction.

4. Transport as soon as possible. All pregnant women should be transported in the left lateral recumbent position unless a back or neck injury is suspected. If so, first secure the mother to a spine board, then tip board and patient as a unit to the left, relieving pressure on the abdominal organs and vena cava. Support the mother with pillows and folded blankets. Be sure to monitor and record vital signs.

5. Provide emotional support. A pregnant woman who is an accident victim will naturally worry about her unborn child. Remind her that the developing baby is well protected in the uterus. Let her know that she is being transported to a medical facility that can take care of her needs and the needs of the unborn child.

CHILDBIRTH AND DEATH

Stillbirths

Some babies die in the womb several hours, days, or even weeks before birth. Such a baby is called **stillborn.**

Patient *ASSESSMENT*

Stillbirth

When a baby has died some time before birth, death is obvious by the presence of blisters, foul odor, skin or tissue deterioration and discoloration, and a softened head. At other times, a baby may be born in pulmonary or cardiac arrest but in otherwise good condition and with the possibility of being resuscitated.

Patient *CARE*

Stillbirth

Emergency care for a stillborn baby is as follows:

1. Stillborn babies who have obviously been dead for some time before birth are not to receive resuscitation.

2. Any other babies who are born in pulmonary or cardiac arrest are to receive basic life support measures.

3. When the baby is alive but respiratory or cardiac arrest appears to be imminent, prepare to provide life support.

Nothing is quite so sad as a baby born dead or one who dies shortly after birth. It is a tragic moment for the parents and other family members. Your thoughtfulness may provide the distraught parents with comfort. In addition, do not lie to the mother. Many death-and-dying experts believe that she should be allowed to view her baby if she so desires. Do not stop her from seeing the dead baby if she wants to.

All resuscitative efforts should be continued until transfer to the hospital. Also, keep accurate records of the time of stillbirth and the care rendered for completion of the fetal death certificate.

Accidental Death of a Pregnant Woman

If a woman in advanced pregnancy dies in an accident and you begin CPR on her immediately, there is a chance of saving the life of the infant. CPR must then be continued until an emergency cesarean section can be performed. Reposition your hands for compressions 1 to 2 inches higher on the sternum to make up for shifting of the heart due to the large fetus. If CPR is delayed 5 to 10 minutes, chances of saving the baby are fair, while a 25-minute delay reduces the chances to almost zero. Continue CPR on the mother until you are relieved in the emergency department.

GYNECOLOGICAL EMERGENCIES

There are several emergencies unique to the reproductive systems of women who are not, or are not necessarily, pregnant.

Vaginal Bleeding

Vaginal bleeding that is not a result of direct trauma or a woman's normal menstrual cycle may indicate a serious gynecological emergency.

Patient ASSESSMENT

Vaginal Bleeding

Since it will be impossible for the EMT-B to determine a specific cause of the bleeding, it is important that all women who have vaginal bleeding be treated as though they have a potentially life-threatening condition. This is especially true if the bleeding is associated with abdominal pain. The most serious complication of vaginal bleeding is hypovolemic shock due to blood loss.

Patient CARE

Vaginal Bleeding

1. Take BSI precautions. Wear gloves, gown, protective eyewear, and mask as indicated.

2. Assure an adequate airway.

3. Assess for signs of shock.

4. Administer high-concentration oxygen by non-rebreather mask.

5. Transport.

Trauma to the External Genitalia

Trauma to a woman's external genitalia can be difficult to care for because of the patient's modesty and the severe pain often involved with such injuries.

Patient ASSESSMENT

Trauma to the External Genitalia

Injuries in this area tend to bleed profusely because of the rich blood supply to the area. Injuries to the female external genitalia are frequently the result of straddle-type injuries.

- In sizing up the scene, observe for mechanisms of injury.
- During initial assessment, look for signs of severe blood loss and shock.

Patient CARE

Trauma to the External Genitalia

1. Control bleeding with direct pressure over a bulky dressing or sanitary pad. (If the patient is alert, she will probably prefer to do this herself.) Do not remove undergarments unless necessary. Do not pack the vagina.

2. If signs of shock are present, treat with high-concentration oxygen.

3. Maintain a professional attitude.

4. Respect the patient's privacy. Remove unneeded bystanders and expose the patient's body only to the extent necessary to provide appropriate care.

Sexual Assault

Situations where a sexual assault has occurred are always a challenge to the EMT-B. Care of the patient must include both medical and psychological considerations. In addition, law enforcement agencies are also frequently involved.

There is no question that the victim of sexual assault is under tremendous stress. You must be prepared to deal with a wide range of emotions that the patient may exhibit. The best approach is to be nonjudgmental and to maintain a professional but compassionate attitude. It is generally preferable that an EMT-B of the same sex as the patient establish rapport and be the primary provider of emergency care.

Patient ASSESSMENT

Sexual Assault

- Since you may be entering a potential crime scene, assure that the scene is safe prior to entering. It may be necessary to "stage" your unit near the scene until it is rendered safe by police.
- During assessment, identify and treat both the medical and the psychological needs of the patient.

Patient CARE

Sexual Assault

1. Provide an open airway.

2. Be careful not to disturb potential criminal evidence unless it is absolutely necessary for patient care.

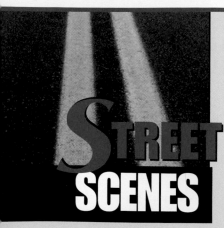

STREET SCENES

Your sleep is interrupted by the tones of the radio and the dispatcher saying "Bravo 3, stand-by for a call." You swing your feet onto the floor and grab the radio. "Go ahead, dispatch," you say.

"Bravo 3, respond to 77 Cherry Tree Lane for a pregnant patient in labor. The other dispatcher is still on the phone with the husband. Additional information to follow."

You and your partner head to the ambulance and start toward the scene. About 3 minutes from the patient's house, the dispatcher tells you that the baby appears to be crowning and the husband is still on the phone getting instructions. You and your partner decide you need a plan. You agree that both the adult and pediatric equipment need to be brought in, as well as the OB kit. You also agree that you will focus on the baby after delivery and your partner will provide care to the mother.

STREET SCENE QUESTIONS

1. What should be the first priority when entering the scene?
2. Should ALS assistance be requested?
3. What questions should you ask the mother or the father?

As you move toward the house, you ask the dispatcher if ALS has responded. You are told they are already en route. When you walk into the room, you see the mother on the bed and the father with the telephone cradled on his shoulder talking to the dispatcher. The father immediately stands aside, and you and your partner see the crowning and realize that the delivery will take place any minute. You put on gloves and set up the OB kit while getting assessment information from the mother. It is her second delivery but it is two weeks early. Labor started about an hour ago, and the pains have been more frequent and very intense. The water broke just before they called 9-1-1. While your partner is obtaining a set of vital signs, the baby starts to deliver. The head comes out and you notice that the umbilical cord is around the baby's neck. You are able to slip it over the baby's head, and the baby continues to deliver. The shoulders and the rest of the baby's body follow quickly.

STREET SCENE QUESTIONS

4. What immediate care should be provided to the newborn?
6. What care should your partner be giving to the mother?

You immediately start down the inverted pyramid for neonate resuscitation. You suction the mouth and then the nose. The baby starts to cry immediately. You dry the baby off and wrap the swaddling blanket around her, making sure that the top of the baby's head is covered. The baby is pink and actively moving. You check the pulse, and it is at least 150 beats per minute. Your partner clamps the cord and makes the cut. You call the dispatcher to log in the time of the delivery and announce that it is a girl. At that time, dispatch reports that ALS has been diverted to a cardiac arrest. After 20 minutes, the placenta still has not delivered and you transport to the hospital without any further delay.

When you arrive back at the station, there is still time to get a couple of hours sleep but you are too excited so you turn on the television.

3. Examine the genitals only if severe bleeding is present.

4. Discourage the patient from bathing, voiding, or cleansing any wounds as this may result in loss of important evidence.

5. Fulfill any reporting requirements that are locally mandated.

PATIENT NAME:	Doris Garfinkel					PATIENT AGE:	32	

CHIEF COMPLAINT

Imminent childbirth

PAST MEDICAL HISTORY

- [ ] None
- [ ] Allergy to _____
- [ ] Hypertension
- [ ] Stroke
- [ ] Seizures
- [ ] Diabetes
- [ ] COPD
- [ ] Cardiac
- [x] Other (List)
- [ ] Asthma

  Second child

Current Medications (List)

  None

V I T A L	TIME	RESP	PULSE	B.P.	MENTAL STATUS	R PUPILS L	SKIN
	0 1 4 5	Rate: **28** [ ] Regular [x] Shallow [ ] Labored	Rate: **100** [x] Regular [ ] Irregular	**130** / **84**	[x] Alert [ ] Voice [ ] Pain [ ] Unresp.	[x] Normal [x] [ ] Dilated [ ] [ ] Constricted [ ] [ ] Sluggish [ ] [ ] No-Reaction [ ]	[ ] Unremarkable [ ] Cool [ ] Pale [ ] Warm [ ] Cyanotic [x] Moist [ ] Flushed [ ] Dry [ ] Jaundiced
S I G N S	0 1 5 7	Rate: **28** [ ] Regular [x] Shallow [ ] Labored	Rate: **100** [x] Regular [ ] Irregular	**138** / **82**	[x] Alert [ ] Voice [ ] Pain [ ] Unresp.	[x] Normal [x] [ ] Dilated [ ] [ ] Constricted [ ] [ ] Sluggish [ ] [ ] No-Reaction [ ]	[ ] Unremarkable [ ] Cool [ ] Pale [ ] Warm [ ] Cyanotic [x] Moist [ ] Flushed [ ] Dry [ ] Jaundiced
	0 2 1 0	Rate: **28** [x] Regular [ ] Shallow [ ] Labored	Rate: **88** [x] Regular [ ] Irregular	**120** / **78**	[x] Alert [ ] Voice [ ] Pain [ ] Unresp.	[x] Normal [x] [ ] Dilated [ ] [ ] Constricted [ ] [ ] Sluggish [ ] [ ] No-Reaction [ ]	[ ] Unremarkable [ ] Cool [ ] Pale [ ] Warm [ ] Cyanotic [x] Moist [ ] Flushed [ ] Dry [ ] Jaundiced

NARRATIVE On arrival, crew met the patient and her husband. They state that the baby is about two weeks early and labor began an hour ago. Labor progressed very quickly and the pains and contractions are very intense and frequent. At the time of the 9-1-1 call, the patient's water broke. Delivery is imminent. A second unit with ALS requested in the event that there are complications, but they were diverted. We assisted with a normal cephalic delivery. The umbilical cord is loosened around the baby's neck and a normal delivery is observed. The baby is suctioned, stimulated, dried, and warmed. The cord is clamped and cut. The baby is placed on the mother's abdomen for transport and warmth. Transport is initiated prior to delivery of the placenta. See Form #107 for PCR on baby.

CHAPTER REVIEW

Summary

Birth is a natural process that usually takes place without complications. The role of the EMT-B at a birth is generally to provide reassurance and to assist the mother in the delivery of her baby. During the normal delivery, the EMT-B will evaluate the mother to determine if there should be immediate transport to a medical facility or if birth is imminent and will take place at the scene. If birth is to take place at the scene, the EMT-B prepares the mother for delivery, assists in the delivery, assesses the newborn, and cares for the newborn and the mother.

Occasionally there will be some complications to delivery, including breech presentation, prolapsed umbilical cord, limb presentation, multiple birth, premature birth, or meconium staining of the amniotic fluid. There may also be predelivery emergencies, or emergencies associated with pregnancy (such as excessive bleeding, ectopic pregnancy, seizures, abortion, or trauma to the pregnant mother) that the EMT-B must be prepared to treat. Stillbirth and death of the mother are difficult emergencies the EMT-B is occasionally called upon to manage, as are gynecological emergencies (such as vaginal bleeding, trauma, or sexual assault).

Key Terms

abortion spontaneous (miscarriage) or induced termination of pregnancy.

abruptio placentae (ab-RUPT-si-o plah-SENT-ta) a condition in which the placenta separates from the uterine wall; a cause of prebirth bleeding.

afterbirth the placenta, membranes of the amniotic sac, part of the umbilical cord, and some tissues from the lining of the uterus that are delivered after the birth of the baby.

amniotic (am-ne-OT-ik) **sac** the "bag of waters" that surrounds the developing fetus.

breech presentation when the baby appears buttocks or both legs first during birth.

cephalic (se-FAL-ik) **presentation** when the baby appears head first during birth. This is the normal presentation.

cervix (SUR-viks) the neck of the uterus at the entrance to the birth canal.

crowning when part of the baby is visible through the vaginal opening.

eclampsia (e-KLAMP-se-ah) a severe complication of pregnancy that produces seizures and coma.

ectopic (ek-TOP-ik) **pregnancy** when implantation of the fertilized egg is not in the body of the uterus, occurring instead in the oviduct (fallopian tube), cervix, or abdominopelvic cavity.

fetus (FE-tus) the baby as he develops in the womb.

induced abortion expulsion of a fetus as a result of deliberate actions taken to stop the pregnancy.

labor the three stages of the delivery of a baby that begin with the contractions of the uterus and end with the expulsion of the placenta.

limb presentation when an infant's limb protrudes from the vagina before the appearance of any other body part.

meconium staining amniotic fluid that is greenish or brownish-yellow rather than clear as a result of fetal defecation; an indication of possible maternal or fetal distress during labor.

miscarriage see *spontaneous abortion*.

multiple birth when more than one baby is born during a single delivery.

perineum (per-i-NE-um) the surface area between the vagina and anus.

placenta (plah-SEN-tah) the organ of pregnancy where exchange of oxygen, foods, and wastes occurs between a mother and fetus.

placenta previa (plah-SEN-tah PRE-vi-ah) a condition in which the placenta is formed in an abnormal location (low in the uterus and close to or over the cervical opening) that will not allow for a normal delivery of the fetus; a cause of excessive prebirth bleeding.

preeclampsia (pre-e-KLAMP-se-ah) a complication of pregnancy where the woman retains large amounts of fluid and has hypertension. She may also experience seizures and/or coma during birth, which is very dangerous to the infant.

premature infant any newborn weighing less than 5½ pounds or born before the 37th week of pregnancy.

prolapsed umbilical cord when the umbilical cord presents first and is squeezed between the vaginal wall and the baby's head.

spontaneous abortion when the fetus and placenta deliver before the 28th week of pregnancy; commonly called a miscarriage.

stillborn born dead.

supine hypotensive syndrome dizziness and a drop in blood pressure caused when the mother is in a supine position and the weight of the uterus, infant, placenta, and amniotic fluid compress the inferior vena cava, reducing return of blood to the heart and cardiac output.

umbilical (um-BIL-i-kal) **cord** the fetal structure containing the blood vessels that carry blood to and from the placenta.

uterus (U-ter-us) the muscular abdominal organ where the fetus develops; the womb.

vagina (vah-JI-nah) the birth canal.

Review Questions

1. Name and describe the anatomical structures of a woman's body that are associated with pregnancy. (pp. 463–464)
2. Describe the three stages of labor. (p. 464)
3. Explain how to evaluate and to prepare the mother for delivery. (pp. 467–469)
4. Name, in the order of the inverted pyramid, the steps that may be taken to resuscitate a newborn infant. (p. 472)
5. Name and describe several possible complications of delivery. (pp. 476–481)
6. Name and describe several possible predelivery emergencies. (pp. 481–484)

Applications

• You are called to respond to a pregnant woman who is in labor. During your evaluation, you find that this is the woman's first pregnancy, the baby's head is not yet crowning, and contractions are 10 minutes apart. You ask the mother if she feels she needs to move her bowels, and she says she does not. Do you prepare for delivery at the scene? Or do you transport the mother to the hospital? Explain your reasoning.

Web Medic

Visit Brady's *Emergency Care* website for direct weblinks. At **www.bradybooks.com/ emergencycare**, you will find information related to the following Chapter 24 topics:

• Female reproductive organs and pregnancy
• Complications of pregnancy and labor

Chapter
Twenty-Five

PUTTING IT ALL TOGETHER FOR THE MEDICAL PATIENT

In previous chapters in this module, you learned how to look for, recognize, and manage a number of medical complaints patients may have. However, each of those chapters assumed the patient had only the problem described in that chapter. What should an EMT-B do when a patient has two or more presenting problems? How should the EMT-B handle situations in which the patient has a chief complaint that is not covered in an EMT-B course? This chapter will help answer these and other questions about applying knowledge and skills from an EMT-B course to the real world.

MULTIPLE MEDICAL COMPLAINTS

Many EMT-Bs feel more comfortable dealing with injuries than illnesses. This may be because it is relatively easy to look at a mechanism of injury, look at the injured patient, and get a good idea of what the patient's problem might be. After all, a deformed leg can only be one of a very few things, such as a fracture or dislocation.

On the other hand, medical conditions present a very different picture. A medical patient's chest pain might be the result of any number of conditions, including myocardial infarction (heart attack), angina, a collapsed lung, a pulmonary embolus (a clot in one of the pulmonary arteries), pneumonia, or plain old heartburn to name just a few. This presents a confusing picture to the EMT-B.

Fortunately, since there are a limited number of interventions an EMT-B can administer, there are also a limited number of decisions that the EMT-B must make. For the medical patient, these decisions are:

- *Airway.* Does the airway need to be cleared with suction? Should the EMT-B position the patient on his side or insert an oral or nasal airway to maintain a patent airway?
- *Breathing.* Should the patient receive high-concentration oxygen by nonre-

breather mask? Should the EMT-B ventilate the patient with oxygen?
- *Circulation.* Is there bleeding that needs to be controlled? Should the patient receive chest compressions? Should the EMT-B apply an AED?
- *Priority determination.* How promptly and rapidly does this patient need transport?
- *Interventions.* Does the EMT-B have any interventions that might help the patient? Specifically, does the patient meet local criteria for assistance with an inhaler, nitroglycerin, or an epinephrine auto-injector; administration of oral glucose or activated charcoal; cooling or warming; talking down or restraining; or assisting in childbirth?

MANAGING THE PATIENT WITH MULTIPLE MEDICAL COMPLAINTS

It can be very challenging for the EMT-B to manage a patient who presents with more than one condition or a familiar condition but under unusual circumstances. When faced with this kind of situation, the EMT-B should assess the patient as usual. Then determine whether the patient meets the criteria for one or more

HOW AND WHY?

Medications can tell you a great deal about the medical problems of patients. This is especially helpful when patients have many conditions at the same time. Go to your Electronic Extras CD for information on common medications.

TOPIC OVERVIEW

In this chapter, you will learn about the following topics:

- Management of patients with more than one medical complaint

- Management of patient conditions not covered in an EMT-B course of your interventions. If there is any reason to believe the patient is at greater risk of harm from the intervention, or that unusual circumstances make the situation difficult to assess, consult medical direction, even if it is not required by your protocols. By consulting on-line medical direction, you will be able to find out which intervention, if any, you should employ.

Typical Calls

The cases below—all in EMS systems where advanced life support is *not* available—demonstrate these principles in action.

Case #1: Overdose in a Patient with Diabetes

You receive a call for a female who has taken an overdose of pills. As you approach the scene, you note that the house is dirty and unkempt but appears to be safe. Your general impression is of a teenage female who looks sleepy. She is awake and answers questions slowly, although she continues to appear drowsy. Her airway is open, and her breathing appears adequate in rate and depth. There is no blood or bleeding visible, and her radial pulse feels rapid and full.

You decide that her condition is serious and requires transport soon, but you have a few minutes to gather more information, which the emergency department will need to institute the proper treatment. From the patient's mother, you learn that the patient is a 16-year-old who had a fight with her boyfriend and then decided to swallow all the pills she could find in the house. To wash the pills down, she had a "couple" of beers. All of this occurred about 10 to 15 minutes ago. The medications include propranolol 80 mg (up to 6 tablets missing), amitriptyline 50 mg (up to 15 tablets missing), and extra-strength acetaminophen 500 mg (up to 50 tablets missing).

Through slurred speech, the patient tells you she feels nauseated but has not vomited. Her last meal was lunch three hours ago. The only medication she is supposed to take is insulin for her diabetes. She refuses to say when she last took her insulin or how much she took. She has no other medical history and has no known medication allergies.

Vital signs are pulse 96 and full, BP 100/70, respirations 14 and adequate, skin warm and dry. Your partner places a nonrebreather mask with 15 liters per minute of oxygen on the patient.

Your standing orders allow you to give one tube of oral glucose to a diabetic with an altered mental status who can swallow without threatening her airway. Your protocols also direct you to call medical direction for conscious overdose patients so that activated charcoal can be considered. Activated charcoal prevents many drugs from being absorbed by the body. You wonder whether you should give the oral glucose now and then call medical direction about the activated charcoal. You decide against doing that, because this case is so unusual and because you are not sure whether oral glucose will work if the patient also receives activated charcoal. You think to yourself that you are glad you will be speaking to a physician in a few minutes anyway.

You contact on-line medical direction. You describe the patient's condition, her history of insulin-dependent diabetes, and the names and amounts of the medications involved in the present emergency. When you ask the doctor whether you should give oral glucose or not, he asks if there is any way to find out what her blood sugar is. Your partner tells you the patient's mother checked prior to your arrival and reports it is 105 mg percent. The doctor is satisfied with this and directs you to withhold oral glucose and to administer 25 grams of activated charcoal orally, if you can get her to swallow without aspirating it. He also advises you to be prepared for the possibility of vomiting and ventricular fibrillation because of the medications involved. You attempt to give the patient the activated charcoal, but she refuses. Otherwise, transport was uneventful.

After you turn over patient care to the emergency department staff, you get a chance to think about the case. Although this patient's condition technically fulfilled the criteria in your standing orders for administration of oral glucose, you wonder if the authors of the protocol ever pictured a situation where the patient had also taken an overdose. You had to consider the possibility that the patient might need activated charcoal. You also did not know whether activated charcoal might prevent the glucose from working or whether the glucose might prevent the activated charcoal from working. For these reasons, it was prudent to consult on-line medical direction before giving the patient something that might end up harming her.

Later, the on-line physician catches you on your way out of the hospital emergency department and tells you he is glad you called in. She is being evaluated now and will be admitted to the hospital.

Case #2 A Surprising Change in a Patient with Chest Pain

You receive a call for a male with chest pain (Figure 25-1). The scene is safe, so you proceed to introduce yourself to the patient and perform an initial assessment. Your general impression is of an older man who appears anxious and uncomfortable. His mental status is alert. His airway is patent, and his breathing appears adequate, although it is a little rapid and shallow. There is no blood or bleeding visible, and his radial pulse feels weak. You decide to assess the patient quickly and get underway to the hospital.

The patient, who is 68, tells you he has had dull substernal pain without radiation for about 15 minutes. It came on at rest. He denies shortness of breath but admits to some nausea. He has a prescription for nitroglycerin, but cannot find the bottle. His medications include ibuprofen, nitroglycerin, and diltiazem. He has a history of arthritis, angina, and high blood pressure. He has no known allergies to medications.

Vital signs are pulse 84 and weak, BP 118/90, respirations 22, skin pale and sweaty. Breath sounds are equal on both sides of his chest.

As your partner puts a nonrebreather mask on the patient, the wife finds the nitroglycerin. Your protocol calls for you to contact on-line medical direction before assisting a patient with his nitro, so you call and speak to a doctor in the emergency department. She advises one sublingual nitro now and another in five minutes, if he still has chest pain and his systolic blood pressure is greater than 100. You help the patient take his nitroglycerin and transport him sitting up. Four minutes later, just after you take his blood pressure, the patient vomits a mixture of material that looks like coffee grounds and bright red blood. You are 15 minutes from the hospital. The patient received some relief after the nitroglycerin and oxygen, but he still has a little bit of pain in his chest. His pulse is 92, weak and regular, BP 102/80, respirations 22, skin pale and sweaty.

The patient fulfills the conditions described by your protocol and the physician you spoke to, but you do not think this is what she expected. You contact her again, inform her of the vomiting and the patient's most recent vital signs, and she directs you to withhold any more nitro for the moment and to inform her of any further changes. The patient's condition and vital signs remain essentially the same for the remainder of the trip, and you turn the patient over to the emergency department staff.

This case began as a very straightforward presentation of chest pain in a patient with a

Figure 25-1 Male patient in his 60s with chest pain.

prescription for nitroglycerin. Then it took a sudden unexpected turn when the patient vomited blood (blood that has been in the stomach for a while frequently looks like coffee grounds when it is vomited). Since you are not familiar with this condition, you ask the emergency physician what happened to this patient.

She explains that the ibuprofen the patient was taking for his arthritis is irritating to the stomach and sometimes causes gastrointestinal bleeding. A patient with angina is sensitive to a decrease in the amount of oxygen getting to his heart. If enough blood is lost, there are not enough red blood cells to carry sufficient oxygen to the heart and, in a patient with angina, this can lead to chest pain. You are grateful for the explanation and relieved, because you had feared the nitro you gave the patient might have caused the bleeding.

The doctor commends you on not going ahead with her original instructions, but instead using good judgment and advising her of the vomited blood. Most of the patient's pain had been relieved by the nitro and oxygen, so she weighed the risks and benefits of another nitro and decided to wait until the patient arrived at the hospital.

Case #3 A Not-So-Simple Allergic Reaction

You receive a call for a pregnant woman stung by a bee. The scene is safe, so you proceed to introduce yourself to the patient and perform an initial assessment. Your general impression is of a woman in her mid-20s who looks a little anxious and who has some hives on her neck and arms. Her mental status is alert. Her airway is patent, and her breathing appears adequate. There is no blood or bleeding visible, and her radial pulse feels weak. You decide that her condition is potentially serious, but that you need more information to determine how urgently you need to transport her.

The patient is a 26-year-old female who is 5 months pregnant with her first child. She was stung 5 minutes ago on her hand by a bee. She is complaining of slight difficulty breathing and itching on her neck and arms.

The patient has a history of allergic reactions to bee stings and has an epinephrine auto-injector, but she does not like needles and was afraid to use it.

As you examine her, you notice that you do not hear any wheezes. She has hives on her neck and arms, but no swelling of the tongue, mouth, face, or neck. There is no stinger visible at the sting site. Vital signs are pulse 88, BP 110/80, respirations 20, skin warm and dry. You have her on high-concentration oxygen by nonrebreather.

Since your protocol requires you to contact on-line medical direction in cases like this one, you contact a physician in the emergency department and advise him of the patient's condition and the availability of an epinephrine auto-injector. He wants you to hold off on the epinephrine auto-injector for the moment, but he also wants you to watch her closely, monitor her vital signs every 5 minutes and report back with any changes in the patient's condition immediately.

About 5 minutes later, you can hear wheezes without a stethoscope. Her difficulty breathing has increased, and the hives have spread over most of her upper body. Vital signs are pulse 104, BP 96/80, respirations 24 and labored, skin warm and dry. When you advise the physician of these changes, he orders use of the epinephrine auto-injector. Five minutes after the epinephrine, the patient's hives have cleared up, you can no longer hear wheezes, and the patient is no longer short of breath. You arrive at the emergency department a few minutes later with the patient looking and feeling much better.

The emergency department is not too busy today, so you get a chance to speak briefly with the physician. He explains he asked you to hold off on using the epinephrine auto-injector because the patient is pregnant and her condition was not initially serious enough to warrant the injection. Epinephrine causes many blood vessels to constrict, including those in the uterus of this pregnant patient. He felt the risk of reducing circulating oxygen to the fetus outweighed the benefit of the epinephrine as long as she had only minor symptoms. Once you advised him of her turn for the worse, the benefit to both mother and baby outweighed the risks. He thanks you for monitoring the patient closely and relaying that important information.

Analysis of the Calls

In each of these cases, the EMT-B was confronted with situations that called for judgment. Most patients you will see will have straightforward complaints, but occasionally you will run into a situation where the usual rules may not be applicable. In these cases, it is essential that you treat any immediate life-threats and then consider the risk to the patient your usual treatment might pose. If the risk appears greater or it is unknown, your best plan of action is to consult on-line medical direction. (See the flowchart in Figure 25-2.)

PATIENT CONDITIONS NOT COVERED IN THE EMT-B COURSE

One of the most important purposes of an EMT-B course is to help you learn when to employ the interventions you have available to you. In the second module of this book, you learned how to detect and treat immediate threats to the airway. Chapters in this module have described the appropriate use of specific interventions for specific problems:

- Assisting a patient in using his own inhaler (respiratory difficulty)
- Assisting a patient in taking his own nitroglycerin (cardiac compromise)
- Application of an automated defibrillator (cardiac arrest)
- Administration of oral glucose (diabetics with altered mental status)
- Assisting a patient in using his own epinephrine auto-injector (allergic reaction)
- Administration of activated charcoal (overdose or poisoning)
- Cooling or warming (environmental emergencies)
- Talking down and restraining (behavioral emergencies)
- Assisting in delivery of an infant (patient in labor)

For a number of reasons, common chief complaints for which EMT-Bs have no specific treatment are not covered in the typical EMT-B course. In each of these conditions, the appropriate course of action for the EMT-B is to assess the patient and provide the appropriate supportive treatment, such as airway management and treatment for shock (hypoperfusion). For example, there is no intervention an EMT-B has available that should be administered specifically for abdominal pain. If the patient with abdominal pain has signs and symptoms of shock

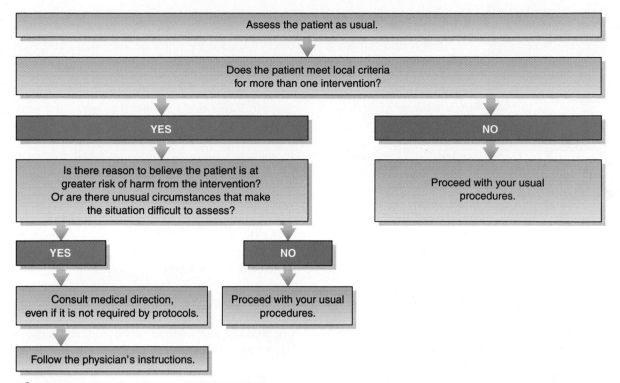

Figure 25-2 Flow chart for decision making.

(hypoperfusion), the patient should be treated for shock. If the patient has a compromised airway, the EMT-B should clear the patient's airway. In neither of these cases did the treatment for the patient depend on the cause of the abdominal pain. There also are no specific EMT-B interventions for patients with post-surgical complications, headache, syncope (fainting), or sickle-cell crisis. In each case, the EMT-B should assess the patient and treat the problems found (control bleeding in a surgical incision that has opened, for instance).

Confronting common problems for which an EMT-B has no treatment can leave the EMT-B feeling lost or inadequate. There are a number of important principles to keep in mind:

- Assess the patient as you learned to do in your EMT-B class.
- Look for and treat the problems for which you have treatments.
- If you work in a system where more advanced providers are available, follow your protocols and procedures for calling for assistance.
- Keep in mind that patients generally do not realize you are providing EMT-B level care, but they do know if you are polite, respectful, and empathetic when you are with them. An air of confidence and

warmth will do wonders to make an anxious patient more comfortable.

An even more alarming situation for an EMT-B, especially a new one, is assessing a patient who tells you his problem is caused by some disease he names and it is one you have never heard of or can even pronounce. In this case, being honest with the patient is usually the best approach. A simple statement like, "I have to admit I'm not familiar with that disease. Could you tell me a little bit about it?" is likely to result in the patient happily informing you about his condition. Most patients will respond very well to this approach. They know you are not a physician, and they do not expect you to be as knowledgeable as one. Often, though not always, the patient is extremely knowledgeable about the condition and the treatment for it. If it is a rare condition, the patient will in all likelihood be very accustomed to explaining it to others (including doctors and nurses).

A very similar situation can arise when the patient is using medical equipment at home that the EMT-B is not familiar with. In this case, the patient or a family member is usually very knowledgeable about the device and its use. You will learn more about high technology treatments at home in Chapter 31, "Infants and Children."

At 3:00 in the morning, your rescue squad is toned-out for a "sick person." Arriving at the residence 6 minutes later, you are met by a woman identifying herself as Mrs. Jones. She tells you that she called 9-1-1 because her husband has been sick with and running a fever. She says he is in the bedroom.

In the bedroom you observe a man lying in bed with a wash cloth on his head. In response to your query, he identifies himself as Wilson Jones, 56 years old. He is alert and verbally responsive. He proceeds to tell you that he has been running a fever for the past 48 hours and that it was his wife, not he, who called 9-1-1. Your assessment reveals a clear airway, respirations of adequate rate and depth, and skin that appears pink, warm, and dry.

STREET SCENE QUESTIONS

1. What pertinent signs or symptoms should you inquire about?

2. What further patient assessment should you perform?

Mr. Jones informs you that he believes he has the "flu." He says he has not been nauseated and he has not vomited. He states he has been eating and drinking normal amounts of fluid. His vital signs include a pulse 80 and regular; blood pressure 150/70; respirations 20 and regular. You determine that Wilson is taking no medications other than an over-the-counter one for his fever. He has no allergies and no significant past medical history. He states he does not want to go to the hospital. Patient denies shortness of breath, chest pain, dizziness, headache, or other complaints.

Contacting medical direction, you are advised that Mr. Jones does not need to go to the emergency department, but instead should contact his personal physician in the morning if symptoms persist. Mr. Jones states he understands and will contact his physician in the morning. You and your partner then leave the residence.

Two hours later, you are once again dispatched to the Jones's residence. Mrs. Jones again meets you at the door, and states that she once again called 9-1-1. She says that her husband was now shaking and it "scared her." Once in the bedroom, you find Mr. Jones still in bed. Though his eyes are open, he is not alert, and responds to verbal commands by groaning. His airway is open and respirations are regular. He is not shaking, but instead repeatedly rolls from his back onto his left side, and then onto his back.

STREET SCENE QUESTIONS

3. What treatment should you provide to Mr. Jones at this time?

You administer high-concentration oxygen by way of a nonrebreather mask. Mr. Jones's vitals include pulse 110 and regular; blood pressure 160/76; respirations 28; skin, hot and dry; pupils, normal. You and your partner place Mr. Jones on your cot, and load him into the ambulance. As you reassess this patient, you find he is now becoming more responsive and wants to know, "What happened?" You arrive at the hospital emergency department with no further medical problems.

PATIENT NAME:	Wilson Jones				PATIENT AGE:	56

CHIEF COMPLAINT		TIME	RESP	PULSE	B.P.	MENTAL STATUS	R PUPILS L	SKIN
Altered mental status	**V I T A L S I G N S**	*0 5 0 7*	Rate: *28* ☒ Regular ☐ Shallow ☐ Labored	Rate: *110* ☒ Regular ☐ Irregular	*160* / *76*	☐ Alert ☑ Voice ☐ Pain ☐ Unresp.	☑ Normal ☑ ☐ Dilated ☐ ☐ Constricted ☐ ☐ Sluggish ☐ ☐ No-Reaction ☐	☐ Unremarkable ☐ Cool ☐ Pale ☑ Warm ☐ Cyanotic ☐ Moist ☐ Flushed ☑ Dry ☐ Jaundiced
PAST MEDICAL HISTORY			Rate: ☐ Regular ☐ Shallow ☐ Labored	Rate: ☐ Regular ☐ Irregular	/	☐ Alert ☐ Voice ☐ Pain ☐ Unresp.	☐ Normal ☐ ☐ Dilated ☐ ☐ Constricted ☐ ☐ Sluggish ☐ ☐ No-Reaction ☐	☐ Unremarkable ☐ Cool ☐ Pale ☐ Warm ☐ Cyanotic ☐ Moist ☐ Flushed ☐ Dry ☐ Jaundiced
☐ None ☐ Allergy to _____ ☐ Hypertension ☐ Stroke ☐ Seizures ☐ Diabetes ☐ COPD ☐ Cardiac ☒ Other (List) ☐ Asthma *Previous EMS call (Run 5428)*			Rate: ☐ Regular ☐ Shallow ☐ Labored	Rate: ☐ Regular ☐ Irregular	/	☐ Alert ☐ Voice ☐ Pain ☐ Unresp.	☐ Normal ☐ ☐ Dilated ☐ ☐ Constricted ☐ ☐ Sluggish ☐ ☐ No-Reaction ☐	☐ Unremarkable ☐ Cool ☐ Pale ☐ Warm ☐ Cyanotic ☐ Moist ☐ Flushed ☐ Dry ☐ Jaundiced
Current Medications (List) *Tylenol*								

NARRATIVE *We initially responded to patient's house earlier this morning (see patient run #5428).*

Past medical history of "flu-like" symptoms for past 48 hours, per patient on previous EMS incident.

No other pertinent medical history. Upon arrival, patient's wife stated she initiated EMS because

husband was "shaking." We observed a 56-year-old male responsive to verbal stimuli by groaning.

Patient has no purposeful movement, although he moves from a supine to left lateral recumbent

position and then back to supine repeatedly. Airway clear; breathing rapid and unlabored; pupils equal

and reactive to light; no vomiting noted; patient unable to ambulate; patient placed on cot by EMS

personnel and high-concentration oxygen initiated. Due to short transport time, no other

treatment/reassessment initiated.

CHAPTER REVIEW

SUMMARY

Most patients you encounter will have straightforward presentations of common problems. When a patient presents with more than one complaint, evaluate the situation, determine any unusual or increased risks from your interventions, and consult on-line medical direction. Similar principles apply to the situation where the patient has a complaint for which you have no specific intervention or a complaint related to a disease you are not familiar with. Assess the patient as you usually do, provide supportive care and consult on-line medical direction as needed.

REVIEW QUESTIONS

1. What are the decisions an EMT-B must make for a medical patient with regard to interventions? (p. 492)
2. What steps should the EMT-B follow when a patient seems to require two interventions? (pp. 492-493)
3. What are the advantages to consulting online medical direction in a difficult medical case? (p. 492)
4. How can an EMT-B learn more about a patient's complaint that is not covered in the EMT-B curriculum? (p. 495)
5. What is an appropriate response on the part of an EMT-B when a patient tells him she has Crohn's disease? (p. 495)

APPLICATIONS

• You are treating a 65-year-old male for carbon monoxide poisoning. He is responsive only to pain, and he is tolerating a nasal airway well. He is breathing adequately, so you apply high-concentration oxygen by nonrebreather mask. His wife tells you that he is not supposed to get any more than 2 liters per minute of oxygen because he has emphysema. What should the EMT-B do? Explain your answer.

Visit Brady's *Emergency Care* website for direct weblinks. At **www.bradybooks.com/ emergencycare**, you will find information related to the following Chapter 25 topics:

- Diabetes

- Allergies in men and women

- Chest pain

Chapter
Twenty-Six

BLEEDING AND SHOCK

*W*ord on the Street

"When patients die, they always die from shock. The seriousness of their injuries and the duration of time that passes until their injuries are treated are key factors that determine how quickly shock develops and how deeply into shock they will go, which greatly impacts whether your treatment will be successful or not. Visualize an injury to any organ. Mentally follow the process from organ failure to body system failure to organism death. When you can do that, you will have a comprehensive knowledge of shock, which will go a long way in helping you improve the care you deliver to the unfortunate victims of trauma."

Mike Smith   MICP, EMS Educator and Author

The leading cause of death in the United States for persons between the ages of 1 and 44 is trauma. As an EMT-Basic, you will be called upon to provide emergency care to victims of traumatic injuries varying in severity from minor to life threatening. It is vital that you learn to recognize the signs and symptoms of serious trauma and shock. Early identification, appropriate care, and expeditious transport contribute greatly to the patient's chance of survival. Understanding the signs, symptoms, and management of bleeding and shock is a vital part of good prehospital care.

CIRCULATORY SYSTEM

Main Components

The circulatory (or cardiovascular) system is responsible for the distribution of blood to all parts of the body. This system has three main components: the heart, blood vessels, and the blood that flows through them. All components must function properly for the system to remain intact. (You may wish to review the information about the heart and the circulatory system in Chapter 4, "The Human Body.")

The heart is a muscular organ that lies within the chest, behind the sternum. Its job is to pump blood, which supplies oxygen and nutrients to the cells of the body. To provide a sufficient supply of oxygen and nutrients to all parts of the body, the heart must pump at an adequate rate and rhythm. The blood is circulated throughout the body through three major types of blood vessel (Figure 26-1):

- *Arteries.* The arteries carry oxygen-rich blood away from the heart. They are under a great deal of pressure during the heart's contractions. (Taking the patient's blood pressure is a means of measuring arterial pressure.) An artery has a thick, muscular wall that enables it to dilate or constrict, depending on the need for oxygen and nutrients of the cells or organ it feeds. (See Figure 26-2.)
- *Capillaries.* Oxygen-rich blood is emptied from the arteries into microscopically small capillaries, which supply every cell of the body. Where capillaries and body cells are in contact, a vital "exchange" takes place. Oxygen and nutrients are given up by the blood and pass through the extremely thin capillary walls into the cells. At the same time, carbon dioxide and other waste products given up by the cells pass through the capillary walls and are taken up by the blood.
- *Veins.* Blood that has been depleted of oxygen and loaded with carbon dioxide and other wastes in the capillaries empties into the veins, which carry it back to the heart. Veins have one-way valves that prevent the blood from flowing in the wrong direction. Blood in a vein is under much less pressure than blood in an artery.

TOPIC OVERVIEW

In this chapter, you will learn about the following topics:

- How to recognize arterial, venous, and capillary bleeding
- When to use BSI precautions with a bleeding patient
- Steps for controlling bleeding
- Signs, symptoms, and care of a patient with internal bleeding
- Signs, symptoms, and care of a patient with shock
- How to use the mechanism of injury to identify potential internal injuries

DOT OBJECTIVES

The adequate circulation of blood throughout the body, which fills the capillaries and supplies the cells and tissues with oxygen and nutrients, is called **perfusion.** If, for some reason, blood is not adequately circulated, some of the cells and organs of the body do not receive adequate supplies of oxygen and dangerous waste products build up. Inadequate perfusion of the body's tissues and organs is called **hypoperfusion,** which is also known as **shock.** (*Hypo-* means "low," so *hypoperfusion* means "low perfusion.")

Recall that the heart, blood vessels, and blood are the three main components of the circulatory system. These components may be likened to a pump, pipes, and fluid in the pipes. For the circulatory system to function properly, all three components must function properly. If any component fails, or "leaks,"

the body will try in various ways to compensate and maintain adequate perfusion. However, if the problem is not corrected and the condition quickly reversed, adequate perfusion cannot be maintained and shock (hypoperfusion) will result.

FUNCTIONS OF THE BLOOD

The blood has several functions. These include:

- *Transportation of gases.* Blood carries inhaled oxygen from the lungs to the body's cells, and it carries carbon dioxide from the body cells back to the lungs where it is then exhaled.

- *Nutrition.* Blood circulates nutrients from the intestines or storage tissues (such as fatty tissue, the liver, and muscle cells) to the other body cells.

- *Excretion.* Blood carries waste products from the cells to organs, such as the kidneys, that excrete (eliminate) them from the body.

- *Protection.* Blood carries antibodies and white blood cells, which help fight disease and infection.

- *Regulation.* Blood carries substances that control the functions of the body, such as hormones, water, salt, enzymes, and chemicals. Blood also helps regulate body temperature by carrying body heat to the lungs and skin surface where it is dissipated.

Figure 26-1   Blood vessels.

A

B

Figure 26-2 An arteriogram of (A) a normal, healthy artery and (B) an artery that has been damaged.

BLEEDING

Severe bleeding, or **hemorrhage,** is the major cause of shock (hypoperfusion). The body contains a certain amount of blood to circulate through the blood vessels. If enough blood volume is lost, perfusion of all cells will not occur. Inadequate perfusion of the body's cells will eventually lead to the death of tissues and organs. The cells and tissues that are the most sensitive to inadequate perfusion are those of the brain, the spinal cord, and the kidneys.

Bleeding, or hemorrhage, is classified as either external or internal, as explained below.

External Bleeding

Whenever bleeding is anticipated or discovered, the use of body substance isolation (BSI) precautions is essential to avoid exposure of the skin and mucous membranes. Blood and open wounds pose a high risk of infection to the EMT-B. Protective gloves must be worn when caring for any bleeding patient. A mask and protective eyewear should also be worn if there is a chance of splattered blood. With profuse or spurting (arterial) bleeding, or if the patient is spitting or coughing blood, masks should be worn. Gowns should be considered if clothing may become contaminated.

While BSI precautions decrease the possibility of exposure to blood and body fluids, you should ALWAYS wash your hands with soap and water immediately after each call. Gloves may develop tears or small holes without your knowing it. Always remove the gloves carefully, turning them inside out as you take them off. This reduces the possibility of blood or fluid on the gloves coming in contact with your hands.

External bleeding may be classified according to which of the three types of blood vessel is injured and losing blood (Figure 26-3):

- Arterial bleeding
- Venous bleeding
- Capillary bleeding

Arterial bleeding is usually bright red in color, because it is still rich in oxygen. It is often rapid and profuse, spurting with each heartbeat, though as the patient's systolic blood pressure drops, the strength of the spurting may decrease. As explained earlier, blood in an artery is under high pressure, and arteries have thick, muscular walls that maintain the pressure. For this reason, arterial bleeding is the most difficult bleeding to control. Control measures may need to continue throughout transport to the hospital.

Venous bleeding is usually dark red or maroon in color, because it has already passed its oxygen to the cells and picked up carbon dioxide and wastes. Bleeding from the veins has a steady flow. It is usually easy to control (although it can be profuse), because veins return blood to the heart under low pressure. Because venous pressure may be lower than atmospheric pressure, large veins may actually suck in debris or air bubbles. Bleeding from the large veins in the neck is an especially serious problem. An air bubble, or embolism, may be carried directly

ARTERIES   VEINS   CAPILLARIES

- Spurting blood
- Pulsating flow
- Bright red color

- Steady, slow flow
- Dark red color

- Slow, even flow

Figure 26-3 Three types of external bleeding.

to the heart, interfering with the regular heart rhythm, or even stopping it completely. An air embolism also can cause damage to the brain or lungs if lodged there.

Capillary bleeding is usually slow and "oozing" due to their small size and low pressure. Most capillary bleeding is considered minor and is easily controlled. It often clots spontaneously, or with minimal treatment. As you would expect, the color of capillary blood is usually somewhere between the bright red of arterial blood and the darker red of venous blood. Capillary bleeding usually results from a minor injury such as a scrape. However, these wounds can easily become contaminated, leading to infection. You may also see capillary bleeding from the edges of more serious wounds.

Severity of External Bleeding

An important skill for the EMT-B to develop is determining the severity of blood loss. The severity of the bleeding is somewhat dependent on the amount of blood lost in relation to the physical size of the patient. While a sudden loss of 1 liter (1000 cc) of blood is considered serious in the average adult, half that amount, or 500 cc, is considered serious in a child. In a one-year-old infant, with a total blood volume of only about 800 cc, a loss of even 150 cc is considered serious.

Severity is dependent on the patient's condition, as well as on the relative amount of blood lost. If, at any time, the patient begins to exhibit signs and symptoms of shock (hypoperfusion), the bleeding is immediately considered serious.

The body's natural response to bleeding is constriction of the injured blood vessel and clotting. However, a serious injury may prevent effective clotting, allowing continued bleeding. Wounds that are large or deep may not clot well. Uncontrolled bleeding or significant blood loss can eventually lead to death.

● Patient *ASSESSMENT*

External Bleeding

It is important for you to learn to estimate the amount of external blood loss in order to predict potential shock (hypoperfusion), triage (prioritize) patients properly, and identify bleeding that must be treated during the initial assessment

It is sometimes difficult to estimate blood loss when the blood has flowed onto the floor or when carpeting or clothing has absorbed it. An exercise that may help you better estimate external blood loss is pouring a pint of liquid on the floor to note its appearance, and soaking an article of clothing in a pint of fluid to note how wet it feels and looks. Since estimating external blood loss is difficult, it is important for you to watch for signs and symptoms of shock (hypoperfusion), which are listed in Table 26-1.

No matter how small blood loss appears to be, if the patient shows any signs or symptoms of shock (hypoperfusion), the bleeding is considered serious. However, do not wait for signs and symptoms to appear before beginning treatment. Any patient with a significant amount of blood loss should be treated to prevent the development of shock. Many of the signs and symptoms of shock appear late in the process. By the time they develop, it may be too late for the patient to recover.

Controlling External Bleeding

The control of external bleeding is one of the most important elements in the prevention and management of shock (hypoperfusion). If bleeding is not controlled, shock will continue to develop and worsen, leading to the death of the patient.

Table 26-1 Signs of Shock

Signs (in order of appearance)	Description
Altered mental status	Altered mental status occurs because the brain is not receiving enough oxygen. The brain is very sensitive to oxygen deficiencies. When it is deprived of oxygen, even slightly, behavioral changes may be noted. These changes may be seen as anxiety, restlessness, or combativeness.
Pale, cool, clammy skin	When the body senses low blood volume, natural mechanisms take over in an attempt to correct the problem. One of these mechanisms is to divert blood from non-vital areas to vital organs. Blood is quickly directed away from the skin to such organs as the brain and heart. This results in the loss of color and temperature in the skin. Infants and children may exhibit capillary refill times of greater than 2 seconds. Note: In neurogenic shock (rare) the skin is typically warm, flushed, and dry because the circulatory system has lost the ability to constrict blood vessels in the skin.
Nausea and vomiting	In the body's continuing effort to keep blood perfusing vital organs, blood is diverted from the digestive system. This causes feelings of nausea and occasionally vomiting.
Vital sign changes	The first vital signs to change are the pulse and respirations: • The pulse will increase in an attempt to pump more blood. As the pulse gradually increases, it becomes weak and thready. • Respirations also increase in an attempt to increase the amount of oxygen in the blood. The respirations will become more shallow and labored as shock progresses. • Blood pressure is one of the last signs to change. When blood pressure drops, the patient is clearly in a state of serious, life-threatening shock. Other signs of shock that you may encounter include thirst, dilated pupils, and in some cases cyanosis around the lips and nail beds.

 Patient *CARE*

External Bleeding

Patient assessment and care always begin with the ABCs. After taking BSI precautions, maintain an open airway, monitor respirations, and ventilate if necessary. Assess circulation by taking a radial pulse; assessing skin color, temperature, and condition; and controlling external bleeding. Severe external bleeding must be identified and controlled during the initial assessment. The major methods of controlling external bleeding are (Scan 26-1):

• Direct pressure
• Elevation
• Pressure points

Other methods include splinting, cold application, and use of the pneumatic anti-shock garment (PASG). Applying a tourniquet is a last resort. Each of these methods will be more thoroughly discussed later in this chapter.

In addition to controlling external bleeding, an important treatment for any trauma patient is oxygen. Blood loss decreases perfusion. This means that less oxygen is delivered to the tissues. The administration of supplemental oxygen will increase the oxygen saturation of the blood that is still in the patient's circulatory system, improving oxygenation of the tissues.

BSI precautions and infection control are mandatory when attempting to control external bleeding. Always wear disposable gloves when caring for the patient and cleaning up after the call. Follow your local infection exposure control plan regarding cleaning and disposal of contaminated bandages, sheets, and other materials and supplies.

CONTROLLING BLEEDING

NOTE: FIRST take BSI precautions.

▲ **1.** Apply direct pressure to a bleeding wound with a gauze pad.

▲ **2.** Elevate a bleeding extremity above the level of the heart.

▲ **3.** If the wound continues to bleed, apply additional dressings over the first one.

▲ **4.** Bandage the dressing in place.

▲ **5.** If a wound to the arm continues to bleed, apply pressure to the brachial artery, or . . .

▲ . . . If a wound to the leg continues to bleed, apply pressure to the femoral artery.

Direct Pressure. The most common and effective way to control external bleeding is by applying direct pressure to the wound. This can be done with your gloved hand, a dressing and your gloved hand, or by a pressure dressing and bandage.

1. Apply pressure to the wound until bleeding is controlled. If the bleeding is mild, use a sterile dressing. If the bleeding is severe or spurting, immediately place your gloved hand directly on the wound. Do not waste time trying to find a dressing (Figure 26-4).

2. Hold the pressure firmly until the bleeding is controlled. Remember your goal of limiting additional blood loss.

3. Once the bleeding has been controlled, bandage a dressing firmly in place to form a pressure dressing (see explanation below).

4. Never remove a dressing once it has been placed on the wound. Removal of a dressing may destroy clotting or cause further injury to the site. If a dressing becomes blood soaked, apply additional dressings on top of it and hold them firmly in place. You may need to continue holding direct pressure on the wound until arrival at the hospital.

Application of a **pressure dressing** will control most external bleeding. Place several gauze pads on the wound. Hold the dressings in place with a self-adhering roller bandage wrapped tightly over the dressings, and above and below the wound site. Enough pressure must be created to control the bleeding.

Warning

After controlling bleeding from an extremity using a pressure dressing, always check for a distal pulse to make sure that the dressing has not been applied too tightly. If you do not feel a pulse, adjust the pressure applied by the dressing to reestablish circulation. Check distal pulses frequently while the patient is in your care.

Dressings should not be removed from the wound. If bleeding continues after a dressing is applied, place additional dressings over the existing one and apply pressure by hand. A tighter bandage (which does not hinder circulation) may be applied. Several types of dressings may be used to control external bleeding (Figure 26-5).

You may be unable to apply an effective pressure dressing to some areas of the body. For example, bleeding from the armpit may require you to hold continuous direct pressure with your gloved hand and a dressing. Remember that direct pressure is usually the quickest and most effective method of controlling external bleeding.

How and Why?

On the average, a healthy person's blood will clot in 6 to 17 minutes. Go to your Electronic Extras CD for more information.

Elevation. Elevation of an injured extremity may be used at the same time as direct pressure. When you elevate an injury above the level of the heart, gravity helps reduce the blood pressure in the

Figure 26-4 In cases of profuse bleeding, do not waste time finding a dressing. Instead, use your gloved hand to apply direct pressure.

Figure 26-5 Various types of dressings.

Chapter 26 • *Bleeding and Shock* **507**

extremity, slowing bleeding. However, do not use this method if you suspect possible musculoskeletal injuries, impaled objects in the extremity, or spine injury.

To use elevation in controlling external bleeding, apply direct pressure to the injury site. Elevate the injured extremity, keeping the injury site above the level of the heart.

Pressure Points. If direct pressure, or direct pressure with elevation, fails to control the external bleeding, your next method is the use of a pressure point. A pressure point is a site where a large artery lies close to the surface of the body and directly over a bone (Figure 26-6). Simply put, any site where a pulse can be felt is a pressure point. In emergency medical care, there are four sites (two on each side) used as pressure points to control profuse bleeding in extremities: the brachial arteries for bleeding from the upper extremities, and the femoral arteries for bleeding from the lower extremities (Figure 26-7).

The pressure-point method of controlling external bleeding should be used only after direct pressure and elevation have failed. To properly use pressure points, you need to know exactly where the points are located and how much pressure to apply. Note that use of the pressure point may not be effective if the wound is at the distal end of the limb. Blood is being sent to this area of the arm from many other smaller arteries.

For bleeding from an upper extremity, apply pressure to a point over the **brachial artery** (Scan 26-1). To find the artery:

1. Hold the patient's arm out at a right angle to his body with the palm of the hand facing up. Do not use force to raise the arm, if the movement causes pain or may aggravate an injury. If it is not possible to raise the arm this far, do the best you can, leaving the arm in the position in which it was found.

2. Locate the groove between the biceps muscle and the upper arm bone (humerus) about midway between the elbow and armpit. Cradle the upper arm in the palm of your hand and position your fingers in this medial groove.

3. Compress the artery against the underlying bone by pressing your finger into the groove. If pressure is properly applied, no radial pulse should be felt.

For bleeding from a lower extremity, apply pressure to a point over the **femoral artery** (Scan 26-1).

Figure 26-6   The use of pressure points can stop profuse bleeding from an arm or leg if direct pressure and elevation fail. The artery is constricted by pressing it firmly against a bone.

Locate the femoral artery on the medial side of the anterior thigh where it joins the lower trunk of the body. You should be able to feel a pulse at a point just below the groin. Place the heel of your hand over the site and apply pressure toward the bone until the bleeding is controlled.

Due to the amount of muscle and tissue in the thigh, you will need to apply more pressure than you apply to the brachial artery pressure point. Even more force will be needed if the patient is very muscular or obese. As with the brachial artery pressure point, if pressure is properly applied, a distal pulse will not be felt. As noted for upper extremity injuries, this method may not control the bleeding of distal wounds.

Splinting. Bleeding associated with a musculoskeletal injury may be controlled by proper splinting of the injury. Since the sharp ends of broken bones may cause tissue and vessel injury, stabilizing them and preventing further movement of the bone ends prevents additional damage. There are several types of splints used for stabilizing injured extremities. (Splinting musculoskeletal injuries will be discussed in detail in Chapter 28.)

Inflatable splints, also called air splints, may be used to control internal and external bleeding from an extremity (Figure 26-8). This type of splint may be used to control bleeding even if there is no suspected bone injury. The splint produces a form of direct pressure. Air splints are useful if there are several wounds to the extremity or one that extends over the length of the extremity. Air splints are most effective for venous and capillary bleeding. They are not usu-

Figure 26-8 Inflatable, or air, splints may be used to help control some internal or external bleeding from an extremity.

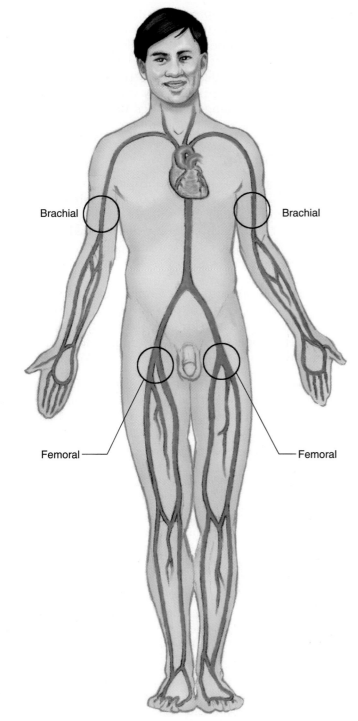

Figure 26-7 Brachial and femoral pressure points.

Brachial

Brachial

Femoral

Femoral

ally effective for the high-pressure bleeding caused by an injured artery—at least not until the arterial pressure has decreased below that of the splint. However, you may use an air splint to maintain pressure on a bleeding wound after other manual methods, such as a pressure dressing, have already controlled the bleeding.

Cold Application. A centuries-old method of controlling bleeding is the application of ice or a cold pack to the injury. The cold minimizes swelling and reduces the bleeding by constricting the blood vessels. Application of cold should not be used alone but in conjunction with other manual techniques. Application of cold will also reduce pain at the injury site.

Warning

Never apply ice or cold packs directly to the skin. This can cause frostbite and further damage to the tissue. Always wrap ice or a cold pack in a cloth or towel before applying it to the skin. Do not leave it in place for longer than 20 minutes at a time.

Pneumatic Anti-Shock Garment (PASG). Although the use of the PASG is controversial, many experts agree that it is useful in controlling bleeding from the areas the garment covers. The PASG controls external bleeding from the lower extremities by direct pressure, similarly to the air splint. It is also useful in providing indirect pressure to help control internal bleeding in the pelvic and abdominal cavities. NEVER inflate only the abdominal section of the PASG. Use of the PASG when there is shock present with a chest wound is generally not advised. Follow your local protocols regarding the use of the PASG or contact medical direction for advice.

If your local protocols call for PASG use, remove the patient's lower outer garments to improve application of the garment and to allow for easier insertion of a urinary catheter later. If clothing cannot be removed, remove the patient's belt and any sharp objects from the pockets. Since transport will be required, place the PASG on the spine board before placing the patient on the PASG. An anti-shock garment should be removed only when a physician is present and under the direction of the physician. Removal should only take place when vital signs have just been monitored and indicate that the patient is stable, and when an operating room is immediately available.

Use of the PASG in the treatment of shock (hypoperfusion) will be discussed later in this chapter.

Tourniquet. A tourniquet is a device that closes off all blood flow to and from an extremity. THE USE OF A TOURNIQUET IS A LAST RESORT. Use is limited to situations when other methods to control LIFE-THREATENING bleeding have failed. Using a tourniquet on an extremity controls life-threatening bleeding, but it is also likely to cause permanent damage to nerves, muscles, and blood vessels and may even cause the loss of the extremity. Tourniquets are rarely needed. Direct pressure, elevation, and pressure points will nearly always control external bleeding.

Tourniquets are most often used on rough-edged amputations. Bleeding from clean-edged amputations usually requires no more than a pressure dressing. The injured blood vessels seal themselves shut as a result of spasms produced by the muscular walls of the vessels. However, in rough-edged amputations caused by crushing or tearing injuries, the vessels do not effectively spasm and close and are likely to bleed heavily. This type of injury may require a tourniquet. Always place the tourniquet as low on the extremity as possible. Attempt bleeding control by direct pressure, elevation, and pressure points before resorting to a tourniquet.

Tourniquets are used on extremity injuries only (Figure 26-9). Do not apply a tourniquet directly over the elbow or knee. The tourniquet should be made of material that is 4 inches wide and 6 to 8 layers thick. Cravats are frequently used for tourniquets. Never use narrow material such as rope or wire that may cut

into the skin. A blood-pressure cuff may be used as a tourniquet (Figure 26-10). Monitor the cuff pressure to be sure the cuff does not gradually deflate.

Once a tourniquet has been applied, do not remove or loosen it unless ordered by medical direction. Loosening a tourniquet may dislodge clots that have formed, resulting in further bleeding. If you must use a tourniquet, keep it in place.

✋ Warning

Remember that the tourniquet is used only as a last resort. The tourniquet should be made of wide material that will not cut into the patient's skin. Use a tourniquet only on extremities, and not directly over joints. Once it is applied, do not remove or loosen it.

While you are applying a tourniquet, have another rescuer apply direct pressure and use a pressure point. This may slow the bleeding until the tourniquet is applied. To properly apply a tourniquet (Figure 26-10), follow these steps:

1. Select a site no farther than 2 inches from the wound. If the wound is on a joint, apply the tourniquet above the joint. The tourniquet should be between the wound and the heart.

2. If using a commercial tourniquet, place the strap around the limb, pull the free end through the buckle or catch, and tighten this end over the pad. Tighten to the point where bleeding is controlled. Do not tighten beyond that point.

If you are using cravats, or triangular bandages, wrap the material around the injured limb and tie a knot over the pad. Slip a pen, stick, or similar device into the knot and rotate to tighten the tourniquet. Tighten to the point that bleeding is controlled; no more. Secure the device in place with tape or by tying with the ends of the cravat. KEEP THE TOURNIQUET IN PLACE. DO NOT LOOSEN OR REMOVE.

3. Attach a notation to the patient to alert other rescuers and hospital staff that a tourniquet has been applied, and the time of the application. Note this on your prehospital care report also. Do not cover the extremity. You must visually monitor the wound site and the effectiveness of the tourniquet. Leave the tourniquet in open view. Advise hospital staff of the application of a tourniquet during your radio report and in person on your arrival at the emergency department.

You may arrive at a scene to find that well-meaning bystanders have already applied a tourniquet to an injury. It may or may not have been necessary. If the EMT-B determines that the bleeding is not se-

Figure 26-9 Application of a tourniquet.

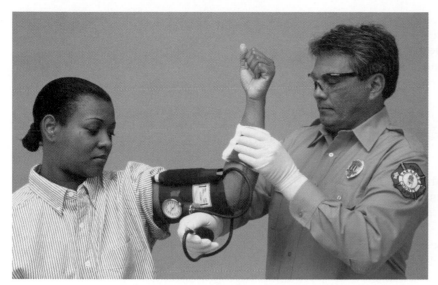

Figure 26-10 A blood-pressure cuff used as a tourniquet.

vere, and other means would control it, medical direction may be contacted about removing the tourniquet. Always follow your local protocols for this situation. If you are directed to remove the tourniquet, have another rescuer apply direct pressure to the wound while the tourniquet is released.

Blood Pressure Cuff. A blood pressure cuff may be used, temporarily, as a tourniquet to control life-threatening arterial bleeding from an extremity while a pressure dressing is applied. Place the cuff above the wound and inflate to approximately 150 mmHg. When the bleeding is controlled, a pressure dressing and bandage are applied. You may then slowly release the pressure in the cuff. Keep the cuff inflated only as long as necessary to secure the pressure dressing and bandage.

Special Situations Involving Bleeding

Bleeding most often occurs from a wound caused by direct trauma (striking or being struck or cut by something, such as in a collision, a fall, a stabbing, or a shooting). However, you may also find external bleeding from other causes, such as bleeding from the ears caused indirectly by a head injury or a nosebleed caused by high blood pressure.

Head Injury. Traumatic injuries resulting in a fractured skull may cause bleeding or loss of cerebrospinal fluid (CSF) from the ears or nose. This fluid loss is not due to direct trauma to the ears or nose. Instead, the head injury results in increased pressure within the skull, which forces fluid out of the cranial cavity. You should not attempt to stop this bleeding or fluid loss. Doing so may increase the pressure in the skull. Do not apply pressure to the ears or nose. Allow the drainage to flow freely, using a gauze pad to collect it.

Nosebleed. Nosebleeds, also called *epistaxis,* may be caused by direct trauma to the nose. However, bleeding from the nose may also be caused by medical problems such as high blood pressure (hypertension). Tiny capillaries in the nose may burst because of increased blood pressure, sinus infection, or digital trauma (nose picking). Controlling bleeding from the nose is sometimes more difficult if the patient is taking certain medications, such as an anticoagulant like Coumadin. To stop a nosebleed, follow these steps:

1. Have the patient sit down and lean forward.

2. Apply or instruct the patient to apply direct pressure to the fleshy portion around the nostrils.

3. Keep the patient calm and quiet.

4. Do not let the patient lean back. This can allow blood to flow down the esophagus to the stomach, resulting in nausea and vomiting.

5. If the patient becomes unconscious or is unable to control his own airway, place the patient in the recovery position (on his side) and be prepared to provide suction and aggressive airway management.

Internal Bleeding

Internal bleeding is bleeding that occurs inside the body. The bleeding itself is not visible, but many of the signs and symptoms are very apparent. There are several reasons why internal bleeding can be very serious:

- Damage to the internal organs and large blood vessels can result in loss of a large quantity of blood in a short period of time.
- Blood loss cannot be seen. While external bleeding is easy to identify, internal bleeding is hidden. Patients may die of blood loss without having any external bleeding.

- Severe internal blood loss may even occur from injuries to the extremities. Sharp bone ends of a fractured femur can cause enough tissue and blood vessel damage to cause shock (hypoperfusion).

● Patient ASSESSMENT

Internal Bleeding

Since internal bleeding is not visible, and may not be obvious, you must identify patients who may have internal bleeding by performing a thorough history and physical exam. Suspicion of internal bleeding and estimates of its severity should be based on the mechanism of injury as well as clinical signs and symptoms. If a patient has a mechanism of injury that suggests the possibility of internal bleeding, treat as though the patient has internal bleeding.

✋ Warning

Treatment for internal injuries will cause no harm if they are not needed. But death may be the result of not treating a patient who needs it.

Blunt trauma is the leading cause of internal injuries and bleeding. Mechanisms of blunt trauma that may cause internal bleeding include:

- Falls
- Motor-vehicle or motorcycle crashes
- Auto-pedestrian collisions
- Blast injuries

Penetrating trauma is also a common cause of internal injuries and bleeding. It is often difficult to judge the severity of the wound even when the size and length of the penetrating object are known. Always assess your patient for exit wounds. Mechanisms of penetrating trauma include:

- Gunshot wounds
- Stab wounds from a knife, ice pick, screwdriver, or similar object
- Impaled objects

Signs of Internal Bleeding

Many of the signs of internal bleeding that you will see are also signs of shock (hypoperfusion). These signs have developed as a result of uncon-trolled internal bleeding. They are late signs, indicating that a life-threatening condition has already developed. If you wait for signs of internal bleeding or shock to develop before beginning treatment, you have waited too long. Signs of internal bleeding are:

- Injuries to the surface of the body, which could indicate underlying injuries
- Bruising (Figure 26-11), swelling, or pain over vital organs (especially in the chest and abdomen). Basic knowledge of anatomy is important for this reason.
- Painful, swollen, or deformed extremities
- Bleeding from the mouth, rectum, vagina, or other body orifice
- A tender, rigid, or distended abdomen
- Vomiting a coffee-ground-like substance or bright red vomitus, indicating the presence of blood. (Red blood is usually "new." Dark blood is usually "old.")
- Dark, tarry stools or bright red blood in the stool
- Signs and symptoms of shock. Remember that the signs listed in Table 26-1 are late signs. They will appear only after internal bleeding has already resulted in significant blood loss.

Remember, your best clue to the possibility of internal bleeding may be the presence of a mechanism of injury that could have caused internal bleeding.

Figure 26-11   Bruising is one sign of internal bleeding.

Internal Bleeding

Care for the patient with internal bleeding centers on the prevention and treatment of shock (hypoperfusion). Definitive treatment for internal bleeding can only take place in the hospital operating room. Patients with suspected internal bleeding must be considered serious, and warrant immediate transport to the hospital.

As with all patients, your first priority is the standard ABCs; that is, ensure an open airway, adequate breathing, and circulation. Patients with internal bleeding may deteriorate quickly. Monitor the ABCs and vital signs often. Be prepared to maintain the patient's airway, to provide or assist ventilations, or to administer CPR as needed.

1. Maintain the ABCs and provide support as needed.

2. Administer high-concentration oxygen by nonrebreather mask, if oxygen administration has not already begun.

3. Control any external bleeding. If you suspect internal bleeding in an injured extremity, apply an appropriate splint.

4. Provide prompt transport to an appropriate medical facility. Internal bleeding must often be controlled in the operating room.

SHOCK (HYPOPERFUSION)

Shock, also known as hypoperfusion, is inadequate tissue perfusion. (Perfusion and hypoperfusion were defined at the beginning of this chapter.) It is the inability of the circulatory system to supply cells with oxygen and nutrients. Hypoperfusion also causes the inadequate removal of waste products from the cells. The result of untreated shock is death.

Causes of Shock

As discussed previously, the circulatory system consists of three components: the heart, blood vessels, and blood. Failure of any of these components—the pumping of the heart, the supply of blood, the integrity of the blood vessels, or the ability of the vessels to dilate and constrict—means that perfusion of the brain, lungs, and other body organs will not be adequate.

Blood vessels can play an important role in the development of shock (if they are *not* functioning properly) or in the body's ability to compensate for shock (if they are functioning properly). Blood vessels can change their diameter, either dilating or constricting. These changes in size are governed by the need for blood in various areas of the body. In an area of the body that is doing more work, blood vessels dilate to allow more blood to flow to that area. At the same time, in another area of the body that is not working as hard, vessels will constrict. For example, if you are running, blood flow to the muscles in the legs increases through dilated arteries. At the same time, blood flow to the digestive system lessens because vessels supplying these organs have been constricted to compensate for the dilation of the arteries in the legs.

Since the amount of blood in the body does not change, this balance between dilation of some vessels and constriction of others is necessary to keep the system full. The same amount of blood is in the body, but it is distributed differently. If all the blood vessels in the body dilated at one time, there would not be enough blood to fill the entire circulatory system. Circulation would fail, and tissues would not be adequately perfused. The result would be the development of shock.

As shock develops, the failure of one component of the system may cause adverse effects on another. If blood is being lost through external bleeding, the heart rate will increase in an effort to circulate the remaining blood to all the tissues. However, the increased heart rate causes increased bleeding. As more blood is lost, the heart tries to compensate by increasing its rate even more. Left untreated, the process continues until the patient dies.

In the early stages of shock, the body attempts to compensate for blood loss. Most of the signs and symptoms of shock are the body's compensating mechanisms attempting to adequately perfuse the tissues. Shock may develop if (1) the heart fails as a pump, or (2) blood volume is lost, or (3) blood vessels dilate, creating a vascular container capacity that is too great to be filled by the available blood.

Severity of Shock

Shock (hypoperfusion) is the body's reaction to decreased blood circulation to the organ systems. It is the result of the inadequate perfusion of tissues with oxygen and nutrients and the inadequate removal of metabolic waste products. If untreated, shock will cause cell and organ malfunction and, finally, it will result in death. Prompt recognition and aggressive treatment are vital to patient survival.

Shock is classified into three categories of severity. These are **compensated shock, decompensated shock,** and **irreversible shock:**

- *Compensated shock.* The body senses the decrease in perfusion and attempts to compensate for it. For

Regardless of the cause, shock is the failure of the circulatory system to provide sufficient blood and oxygen to all the vital tissues of the body. The three major types of shock are **hypovolemic shock, cardiogenic shock,** and **neurogenic shock:**

• *Hypovolemic shock.* This is the type of shock most commonly seen by EMT-Bs. When it is caused by uncontrolled bleeding, or hemorrhage, it can be called **hemorrhagic shock.** The bleeding can be internal, external, or a combination of both. Hypovolemic shock may also be caused by burns or crush injuries, where plasma is lost.

• *Cardiogenic shock.* Patients suffering a myocardial infarction, or heart attack, may develop shock from the inadequate pumping of blood by the heart. The strength of the heart's contractions may be decreased because of the damage to the heart muscle. Or the heart's electrical system may be malfunctioning, causing a heartbeat that is too slow, too fast, or irregular. Other cardiac problems, such as congestive heart failure, may also cause shock. Watch for low blood pressure, edema in the feet and ankles, and other signs of heart failure. (Review Chapter 18, "Cardiac Emergencies.")

• *Neurogenic shock.* Shock may result from the uncontrolled dilation of blood vessels due to nerve paralysis caused by spinal-cord injuries. While there is no actual blood loss, the dilation of the blood vessels increases the capacity of the circulatory system to the point where the available blood can no longer adequately fill it. *Sepsis* (massive infection) or an *anaphylactic* (severe allergic) reaction may also cause neurogenic shock. Neurogenic shock is seen only occasionally in the field.

Keep in mind that, as an EMT-B, you do not need to diagnose the type of shock. Instead, you must recognize and treat for shock whenever there is a mechanism of injury or signs that indicate the possibility of shock.

a time, the body's compensating mechanisms work, and blood pressure is maintained. Some early signs of shock are actually the body's compensating mechanisms at work. You will note an increased heart rate (to increase blood flow) and increased respirations (to increase oxygenation of the blood). Constriction of the peripheral circulation (to redirect blood to the vital core organs) results in pale, cool skin and, in infants and children, increased capillary refill time.

• *Decompensated shock.* At the point when the body can no longer compensate for the low blood vol-

ume or lack of perfusion, decompensated shock begins. Late signs of shock, such as falling blood pressure, develop.

• *Irreversible shock.* Irreversible shock exists when the body has lost the battle to maintain perfusion to the organ systems. Cell damage occurs, especially in the liver and kidneys. Even if adequate vital signs can be restored, the patient may die days later due to the failure of irreparably damaged organs.

Patient ASSESSMENT

Shock (Hypoperfusion)

Many of the signs and symptoms of shock are the same no matter what the cause (hypovolemic, cardiogenic, or neurogenic). The symptoms follow a logical progression as shock develops and worsens. The signs and symptoms, in the order they appear, are as follows (Table 26-1):

• *Altered mental status.* The brain is very sensitive to any decrease in oxygen supply. When the brain is deprived of oxygen, even slightly, mental and behavioral changes may be seen. These may include anxiety, restlessness, and combativeness.

• *Pale, cool, clammy skin.* When the body senses inadequate tissue perfusion, it attempts to correct the problem by diverting, or shunting, blood from non-vital areas to the vital organs. Blood is quickly directed away from the skin and sent to organs such as the heart and brain. This results in loss of skin color and temperature. Infants and young children may have a capillary refill time of greater than 2 seconds. (Delayed capillary refill time is considered an unreliable sign of shock in patients over the age of 5 when capillary refill time can more readily be influenced by other factors.) Note that in neurogenic shock (rare) the skin is typically warm, flushed, and dry because the circulatory system has lost the ability to constrict blood vessels in the skin.

• *Nausea and vomiting.* In the body's efforts to direct blood to the vital organs, blood is diverted from the digestive system, resulting in nausea and sometimes vomiting.

• *Vital sign changes.* The first vital signs to change are the respiratory and pulse rates:

– The pulse will increase in an attempt to pump more blood. As it continues to increase and blood loss worsens, the pulse becomes weak and thready.

– Respirations increase in an attempt to raise the oxygen saturation of the blood left in the system. As shock progresses, respirations become more rapid, labored, shallow, and sometimes irregular.

– Blood pressure drops because the body's compensating mechanisms can no longer keep up with the decrease in perfusion or blood loss. Decreased blood pressure is a LATE sign of shock. By the time the blood pressure drops, the patient is in a truly life-threatening condition.

• *Other signs.* Other signs of shock include thirst, dilated pupils, and sometimes cyanosis around the lips and nail beds.

Pediatric Notes

Infants and children present a special problem when assessing for shock. They have such efficient compensating mechanisms that they can maintain a normal blood pressure until over half of their blood volume is gone. By the time their blood pressure drops, they are already near death. Shock must be considered and cared for early. Do not wait for signs of shock to appear.

Emergency Care

Emergency care for the patient in shock includes airway maintenance and the administration of high-concentration oxygen. Increasing the oxygen saturation of the blood will improve oxygen supply to the tissues. You must also attempt to stop what is causing the shock, such as external bleeding, and attempt to maintain perfusion.

Remember that TRANSPORTATION IS AN INTERVENTION. Your most significant treatment for the shock patient may be early recognition of the problem and prompt transportation to a hospital where the patient will receive definitive care. A term frequently used in relation to trauma care is the **golden hour.** This term refers to the optimum limit of 1 hour from the time the patient's injury occurs until surgery takes place at a hospital.

Note that the clock begins running at the time of injury, not the time of your arrival on scene. If the patient is not quickly found, or you have a long response time to the scene, much of the golden hour may have already ticked away. Studies have shown that survival rates from traumatic injuries are best if needed surgery takes place within this first hour. Survival rates rapidly decrease thereafter. Your goal in caring for trauma and shock patients is to limit on-scene time and provide immediate transportation to the hospital. Be sure to alert the receiving hospital as soon as possible, as they may need to call in a sur-

geon. The clock does not stop with the patient's arrival at the hospital. It stops in the operating room.

The goal for on-scene time when caring for a trauma or shock patient is a maximum of 10 minutes (unless lengthy extrication is required). This on-scene time limit is referred to as the **platinum ten minutes.** In order to meet the golden hour, procedures done at the scene must be kept to a minimum. In patients showing signs of shock, or a mechanism of injury that suggests the possibility, some elements of patient assessment, such as detailed exams and treatments, are best done in the ambulance en route to the hospital. On-scene assessment and care should consist of the ABCs with spinal precautions, a rapid trauma exam, immobilization, and moving the patient to the ambulance. Always drive safely and responsibly to the hospital no matter how serious your patient may be.

Patient *CARE*

Shock (Hypoperfusion)

Care for shock is similar to the care for bleeding described earlier. Remember BSI precautions when caring for any patient who is bleeding externally. The emergency care steps for shock (Scan 26-2) are as follows:

1. Maintain an open airway and assess the respiratory rate. If the patient is breathing adequately, apply high-concentration oxygen by nonrebreather mask. Assist ventilations or perform CPR if necessary.

2. Control any external bleeding.

3. Apply and inflate the pneumatic anti-shock garment (PASG) if approved or ordered by your local medical direction (Scan 26-3). The PASG is usually indicated for bleeding in areas covered by the garment, pelvic injury, and some abdominal trauma. Always follow your local protocols for use of the PASG.

Use of the PASG is usually contraindicated in cardiogenic shock, or if there are abnormal lung sounds. Special consideration should be taken if your patient has bleeding in areas not covered by the garment. Use of the PASG when there is shock in the presence of a chest wound is generally not advised. If your female patient is pregnant, inflate only the leg sections. If your patient is a child, it is recommended that only the leg sections be inflated. This is because the top of the abdominal section of the pediatric-size garment often covers the lower portion of a child's chest, which can interfere with the child's respirations.

MANAGING SHOCK

NOTE: FIRST take BSI precautions.

▲ **1.** Maintain an open airway, and give high-concentration oxygen by nonrebreather. Control external bleeding. Assist ventilations and perform CPR, if needed.

▲ **2.** If there is no serious injury, elevate the patient's legs 8 to 12 inches, or . . .

▲ . . . If there is any possibility of spine injury, position the patient with NO elevation of the extremities.

▲ **3.** Place the patient on a spine board to splint the entire body. Splinting of bone and joint injuries should be done en route.

▲ **4.** Protect the patient from heat loss.

▲ **5.** Transport immediately.

APPLYING THE ANTI-SHOCK GARMENT

Follow local protocols regarding application and inflation.

▲ Pneumatic anti-shock garment and inflation pump.

▲ **1.** Unfold the garment and lay it flat on a backboard. It should be free of wrinkles.

▲ **4.** Enclose the other leg, securing the Velcro straps.

▲ **2.** Log roll the patient onto the garment, or slide it under him. The upper edge must be just below the patient's bottom rib.

▲ **5.** Enclose the abdomen and pelvis, securing the Velcro straps.

▲ **3.** Enclose one leg, securing the Velcro straps.

▲ **6.** Check the tubes leading to the compartments and the pump.

(continued)

▲ **7.** Open the stopcocks to the legs and close the abdominal compartment stopcock.

▲ **8.** Use the pump to inflate the lower compartments simultaneously. Inflate until the Velcro makes a crackling noise.

▲ **9.** Close the stopcocks.

▲ **10.** Check the patient's blood pressure.

▲ **11.** Check both extremities for distal pulse.

▲ **12.** If systolic BP is still below 90 mmHg, open the stopcock and inflate the abdominal compartment. Close the stopcock.

Monitor and record vital signs every 5 minutes. If the garment loses pressure, add air as needed. Some protocols call for the inflation of all three compartments of the garment simultaneously. Always follow local protocols. Some systems require direct medical direction to inflate.

Note: Patient's clothing remains on for demonstration purposes. In actual use, clothing should be removed.

4. If there is no possibility of spine injury, elevate the legs 8 to 12 inches. This position will assist the body in maintaining perfusion to the vital organs. Elevation is not necessary if you have applied and inflated the PASG.

5. Splint any suspected bone injuries or joint injuries. If your patient is in shock, do not use your valuable on-scene time for this. Splints should be applied en route to the hospital. Do not take time to individually splint multiple injuries. Splint the entire body by securing the patient to a long spine board. This will adequately stabilize the injuries until further care can be given.

6. Prevent loss of body heat by covering the patient with a blanket.

7. Transport the patient immediately. Detailed exams and care procedures should be done en route to the hospital. Notify the receiving hospital as soon as possible. Give them information on the patient's injuries and condition. Contact medical direction if necessary. If your on-scene time is extended due to extrication, or your transport time to the hospital is lengthy, request an ALS intercept if available. This may be a ground ambulance or a helicopter service. If you have the patient loaded in your ambulance,

begin transport and ask that the ALS unit intercept your unit en route. Time is of the essence.

8. If the patient is conscious, speak calmly and reassuringly throughout assessment, care, and transport. Fear increases the body's work and worsens developing shock.

Documentation Tip— Bleeding and Shock

When giving your report to the hospital by radio, and writing the narrative portion of your prehospital care report, it is important to "paint a picture" of your patient and the incident. At the scene, you are the eyes and ears for the emergency department physician. You see things that the hospital staff cannot, such as the mechanism of injury (e.g., the condition of the vehicle at the crash scene) and the amount of external blood loss. Be sure to describe in detail significant things you saw on scene. Many EMS personnel now carry an instant-type camera in their vehicles. The adage "a picture is worth a thousand words" is very true in EMS. Photos taken at the scene may give the emergency department physician much more insight into the patient's condition.

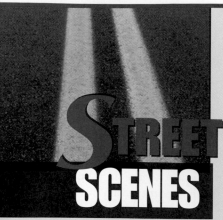

STREET SCENES

Arnold Johnson likes to do odd jobs around the house. Today's project is to fix a loose shelf in the kitchen. He gets out his ladder and tools and starts to work. As he reaches to hammer his first nail, he loses his footing and falls a few feet, hitting his left side on the corner of the kitchen table. It hurts but he goes back to finish the shelf. After a few minutes, he realizes he is in considerable discomfort. As the pain increases and Arnold starts to feel worse, he knows something is wrong and calls 9-1-1. Your ambulance is dispatched with a First Response unit from the fire department, Squad 31, to a 46-year-old male with injuries from a fall. Squad 31 is on scene first, gathering a history and taking a set of vital signs. You arrive about three minutes later. Mr. Johnson is sitting in a chair and looks anxious.

STREET SCENE QUESTIONS

1. What is the priority for this patient? Does an initial assessment still need to be done?

2. What assessment information do you want to receive from Squad 31?

3. Is the mechanism of injury important information for this patient?

You approach the patient as your partner gets the First Responder information. You notice that Mr. Johnson seems pale and with an increased respiratory rate. Your partner gives you the patient history from Squad 31, including their impression that the patient may have broken some ribs. The First Responders report the following vital signs: a thready pulse of 110, respiratory rate of 24 and labored, and a blood pressure of 130/85. As you move on to the focused assessment, your partner prepares the stretcher. You are becoming more concerned. You ask the wife if this is his normal color and she tells you he is very pale. At that point, the patient tells you he feels nauseated and thinks he might throw up.

STREET SCENE QUESTIONS

4. What is the treatment priority for this patient?

5. How often should you get a new set of vital signs?

You load the patient on the stretcher, ask him how he feels, and notice he is not as alert as when you arrived on the scene about 10 minutes ago. You administer O_2 by way of nonrebreather and move toward the ambulance, concerned that this patient may be bleeding internally. Once en route to the hospital, you get another set of vital signs and realize the pulse is weak and increased by 10 beats per minute. The respiratory rate is now 28 and seems more labored. You do a detailed assessment of the abdomen, and the patient reacts with tenderness in the left upper quadrant. The closest hospital is a trauma center, and you tell your partner this is a high priority. You continue patient care with 15 liters per minute of O_2 by nonrebreather and keep the patient warm. Another set of vital signs is taken, followed by a radio report to the hospital. You end the transmission by advising ETA in 7 minutes.

A short time after you give your prehospital care report to emergency department personnel, you overhear a surgeon turn to a nurse and quietly say, "Get an operating room set up. This patient likely has a severe spleen injury."

| PATIENT NAME: | Arnold Johnson | | | | | PATIENT AGE: | 46 |

CHIEF COMPLAINT		TIME	RESP	PULSE	B.P.	MENTAL STATUS	R PUPILS L	SKIN
Tenderness LUQ	V I T A L S I G N S	0922	Rate: **24** ☐ Regular ☐ Shallow ☒ Labored	Rate: **110** ☒ Regular ☐ Irregular	**130** / **85**	☒ Alert ☐ Voice ☐ Pain ☐ Unresp.	☑ Normal ☑ ☐ Dilated ☐ Constricted ☐ Sluggish ☐ No-Reaction	☐ Unremarkable ☐ Cool ☑ Pale ☐ Warm ☐ Cyanotic ☑ Moist ☐ Flushed ☐ Dry ☐ Jaundiced
PAST MEDICAL HISTORY		0928	Rate: **28** ☐ Regular ☐ Shallow ☒ Labored	Rate: **120** ☒ Regular ☐ Irregular	**124** / **80**	☐ Alert ☑ Voice ☐ Pain ☐ Unresp.	☑ Normal ☑ ☐ Dilated ☐ Constricted ☐ Sluggish ☐ No-Reaction	☐ Unremarkable ☑ Cool ☑ Pale ☐ Warm ☐ Cyanotic ☑ Moist ☐ Flushed ☐ Dry ☐ Jaundiced
☒ None ☐ Allergy to _____ ☐ Hypertension ☐ Stroke ☐ Seizures ☐ Diabetes ☐ COPD ☐ Cardiac ☐ Other (List) ☐ Asthma		0935	Rate: **28** ☐ Regular ☐ Shallow ☒ Labored	Rate: **120** ☒ Regular ☐ Irregular	**118** / **78**	☐ Alert ☑ Voice ☐ Pain ☐ Unresp.	☑ Normal ☑ ☐ Dilated ☐ Constricted ☐ Sluggish ☐ No-Reaction	☐ Unremarkable ☑ Cool ☑ Pale ☐ Warm ☐ Cyanotic ☑ Moist ☐ Flushed ☐ Dry ☐ Jaundiced

Current Medications (List)
None

NARRATIVE Our patient states that he fell several feet while standing on a ladder. While falling, he struck his left side on the edge of a protruding kitchen table. Patient denies striking his head, neck, or back. He denies any loss of consciousness. 0922 vital signs were reported by First Responders. Patient is now ashen, respiration has become more rapid and labored, and pulse has become weak and more rapid. Patient has a decreasing level of responsiveness, and is becoming nauseated. Our physical exam reveals a very tender LUQ. Patient placed on 15 LPM via nonrebreather. Monitored and managed patient's body temperature en route to trauma center.

CHAPTER REVIEW

SUMMARY

Blood loss can be external or internal. External bleeding can be controlled by direct pressure, elevation, and the use of pressure points. Emergency care for internal bleeding is based on the prevention and treatment of shock.

Shock is usually first seen in a patient as restlessness or anxiety. Skin becomes pale, and the pulse and respirations increase. If shock remains uncontrolled, the patient's blood pressure begins to fall. A decrease in blood pressure is a late sign of shock. Signs and symptoms of shock may not be evident early in the call, so treatment based on the mechanism of injury may be life-saving.

Treat shock by airway maintenance, administration of high-concentration oxygen, controlling bleeding, and keeping the patient warm. One of the most important treatments is early recognition of shock and immediate transport to a hospital.

KEY TERMS

arterial bleeding bleeding from an artery, which is characterized by bright red blood and as rapid, profuse, and difficult to control.

brachial (BRAY-ke-al) **artery** the major artery of the upper arm.

capillary bleeding bleeding from capillaries, which is characterized by a slow, oozing flow of blood.

cardiogenic shock shock, or lack of perfusion, brought on not by blood loss, but by inadequate pumping action of the heart. It is often the result of a heart attack or congestive heart failure.

compensated shock when the patient is developing shock but the body is still able to maintain perfusion. See *shock*.

decompensated shock occurs when the body can no longer compensate for low blood volume or lack of perfusion. Late signs such as decreasing blood pressure become evident. See *shock*.

femoral (FEM-or-al) **artery** the major artery supplying the thigh.

golden hour refers to the optimum limit of one hour between time of injury and surgery at the hospital.

hemorrhage (HEM-o-rej) bleeding, especially severe bleeding.

hemorrhagic (HEM-or-AJ-ik) **shock** shock resulting from blood loss.

hypoperfusion (HI-po-per-FEW-zhun) inability of the body to adequately circulate blood to the body's cells to supply them with oxygen and nutrients. See also *shock*.

hypovolemic (HI-po-vo-LE-mik) **shock** shock resulting from blood or fluid loss.

irreversible shock when the body has lost the battle to maintain perfusion to vital organs. Even if adequate vital signs return, the patient may die days later due to organ failure.

neurogenic shock hypoperfusion due to nerve paralysis (sometimes caused by spinal cord injuries) resulting in the dilation of blood vessels that increases the volume of the circulatory system beyond the point where it can be filled.

perfusion the supply of oxygen to and removal of wastes from the cells and tissues of the body as a result of the flow of blood through the capillaries.

platinum ten minutes refers to an optimum limit of ten minutes at the scene with a serious trauma patient.

pressure dressing a bulky dressing held in position with a tightly wrapped bandage to apply pressure to help control bleeding.

pressure point a site where a main artery lies near the surface of the body and directly over a bone. Pressure on such a point can stop distal bleeding.

shock also known as *hypoperfusion*. The inability of the body to adequately circulate blood to the body's cells to supply them with oxygen and nutrients. A life-threatening condition.

tourniquet (TURN-i-ket) a device used for bleeding control that constricts all blood flow to and from an extremity.

venous bleeding bleeding from a vein, which is characterized by dark red or maroon blood and as a steady flow, easy to control.

Review Questions

1. Name the three main types of blood vessels, and describe the type of bleeding you would expect to see from each one. (pp. 501, 503–504)
2. List the patient care steps for external bleeding control. (p. 505)
3. Define *perfusion* and *hypoperfusion*. (p. 502)
4. List the signs and symptoms of shock. Which would you expect to see early? Which are late signs? Explain what causes each of them. (pp. 514–515)
5. List the three major types of shock and what causes each one. (pp. 513–514)
6. List the emergency care steps for treating a patient in shock. (pp. 515, 519)
7. Define the "golden hour" and the "platinum ten minutes." (p. 515)

Applications

• A patient has been involved in a motor-vehicle crash. There is considerable damage to his vehicle. The steering column and wheel are badly deformed. The patient complains of a "sore chest." You note no external bleeding. The patient's vital signs are pulse 116, respirations 20, blood pressure 106/70. How would you proceed to assess and care for this patient?

Web Medic

Visit Brady's *Emergency Care* website for direct weblinks. At **www.bradybooks.com/emergencycare**, you will find information related to the following Chapter 26 topics:

- Bleeding and shock
- Hemophilia

Chapter
Twenty-Seven

SOFT-TISSUE INJURIES

EMT-Bs are frequently called to deal with injuries to the soft tissues of the body. These injuries may range from minor scrapes and bruises to life-threatening injuries to the chest and abdomen. It is the responsibility of the EMT-B to identify and treat each of these injuries skillfully and professionally. Many soft-tissue injuries are open wounds, which can be very upsetting to the patient. Your emotional care and demeanor will mean a great deal. Overall, the assessment and care of the patient with a soft-tissue injury will be a challenging part of your responsibilities as an EMT-B.

SOFT TISSUES

The soft tissues of the body include the skin, fatty tissues, muscles, blood vessels, fibrous tissues, membranes (tissues that line or cover organs), glands, and nerves (Figure 27-1). Teeth, bones, and cartilage are considered hard tissues.

The most obvious soft-tissue injuries involve the skin (Figure 27-2). Most people do not think of the skin as a body organ, but it is. In fact, it is the largest organ of the human body. The skin's total surface area is over 20 square feet. The major functions of the skin include:

- *Protection.* The skin is a barrier that keeps out microorganisms (germs), debris, and unwanted chemicals. Underlying tissues and organs are protected from environmental contact.
- *Water balance.* The skin helps prevent water loss and stops environmental water from entering the body. This helps preserve the chemical balance of body fluids and tissues.
- *Temperature regulation.* Blood vessels in the skin can dilate (increase in diameter) to carry more blood to the skin, allowing heat to radiate away from the body. When the body needs to conserve heat, these vessels constrict (decrease in diameter) to prevent heat loss. The sweat glands found in the skin produce perspiration, which will evaporate and help cool the body. The fat that is part of the skin serves as a thermal insulator.
- *Excretion.* Salts, carbon dioxide, and excess water can be released through the skin.
- *Shock (impact) absorption.* The skin and its layers of fat help protect the underlying organs from minor impacts and pressures.

The skin has three major layers: the epidermis, the dermis, and the subcutaneous layer. The outer layer of the skin is the **epidermis.** The outermost epidermis is composed of dead cells, which are rubbed off or sloughed off and are replaced. The pigment granules of the skin and living cells are found deeper in the epidermis. The cells of the innermost portion are actively dividing, replacing the dead cells of the outer layers. The epidermis contains no blood vessels or nerves. Except for certain types of burns and injuries due to cold, injuries of the epidermis present few problems in EMT-B-level care.

The layer of skin below the epidermis is the **dermis.** This layer is rich with blood vessels, nerves, and

HOW AND WHY?

Although the process can be slow, the skin can heal itself effectively even after considerable damage has occurred. Go to your Electronic Extras CD to learn about the four stages of skin regeneration.

TOPIC OVERVIEW

In this chapter, you will learn about the following topics:

- Emergency care for burns, amputations, chest and abdominal wounds, impaled objects, and both open and closed soft-tissue injuries

- How to recognize the different types of burns

- How to dress and bandage wounds

DOT OBJECTIVES

---

specialized structures such as sweat glands, sebaceous (oil) glands, and hair follicles. Specialized nerve endings in the dermis are involved with the senses of touch, cold, heat, and pain. Once the dermis is opened to the outside world, contamination and infection become major problems. Such wounds can be serious, accompanied by profuse bleeding and intense pain.

The layers of fat and soft tissue below the dermis are called the **subcutaneous layers.** Shock absorption and insulation are major functions of this layer. Again, when these layers are injured there are the problems of tissue and bloodstream contamination, bleeding, and pain.

Soft-tissue injuries are generally classified as closed wounds or open wounds.

CLOSED WOUNDS

A **closed wound** is an internal injury; that is, there is no open pathway from the outside to the injured site. These wounds usually result from the impact of a blunt object. Although the skin itself may not be broken, there may be extensively crushed tissues beneath it. Closed wounds can be simple bruises, internal lacerations (cuts), and internal punctures caused by fractured bones, crushing forces, or the rupture (bursting open) of internal organs (Figure 27-3). Internal bleeding from a closed wound can range from minor to life threatening.

Types of Closed Wounds

There are three types of closed wound: contusions, hematomas, and crush injuries. A **contusion** is a bruise, the most frequently encountered type of

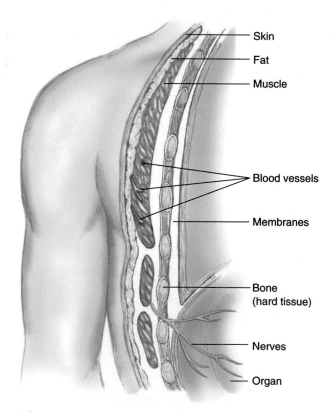

Figure 27-1 Soft tissues.

Skin
Fat
Muscle
Blood vessels
Membranes
Bone (hard tissue)
Nerves
Organ

23. Describe the steps in applying a pressure dressing. (p. 556)

24. Establish the relationship between airway management and the patient with chest injury, burns, and blunt and penetrating injuries. (pp. 529, 533, 534, 536, 538, 540, 542, 544, 545, 548, 550, 553, 554)

25. Describe the effects of improperly applied dressings, splints, and tourniquets. (pp. 556–560)

26. Describe the emergency medical care of a patient with an impaled object. (pp. 535–537)

27. Describe the emergency medical care of a patient with an amputation. (p. 538)

28. Describe the emergency care for a chemical burn. (pp. 551, 553)

29. Describe the emergency care for an electrical burn. (pp. 554–555)

✔ **Skills**

1. Demonstrate the steps in emergency medical care of closed soft-tissue injuries.

2. Demonstrate the steps in emergency medical care of open soft-tissue injuries.

3. Demonstrate the steps in emergency medical care of a patient with an open chest wound.

4. Demonstrate the steps in emergency medical care of a patient with open abdominal wounds.

5. Demonstrate the steps in emergency medical care of a patient with an impaled object.

6. Demonstrate the steps in emergency medical care of a patient with an amputation.

7. Demonstrate the steps in emergency medical care of an amputated part.

8. Demonstrate the steps in emergency medical care of a patient with superficial burns.

9. Demonstrate the steps in emergency medical care of a patient with partial thickness burns.

10. Demonstrate the steps in emergency medical care of a patient with full thickness burns.

11. Demonstrate the steps in emergency medical care of a patient with a chemical burn.

12. Demonstrate completing a prehospital care report for patients with soft-tissue injuries.

Figure 27-2 The skin.

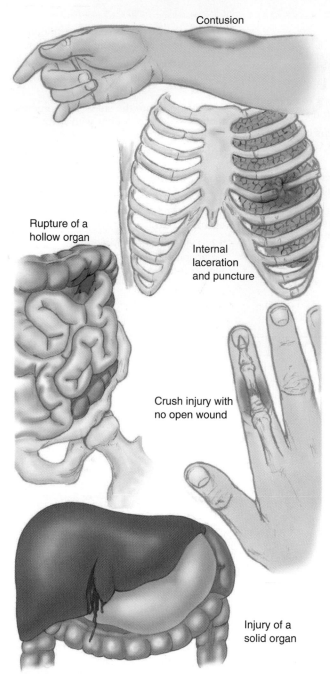

Contusion

Rupture of a
hollow organ

Internal
laceration
and puncture

Crush injury with
no open wound

Injury of a
solid organ

Figure 27-3   Closed wounds.

Figure 27-4   Contusions are the most common type of closed wound.

Blood almost always collects at the injury site. This results in a **hematoma.** A hematoma differs from a contusion in that hematomas involve a larger amount of tissue damage, including damage to larger blood vessels with greater blood loss. As much as a liter of blood may be lost in a hematoma.

Force can be transmitted from the body's exterior to its internal structures, even when the skin remains intact and even when the only indication of injury is a simple bruise. This force can cause the internal organs to be crushed or ruptured, bleeding internally. When this happens, it is called a **crush injury.** Solid organs such as the liver and spleen normally contain considerable amounts of blood. When crushed, they bleed severely and cause shock. Contents of hollow organs, such as digested food or urine, can leak into the body cavities, causing severe inflammation and tissue damage.

Patient *ASSESSMENT*

Closed Wounds

Bruising may be an indication of internal injuries and related internal bleeding (Table 27-1). In addition, consider the possibility of closed soft-tissue injuries whenever there is swelling, pain, or deformity, and a mechanism of blunt trauma. Always consider the mechanism of injury (MOI) when you examine a patient with a closed wound. Crush injuries may be difficult or impossible to identify during assessment, so you must rely on the MOI. Patients with a significant MOI should be considered to have internal bleeding and shock until they are ruled out in the emergency department.

closed wound (Figure 27-4). In a contusion, the epidermis remains intact, but cells and blood vessels in the dermis are damaged. A variable amount of bleeding occurs at the time of injury and may continue for a few hours. There is pain, swelling, and discoloration at the wound site. Swelling and discoloration may occur immediately or may be delayed as much as 24 to 48 hours. The swelling is caused by a collection of blood under the skin or within the damaged tissues. Other organs such as the kidneys or brain may also be contused.

Table 27-1 Contusions (Bruises) as Signs of Soft-Tissue Injury

Sign	Indicates
Large bruise or bruised areas directly over body organs such as the spleen, liver, or kidneys	Possible injury to underlying organs
Swelling or deformity at site of bruise	Possible underlying fracture
Bruise on the head or neck	Possible injury to the cervical spine or brain. Search for blood in the mouth, nose, and ears.
Bruise on the trunk or signs of damage to the ribs or sternum	Possible chest injury. Determine if the patient is coughing up frothy red blood, which may indicate a punctured lung, and assess for difficult breathing. Use your stethoscope to listen for equal air entry and any unusual breath sounds.
Bruise on the abdomen	Possible injury to the abdominal organs. Look to see if the patient has vomited. If so, is there any substance in the vomitus that looks like coffee grounds (partially digested blood)? Palpate to detect if patient's abdomen is rigid or tender.

Note: Treatment for internal bleeding is discussed in Chapter 26; treatment of head injury in Chapter 29; treatment of chest and abdominal injuries in this chapter.

Figure 27-5 Administer high-concentration oxygen and emergency care for shock.

Patient CARE

Closed Wounds

Take the appropriate BSI precautions and follow these steps for emergency care of a patient with closed wounds (Figure 27-5):

1. Manage the patient's airway, breathing, and circulation. Apply high-concentration oxygen by nonrebreather mask.

2. MANAGE AS IF THERE IS INTERNAL BLEEDING and PROVIDE CARE FOR SHOCK, if you believe that there is any possibility of internal injuries.

3. Splint extremities that are painful, swollen, or deformed.

4. Stay alert for the patient to vomit.

5. Continue to monitor the patient for the development of shock and transport as soon as possible.

OPEN WOUNDS

An **open wound** is an injury in which the skin is interrupted, or broken, exposing the tissues underneath. The interruption can come from the outside, as a laceration, or from the inside when a fractured bone end tears outward through the skin.

Types of Open Wounds

Abrasions

The classification of **abrasion** includes simple scrapes and scratches in which the outer layer of the skin is damaged but all the layers are not penetrated (Figure 27-6). Skinned elbows and knees, "road rash," "mat burns," "rug burns," and "brush burns" are examples of abrasions. There may be no detectable bleeding or only the minor ooze of blood from capillary beds. The patient may be experiencing great pain, even if the injury is minor. Because of dirt or other substances ground into the skin, the opportunity for infection is great.

Lacerations

A **laceration** is a cut. It may be smooth or jagged (Figure 27-7). This type of wound is often caused by an object with a sharp edge, such as a razor blade, broken glass, or a jagged piece of metal. However, a laceration can also result from a severe blow or impact with a blunt object. If the laceration has rough edges, it may tend to fall together and obstruct the view as you try to determine the wound depth. It is usually impossible to look at the outside of a laceration and determine the extent of the damage to underlying tissues. If significant blood vessels have been torn, bleeding will be considerable. Sometimes the bleeding is partially controlled when blood vessels are stretched and torn. This is due to the natural retraction and constriction of the cut ends that aid in rapid clot formation.

A

B

Figure 27-7 Some lacerations have smooth edges (A), and some have jagged edges (B).

Figure 27-6 Abrasions are usually the least serious type of open wound.

Punctures

When a sharp, pointed object passes through the skin or other tissue, a **puncture wound** has occurred. Typically, puncture wounds are caused by objects such as nails, ice picks, splinters, or knives (Figure 27-8). Often, there is no severe external bleeding, but internal bleeding may be profuse. The threat of contamination must always be seriously considered.

There are two types of puncture wounds. A *penetrating puncture wound* can be shallow or deep

HOW AND WHY?

While you won't be stitching patients, knowledge of how and why stitching is done may help you understand wound care better. Go to your Electronic Extras CD for more information.

A

Avulsions

In an **avulsion,** flaps of skin and tissues are torn loose or pulled off completely (Figure 27-11). When the tip of the nose is cut or torn off, this is an avulsion. The same applies to the external ear. A *degloving avulsion* occurs when the hand is caught in a roller. In this type of accident, the skin is stripped off like a glove. An eye pulled from its socket (extruded) is a form of avulsion. The term *avulsed* is used in reporting the wound, as in "an avulsed eye," or "an avulsed ear." When tissue is avulsed, it is cut off from its oxygen supply and will soon die.

B

A

Figure 27-8 (A) A penetrating puncture wound and (B) a perforating puncture wound.

(Figures 27-8 and Figure 27-9). In either case, tissues and blood vessels are injured. A *perforating puncture wound* has both an entrance wound and an exit wound (Figure 27-10). The object causing the injury passes through the body and out again. In many cases, the exit wound is more serious than the entrance wound. A "through-and-through" gunshot wound is an example of a perforating puncture wound.

Figure 27-9 (A) A penetrating puncture wound, external view, and (B) an x-ray of the same wound.

B

A

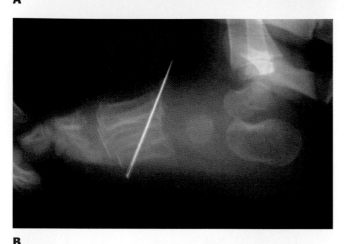

B

Figure 27-10 This perforating puncture wound has both an entry wound (at the bottom of the foot) and an exit wound (the top of the foot).

Amputations

The extremities are sometimes subject to **amputation.** The fingers, toes, hands, feet, or limbs are completely cut through or torn off (Figure 27-12). Jagged skin and bone edges can sometimes be observed. There may be massive bleeding; or the force that amputates a limb may close off torn blood vessels, limiting the amount of bleeding. Often, blood vessels collapse, or they retract and curl up, which limits bleeding from the wound site.

Crush Injuries

Crush injuries were discussed earlier in this chapter as closed wounds, but crush injuries also can be open wounds. An open crush injury can result when an extremity is caught between heavy items, such as pieces of machinery. Blood vessels, nerves, and muscles are involved and swelling may be a major prob-

Figure 27-11 (A) An avulsion, (B) an avulsion injury that caused a degloving, and (C) an avulsion of male genitalia.

A

B

C

A

B

Figure 27-12 Amputation at the wrist.

lem with resulting loss of blood supply distally. Bones are fractured and may protrude through the wound site. Soft tissues and internal organs can be crushed to produce profuse bleeding, both externally and internally (Figure 27-13).

Figure 27-13 An open crush injury.

Emergency Care for Open Wounds

Open wounds require strict attention to BSI precautions. In addition to wearing gloves, a gown and protective eyewear may also be required. Remember to properly dispose of all soiled materials and wash your hands after each call.

Patient ASSESSMENT

Open Wounds

Airway, breathing, circulation, and severe bleeding are identified and treated in the initial assessment. Once the initial assessment and the appropriate physical examination have been completed, care for the individual wounds begins.

Patient CARE

Open Wounds

The steps listed below are general guidelines for the emergency care of open wounds. Steps for specific kinds of open wounds are detailed on the following pages.

1. Expose the wound. Clothing that covers a soft-tissue injury must be lifted, cut, or split away. For some articles of clothing, this is best done with scissors or a seam cutter. Do not attempt to remove clothing in the usual manner, which can aggravate existing injuries and cause additional damage and pain.

2. Clean the wound surface. Do not try to pick embedded particles and debris from the wound. Simply remove large pieces of foreign matter from the surface. When possible, use a piece of sterile dressing to brush away large debris while protecting the wound from contact with your soiled gloves. Do not spend much time cleaning the wound. Control of bleeding is the priority.

3. Control bleeding. Start with direct pressure, or direct pressure and elevation. When necessary, employ pressure point procedures. Remember, a tourniquet is used only as a last resort (see Chapter 26, "Bleeding and Shock").

4. For all serious wounds, provide care for shock, including administration of high-concentration oxygen (see Chapter 26, "Bleeding and Shock").

5. Prevent further contamination. Use a sterile dressing. When none is available, use the cleanest cloth material at the scene.

6. Bandage the dressing in place after bleeding has been controlled. If an extremity is involved, check for a distal pulse to make certain that circulation has not been interrupted by the application of a tight bandage. With the exception of a pressure dressing, bleeding must be controlled before bandaging is started. Periodically recheck the bandage to make certain that bleeding has not restarted.

7. Keep the patient lying still. Any movement will increase circulation and could restart bleeding.

8. Reassure the patient. This will help ease the patient's emotional response and perhaps lower his pulse rate and blood pressure. In some cases this may help to reduce the bleeding rate. Also, a patient who feels reassured will usually be more willing to lie still, reducing the chances of restarting bleeding.

Treating Abrasions and Lacerations

In treating abrasions, take care to reduce wound contamination. Bleeding from a long, deep laceration may be difficult to control, but direct pressure over a dressing usually works well. The air-inflated splint can be useful in the management of this type of wound when it is applied over a dressing. Do not pull apart the edges of a laceration in an effort to see into the wound.

Most lacerations can be cared for by bandaging a dressing in place. Some EMS systems recommend using a butterfly bandage for minor lacerations. (A *butterfly bandage* is made up of thin strips of adhesive bandaging and is designed to bring the sides of a laceration together.) Bandage a gauze dressing over the butterfly strip.

Note

Do not underestimate the effects of a laceration. When evaluating a laceration, check the pulse, as well as motor and sensory function, distal to the injury. The patient may need stitches, plastic surgery, or a tetanus shot at the hospital, so do not put on butterfly bandages and leave the patient at the scene. Serious infection or scarring could result.

Treating Puncture Wounds

Use caution when caring for puncture wounds. An object that appears to be embedded only in the skin may actually go all the way to the bone. In such cases, it is possible that the patient may not have any serious pain. Even an apparently moderate puncture wound may cause extensive internal injury with serious internal bleeding. What appears at first to be a simple, shallow puncture wound may be only part of the problem. There also could be a severe exit wound that requires immediate care, so be sure to search for one.

Gunshot wounds are puncture wounds that can fracture bones and cause extensive soft-tissue and organ injury. The seriousness of the wound cannot be determined by the caliber of the bullet or the point of entry and exit. The bullet may have tumbled through tissues, been deflected off a bone, fragmented, or exploded inside the body (Figure 27-14). All bullet wounds are considered serious. If the bullet has penetrated the body, you must assume that there is considerable internal injury. Close-range shootings often have burns around the entry wound. Remember that any gunshot wound to the face, no matter how minor, can create airway problems. Air guns fired at close range can cause serious damage by injecting air into the tissues.

All stab wounds should be considered serious, especially when they involve the head, neck, chest, abdomen, or groin.

Care for a patient with a moderate or serious puncture wound includes these steps:

1. Reassure the alert patient. Such wounds can be frightening.

2. Search for an exit wound, especially when there is a gunshot wound. Control bleeding and provide adequate wound treatment to both the entry and exit wounds.

3. Assess the need for basic life support whenever there is a gunshot wound. Care for shock, administering oxygen at a high concentration.

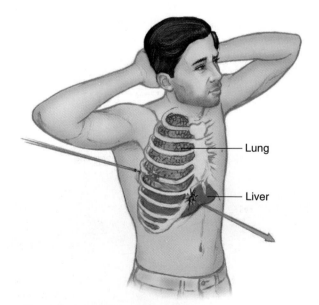

Figure 27-14 Bullets travel an unpredictable path once inside the body and can cause damage to multiple organs and bones.

4. Immobilize the spine when the patient's head, neck, or torso is involved.

5. Transport the patient. If the object that caused the puncture wound is available, take it to the emergency department for examination also.

Treating Impaled Objects

A puncture wound may contain an impaled object. The object may be a knife, a fence post or guard rail, a shard of glass, or even a wooden stick, piercing any part of the body. Even though it is rare, you may be confronted with an impaled object that is long enough to make transport impossible unless the object is shortened. In such cases, contact the emergency department physician for specific directions. Usually, someone must hold the object, keeping it very stable, while you gently saw through it at the desired length. A fine-toothed saw with rigid blade support (e.g., a hack saw or reciprocating saw) should be used. In some cases, you may need to leave the object in place as found. The challenge in these cases is stabilization of the object.

In general, when caring for a patient with a puncture wound involving an impaled object, DO NOT REMOVE THE IMPALED OBJECT. The object may be plugging bleeding from a major artery while it is in place. To remove it may cause severe bleeding when the pressure is released. Removal of the object also may cause further injury to nerves, muscles, and other soft tissues. Any movement of the impaled object at the skin's surface will be magnified several times in the inner tissues. Proceed as follows:

1. Expose the wound area. Cut away clothing, taking great care not to disturb the object. Do not attempt to lift clothing over the object; you may accidentally move it. Long impaled objects may have to be stabilized by hand during exposure, bleeding control, and dressing.

2. Control profuse bleeding by direct pressure if possible. Be careful to position your gloved hands on either side of the object and exert pressure downward. *Do not put pressure on the object.* Apply pressure with great care if the object has a cutting edge, such as a knife or a shard of glass; otherwise, you may cause additional injury to the patient. Be careful not to injure your hands or damage your gloves.

3. While you continue to stabilize the object and control bleeding, have another trained rescuer place several layers of bulky dressing around the injury site so that the dressings surround the object on all sides (Figure 27-15). Manual stabilization must continue until the stabilizing dressings are secured in place.

A

B

Figure 27-15 Stabilize an impaled object with a bulky dressing.

Have the other rescuer begin by placing folded universal pads, sanitary napkins, or some other bulky dressing material on opposite sides of the object. For long or large objects, folded towels, blankets, or pillows may have to be used in place of dressing pads. Remove your hands from under the pads. Place them on top and apply pressure as each layer is placed in position. The next layer of pads should be placed on opposite sides of the object, perpendicular to the first layer. Continue this process until as much of the object as possible has been stabilized.

Once bandaged in place, the dressings will stabilize the object and exert downward pressure on bleeding vessels. Keep in mind that there is a limited amount of time that can be given to stabilizing an impaled object. Stay in contact with the medical director for directions and recommendations.

4. Secure the dressings in place. Adhesive strips may hold the dressings in place. However, blood around the wound site, sweat, and body movements may not allow you to use tape. Triangular bandages folded into strips (cravats) can be applied by tying one above and one below the impaled object. The cravats should be wide (no less than 4 inches in width once folded). A thin rigid splint can be used to push the cravats under the patient's back when they are needed to care for objects impaled in the trunk of the body.

5. Care for shock. Provide oxygen at the highest possible concentration. When appropriate, oxygen administration and heat conservation measures should be accomplished as soon as possible. When working by yourself, these may have to be delayed while you attempt to control bleeding.

6. Keep the patient at rest. Position the patient for minimum stress. If possible, immobilize the affected area, for example with a splint or a spine board. Provide emotional support.

7. Transport the patient carefully and as soon as possible. Avoid any movement that may jar, loosen, or dislodge the object. If the object was removed by bystanders before you arrived, bring it to the hospital for examination.

8. Reassure the patient throughout all aspects of care. An alert patient with an impaled object is usually very frightened.

Object Impaled in the Cheek. A dangerous situation exists when the cheek has been penetrated by a foreign object. First, the object may go into the oral cavity and create an airway obstruction, or it may stay impaled in the cheek wall but work its way free and enter the oral cavity later. Second, when the cheek wall is perforated, bleeding into the mouth and throat can be profuse and interfere with breathing, or it may make the patient nauseated and induce vomiting. External wound care will not stop the flow of blood into the mouth.

If you find a patient with an object impaled in the cheek, you should (Figure 27-16):

1. Examine the wound site. Gently inspect both the external cheek and the inside of the mouth. Use your penlight and look into the patient's mouth. If need be, carefully use your gloved fingers to probe the inside cheek to determine if the object has passed through the cheek wall. This is best done with a dressing pad used to protect your fingers and any wound you touch.

2. Remove the object, IF you find perforation and you can SEE BOTH ENDS of the object. Pull it out in the direction that it entered the cheek. If this cannot be done easily, leave the object in place. Do not twist the object. OR IF you find perforation but the tip of the object is also IMPALED INTO A DEEPER STRUCTURE (e.g., the palate), STABILIZE THE OBJECT. Do not try to remove it.

3. Position the patient. Make certain that you allow for drainage (the possibility of spine injuries may require you to immobilize the head, neck, and

Figure 27-16 Removing an impaled object from the cheek.

spine first, then tilt the patient and the spine board as a unit).

4. Monitor the patient's airway, once the object is removed or stabilized. *Be prepared to suction as necessary.* Keep in mind that an object penetrating the cheek wall also may have caused teeth or dentures to break, creating potential airway obstruction. Pay close attention, especially if the patient is not alert. Blood in the patient's mouth can compromise the airway.

5. Dress the outside of the wound using a pressure dressing and bandage or apply a sterile dressing and use direct hand pressure to control the bleeding. You may be able to place gauze on the inside of the cheek to help control bleeding into the mouth, but only if the patient is alert and cooperative. Monitor the patient's mental status closely, and make sure the dressing does not work its way into the airway.

6. Provide oxygen and care for shock. You may have to use a nasal cannula if constant suctioning is required. If any dressing materials are placed in the patient's mouth, use of standard face masks can be dangerous unless you leave 3 to 4 inches of the dressing outside of the patient's mouth.

Puncture Wound or Object Impaled in the Eye. Use loose dressings for a puncture wound to the eye with no impaled object. If you find an object impaled in the eye, you should (Figure 27-17):

1. Stabilize the object. Place a roll of 3-inch gauze bandage or folded 4 × 4s on either side of the object, along the vertical axis of the head in a manner that will stabilize the object.

2. Apply rigid protection. Fit a disposable paper drinking cup or paper cone over the impaled object and allow it to come to rest on the dressing rolls.

A

B

Figure 27-17 Managing a patient with an object impaled in the eye.

Do not allow it to touch the object. Do not use a Styrofoam cup, which can flake.

3. Have another rescuer stabilize the dressings and cup while you secure them in place with a self-adherent roller bandage or with a wrapping of gauze. Do not secure the bandage on top of the cup.

4. Dress and bandage the uninjured eye. This will help to reduce sympathetic eye movements.

5. Provide oxygen and care for shock.

6. Reassure the patient and provide emotional support.

The above method can also be used as a pressure dressing to control bleeding in the area of the eye.

An alternative to the above method calls for the rescuer to make a thick dressing with several layers of sterile gauze pads or universal dressings. A hole is cut in the center of this pad, approximately the size of the impaled object. The rescuer then carefully passes this dressing over the impaled object and po-

sitions the pad so that the impaled object is centered in the opening. The rest of the procedure remains the same as previously described. If your EMS system has you use this technique, remember that you must take great care not to touch the object as the dressing is set in place.

Treating Avulsions

Emergency care for avulsions requires the application of large, bulky pressure dressings. In addition, you should make every effort to preserve any avulsed parts and transport them to the medical facility along with the patient. It may be possible to surgically restore the part or to use it for skin grafts.

In cases in which flaps of skin have been torn loose but not off, follow these steps:

1. Clean the wound surface.

2. Fold the skin back to its normal position as gently as possible.

3. Control bleeding and dress the wound using bulky pressure dressings.

Should skin or another body part be torn from the body, control bleeding and dress the wound using a bulky pressure dressing. Save the avulsed part by wrapping it in a dry sterile gauze dressing secured in place by self-adherent roller bandage. Then place it in a plastic bag, plastic wrap, or aluminum foil, in accordance with local protocol. If none of these items is available at the scene, wrap the avulsed part in a lint-free, dry sterile dressing. (Some research suggests that the sterile wrap should be soaked in sterile saline to make a moist dressing. Follow local protocols.)

Make certain that you label the avulsed part with what it is, the patient's name and date, and the time the part was wrapped and bagged. Your records should show the approximate time of the avulsion. Be sure to keep the part as cool as possible, without freezing it, by placing it in a cooler or any other available container so that it is on top of a cold pack or a SEALED bag of ice. Do not use dry ice. Do not immerse the avulsed part in ice, cooled water, or saline. Label the container the same as the label used for the saved part.

Remember

Serious avulsions can be frightening. You must reassure the patient.

Note

The care of avulsed tissues is directed by local protocols, which are often written to match the reimplantation procedures of the hospitals in your EMS system. Some EMS systems prefer that the dressing used to wrap the avulsed part be moistened with sterile normal saline (sterile distilled water is not recommended). This saline must be from a fresh sterile source. Keep in mind that once a sterile source of saline has been opened, it is no longer considered sterile. Take great care if you use this method, since the saline may carry microorganisms from your gloved hand through the dressing to the avulsed part.

Treating Amputations

Never complete an amputation. As in other external bleeding situations, the most effective method to control bleeding is a snug pressure dressing:

1. Apply the pressure dressing. Place it over the stump.

2. Use pressure points to control bleeding. A tourniquet should not be applied unless other methods used to control bleeding have failed.

3. Care for the amputated part. When possible, wrap it in a sterile dressing and secure the dressing with self-adhesive gauze bandage. Wrap or bag the amputated part in a plastic bag and place the bag in a pan with water kept cool by cold packs. Do not immerse the amputated part directly in water or saline. Do not let the part come in direct contact with ice or it may freeze.

Wounds to the Neck

Because large arteries and veins lie close to the surface of the neck, the potential for serious bleeding from an open wound is great. Since the pressure in a large vein is likely to be lower than atmospheric pressure, the possibility of an **air embolus** (air bubble) being sucked in through a vein is also great. An air embolus can be carried to the heart and interfere with the heart's ability to circulate blood or actually cause cardiac arrest. The treatment of neck veins is aimed at stopping bleeding and preventing an embolus from entering the circulation.

Patient ASSESSMENT

Open Neck Wound

An injury that has severed a major artery or vein of the neck will produce severe bleeding. Arterial bleeding will be profuse, with bright red blood spurting from the wound. Venous bleeding will be profuse with dark red to maroon-colored blood flowing steadily from the wound.

Patient CARE

Open Neck Wound

Follow these steps for providing emergency care to a patient with an open neck wound (Scan 27-1):

1. Assure an open airway.

2. Place your gloved hand over the wound.

3. Apply an occlusive dressing to the wound. The dressing should be a thick material that will not be sucked into the wound and must extend 2 inches past the sides of the wound.

4. Place a dressing over the occlusive dressing.

5. Apply pressure as needed to stop the bleeding. Be careful not to compress both carotid arteries at once.

6. Once bleeding has stopped, bandage the dressing in place. Take care not to restrict the airway or the arteries and veins of the neck.

7. If the mechanism of injury could have caused cervical injury, immobilize the spine.

Chest Injuries

The chest can be injured in a number of ways, including by blunt trauma, penetrating objects, and compression:

- *Blunt trauma.* A blow to the chest can fracture the ribs, the sternum, and the costal (rib) cartilages. Whole sections of the chest can collapse. With severe blunt trauma, the lungs and airway can be damaged and the great vessels (aorta and venae cavae) and the heart may be seriously injured.
- *Penetrating objects.* Bullets, knives, pieces of metal or glass, steel rods, pipes, and various other objects can penetrate the chest wall, damaging internal organs and impairing respiration.
- *Compression.* This results from severe blunt trauma in which the chest is rapidly compressed, as when a driver in a motor-vehicle collision strikes his chest on the steering column. The heart can be severely squeezed, the lungs can be ruptured, and the sternum and ribs can be fractured.

Chest injuries are classified as closed or open. In a closed chest injury, the skin is not broken, leading many people to think that the damage done is not serious. However, such injuries, sustained through blunt trauma and compression injuries, can cause contusions and lacerations of the heart, lungs, and great vessels.

DRESSING AN OPEN NECK WOUND

FIRST take BSI precautions.

▲ **1.** Do not delay! Place your gloved palm over the wound.

▲ **2.** Place an occlusive dressing over the wound. It must be heavy plastic, sized to be 2 inches larger in diameter than the wound site.

▲ **3.** Place a gauze dressing over the occlusive dressing. (A gauze roll can be placed between the trachea and the dressing to help keep pressure off the airway.)

▲ **4.** Bring a bandage over the dressing and wrap it in a figure-eight configuration, winding the bandage under the arm opposite the wound. Never wind the bandage around the neck.

NOTE: For demonstration purposes, the patient is upright.

When the skin is broken, the patient has an open wound. However, the term *open chest wound* usually means that the chest wall is penetrated, as for example by a bullet or a knife blade. An object can pass through the wall from the outside, or a fractured and displaced rib can penetrate the chest wall from within. The heart, lungs, and great vessels can be injured at the same time the chest wall is penetrated. It may be difficult to tell if the chest cavity has been penetrated by looking at the wound. Do not open the wound to determine its depth. Specific signs (see below) will indicate possible open chest injury.

You must consider all open wounds to the chest to be life threatening. Open chest wounds are usually penetrating or perforating puncture wounds. A penetrating puncture wound is one that penetrates the chest wall once; a perforating puncture wound has both an entrance and an exit wound as, for example, many gunshot wounds. An object producing a wound may remain impaled in the chest, or the wound may be completely open.

When air enters the chest cavity, the delicate pressure balance within the chest cavity is destroyed. This causes the lung on the injured side to collapse. (Injuries associated with air in the chest cavity are discussed in more detail under "Chest Injury Complications" on the following pages.)

Patient ASSESSMENT

Open Chest Wound

The term sucking chest wound is used when the chest cavity is open to the atmosphere. Each time the patient breathes, air can be sucked into the opening. This patient will develop severe difficulty breathing. Signs include:

- A wound to the chest
- There may or may not be the characteristic sucking sound associated with an open chest wound.

- The patient may be gasping for air.

Keep in mind that the object penetrating the chest wall may have seriously damaged a lung, major blood vessel, or the heart itself.

Patient CARE

Open Chest Wound

An open chest wound is a TRUE EMERGENCY that requires rapid initial care and immediate transport to a medical facility. Follow these steps:

1. Maintain an open airway. Provide basic life support if necessary.

2. Seal the open chest wound as quickly as possible. If need be, use your gloved hand. Do not delay sealing the wound to find an occlusive dressing.

3. Apply an occlusive dressing to seal the wound. When possible, the dressing should be at least 2 inches wider than the wound. If there is an exit wound in the chest, apply an occlusive dressing over this wound too. Follow your local protocols as to whether this should be an occlusive dressing that is sealed on all four sides or a flutter-valve dressing with one corner or side unsealed. These dressings will be discussed in detail later under "Occlusive and Flutter-Valve Dressings."

4. Administer a high concentration of oxygen.

5. Care for shock.

6. Transport as soon as possible. Unless other injuries prevent you from doing so, keep the patient positioned on the injured side. This allows the uninjured lung to expand without restriction.

7. Consider advanced life support intercept if it will not delay the patient's arrival at the hospital.

CHEST INJURY COMPLICATIONS

In trauma to the chest, the lungs, heart, and great blood vessels can be injured, causing serious complications. The information that follows on the conditions known as pneumothorax, tension pneumothorax, hemothorax, hemopneumothorax, traumatic asphyxia, and cardiac

tamponade is provided as general background. As an EMT-B, you do not need to be able to diagnose these specific complications of chest injury, but it is important to be aware of general signs and symptoms and the emergency care steps to be taken whenever such complications are suspected.

• *Pneumothorax and tension pneumothorax.* Pneumothorax occurs when the lung collapses as a result of air that has

entered the chest cavity. The air can enter through an external wound (Figure 27-18), or the air may come out of a punctured lung, or both. Especially critical is tension pneumothorax, which is most often found with a closed chest injury or after a sealed occlusive dressing has been applied to an open chest wound. The lung may be punctured by a broken rib or other cause. If there is no opening to the outside of the chest, air that leaks from the lung has no avenue of escape.

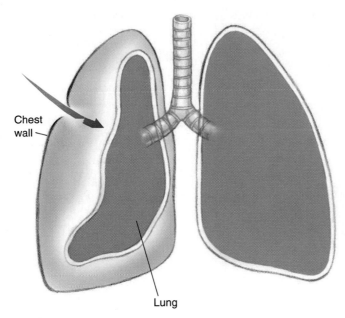

Figure 27-18 Air can enter the chest cavity through a puncture in the chest wall. This can cause a collapse of a lung and impaired breathing.

It builds up in the chest cavity and puts pressure on the heart, great blood vessels, and the unaffected lung, reducing cardiac output and the ability of the lungs to oxygenate the blood.

• *Hemothorax and hemopneumothorax* (Figure 27-19). Hemothorax is a condition in which the chest cavity fills with blood. With hemopneumothorax, the chest cavity fills with both blood and air. It is easy to compare these two complications with pneumothorax, if you remember that *pneumo* means "air" and

hemo means "blood." In pneumothorax, there is a buildup of air in the thorax. In hemothorax and hemopneumothorax, blood creates or adds to the pressure buildup.

Hemothorax can be caused when lacerations within the chest cavity are produced by penetrating objects or fractured ribs. Blood will flow into the space around the lung, the lung may collapse, and the patient will experience a loss of blood leading to shock. Hemopneumothorax is a combination of blood and air, usually producing the same results: a collapsed lung and loss of blood leading to shock.

• *Traumatic asphyxia.* Traumatic asphyxia is associated with sudden compression of the chest. When this occurs, the sternum and the ribs exert severe pressure on the heart and lungs, forcing blood out of the right atrium and up into the jugular veins in the neck. The pressure of the blood being forced into the head and neck will usually result in blood vessels rupturing, causing extensive bruising of the face and neck (Figure 27-20).

• *Cardiac tamponade.* When an injury to the heart causes blood to flow into the surrounding pericardial sac, the condition produced is cardiac tamponade. The heart's unyielding sac fills with blood and compresses the chambers of the heart to a point where they will no longer fill adequately, backing up blood into the veins.

PNEUMOTHORAX **HEMOTHORAX** **HEMOPNEUMOTHORAX**

Figure 27-19 Conditions produced by chest injuries.

Figure 27-20 A patient suffering traumatic asphyxia.

- Steadily decreasing pulse pressure. (Pulse pressure is the difference between systolic and diastolic readings.)

Patient CARE

Chest Injury Complications

The treatment for any type of chest injury complication is the same:

1. Maintain an open airway. Be prepared to apply suction.

2. Administer a high concentration of oxygen.

3. Follow local protocols as to the preferred type of dressing for any open wound.

4. Care for shock.

5. Transport as soon as possible.

6. Consider advanced life support intercept if it will not delay the patient's arrival at the hospital. Advanced life support personnel can perform procedures such as chest decompression that can greatly benefit a patient suffering chest injury complications.

Signs of hemothorax or hemopneumothorax

- Signs of pneumothorax plus coughed-up frothy red blood

Signs of traumatic asphyxia
- Distended neck veins
- Head, neck, and shoulders appearing dark blue or purple

- Eyes may be bloodshot and bulging
- Tongue and lips may appear swollen and blue
- Chest deformity may be present

Signs of cardiac tamponade
- Distended neck veins
- Very weak pulse
- Low blood pressure

Occlusive and Flutter-Valve Dressings

There are two methods commonly used for dressing an open chest wound. One approach, recommended in many local protocols, calls for taping the occlusive dressing in place, leaving a corner of the dressing unsealed (Figure 27-21). (Some EMS systems now recommend leaving one entire side unsealed.) As the patient inhales, the dressing will seal the wound. As the patient exhales, the free corner or edge will act as a flutter valve to release air that is trapped in the chest cavity. A traditional approach, still recommended in many local protocols, calls for sealing all four edges (Figure 27-22), the last edge being sealed when the patient forcefully exhales. If the seal is effective, respirations will be partially stabilized.

The danger of a pneumothorax developing into a tension pneumothorax, as discussed earlier, is the reason why many medical authorities now recommend the flutter-valve occlusive dressing instead of the traditional occlusive dressing (Figure 27-23). If, instead, your local protocols recommend that you treat a sucking chest wound with a traditional dressing sealed on all four sides and you find that the patient worsens rapidly, you will have to lift a corner of the seal to let air escape. (The patient should respond almost immediately as pressure is released around the heart, great blood vessels, and uninjured lung.) Then you must reseal the wound and monitor the patient. You may have to unseal and reseal the wound several times during transport.

You may have to maintain hand pressure over the occlusive dressing en route to the hospital. The tape also may not stick well to bloody skin or to skin that is sweaty from shock.

Caution

Once a chest wound is sealed, you must continue to monitor the patient and stay alert for complications. Even if you use a flutter valve, you still must monitor the patient for this condition. The free corner or edge of the dressing may stick to the chest or the dressing may be drawn into the wound, causing the valve to fail.

On inspiration, dressing seals wound, preventing air entry

Collapsed lung

Expiration allows trapped air to escape through untaped section of dressing

Figure 27-21 Creating a flutter valve to allow air to escape from the chest cavity.

Figure 27-22 Sealing all four edges of an occlusive dressing.

Note that if a commercial occlusive dressing is not available, you may have to improvise. Most ambulances carry sterile disposable items that are wrapped in plastic. The inside surface of the plastic is sterile. If you do not have an occlusive dressing, use one of these wrappers or an IV bag. Keep in mind that household plastic wrap is not thick enough to make an effective occlusive dressing for an open chest wound. If nothing else is available, household wrap can be used, but it must be folded several times to be of the proper thickness. Even then, it may fail. If there is no other choice, aluminum foil may be used to make the seal. Be careful, however, as foil edges may lacerate skin and may tear when lifted to release pressure.

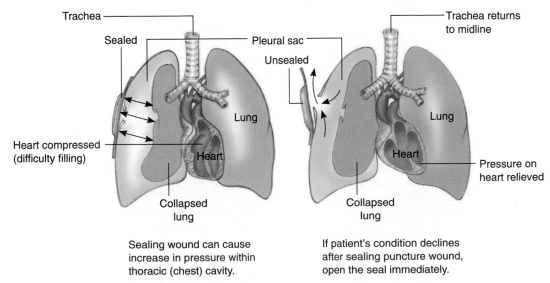

Figure 27-23 Sealing an open chest wound may cause a dangerous increase in pressure. If the patient's condition worsens, release the seal to allow pressure to escape. Then reseal.

Documentation Tips— Open Chest Wounds

With an open chest wound, be sure to document the patient's response to treatment. After application of the occlusive dressing, record any changes—whether improvements or deteriorations—in respiratory difficulty, breath sounds, chest wall movement, color, and signs of shock.

Abdominal Injuries

Abdominal injuries can be open or closed, with a closed injury usually due to blunt trauma. Internal bleeding can be severe if organs and major blood vessels are lacerated or ruptured. Very serious and painful reactions can occur when the hollow organs are ruptured and their contents leak into the abdominal cavity. Penetrating wounds to the abdomen can be caused by objects such as knives, ice picks, arrows, and the broken glass and twisted metal of vehicular collisions and structural accidents. Very serious perforating wounds can be caused by bullets, even when the bullet is small caliber. Open wounds of the abdomen may be so large and deep that organs protrude through the wound opening. This is known as an **evisceration.**

Patient *ASSESSMENT*

Abdominal Injury

Gunshot wounds without exit wounds can cause serious abdominal damage, just as those with exit wounds do. A misconception about bullet wounds is that internal damage can be assessed easily. On the contrary, any projectile entering the body can be deflected, or it can explode and send out pieces in many directions. Do not believe that only the structures directly under the entrance wound have been injured. Also, keep in mind that the pathway of a bullet between entrance wound and exit wound is seldom a straight line.

Complicating the problem even more is the fact that penetrating abdominal wounds can be associated with wounds in adjacent areas of the body. For example, a bullet can enter the chest cavity, pierce the diaphragm, and cause widespread damage in the abdomen. A complete patient assessment is essential in determining the probable extent of injuries. *Always assess for an exit wound.*

Signs and symptoms of abdominal injury include:

- Pain, often starting as mild pain then rapidly becoming intolerable
- Cramps

- Nausea
- Weakness
- Thirst
- Obvious lacerations and puncture wounds to the abdomen
- Lacerations and puncture wounds to the pelvis and middle and lower back or chest wounds near the diaphragm
- Indications of blunt trauma, such as a large bruised area or an intense bruise on the abdomen
- Indications of developing shock, including restlessness; pale, cool, and clammy skin; rapid shallow breathing; a rapid pulse; and low blood pressure. (Sometimes patients with abdominal injury who are in extreme pain show an initial elevated blood pressure.)
- Coughing up or vomiting blood. The vomitus may contain a substance that looks like coffee grounds (partially digested blood).
- Rigid and/or tender abdomen. The patient tries to protect the abdomen (guarded abdomen).
- Distended abdomen
- The patient tries to lie very still, with the legs drawn up in an effort to reduce the tension on the abdominal muscles.

Patient *CARE*

Abdominal Injury

Some emergency care steps apply to both closed and open abdominal injuries. Some additional care steps are necessary for open abdominal injuries.

For both closed and open abdominal injuries

1. Stay alert for vomiting and keep the airway open.

2. Place the patient on his back, legs flexed at the knees, to reduce pain by relaxing abdominal muscles.

3. Administer a high concentration of oxygen.

4. Care for shock.

5. Apply anti-shock garments, if indicated and local protocols recommend.

6. Give nothing to the patient by mouth. This may induce vomiting or pass through open wounds in the esophagus, stomach, or intestine and enter the abdominal cavity.

7. Constantly monitor vital signs.

8. Transport as soon as possible.

Additional steps for open abdominal injuries

9. Control external bleeding and dress all open wounds.

10. Do not touch or try to replace any eviscerated, or exposed, organs. Apply a sterile dressing moistened with sterile saline over the wound site before you apply an occlusive dressing. Maintain warmth by placing layers of bulky dressing or a lint-free towel over the occlusive dressing (Scan 27-2).

Warning

Do not use aluminum foil. Aluminum foil occlusive dressings have been known to cut eviscerated organs.

11. Do not remove any impaled objects. Stabilize impaled objects with bulky dressings that are bandaged in place. Leave the patient's legs in the position in which you found them to avoid muscular movement that may move the impaled object.

Burns

Most people think of burns as injuries to the skin, but burns can do much more. Burn injuries often involve structures below the skin, including muscles, bones, nerves, and blood vessels. Burns can injure the eyes beyond repair. Respiratory system structures can be damaged, producing airway obstruction due to tissue swelling, even respiratory failure and respiratory arrest. In addition to the physical damage caused by burns, patients often suffer emotional and psychological problems that begin at the emergency scene and may last a lifetime.

When caring for a burn patient, always think beyond the burn. For example, a medical emergency or accident may have led to the burn. The patient may have had a heart attack while smoking a cigarette, and the unattended cigarette caused a fire. During the patient assessment, the EMT-B should detect the heart problem even though the burn may be the most obvious injury. Conversely, a fire or burn may cause or aggravate another injury or medical condition. Someone trying to escape a fire may fall and suffer spine damage and fractures. The EMT-B should detect not only the burn but the spine damage and fractures as well.

Remember

Patient assessment should not be neglected in order to immediately begin burn care.

Burns

When your patient has been burned, patient assessment involves classifying, then evaluating, the burns. Burns can be classified and evaluated in three ways:

- By agent and source
- By depth
- By severity

All three are important in deciding the urgency and the kind of emergency care the burn requires. These classifications are discussed in detail below.

Classifying Burns by Agent and Source

Burns can be classified according to the agent causing the burn (e.g., chemicals or electricity). Noting the source of the burn (e.g., dry lime or alternating current) can make the classification more specific. You should report the agent and also, when practical, the source of the agent (Table 27-2). For example, a burn can be reported as "chemical burns from contact with dry lime."

Never assume the agent or source of the burn. What may appear to be a thermal burn could in fact be caused by radiation. You may find minor thermal burns on the patient's face and forget to consider light burns to the eyes. Always gather information from your observations of the scene, bystanders' reports, and the patient interview.

Classifying Burns by Depth

Burns involving the skin are classified as superficial, partial-thickness, and full-thickness burns (Figure 27-24). These classifications are also sometimes called first-degree, second-degree, and third-degree burns, with first-degree burns corresponding to superficial burns, and so on, as described below (Figure 27-25):

- *Superficial burn.* This burn involves only the epidermis (the outer layer of the skin). It is characterized by reddening of the skin and perhaps some swelling. An example is a sunburn. The patient will usually complain about pain (sometimes severe) at the site. The burn will heal of its own accord, without scarring. Superficial burns are also called first-degree burns.

- *Partial-thickness burn.* In this type of burn, the epidermis is burned through and the dermis (the second layer of the skin) is damaged, but the burn does not pass through to underlying tissues. There will be deep intense pain, noticeable reddening, blisters, and a mottled (spotted) appearance to the skin. Burns of this type cause swelling and blistering

Chapter 27 • *Soft-Tissue Injuries* **545**

DRESSING AN OPEN ABDOMINAL WOUND

FIRST take BSI precautions.

▲ Open abdominal wound with evisceration.

▲ **1.** Cut away clothing from wound.

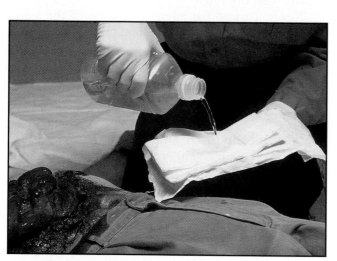

▲ **2.** Soak a dressing with sterile saline.

▲ **3.** Place the moist dressing over the wound.

▶ **4.** Apply an occlusive dressing over the moist dressing if local protocols recommend that you do so.

▶ **5.** Cover the dressed wound to maintain warmth. Secure the covering with tape or cravats tied above and below the position of the exposed organ.

Table 27-2 Agents and Sources of Burns

Agents	Sources
Thermal	Flame; radiation; excessive heat from fire, steam, hot liquids, hot objects
Chemicals	Various acids, bases, caustics
Electricity	Alternating current, direct current, lightning
Light (typically involving the eyes)	Intense light sources, ultraviolet light (includes sunlight)
Radiation	Usually from nuclear sources; ultraviolet light can also be considered a source of radiation burns.

for 48 hours after the injury, as plasma and tissue fluids are released and rise to the top layer of skin. When treated with reasonable care, partial-thickness burns will heal themselves, producing very little scarring. Partial-thickness burns are also called second-degree burns.

Figure 27-24 Burns are classified by depth.

Superficial — Skin reddened

Partial thickness — Blisters

Full thickness — Charring

Epidermis
Dermis
Fat
Muscle

• *Full-thickness burn.* This is a burn in which all the layers of the skin are damaged. Some full-thickness burns are difficult to tell from partial-thickness burns; however, there are usually areas that are charred black or brown or areas that are dry and white. The patient may complain of severe pain, or if enough nerves have been damaged, he may not feel any pain at all (except at the periphery of the burn where adjoining partial-thickness burns may be causing pain). This type of burn may require skin grafting. As these burns heal, dense scars form. Full-thickness burns damage all layers of the skin and additionally may damage subcutaneous tissue, muscle, bone, and underlying organs. These burns are sometimes called third-degree burns.

Determining Severity of Burns

When determining the severity of a burn, consider the following factors:

• Agent or source of the burn
• Body regions burned
• Depth of the burn
• Extent of the burn
• Age of the patient
• Other illness and injuries

The agent or source of the burn can be significant in terms of patient assessment. A burn caused by electrical current may cause only small areas of skin injury but pose a great risk of severe internal injuries. Chemical burns are of special concern since the chemical may remain on the skin and continue to burn for hours or even days, eventually entering the bloodstream. This is sometimes the case with certain alkaline chemicals.

A

B

C

Figure 27-25 (A) A superficial burn, (B) a partial-thickness burn, and (C) a full-thickness burn.

Figure 27-26 A singed mustache and burns to the tip of the tongue signal danger of airway burns or burns to the eyes.

When you are considering the body regions burned, keep in mind that any burn to the face is of special concern since it may involve injury to the airway or the eyes (Figure 27-26). The hands and feet also are areas of concern because scarring may cause loss of movement of fingers or toes. Special care is required to reduce aggravation to these injury sites when moving the patient and to prevent the damaged tissues from sticking to one another. When the groin, genitalia, buttocks, or medial thighs are burned, potential bacterial contamination can be far more serious than the initial damage to the tissues. Note that circumferential burns (burns that encircle the body or a body part) can be very serious because they constrict the skin and, when they occur to an extremity, they can interrupt circulation to the distal tissues. In addition, the burn healing process can be very complicated. This is particularly true when circumferential burns occur to joints, the chest, and abdomen where the encircling scarring tends to limit normal functions.

The depth of the burn is important to determining severity. In partial-thickness and full-thickness burns, the outer layer of the skin is penetrated. This can lead to contamination of exposed tissues and the invasion of the circulatory system by harmful chemicals and microorganisms.

You also will need to estimate roughly the extent of the burn area. The amount of skin surface involved can be calculated quickly by using the **rule of nines** (Figure 27-27). For an adult, each of the following areas represents 9% of the body surface: head and neck, each upper extremity, chest, abdomen, upper back, lower back and buttocks, the front of each lower extremity, and the back of each lower extremity. These make up 99% of the body's surface.

Figure 27-27   Rule of nines.

The remaining 1% is assigned to the genital region.

In the rule of nines, the percentages are modified for infants and young children, whose heads are much larger in relationship to the rest of the body than adults' heads are. An infant's or young child's head and neck are counted as 18%; each upper extremity, 9%; chest and abdomen, 18%; the entire back, 18%; each lower extremity, 14%; and the genital region, 1%. (This adds up to 101%, but it is only used to give a rough determination. Some systems count each lower limb as 13.5% to achieve an even 100%.)

An alternative way to estimate the extent of a burn is the **rule of palm,** which uses the patient's hand to approximate the surface area. The rule of palm can be applied to any patient—infant, child, or adult. Since the palm of the hand equals about 1% of the body's surface area, mentally compare the patient's palm with the size of the burn to estimate its extent. (For example, a burn the size of five palms = 5% of the body.) The rule of palm may be easier to apply to smaller or localized burns, the rule of nines to larger or more widespread burns.

The age of the patient is a major factor in considering the severity of burns. Infants, children under age 5, and adults over age 55, because of their anatomy and physiology, have the most severe responses to burns and the greatest risk of death. They also have different healing patterns than other age groups.

Geriatric Notes

Burn intensity and body-area involvement that would be minor to moderate in a young adult could be fatal for an aged person. In late adulthood, the body's ability to cope with injury is reduced by aging tissues and failing body systems. The ability of tissues to heal from any injury is lessened and the time of healing is increased.

When determining the severity of a burn, you also must consider the other illnesses and injuries a patient may have. Obviously, a patient with an existing respiratory illness will be especially vulnerable to exposure to heated air or chemical vapors. Likewise, the stress of a fire or other environmental emergency will be of particular concern for patients with heart disease. Patients with respiratory ailments, heart disease, or diabetes will react more severely to burn damage. What may be a minor burn for a healthy adult could be of major significance to a patient with a pre-existing medical condition. Similarly, the stress of a burn added to other injuries sustained during the emergency may lead to shock or other life-threatening problems that would not have resulted from the non-burn injuries or the burn alone.

Note

All burns are to be treated as more serious if accompanied by other injuries or medical problems. If you discover that the patient has a decreased blood pressure, always assume that he has other serious injuries. Attempt to determine the patient's problem through standard assessment techniques.

Table 27-3   Classification of Burn Severity: Adults

Classifications by Thickness, Percent of Body Surface Area, and Complicating Factors

Minor Burns
- Full-thickness burns of less than 2%, excluding face, hands, feet, genitalia, or respiratory tract
- Partial-thickness burns of less than 15%
- Superficial burns of 50% or less

Moderate Burns
- Full-thickness burns of 2% to 10%, excluding face, hands, feet, genitalia, or respiratory tract
- Partial-thickness burns of 15% to 30%
- Superficial burns that involve more than 50%

Critical Burns
- All burns complicated by injuries of the respiratory tract, other soft-tissue injuries, and injuries of the bones
- Partial- or full-thickness burns involving the face, hands, feet, genitalia, or respiratory tract
- Full-thickness burns of more than 10%
- Partial-thickness burns of more than 30%
- Burns complicated by musculoskeletal injuries
- Circumferential burns

Note: Burns which, by the above classification, are moderate should be considered critical in a person less than 5 or greater than 55 years of age. See Table 27-4 for classifications for children less than 5 years of age.

Classifying Burns by Severity

Burns must be classified as to severity to determine the order and type of care and order of transport and to provide maximum information to the emergency department. In some cases, the severity of the burn may determine if the patient is to be taken directly to a hospital with special burn-care facilities. For most adults, use the classifications in Table 27-3.

Geriatric Notes

Note that burns usually classified as moderate are considered critical in adults over 55 years of age.

Pediatric Notes

Burns pose greater risks to infants and children. This is because their body surface area is greater in relation to their total body size. This results in greater fluid and heat loss than would be found in an adult patient. Infants have a higher risk of shock, airway problems, and hypothermia from burns. Additionally, the classification of burn severity differs in patients less than 5 years of age as shown in Table 27-4. When a child has been burned, consider the possibility of child abuse.

Table 27-4   Classification of Burn Severity: Children Less Than 5 Years of Age

Classifications by Thickness and Percent of Body Surface Area

Minor Burns
- Partial-thickness burns of less than 10% of body surface

Moderate Burns
- Partial-thickness burns of 10% to 20% of body surface

Critical Burns
- Full-thickness burns or partial-thickness burns of more than 20% of body surface

Figure 27-28 Chemical burns to the eyes.

Emergency Care for Burns

There are special approaches to the care of thermal burns, general chemical burns, and chemical burns to the eyes (Figure 27-28).

● Patient *CARE*

Thermal Burns

As an EMT-B you will have to care for thermal burns caused by scalding liquids, steam, contact with hot objects, flames, flaming liquids and gases. Sunburn can also be severe in infants and young children, who may have other heat-related injuries.

The steps for basic care of thermal burns are given in Table 27-5. Currently, dry sterile dressings are recommended by the national EMT-B curriculum for all burns. The standing orders for burn care are the decision of your EMS medical director and the regional EMS system. Some EMS systems state that all partial-thickness and full-thickness burns are to be wrapped with dry sterile dressing or a burn sheet, while some burn centers recommend moist dressings for partial-thickness burns to less than 10% of the body and dry dressings for more severe cases. The latter protocol is now being adopted by most EMS systems.

Note that EMT-Bs must manage burns correctly until the patient can be transferred to the care of the staff of a medical facility. Never apply ointments, sprays, or butter (which would trap the heat against the burn site and have to be scraped off by the hospital staff). Do not break blisters. Do not apply ice to any burn (it can cause tissue damage). Keep the burn site clean to prevent infection. Keep the patient warm, as the temperature regulation function of the skin may be affected by the burn.

● Safety Note

Do not attempt to rescue persons trapped by fire unless you are trained to do so and have the equipment and personnel required. The simple act of opening a door might cost you your life. In some fires, opening a door or window may greatly intensify the fire or even cause an explosion.

● Patient *CARE*

Chemical Burns

Chemical burns require immediate care. It is hoped that people at the scene will begin this care before you arrive. At many industrial sites, workers and First Responders are trained to provide initial care for accidents involving the chemicals in use. Most major industries have emergency deluge-type safety showers to wash dangerous chemicals from the body. This will not always be the case. Be prepared for situations in which nothing has been done and there is no running water near the scene.

Emergency care for a patient with chemical burns includes the following (Figure 27-29):

1. The primary care procedure is to WASH away the chemical with flowing water. If a dry chemical is involved, BRUSH away as much of the chemical as possible and then flush the skin. Simply wetting the burn site is not enough. Continuous flooding of the affected area is required, using a copious but gentle flow of water. Avoid hard sprays that may damage badly burned tissues. Continue to wash the area for at least 20 minutes, and continue the process en route to the hospital. Remove contaminated clothing, shoes, socks, and jewelry from the patient as

Table 27-5 Care for Thermal Burns

1. STOP THE BURNING PROCESS!
   Flame—Wet down, smother, then remove clothing.
   Semi-solid (grease, tar, wax)—Cool with water. **Do not** remove substance.
2. Ensure an open airway. Assess breathing.
3. Look for signs of airway injury: soot deposits, burnt nasal hair, facial burns.
4. Complete the initial assessment.
5. Treat for shock. Provide high-concentration oxygen. Treat serious injuries.
6. Evaluate burns by depth (see below), extent (rule of nines or rule of palm), and severity.

Depth of Burn	Outer Skin Layer Is Burned	Second Skin Layer Is Burned	Tissue Below Skin Is Burned	Color Changes	Pain	Blisters
Superficial	Yes	No	No	Red	Yes	No
Partial-thickness	Yes	Yes	No	Deep red	Yes	Yes
Full-thickness	Yes	Yes	Yes	Charred black or white	Yes/No	Yes/No

7. **Do not** clear debris. Remove clothing and jewelry.
8. Wrap with dry sterile dressing.
9. Burns to hands or feet—Remove rings or jewelry that may constrict with swelling. Separate fingers or toes with sterile gauze pads.

   Burns to the eyes—Do not open eyelids if burned. Be certain burn is thermal, not chemical. Apply sterile gauze pads to **both** eyes to prevent sympathetic movement. (If burn is chemical, flush eyes for 20 minutes en route to hospital.)

FOLLOW LOCAL BURN CENTER PROTOCOLS, AND TRANSPORT ALL BURN PATIENTS AS SOON AS POSSIBLE.

A

B

Figure 27-29 For a chemical burn, (A) brush away dry powders, and then (B) flood the area with water.

you apply the wash. *Do not contaminate skin that has not been in contact with the chemical.*

Warning

Protect yourself during the washing process. Wear protective gloves and eyewear and control the wash to avoid splashing.

2. Apply a sterile dressing or burn sheet.

3. Treat for shock.

4. Transport.

Continue to be on the alert for delayed reactions that may cause renewed pain or interfere with the patient's ability to breathe. Should the patient complain of increased burning or irritation, wash the burned areas again with flowing water for several minutes.

● Patient *CARE*

Chemical Burns to the Eyes

A corrosive chemical can burn the globe of a person's eye before he can react and close the eyelid. Even with the lid shut, chemicals can seep through onto the globe.

To care for chemical burns to the eye, you should take the following steps:

1. IMMEDIATELY flood the eyes with water. Often the burn will involve areas of the face as well as the eye. When this is the case, flood the entire area. Avoid washing chemicals back into the eye or into an unaffected eye (Figure 27-30).

2. Keep running water from a faucet, low-pressure hose, bucket, cup, bottle, rubber bulb syringe, IV setup, or other such source flowing into the burned eye. The flow should be from the medial (nasal) corner of the eye to the lateral corner. Since the patient's natural reaction will be to keep the eyes tightly shut, you may have to hold the eyelids open.

3. Start transport and continue washing the eye for at least 20 minutes or until arrival at the medical facility.

4. After washing the eye, cover both eyes with moistened pads.

5. Wash the patient's eyes for 5 more minutes if he begins to complain about renewed burning sensations or irritation.

Warning

Do not use neutralizers such as vinegar or baking soda in a patient's eyes.

● Patient *CARE*

Specific Chemical Burns

When possible, find out the exact chemical or mixture of chemicals that were involved in the accident. Some special chemical burns require specific care procedures.

• *Mixed or strong acids or unidentified substances.* Many of the chemicals used in industrial processes are mixed acids. Their combined action can be immediate and severe. The pain produced from the initial chemical burn may mask any pain being caused by renewed burning due to small concentrations left on the skin.

When the chemical is a strong acid (e.g., hydrochloric acid or sulfuric acid), a combination of acids, or an unknown, play it safe and continue washing even after the patient claims he is no longer experiencing pain.

• *Dry lime.* If dry lime is the burn agent, do not wash the burn site with water. To do so will create a corrosive liquid. Brush the dry lime from the patient's skin, hair, and clothing. Make certain that you do not contaminate the eyes or airway.

Use water only after the lime has been brushed from the body, contaminated clothing and jewelry have been removed, and the process of washing can be done quickly and continuously with running water.

• *Carbolic acid (phenol).* Carbolic acid does not mix with water. When available, use alcohol for the initial wash of unbroken skin, followed by a long steady wash with water. (Follow local protocols.)

• *Sulfuric acid.* Heat is produced when water is added to concentrated sulfuric acid, but it is still preferable to wash rather than leave the contaminant on the skin.

• *Hydrofluoric acid.* This acid is used for etching glass and in many other manufacturing processes. Burns from it may be delayed, so treat all patients who may have come into contact with the chemical, even if burns are not in evidence. Flood with water. Do not delay care and transport to find neutralizing agents. (Follow local protocols.)

• *Inhaled vapors.* Whenever a patient is exposed to a caustic chemical and may have inhaled the vapors, provide a high concentration of oxygen (humidified, if available) and transport as soon as possible. This is very important when the chemical is an acid that is known to vaporize at standard environmental temperatures. (Examples include hydrochloric acid and sulfuric acid.)

Some scenes where chemical burns have taken place can be very hazardous. Always evaluate the scene. There may be large pools of dangerous chemicals around the patient. Acids could be spurting from containers. Toxic fumes may be present. If the scene will place you in danger, do not attempt a rescue unless you have been trained for such a situation and have the needed equipment and personnel at the scene.

Electrical Injuries

Electric current, including lightning, can cause severe damage to the body. The skin is burned where the energy enters the body and where it flows into a ground. Along the path of this flow, tissues are damaged due to heat. In addition, significant chemical changes take place in the nerves, heart, and muscles, and body processes are disrupted or may completely shut down.

Safety Note

The scenes of injuries due to electricity are often very hazardous. Assume that the source of electricity is still active unless a qualified person tells you that the power has been turned off. Do not attempt a rescue unless you have been trained to do this kind of rescue and have the necessary equipment and personnel. For information about electrical hazards at the scene of a vehicle collision, see Chapter 7, "Scene Size-up," and Chapter 33, "Gaining Access and Rescue Operations."

Patient *ASSESSMENT*

Electrical Injuries

The victim of an electrical accident may have any or all of the following signs and symptoms (Figure 27-31):

- Burns where the energy enters and exits the body
- Disrupted nerve pathways displayed as paralysis
- Muscle tenderness, with or without muscular twitching
- Respiratory difficulties or respiratory arrest
- Irregular heartbeat or cardiac arrest
- Elevated blood pressure or low blood pressure with the signs and symptoms of shock

Figure 27-30 Emergency care of chemical burns to the eye.

- Restlessness or irritability if conscious, or loss of consciousness
- Visual difficulties
- Fractured bones and dislocations from severe muscle contractions or from falling. This can include the spinal column.
- Seizures (in severe cases)

Patient *CARE*

Electrical Injuries

Follow the steps below to provide emergency care to a patient with electrical injuries:

Warning

Make certain that you and the patient are in a SAFE ZONE (not in contact with any electrical source and outside the area where downed or broken wires or other sources of electricity can reach you).

1. Provide airway care. Electrical shock may cause severe swelling along the airway.

2. Provide basic cardiac life support as required. Since cardiac rhythm disturbances are common, be prepared to perform defibrillation if necessary.

3. Care for shock and administer high-concentration oxygen.

4. Care for spine injuries, head injuries, and severe fractures. All serious electrical shock patients should be fully immobilized because electrical current can cause severe muscular contraction. Also, the patient may have been thrown by a high-voltage

Swollen tongue may obstruct airway

Irregular heartbeat or cardiac arrest

Muscle tenderness and possible twitching

Restless or irritable loss of consciousness

Problems of vision

Paralysis

Difficult breathing or respiratory arrest

ENTRY BURN

Possible convulsions

Elevated blood pressure

Fractured bones

EXIT BURN

Figure 27-31   Injuries due to electrical shock (top), and detail of entry and exit burns (bottom).

current. In either case, there is the possibility of spine injury that requires immobilization.

5. Evaluate electrical burns, looking for at least two external burn sites: contact with the energy source and contact with a ground.

6. Cool the burn areas and smoldering clothing the same as you would for a flame burn.

7. Apply dry sterile dressings to the burn sites.

8. Transport as soon as possible. Some problems have a slow onset. If there are burns, there also may be more serious hidden problems. In any case of electrical shock, heart problems may develop.

Remember that the major problem caused by electrical shock is usually not the burn. Respiratory and cardiac arrest are real possibilities. Be prepared to provide basic cardiac life support measures with automated defibrillation.

In the narrative portion of your prehospital care report, be sure to include things you have observed at the scene that hospital personnel will not be able to see. For example, note the source and agent of the burn, such as "thermal burns from hot radiator," "chemical burns from contact with hydrochloric acid," or "electrical burns from contact with household alternating current." If possible, note the exact chemical or mixture of chemicals involved in a chemical burn. If safe for you to do so, copy exact information from a label or describe the container of the chemical if it is too large or unsafe to bring along to the hospital.

Dressing and Bandaging

Most cases of open wound care require the application of a dressing and a bandage (Scan 27-3). A **dressing** is any material applied to a wound in an effort to control bleeding and prevent further contamination. Dressings should be sterile. A **bandage** is any material used to hold a dressing in place. Bandages need not be sterile (Figure 27-32).

Warning

Be certain to wear disposable gloves and other barrier devices to avoid contact with the patient's blood and body fluids. Follow infection control procedures.

Various dressings are carried in emergency care kits. These dressings should be sterile, meaning that all microorganisms and spores that can grow into active organisms have been killed. Dressings also should be aseptic, meaning that all dirt and foreign debris have been removed. In emergency situations, when commercially prepared dressings are not available, clean cloth, towels, sheets, handkerchiefs, and other similar materials may be suitable alternatives.

The most popular dressings are individually wrapped sterile gauze pads, typically 4 inches square. A variety of sizes are available, referred to according to size in inches, such as 2 × 2s, 4 × 4s, 5 × 9s, and 8 × 10s.

Large bulky dressings, such as the multi-trauma or **universal dressing,** are available when bulk is required for profuse bleeding or when a large wound must be covered. These dressings are especially useful for stabilizing impaled objects. Sanitary napkins can sometimes be used in place of the standard bulky dressings. Although not sterile, they are separately wrapped and have very clean surfaces. (Do not apply any adhesive surface of the napkin directly to the wound.) Of course, bulky dressings can be made by building up layers of gauze pads.

A pressure dressing is used to control bleeding. Gauze pads are placed on the wound and a bulky dressing is placed over the pads. A self-adherent roller bandage is wrapped tightly over the dressing and above and below the wound. Distal pulse must be checked and frequently rechecked, and you may need to readjust the pressure to ensure distal circulation.

An **occlusive dressing** is used when it is necessary to form an airtight seal. This is done when caring for open wounds to the abdomen, for external bleeding from large neck veins, and for open wounds to the chest. Sterile, commercially prepared occlusive dressings are available in two different forms. There are plastic wrap and petroleum-gel-impregnated gauze occlusive dressings. Local protocols vary as to which form to use. Nonsterile wrap and foil also can be used in emergency situations. In emergencies, EMT-Bs have been known to fashion

A

B

Figure 27-32 (A) Dressings cover wounds, and (B) bandages hold dressings in place.

DRESSING AND BANDAGING

NOTE: Unless they are burned, always leave fingertips or toes showing to assess circulation.

▲ **FOREHEAD OR EAR** (no skull injury). Place dressing and secure with self-adherent roller bandage.

▲ **ELBOW OR KNEE.** Place dressing and secure with cravat or roller bandage. Apply roller bandage in figure-eight pattern.

▲ **FOREARM OR LEG.** Place dressing and secure with roller bandage, distal to proximal. Better protection is offered if palm or sole is wrapped.

▲ **HAND.** Place dressing, wrap with roller bandages, and secure at wrist. When possible, bandage in position of function.

▲ **SHOULDER.** Place dressing and secure with figure-eight of cravat or roller dressing. Pad under knot if cravat is used.

▲ **HIP.** Place bandage and large dressing to cover hip. Secure with first cravat around waist and second cravat around thigh on injured side.

557

occlusive dressings from plastic credit cards, plastic bags, aluminum foil wrappers, and defibrillator pads.

Warning

Some EMS systems report that aluminum foil has caused lacerations of exposed abdominal organs.

Large dressings are sometimes needed in emergency care. Sterile, disposable burn sheets are commercially available. Bed sheets can be sterilized and kept in plastic wrappers to be later used as dressings. These sheets can make effective burn dressings or may be used in some cases to cover exposed abdominal organs.

Bandages are provided in a wide variety of types. The preferred bandage is the self-adhering, form-fitting roller bandage (Figure 27-33). It eliminates the need to know many specialized bandaging techniques developed for use with ordinary gauze roller bandages.

Dressings can be secured using adhering or non-adhering gauze roller bandage, triangular bandages, strips of adhesive tape, or an air splint. In a situation where one of these is not available, you can use strips of cloth, handkerchiefs, and other such materials. Elastic bandages that are used in the general care of strains and sprains should not be used to hold dressings in place. They can become constricting bands, interfering with circulation. This is very likely to occur as the tissues around the wound site begin to swell after the elastic bandage is in place.

Patient *CARE*

Dressing Open Wounds

The following rules apply to the general dressing of wounds (Figure 27-34):

1. Take BSI precautions.

2. Expose the wound. Cut away any clothing so the entire wound is exposed.

3. Use sterile or very clean materials. Avoid touching the dressing in the area that will come into contact with the wound. Grasp the dressing by the corner, taking it directly from its protective pack, and place it on the wound.

4. Cover the entire wound. The entire surface of the wound and the immediate surrounding areas should be covered.

5. Control bleeding. With the exception of the pressure dressing, a dressing should not be bandaged into place if it has not controlled the bleeding.

A

B

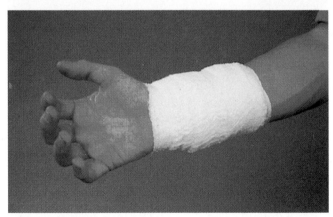

C

Figure 27-33 To apply a self-adhering roller bandage, (A) secure it with several overlapping wraps, (B) keep it snug, and (C) cut and tape or tie it in place.

You should continue to apply dressings and pressure as needed for the proper control of bleeding.

6. Do not remove dressings. Once a dressing has been applied to a wound, it must remain in place. Bleeding may restart and tissues at the wound site may be injured if the dressing is removed. If the bleeding continues, put new dressings over the blood-soaked ones.

A

B

C

D

Figure 27-34 To dress an open wound, (A) expose the wound site, (B) control bleeding, (C) dress and bandage the wound, and (D) keep the patient at rest.

There is an exception to the rule prohibiting the removal of dressings. If a bulky dressing has become blood-soaked, it may be necessary to remove the dressing so that direct pressure can be reestablished or a new bulky dressing can be added and a pressure dressing created. Protection for the wound site is better maintained if one or more gauze pads are placed over the injured tissues before placing the bulky dressing. This will allow for the removal of a bulky dressing without disturbing the wound.

Patient *CARE*

Bandaging Open Wounds

The following rules apply to general bandaging:

1. Do not bandage too tightly. All dressings should be held snugly in place, but they must not restrict the blood supply to the affected part.

2. Do not bandage too loosely. Hold the dressing by bandaging snugly, so the dressing does not move around or slip from the wound. Loose bandaging is a common error in emergency care.

3. Do not leave loose ends. Any loose ends of gauze, tape, or cloth may get caught on objects when the patient is moved.

4. Do not cover the tips of fingers and toes. When bandaging the extremities, leave the fingers and toes exposed whenever possible to observe skin color changes that indicate a change in circulation and to allow for easier neurologic reassessment. Pain, pale or blue-colored skin, cold skin, numbness, and tingling are all indications that a bandage may be too tight. The exception is burned fingers or toes, which have to be covered.

5. Cover all edges of the dressing. This will help to reduce additional contamination. The flutter-valve dressing for an open chest wound is an exception (see earlier in this chapter).

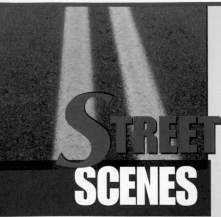

STREET SCENES

Late Sunday evening you respond to #4 Mountain View Apartments. You and your partner are met by the manager and a security guard, who lead you to Mary, a 42-year-old female sitting in a chair in the manager's office with a thick towel wrapped around her right forearm. BSI precautions are in place. "Hi, my name's Jim Morrow," you say, "and I'm with the ambulance service. What happened?" You note the trail of blood spots on the floor leading to an outside door.

"I locked myself out of my apartment. So, I wrapped my coat around my arm and broke the glass window above my kitchen sink. I thought the coat would protect me," she tells you, "but I was wrong."

STREET SCENE QUESTIONS

1. What is your general impression of this patient?
2. What priority would you assign to her?
3. What interventions are appropriate at this time?

Your general impression is of an alert female patient holding a blood-soaked towel to her right forearm. Initial assessment shows her airway open and clear, respirations normal, and a regular pulse in her right wrist. You assign her a low transport priority.

You ask Norma, your partner, to go to Mary's apartment accompanied by the security guard to see if she can learn anything more about the mechanism of injury. Meanwhile, you observe that the bleeding is being controlled, and begin a focused history and physical exam. You gently remove the towel from her arm and note there is no active bleeding from a

smooth and deep laceration with muscle and tendons visible. You carefully apply a dressing.

There were no other injuries or medical problems present. You do, however, detect an odor of alcohol on Mary's breath. "Have you had any alcohol today?" you ask.

"Yes, I drank two beers about three hours ago. That's all!" she exclaims. However, you figure with the odor on her breath, she must have had more than two beers. Focusing on her right arm, you find pulses still present in that extremity. She is also able to feel your finger touch her palm. However, when asked to wiggle her fingers, the ring and little fingers remain motionless. She also tells you it hurts to move her fingers. Norma returns and tells you there is a pool of blood on Mary's patio.

STREET SCENE QUESTIONS

4. Would you change the priority of transport of this patient based on what you now know? Why or why not?
5. What interventions are appropriate for this patient?

While you continue with the patient history, Norma obtains baseline vital signs. You learn Mary is taking thyroid medication and a blood-thinner for a medical condition. You ask when her last tetanus shot had been. She tells you she cannot remember.

Norma informs you that Mary's pulse is equal in both extremities at a rate of 128 and regular; her blood pressure is 156/94; her respirations are 24 and unlabored; pupils are equal and reactive to light; and her skin is warm, dry, and a normal color.

You contact medical direction, concerned about the loss of movement in her affected extremity. The doctor tells you that you should stabilize Mary's arm with a sling.

You apply a sling, reassess vitals, and find no significant changes. Reassessing pulse, motor func-

Two special problems occur when bandaging an extremity. First, point pressure can occur if you bandage around a very small area. It is best to wrap a large area, ensuring a steady, uniform pressure. Apply the bandage from the smaller diameter of the limb to the larger diameter (distal to proximal) to help ensure proper pressure and contact. Second, the

joints have to be considered. You can bandage across a joint, but do not bend the limb once the bandage is in place. To do so may restrict circulation, loosen the dressing and bandage, or both. In some cases, it may be necessary to apply an inflatable or rigid splint, or to use a sling and swathe to prevent movement of the joint.

PATIENT NAME: Mary Brighton   **PATIENT AGE:** 42

CHIEF COMPLAINT

"wrapped coat around arm and broke glass window"

PAST MEDICAL HISTORY

- [ ] None
- [ ] Allergy to _____
- [ ] Hypertension   [ ] Stroke
- [ ] Seizures   [ ] Diabetes
- [ ] COPD   [ ] Cardiac
- [x] Other (List)   [ ] Asthma
  - Thyroid problems

Current Medications (List)
  - Synthroid, Coumadin

VITAL SIGNS

TIME	RESP	PULSE	B.P.	MENTAL STATUS	R PUPILS L	SKIN
2355	Rate: 24 / [x] Regular / [ ] Shallow / [ ] Labored	Rate: 128 / [x] Regular / [ ] Irregular	156 / 94	[x] Alert / [ ] Voice / [ ] Pain / [ ] Unresp.	[x] Normal [x] / [ ] Dilated [ ] / [ ] Constricted [ ] / [ ] Sluggish [ ] / [ ] No-Reaction [ ]	[x] Unremarkable / [ ] Cool [ ] Pale / [ ] Warm [ ] Cyanotic / [ ] Moist [ ] Flushed / [ ] Dry [ ] Jaundiced
0005	Rate: 26 / [x] Regular / [ ] Shallow / [ ] Labored	Rate: 126 / [x] Regular / [ ] Irregular	152 / 96	[x] Alert / [ ] Voice / [ ] Pain / [ ] Unresp.	[x] Normal [x] / [ ] Dilated [ ] / [ ] Constricted [ ] / [ ] Sluggish [ ] / [ ] No-Reaction [ ]	[x] Unremarkable / [ ] Cool [ ] Pale / [ ] Warm [ ] Cyanotic / [ ] Moist [ ] Flushed / [ ] Dry [ ] Jaundiced
0011	Rate: 24 / [x] Regular / [ ] Shallow / [ ] Labored	Rate: 128 / [x] Regular / [ ] Irregular	156 / 94	[x] Alert / [ ] Voice / [ ] Pain / [ ] Unresp.	[x] Normal [x] / [ ] Dilated [ ] / [ ] Constricted [ ] / [ ] Sluggish [ ] / [ ] No-Reaction [ ]	[x] Unremarkable / [ ] Cool [ ] Pale / [ ] Warm [ ] Cyanotic / [ ] Moist [ ] Flushed / [ ] Dry [ ] Jaundiced

NARRATIVE Upon arrival, noted patient sitting upright in a chair in the manager's office of apartment complex. Patient was alert and oriented, with a large towel wrapped around her right forearm. Blood had soaked through the towel, and spots of blood noted on floor. Further investigation revealed a pool of blood approx. 12" in diameter on patient's patio. Patient attempted to break into her own apartment by breaking glass window; suffered a laceration with muscle and tendons visible. Upon EMS arrival, bleeding arrested by direct pressure. Patient has pulse and sensation, but unable to move fourth and fifth digits on affected limb. She c/o pain when moving fingers. Patient denies any other pain/medical problems at this time other than aforementioned. Patient states she had "two beers 3 hours ago"; significant fruity odor apparent on breath. Patient's extremity dressed, bandaged, and stabilized with a sling. Medical direction established and advised EMS to transport immediately to appropriate facility. No significant change noted en route. O$_2$ administered via nonrebreather at 15 LPM.

tion, and sensation, you find Mary still unable to move her fourth and fifth digits on her right hand. You place her on your cot, load her into the ambu-lance, and transport her to the closest facility, moni-toring her condition throughout the 15-minute ride. You find no other significant changes occurring.

CHAPTER REVIEW

SUMMARY

Injuries to the soft tissues of the body are common calls for the EMT-B. Soft-tissue injuries may be closed (internal, with no pathway to the outside) or open (an injury in which the skin is interrupted, exposing the tissues below). An open chest or abdominal wound is considered to be one that penetrates not only the skin but the chest or abdominal wall to expose internal organs. Closed injuries include contusions (bruises), hematomas, and crush injuries. Open wounds include abrasions, lacerations, punctures, avulsions, amputations, and crush injuries. Open neck, chest, and abdominal wounds are life threatening.

For open wounds, expose the wound, control bleeding, and prevent further contamination. For an open neck, chest, or abdominal wound apply an occlusive dressing. For both open and closed injuries, take appropriate BSI precautions, note the mechanism of injury, protect the patient's airway and breathing, administer high-concentration oxygen by nonrebreather mask, treat for shock, and transport.

Burn severity is determined by considering the source of the burn, body regions burned, depth of burn (superficial, partial-thickness, and full-thickness), extent of burn (by rule of nines or rule of palm), age of patient (children under 5 and adults over 55 react most severely), and other patient illnesses or injuries. Care for burns includes stopping the burning process (water for a thermal burn, brushing away chemicals), covering a thermal burn with a dry sterile dressing, flushing a chemical burn with sterile water, protection of the airway, administration of oxygen, treatment for shock, and transport.

For treatment of electrical injuries, be sure that you and the patient are in a safe zone away from possible contact with electrical sources. Protect airway, breathing, and circulation. Be prepared to care for respiratory or cardiac arrest. Treat for shock, care for burns, and transport.

KEY TERMS

abrasion (ab-RAY-zhun) a scratch or scrape.

air embolus (EM-bo-lus) a bubble of air in the bloodstream.

amputation (am-pyu-TAY-shun) the surgical removal or traumatic severing of a body part, usually an extremity.

avulsion (ah-VUL-shun) the tearing away or tearing off of a piece or flap of skin or other soft tissue. This term also may be used for an eye pulled from its socket or a tooth dislodged from its socket.

bandage any material used to hold a dressing in place.

closed wound an internal injury with no open pathway from the outside.

contusion (kun-TU-zhun) a bruise.

crush injury an injury caused when force is transmitted from the body's exterior to its internal structures. Bones can be broken, muscles, nerves and tissues damaged, and internal organs ruptured, causing internal bleeding.

dermis (DER-mis) the inner (second) layer of the skin found beneath the epidermis. It is rich in blood vessels and nerves.

dressing any material (preferably sterile) used to cover a wound that will help control bleeding and help prevent additional contamination.

epidermis (ep-i-DER-mis) the outer layer of the skin.

evisceration (e-vis-er-AY-shun) an intestine or other internal organ protruding through a wound in the abdomen.

full-thickness burn a burn in which all the layers of the skin are damaged. There are usually areas that are charred black or areas that are dry and white. Also called a *third-degree burn*.

hematoma (hem-ah-TO-mah) a swelling caused by the collection of blood under the skin or in damaged tissues as a result of an injured or broken blood vessel.

laceration (las-er-AY-shun) a cut.

occlusive dressing any dressing that forms an airtight seal.

open wound an injury in which the skin is interrupted, exposing the tissue beneath.

partial-thickness burn a burn in which the epidermis (first layer of skin) is burned through and the dermis (second layer) is damaged. Burns of this type cause reddening, blistering, and a mottled appearance. Also called a *second-degree burn*.

puncture wound an open wound that tears through the skin and destroys underlying tissues. A penetrating puncture wound can be shallow or deep. A perforating puncture wound has both an entrance and an exit wound.

rule of nines a method for estimating the extent of a burn. For an adult, each of the following areas represents 9% of the body surface: the head and neck, each upper extremity, the chest, the abdomen, the upper back, the lower back and buttocks, the front of each lower extremity, and the back of each lower extremity. The remaining 1% is assigned to the genital region. For an infant or child the percentages are modified so that 18% is assigned to the head, 14% to each lower extremity.

rule of palm a method for estimating the extent of a burn. The palm of the patient's hand, which equals about 1% of the body's surface area, is compared with the patient's burn to estimate its size.

subcutaneous (SUB-ku-TAY-ne-us) **layers** the layers of fat and soft tissues found below the dermis.

sucking chest wound an open chest wound in which air is "sucked" into the chest cavity.

superficial burn a burn that involves only the epidermis, the outer layer of the skin. It is characterized by reddening of the skin and perhaps some swelling. An example is a sunburn. Also called a *first-degree burn*.

universal dressing a bulky dressing.

REVIEW QUESTIONS

1. List three types of closed soft-tissue injury. (pp. 526, 528)
2. List four types of open soft-tissue injury. (pp. 530–532)
3. Describe the care for an open wound to the chest. (p. 540)
4. Describe the care for impaled objects in the eye. (pp. 536–537)
5. Explain when you would remove an object impaled in the cheek and when you would, instead, stabilize an object impaled in the cheek. (p. 536)
6. Describe the three classifications (depths) of burns. (pp. 545, 547)
7. Differentiate between a dressing and a bandage. (p. 556)
8. List the qualities and purpose of an effective bandage. How could you tell if a bandage were improperly applied? (pp. 556, 558–560)

APPLICATIONS

• You have been caring for a patient who shot himself in the chest with a nail gun. You applied an occlusive dressing around the wound. The patient is now suddenly beginning to deteriorate. He is having extreme difficulty breathing and his color has worsened. Breath sounds have become almost totally absent on the side with the impaled nail. What complication might you suspect is causing his worsening condition? How could this be corrected?

WEB MEDIC

Visit Brady's *Emergency Care* website for direct weblinks. At **www.bradybooks.com/emergencycare**, you will find information related to the following Chapter 27 topics:

• Dog bites

• Anatomy of the skin

• Thunder and lightning storm safety

Chapter
Twenty-Eight

MUSCULO-SKELETAL INJURIES

*W*ord on the Street

"I'm a paramedic instructor, so I'm supposed to know everything, right? Well, it's what you learn after you think you know it all that counts. I remember an elderly woman who presented to me with classic stroke signs: altered mental status, slurred speech, right-sided weakness. I did all the routine stroke stuff: oxygen and so on. When we went to move her, however, I discovered two obviously fractured wrists, probably from trying to break her fall. After all these years and all these calls, those two fractures remind me never to allow tunnel vision to blind me to the possibility of other problems."

Dick Cherry   EMT-P and Paramedic Instructor

Musculoskeletal injuries are common. As an EMT, you will be called upon to treat injuries to muscles and bones, which range from minor to life threatening. Many musculoskeletal injuries can have a grotesque appearance. You will be called upon to fully evaluate the patient and not be distracted from life-threatening injuries by a deformed limb.

MUSCULOSKELETAL SYSTEM

The musculoskeletal system is composed of all the bones, joints, and muscles of the body, as well as cartilage, tendons, and ligaments. As an EMT-B, you do not need to know every structure found in the body. However, you do need to remember how complex the structures are and how damage may be done to soft tissues in case of injury. Examine the skeleton and its major divisions in Figures 28-1 and 28-2. Also review the musculoskeletal system in Chapter 4, "The Human Body."

In this chapter, we will pay special attention to the **extremities**—the portions of the skeleton that include the clavicles, scapulae, arms, wrists, and hands (upper extremities, Figure 28-3) and the pelvis, thighs, legs, ankles, and feet (lower extremities, Figure 28-4).

Anatomy of Bone

Bones are formed of dense connective tissue. As components of the skeleton, they provide the body's framework. They are strong to provide support and protection for the internal organs, but they are also flexible to withstand stress. The bones store salts and metabolic materials and provide a site for the production of red blood cells. **Joints** are the places where bones articulate, or meet, and are a critical element in the body's ability to move.

Generally, bones are classified according to their appearance—long, short, flat, and irregular (Figure 28-5). The bones found in the arm and thigh are examples of long bones. The major short bones of the body are in the hands and feet. Among the flat bones are the sternum, shoulder blades, and ribs. The vertebrae of the spinal column are examples of irregular bones.

The outward appearance of a typical long bone creates the impression that it is a simple, rigid structure made of the same material throughout. Actually, it is quite complex. Most people are aware that bone contains calcium, which helps to make it very hard. Bone also contains protein fibers that make it somewhat flexible. The strength of our bones is a combination of this hardness and flexibility. As we age, less protein is formed in the bones, less calcium is stored, and as a result, bones become brittle and break more easily.

Bones are covered by a strong, white, fibrous material called the *periosteum*. Blood vessels and nerves pass through this membrane as they enter and leave the bone. When bone is exposed as a result of injury, the periosteum becomes visible. You may see fragments of bones and foreign objects on this covering, but do not remove them. If they have pierced the periosteum, the objects may be held firmly in place and offer a great resistance to any pulling or

HOW AND WHY?

Bones in our bodies contain a soft material called "marrow," some of which actually creates red blood cells. Go to your Electronic Extras CD for more about bones.

TOPIC OVERVIEW

In this chapter, you will learn about the following topics:

- Major bones and regions of the musculoskeletal system
- How to identify open and closed extremity injuries
- Purposes and general procedures for splinting
- How to splint injured extremities

✔ **Knowledge and Attitude**

1. Describe the function of the muscular system. (pp. 565, 567)

2. Describe the function of the skeletal system. (pp. 565, 567)

3. List the major bones or bone groupings of the spinal column, the thorax, the upper extremities, and the lower extremities. (pp. 566, 568, 569)

4. Differentiate between an open and a closed painful, swollen, deformed extremity. (p. 572)

5. State the reasons for splinting. (p. 574)

6. List the general rules of splinting. (pp. 575–576) (Scans 28-1 through 28-3, pp. 577–581)

7. List the complications of splinting. (p. 576)

8. List the emergency medical care for a patient with a painful, swollen, deformed extremity. (pp. 573–574)

9. Explain the rationale for splinting at the scene versus load and go. (pp. 574, 575)

10. Explain the rationale for immobilization of the painful, swollen, deformed extremity. (pp. 574–576) (Scans 28-4 through 28-17, pp. 588–607)

✔ **Skills**

1. Demonstrate the emergency medical care of a patient with a painful, swollen, deformed extremity.

2. Demonstrate completing a prehospital care report for patients with musculoskeletal injuries.

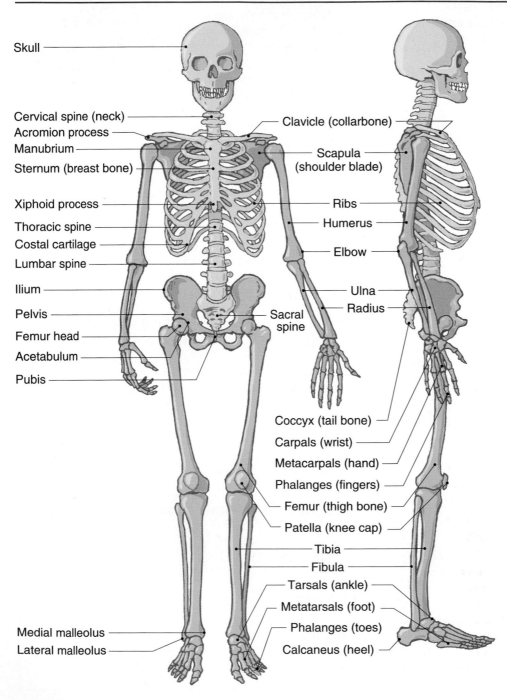

Skull
Cervical spine (neck)
Acromion process
Manubrium
Sternum (breast bone)
Xiphoid process
Thoracic spine
Costal cartilage
Lumbar spine
Ilium
Pelvis
Femur head
Acetabulum
Pubis
Medial malleolus
Lateral malleolus

Clavicle (collarbone)
Scapula (shoulder blade)
Ribs
Humerus
Elbow
Ulna
Radius
Sacral spine
Coccyx (tail bone)
Carpals (wrist)
Metacarpals (hand)
Phalanges (fingers)
Femur (thigh bone)
Patella (knee cap)
Tibia
Fibula
Tarsals (ankle)
Metatarsals (foot)
Phalanges (toes)
Calcaneus (heel)

Figure 28-1 Human skeleton.

AXIAL   **APPENDICULAR**

Figure 28-2   Two major divisions of the human skeleton.

sweeping efforts. In addition, you will not be able to tell if the object has entered the bone or is impaled in an underlying blood vessel or nerve.

The shafts of bones appear to be straight, but each bone has its own unique curvature. When the end of a bone is involved in forming a ball-and-socket joint, it will be rounded to allow for rotational movement. This rounded end is called the head of the bone. It is connected to the shaft by the neck. Bone marrow, which is contained in the center of bones, is the site of red blood cell production.

Self-Healing Nature of Bone

The most common bone injury is a break, or **fracture** (Figure 28-6). The first effects of an injury to bone are swelling of soft tissue and the formation of a blood clot in the area of the fracture. Both the swelling and the clotting are due to the destruction of blood vessels in the periosteum and the bone, and to loss of blood from adjacent damaged vessels.

Interruption of the blood supply causes death to the cells at the injury site. Cells a little farther from the fracture remain intact and, within a few hours, begin to divide rapidly. They soon grow together to form a mass of tissue that completely surrounds the fracture site. New bone is generated from this mass to eventually heal the damaged bone. The whole process can take weeks or months, depending on the bone that has been fractured, the type of fracture, and the health and age of the patient.

It is therefore very important for a broken bone to be immobilized quickly and remain immobilized to heal properly. Should the fractured bone be mishandled early in care, more soft tissue may be damaged, which would require a longer period for the formation of a tissue mass and replacement of bone. If the bone ends are disturbed during regeneration, proper healing will not take place and a permanent disability may result. In children, the majority of growth of a long bone occurs in the area known as the growth plate, which is near the ends of the shaft. If a fracture in this area is not properly handled, the child may grow up with one limb shorter than the other.

Muscles, Cartilage, Ligaments, and Tendons

In addition to bones, the elements of the musculoskeletal system are the muscles, cartilage, ligaments, and tendons. **Muscles** are the tissues or fibers that cause movement of body parts or organs. There are three kinds of muscles: skeletal (voluntary), smooth (involuntary), and cardiac (myocardium) (Figure 28-7). Smooth, or involuntary, muscles are found in the walls of organs and digestive structures. These are the muscles that move food through the digestive system. Cardiac muscle is found in the walls of the heart. The muscles that are of chief concern in trauma and musculoskeletal injury are the skeletal, or voluntary, muscles. These are the muscles that control all conscious or deliberate motions. The skeletal or voluntary muscles include all the muscles that are connected to bones as well as the muscles in the tongue, pharynx, and upper esophagus.

Cartilage is connective tissue that covers the outside of the bone ends (epiphysis) and acts as a surface for articulation, allowing for smooth movement at joints. Cartilage, which is less rigid than bone, forms or helps to form some of the more flexible structures of the body, such as the septum of the nose (the wall between the nostrils), the external ear, the trachea, and the connections between ribs and sternum (breastbone).

Tendons are bands of connective tissue that bind the muscles to bones. The tendons allow for the power of movement across the joints. **Ligaments** are connective tissue that supports joints by attaching the

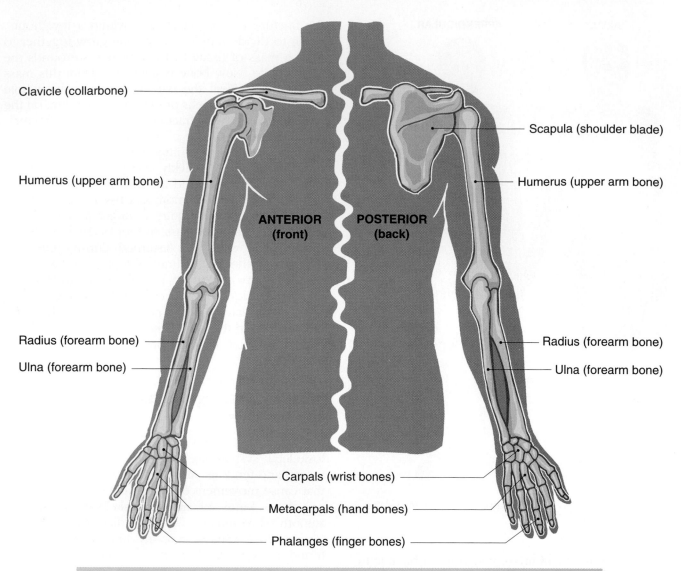

Clavicle (collarbone)

Scapula (shoulder blade)

Humerus (upper arm bone)

Humerus (upper arm bone)

ANTERIOR (front)

POSTERIOR (back)

Radius (forearm bone)

Radius (forearm bone)

Ulna (forearm bone)

Ulna (forearm bone)

Carpals (wrist bones)

Metacarpals (hand bones)

Phalanges (finger bones)

THE UPPER EXTREMITIES

COMMON NAME	ANATOMICAL NAME
Shoulder girdle	Pectoral girdle (PEK-tor-al): clavicle, scapula, and head of humerus
Collarbone (1/side)	Clavicle (KLAV-i-kul)
Shoulder blade (1/side)	Scapula (SKAP-u-lah)
Arm bone (1/limb, from shoulder to elbow)	Humerus (HU-mer-us)
Forearm bones (2/limb, from elbow to wrist: 1/medial, 1/lateral)	Ulna (UL-nah)–medial Radius (RAY-de-us)–lateral
Wrist bones (8/wrist)	Carpals (KAR-pals)
Hand bones (5/palm, palm bones)	Metacarpals (meta-KAR-pals)
Finger bones (14/hand)	Phalanges (fah-LAN-jez)

Figure 28-3 Bones of the upper extremities.

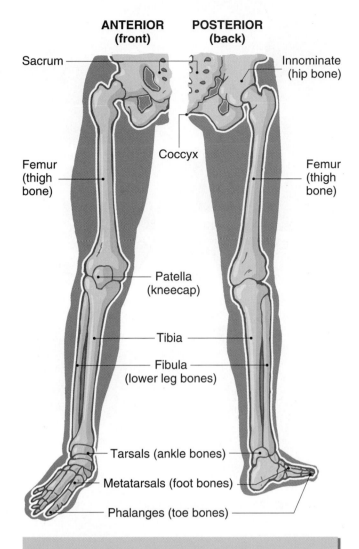

ANTERIOR (front)   **POSTERIOR (back)**

Sacrum

Innominate (hip bone)

Coccyx

Femur (thigh bone)

Femur (thigh bone)

Patella (kneecap)

Tibia

Fibula (lower leg bones)

Tarsals (ankle bones)

Metatarsals (foot bones)

Phalanges (toe bones)

THE LOWER EXTREMITIES

COMMON NAME	ANATOMICAL NAME
Pelvic girdle (pelvis or hips)	Innominate on each side made up of the fused ilium, ischium, and pubis bones, as well as sacrum and coccyx posteriorly
Thigh bone (1/limb)	Femur (FE-mer)
Kneecap (1/limb)	Patella (pah-TEL-lah)
Leg bones (shin bones, 2/leg, 1 medial, 1 lateral)	Tibia (TIB-e-ah) – medial
	Fibula (FIB-yo-lah) – lateral
Ankle bones (7/foot)	Tarsals (TAR-sals)
Foot bones (5/foot)	Metatarsals (meta-TAR-sals)
Toe bones (14/foot. Some people have two bones in their little toe, others may have three.)	Phalanges (fah-LAN-jez)

Figure 28-4   Bones of the lower extremities.

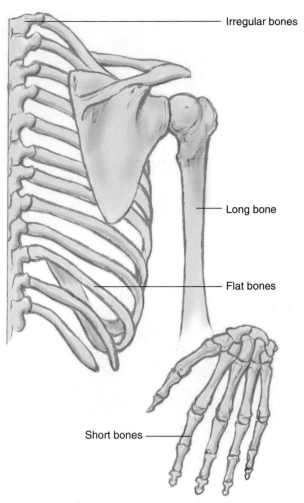

Irregular bones

Long bone

Flat bones

Short bones

Figure 28-5   Bones are classified by shape.

bone ends and allowing for a stable range of motion. Two mnemonics can help you distinguish between the connective functions of tendons and ligaments: MTB = muscle-tendon-bone; BLB = bone-ligament-bone (Figure 28-8).

GENERAL GUIDELINES FOR EMERGENCY CARE

Mechanisms of Musculoskeletal Injury

There are basically three types of mechanisms that cause musculoskeletal injuries: direct force, indirect force, and twisting force (Figure 28-9). An example of direct force is a person being struck by an automobile, causing crushed tissue and fractures. Twisting or rotational forces can cause stretching or tearing of muscles and ligaments, as well as broken

A

B

Figure 28-6 A broken wrist (A) can be definitively diagnosed by an x-ray (B).

Skeletal muscle

Cardiac muscle

Smooth muscle

Figure 28-7 Three types of muscles.

Muscle

Bone

Tendon

Ligament

Bone

Figure 28-8 Tendons tie muscle to bone. Ligaments tie bone to bone.

Indirect force

Direct force

Severe twisting force

Figure 28-9 Three basic types of mechanisms of musculoskeletal injury.

bones, such as occur when a ski digs into the snow while the skier's body rotates. Sporting activities such as football, basketball, soccer, in-line skating, skiing, snowboarding, and wrestling—in addition to motor-vehicle collisions—account for many musculoskeletal injuries.

It is easy to see how direct forces cause injuries, but an indirect force can be just as powerful. For example, a well known injury pattern occurs when people fall from heights and land on their feet. The direct forces cause injuries to the feet and ankles, while indirect forces usually cause injuries to the knees, femurs, pelvis, and spinal column. In fact, most injuries to the upper extremities are caused by forces applied to an outstretched arm. In the course of a fall, the person reaches out with an arm in an effort to break the fall and, in doing so, often breaks the radius, ulna, or clavicle, or dislocates the shoulder.

Painful, Swollen, or Deformed Extremity

Unless there is very obvious deformity, it is not possible or even important for you to decide if a patient's injury is a fracture, dislocation, sprain, or severe bruise. Most patients simply present with pain, swelling, and—sometimes—deformity. It will take an X-ray or other imaging process to diagnose the injury precisely (Figure 28-10). So in the field the worst must be assumed, and patients with a painful, swollen, or deformed extremity should be treated as though they have a fracture. Though most fractures are not life threatening, remember that bones are living tissue. Even in simple uncomplicated fractures, bones bleed. For example, a simple closed tibia-fibula fracture typically causes a 1-pint (500 cc) blood loss. Fractures of the femur typically cause a 2-pint (1,000 cc) blood loss, and pelvic fractures

A

B

Figure 28-10   (A) Some fractures are severe and obvious during external exams, while (B) others are subtle and difficult to detect without an x-ray.

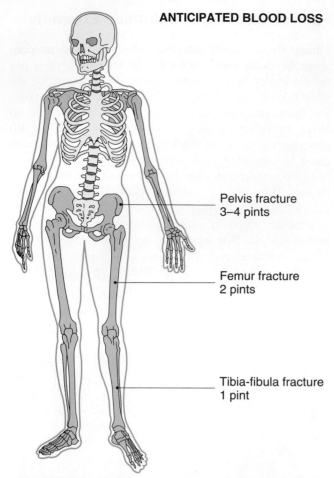

Pelvis fracture
3–4 pints

Femur fracture
2 pints

Tibia-fibula fracture
1 pint

Figure 28-11 Bones bleed. In fact, there may be considerable blood loss, even from an uncomplicated closed fracture.

cause a 3- to 4-pint (1,500-2,000 cc) blood loss (Figure 28-11).

In World War I, the battlefield death rate from a closed fracture of the femur was about 80%, because of complications such as blood loss. Two surgeons noticed that large muscle groups in the thigh go into spasms (contract, or shrink), forcing the broken femoral ends to override each other, injuring the blood vessels. To correct the problem, they invented the **traction splint,** a splint that applies constant pull along the length of the leg to help stabilize the fractured bone and reduce muscle spasms. With early application of a traction splint, the mortality rate from femur fractures dropped to under 20% (and much lower today).

Remember that splinting a painful, swollen, or deformed extremity can prevent additional blood loss, pain, and complications from nerve and blood vessel injury. Therefore, treat for the worst (a fracture) and immobilize. Physicians in the hospital will diagnose the actual injury by using an X-ray.

While it is not important for you to attempt to diagnose the underlying problem, it may be helpful for you to know the terminology health professionals use to define various musculoskeletal injuries.

- *Fracture.* A **fracture** is any break in a bone (Figure 28-12). Fractures can be classified as open or closed, and by the way a bone is broken, such as *comminuted* if broken in several places, or *greenstick* if the break is incomplete, or *angulated* if the broken bone is bent at an angle.
- *Dislocation.* The disruption or "coming apart" of a joint is called a **dislocation**. In order for a joint to dislocate, the soft tissue of the joint capsule and ligaments must be stretched beyond the normal range of motion and torn.
- *Sprain.* A **sprain** is caused by the stretching and tearing of ligaments. It is most commonly associated with joint injuries.
- *Strain.* A **strain** is a muscle injury caused by over-stretching or over-exertion of the muscle.

A **closed extremity injury** is one in which the skin is not broken. An **open extremity injury** is one in which the skin has been broken or torn through from the inside by the injured bone or from the outside by something that has caused a penetrating wound with associated injury to the bone. An open injury is a serious situation because of the increased likelihood of infection.

While many closed injuries can be handled simply in the hospital emergency department, all patients with open fractures require surgery. Proper splinting and prehospital care of musculoskeletal injuries help prevent closed injuries from becoming open ones.

Closed

Open

ANGULATED FRACTURES

Figure 28-12 Injuries to the bones may be open or closed and angulated.

Assessment of Musculoskeletal Injuries

Examination involves your senses and the skills of inspection (looking), palpation (feeling), and auscultation (listening). One of the basic principles of assessment is that it is difficult to do a proper examination on patients when they are fully clothed. However, it often is difficult, impractical, or inadvisable to completely disrobe or cut away a patient's clothing due to weather, the patient's modesty, or patient refusal. A good rule of thumb is cut or remove clothing according to the environment and severity of the situation.

In cases of severe extremity trauma, injuries can be very obvious. However, when treating trauma patients, *your priority must be to rapidly identify and treat life-threatening conditions first.* Do not let a grotesque but relatively minor extremity injury sidetrack you—or the patient. The pain or terrible appearance of an extremity injury may distract the patient from awareness of other injuries or symptoms. Be sure to assess the patient fully and ask appropriate questions to avoid missing another injury. After your initial assessment and focused exam rules out obvious life-threatening airway, breathing, or circulation problems and injuries to the head, spine, chest, and abdomen, focus your attention on musculoskeletal injuries to the extremities.

● Patient *ASSESSMENT*

Musculoskeletal Injuries

Signs and symptoms of musculoskeletal injuries in a patient include the following:

- *Pain and tenderness.* The patient with a painful, swollen, or deformed extremity experiences pain when the injured part is touched or moved. Generally, a patient will hold the injured part still, or guard it, in an effort to minimize pain. When examining a conscious patient, ask him to point to the location of pain if possible. Then, initially avoiding that location, carefully examine the injured part to assess if there are any other painful or injured areas. With unresponsive patients, suspicion of injury must be based on other physical findings.

- *Deformity or angulation.* The force of trauma causes bones to fracture and become deformed, or angulated, out of anatomical position. Note that with joint injuries, sometimes the deformity is subtle. When in doubt, look at the uninjured side and compare it to the injured one.

- *Grating,* or **crepitus**. This is a sound or feeling caused by broken bone ends rubbing together. It

can be painful for the patient. Never intentionally cause crepitus. The patient may report grating noises or sensations that occurred prior to your arrival and examination.

- *Swelling.* When bones break and soft tissue is torn, bleeding occurs causing swelling that may increase the proportions of a deformity. Rings, watches, and other jewelry can easily constrict and injure underlying tissue. Therefore, slide or cut them off as soon as possible if swelling is likely to occur.

- *Bruising.* Ecchymosis, or large black-and-blue discoloration of the skin, indicates an underlying injury that may be hours or days old. Obvious bruises indicate the need for splinting.

- *Exposed bone ends.* Bone ends protruding through the skin indicate a fracture and the need for splinting. Again, the more gruesome the appearance of the extremity, the greater the temptation to treat that injury first. Remember to care for life-threatening injuries first. Extremity injuries rarely kill patients.

- *Joints locked into position.* When joints are dislocated, they may lock into normal or abnormal anatomical positions. Joint injuries must usually be splinted as found.

- *Nerve and blood-vessel compromise.* Examine for pulses, sensation, and movement distal to the injury site. This must be accomplished *before* and *after* splinting. Check for nerve injury by asking the patient if he can sense your touch and can move all fingers or toes. Any problem of sensation or movement must be noted. Then feel for pulses in the wrist (radial), ankle (posterior tibial), or foot (dorsalis pedis). Obviously, to accurately examine for sensation, movement, and pulses, the patient's gloves and footwear must be removed.

Another method of assessing compromise to an extremity when a musculoskeletal injury is suspected is to learn and follow the "five p's." They are: pain or tenderness; pallor, pale skin, or poor capillary refill; paresthesia, or the sensation of "pins and needles"; pulses diminished or absent in the injured extremity; and paralysis or the inability to move.

● Patient *CARE*

Musculoskeletal Injuries

Emergency care of a patient with musculoskeletal injuries includes the following:

1. Take and maintain appropriate BSI precautions.

2. Perform the initial assessment. Remember, do not get distracted from your initial assessment and from determining patient priority by a dramatic-looking or painful extremity injury. Keep in mind, however, that multiple fractures, especially to the femurs, can cause life-threatening external or internal bleeding.

3. During the rapid trauma exam, apply a cervical collar if spine injury is suspected.

4. After life-threatening conditions have been addressed, all patients with a painful, swollen, or deformed extremity must be splinted. For a low-priority (stable) patient, splint individual injuries before transport. For a high-priority (unstable) patient, immobilize the whole body on a long spine board, then "load and go." If time and the patient's condition permit, you may be able to splint a specific injury en route.

5. If appropriate, cover open wounds with sterile dressings, elevate the extremity, and apply a cold pack to the area to help reduce swelling.

Remember

If an initial assessment reveals that your patient is unstable, managing extremity injuries becomes a low priority. An unstable patient with "load and go" problems must have the ABCs managed and the entire body splinted or immobilized on a long spine board. Do not take time to splint each injury individually. It is not in the patient's best interest to waste the "Golden Hour" treating minor injuries and delivering a perfectly packaged but unsavable patient to the hospital.

Splinting

Emergency care for all painful, swollen, or deformed extremities is splinting. *For any splint to be effective, it must immobilize adjacent joints and bone ends.* Effective splinting minimizes the movement of disrupted joints and broken bone ends, and it decreases the patient's pain. It helps prevent additional injury to soft tissues such as nerves, arteries, veins, and muscles. It can prevent a closed fracture from becoming an open fracture, a much more serious condition, and it can help to minimize blood loss. In the case of the spine, splinting on a backboard prevents injury to the spinal cord and helps to prevent permanent paralysis.

Realignment of the Deformed Extremity

The object of realignment (straightening) is to assist in restoring effective circulation to the extremity and to fit it to a splint. Some injuries, such as a Colles fracture of the wrist, may be completely splintable because they are only slightly deformed. In this case, the only reason to attempt realignment would be to

restore circulation to the hand if it appeared to be cyanotic or lacked pulses.

The thought of realigning an angulated injury can be a frightening one. However, remember these points:

- If the extremity is not realigned, the splint may be ineffective, causing increased pain and possible further injury (including an open fracture) during transportation.
- If the extremity is not realigned, the chance of nerves, arteries, and veins being compromised increases. When distal circulation is compromised or shut down, tissues beyond the injury become starved for oxygen and die.
- Pain is only increased for a moment during realignment under traction. Pain is reduced by effective splinting.

Due to the size and weight of extremities, attempting to splint one in the deformed position is usually futile and only increases the chance of its becoming an open fracture. When angulated injuries to the tibia or fibula, femur, radius or ulna, or humerus cannot be fit into a rigid splint, realign the bone. Also realign a long bone when the distal extremity is cyanotic or lacks pulses, indicating compromised circulation.

The general guidelines for realigning an extremity are as follows (Figure 28-13):

1. One EMT-B grasps the distal extremity, while a partner places one hand above and one hand below the injury site.

2. The partner supports the site while the first EMT-B pulls gentle **manual traction** in the direction of the long axis of the extremity. If resistance is felt or if it appears that bone ends will come through the skin, stop realignment and splint the extremity in the position found.

3. If no resistance is felt, maintain gentle traction until the extremity is properly splinted.

Generally, injuries to joints should be splinted in the position found unless the distal extremity is cyanotic or lacks pulses. If so, an attempt should be made to align the joint to a neutral anatomical position using gentle traction, provided that no resistance is felt.

Strategies for Splinting

Effective splinting may require some ingenuity. Even though you carry different types of splinting devices, many situations will require you to improvise. In a pinch, you can use pillows or rolled blankets as soft splints. For rigid splints you can use a piece of lumber, cardboard, a rolled newspaper, an umbrella, a

Figure 28-13 Aligning an extremity.

cane, a broom handle, a catcher's shin guard, or a tongue depressor for a finger. A bystander can often rummage through his car trunk and find something suitable.

Splints carried on EMS units come in three basic types: rigid splints, formable splints, and traction splints (Figure 28-14). Rigid splints require the limb to be moved to the anatomical position. They tend to provide the greatest support and are ideally used to splint long-bone injuries. Examples are cardboard,

Figure 28-14 Splints and accessories for musculoskeletal injuries.

wood, pneumatic splints such as air splints and vacuum splints, and the pneumatic anti-shock garment. Formable splints are capable of being molded to different angles and generally allow for considerable movement. They are most commonly used to immobilize joint injuries in the position found. Examples are pillow and blanket splints. Traction splints are used specifically for femur fractures.

Regardless of the method of splinting, general rules that apply to all types of immobilization are as follows:

- *Expose the injury site.* Before moving the injured extremity, expose the area and control any bleeding.
- *Assess distal PMS.* Because complications of musculoskeletal injury include nerve and blood vessel injury, assess and record distal pulse, motor function, and sensation (PMS) both before and after splinting. (Review Scan 10-5 in Chapter 10, which illustrates how to assess distal function.)
- *Align long-bone injuries to anatomical position* under gentle traction, if severe deformity exists or distal circulation is compromised.
- *Do not push protruding bones back into place.* However, when you realign deformed open injuries, they can slip back into position under traction.
- *Immobilize both the injury site and adjacent joints.* In order for splints to be effective, they must keep the injury site and the joints above and below still. (If it is the joint that is injured, splint to immobilize the joint and the adjacent bones.)
- *Splint before moving the patient* to a stretcher or other location, if possible. A good rule of thumb is "least handling causes least damage." Sometimes patients must be extricated from where they are before ideal splinting techniques can occur. Attempt to immobilize the extremity as well as you can. (For example, prior to extrication, the injured extremity might be immobilized to the uninjured one.)
- *Pad the voids.* Many rigid splints do not conform to body curves and allow too much movement of the limb. Pad the voids, or spaces between the body part and the splint, to increase patient comfort and ensure proper immobilization.
- *Choose a method of splinting,* which is always dictated by the severity of the patient's condition and priority decision. If the patient is a high priority for "load and go" transport, choose a fast method of splinting. If the patient is a low priority for transport, choose a slower-but-better splinting method. The methods of splinting from slowest to fastest are: each site is individually splinted (slowest but

best); the limb is secured to the torso or an unin-jured leg (a bit faster, but second choice to indi-vidual splints); and the entire body is secured to a spine board (fastest, but only better than no splint at all).

- *Care for life-threatening problems first.* If the pa-tient is unstable, do not waste time with splinting. You can align the injuries in anatomical position and immobilize the whole body to a long spine board.

Documentation Tip– Realigning an Extremity

When realigning an open extremity injury, be sure to make a note on the prehospital care re-port—and verbally report to the emergency depart-ment staff—if bone ends initially protruded from the open wound and slipped back into position, and out of sight, during realignment.

Hazards of Splinting

By far the most serious hazard of splinting is "splint-ing someone to death": splinting before life-threatening conditions are addressed, or spending time splinting a high-priority patient instead of immediately getting the patient into the ambulance and to the hospital. Always assure airway, breathing, and circulation be-fore going on to care for other injuries. Remember, the method of splinting is always dictated by the severity of the patient's condition and by the priority for transportation.

Other hazards include improper or inadequate splinting. If a splint is applied too tightly, it can com-press soft tissue and injure nerves, blood vessels, and muscles. If it is applied too loosely or inappropri-ately, it will allow so much movement that further soft-tissue injury or an open fracture may occur. In addition, because rescue workers may be insecure about realigning a deformed injury, they may attempt to splint it in a deformed position and actually do more harm than good. Remember, it can be very dif-ficult to splint deformed long-bone injuries well enough to prevent excessive movement.

Splinting Long-Bone and Joint Injuries

Before you start the splinting process, select a splint appropriate to the severity of the patient's condition and method of transportation. Be sure to have cravats, padding, and roller bandages immediately at hand.

The splinting of joints usually requires consider-able ingenuity. In most cases formable splints are used to splint the extremity in the position it is found. If the distal extremity is pulseless or cyanotic, an attempt should be made to align it to anatomical position using gentle traction. As with long-bone

splinting, get all of your equipment ready before starting the splinting process.

To splint long-bone or joint injuries, follow these guidelines (Scans 28-1 and 28-2):

1. Take appropriate BSI precautions and, if pos-sible, expose the area to be splinted.

2. Manually stabilize the injury site. This can be done either by you or by a helper.

3. Assess pulses and circulation, motor function, and sensation (PMS). Check for pulses and see if the patient can feel your touch distal to the injury. Ask the patient to wiggle the fingers or toes, grasp your fingers, or push feet against your hands.

4. Realign the injury if deformed or if the distal extremity is cyanotic or pulseless. Be sure to attempt to realign an injured joint only if the distal extremity is pulseless or cyanotic.

5. Measure or adjust the splint and move it into position under or alongside the limb. Maintain man-ual stabilization or traction during positioning and until the splinting procedure is complete.

6. Apply and secure the splint to immobilize adja-cent joints and injury site.

7. Reassess PMS distal to the injury.

Traction Splint

An injury to the femur is an exception to the general guidelines for splinting long-bone and joint injuries. The major problem with femur fractures is the ten-dency for the large muscle groups of the thigh (quad-riceps and hamstrings) to go into spasm, forcing the bone ends to override each other, causing pain and further soft-tissue injury. A traction splint counteracts the muscle spasms and greatly reduces the pain.

Traction splints come in two basic varieties: bipo-lar and unipolar. A bipolar splint cradles the leg be-tween two metal rods; a unipolar splint has a single metal rod that is placed alongside the leg. Examples of the bipolar splint are the half-ring splint, Hare, and Fernotrac. Examples of the unipolar splint are the Sager and the Kendrick traction devices. (The Fer-notrac, Sager, and Kendrick traction devices are illus-trated at the end of this chapter.)

One of the most common questions is "How much traction should I pull?" An answer commonly given is "Pull enough traction to give the patient some relief from the pain." This answer can be misleading. When the thigh muscles begin to spasm and the bones begin to override, the patient is in real pain. When manual or mechanical traction is applied, you are pulling against a muscle spasm, and that hurts too. Most patients do not begin to feel relief with the trac-tion splint until it has been applied for several min-utes and the muscle spasm begins to subside. (With

IMMOBILIZING A LONG BONE

FIRST take BSI precautions.

▲ **1.** Manually stabilize the injured limb.

▲ **2.** Assess distal pulse, motor function, and sensation (PMS).

▲ **3.** Measure the splint. It should extend several inches beyond joints above and below injury.

▲ **4.** Apply splint and immobilize joints above and below injury.

(continued)

▲ **5.** Secure the entire injured extremity.

▲ **6.** Secure foot in position of function. . . .

▲ . . . Or if splinting an arm, secure hand in position of function. This is the position the hand would be in if the patient were holding a palm-sized ball. A roll of bandage can be placed in the patient's hand to help maintain the position of function.

▲ **7.** Reassess distal PMS function.

IMMOBILIZING A JOINT

FIRST take BSI precautions.

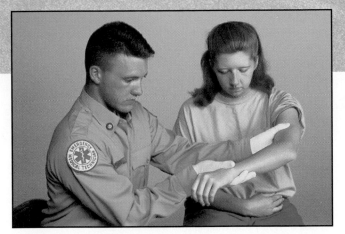

▲ **1.** Manually stabilize the injured limb.

▲ **2.** Assess distal pulse, motor function, and sensation (PMS).

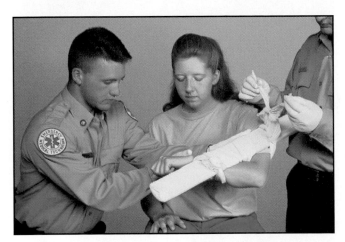

▲ **3.** Select proper splint material. Immobilize site of injury and bones above and below.

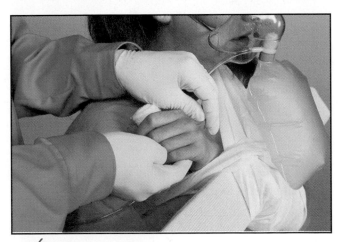

▲ **4.** Reassess distal PMS function.

APPLYING A TRACTION SPLINT

FIRST take BSI precautions.

▲ **1.** Manually stabilize the injured leg, and assess distal pulse, motor function, and sensation (PMS).

▲ **2.** Apply and maintain manual traction.

▲ **3.** Measure the splint.

▲ **4.** Apply proximal securing device (e.g., ischial strap).

▲ **5.** Apply distal securing device (e.g., ankle hitch).

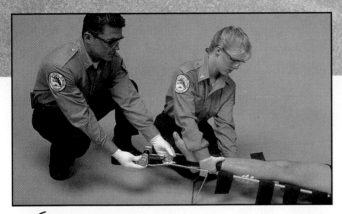

▲ **6.** Apply mechanical traction.

▲ **7.** Position and secure support straps.

▲ **8.** Reassess distal PMS function.

▲ **9.** Secure patient's torso and traction splint to long board for transport.

the Sager splint, traction can be measured. The amount of traction applied should be roughly 10% of the patient's body weight and not exceed 15 pounds.) With a bipolar splint, firm traction should be applied to align the limb. Exert and maintain a firm pull to prevent bones from continuing to override.

No traction splint applied in the field pulls true traction. All exert "counter traction." The splint pulls on an ankle hitch and the splint frame is anchored against the pelvis. Once anchored, a pull is felt on the leg. With bipolar splints, any movement of the pelvis off the ground causes a shifting of the splint and loss of traction. Unipolar splints, such as the Sager, are anchored against the pubis between the legs and are less apt to shift during patient movement and cause a loss of traction.

The indications for a traction splint are a painful, swollen, deformed mid-thigh with no joint or lower leg injury. A traction splint is contraindicated if there is a pelvis, hip, or knee injury, if there is an avulsion or partial amputation where traction could separate the extremity, or if there is an injury to the lower third of the leg that would interfere with the ankle hitch.

General guidelines for the application of a traction splint are as follows (Scan 28-3):

1. Take BSI precautions and, if possible, expose the area to be splinted.

2. Manually stabilize the leg and apply manual traction.

3. Assess PMS distal to the injury.

4. Adjust the splint to the proper length, and position it at or under the injured leg.

5. Apply the proximal securing device (ischial strap).

6. Apply the distal securing device (ankle hitch).

7. Apply mechanical traction.

8. Position and secure support straps.

9. Re-evaluate the proximal and distal securing devices, and reassess PMS distal to the injury.

10. Secure the patient's torso and the traction splint to a long spine board to immobilize the hip and to prevent movement of the splint.

When possible, use three rescuers to apply a traction splint. One can support the injury site when the limb is lifted to position the traction splint.

Note

Most of the traction splints in use today require that the patient's shoe be removed for proper traction splinting. With some older splints, the patient's shoe may remain in place if neurologic and pulse assessment is possible, if the shoe will not prevent the ankle hitch from being properly placed, and if the shoe will not slip off after mechanical traction (tension) is applied.

EMERGENCY CARE OF SPECIFIC INJURIES

The specific injuries described in this section are usually identified as fractures or dislocations. Remember that you do not need to determine the exact nature of an extremity injury. You will immobilize any painful, swollen, or deformed extremity. Specific techniques are discussed on the following pages and illustrated in Scans 28-4 through 28-17.

Upper Extremity Injuries

Shoulder Girdle Injuries

Signs and symptoms of an injury to the shoulder girdle include:

• Pain in the shoulder may indicate several types of injury. Look for specific signs.

• A dropped shoulder, with the patient holding the arm of his injured side against the chest, often indicates a fracture of the clavicle.

• A severe blow to the back over the scapula may cause a fracture of that bone. (All the bones of the shoulder girdle can be felt except the scapula. Only the superior ridge of the scapula, called its spine, can be easily palpated. Injury to the scapula is rare but must be considered if there are indications of a severe blow at the site of this bone.)

Check the entire shoulder girdle. Check for deformity where the clavicle attaches to the sternum. Feel for deformity where the clavicle joins the scapula. Feel and look along the entire clavicle for deformity. Note if the head of the humerus can be felt or moves in front of the shoul-

der. This is a sign of possible anterior dislocation, which may be due to a fracture.

Patient CARE

Shoulder Girdle Injuries

Emergency care of a patient with a shoulder-girdle injury includes the following:

1. Assess distal PMS function. If distal PMS function is impaired, immobilize and transport as soon as possible, notifying the receiving facility.

2. It is not practical to use a rigid splint for injuries to the clavicle, scapula, or the head of the humerus. Use a sling and swathe (Scan 28-4). If there is possible cervical-spine injury, do not tie a sling around the patient's neck.

3. If there is evidence of a possible anterior dislocation of the head of the humerus (the bone head is pushed toward the front of the body), place a thin pillow between the patient's arm and chest before applying the sling and swathe.

4. Do not attempt to straighten or reduce any dislocations.

5. Reassess distal PMS function.

Note: Sometimes a dislocated shoulder will reduce itself (the displaced head of the humerus "pops back into place"). When this happens, check for distal PMS function. Apply a sling and swathe and transport the patient. The patient must be seen by a physician.

Documentation Tip—Self-Reduction of Shoulder Dislocation

If a dislocated shoulder appears to go back into place, be certain to note the self-reduction on the report form. Also report the event to the emergency department staff to be sure they are aware of the previous dislocation.

Lower Extremity Injuries

 Patient *ASSESSMENT*

Pelvic Injuries

Fractures of the pelvis may occur with falls, in motor-vehicle collisions, or when a person is crushed by being squeezed between two objects. Pelvic fractures may be the result of direct or indirect force. Signs and symptoms of a pelvic injury in a patient include:

- Complaint of pain in pelvis, hips, groin, or back. This may be the only indication, but it is significant if the mechanism of injury indicates possible fracture. Usually, obvious deformity is associated with the pain.
- Painful reaction when pressure is applied to the iliac crests (wings of the pelvis) or to the pubic bones.
- Patient complains that he cannot lift his legs when lying on his back. (Do not test for this, but do check for sensation.)
- Foot on the injured side may turn outward (lateral rotation). This also may indicate a hip fracture.

- Patient has an unexplained pressure on the urinary bladder and the feeling of having to empty the bladder.

Warning: Indications of pelvic fractures mean that there may be serious damage to internal organs, blood vessels, and nerves. Internal bleeding may be profuse and lead to shock. Any force strong enough to fracture the pelvis also can cause injury to the spine.

Patient *CARE*

Pelvic Injuries

Note: It may be very difficult to tell a fractured pelvis from a fracture of the upper femur. When there is doubt, care for the patient as if there is a pelvic fracture to protect blood vessels and nerves associated with the joint. Remember, there may be spinal injuries.

Emergency care includes the following:

1. Move the patient as little as possible. Any emergency move should be done so that the patient moves as a unit. Never lift the patient with the pelvis unsupported. *Warning: do not use a log roll to move a patient with a suspected pelvic fracture.*

2. Determine PMS function distal to the injury site.

3. Straighten the patient's lower limbs into the anatomical position, if there are no injuries to the hip joints and lower limbs and if it is possible to do so without meeting resistance or causing excessive pain.

4. Prevent additional injury to the pelvis by stabilizing the lower limbs. Place a folded blanket between the patient's legs, from the groin to the feet, and bind them together with wide cravats. Thin rigid splints can be used to push the cravats under the patient. The cravats can then be adjusted for proper placement at the upper thigh, above the knee, below the knee, and above the ankle.

5. Apply a pneumatic anti-shock garment (PASG) to stabilize the pelvis in a patient with hypotension (blood pressure below 90).

6. Assume that there are spinal injuries. Immobilize the patient on a long spine board. When securing the patient, avoid placing the straps or ties over the pelvic area.

7. Reassess distal PMS function.

8. Care for shock, providing a high concentration of oxygen.

9. Transport the patient as soon as possible.

10. Monitor vital signs.

Once the patient is in the ambulance and prepared for transport, some EMT-Bs are allowed to make adjustments to improve patient comfort and reduce muscle spasms of the abdomen and lower limb. This can be done by gently flexing the patient's legs and placing a pillow under the knees. If you are allowed to follow this protocol, be extremely careful not to move the spine, since the patient may have associated spinal injuries.

The pneumatic anti-shock garment (PASG) is strongly indicated for splinting a suspected pelvic fracture in a patient with hypotension (blood pressure below 90). Some EMS systems also use the anti-shock garment for splinting hip, femoral, and multiple leg fractures. An anti-shock garment is to be applied in accordance with local protocols. In many localities, application requires an order from a physician. (Review Chapter 26, Scan 26-3, "Applying the Anti-Shock Garment.")

When pelvic fracture is a possibility, always be alert for shock and possible injuries to internal organs. Always take vital signs before applying an anti-shock garment and monitor the vital signs every 5 minutes thereafter.

Patient *ASSESSMENT*

Hip Dislocation

A hip dislocation occurs when the head of the femur is pulled or pushed from its pelvic socket. It is difficult to tell a hip dislocation from a fracture of the proximal (uppermost portion of the) femur. Conscious patients will complain of intense pain with both types of injury. Patients who have had a surgical replacement of the hip joint are at increased risk of hip dislocation. The hip can be dislocated either anteriorly or posteriorly.

Signs and symptoms of a hip dislocation include:

• *Anterior hip dislocation.* The patient's entire lower limb is rotated outward and the hip is usually flexed.

• *Posterior hip dislocation* (most common). The patient's leg is rotated inward, the hip is flexed, and the knee is bent. The foot may hang loose (foot drop), and the patient is unable to flex the foot or lift the toes. Often, there is a lack of sensation in the limb. These signs indicate possible damage, caused by the dislocated femoral head, to the sciatic nerve, the major nerve that extends from the lower spine to the posterior thigh. This injury often occurs when a person's knees strike the dashboard during a motor-vehicle collision.

● Patient *CARE*

Hip Dislocation

Emergency care of a patient with a hip dislocation includes:

1. Assess distal PMS function.

2. Move the patient onto a long spine board. Some systems use a scoop-style stretcher. When this device is used, the limb should be immobilized.

3. Immobilize the limb with pillows or rolled blankets.

4. Secure the patient to the long spine board with straps or cravats.

5. Reassess distal PMS function. If there is a pulse, motor, or sensory problem, notify medical direction and transport immediately.

6. Care for shock, providing a high concentration of oxygen.

7. Transport carefully, monitor vital signs, and continue to check for nerve and circulation impairment.

Note that if you find a painful, swollen, or deformed thigh and the leg is flexed and will not straighten, the patient may also have a fractured femur.

Documentation Tip—Self-Reduction of Hip Dislocation

If the head of the femur slides or pops back into place, note this self-reduction of the dislocation on the patient form and report the event to the hospital emergency department staff so that the previous dislocation does not go unnoticed.

● Patient *ASSESSMENT*

Hip Fracture

As noted earlier, a hip fracture is a fracture of the proximal femur, not the pelvis. The fracture can occur to the femoral head, the femoral neck, or at the portion of the femur just below the neck of the bone.

Signs and symptoms of a hip fracture include the following:

• Pain is localized, but some patients complain of pain in the knee.

• Sometimes the patient is sensitive to pressure exerted on the lateral prominence of the hip (greater trochanter).

• Surrounding tissues are discolored. Discoloration may be delayed.

• Swelling may be evident.

• Patient is unable to move limb while on his back.

• Patient complains about being unable to stand.

• Foot on injured side usually turns outward; however, it may rotate inward (rarely).

• Injured limb may appear shorter.

G Geriatric Notes

Direct force (as occurs in a motor-vehicle collision) and twisting forces (as may occur in falls) can cause a hip fracture. Elderly people are more susceptible to this type of injury because of brittle bones or bones weakened by disease.

● Patient *CARE*

Hip Fracture

Be certain to assess distal PMS function before and after splinting and during transport. The patient should be managed for shock and receive oxygen at a high concentration. It is recommended that the patient be placed on a long spine board or orthopedic stretcher after splinting.

A

B

Figure 28-15   For a patient with a hip or pelvic injury, (A) bind the legs together or (B) splint with a padded long board. Apply an anti-shock garment, if local protocols indicate.

One of the following emergency care methods can be used to stabilize a hip fracture (Figure 28-15):

• *Bind the legs together.* Place a folded blanket between the patient's legs and bind the legs together with wide straps, Velcro-equipped straps, or wide cravats. Carefully place the patient on a long spine board and use pillows to support the lower limbs. Secure the patient to the board. An orthopedic stretcher can be used in place of the long spine board.

• *Padded boards.* Use thin splints to push cravats or straps under the patient at the natural voids (such as the small of the back and back of the knees) and readjust them so that they will pass across the chest, the abdomen just below the belt, below the crotch, above and below the knee, and at the ankle. Splint with two long padded boards. Ideally, one should be long enough to extend from the patient's armpit to beyond the foot. The other should be long enough to extend from the crotch to beyond the foot. Cushion with padding in the armpit and crotch and pad all voids created at the ankle and knee. Secure the boards with the cravats or straps.

• Apply an anti-shock garment, if local protocols indicate.

● Patient ASSESSMENT

Femoral Shaft Fracture

Because the femur is a large, strong bone, considerable force is necessary to cause a fracture of the femoral shaft. Remember also that muscle contractions can cause bone ends to ride over each other. The bone ends may or may not protrude from an open wound. Never assume that a wound on the thigh is of external origin because you do not see bone ends. Always check for signs and symptoms that this may be an open fracture.

Signs and symptoms of a femoral shaft fracture include:

• Pain, often intense

• Often there will be an open fracture with deformity and sometimes with the end of the bone protruding through the wound. When the injury is a closed fracture, often there will be deformity with possible severe angulation.

• Injured limb may appear to be shortened because the contraction of the thigh muscles caused the bone ends to override each other.

Pediatric Notes

When traction-splinting thigh injuries in children, be sure to use appropriately-sized splints. **Warning:** Studies of mechanisms of injury indicate that infants and children with fractured femurs often have injury to internal organs.

● Patient CARE

Femoral Shaft Fracture

Emergency care of a patient with a femoral shaft fracture includes:

1. Control any bleeding by applying direct pressure (avoiding the possible fracture site) forcefully enough to overcome the barrier of muscle mass. The femoral artery pressure point may be used.

2. As soon as possible, manage the patient for shock (hypoperfusion) and provide high-concentration oxygen.

3. Assess distal PMS function.

4. Apply a traction splint. If a traction splint is not available, bind the legs together after placing them in the anatomical position.

5. Reassess distal PMS function.

Warning: The traction splint should not be applied if you suspect that there may be additional injuries or fractures to the area of the knee or tibia/fibula of the same limb.

If local protocols permit, an anti-shock garment may be used if there are multiple leg fractures. It is not, however, a good splint for the lower leg since it does not immobilize the ankle.

● Patient ASSESSMENT

Knee Injury

The knee is a joint and not a single bone. Fractures can occur to the distal femur, to the proximal tibia and fibula, and to the patella (kneecap). Signs and symptoms of a knee injury include:

• Pain and tenderness

• Swelling

• Deformity with obvious swelling

● Patient CARE

Knee Injury

There are two general emergency care methods of immobilizing the knee—one if the knee is bent, the other if it is straight:

• *Knee is bent.* Assess distal PMS function. Immobilize in the position in which the leg is found. Tie two padded board splints to the thigh and above the ankle so that the knee is held in position. A pillow can be used to support the leg. Reassess distal PMS function. (See Scan 28-13.)

• *Knee is straight or returned to anatomical position.* Assess distal PMS function. Immobilize with two padded board splints or a single padded splint. When using two padded boards, one medial and one lateral offer the best support. Remember to pad the voids created at the knee and ankle. Reassess distal PMS function. (See Scans 28-14 and 28-15.)

Do not confuse a knee dislocation with a patella dislocation. The patella can become displaced by ligament damage when the lower leg and knee are twisted, as in a skiing or racquetball accident. A knee dislocation occurs when the tibia itself is forced either anteriorly or posteriorly in relation to the distal femur. Always check for a distal pulse, since the dislocated knee joint can compress the popliteal artery and stop the major blood supply to the lower leg. If there is no pulse, this is a true emergency. Contact medical direction for permission to gently move the lower leg anteriorly to allow for a pulse, and transport immediately.

What may appear to be a dislocation may prove to be a fracture or a combined fracture and dislocation. Even if you believe that the patient has suffered a dislocated patella and the kneecap has repositioned itself, realize that other damage may be hidden. Whether you suspect a fracture, a dislocation, a sprain, or a strain, always splint and transport.

Once splinting is done, monitor the patient. If there is a loss of distal PMS function, or if the foot becomes discolored (white, mottled, or blue) and turns cold, transport the patient without delay. Notify medical direction while en route.

Tibia or Fibula Injury

Signs and symptoms of a tibia or fibula injury include:

*   Pain and tenderness
*   Swelling
*   Possible deformity (You might expect to see a deformity of the lower leg when the tibia or fibula is fractured. However, such deformity is often absent.)

Tibia or Fibula Injury

Emergency care of a patient with a tibia or fibula injury includes providing care for shock and administering high-concentration oxygen. Because immobilizing the leg can help to relieve pain and control bleeding, apply a splint using one of methods listed below. Remember to assess distal PMS function before and after application.

*   *Air-inflated splint.* Apply an air-inflated splint (Figure 28-16). Slide the uninflated splint over your hand and gather it in place until the lower edge clears your wrist. Using your free hand, grasp the patient's foot and leg just above the injury site. While maintaining manual traction, have your partner slide the splint over your hand and onto the injured leg. Your partner must make sure that the splint is relatively wrinkle free and that it covers the injury site. Continue to maintain traction while your partner inflates the splint. Test to see if you can cause a slight dent in the plastic with fingertip pressure. Remember to check periodically to see that the pressure in the splint has remained adequate and has not decreased or increased.
*   *Two-splint method.* You can immobilize the fracture using two rigid board splints (Scan 28-16).

*   *Single splint with ankle hitch.* A single splint with an ankle hitch can be applied (Scan 28-17).

Ankle or Foot Injury

Sprains (torn ligaments) and fractures are the most common musculoskeletal injuries to the ankle and foot. It is often difficult to distinguish between them, so always treat for a fracture. Signs and symptoms of an ankle or foot injury include:

*   Pain
*   Swelling
*   Possible deformity

Ankle or Foot Injury

Long splints, extending from above the knee to beyond the foot, can be used. However, soft splinting is an effective, rapid method and is recommended for most patients (Figure 28-17). To soft splint, you should follow the emergency care steps described below:

1. Assess distal PMS function.

2. Stabilize the limb. Remove the patient's shoe if possible, but only if it removes easily and can be done with no movement to the ankle.

3. Lift the limb, but do not apply manual traction (tension).

4. Place three cravats on the floor under the ankle. Then place a pillow lengthwise under the ankle on top of the cravats. The pillow should extend 6 inches beyond the foot.

5. Gently lower the limb onto the pillow, taking care not to change the position of the ankle. Stabilize by tying the cravats, and adjust them so they are at the top of the pillow, midway, and at the heel.

6. Tie the pillow to the ankle and foot.

7. Tie a fourth cravat loosely at the arch of the foot.

8. Elevate with a second pillow or blanket. Reassess distal PMS function.

Figure 28-16 An air splint may be used for a lower leg injury.

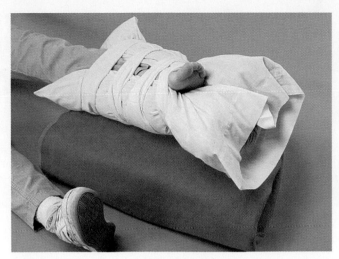

Figure 28-17 A pillow splint may be used for an injured ankle.

9. Care for shock (hypoperfusion) if needed.

10. Apply an ice pack to the injury site to reduce bleeding and swelling, if appropriate. Do not apply the ice pack directly to the skin.

Note that a commercial splint with a foot and leg that extends above the knee may be better than a pillow since it will immobilize the knee, the joint adjacent to the ankle.

Documentation Tip—Painful, Swollen, Deformed Extremities

When caring for a painful, swollen, deformed extremity, always check and record distal pulses, motor function, and sensation both before and after splinting. If the hospital staff discovers that PMS function is impaired, they will need to know if this occurred before splinting, as a possible result of splinting, or did not occur until after the patient was at the hospital. Documenting this information not only contributes to good patient care but can also protect you from charges that the function of the limb was impaired by incorrect splinting or other prehospital procedures.

APPLYING A SLING AND SWATHE

A sling is a triangular bandage used to support the shoulder and arm. Once the patient's arm is placed in a sling, a swathe can be used to hold the arm against the side of the chest. Commercial slings are available. Velcro straps can be used to form a swathe. Use whatever materials you have on hand, provided they will not cut into the patient. Also, remember to assess distal pulse, motor function, and sensation both before and after immobilizing or splinting an extremity.

▲ **1.** Prepare the sling by folding cloth into a triangle.

▲ **2.** Position the sling over the top of the patient's chest as shown. Fold the injured arm across her chest. Or . . .

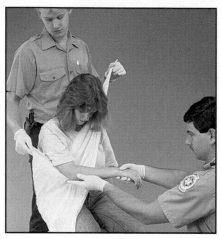

▲ . . . If the patient cannot hold her arm, have someone assist until you tie the sling.

▲ **3.** Extend one point of the triangle behind the elbow on the injured side.

▲ **4.** Take the bottom point and bring it up over the patient's arm. Then take it over the top of the injured shoulder.

▲ **5.** If appropriate, draw up the ends of the sling so that the patient's hand is about 4 inches above the elbow.

▲ **6.** Tie the two ends of the sling together, making sure that the knot does not press against the back of the patient's neck. The area can be padded with bulky dressings.

▲ **7.** Check to be sure you have left the patient's fingertips exposed.

▲ Then assess distal pulse, motor function, and sensation (PMS). If the pulse has been lost, take off the sling and repeat the procedure. Then check again.

▲ **8.** To form a pocket for the patient's elbow, take hold of the point of material at the elbow and fold it forward, pinning it to the front of the sling. Or . . .

▲ . . . If you do not have a pin, twist the excess material and tie a knot in the point.

▲ **9.** Form a swathe from a second piece of material. Tie it around the chest and the injured arm, over the sling. Do not place it over the patient's arm on the uninjured side.

▲ **10.** Reassess distal pulse, motor function, and sensation (PMS). Treat for shock, and provide high-concentration oxygen. Take vital signs. Perform detailed and ongoing assessments as appropriate.

NOTE: If the patient has a cervical-spine injury, do not tie the sling around her neck.

SPLINTING AN INJURED HUMERUS

NOTE: Assess distal pulse, motor function, and sensation both before and after immobilizing or splinting an extremity.

Signs: Injury to the humerus can take place at the proximal end (shoulder), along the shaft of the bone, or at the distal end (elbow). Deformity is the key sign used to detect fractures to this bone in any of these locations; however, assess for all signs of skeletal injury, including pain or swelling. Follow the rules and procedures for care of an injured extremity.

▲ **Variation One:** Apply a sling and swathe. If you have only enough material for a swathe, bind the patient's upper arm to her body, taking great care not to cut off circulation to the forearm.

▲ **Variation Two:** If you have only a short length of material to use as a sling, apply it so that it supports the wrist only.

WARNING Before applying a sling and swathe to care for injuries to the humerus, check for distal pulse, motor function, and sensation (PMS). If you do not feel a pulse, attempt to straighten any slight angulation if the patient has a closed fracture (follow local protocol). Otherwise, prepare for immediate immobilization and transport. Should straightening of the angulation fail to restore the pulse or function, splint with a medium board splint, keeping the forearm extended. If there is no sign of circulation or sensory or motor function, you will have to attempt a second splinting. If this fails to restore distal function, transport immediately. Do not try to straighten angulation of the humerus if there are any signs of fracture or dislocation of the shoulder or elbow.

SPLINTING ARM AND ELBOW INJURIES

NOTE: Assess distal pulse, motor function, and sensation both before and after immobilizing or splinting an extremity.

The elbow is a joint and not a bone. It is composed of the distal humerus and the proximal ulna and radius, forming a hinge joint. You will have to decide if the injury is truly to the elbow. The location of deformity and tenderness will direct you to the injury site.

Care: If there is a distal pulse, the dislocated elbow should be immobilized in the position in which it is found. The joint has too many nerves and blood vessels to risk movement. When a distal pulse is absent, make one attempt to slightly reposition the limb after contacting medical direction. Do not force the limb into anatomical position.

Elbow in or Returned to Bent Position

▲ **1.** Move the limb only if necessary for splinting or if pulse is absent. STOP if you meet resistance or significantly increase the pain.

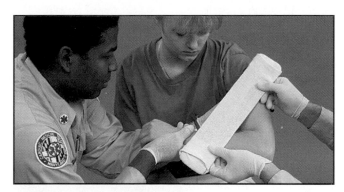

▲ **2.** Use a padded board splint that will extend 2 to 6 inches beyond the arm and wrist when placed diagonally.

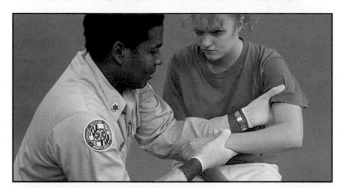

▲ **3.** Place the splint so it is just proximal to the elbow and wrist. Use cravats to secure it to the forearm, then the arm.

▲ **4.** A wrist sling can be applied to support the limb. Keep the elbow exposed. Apply a swathe if possible.

(continued)

Elbow in a Straight Position

▲ **1.** Assess distal pulse, motor function, and sensation (PMS).

▲ **2.** Use a padded board splint that extends from under the armpit to a point past the fingertips. Pad the armpit.

▲ **3.** Place a roll of bandages in the patient's hand to help maintain position of function. Place padded side of board against medial side of limb. Pad all voids.

▲ **4.** Secure the splint. Leave the patient's fingertips exposed.

▲ **5.** Place pads between patient's side and the splint.

▲ **6.** Secure splinted limb to body with two cravats. Avoid placing the cravats over suspected injury site. Reassess distal pulse, motor function, and sensation (PMS).

SPLINTING
FOREARM, WRIST, AND HAND

NOTE: Assess distal pulse, motor function, and sensation both before and after immobilizing or splinting an extremity.

Signs:

- *Forearm*. Deformity and tenderness. If only one bone is broken, deformity may be minor or absent.
- *Wrist*. Deformity and tenderness.
- *Hand*. Deformity and pain. Dislocated fingers are obvious.

Care: Injuries occurring to the forearm, wrist, or hand can be splinted using a padded rigid splint that extends from the elbow past the fingertips. The patient's elbow, forearm, wrist, and hand all need the support of the splint. Tension must be provided throughout the splinting. A roll of bandage should be placed in the hand to ensure the position of function. After rigid splinting, apply a sling and swathe.

Alternative Care: Injuries to the hand and wrist can be cared for with soft splinting by placing a roll of bandage in the hand to maintain position of function, then tying the forearm, wrist, and hand into the fold of one pillow or between two pillows. An injured finger can be taped to an adjacent uninjured finger or splinted with a tongue depressor. Some emergency department physicians prefer that care be limited to a wrap of soft bandages. *Do not* try to "pop" dislocated fingers back into place.

APPLYING AN AIR SPLINT

NOTE: Assess distal pulse, motor function, and sensation both before and after immobilizing or splinting an extremity.

▲ **1.** Slide the inflated splint up your forearm, well above the wrist. Use this same hand to grasp the hand of the patient's injured limb as though you were going to shake hands and apply steady tension.

▲ **2.** While you support his arm, your partner gently slides the splint over your hand and onto the patient's injured limb. The lower edge of the splint should be just above his knuckles. Make sure the splint is free of wrinkles.

▲ **3.** Continue to support the arm while your partner inflates the splint by mouth to a point where you can make a slight dent in the plastic when you press it with your thumb.

▲ **4.** Continue to assess distal pulse, motor function, and sensation (PMS).

WARNING Air-inflated splints may leak. When applied in cold weather, an inflatable splint will expand when the patient is moved to a warmer place. Variations in pressure also occur if the patient is moved to a different altitude. Frequently monitor the pressure in the splint with your fingertip. Air-inflated splints may stick to the patient's skin in hot weather.

PREPARING THE FERNOTRAC TRACTION SPLINT

NOTE: Assess distal pulse, motor function, and sensation (PMS) both before and after immobilizing or splinting an extremity.

Ischial pad

Ischial (pubic or groin) strap

Support straps (4)

Collett sleeve (locking device)

Ankle strap with Velcro®

Bend

Traction ratchet

O- or D-ring

Velcro® Fastener strap

Traction strap

S-hook

Heel stand

▲ Fernotrac Traction Splint.

▲ **1.** Loosen the sleeve locking device.

▲ **2.** Place the splint next to uninjured leg, ischial pad next to iliac crest.

▲ **3.** Hold top and move bottom until bend is at heel.

▲ **4.** Lock sleeve.

(continued)

▲ **5.** Open support straps.

Ischial strap
Top strap
Above knee
Below knee
Mid calf

▲ **6.** Place straps under splint.

▲ **7.** Release ischial strap. Attached ends should be next to ischial pad.

▲ **8.** Pull release ring on ratchet and . . .

▲ . . . Release the traction strap.

▲ **9.** Extend and position heel stand after splint is in position under patient.

Note: Traction splints vary depending on the manufacturer. Some splints in use are measured by placing the ring at the level of the bony prominence that can be felt in the middle of each buttock (ischial tuberosity) and the distal end of the splint placed 8 to 10 inches beyond the foot. Learn to use the equipment supplied in your area and keep up to date with new equipment as it is approved for use.

TRACTION SPLINTING

NOTE: Assess distal pulse, motor function, and sensation both before and after immobilizing or splinting an extremity.

▲ **1.** Some systems attach the ankle hitch prior to applying manual traction (tension). EMT-B #1 should apply the hitch while EMT-B #2 stabilizes the patient's limb.

▲ **2.** While EMT-B #1 applies manual traction (tension), EMT-B #2 can position the splint. Note . . .

▲ . . . Some systems allow manual traction to be applied by grasping the D-ring and ankle.

▲ **3.** EMT-B #1 maintains manual traction (tension) and lowers the limb onto the cradles of the splint.

(continued)

597

▲ **4.** While EMT-B #1 maintains manual traction, EMT-B #2 applies padding to the groin area before securing the ischial strap. Note: Some EMS systems do not apply padding in order to reduce slippage.

▲ **5.** EMT-B #2 secures the ischial strap.

▲ **6.** EMT-B #2 connects the ankle hitch to the windlass and tightens the ratchet to equal manual traction (tension).

▲ **7.** EMT-B #2 secures the cradle straps.

APPLYING THE SAGER TRACTION SPLINT

NOTE: Assess distal pulse, motor function, and sensation both before and after immobilizing or splinting an extremity.

▲ **1.** Place the splint medially.

▲ **2.** The length of the splint should be from groin to 4 inches below the heel. Unlock clasp to extend splint.

▲ **3.** Secure thigh strap.

▲ **4.** Wrap ankle harness above ankle (malleoli) and secure it under heel.

▲ **5.** Release lock and extend splint to achieve desired traction (in pounds on pulley wheel).

▲ **6.** Secure straps at thigh, lower thigh and knee, and lower leg. Strap ankles and feet together. Secure patient to spine board.

APPLYING THE KENDRICK TRACTION DEVICE

NOTE: Assess distal pulse, motor function, and sensation both before and after immobilizing or splinting an extremity.

▲ Components of the Kendrick traction device

▲ **1.** Apply ankle hitch snugly just above the ankle.

▲ **2.** Apply thigh strap with traction pole receptacle at belt line or pelvic crest.

▲ **3.** Size pole so that one section extends beyond the patient's foot.

▲ **4.** Insert pole ends into traction pole receptacle.

▲ **5.** Secure elastic strap around knee.

▲ **6.** Apply traction by pulling red tab.

▲ **7.** Apply elastic straps over thigh and lower leg.

▲ **8.** Secure patient's torso and traction splint to long board for transport.

TWO-SPLINT METHOD—BENT KNEE

NOTE: Assess distal pulse, motor function, and sensation (PMS) both before and after immobilizing or splinting an extremity.

If there is a distal pulse and nerve function, or the limb cannot be straightened without meeting resistance or causing severe pain, knee injuries should be splinted with the knee in the position in which it is found.

▲ **1.** Assess distal PMS function.

▲ **2.** Stabilize the knee above and below the injury site.

▲ **3.** Place the padded side of the splints next to the injured extremity. Note that they should be equal in length and extend 6-12 inches beyond the mid thigh and mid calf.

▲ **4.** Place a cravat through the knee void and tie the boards together.

▲ **5.** Using a figure-eight configuration, secure one cravat to the ankle and the boards, the second cravat to the thigh and the boards. Reassess distal PMS function.

ONE-SPLINT METHOD–STRAIGHT KNEE

NOTE: Assess distal pulse, motor function, and sensation both before and after immobilizing or splinting an extremity.

▲ **1.** Assess distal PMS function.

▲ **2.** Stabilize. The padded board splint should extend from buttocks to 4 inches beyond heel.

▲ **3.** Maintain stabilization and lift limb.

▲ **4.** Place splint along posterior of limb.

▲ **5.** Pad the voids.

▲ **6.** Use a 6-inch roller bandage or cravats to secure injured leg to splint.

(continued)

▲ **7.** Place folded blanket between legs, groin to feet.

▲ **8.** Tie thighs, calves, and ankles together. Do not tie the knot over the injured limb.

▲ **9.** Reassess distal PMS function.

▲ **10.** Provide emergency care for shock, and continue to administer high-concentration oxygen.

▲ **11.** Monitor distal pulse and vital signs.

TWO-SPLINT METHOD—STRAIGHT KNEE

NOTE: Assess distal pulse, motor function, and sensation both before and after immobilizing or splinting an extremity.

▲ **1.** Stabilize the injured limb, and assess distal PMS function.

▲ **2.** Measure the padded board splints, medial from groin, lateral from iliac crest, both to 4 inches beyond foot.

▲ **3.** Position the splints.

▲ **4.** Pad the groin.

▲ **5.** Secure splints at thigh, above and below knee, and at mid calf. Pad all voids.

▲ **6.** Cross and tie two cravats at the ankle or hitch the ankle.

NOTE: Reassess distal PMS function, care for shock, and provide high-concentration oxygen.

TWO-SPLINT METHOD—LEG INJURIES

NOTE: Assess distal pulse, motor function, and sensation both before and after immobilizing or splinting an extremity.

▲ **1.** Measure the splints. They should extend above the knee and below the ankle.

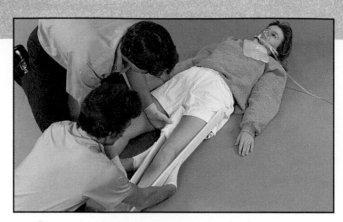

▲ **2.** Apply manual traction (tension) and place one splint medially and one laterally. Padding is toward the leg.

▲ **3.** Secure splints, padding voids.

▲ **4.** Reassess distal PMS function.

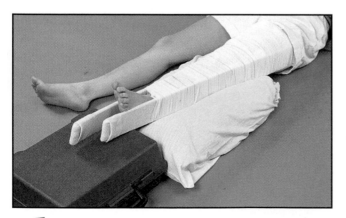

▲ **5.** Elevate the immobilized limb.

▲ **6.** Provide emergency care for shock, and administer high-concentration oxygen. Transport on a long spine board.

ONE-SPLINT METHOD–LEG INJURIES

NOTE: Assess distal pulse, motor function, and sensation both before and after immobilizing or splinting an extremity.

▲ **1.** Measure splint, which should extend from mid thigh to 4 inches below ankle.

▲ **2.** Apply manual traction (tension), and lift limb 10 inches off ground.

▲ **3.** Place splint along the posterior of the limb, from mid thigh.

▲ **4.** Secure the splint to the injured leg.

NOTE: Reassess distal PMS function. Elevate the injured limb, care for shock, and continue to administer a high concentration of oxygen.

STREET SCENES

You and your crew arrive for duty at the firehouse when you are called out for a "fall injury." A police unit is already on scene. They inform you that it is safe. Exiting your engine and taking BSI precautions, you observe a tall woman in her 20s in jogging clothes, leaning on the front hood of a car. She is wincing. The police officer standing next to her approaches and introduces you to your patient.

"How're you doing?" you ask. "My name's Len."

"Hi Len, I'm Desta," she replies.

Your initial assessment reveals that Desta has a good airway and that she is breathing fine. "What happened, Desta, and why did you call EMS this morning?"

"I fell off that wall while trying to climb over it," she answers, simultaneously pointing to a 4-foot rock wall approximately 100 feet away. "When I landed, I heard something crack in my right leg. I hopped on one foot to this car, and called for help." You quickly make a mental note that the surface she landed on is asphalt.

STREET SCENE QUESTIONS

1. What priority would you assign to this patient? Why?

2. How would you continue your assessment?

Desta's mental status seems normal. There are no signs of bleeding anywhere on her body. You assign a low priority to her, and continue your assessment by performing a focused history and physical exam. Desta tells you that she is taking no medications. You ask if she has any allergies and she replies smiling, "Rock walls, apparently." She laughs, then suddenly grimaces in pain as she unintentionally shifts her weight onto her right leg.

Baseline vitals are obtained and you learn Desta's pulse is 88 and regular, respirations are 16 and unlabored, and blood pressure is 108/72. Her pupils are equal and reactive. She states she has no pain anywhere but in her lower right leg.

STREET SCENE QUESTIONS

3. What signs might you expect to find with a broken long bone?

4. What are your major concerns with possible broken bones in the extremities?

You assist Desta from her standing position onto your cot, carefully supporting her right leg. Then you expose the extremity. About 2 inches above the ankle, you observe swelling and a noticeable, unnatural curve to her leg. The skin is not broken. You are concerned that she might have nerve and muscle damage below the injury, but she is able to move her toes and feel you touch her foot. You also detect a pulse below the injury site.

STREET SCENE QUESTIONS

5. What interventions are appropriate for this patient?

PATIENT NAME: Modesta Salerno   **PATIENT AGE:** 24

CHIEF COMPLAINT

Pain in lower right extremity

PAST MEDICAL HISTORY

- [x] None
- [ ] Allergy to _____
- [ ] Hypertension
- [ ] Seizures
- [ ] COPD
- [ ] Other (List)
- [ ] Stroke
- [ ] Diabetes
- [ ] Cardiac
- [ ] Asthma

Current Medications (List)

_____

VITAL SIGNS

TIME	RESP	PULSE	B.P.	MENTAL STATUS	R PUPILS L	SKIN
0630	Rate: 16 [x] Regular [ ] Shallow [ ] Labored	Rate: 88 [x] Regular [ ] Irregular	108 / 72	[x] Alert [ ] Voice [ ] Pain [ ] Unresp.	[x] Normal [x] / [ ] Dilated [ ] / [ ] Constricted / [ ] Sluggish / [ ] No-Reaction	[x] Unremarkable [ ] Cool [ ] Pale [ ] Warm [ ] Cyanotic [ ] Moist [ ] Flushed [ ] Dry [ ] Jaundiced
0640	Rate: 16 [x] Regular [ ] Shallow [ ] Labored	Rate: 86 [x] Regular [ ] Irregular	108 / 72	[x] Alert [ ] Voice [ ] Pain [ ] Unresp.	[x] Normal [x] / [ ] Dilated [ ] / [ ] Constricted / [ ] Sluggish / [ ] No-Reaction	[x] Unremarkable [ ] Cool [ ] Pale [ ] Warm [ ] Cyanotic [ ] Moist [ ] Flushed [ ] Dry [ ] Jaundiced
	Rate: [ ] Regular [ ] Shallow [ ] Labored	Rate: [ ] Regular [ ] Irregular	/	[ ] Alert [ ] Voice [ ] Pain [ ] Unresp.	[ ] Normal [ ] Dilated [ ] Constricted [ ] Sluggish [ ] No-Reaction	[ ] Unremarkable [ ] Cool [ ] Pale [ ] Warm [ ] Cyanotic [ ] Moist [ ] Flushed [ ] Dry [ ] Jaundiced

NARRATIVE

Upon arrival, noted a 24-year-old female patient leaning back onto the hood of a car. States she attempted to climb over an approximately 4-foot rock wall when she fell, landing on an asphalt surface. She states she heard a "crack" as she landed. Focused physical exam reveals no bleeding. Trauma isolated to lower right tibia/fibula. Noted swelling and tenderness, as well as an unnatural curve to extremity approximately 2 inches above ankle. Good pulse, motor function, and sensation before and after application of full-leg air splint. No change noted during transport.

A member of your crew brings a splint, which provides immobilization in the joint above and below the injury site. You maintain manual traction, being careful not to move the extremity unnecessarily, and apply the splint. After application, the patient states the leg feels more secure. You reassess her vitals as well as pulses, motor function, and sensation below the injury site. Everything appears to be normal. During transport, you continue to check distal pulses, motor function, and sensation on the affected extremity. Transport to the hospital is uneventful.

CHAPTER REVIEW

Summary

Injuries to bones and joints should be splinted prior to moving the patient. If life-threatening injuries exist, address them first and, if the patient is a high priority for transport, immobilize the whole patient on a long spine board. When time and the patient's condition permit, proper splinting of a bone or joint injury can prevent further damage to soft tissues, organs, nerves, and muscles, and it can keep a closed injury from becoming an open one. It also can help to control the pain and bleeding associated with the injury, and prevent permanent damage or disability.

Key Terms

bones hard but flexible living structures that provide support for the body and protection to vital organs. Types of bones are long, short, flat, and irregular. The typical long bone has a cylindrical shaft and a rounded end or *head,* which is connected to the shaft by the *neck.*

cartilage tough tissue that covers the joint ends of bones and helps to form certain body parts such as the ear.

closed extremity injury an injury to an extremity with no associated opening in the skin.

crepitus (KREP-i-tus) a grating sensation or sound made when fractured bone ends rub together.

dislocation the disruption or "coming apart" of a joint.

extremities (ex-TREM-i-teez) the portions of the skeleton that include the clavicles, scapulae, arms, wrists, and hands (upper extremities) and the pelvis, thighs, legs, ankles, and feet (lower extremities).

fracture (FRAK-cher) any break in a bone.

joints places where bones articulate, or meet.

ligaments connective tissues that connect bone to bone.

manual traction the process of applying tension to straighten and realign a fractured limb before splinting. Also called *tension.*

muscles tissues or fibers that cause movement of body parts and organs.

open extremity injury an extremity injury in which the skin has been broken or torn through from the inside by an injured bone or from the outside by something that has caused a penetrating wound with associated injury to the bone.

sprain the stretching and tearing of ligaments.

strain muscle injury resulting from over-stretching or over-exertion of the muscle.

tendons tissues that connect muscle to bone.

traction splint a special splint that applies constant pull along the length of a lower extremity to help stabilize the fractured bone and to reduce muscle spasm in the limb. Traction splints are used primarily on femoral shaft fractures.

Review Questions

1. Describe the basic anatomy of bone and its purposes. (pp. 565, 567)
2. Identify the signs and symptoms of musculoskeletal injury. (p. 573)
3. Describe basic emergency care for painful, swollen, deformed extremities, including general guidelines for splinting long bones and joints. (pp. 573–576)
4. Explain why angulated deformed injuries to the long bones should be realigned to anatomical position. (p. 574)
5. List the basic principles of splinting. (p. 575)
6. Describe the hazards of splinting. (p. 576)
7. Describe the basic types of splints carried on ambulances. (p. 575)

APPLICATIONS

- A hiker drives his boot under an old tree root and is tossed head over heels down the slope of a small hill. When he finally comes to rest, his left leg is bent below the knee at an unusual angle. Your initial assessment shows an alert adult male, guarding a grossly deformed left leg. He hasn't lost consciousness and has no other pain. You find he has a strong radial pulse, normal skin, and no bleeding. How should you proceed?

WEB MEDIC

Visit Brady's *Emergency Care* website for direct weblinks. At **www.bradybooks.com/ emergencycare**, you will find information related to the following Chapter 28 topics:

- Bone injuries

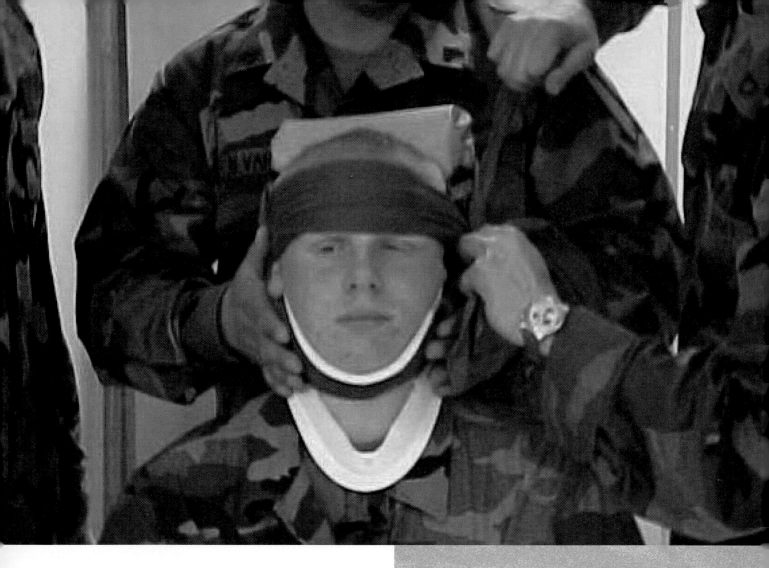

Chapter
Twenty-Nine

INJURIES TO THE HEAD AND SPINE

*W*ord on the Street

"The best care that can be provided to a head- or spine-injured patient by an EMT-B is proper stabilization and immobilization of the spine. I am hindered by poor technique, if I arrive on scene and have to do the backboarding all over again before I can start my advanced treatment or move the patient up the embankment or down the stairs. Improper spinal immobilization hinders care, creates longer scene and transport times, and can permanently paralyze a patient. Learning good habits now and insisting on them from your partners will positively impact your patients, your provider service, and your advanced care partners."

Heather Davis MS, NREMT–P, EMS Educator

You have probably noticed that throughout the earlier chapters of this book, there have been many cautions for patients with possible injuries to the head and spine. This is because injuries to these areas are extremely serious and may result in severe permanent disability or death if improperly treated or missed during your assessment. Second only to proper assessment and care of the ABCs, proper assessment and care for head and spine injuries will be your most important responsibility as an EMT-B.

NERVOUS AND SKELETAL SYSTEMS

The following segments briefly review the anatomy of the nervous system, head, and spine. For more information, review Chapter 4, "The Human Body."

Nervous System

The major components of the **nervous system** are the brain and the spinal cord. The nervous system provides overall control of thought, sensations, and motor functions. The skeletal system provides support and protection. The skull protects the brain, while the bones of the spine protect the spinal cord (Figure 29-1). Whenever the skull or the spine is injured, suspect nervous system damage as well.

The nervous system (Figure 29-2) is divided into two sub-systems: the central nervous system and the peripheral nervous system. The **central nervous system** consists of the brain and the spinal cord. The **peripheral nervous system** includes the pairs of nerves that enter and exit the spinal cord between each pair of vertebrae, the 12 pairs of cranial nerves that travel from the brain without passing through the spinal cord, and all of the body's other motor and sensory nerves. (See Figure 29-3.)

Messages from the body to the brain are carried by sensory nerves. Messages from the brain to the muscles are carried by motor nerves. These nerves control voluntary movements, or those we consciously control such as running or grasping. As the nerves exit the brain, prior to traveling down the spinal cord, they cross over to the opposite side of the body. This is why an injury to the left side of the brain may produce effects such as weakness or lack of sensation on the right side of the body.

Some nerves control involuntary functions—those we do not consciously control—including heartbeat, breathing, control of the diameter of your vessels, control of the round sphincter muscles closing your bladder and bowel, and digestion. These nerves are part of the **autonomic nervous system** (autonomic means automatic).

The brain is the master organ of life. Messages from all over the body are received by the brain, which determines the body's response. The brain sends messages to the muscles so that we can move, or to a particular organ so that it will carry out a desired function. (For example, it may tell the adrenal gland to dump epinephrine into the blood stream, which increases heart rate.) Any major head injury can damage the brain, causing vital body functions to fail.

The spinal cord is a relay between most of the body and the brain. A large number of the messages to and from the brain are sent through the spinal cord. Damage to the cord can isolate a part of the body from the brain. Function of this region can be lost, possibly forever.

TOPIC OVERVIEW

In this chapter, you will learn about the following topics:

- Identification of mechanisms of head and spine injury

- Stabilization of the cervical spine

- Application of a cervical spine immobilization device

- How and when to perform a rapid extrication

- Immobilization using short and long backboards

- Procedures for helmet removal

DOT OBJECTIVES

The healing power of nerve tissue is limited. This is especially true in certain areas. If nerve tissue in the brain or spinal cord is damaged, to a certain extent function is lost and cannot be restored. As an EMT-B, your initial care will often prevent additional damage to the brain, spinal cord, and major nerves of the body.

Anatomy of the Head

The skull is made up of the **cranium** and the facial bones (Figure 29-4). The cranium is the portion of the skull that encloses the brain. It is formed by the forehead, top, back, and upper sides of the skull. The cranial floor is the inferior wall of the brain case,

Figure 29-1 Enhanced color spinal cord.

23. Explain the preferred methods to remove a helmet. (pp. 638, 642)

24. Discuss alternative methods for removal of a helmet. (pp. 638, 642) (Scan 29-6, pp. 643–644)

25. Describe how the patient's head is stabilized to remove the helmet. (pp. 643–644)

26. Differentiate how the head is stabilized with a helmet compared to without a helmet. (pp. 643–644)

27. Explain the rationale for immobilization of the entire spine when a cervical spine injury is suspected. (pp. 623–624)

28. Explain the rationale for utilizing immobilization methods apart from the straps on the cot. (pp. 623, 634, 642) (Scan 29-7, p. 645)

29. Explain the rationale for utilizing a short spine immobilization device when moving a patient from the sitting to supine position. (pp. 626, 630, 633)

30. Explain the rationale for utilizing rapid extrication approaches only when they indeed will make the difference between life and death. (pp. 626, 630, 633)

31. Defend the reasons for leaving a helmet in place for transport of a patient. (pp. 638, 642)

32. Defend the reasons for removal of a helmet prior to transport of a patient. (pp. 638, 642)

✔ Skills

1. Demonstrate opening the airway in a patient with suspected spinal cord injury.

2. Demonstrate evaluating a responsive patient with a suspected spinal cord injury.

3. Demonstrate stabilization of the cervical spine.

4. Demonstrate the four person log roll for a patient with a suspected spinal cord injury.

5. Demonstrate how to log roll a patient with a suspected spinal cord injury using two people.

6. Demonstrate securing a patient to a long spine board.

7. Demonstrate using the short board immobilization technique.

8. Demonstrate the procedure for rapid extrication.

9. Demonstrate preferred methods for stabilization of a helmet.

10. Demonstrate helmet removal techniques.

11. Demonstrate alternative methods for stabilization of a helmet.

12. Demonstrate completing a prehospital care report for patients with head and spinal injuries.

---

the bony floor beneath the brain. The cranial bones are fused together to form immovable joints.

There are 14 irregularly shaped bones forming the face. The facial bones are fused into immovable joints, except for the **mandible.** It joins on each side of the cranium with a **temporal bone** to form the **temporomandibular joint.** This joint is sometimes referred to as the TM joint.

The upper jaw is made up of two fused bones called the **maxillae.** Each is known as a *maxilla.* The upper third, or bridge, of the nose contains two **nasal bones.** There is a cheek bone on each side of the skull. The cheek bone can be called the **malar** or the *zygomatic* bone. The malars and the maxillae form a portion of the **orbits** (sockets) of the eyes.

The brain is held within the skull. The spinal cord exits the base of the brain and leaves the skull through a large hole where the spinal column is attached. The brain is bathed in a fluid called **cerebrospinal fluid (CSF).** This fluid also circulates down the spine around the spinal cord.

Anatomy of the Spine

The spine is made up of 33 irregularly shaped bones, called **vertebrae** (singular *vertebra*), which sit one on top of another to form the spinal column. Each vertebra has a **spinous process,** a bony bump you can feel on a person's back. Every vertebra has a hollow space like the hole in a donut. These hollow spaces form a channel that runs the length of the spinal column and contains the spinal cord, which is cushioned by the cerebrospinal fluid.

The vertebrae are divided into five areas (shown in Figure 29-5). From top to bottom, they are: 7 cervical (in the neck), 12 thoracic (to which the ribs attach), 5 lumbar (mid back), 5 sacral (lower back), and 4 coccygeal (in the coccyx, or tailbone). Both the sacral and coccygeal vertebrae are fused together, forming the posterior portion of the pelvis.

INJURIES TO THE BRAIN AND SKULL

Scalp Injuries

The scalp has many blood vessels, so any scalp injury may bleed profusely. Control bleeding with direct pressure. Dress and bandage as you would other soft-tissue injuries. Be careful about applying direct pressure when there is a possible skull injury. Do not apply pressure if the injury site shows bone fragments or depression of the bone or if the brain is exposed. Instead, use a loose gauze dressing.

Skull Injuries

Skull injuries include fractures to the cranium and the face. If severe enough, there can also be injuries to the brain.

Skull injuries can be either open or closed. With most injuries, the words *open* and *closed* refer to

THE NERVOUS SYSTEM

CENTRAL NERVOUS SYSTEM
Controls all basic bodily functions, and responds to external changes

PERIPHERAL NERVOUS SYSTEM
Provides a complete network of motor and sensory nerve fibers connecting the central nervous system to the rest of the body

Figure 29-2 Nervous system.

Figure 29-3 The neuron is the specialized nerve cell that transmits the nervous system impulses throughout the body.

jury is open or closed. It is safest to assume that there may be an open head injury beneath any contusion or laceration of the scalp.

Brain Injuries

Brain injuries can be classified as direct or indirect. Direct injuries to the brain can occur in open head

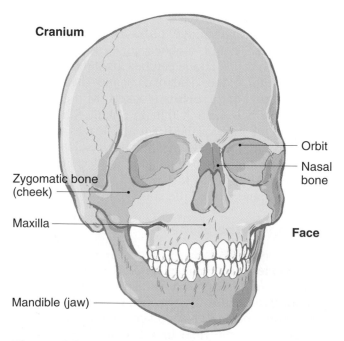

Figure 29-4 Skull: cranium and face.

whether or not the skin and its underlying tissues have been broken. With head injuries, the words *open* and *closed* refer to the cranial bones. When the bones of the cranium are fractured, and the overlying scalp is lacerated, the patient has an *open head injury.* If the scalp is lacerated but the cranium is intact, it is considered to be a *closed head injury.* In practice, you may not be able to determine if a head in-

Figure 29-5 Divisions of spinal column.

Cervical

Thoracic

Lumbar

Sacral

Coccyx

injuries, with the brain being lacerated, punctured, or bruised by the broken bones or by foreign objects. Indirect injuries to the brain may occur with either closed or open head injuries. In an indirect injury, the shock of impact on the skull is transferred to the brain. Indirect injuries to the brain include concussions and contusions.

 Note

> Whenever you suspect skull or brain injury, also suspect spine injury.

Patient *ASSESSMENT*

Skull Fractures and Brain Injuries

The signs of skull fracture and of brain injury are very similar, as listed below (Figure 29-6):

- Visible bone fragments and perhaps bits of brain tissue are the most obvious signs of skull fracture, but most skull fractures do not produce these signs.
- Altered mental status. Check mental status by using the AVPU scale (alert, responsive to verbal stimulus, responsive to painful stimulus, unresponsive). If the patient is alert, check for orientation to person, place, and time. Some EMS agencies also use the Glasgow Coma Scale (discussed later).
- Deep laceration or severe bruise or hematoma to the scalp or forehead. Do not probe or separate the wound opening to determine wound depth.
- Depressions or deformity of the skull, large swellings ("goose eggs"), or anything unusual about the shape of the cranium

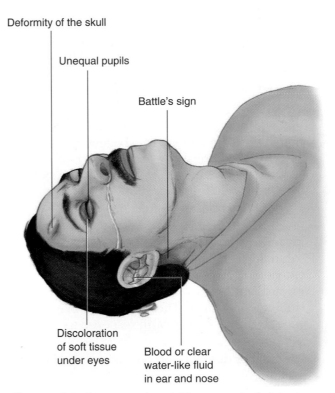

Deformity of the skull

Unequal pupils

Battle's sign

Discoloration of soft tissue under eyes

Blood or clear water-like fluid in ear and nose

Figure 29-6 Signs of cranial fracture or brain injury.

- Severe pain at the site of a head injury. Pain may range from a headache to severe discomfort. Do not palpate the injury site with your fingertips as you may push bone fragments into the injury.
- "Battle's sign," a bruise behind the ear
- Pupils unequal or unreactive to light (Figure 29-7)
- "Raccoon eyes," black eyes, or discoloration of the soft tissues under both eyes
- One eye that appears to be sunken
- Bleeding from the ears and/or nose
- Clear fluid flowing from ears and/or nose
- Personality change, ranging from irritable to irrational behavior (a major sign)
- Increased blood pressure and decreased pulse rate (Cushing's syndrome)

Figure 29-7 Unequal pupils.

- Irregular breathing patterns
- Temperature increase (late sign due to inflammation, infection, or damage to temperature-regulating centers)
- Blurred or multiple-image vision in one or both eyes
- Impaired hearing or ringing in the ears
- Equilibrium problems. The patient may be unable to stand still with his eyes closed or may stumble when attempting to walk. (Do not test for this.)
- Forceful or projectile vomiting
- Posturing. The patient may exhibit neurological posturing, such as flexing arms and wrists and extending legs and feet (decorticate posture) or extending arms with the shoulders rotated inward and wrists flexed, legs extended (decerebrate posture). These postures may be assumed spontaneously or in response to a painful stimulus.
- Paralysis or disability on one side of the body
- Seizures
- Deteriorating vital signs

Note that shock (hypoperfusion) from blood loss is generally not a sign of head injury, except in infants. There simply is not enough room within the adult skull to permit enough bleeding to cause shock. If there is head injury with shock, look for indications of blood loss somewhere else on the body.

With so many factors to consider, possible skull or brain injury can be very difficult to determine definitively. Therefore, assume skull or brain injury when the mechanism of injury and the location of the injury indicate a possible head injury.

✋ Note

Some of the signs of brain injury can mimic intoxication from alcohol or the effects of other drugs. Never assume intoxication or drug abuse without assessment.

⬤ Patient *CARE*

Skull Fractures and Brain Injuries

Emergency care of a patient with skull fractures and brain injuries include the following:

1. Take appropriate BSI precautions.

2. Assume spine injury. Provide manual stabilization of the head on first patient contact, and use the jaw-thrust maneuver to open the airway. For the unconscious patient, insert an oropharyngeal airway without hyperextending the neck. Have suctioning equipment ready, since these patients are prone to vomiting.

3. Monitor the conscious patient for changes in breathing. Provide artificial ventilations, if breathing is inadequate.

4. Apply a rigid cervical collar, immobilize the neck and spine and, if appropriate, determine the method of extrication, either normal or rapid (discussed later in this chapter).

5. Administer high-concentration oxygen by nonrebreather mask, and evaluate the need for artificial ventilations with supplemental oxygen. This is critical should there be any brain damage. In some EMS systems, if the patient shows signs of a brain injury (such as, increased blood pressure with decreased pulse, altered mental status), EMT-Bs are instructed to hyperventilate the patient with supplemental oxygen at the rate of at least 25 ventilations per minute. Hyperventilation will help reduce brain tissue swelling by lowering carbon dioxide levels and raising oxygen levels. Follow your local protocol.

6. Control bleeding. Do not apply direct pressure if the injury site shows bone fragments or depression of the bone or if the brain is exposed. Do not attempt to stop the flow of blood or cerebrospinal fluid from the ears or the nose. If the skull is fractured, you may increase intracranial pressure and the risk of infection. Instead, use a loose gauze dressing.

7. Keep the patient at rest. This can be critical.

8. Talk to the conscious patient, providing emotional support. Ask the patient questions so that he will have to concentrate. This procedure also will help you to detect changes in the patient's mental status.

9. Dress and bandage open wounds. Stabilize any penetrating objects. (Do not remove any objects or fragments of bone.)

10. Manage the patient for shock even if signs of shock are not yet present. However, do not elevate the legs unless signs of shock are present and your local protocols permit. Avoid overheating.

11. Be prepared for vomiting. Have a suction unit ready for use.

12. Transport the patient promptly.

13. Monitor vital signs every 5 minutes en route to the hospital.

If you are not certain of the severity of the patient's injuries, or if there is evidence of cervical-spine injury, or if the patient with a head injury is unconscious, then the patient must be immobilized to a long spine board. With the entire head, neck, and body rigidly immobilized, the patient may be rotated into a lateral recumbent position so that blood and saliva can drain freely. If the patient vomits, the vomitus is less likely to cause an airway obstruction or be aspirated (breathed into the lungs). Some patients with a head injury will vomit without warning. Many vomit without first experiencing nausea. If injuries prevent such positioning, constant monitoring and frequent suctioning are required.

Types of Brain Injuries

As an EMT-B, you do not need to understand brain injuries in order to assess and care for your patient, but the following will provide some background information on brain injuries.

A **concussion** (Figure 29-8) may be so mild that the patient is unaware of the injury. When a person strikes his head in a fall, or is struck by a blunt object, a certain amount of the force is transferred through the skull to the brain. Usually there is no detectable damage to the brain and the patient may or may not become unconscious. Most patients with a concussion will feel a little "groggy" after receiving a blow to the head. Headache is common. If there is a loss of consciousness, it usually lasts only a short time and does not tend to recur. Sometimes, after a head blow, bystanders will say the patient "just sat there staring off into space for a few minutes." Some loss of memory (amnesia) of the events surrounding the accident is fairly common. A common saying is that the fighter did not see the punch that did him in. Actually, he probably did see the punch but then forgot it. However, long-term memory loss associated with concussion is rare.

A bruised brain, or **contusion,** can occur with closed head injuries, when the force of the blow is great enough to rupture blood vessels on or within the brain. A contusion is often caused by a collision or blow that causes the brain to hit the inside of the skull, bounce off the opposite side, and then rebound to strike the first side of the skull again. When the bruising of the brain occurs on the side of the blow, it is called a *coup;* when it occurs on the side opposite the blow, it is called a *contrecoup.*

A laceration, or cut, to the brain can occur from the same forces that might cause a contusion. The inner skull has many sharp, bony ridges that can lacerate a moving brain. A laceration or a puncture wound can also be caused by an object penetrating the cranium.

A **hematoma** is a collection of blood within tissue. A hematoma inside the cranium is named according to its location. It may be located inside or outside the dura, the brain's protective outer covering (Figure 29-9), or within the brain itself. A *subdural hematoma* is a collection of blood between the brain and the dura. An *epidural hematoma* is blood between the dura and the skull. An *intracerebral hematoma* occurs when blood pools within the brain (Figure 29-10).

Head injury is made worse by several problems. There is limited room for expansion inside the hard skull. When a hematoma develops, pressure inside the skull increases, making it difficult for normal blood flow to enter the head. To meet this challenge, the blood pressure is forced to increase. As a result of decreased blood flow, the brain becomes starved for oxygen and high in waste carbon dioxide, causing even more swelling. Finally, head injury may cause decreased respiratory effort, which further worsens oxygen starvation and swelling in the brain.

CONCUSSION
• Mild injury, usually with no detectable brain damage
• May have brief loss of consciousness
• Headache, grogginess, and short-term memory loss common

CONTUSION
• Unconsciousness or decreased level of responsiveness
• Bruising of brain tissue

Figure 29-8 Closed head injuries.

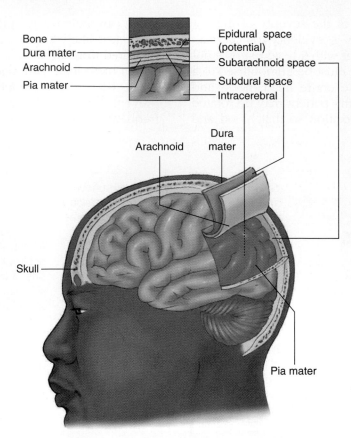

Figure 29-9 Meninges (covering layers) of the brain.

CRANIAL HEMATOMAS

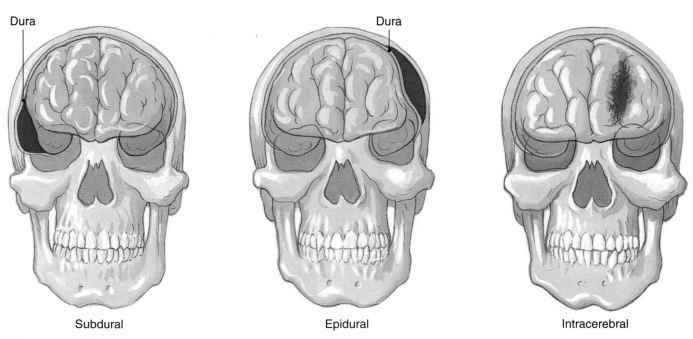

Subdural   Epidural   Intracerebral

Figure 29-10 Hematomas within the cranium.

GLASGOW COMA SCALE

All head-injury patients must be constantly monitored during transport. Be prepared in case the patient vomits or has a seizure.

What you observe and report can have a great bearing on the initial actions that will be taken by the emergency department staff. The early signs of deterioration are subtle changes in mental status that may be overlooked if you are not watching for them.

Some EMS agencies use the Glasgow Coma Scale (GCS) (Figure 29-11), in addition to AVPU, for ongoing neurological assessment. Some systems would immediately transport a patient with a GCS score of 8 or less directly to the trauma center if they are within 30 minutes transport time. When using this score, keep the following considerations in mind:

• *Eye opening.* Spontaneous eye opening means that the patient opens his eyes without your having to do anything. If his eyes are closed, say "Open your eyes" to see if he will obey. Try a normal level of voice. If this fails, shout the command. Should the patient's eyes remain closed, apply an accepted painful stimulus (such as pinch a toe, scratch the palm or sole, rub the sternum). Note any eye injuries or injuries to the face that prevent the patient from opening the eyes. If the injuries are more than minor ones, do not ask the patient to open his eyes.

• *Verbal response.* When evaluating the patient's verbal responses, use the following criteria:

– *Oriented.* The patient, once aroused, can tell you who he is, where he is, and the day of the week. A person who can answer all three of these questions appropriately is said to be alert on the AVPU scale.

– *Confused.* The patient cannot answer the above questions, but he can speak in phrases and sentences.

– *Inappropriate words.* The patient says or shouts a word or several words at a time. Usually this requires physical stimulation. The words do not fit the situation or a particular question. Often, the patient curses.

– *Incomprehensible sounds.* The patient responds with mumbling, moans, or groans.

– *No verbal response.* Repeated stimulation, verbal and physical, does not cause the patient to speak or make any sounds.

• *Motor response.* The following are the criteria used to evaluate motor response:

– *Obeys command.* The patient must be able to understand your instruction and carry out the request. For example, you may ask the patient (when appropriate) to hold up two fingers.

– *Localizes pain.* Should the patient fail to respond to your commands, apply pressure to one of the nail beds for 5 seconds or firm pressure to the sternum. Note if the patient attempts to remove your hand. Do not apply pressure over an injury site. Do not apply pressure to the sternum if the patient is experiencing difficulty breathing.

– *Withdraws,* after painful stimulation. Note if the elbow flexes, if the patient moves slowly, if there is the appearance of stiffness, if he holds

GLASGOW COMA SCALE

Eye Opening	Spontaneous	4	
	To Voice	3	
	To Pain	2	
	None	1	
Verbal Response	Oriented	5	
	Confused	4	
	Inappropriate Words	3	
	Incomprehensible Sounds	2	
	None	1	
Motor Response	Obeys Command	6	
	Localizes Pain	5	
	Withdraw (pain)	4	
	Flexion (pain)	3	
	Extension (pain)	2	
	None	1	
Glasgow Coma Score Total			

TOTAL GLASGOW COMA SCALE POINTS	CONVERSION = APPROXIMATELY ONE-THIRD TOTAL VALUE
14-15=5	
11-13=4	
8-10=3	
5-7=2	
3-4=1	

| **Neurologic Assessment** | |

Figure 29-11 Glasgow Coma Scale.

his forearm and hand against the body, or if the limbs on one side of the body appear to be paralyzed (hemiplegic position).

– *Posturing,* after painful stimulation. Note if the legs and arms extend, if there is apparent stiffness with these moves, and if there is an internal rotation of the shoulder and forearm.

– *No motor response to pain.* Repeated painful stimulation does not cause the patient to grimace or make any motions.

Note: Do not spend time at the scene calculating a GCS score unless your system requires it.

Cranial Injuries with Impaled Objects

If there is an object impaled in the cranium, do not remove it. Instead, stabilize the object in place with bulky dressings. (See information on stabilizing impaled objects in Chapter 27, "Soft-Tissue Injuries.") This, with care in handling, will minimize accidental movement of the object.

A lengthy impaled object can make transporting the patient impossible until the object is cut or shortened. Pad around the object with bulky dressings, then carefully (and rigidly) stabilize the object on both sides of where the cut will be made. Cutting should be done with a tool that will not cause the object to move or vibrate when it is finally severed. A hand hacksaw with a fine-tooth blade can be carefully controlled and produces only a small amount of heat. In any case in which you may have to cut an impaled object, seek advice from medical direction or the emergency department physician.

Injuries to the Face and Jaw

Facial fractures are usually caused by an impact, as when a child is struck in the face by a baseball bat or when someone is thrown against a windshield. Bone fragments may lodge in the back of the pharynx and cause airway obstruction. So may blood, blood clots, dislodged teeth, or a separated palate. Signs of a facial fracture are shown in Figure 29-12.

The mandible is subject to dislocation as well as to fracture. As with any facial injury, there may be pain, discoloration, swelling, and facial distortion. In addition, when the mandible is injured or dislocated, the patient may be unable to move the lower jaw or may have difficulty speaking. There may be an improper alignment of the upper and lower teeth and bleeding around the teeth.

The primary concern with facial fractures is the patient's airway (Figure 29-13). Be prepared to suction to remove debris and blood from the airway. Because of possible spinal injury, use the jaw-thrust maneuver to open the airway. Control profuse bleeding. (See Chapter 27, "Soft-Tissue Injuries," for care of an object impaled in the cheek.) Apply a rigid collar and immobilize the patient on a spine board. If possible, position the patient for drainage from the mouth. Care for shock.

Remember

The face is part of the skull. Brain injury may accompany a blow of sufficient force to

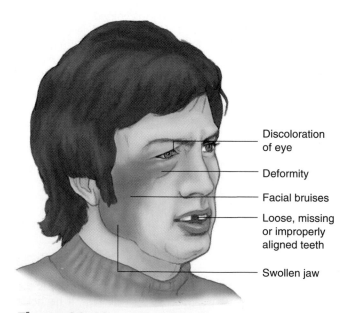

Discoloration of eye

Deformity

Facial bruises

Loose, missing or improperly aligned teeth

Swollen jaw

Figure 29-12   Signs of facial fracture.

KEEP AIRWAY OPEN AND STOP BLEEDING

FORCE

Bone fractures cause airway obstruction

Blood clots, bone fragments, and teeth form obstructions.

Figure 29-13   Complications of facial fracture.

the face. Treat this patient as you would any patient with a suspected skull or brain injury.

Nontraumatic Brain Injuries

Many of the signs of brain injury may be caused by an internal brain event such as a hemorrhage or blood clot. (See the information on stroke in Chapter 19.) The signs of nontraumatic (not caused by external trauma) brain injury will be the same as those for a traumatic injury, except that there will be no evidence of trauma and no mechanism of injury.

INJURIES TO THE SPINE

Injuries to the spine must be considered whenever there is serious trauma to any part of the body. Spine injury can be associated with head, neck, and back injuries—and also with chest, abdominal, and pelvic injuries. Even injuries to the upper and lower extremities can be caused by forces intense enough to also produce spine injury.

As an EMT-B, you should "uptriage," or overtreat, patients with potential spine injuries because you cannot rule out a spine injury in the field and because the costs in terms of pain, suffering, disability, and dollars are very high when a spine-injured patient is unintentionally made worse by failure to immobilize the spine.

Injuries to the spinal column include fractures with and without bone displacement, dislocations, muscular strains, and disk injury including compression. The vertebral column may be injured without damage to the spinal cord or spinal nerves. For example, a fractured coccyx is below the level of the spinal cord. Muscular strains are relatively simple injuries. However, when displaced fractures or dislocations occur, the cord, disk, and spinal nerves may be severely injured.

Mechanisms of Injury

A simple rule of thumb is: If the mechanism of injury exerts great force on the upper body (Figure 29-14) or if there is any soft-tissue damage to the head, face, or neck due to trauma (such as from being thrown against a dashboard), assume possible cervical-spine injury. Any blunt trauma above the clavicles may damage the cervical spine.

Some parts of the spine are more susceptible to injury than others. Because it is somewhat splinted by the attached ribs, the thoracic spine is not usually damaged except in the most violent accidents or in gunshot wounds. The pelvic-sacral spine attachment helps to protect the sacrum in the same way. However, the cervical and lumbar vertebrae are suscepti-

Figure 29-14   Mechanisms of injury to the upper body.

ble to injury because they are not supported by other bony structures.

The spine is most often injured by compression or excessive flexion, extension, or rotation from falls, diving accidents, and motor-vehicle collisions. Spine injuries in EMS workers often result from not adhering to the proper lifting techniques, causing lateral bending or disk injuries. When the spine is excessively pulled, it can cause a "distraction" injury. This is the mechanism of spine injury that occurs in a hanging. Years ago, rescuers were taught to pull traction on the neck of an injured patient sitting in an automobile. This actually had the potential to cause injury, so today EMT-Bs are taught to manually stabilize the head and neck, or hold it still.

Maintain a high degree of suspicion of a potential spine injury when your patient is a victim of a motor-vehicle or motorcycle collision, was struck by a vehicle, received blunt injury to the spine or above the clavicles, was involved in a diving accident, was found hanging by his neck, or was found unconscious due to trauma.

HOW AND WHY?

Injuries to the spine can cause paralysis. But have you ever wondered why some spine injuries cause paralysis and others do not? Go to your Electronic Extras CD for more information.

The adult skull weighs more than 17 pounds and rests on a very small area of the cervical spine (like a pumpkin on a broom handle). Motor-vehicle collisions produce violent whiplash injuries because of the speed and sudden deceleration of the vehicle (Figure 29-15). When a vehicle strikes another vehicle or a fixed object head on, the neck can whip quickly back and forth. The vehicle decelerates abruptly, but the head continues to travel forward at the same speed that the vehicle was traveling, even though the body is held by seat restraints. This neck movement may exceed the normal range of motion. Virtually the same thing occurs when the vehicle is struck from behind.

A fall can generate enough force to fracture or dislocate vertebrae. Assume that any fall three times the patient's height or with enough force to cause open fractures to the ankles will also be accompanied by a spine injury. Needless disability has been caused when head injuries or other injuries resulting from a fall were noted and cared for but spinal injuries were overlooked.

Today more and more people are participating in sports of all kinds: in-line skating, mountain biking, surfing, rock climbing, and others too numerous to mention. Many sports accidents can cause spine injury. A sledding or skiing accident can hurl a person into a tree or other fixed object, twisting or compressing the spinal column. There may be no open wound or fracture of an extremity, or signs of injury may be hidden by bulky clothing. As a result, improper care may be rendered as the victim with a possible spinal injury is placed on a stretcher without adequate examination and immobilization.

Diving accidents often produce injury to the cervical spine. When the diver strikes the diving board, the side or bottom of the pool, or an underwater object, the head can be severely forced beyond its normal limits of motion (flexion, extension, or compression). Cervical vertebrae may be fractured or dislocated, ligaments may be severely sprained, and the spinal cord may be compressed or otherwise traumatized in the cervical region and at other spots along the cord.

Football and other contact sports can cause accidents severe enough to produce spinal injury. Spear tackling, using the head, has been outlawed in grade schools and high schools for a number of years due to the incidence of cervical compression fractures. Whenever a game involves player contact or falling to the ground, be on the alert for spinal injury.

Patient ASSESSMENT

Spinal Injury

The most common causes of spinal-cord injury are motor-vehicle collisions, falls, diving accidents, and gunshot wounds. You must do a complete assessment of the patient. Assume that all unconscious trauma patients have spinal injury.

Geriatric Notes

Keep in mind that fractured spines in the elderly are often caused by falls or spontaneous fractures of brittle bones that, in turn, cause falls.

Whenever in doubt, assume that there are spine injuries and immobilize torso, head, and neck. Signs and symptoms of spine injury include:

- *Paralysis of the extremities.* PARALYSIS OF THE EXTREMITIES IS PROBABLY THE MOST RELIABLE SIGN OF SPINAL-CORD INJURY IN CONSCIOUS PATIENTS.

- *Pain without movement.* The pain is not always constant and may occur anywhere from the top of the head to the buttocks. Pain in the leg is common for certain types of injury to the lower spine. Other painful injuries can mask this symptom of spinal injury.

- *Pain with movement.* The patient normally tries to lie perfectly still to prevent pain. Do not ask the patient to move just to determine if it will cause pain. However, if the patient complains of pain in the neck or back experienced with voluntary movements, including spinal pain with

Figure 29-15 Usually, whiplash is caused by a poorly adjusted or absent head rest during a rear-end collision.

movement in apparently uninjured shoulders and legs, this is a good indicator of possible spinal injury.

- *Tenderness anywhere along the spine.* Gentle palpation of the injury site, when accessible, may reveal point tenderness.

The above signs and symptoms are reliable indicators of possible spinal injury in the conscious patient. If any one of them is present, you have sufficient reason to immobilize the patient. In the field, it is not possible to rule out spinal injury even when the patient has no pain and is able to move his limbs. The mechanism of injury alone may be the deciding factor. Additional signs of spinal injury may include:

- *Impaired breathing.* Watch the patient breathe. If there is only a slight movement of the abdomen, with little or no movement of the chest, it is safe to assume that the patient is breathing with the diaphragm alone (diaphragmatic breathing). This is also true if there is a reversal of normal breathing patterns with the rib cage collapsing on inspiration and rising on expiration. Damage to the nerves that control the movement of the rib cage can cause this breathing pattern. The nerves that control the diaphragm are located high in the cervical area and are often unharmed, but the intercostal (between-the-ribs) nerves that control the chest muscles are often damaged in cervical and thoracic injuries. As a result, when the diaphragm moves downward to pull in air, the ribs, instead of expanding, collapse. When the diaphragm relaxes and air is expelled, the rib cage rises—the opposite of the normal pattern.

  Impaired breathing is characteristic of spinal-cord injury. Check abdominal movement from the side by placing your hand on the patient's abdomen and looking for reversed movements during respiration. Panting due to respiratory insufficiency may develop.

- *Deformity.* Removing clothing to check for deformity of the spine is not recommended. OBVIOUS SPINAL DEFORMITIES ARE RARE. However, if you note a gap between the spinous processes (bony extensions) of the vertebrae, or if you can feel a broken spinous process, you must consider the patient to have serious spinal injuries. It is also possible to feel tight muscles in spasm.

- *Priapism.* Persistent erection of the penis is a sign of spinal injury affecting nerves to the external genitalia.

- *Posturing.* In some cases of spinal injury, motor-nerve pathways to the muscles that extend the arm can be interrupted, but those that lead to the muscles that bend the elbow and lift the arm remain functional. The patient may be found on his back, with the arms extended above the head, which may indicate a cervical-spine injury. Arms flexed across the chest or extended along the sides with wrists flexed also signals spinal injury.

- *Loss of bowel or bladder control* may indicate spinal injury.

- *Nerve impairment to the extremities.* The patient may experience loss of use, weakness, numbness, tingling, or loss of feeling in the upper and/or lower extremities—especially below the suspected level of the injury.

- *Severe spinal shock.* This kind of shock (neurogenic shock) can be caused by the failure of the nervous system to control the diameter of blood vessels. The pulse rate may be normal because a message to "speed up" the heart may be prevented from getting to the heart due to the cord injury.

- *Soft-tissue injuries associated with trauma.* Traumatic soft-tissue injuries to the head and neck may signal injury of the cervical spine. Traumatic soft-tissue injuries to the shoulders, back, or abdomen may signal injury of the thoracic or lumbar spine. Traumatic soft-tissue injuries to the lower extremities may signal injury of the lumbar or sacral spine.

Remember

The ability to walk, move the extremities, feel sensation, or a lack of pain in the spinal area does not rule out the possibility of spinal-column or spinal-cord injury.

Assessment strategies for a responsive patient with suspected spinal injury include the following:

- Ascertain the mechanism of injury.
- Ask these questions (and tell the patient not to move while answering):
  - What happened?
  - Where does it hurt? Does your neck or back hurt?
  - Can you move your hands and feet?
  - Can you feel me touching (lightly) your fingers? Your toes?
  - Do you feel "pins and needles" (tingling) in your legs? Anywhere?
- Inspect for contusions, deformities, lacerations, punctures, penetrations, swelling.
- Palpate for tenderness or deformity.

- Assess equality of strength in the extremities by checking hand grip or pushing against the patient's hands and feet.

  Assessment strategies for an unresponsive patient with suspected spinal injury include the following:

- Ascertain from bystanders the mechanism of injury and information about the patient's mental status prior to your arrival.
- Inspect for contusions, deformities, lacerations, punctures, penetrations, swelling.
- Palpate for area of tenderness (some unresponsive patients will withdraw from or react to pain) or deformity.

Note: Do not spend much time trying to rule out spinal injury in an unresponsive patient. If there is a mechanism of injury associated with spinal injury, immobilize the patient and treat as if there is a spinal injury.

● Patient *CARE*

Spinal Injury

Regardless of where the apparent spinal injury is located on the cord, care is the same. Perform the initial assessment and rapid trauma exam and determine the patient's priority, since this will be important in deciding how to immobilize him (Figure 29-16).

For all patients with possible spinal injury, and for all accident victims when there is doubt as to the extent of injury, emergency care includes the following:

1. Provide manual in-line stabilization for the head and neck on first patient contact. Place the head in a neutral in-line position unless the patient complains of pain or the head is not easily moved into that position. If that is the case, steady the head in the position found. Maintain manual stabilization until the patient is properly secured to a backboard.

2. Assess airway, breathing, and circulation. If necessary, open and control the airway with the jaw-thrust maneuver, maintaining in-line stabilization of the head.

3. In your rapid trauma exam, assess the head and neck, then apply a rigid cervical collar. Make sure the collar is properly sized. A wrong-size collar may do more harm than good by hyperextending the neck if too large or allowing flexion if too small. Also make sure the collar is not applied in a way that will obstruct the airway. Maintain manual stabi-

lization even after the collar is in place until the patient is secured to a backboard, since no collar completely restricts motion.

● Pediatric Notes

For an infant or child, be sure to use a pediatric-sized collar. If you do not have the right pediatric size, use a rolled towel, maintaining manual support of the infant's or child's head.

4. Quickly assess sensory and motor function in all four extremities if the patient is responsive.

5. Based on the patient's priority, apply the appropriate spinal immobilization device at the appropriate speed. (Scans 29-1 through 29-8 are provided in this chapter in order to demonstrate the proper procedure to use based upon the condition of the patient and the position in which the patient is found.)

6. If the patient has paralysis or weakness of the extremities, administer high-concentration oxygen via nonrebreather mask and evaluate the need for artificial ventilations with supplemental oxygen. This is critical should there be any cord damage.

7. Reassess sensory and motor function in all four extremities if the patient is responsive.

▌IMMOBILIZATION ISSUES

Tips for Applying a Cervical Collar

Cervical spine immobilization devices, or rigid extrication collars, are designed to limit flexion, extension, and lateral movement when combined with an immobilization device such as a long backboard or a vest-style device. Even though there have been marked improvements in collars, there is still no collar that completely eliminates movement of the spine. For this reason, when applying a collar, always manually maintain the neck and head in a neutral position in alignment with the rest of the body.

Review the information on manual stabilization in Chapter 8 and on cervical-collar sizing and application in Chapter 10.

Tips for Immobilizing a Seated Patient

When a patient is found in a sitting position, you will need to decide his priority. If the patient is stable and a low priority, use the normal procedure for spinal immobilization as shown in Scan 29-1. In such situations, where time is not of the essence, the patient must be secured to a short spine board or extrication

EXTRICATION AND IMMOBILIZATION PROCEDURE DECISIONS

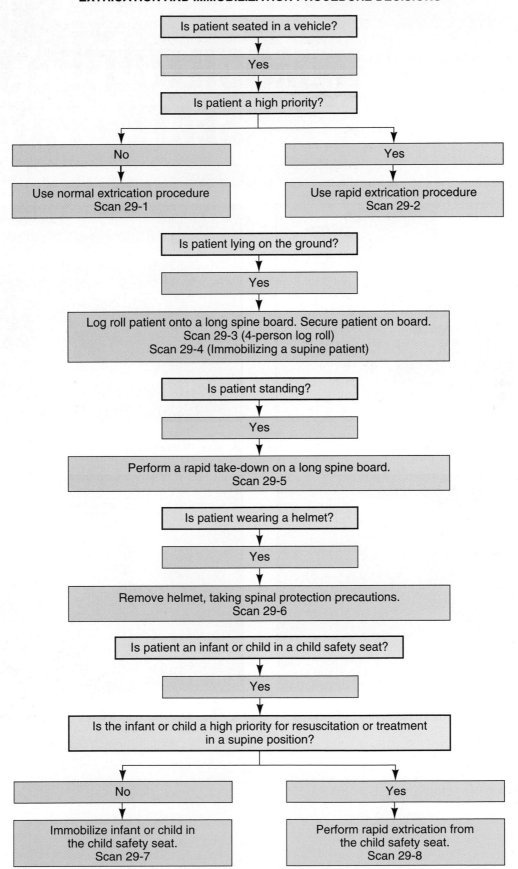

Figure 29-16 Choose appropriate extrication and immobilization procedures.

SPINAL IMMOBILIZATION OF A SEATED PATIENT

FIRST take BSI precautions.

▲ **1.** Select an immobilization device.

▲ **2.** Manually stabilize patient's head in neutral, in-line position.

▲ **3.** Assess distal pulse, motor function, and sensation (PMS).

▲ **4.** Apply the appropriately sized extrication collar.

(continued)

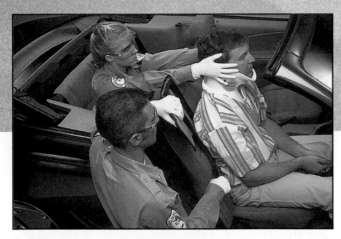

▲ **5.** Position immobilization device behind patient.

▲ **6.** Secure device to patient's torso.

▲ **7.** Evaluate and pad behind patient's head as necessary. Secure patient's head to device.

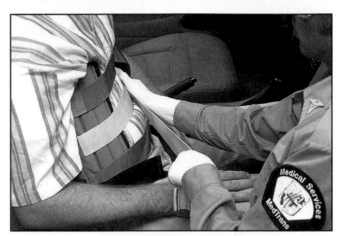

▲ **8.** Evaluate and adjust straps. They must be tight enough so device does not move up, down, left, or right excessively, but not so tight as to restrict patient's breathing.

▲ **9.** As needed, secure patient's wrists and legs.

▲ **10.** Reassess distal pulse, motor function, and sensation (PMS), and transfer the patient to the long board.

vest that will immobilize the head, neck, and torso until he can be transferred to a long spine board.

In high-priority situations when there is not enough time to apply a short board or extrication vest—or if the patient must be moved rapidly because of dangers at the scene or to provide access to other potentially more seriously injured patients—the patient should be immobilized manually while moving him onto the long spine board. This rapid extrication technique is shown in Scan 29-2.

The normal extrication technique is as follows: The patient's head and neck are manually stabilized during initial assessment. After the head and neck are assessed in the rapid trauma exam, a rigid collar is applied. Then the patient is secured to a short spine board or extrication vest.

A short spine board (Figure 29-17) is just a shortened version of a long spine board. It is the original extrication device and has been used for many years. It is used less frequently now, because today's contoured automobile seat backs do not accommodate a flat board. Also, the short spine board is often too wide and too high to be used effectively in a small car.

A vest-style extrication device (such as the one shown in Figure 29-18) is a flexible piece of equipment useful for immobilizing patients with possible injury to the cervical spine. It can be used when the patient is found in a bucket seat, in a short compact car seat, in a seat with a contoured back, or in a confined space. It is also useful when the short spine board cannot be inserted into a car because of obstructions. A number of commercial vest-style extrication devices such as the KED, Kansas Backboard, XP-1, and LSP Halfback Vest, are available. Use the devices approved by your EMS system.

A particular sequence must be followed in all applications, whether of a short spine board or a flexible extrication device. That sequence is: secure the torso first and the head last. This assures greater sta-

Figure 29-18   Ferno KED (Kendrick Extrication Device).

bility during the strapping process and may help prevent compression of the cervical spine. If the patient has suffered abdominal injuries or displays diaphragmatic breathing that prevents adequate securing of the torso, the torso straps will still be needed but care must be taken so as not to interfere with breathing.

There are a number of special considerations when applying a short board to the patient:

- Assessment of the back, shoulder blades, arms, or collarbones must be done before the device is placed against the patient.
- The EMT-B applying the board must angle it, without striking or jarring, to fit between the arms of the rescuer who is stabilizing the head from behind the patient.
- To provide full cervical support, the uppermost holes must be level with the patient's shoulders. The base of the board should not extend past the coccyx.
- Never place a chin cup or chin strap on the patient, which can prevent him from opening his mouth if he has to vomit.
- Avoid applying the first torso strap too tightly. This could aggravate an abdominal injury or limit respirations for the diaphragmatic breathing patient.
- Some buckles have quick-release mechanisms. Be careful not to accidentally loosen these buckles when moving the patient.
- Do not pad between collar and board. This will create a pivot point that may cause the hyperextension of the cervical spine when the head is secured. Instead, pad the occipital region, but only enough to fill any void. This will help keep the head in a neutral position. Sometimes when the shoulders are rolled back to the board, the head will come back to the board far enough so padding is not needed. Never use excessive

Figure 29-17   Short spine board.

RAPID EXTRICATION PROCEDURE FOR HIGH-PRIORITY PATIENTS ONLY

Note: In the photos, the roof of the vehicle has been removed to allow for easier illustration of the positions of the EMT-Bs. In most cases, this procedure will be done and should be practiced with the roof intact.

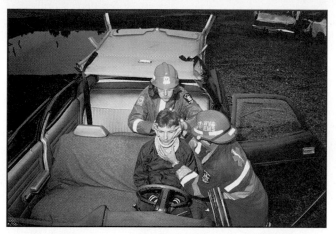

▲ **1.** Manually stabilize the patient's head and neck and have a second EMT-B apply a cervical collar.

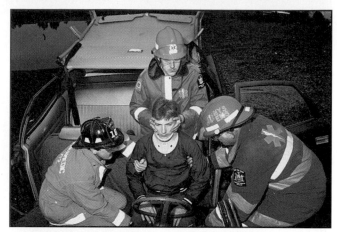

▲ **2.** At the direction of the EMT-B stabilizing the head and neck, two EMT-Bs each lift the patient by the armpits and buttocks/thighs just enough for a bystander or additional rescuer to slide a long spine board between the patient and the vehicle seat.

▲ **3.** The EMT-Bs reposition their hands so the EMT-B on the front seat inside the vehicle holds the patient's legs and pelvis, while the EMT-B outside the vehicle holds the upper chest and arms.

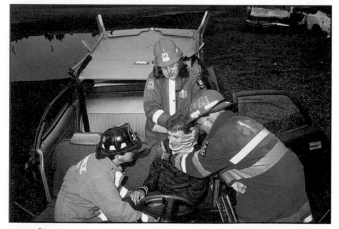

▲ **4.** At the direction of the EMT-B holding the head and neck, carefully turn the patient a quarter turn so his back is facing the side door of the vehicle.

(continued)

▲ **5.** The EMT-B who was holding the pelvis temporarily holds the chest so the EMT-B who was holding the chest can take over head and neck stabilization. The EMT-B in the back seat can then reach over the seat and assist with the chest, and the EMT-B inside on the front seat can move his hands back to the pelvis.

▲ **6.** At the direction of the EMT-B at the head and neck, gently lower the patient to the spine board. **Note:** Sometimes it may be necessary to move the patient inside the vehicle a few inches so there is ample room to lay him down without touching the upper door opening.

▲ **7.** As a bystander or additional rescuer holds the end of the spine board, the EMT-Bs slide the patient to the head end of the board.

▲ **8.** Quickly apply straps to the patient's chest, pelvis, and legs and remove the patient to a stretcher or the ground, under the direction of the EMT-B stabilizing the head and neck. **Note:** Since the patient's head is not yet fully immobilized (it is only being manually held stable by the EMT-B and collar), DO NOT walk more than a few steps with the patient. Once on stable ground or the stretcher, apply a head immobilizer or blanket roll and wide tape.

▲ As you move the patient from a sitting to a supine position, her spine must not bend, twist, or get jolted. Handle her very gently, and make sure you have enough assistance to perform the move correctly.

Note: The rapid extrication procedure is only for critical or unstable high-priority patients who must be moved in less time than would be required to apply a short spine board or extrication vest inside the vehicle before moving the patient to the long spine board. (Scan 29-1)

Figure 29-19   Seated patient, "packaged."

padding behind the head, because when the patient is placed in a supine position, the shoulders will fall back but the head will not be able to. This will place the patient in an undesirable position of flexion.

- Follow the instructions of the manufacturer of the device you are using.

- After applying the short spine board, the packaging of the patient will be completed as shown in Figure 29-19.

Tips for Applying a Long Backboard

The following tips relate to immobilization of the supine patient:

- You will need to log roll the patient to apply the long backboard (Scans 29-3 and 29-4). This procedure must be done carefully, keeping the spine in alignment. Quickly assess the posterior body before rolling the patient back onto the board.

Whenever a move is done involving neck stabilization, the EMT-B holding the head calls for the move ("We will turn on three: One . . . two . . . three").

- Pad voids between the patient's head and torso and the board. Be careful not to cause extra movement or to move the patient's spine out of alignment.

- When a patient is secured to a long spine board (Figure 29-20), the head is secured last. Strapping is easier with Velcro or speed-clip straps.

- Additional immobilization for the head and neck can be provided with light foam-filled cushions, a

Figure 29-20   Long spine board with head immobilizer.

commercial head immobilization device (such as the Ferno Washington head immobilizer, or Bashaw CID, or the Laerdal Head Bed), or a blanket roll (Figure 29-21). If used, these are applied after securing the patient's body to the long backboard. Secure the head with 3-inch hypoallergenic adhesive tape. The tape offers support, especially if the patient and board are to be tilted to allow for drainage. However, blood on the patient's skin and hair may make using tape impractical. You should learn to use cravats or self-adhering roller bandages as a backup method. Do not tape or tie the cravats across the patient's eyes.

- If the patient is a full-term pregnant woman, after immobilizing on the back board, tilt the board to the left by propping up the right side to minimize the effect of the uterus compressing the vena cava and causing hypotension and dizziness.

- Unless the spine board has straps specifically intended to criss-cross the shoulders and chest, it is

best to strap across the upper chest including the arms, the pelvis excluding the hands, and the thighs. If you will need to stand the patient up to carry him out of a tight building, up a basement stairwell, or into a small elevator, make sure the straps are secure under the arm pits and tight on the thighs.

Pediatric Notes

When immobilizing a 6-year-old or younger child, provide padding beneath the shoulder blades to compensate for the large head. Pad from shoulders to toes as needed to establish a neutral position.

If you do not carry a pediatric long spine immobilization device, then practice immobilizing children using adult equipment and lots of towels or blankets to pad around the child. EMT-Bs are usually very good at improvising. In this case, however, the first time you improvise should be in the classroom so you will be quick in the field!

- If your service transports to a helicopter, make sure that your backboard fits. There are some restrictions on the size or taper of the long backboard, depending on the helicopter's loading configuration, so find this out ahead of time.

- For a water rescue or diving injury there are various specialty backboards, such as the Miller board, that are designed to float up beneath the patient and use Velcro closures for ease of application.

Tips for Dealing with a Standing Patient

When you approach a vehicle and see the tell-tale spider-web-cracked windshield, you know whoever sat behind that crack needs full spinal immobilization. Sometimes this patient is up and walking around at the collision scene. He still has the potential for a spine injury but may not yet have dislocated the fracture or ligament injury site. It would be dangerous to have him sit down or lie down on your long backboard, so instead use a backboard to carefully but rapidly take him down to the supine position without compromising his spine.

Some EMS providers advocate strapping the patient onto the long board while the patient is standing. However, this is often not practical in the field. (It works in the classroom because the simulated patients are not in shock, intoxicated, head injured, combative, or just dizzy!)

The easiest technique is the rapid takedown which, like all skills in this text, should be demonstrated by a qualified instructor and practiced in the classroom prior to use in the field. The procedure

A

B

Figure 29-21 (A) Ferno head immobilizer and (B) disposable head immobilizer.

FOUR-RESCUER LOG ROLL

FIRST take BSI precautions.

▲ **1.** Stabilize the head and neck. Apply a rigid cervical collar.

▲ **2.** Place the board parallel to the patient.

▲ **3.** Have three rescuers kneel at the patient's side opposite the board, leaving room to roll the patient toward them. Place rescuers at the shoulder, waist, and knee. One EMT-B will continue to stabilize the head, while the others reach across the patient to position their hands properly.

▲ **4.** The EMT-B at the head and neck directs the others to roll the patient as a unit.

▲ **5.** The EMT-B at the patient's waist grips the spine board and pulls it into position against the patient. (This can be done by a fifth rescuer.)

▲ **6.** Roll the patient as a unit onto the board.

SPINAL IMMOBILIZATION OF A SUPINE PATIENT

FIRST take BSI precautions.

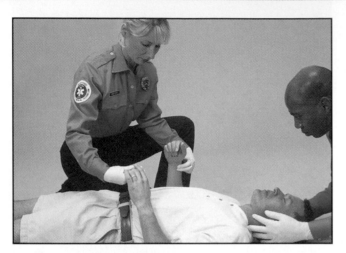

▲ **1.** Place head in neutral, in-line position and maintain manual stabilization of the head and neck. Assess distal pulse, motor function, and sensation (PMS).

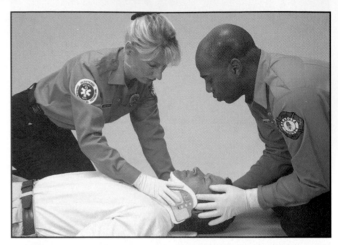

▲ **2.** Apply an appropriately sized rigid cervical collar.

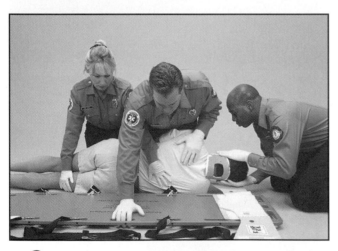

▲ **3.** Position an immobilization device.

▲ **4.** Move patient onto the device without compromising the integrity of the spine. Once the patient is in position, apply padding to voids between torso and board.

▲ **5.** Secure the patient's torso to the board first.

▲ **6.** Then the patient's legs.

▲ **7.** Pad and immobilize the patient's head last.

▲ **8.** Reassess the patient's distal pulse, motor function, and sensation (PMS).

Figure 29-22 Standing takedown at the scene of an emergency.

takes three EMT-Bs, a set of collars, and a long backboard. (See Figure 29-22 and Scan 29-5.)

Patient Found Wearing a Helmet

Helmets are worn in many sporting events and by many motorcycle riders. Even ski resorts are starting to advocate the use of helmets. Sporting helmets are typically open in the front, making it easier to access the patient's airway than with a motorcycle helmet, which has a shield and often a full face section that is not removable.

Face, neck, and spine care and airway management or resuscitation may call for the removal of the helmet, especially if the helmet will prevent you from reaching the patient's mouth or nose. If the helmet is left on, shields can be lifted and face guards removed. One EMT-B must manually steady the patient's head and neck while the other cuts, snaps off, or unscrews the guard. Do not attempt to remove a helmet if doing so causes increased pain, or if the helmet proves difficult to remove, unless there is a possible airway obstruction or ventilatory assistance must be provided. Indications for leaving the helmet in place or for removing the helmet are summarized below:

Indications for Leaving the Helmet in Place
- Helmet fits snugly, allowing little or no movement of the patient's head within the helmet.
- There are absolutely no impending airway or breathing problems nor any reason to resuscitate or hyperventilate the patient.

- Removal would cause further injury.
- Proper spinal immobilization can be done with the helmet in place.
- There is no interference with the EMT-B's ability to assess the airway or breathing.

Indications for Removing the Helmet
- Helmet interferes with ability to assess and manage airway and breathing.
- Helmet is improperly fitted, allowing excessive head movement.
- Helmet interferes with immobilization.
- Cardiac arrest.

Many experienced EMS providers put the controversy of removal versus non-removal into the following perspective: If your child's neck were injured in a football accident, would you want the trainer and the EMT-B to work together carefully to remove the helmet at the scene, or would you prefer this be left to emergency department personnel who probably will not have the help of the trainer nor the benefit of lots of practice in the helmet removal technique?

Note that if a football player is wearing shoulder pads and you remove his helmet, you should either remove the pads or pad behind the head to make up for the fact that his shoulders are off the ground. This will prevent the head from falling into a hyperextended position when the helmet is removed and the head is slowly lowered to the ground.

When a helmet must be removed, it is a two-rescuer procedure, as shown in Scan 29-6.

RAPID TAKEDOWN OF A STANDING PATIENT

FIRST take BSI precautions.

▲ **1.** Position your tallest crew member (EMT-B #1) behind patient and have him manually stabilize the head and neck. His hands should not leave the patient's head until entire procedure is complete and head is secured to the long spine board.

▲ **2.** EMT-B #2 applies a properly sized cervical collar to patient. EMT-B #1 continues manual stabilization (collar aids, but does not replace manual stabilization).

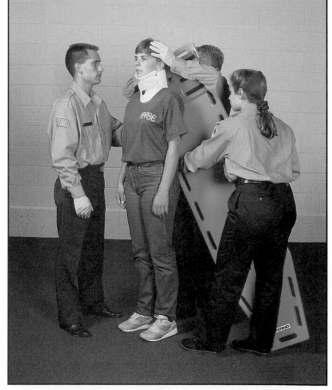

▲ **3.** EMT-B #1 continues manual stabilization, as EMT-B #2 and another rescuer position a long spine board behind the patient, being careful not to disturb EMT-B #1's manual stabilization of patient's head and neck. It will help if EMT-B #1 spreads elbows to give the other rescuers more room to maneuver the spine board.

(continued)

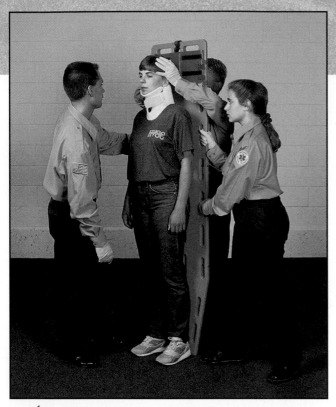

▲ **4.** EMT-B #1 continues manual stabilization. EMT-B #2 looks at the spine board from the front of the patient and does any necessary repositioning to be sure it is centered behind the patient.

▲ **5.** EMT-B #1 continues manual stabilization. EMT-B #2 and third rescuer reach arm that is nearest patient under patient's armpits and grasp the spine board. (Once the board is tilted down, patient will actually be temporarily suspended by armpits.) To keep patient's arms secure, they will use other hand to grasp patient's arm just above elbow and hold it against patient's body.

▲ **6.** EMT-B #2 and third rescuer, when reaching under patient's armpits, must grasp a handhold on the spine board at patient's armpit level or higher.

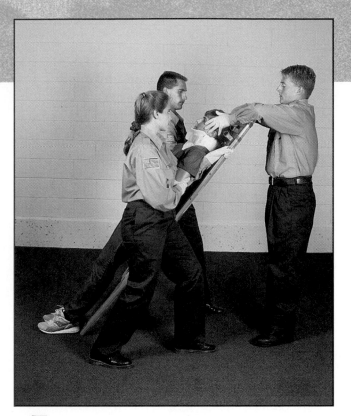

▲ **7.** EMT-B #1 continues manual stabilization. EMT-B #2 and third rescuer maintain their grasp on the spine board and patient. EMT-B #1 explains to patient what is going to happen, then gives signal to begin slowly tilting board and patient to the ground. As board is lowered, EMT-B #1 walks backward and crouches, keeping up with the board as it is lowered and allowing patient's head to slowly move back to the neutral position against the board. EMT-B #1 must accomplish all this without holding back or slowing the lowering of the board. EMT-B #1 may need to rotate somewhat so that, once the board is almost flat, he is holding the head down on the board. Once the patient's head comes in contact with the board, it must not be allowed to leave the board, to avoid flexing the neck. The job of the two rescuers doing the lowering is to control it so that it is slow and even on both sides. They should also move into a squatting position as they lower the board to avoid injuring their backs.

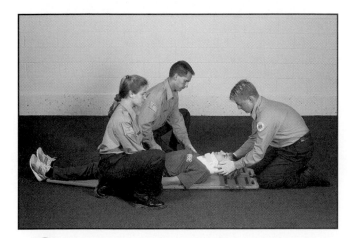

▲ **8.** EMT-B #1 maintains manual in-line stabilization throughout the procedure.

Pediatric Notes

Occasionally, EMT-Bs are confronted at a motor-vehicle collision with an infant or young child who was riding in a child safety seat. Placing a child in a supine position with the legs elevated, as you will need to do if you are going to tip the seat backward and move the child onto a spine board, places a great deal of pressure on the abdominal organs and diaphragm, making respiration difficult. So, provided the patient is not in need of immediate resuscitative measures, or for any other reason needs to be placed in the supine position, it makes sense to let the child remain sitting upright and use the child safety seat as an immobilization device.

The key decision on whether to immobilize the child in the seat or to rapidly remove the child from the seat onto a spine board is based upon the patient's priority and need to be in a supine position.

The procedure for immobilization in the child safety seat is described in Scan 29-7 and the procedure for rapid extrication from the car seat is shown in Scan 29-8.

Documentation Tip— Injuries to the Head and Spine

In documenting a possible head or spine injury, it is critical to note whether the patient lost consciousness, even if only briefly. If the patient did not lose consciousness, be sure to document that fact as a pertinent negative.

Also be sure to document carefully the patient's mental status. If the patient is responsive, note his orientation to person, place, and time. Carefully document any changes in the patient's mental status throughout assessment, treatment, and transport.

REMOVING A HELMET FROM AN INJURED PATIENT

▲ **1.** EMT-B #1 is positioned at the top of the patient's head and maintains manual stabilization. Two hands hold the helmet stable while the fingertips hold the lower jaw.

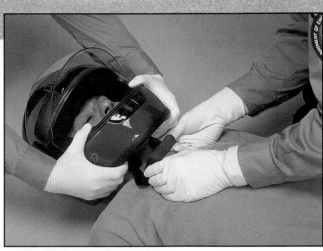

▲ **2.** EMT-B #2 opens, cuts, or removes the chin strap.

▲ **3.** EMT-B #2 then places one hand on the patient's mandible and, using the other hand, reaches in behind the neck and stabilizes the occipital region. Using the combination of the hand in front of the chin and the hand behind the neck, EMT-B #2 should be able to hold the head securely. If the patient has glasses on, they should be removed now, prior to removal of the helmet.

▲ **4.** EMT-B #1 can now release manual stabilization and slowly remove the helmet. The lower sides, or ear cups, of the helmet will have to be gently pulled out to clear the ears.

(continued)

▲ **5.** The helmet should come off straight with no backward tilting. A full-face helmet may need to be tilted just enough for the chin guard to clear the nose. EMT-B #2 must support and prevent the head from moving as the helmet is removed.

▲ **6.** EMT-B #1, after removing the helmet, re-establishes manual stabilization and maintains an open airway by using the jaw-thrust.

Helmet Removal—Alternative Method

▲ **1.** EMT-B #1 applies manual stabilization with the patient's neck in neutral position.

▲ **2.** EMT-B #2 removes the chin strap.

▲ **3.** EMT-B #2 removes the helmet, pulling out on each side to clear the ears.

▲ **4.** EMT-B #1 maintains manual stabilization as EMT-B #2 applies a cervical collar.

Note: If the patient has shoulder pads and you are removing a football helmet, remember to remove the shoulder pads or pad behind the head to keep it aligned with the padded shoulders. With either helmet-removal method, manual stabilization must be maintained until the patient is secured to a long spine board with full immobilization of the head.

IMMOBILIZING IN A CHILD SAFETY SEAT

▲ **1.** EMT-B #1 stabilizes car seat in upright position, applies manual stabilization to the head and neck . . .

▲ . . . as EMT-B #2 prepares equipment, then applies cervical collar, or improvises with rolled hand towel for the newborn or infant.

▲ **2.** As EMT-B #1 maintains manual stabilization, EMT-B #2 places small blanket or towel on child's lap, then straps or uses wide tape to secure pelvis and chest area to seat.

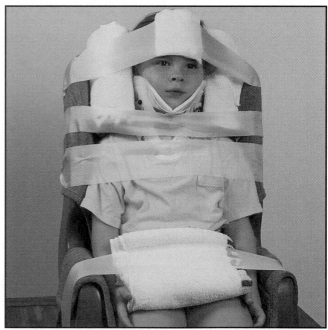

▲ **3.** EMT-B #1 maintains manual stabilization, as patient and seat are carried to ambulance and strapped onto stretcher with stretcher head raised. EMT-B #2 places a towel roll on both sides of head to fill voids, tapes forehead in place, then tapes across collar or maxilla. (Avoid taping chin, which would place pressure on child's neck.)

RAPID EXTRICATION FROM A CHILD SAFETY SEAT

▲ **1.** EMT-B #1 stabilizes car seat in upright position, applies manual stabilization of the head and neck. EMT-B #2 prepares equipment, and then loosens or cuts the seat straps and raises the front guard.

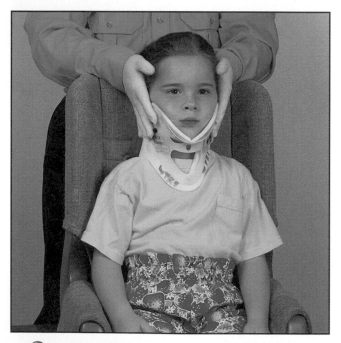

▲ **2.** Cervical collar is applied to patient as EMT-B #1 maintains manual stabilization of the head and neck.

▲ **3.** As EMT-B #1 maintains manual stabilization, EMT-B #2 places child safety seat on center of backboard and slowly tilts it into supine position. EMT-Bs are careful not to let child slide out of chair. For child with large head, place a towel under area where shoulders will eventually be placed on the board to prevent head from tilting forward.

▲ **4.** EMT-B #1 maintains manual stabilization and calls for a coordinated long axis move onto backboard.

▶ **5.** EMT-B #1 maintains manual stabilization, as move onto board is completed, with child's shoulders over the folded towel.

▲ **6.** EMT-B #1 maintains manual stabilization, as EMT-B #2 places rolled towels or blankets on both sides of patient.

▲ **7.** EMT-B #1 maintains manual stabilization, as EMT-B #2 straps or tapes patient to board at level of upper chest, pelvis, and lower legs. DO NOT STRAP ACROSS ABDOMEN.

▲ **8.** EMT-B #1 maintains manual stabilization, as EMT-B #2 places rolled towels on both sides of head, then tapes head securely in place across forehead and maxilla or cervical collar. DO NOT TAPE ACROSS CHIN TO AVOID PRESSURE ON NECK.

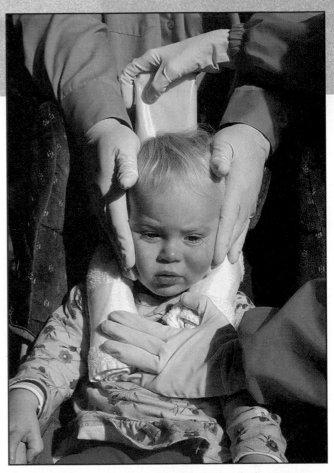

▲ The newborn and infant procedure is exactly the same as for a child, except that an armboard is inserted behind the child in Step 2. If the infant is very small, the armboard may actually be used as the spine board.

You and your partner are dispatched to the city park for a head injury. Arriving on scene, you determine the scene is safe and observe a group of teenage boys huddled around a person who is lying on the ground. Taking BSI precautions, you grab your equipment and approach the patient. Your partner asks, "What happened?"

"We were jumping ramps on our bicycles when Lee tried to do a flip," states one of the boys. "He hit the ground head first. I told that fool he should be wearing a helmet!" You observe a young male lying supine on the asphalt parking lot, eyes closed, with blood oozing from the top of his head from what appears to be an abrasion.

One of the boys identifies himself as Lee's brother and tells you that Lee is 13 years old. He states he lives just around the corner. You ask if his mother is home and he says she is. You ask him to go tell his mother what happened and to come to the park immediately.

STREET SCENE QUESTIONS

1. What is your general impression of this patient?
2. What immediate treatment should be provided?

Your general impression is of an unconscious male with a head and possible spine injury, so your partner provides manual stabilization of the head and neck. Lee's airway is patent, he is breathing normally, and you observe no other bleeding other than the laceration on the top of his head. You decide this is a high-priority trauma patient.

"Lee," you call out. "Lee, can you hear me?"

Lee opens his eyes and asks, "What happened?" Though the patient responds to verbal stimuli, it is apparent that he does not know what happened. He is able to tell you what day it is (Saturday), but not the date.

"Lee, I am going to give you a number to remember. It's number 51. Can you say that?" you ask.

He replies, "51." About this time, Lee's mother arrives. You briefly recount what you know. She seems concerned, but not overly upset. You apply a rigid collar to further restrict the motion of the patient's neck. You learn that Lee is on no medications, has no allergies, and no medical history. He ate lunch two hours before. You obtain baseline vitals and find his pulse is 80 and normal; respirations are 24 and unlabored; BP is 108/74; skin is pink, warm, and dry; and pupils are equal and reactive to light.

STREET SCENE QUESTIONS

3. How should you monitor changing levels of responsiveness in a patient with a head injury?

"Lee, tell me what day it is today. Then tell me that number I asked you to keep in mind," you say.

"Saturday. But what number?" he responds.

You place Lee on a nonrebreather mask at 10 liters per minute, and also apply a loose dressing to the abrasion on his forehead. There is no other sign of injury on his body. Lee denies any neck pain and has good pulses, motor function, and sensation in all extremities.

The fire department rescue squad is now on scene, and they help you restrict motion of the patient's neck and spine by securing Lee to a rigid board. Lee continues to have good pulses, motor function, and sensation in all extremities. When asked to recall the number again, he states, "I think it was 37." You tell him it is "51" and ask him to repeat it. "51," he says.

On-line medical direction has no other orders for you, but tells you to keep an eye on his airway and mental status. You allow his mother to ride in the ambulance with you. You assess vitals once more en route, noting no significant changes. You once again ask Lee what day and what number and this time he looks at you and says "Saturday, and I think it's 51." You tell him he's correct. He groans and states he has a headache. The rest of the transport is uneventful.

PATIENT NAME: *Lee Zhu*   **PATIENT AGE:** *13*

CHIEF COMPLAINT		TIME	RESP	PULSE	B.P.	MENTAL STATUS	R PUPILS L	SKIN
Loss of consciousness	V I T A L	1 8 3 0	Rate: *24* ☒ Regular ☐ Shallow ☐ Labored	Rate: *80* ☒ Regular ☐ Irregular	*108* / *74*	☐ Alert ☑ Voice ☐ Pain ☐ Unresp.	☑ Normal ☑ ☐ Dilated ☐ ☐ Constricted ☐ ☐ Sluggish ☐ ☐ No-Reaction ☐	☑ Unremarkable ☐ Cool ☐ Pale ☐ Warm ☐ Cyanotic ☐ Moist ☐ Flushed ☐ Dry ☐ Jaundiced
PAST MEDICAL HISTORY	S	1 8 3 5	Rate: *24* ☒ Regular ☐ Shallow ☐ Labored	Rate: *83* ☒ Regular ☐ Irregular	*110* / *74*	☐ Alert ☑ Voice ☐ Pain ☐ Unresp.	☑ Normal ☑ ☐ Dilated ☐ ☐ Constricted ☐ ☐ Sluggish ☐ ☐ No-Reaction ☐	☑ Unremarkable ☐ Cool ☐ Pale ☐ Warm ☐ Cyanotic ☐ Moist ☐ Flushed ☐ Dry ☐ Jaundiced
☒ None ☐ Allergy to _____ ☐ Hypertension ☐ Stroke ☐ Seizures ☐ Diabetes ☐ COPD ☐ Cardiac ☐ Other (List) ☐ Asthma	I G N S	1 8 4 0	Rate: *25* ☒ Regular ☐ Shallow ☐ Labored	Rate: *85* ☒ Regular ☐ Irregular	*108* / *76*	☑ Alert ☐ Voice ☐ Pain ☐ Unresp.	☑ Normal ☑ ☐ Dilated ☐ ☐ Constricted ☐ ☐ Sluggish ☐ ☐ No-Reaction ☐	☑ Unremarkable ☐ Cool ☐ Pale ☐ Warm ☐ Cyanotic ☐ Moist ☐ Flushed ☐ Dry ☐ Jaundiced

Current Medications (List) _____

NARRATIVE   *13-year-old male rode bicycle and jumped off ramp approx. 3 feet high at approx. 15 mph; landed on head; no helmet; landed on asphalt surface. Apparent loss of consciousness; responded to verbal; oriented to person, place, and day. Patient given number 51 to recall, but unable to recall that number while on scene. Airway, breathing, and circulation normal. Abrasion noted on forehead approx. 2" above bridge of the nose with minimal bleeding. Patient denies neck and back pain; good pulse/motor function/sensation in all four extremities. Mother arrived on scene approx. 10 minutes post EMS arrival; related history and other pertinent information as well as permission to treat.*

Treatment: manual stabilization of C-spine with rigid collar and full spinal motion restriction; nonrebreather at 10 LPM; vitals; dressing for abrasion; on-line medical direction established; transport uneventful.

Reassess: En route, patient able to recall number 51 for first time; c/o headache. No change.

CHAPTER REVIEW

SUMMARY

It is important to maintain a high index of suspicion for head or spine injury whenever there is a relevant mechanism of injury. When there is a head injury, assume a brain injury as well as a spine injury. Provide high-concentration oxygen, immobilize, and transport.

Assume a spine injury whenever there is a mechanism of injury of sufficient force or an injury to the head, neck, or upper body. Provide manual stabiliza-

tion of the head and neck and apply a cervical collar, continuing manual stabilization until the patient is fully immobilized on a long spine board.

In the event of a suspected head or spine injury, ascertain if there has been a loss of consciousness, however brief, and carefully assess the patient's mental status, including orientation to person, place, and time. Monitor and document any changes in the patient's mental status.

KEY TERMS

autonomic nervous system controls involuntary functions.

central nervous system the brain and the spinal cord.

cerebrospinal (suh-RE-bro-SPI-nal) **fluid (CSF)** the fluid that surrounds the brain and spinal cord.

concussion mild closed head injury without detectable damage to the brain. Complete recovery is usually expected.

contusion in brain injuries, a bruised brain caused when the force of a blow to the head is great enough to rupture blood vessels.

cranium (KRAY-ne-um) the bony structure making up the forehead, top, back, and upper sides of the skull.

hematoma (HE-mah-TO-mah) in a head injury, a collection of blood within the skull or brain.

malar (MAY-lar) the cheek bone, also called the *zygomatic bone.*

mandible (MAN-di-bl) the lower jaw bone.

maxillae (mak-SIL-e) the two fused bones forming the upper jaw.

nasal (NAY-zul) **bones** the bones that form the upper third, or bridge, of the nose.

nervous system provides overall control of thought, sensation, and the voluntary and involuntary motor functions of the body. The major components of the nervous system are the brain and the spinal cord.

orbits the bony structures around the eyes; the eye sockets.

peripheral nervous system the nerves that enter and exit the spinal cord between the vertebrae and the twelve pairs of cranial nerves that travel between the brain and organs without passing through the spinal cord, and all of the body's other motor and sensory nerves.

spinous (SPI-nus) **process** the bony bump on a vertebra.

temporal (TEM-po-ral) **bone** bone that forms part of the side of the skull and floor of the cranial cavity. There is a right and a left temporal bone.

temporomandibular (TEM-po-ro-mand-DIB-yuh-lar) **joint** the movable joint formed between the mandible and the temporal bone, also called the *TM joint.*

vertebrae (VERT-uh-bray) the bones of the spinal column (singular *vertebra*).

REVIEW QUESTIONS

1. Name the two components of the nervous system and discuss their functions. (p. 613)

2. List five signs of a brain injury and explain why mechanism of injury is important in determining possible brain injury. (pp. 616–618)

3. Describe the appropriate emergency treatment of a patient with possible head or brain injury. (pp. 618–619)
4. List five mechanisms of injury that would support suspicion of a spine injury. (pp. 623–624)

5. Describe the appropriate emergency care for a patient with a possible spine injury. (p. 626)

APPLICATIONS

- You are called to the scene of a motor-vehicle collision. After assuring scene safety and taking BSI precautions, you approach the car, which has struck a bridge abutment, and note a deformed steering wheel. The driver's side door is open and, out on the middle of the bridge, you see a person you presume to be the driver wandering erratically toward the opposite side of the bridge. How should you proceed?

WEB MEDIC

Visit Brady's *Emergency Care* website for direct weblinks. At **www.bradybooks.com/ emergencycare**, you will find information related to the following Chapter 29 topics:

- Brain injuries
- Spinal injuries

Chapter
Thirty

PUTTING IT ALL TOGETHER FOR THE TRAUMA PATIENT

*W*ord on the Street

"I remember distinctly the first time I was in charge of a multiple-trauma patient, even though it was more than 20 years ago. I remember the girl's name and age, the bathing suit she was wearing to go swimming in after her senior prom, and the location where her car had rolled several times and ejected her. I remember feeling helpless, because in none of my training had anyone ever described how to handle a patient with multiple injuries. I vowed not to let it happen again and learned all I could about management of patients with multiple trauma."

Mike O'Keefe EMT-P, Textbook Author

In Chapter 7, "Scene Size-up," you learned about mechanism of injury. Although using a mechanism of injury to predict specific injuries is not yet an exact science, you learned that you can still gain important information about the amount of force involved, the directions of those forces, and the obstacles the patient might have struck. This can give you a general indication of the severity of injury to expect.

Then in the last few chapters, you learned how to manage those injuries. In each case, there was an assumption that the patient had *at most* one other problem. (For example, the presence of a head injury would lead you to suspect a spine injury.) This is often true, but not always. Although the number of deaths from vehicular trauma is decreasing, EMT-Bs must be prepared for situations where the patient has multiple injuries, also known as "multiple trauma."

MULTIPLE TRAUMA

The multiple-trauma patient has more than one serious injury. For example, a patient with crush injuries to the chest and a painful, swollen, deformed extremity is a multiple-trauma patient. Although multiple internal organs may be involved, a patient who has a crush injury to the chest, and no other apparent injuries, is not a multiple-trauma patient.

When the mechanism of injury suggests that your patient has more than one injury, decisions beyond what are called for on more typical EMS runs become necessary. For example, consider the patient who is reported to have an angulated forearm: your initial assessment reveals him to be unresponsive with the airway partially occluded by his tongue. Do you spend the time applying a rigid splint to the limb? The answer in this case is no. This patient has life-threatening injuries that can only be treated in a hospital emergency department or operating room. Spending additional time at the scene to treat an injury that is not life threatening may reduce the patient's chances of survival. Now consider an alert patient with no signs or symptoms of shock who has pain and tenderness in the middle of his thigh as well as an angulated forearm? In this case, the patient is stable enough to allow you a few minutes to apply a splint and prevent further injury. In each of these two examples, an EMT's actions should be intended to provide the most benefit to the patient, while at the same time, reducing the risk as much as possible.

These decisions are made easier when your crew works well together, each member knowing what to expect from another. This is called *teamwork*. Crew members also must be aware of the importance of moving a multiple-trauma patient to definitive care as soon as possible, since it is rarely possible for EMS providers (even EMT-Paramedics) to truly stabilize a trauma patient in the field. This is called *timing*. Finally, the appropriate destination must be chosen for the patient—*transport*. In areas where some hospitals are designated trauma centers, it is important that protocols specify which patients need to be taken there and when it is (and is not) appropriate for EMS to bypass another hospital.

Integrating the three "Ts"—*teamwork, timing,* and *transport*—into your management of a multiple-

TOPIC OVERVIEW

In this chapter, you will learn about the following topics:

- How to balance the critical trauma patient's need for prompt transport against the time needed to treat all of the patient's injuries at the scene

- How to select the critical interventions to implement at the scene of a multiple-trauma patient

- How to choose an appropriate destination for a critical trauma patient

*Note: There are no objectives in the
national standard curriculum that
pertain to the material in this chapter.*

trauma patient will help things go smoother and
more efficiently for the patient.

MANAGING THE MULTIPLE-TRAUMA PATIENT

HOW AND WHY?

The mechanism of injury may be used as an indicator of injury potential in a crash. Go to your Electronic Extras CD for information on crash tests done on automobiles at various speeds.

The following scenario describes a typical multiple-trauma call. As you read, ask yourself these questions: When does the EMT-B recognize that the patient has multiple injuries? What is his first decision about managing those injuries, and why do you think he made it? What priorities does he set for his patient?

A Typical Call

You receive a call for a motorcyclist who was hit by a car. The scene is safe, so you approach the patient, an adult male you estimate to be about 25 years old, who appears unresponsive in a pool of blood on the road. Police point about 20 feet away to the motorcycle he was riding.

The patient responds purposefully to a painful stimulus; that is, he tries to push your hand away. He is making gurgling sounds with each breath, so you suction some blood out of his airway. He also is making snoring sounds, so you insert an oropharyngeal airway, which he tolerates and which eliminates the snoring sounds. His breathing is shallow and labored at a rate of about 30, so you have your partner ventilate him with a bag-valve mask and high-concentration oxygen as she simultaneously stabilizes his head with her knees.

There is a pool of blood around the patient's left thigh, which appears angulated. You quickly cut away the left leg of his pants so you can apply direct pressure with a sterile dressing and a pressure bandage to an apparent compound angulated midshaft femur fracture. The patient's radial pulse is rapid and weak. Skin is pale and sweaty.

You assign this patient a high priority for rapid treatment and transport based on mechanism of injury,

altered mental status, and presence of shock (hypoperfusion). You cannot request ALS back-up, because you work in a BLS system.

You perform a rapid trauma assessment. At the same time, a firefighter with whom you have worked before gets a long backboard and the other equipment necessary to immobilize the patient. By the time he returns, you have finished the rapid trauma assessment and gained the following information: a hematoma (lump) is present on the left side of the patient's head, neck veins are flat, there is no deformity of the cervical spine, breath sounds are decreased on the left side of his chest, his abdomen is soft, pelvis seems stable, there is an obvious compound angulated midshaft femur fracture on the left side, there are some non-bleeding lacerations on the left forearm and lower leg, and pulses are weak but palpable in all extremities.

With a cervical collar in place on the patient, you roll him as a unit and examine his spine and posterior trunk. You find no further injuries. You roll him down on the board, taking care to move the injured leg as little as possible once it is in the anatomical position.

As you quickly immobilize the patient on the board (using the board as a splint for the fractured femur), you make sure the firefighter is available to drive the ambulance so you and your partner can tend to the patient in back. You make sure the firefighter knows you are to go to the trauma center, not the community hospital that is five minutes closer. Your protocols specify that you are to go directly to the trauma center under conditions such as these because of the comprehensive care available there.

You move the patient and board onto the stretcher and into the ambulance, making sure your partner is able to continue ventilating him during the move. Once inside the patient compartment, you repeat the initial assessment. Your general impression is of a young adult male with multiple injuries. His mental status remains unchanged: he again tries to brush your hand away when you apply a painful stimulus. His tongue is prevented from obstructing his airway by an oropharyngeal airway. There is a little bit of gurgling when you listen carefully, so you suction some more blood out of his mouth. There are now no abnormal sounds as your partner ventilates him. Oxygen is flowing, and you see the patient's chest rise with each breath. The pressure dressing you applied to the open thigh wound has not bled through, and you see no other wounds that are bleeding. Radial pulse is rapid and weak. The patient is still a high priority.

With a second initial assessment completed, you call the trauma center and notify them of the patient's condition and your estimated time of arrival (10 minutes). You tell them you will give them vital signs as soon as you get them. With the hospital preparing for the patient's arrival, you turn to obtaining vital signs. Pulse is 108, weak and regular, BP 100/80, respirations assisted at 12 per minute, skin pale and sweaty. You relay this information to the trauma center (Figure 30-1).

You have a few minutes before you arrive, so you check with your partner to make sure she is still able to ventilate the patient well before you perform a detailed physical exam. You find equal pupils that are slow to react, a hematoma (lump) on the left side of his head, nothing unusual in or behind the ears, deformity on both sides of his mandible (you conclude this is what is causing the bleeding into his airway), flat neck veins (you are unable to palpate the cervical spine because the cervical collar is in place), breath sounds are still decreased on the left side of his chest, his abdomen seems to be firmer than before, pelvis seems stable, there is an obvious compound midshaft femur fracture on the left side (it is no longer angulated because you straightened it out when you put the patient on the board), and there are some non-bleeding lacerations on the left forearm and lower leg. It is more difficult now to palpate peripheral pulses.

You would like to apply a traction splint, but realize you do not have enough time or personnel. With just a few minutes before you arrive at the trauma center, you repeat the initial assessment one more time. The patient still responds purposefully to painful stimuli, but now he also opens his eyes briefly when you apply it. You find no other changes. You get another set of vital signs: pulse 120, BP 90 by palpation, respirations assisted at 12 per minute, skin pale and sweaty.

You arrive at the emergency department and give a report to the team as you transfer your patient to their bed. The patient's mental status continues to improve in the emergency department. Soon, the staff stops ventilating him and removes the airway. The patient becomes conscious, although confused and disoriented. The staff stabilizes his vital signs for the moment. There will be a slight delay before the patient leaves the emergency department for further tests, so the staff asks you and your partner to apply a traction splint to the patient's fractured femur. You are able to do so quickly and efficiently. The patient goes off for further tests and surgery.

Later you learn that the patient had a cerebral contusion (bruise of the brain), bilateral fracture of the mandible, left hemothorax (blood in the left side of the chest cavity), and a fractured femur.

After a lengthy stay, the patient is able to walk out of the hospital with some temporary assistance from a pair of crutches.

Analysis of the Call

The scenario above is an example of a patient who has critical injuries. Immediate threats to his life included shock (hypoperfusion) and bleeding into an airway that was partially obstructed by his tongue. Other serious injuries included an apparent head injury, inadequate ventilation, a presumed chest injury, a mandible injury, a compound angulated femur fracture, and a suspected spine injury (based on mechanism of injury). The EMT-B in the scenario gave his patient the best possible chance of survival by following the priorities determined by his assessments.

The initial assessment revealed several immediate threats to life that the EMT-B could do something about:

- The airway was partially obstructed by blood, which he suctioned.
- The patient's tongue was partially blocking the airway, causing snoring sounds with breathing, for which he inserted an artificial airway.
- Breathing was shallow and labored at a rate of about 30, which described inadequate ventilation, for which the EMT-B's partner instituted assisted ventilations with high-concentration oxygen.

The EMT-B then picked up on the seriousness of the patient's condition and made the decision not to treat some injuries the way he ordinarily would. That is, normally he would have applied a traction splint and dressed and bandaged the limb lacerations. Although it was tempting to do so, he realized this would delay transport for a patient

Figure 30-1 Unresponsive adult male patient, victim of a motorcycle-passenger vehicle collision.

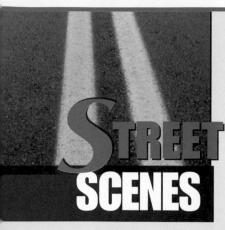

At 9:15 a.m. your BLS ambulance is dispatched to a high-speed intersection for a motor-vehicle crash. While responding, you are advised by dispatch that she has had several 9-1-1 calls regarding this crash and that there are two vehicles involved. As you arrive on scene, you observe that a full-size pick-up truck apparently struck a smaller compact vehicle head on. Your partner strategically places the ambulance to protect the scene. You notice two occupants slumped over inside the small vehicle, which has fluid draining from under the engine.

STREET SCENE QUESTIONS

1. What is your initial impression of the crash?
2. What additional resources will be necessary on scene?

The driver of the pick-up truck walks over to you and says that he bumped his head but he feels okay. Since he can walk and talk, you move toward the smaller car. As you approach, you note that both airbags have deployed and that the leaking fluid appears to be antifreeze, which does not pose a danger. You call for additional ambulances and make sure the police are en route. The male driver is wearing a full shoulder and lap restraint and appears conscious but "dazed." You notice his unrestrained passenger lying on her left side across the console motionless. Your initial assessment of the passenger reveals an approximately 25-year-old female responding to verbal stimuli, verbally abusive, and unaware of her surroundings. She is crying and complaining of pain to her right arm. Her airway appears clear as you notice she has sustained severe facial trauma. Her respirations appear slightly labored and shallow. You note a strong and rapid radial pulse and warm and dry skin.

STREET SCENE QUESTIONS

3. Which patient should be transported first?
4. What is your critical decision regarding the female patient?
5. What critical interventions should you perform on-scene?

You realize that the woman is the priority because of her altered mental status and labored respirations. She has a large laceration, which extends from her upper lip up through her hair line, and you observe angulation to her right humerus. Because of the mechanism of injury and the patient's current status, you decide to perform a rapid extrication. You place a cervical collar on her and spin her onto a board. When she yells, "My baby! Don't hurt my baby!," you note her large abdomen, which is consistent with pregnancy. You move her to the ambulance with 15 liters of oxygen by nonrebreather in place.

Once in the ambulance, you suction blood that has begun to drain into her mouth from the facial laceration. Her initial vital signs show a pulse rate of 122, slightly labored respirations at a rate of 28, and a blood pressure of 142/94. Her pupils appear equal and reactive, and you notice no fluid exiting the ears. Her neck veins are flat and her trachea appears midline. You expose the patient, auscultate lung sounds, and find the right side sounds diminished, coinciding with tenderness to the right side of her chest. As you assess her large abdomen, she winces and again yells about her baby. You recheck her arm and notice angulation and crepitus. You align it and secure her arm alongside her torso, which acts as a splint. Her remaining extremities appear unremarkable. Your patient's level of responsiveness is not reliable enough for a medical history, but you notice she is wearing a medical identification tag, which states she is allergic to sulfa medication.

STREET SCENE QUESTIONS

6. What further information would you like to attain about the female patient?
7. To what type of receiving facility should your patient be transported?

PATIENT NAME: *Jan Jackson* **PATIENT AGE:** *Approx. 25*

CHIEF COMPLAINT

Multi-trauma

PAST MEDICAL HISTORY

- [ ] None
- [x] Allergy to *Sulfa*
- [ ] Hypertension [ ] Stroke
- [ ] Seizures [ ] Diabetes
- [ ] COPD [ ] Cardiac
- [ ] Other (List) [ ] Asthma

Unknown

Current Medications (List)

Unknown

VITAL SIGNS

TIME	RESP	PULSE	B.P.	MENTAL STATUS	R PUPILS L	SKIN
0922	Rate: *28* / [ ] Regular / [x] Shallow / [x] Labored	Rate: *122* / [x] Regular / [ ] Irregular	*142* / *94*	[ ] Alert / [x] Voice / [ ] Pain / [ ] Unresp.	[x] Normal [x] / [ ] Dilated / [ ] Constricted / [ ] Sluggish / [ ] No-Reaction	[ ] Unremarkable / [ ] Cool [ ] Pale / [x] Warm [ ] Cyanotic / [ ] Moist [ ] Flushed / [x] Dry [ ] Jaundiced
0927	Rate: *28* / [ ] Regular / [x] Shallow / [x] Labored	Rate: *128* / [x] Regular / [ ] Irregular	*122* / *86*	[ ] Alert / [x] Voice / [ ] Pain / [ ] Unresp.	[x] Normal [x] / [ ] Dilated / [ ] Constricted / [ ] Sluggish / [ ] No-Reaction	[ ] Unremarkable / [ ] Cool [ ] Pale / [x] Warm [ ] Cyanotic / [ ] Moist [ ] Flushed / [x] Dry [ ] Jaundiced
	Rate: / [ ] Regular / [ ] Shallow / [ ] Labored	Rate: / [ ] Regular / [ ] Irregular	/	[ ] Alert / [ ] Voice / [ ] Pain / [ ] Unresp.	[ ] Normal / [ ] Dilated / [ ] Constricted / [ ] Sluggish / [ ] No-Reaction	[ ] Unremarkable / [ ] Cool [ ] Pale / [ ] Warm [ ] Cyanotic / [ ] Moist [ ] Flushed / [ ] Dry [ ] Jaundiced

NARRATIVE

Responded to a motor-vehicle collision at Algonquin intersection. Upon arrival, found approximately 25-year-old female lying left lateral recumbent across center of vehicle. Patient appeared to be the unrestrained passenger of compact vehicle that received head-on impact from full-size pick-up truck travelling approx. 45 mph. Airbags were deployed. Initial assessment showed patient responsive to verbal stimuli but unaware of surroundings and unable to recall incident. Obvious bleeding noted to facial region with no apparent compromise to airway. Skin warm and dry. Rapidly extricated patient onto spine board and immobilized with straps, c-collar, and head blocks and initiated high-flow O$_2$ and rapid transport. Change in patient position (recumbent on backboard) required constant suctioning of airway from facial laceration (full thickness from patient's upper lip to unknown point on top of head). Head, ears, eyes, nose, and throat clear except for facial laceration. Neck/trachea unremarkable. Chest—noted point tenderness to right axial chest wall with accompanied diminished lung sounds to that side; left side normal. Abdomen is tender to touch in all four quadrants, with possible pregnancy noted. Padding placed under right side of backboard to displace patient to left. Deformed right humerus splinted in place. Pulses, motor function, and sensation intact x 4. Contacted the emergency department and received orders to divert to nearest Level One trauma center. Upon arrival, updated the waiting staff and transferred patient and care. No changes at the time.

While en route to the hospital, you notice the patient's heart rate has increased to 128, her blood pressure has fallen to 122/86, and she is now guarding her abdomen with her left arm. You place padding under the right side of the backboard, which moves the patient onto her left side. This prevents the baby from compressing the vena cava, which could lower blood pressure. You have contacted medical direction and have been advised to transport the patient to the nearest trauma center. Upon arrival at the trauma center, you update the staff and transfer the patient to their care.

who might have very little time to waste. A patient who has bleeding into his airway does not have any time to spare. Accordingly, he used a backboard as a universal splint for the femur and did not bandage the lacerations because they were not bleeding.

Some might say the EMT-B in the scenario was wrong and should have applied the traction splint in the field. After all, the emergency department staff later asked him to do it, right? In fact, the EMT-B showed good judgment. The appropriate place to apply a traction splint to this patient was in the emergency department, not in the field. When the emergency department staff asked him to apply the splint, it was because the patient was stable enough (and because the EMT-B was more familiar with the device than they were). If the patient's condition had not improved, they would not have asked him to put the splint on. Instead, the patient would have been whisked away for surgery or further tests.

There were two ways in which the EMT-B showed good judgment: he postponed taking vital signs, and he gave the hospital staff time to prepare. That is, the patient was ready to be put in the ambulance before the EMT-B was able to get vital signs, so he appropriately postponed taking them until they were en route. As tempting as it might be to complete an assessment all at once, the EMT-B realized that vital signs were not going to change anything he could do and taking them would delay transport. He also called the hospital and gave them an admittedly incomplete report so that they could prepare properly. He made sure to tell them he would get vital signs as soon as possible and then he did. This gave the hospital some additional time to notify the trauma team.

General Principles of Multiple-Trauma Management

Prepare for a call to a multiple-trauma patient by practicing for it. If you are on a regular crew, determine roles beforehand. For example, someone should be designated to manually immobilize the patient's head and, if necessary, ventilate with a bag-valve mask. Depending on the number of people available, you may have to have each person doing several roles. En route to the call, if you have reason to believe you might care for a multiple-trauma patient, review the roles each person will have.

At the scene, follow the steps of assessment as you learned them in your EMT-B course. Follow the priorities you discover in your initial assessment (airway, breathing, and circulation). Then balance the need for scene interventions with the time needed to perform them. As you may recall, the concept of the "golden hour" refers to the need for critical trauma pa-

tients to get to surgery within one hour of injury (not one hour from when you get to the patient). Although the time the patient has to get to surgery has not been scientifically proven to be an hour, the concept is still a useful one in avoiding delays at the scene.

For most critical patients, limit scene treatment to:

- Suctioning the airway
- Inserting an oral or nasal airway
- Restoring a patent airway by sealing a sucking chest wound
- Ventilating with a bag-valve mask
- Administering high-concentration oxygen
- Controlling bleeding
- Immobilizing the patient with a cervical collar and a long backboard
- Inflating a pneumatic anti-shock garment (in areas where it is used) at the scene or en route according to local protocol

Principles of multiple-trauma management also include the following:

- *Scene safety is paramount.* Different kinds of trauma tend to have different kinds of dangers. Blunt trauma, more common in rural and suburban areas, can be associated with such dangers as bent power poles, leaking fuel, sharp glass and metal edges, and passing traffic. Penetrating trauma, such as stab wounds and gunshot wounds, tend to occur more commonly in urban areas. Risks you will need to consider include presence of the assailant (especially one who is upset because you are trying to save a person he tried to kill), presence of multiple weapons (on the victim, assailant, and bystanders), absent or delayed police response, and angry crowds.

- *Assure an open airway.* If you are unable to ventilate your patient without assistance, try other approaches until you find one that works. You might get another person to assist you en route or you might have to switch places with your partner. Other alternatives include using a different device to ventilate, such as a pocket mask with supplemental oxygen, or you and your partner may have to work together to ventilate the patient.

- *Perform urgent or emergency moves as necessary.* For example, if a critical patient is sitting in a vehicle, you will need to perform a rapid extrication.

- *Adapt to the situation.* When a patient is trapped, for example, and part of the patient's body is not accessible, assess as much of him as you can. Keep in mind that when he is extricated you will need to perform a complete examination.

For a multiple-trauma patient, your overall goal is to treat immediate threats to life, which you can treat with prompt transportation to a facility that will provide definitive care (or as close to it as is available). Guard against the temptation in these cases to spend time at the scene treating all of the patient's injuries and immobilizing him perfectly. It is not good patient care to arrive at the hospital with the best packaged corpse in the world.

CHAPTER REVIEW

SUMMARY

The multiple-trauma patient has conflicting needs. He requires treatment of his injuries at the same time that he requires prompt transport to a facility that can provide definitive treatment. The EMT-B must balance and meet these competing needs in a way that provides the most benefit for the patient. Teamwork, timing, and transport are important elements in a plan to provide quality trauma care. Practice and planning are also essential if a critical trauma patient is to get the care he needs in the field and in the hospital.

REVIEW QUESTIONS

1. What considerations must the EMT-B weigh when considering whether to perform an intervention at the scene? (pp. 658-659)
2. What are the interventions that should generally be performed for a critical trauma patient at the scene? (p. 658)
3. When might it be appropriate for EMT-Bs to bypass a closer hospital for a trauma center? (p. 653)
4. What are the three "Ts" of multiple trauma patient management? (p. 653)
5. When might it be appropriate not to apply a traction splint in the field to an obviously fractured femur? (p. 658)

APPLICATIONS

A controversy exists regarding whether patients with penetrating trauma, such as stab and gunshot wounds, should have spine immobilization before transport.

• What factors would have to be considered in this type of case?
• What do your local protocols say about this topic?

WEBMEDIC

Visit Brady's *Emergency Care* website for direct weblinks. At **www.bradybooks.com/emergencycare**, you will find information related to the following Chapter 30 topics:

• Motorcycle safety

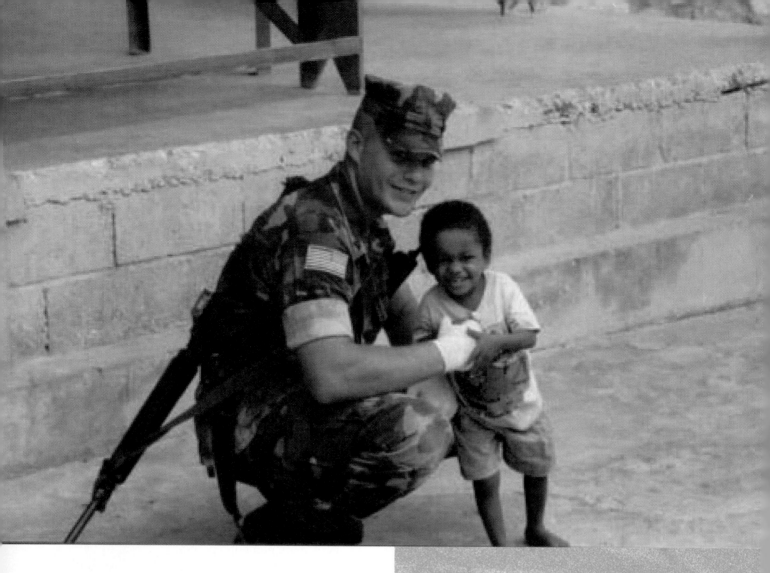

Chapter
Thirty-One

INFANTS AND CHILDREN

*W*ord on the Street

"Although these small patients can raise a significant amount of anxiety, especially when very sick or traumatized, most EMTs meet this challenge well. I've seen many provide excellent care on 'kid calls,' and then admit afterwards they had been very apprehensive. What seems to have made a difference to them is they continually focused assessment and treatment on the ABC agenda. After the calls, these high quality EMS providers also take time for debriefing with a colleague or the medical director. Yet, what stands out in my mind is how well most EMTs—even the anxious ones—handle calls for children."

Andrew Stern NREMT-P
Paramedic/Flight Medic and Educator

The principles of managing the pediatric patient are similar to those for an injured or ill adult. Yet children are not just little adults. The EMT-B must be aware of the special characteristics of pediatric patients as well as some of the medical and trauma problems to which they are susceptible.

DEVELOPMENTAL CHARACTERISTICS OF INFANTS AND CHILDREN

Some important differences should be kept in mind when you are caring for a young patient. For example, since young children do not like to be separated from their parents, you will want to let the child sit in the parent's lap, if possible, during assessment and treatment (Figure 31-1). Some of the special psychological and social characteristics of infants and children and the implications for care are summarized in Table 31-1. Key anatomical and physiological characteristics and their potential impact on care are summarized in Table 31-2. For additional discussion of the developmental characteristics of infants and children, you may also want to review Chapter 13, "Pediatric, Adolescent, and Geriatric Assessment."

SPECIAL CONCERNS IN PEDIATRIC CARE

Like adults, infants and children may be subject to either medical problems or trauma. Concerns that frequently apply to both medical emergencies and trauma are: airway maintenance, providing supplemental oxygen, supporting ventilations, caring for shock, and protecting the infant or child from hypothermia (Figure 31-2).

Maintaining an Open Airway

Just as with an adult, it is important to position the child's head and neck to align and open the airway. It is important not to hyperextend or to permit flexion of a child's neck. The child's head should be positioned in a more neutral position than an adult's because of the danger of closing the airway when the neck is flexed or hyperextended. Placing a folded towel under the shoulders of a young infant or child will help to keep the airway aligned (Figure 31-3). To achieve the proper position, perform a head-tilt, chin-lift if there is no trauma, a jaw-thrust with spinal immobilization if trauma is suspected.

Be prepared to suction the airway as needed. Use suction catheters that are sized for infant and child patients. Do not touch the back of the patient's throat, as this may activate the gag reflex, causing vomiting. It is also possible to stimulate the vagus nerve in the back of the throat, which can slow the heart rate. Do not suction for more than a few seconds at a time, as cutting off the body's oxygen supply is especially dangerous to infants and children, causing cardiac arrest more quickly than in adults. You may hyperventilate the patient (provide ventilations at a faster-than-normal rate) before and after suctioning.

As with adults, the tongues of infants and children are likely to slide back into the pharynx and block the airway. In fact, airway blockage by the tongue is even more likely with infants and children because their tongues are proportionately larger compared to the size of the mouth and pharynx. If the patient is unconscious and does not have a gag reflex, you may insert an oropharyngeal airway to prevent the tongue from blocking the airway.

To insert an oropharyngeal airway, insert a tongue depressor to the base of the tongue. Push down against the tongue while lifting the jaw upward. Then insert the oropharyngeal airway. An important difference

TOPIC OVERVIEW

In this chapter, you will learn about the following topics:

- Ways of dealing with children of different ages

- Differences in anatomy between children and adults

- How to identify and treat respiratory conditions in infants and children

- Differences between children and adults when identifying and dealing with shock and trauma

DOT OBJECTIVES

✔ Knowledge and Attitude

1. Identify the developmental considerations for the following age groups: (pp. 661, 663, 664)

– infants

– toddlers

– preschool

– school age

– adolescent

2. Describe differences in anatomy and physiology of the infant, child, and adult patient. (p. 664)

3. Differentiate the response of the ill or injured infant or child (age specific) from that of an adult. (p. 663)

4. Indicate various causes of respiratory emergencies. (pp. 669–671)

5. Differentiate between respiratory distress and respiratory failure. (pp. 669–671)

6. List the steps in the management of foreign body airway obstruction. (pp. 662, 665–666)

7. Summarize emergency medical care strategies for respiratory distress and respiratory failure. (pp. 669–671)

8. Identify the signs and symptoms of shock (hypoperfusion) in the infant and child patient. (pp. 666–668)

9. Describe the methods of determining end organ perfusion in the infant and child patient. (pp. 666–668)

10. State the usual cause of cardiac arrest in infants and children versus adults. (pp. 669–671)

11. List the common causes of seizures in the infant and child patient. (p. 673)

12. Describe the management of seizures in the infant and child patient. (p. 673)

13. Differentiate between the injury patterns in adults, infants, and children. (pp. 676–677)

14. Discuss the field management of the infant and child trauma patient. (pp. 677–678)

15. Summarize the indicators of possible child abuse and neglect. (pp. 678–680)

16. Describe the medical/legal responsibilities in suspected child abuse. (pp. 678–680)

17. Recognize the need for EMT-Basic debriefing following a difficult infant or child transport. (p. 684)

18. Explain the rationale for having knowledge and skills appropriate for dealing with the infant and child patient. (p. 661)

19. Attend to the feelings of the family when dealing with an ill or injured infant or child. (pp. 676, 681)

20. Understand the provider's own response (emotional) to caring for infants or children. (p. 684)

✔ Skills

1. Demonstrate the techniques of foreign body airway obstruction removal in the infant.

2. Demonstrate the techniques of foreign body airway obstruction removal in the child.

3. Demonstrate bag-valve-mask artificial ventilations for the infant.

4. Demonstrate bag-valve-mask artificial ventilations for the child.

5. Demonstrate oxygen delivery for the infant and child.

Figure 31-1   If at all possible, let a young child sit in the parent's lap during assessment and care.

to note is that when an oropharyngeal airway is inserted in an adult, it is inserted with the tip pointing toward the roof of the mouth, then rotated 180 degrees into position. For an infant or child, the oropharyngeal airway is inserted with tip pointing toward the tongue and throat, in the same position it will be in after insertion (Figure 31-4).

Clearing an Airway Obstruction

Infants and children are naturally curious. They explore their environment and often put things in their mouths. They can easily choke on a foreign object as well as on a piece of food.

An airway obstruction can be partial or complete. With many partial obstructions, the child is still able to breathe and get enough oxygen. With other partial obstructions or with complete obstruction of the airway, the supply of air is cut off to a significant extent or completely. The assessment and care summaries in this chapter detail how to determine if an obstruction is partial or complete and how to manage an obstruction.

Table 31-1 Psychological and Social Characteristics of Infants and Children

Infant	Toddler	Preschool	School Age	Adolescent
Birth to 1 Year	**1 to 3 Years**	**3 to 6 Years**	**6 to 12 Years**	**12 to 18 Years**
Has minimal stranger anxiety				
Needs to be kept warm (warm hands and stethoscope before use)				
Fears having head or face touched by strangers (examine heart and lungs first, head last, to build confidence)				
Does not like being separated from parents (have patient sit on parent's lap)				
Feels suffocated by oxygen mask (try "blow-by" method)				
	Fears needles and instruments (explain what you are doing; reassure)			
	Thinks injury or illness is punishment for being bad (assure this is not true)			
	Fears pain (do not lie to patient, but reassure)			
		Fears blood (explain and reassure)		
		Fears permanent injury (do not lie to patient, but reassure)		
		Is modest (protect privacy)		
			Fears disfigurement (do not lie to patient, but reassure)	
				Sensitive to violations of dignity (talk to as if to an adult; assess away from parents; have same-sex EMT-B examine if possible)

Table 31-2 Anatomical and Physiological Characteristics of Infants and Children

Anatomical and Physiological Differences Compared to Adults	Potential Impact on Assessment and Care
Tongue proportionally larger	More likely to block airway
Smaller airway structures	More easily blocked
Abundant secretions	Can block the airway
Deciduous (baby) teeth	Easily dislodged; can block the airway
Flat nose and face	Difficult to obtain good face mask seal
Head heavier relative to body and less-developed neck structures and muscles	Head may be propelled more forcefully than body, creating a higher incidence of head injury
Fontanelle and open sutures (soft spots) palpable on top of young infant's head	Bulging fontanelle can be a sign of intracranial pressure (but may be normal if infant is crying); sunken fontanelle may indicate dehydration
Thinner, softer brain tissue	Susceptible to serious brain trauma
Head larger in proportion to body	Tips forward when supine, causing flexion of neck, making neutral alignment of airway difficult
Shorter, narrower, more elastic (flexible) trachea	Can close off trachea with hyperextension of neck
Short neck	Difficult to stabilize or immobilize
Abdominal breathers	Difficult to evaluate breathing
Faster respiratory rate	Muscles easily fatigue, causing respiratory distress
Newborns breathe primarily through the nose (obligate nose breathers)	May not automatically open mouth to breathe if nose is blocked; airway more easily blocked
Larger body surface relative to body mass	Prone to hypothermia
Thinner skin	More sensitive to effects of burns
Softer bones	More flexible, less easily fractured; traumatic forces may be transmitted to, and injure, internal organs without fracturing ribs or other bones
More flexible ribs	Traumatic forces may be transmitted to chest cavity without fracturing ribs; lungs easily damaged with trauma
Spleen and liver more exposed	Injury likely with significant force to abdomen

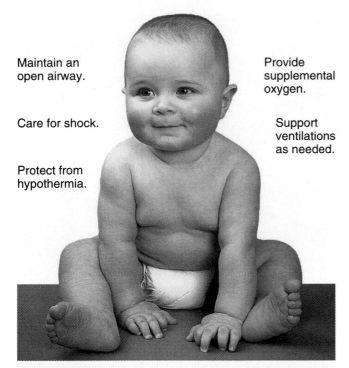

Maintain an open airway.

Care for shock.

Protect from hypothermia.

Provide supplemental oxygen.

Support ventilations as needed.

Figure 31-2 Some special considerations apply to a variety of pediatric medical and trauma emergencies.

● Patient *ASSESSMENT*

Partial Airway Obstruction

Signs of a partial airway obstruction in a pediatric patient include the following:

- Noisy breathing (stridor, crowing)
- Retractions of the muscles around the ribs and sternum when inhaling
- Skin is still pink
- Peripheral perfusion is satisfactory (capillary refill under 2 seconds in a child 5 years old or less)
- Still alert, not unconscious

Figure 31-3 Place a folded towel under the young patient's shoulders to keep the airway aligned.

● Patient *CARE*

Partial Airway Obstruction

Emergency care of a pediatric patient with a partial airway obstruction is as follows:

1. Allow the child to assume a position of comfort, sitting up, not lying down. Assist an infant or younger child into a sitting position. Allow child to sit on parent's lap.

2. Offer high-concentration oxygen by pediatric nonrebreather mask or blow-by technique (described later in this chapter).

3. Transport.

4. Do not agitate the child. Do a limited exam. Do not assess blood pressure.

● Patient *ASSESSMENT*

Complete Airway Obstruction or Partial Obstruction with No Crying or Speaking and Cyanosis

The obstruction may be complete, or a partial obstruction may be severe enough to prevent adequate intake of oxygen. Signs include:

- Cyanosis
- Child's cough becomes ineffective; child cannot cry or speak
- Increased respiratory difficulty accompanied by stridor or respiratory arrest
- Altered mental status or child has lost or loses consciousness

Figure 31-4 Unlike in an adult, the oropharyngeal airway is inserted in the same position it will be in after insertion.

Patient *CARE*

Complete Airway Obstruction or Partial Obstruction with No Crying or Speaking and Cyanosis

Follow the steps below for emergency care:

1. Perform airway clearance techniques. For infants less than 1 year old, alternate back blows and chest thrusts (Figure 31-5) and use finger sweeps to remove visible objects (no blind sweeps). For children older than 1 year, provide abdominal thrusts and finger sweeps to remove visible objects. (Airway clearance sequences are summarized in Table 31-3.)

2. Attempt artificial ventilations with a pocket mask or bag-valve-mask unit in the appropriate pediatric size and supplemental oxygen. (See Table 31-4.)

Providing Supplemental Oxygen and Ventilations

As for adults, high-concentration oxygen should be administered to children in respiratory distress or with inadequate respirations or with possible shock. Hypoxia (oxygen starvation) is the underlying reason for many of the most serious medical problems with children. Inadequate oxygen will have immediate effects on the heart rate and the brain, as shown by a slowed heart rate and an altered mental status.

However, infants and young children are often afraid of an oxygen mask. For these patients, try a "blow-by" technique. That is, have a parent hold the oxygen tubing or the pediatric nonrebreather mask 2 inches from the patient's face so the oxygen will pass over the face and be inhaled. Some children respond well when the tubing is pushed through the bottom of a paper cup, especially if the cup is colorful or has a picture drawn inside it. Hand the cup to the child or ask a parent to hold it. Infants and young children instinctively explore new things by bringing them up to their mouths. As the patient handles and explores the cup, he will breathe in the oxygen (Figure 31-6). Do not use a Styrofoam cup. Styrofoam will flake and the particles can be inhaled.

Artificial ventilations should be provided at the rate of 20 per minute (one every 3 seconds) for an infant or child under 8 years of age, at 12 per minute (one every 5 seconds) if the child is over 8 years. Use a pocket face mask or a bag-valve-mask unit in the correct infant or child size. Follow these guidelines when ventilating the infant or child patient:

- Avoid breathing too hard through the pocket face mask or using excessive bag pressure and volume. Use only enough force to make the chest rise.

A

B

Figure 31-5   For a complete airway obstruction in an infant, (A) alternate back blows with (B) chest thrusts.

- Use properly sized face masks to assure a good mask seal.
- Flow-restricted, oxygen-powered ventilation devices are contraindicated in infants and children.
- If ventilation is not successful in raising the patient's chest, perform procedures for clearing an obstructed airway. Then try to ventilate again. (Review Tables 31-3 and 31-4.)

Caring for Shock (Hypoperfusion)

Shock is another term for hypoperfusion, or the inadequate circulation of blood and oxygen throughout the body. One common cause of shock in

Table 31-3 Pediatric Airway Clearance Sequences

	Child Over 8 Years	Child 1 to 8 Years	Infant Birth to 1 Year
Conscious	Ask, "Are you choking?" Perform Heimlich maneuver.	Ask, "Are you choking?" Perform Heimlich maneuver.	Observe signs of choking (small objects or food, wheezing, agitation, blue color, not breathing). Series of 5 back blows, 5 chest thrusts
Loses consciousness during procedure	Assist patient to floor. If alone, call for help, then . . . Open airway with tongue-jaw lift. Perform finger sweeps. Attempt to ventilate. If unsuccessful, reposition head and attempt to ventilate again. If unsuccessful, perform Heimlich maneuver. (Repeat as needed.)	Assist patient to floor. Open airway with tongue-jaw lift. Remove visible objects. (NO blind sweeps.) Attempt to ventilate. If unsuccessful, reposition head and attempt to ventilate again. If unsuccessful, perform Heimlich maneuver. (Repeat as needed.) If alone, call for help after 1 minute.	Open airway with tongue-jaw lift. Remove visible objects. (NO blind sweeps.) Attempt to ventilate. If unsuccessful, reposition head and attempt to ventilate again. If unsuccessful, perform 5 back blows and 5 chest thrusts. (Repeat as needed.) If alone, call for help after 1 minute.
Unconscious when found	Establish unresponsiveness. If alone, call for help, then . . . Open airway. Attempt to ventilate. If unsuccessful, reposition head and attempt to ventilate again. If unsuccessful, perform Heimlich maneuver and finger sweeps. (Repeat as needed.)	Establish unresponsiveness. Open airway. Attempt to ventilate. If unsuccessful, reposition head and attempt to ventilate again. If unsuccessful, perform Heimlich maneuver. Remove visible objects. (NO blind sweeps.) (Repeat as needed.) If alone, call for help after 1 minute.	Establish unresponsiveness. Open airway. Attempt to ventilate. If unsuccessful, reposition head and attempt to ventilate again. If unsuccessful, perform 5 back blows and 5 chest thrusts. Remove visible objects. (NO blind sweeps.) (Repeat as needed.) If alone, call for help after 1 minute.

adults—a failure of heart function or of the cardiovascular system—is rare in infants and children. Common causes of shock in infants and children include:

- Diarrhea and/or vomiting with resulting dehydration
- Infection
- Trauma (especially abdominal injuries)
- Blood loss

Less common causes include:

- Allergic reactions
- Poisoning
- Cardiac events (rare)

It is important to remember that infants and children have a small volume of blood compared to adults (approximately 8% of the total body weight). Bleeding that would not be dangerous in an adult may be serious in an infant or child. Shock can

Table 31-4 Artificial Ventilation

	Over 8 Years	1 to 8 Years	Birth to 1 Year
Ventilation duration	2 sec	1 to 1½ sec	1 to 1½ sec
Ventilation rate	10-12 breaths/min	20 breaths/min	20 breaths/min

Figure 31-6 You can deliver oxygen to an infant using the blow-by method.

develop in the small child who has a laceration to the scalp (with its many blood vessels), or in the 3-year-old who loses as little as a cup of blood.

The most important thing to understand about shock in infants and children is that their bodies are able to compensate for it for a long time. Then the compensating mechanisms fail, at approximately 30% blood loss, and decompensated shock develops very rapidly. This means that a child may appear to be fine, then "go sour" in a hurry. This is in contrast to the adult patient in whom decompensated shock develops earlier and more gradually, making it easier to assess and treat than in a child.

The definitive care for shock takes place at the hospital (usually in the operating room). Since infants and children are prone to go into decompensated shock so suddenly, IT IS IMPORTANT NOT TO WAIT FOR SIGNS OF DECOMPENSATED SHOCK TO DE-

VELOP. Instead, in any situation in which shock is a possibility, provide oxygen (which boosts the supply of oxygen to poorly perfused tissues and helps keep up heart function) and transport as quickly as possible.

The signs and emergency treatment of shock (Figure 31-7) are detailed below.

Patient ASSESSMENT

Shock

Signs of shock in pediatric patients include the following:

- Rapid respiratory rate
- Pale, cool, clammy skin
- Weak or absent peripheral pulses
- Delayed capillary refill, more than 2 seconds (in a child 5 years or younger)
- Decreased urine output (Ask parents about diaper wetting; look at diaper.)
- Mental status changes
- Absence of tears, even when crying

Patient CARE

Shock

Follow these steps for emergency care:

1. Assure an open airway.

2. Provide high-concentration oxygen. Be prepared to artificially ventilate.

3. Manage external bleeding, if present.

4. Elevate legs if there is no trauma.

5. Keep warm.

6. Transport immediately. Perform any additional assessment and treatments en route.

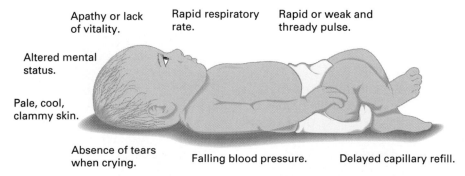

Apathy or lack of vitality.

Rapid respiratory rate.

Rapid or weak and thready pulse.

Altered mental status.

Pale, cool, clammy skin.

Absence of tears when crying.

Falling blood pressure.

Delayed capillary refill.

Figure 31-7 Signs of shock in an infant or child.

Protecting Against Hypothermia

Hypothermia, or cooling of the body temperature, is a condition that in extreme cases is life threatening. People lose heat more readily if their clothes are wet, if they are exposed to wind, or if they are submerged in cold water. The body attempts to compensate for a decrease in body temperature, but as these compensatory functions begin to fail, the core body temperature drops. Because children have a large surface area in proportion to their body mass, exposure to cool weather and water can result in hypothermia more easily than with adults. So hypothermia is always a concern with a pediatric patient.

Other causes of hypothermia, in children as well as in adults, include ingestion of alcohol or drugs that dilate peripheral vessels and cause loss of body heat; metabolic problems such as hypoglycemia; brain disorders that interfere with temperature regulation; severe infection or sepsis; and shock.

Hypothermia may be a concern in both medical and trauma emergencies. For example, a sick child in a cool room or in sheets or nightclothes that have become wet from perspiration or loss of bladder control may be hypothermic. When trauma occurs outdoors, caregivers attending to injuries may forget to protect the patient from a cool or damp environment, and may exacerbate the situation by exposing the patient's body during the physical exam.

Field care for children is the same as for adults. It is important to keep the patient warm. Cover the patient to avoid further loss of body heat. Special attention should be paid to covering the head, as the head is a major area of heat loss. Consult medical direction for advice on active rewarming by application of hot water bottles or other heat sources to the body if the patient is awake and responding appropriately. Avoid rough handling and inserting anything in the mouth as these actions may cause ventricular fibrillation or cardiac arrest in the severely hypothermic child. Suction very gently if suctioning is necessary, being alert to the possibility of cardiac arrest.

MEDICAL EMERGENCIES

Respiratory Disorders

Respiratory disorders are a great concern in infants and children. For example, it is important to remember that while cardiac arrest in the adult is likely to be caused by a heart problem, the likeliest cause of cardiac arrest in a child, other than trauma, is respiratory failure. For the pediatric patient, it is important to distinguish whether the probable cause of breathing difficulty is an airway obstruction or a respiratory disease, because the care will be very different. The care that you would give for an airway obstruction can be lethal in a child with a respiratory disease. Also, because respiratory problems can have such serious consequences in infants and children, it is critical to be alert for early signs of respiratory distress.

Differentiating Airway Obstruction from Respiratory Disease

In infants and children, it is especially important to try to distinguish between an airway obstruction and an airway disease. Many of the signs of an airway obstruction are the same as the signs of airway respiratory disease, since respiratory infection or disease will also often swell and obstruct the airway passages.

With some of these diseases, it is dangerous to perform finger sweeps or to place a tongue depressor or any other instrument in the patient's mouth or pharynx because this may set off spasms along the airway. Do not attempt to clear the airway of a foreign obstruction unless it is clear that this is the problem—that is, the child has been observed ingesting a foreign object or the signs of such ingestion are clear.

In general, with suspected airway diseases you should transport as quickly as possible if you see or hear wheezing, breathing effort on exhalation, or rapid breathing.

Respiratory Distress

There are a number of respiratory diseases or disorders an infant or child may have that will cause respiratory distress, including serious ones like epiglottitis, and less serious ones like a cold. It is not easy to determine which respiratory problem the child may have. Many signs and symptoms are similar, and age ranges for occurrence overlap.

As an EMT-B, you do not need to decide what respiratory disorder a child is suffering from. Instead, follow the guidelines below for recognizing and managing respiratory distress. It is especially important to recognize the signs of early respiratory distress and treat it before it advances to a life-threatening stage or to respiratory arrest.

FYI

RESPIRATORY DISEASES

Two illnesses that sometimes cause airway problems in children are croup and epiglottitis.

Croup

Croup is caused by a group of viral illnesses that result in inflammation of the larynx, trachea, and bronchi. It is typically an illness of children 6 months to about 4 years of age that often occurs at night. This problem sometimes follows a cold or other respiratory infection. Tissues in the airway (particularly the upper airway) become swollen and restrict the passage of air.

 Patient *ASSESSMENT*

Croup

During the day, the child usually will have these signs:

* Mild fever
* Some hoarseness

At night, the child's condition will worsen and he or she will develop:

* A loud "seal bark" cough
* Difficulty breathing
* Signs of respiratory distress including nasal flaring, retraction of the muscles between the ribs, tugging at the throat
* Restlessness
* Paleness with cyanosis

Patient *CARE*

Croup

Emergency care of a pediatric patient with croup is as follows:

1. Place the patient in a position of comfort (usually sitting up).

2. Administer high-concentration oxygen. When possible, this should be from a humidified source.

3. Walking to the ambulance in the cool night air may provide relief as the cool air reduces the edema in the airway tissues.

4. Do not delay transport unless ordered to do so by medical direction.

Epiglottitis

Epiglottitis is most commonly caused by a bacterial infection that produces swelling of the epiglottis and partial airway obstruction. The typical patient will be between 3 and 7 years old. Although epiglottitis has become much less common with the development of vaccines, it is a life-threatening illness that must be suspected when treating any child with stridor (a high-pitched sound caused by air moving through narrowed passageways).

Patient *ASSESSMENT*

Epiglottitis

Signs include:

* A sudden onset of high fever
* Painful swallowing (the child often will drool to avoid swallowing)
* Patient will assume a "tripod" position, sitting upright and leaning forward with the chin thrust outward (sniffing position) and the mouth wide open in an effort to maintain a wide airway opening.
* Patient will sit very still, but the muscles will work hard to breathe, and the child can tire quickly from the effort.
* Child appears more generally ill than with croup.

Note: All cases of epiglottitis must be considered life threatening, no matter how early the detection.

Patient *CARE*

Epiglottitis

Emergency care for the pediatric patient with epiglottitis is as follows:

1. Immediately transport the child, with the child sitting on the parent's lap.

2. Provide high-concentration oxygen from a humidified source. Do not increase the child's anxiety. If he or she resists the mask, let the parent hold it in front of the child's face.

3. Constantly monitor the child for respiratory distress or arrest and be ready to resuscitate.

4. DO NOT PLACE ANYTHING INTO THE CHILD'S MOUTH, including a thermometer, tongue blade, or oral airway. To do so may set off spasms along the upper airway that will totally obstruct the airway.

The child will not want to lie down, and you should not force him to do so. The child must be handled gently, since rough handling and stress could lead to a total airway obstruction from spasms of the larynx and swelling tissues.

Patient *ASSESSMENT*

Respiratory Distress

Gather information quickly from the parents and do a rapid assessment of the child. Unless there are clear indications of foreign body airway obstruction, do not put a tongue depressor in the child's mouth to examine the airway. This may cause spasms that can totally obstruct the airway. Rely on any of the following signs of early respiratory distress (Figure 31-8):

* Nasal flaring
* Retraction of the muscles above, below, and between the sternum and ribs
* Use of abdominal muscles
* Stridor (high-pitched, harsh sound)
* Audible wheezing
* Grunting
* Breathing rate greater than 60

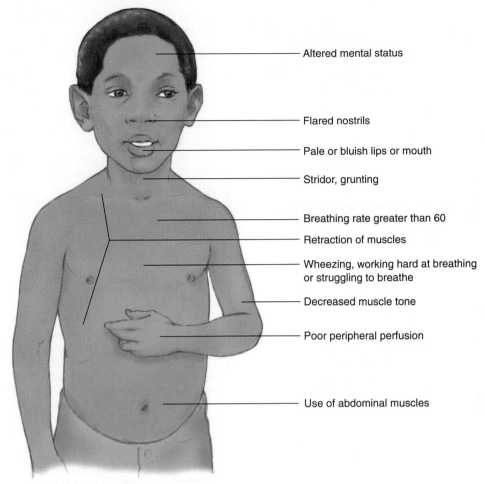

Altered mental status

Flared nostrils

Pale or bluish lips or mouth

Stridor, grunting

Breathing rate greater than 60

Retraction of muscles

Wheezing, working hard at breathing or struggling to breathe

Decreased muscle tone

Poor peripheral perfusion

Use of abdominal muscles

Figure 31-8   Signs of respiratory distress

In addition to the above signs of early respiratory distress, watch for these additional signs:

- Cyanosis
- Decreased muscle tone
- Poor peripheral perfusion (capillary refill greater than 2 seconds)
- Altered mental status
- Decreased heart rate (a late sign)

Patient *CARE*

Respiratory Distress

PROVIDE OXYGEN TO ALL CHILDREN WITH RESPIRATORY EMERGENCIES. For children in early respiratory distress:

- Provide oxygen by pediatric nonrebreather mask or blow-by technique.

For children in severe respiratory distress (those with respiratory distress and altered mental status, cyanosis even when oxygen is administered, poor muscle tone, or inadequate breathing):

- Provide assisted ventilations with pediatric pocket mask or bag-valve mask and supplemental oxygen.

For children in respiratory arrest:

- Ventilate with pediatric pocket mask or bag-valve mask and supplemental oxygen.

ALL RESPIRATORY DISORDERS IN CHILDREN MUST BE TAKEN SERIOUSLY. RESPIRATORY DISEASE IS THE PRIMARY CAUSE OF CARDIAC ARREST NOT DUE TO TRAUMA. If you treat the respiratory system, the heart will also respond. The EMT-B's primary concern when caring for infants and children with respiratory problems, whether medical or trauma related, is to establish and maintain an open airway. About one-third of all pediatric trauma deaths are related to airway mismanagement.

Fever

Above-normal body temperature is one of the most important signs of an existing or impending acute illness. Fever usually accompanies infections (ear infections are common) as well as such childhood diseases as chicken pox, mononucleosis, pneumonia, epiglottitis, and meningitis. The fever also may be due to heat exposure, any infection, or some other noninfectious disease problem.

● Patient ASSESSMENT

Fever

Never regard a fever as unimportant. Parents may have an opinion about what they believe may be the problem, but the EMT-B is not qualified to diagnose or determine what is likely to happen over the next few hours.

Use relative skin temperature as a sign. Generally oral or rectal temperatures are not taken in the prehospital setting unless permitted by local medical direction. Either a skin thermometer or information provided by the parents should be used for determining the patient's temperature. The ungloved back of your hand applied to the patient's forehead or to the abdomen beneath the clothing is another way to determine relative skin temperature. A high relative skin temperature is always enough reason to transport and seek medical opinion. Other signs include:

- Fever with a rash is a sign of a potentially serious condition.
- A seizure or seizures may accompany a high fever.

● Patient CARE

Fever

Children can tolerate a high temperature, and only a small percent will have a seizure due to fever (febrile seizure). It is the rapid rise in temperature rather than the temperature itself that causes seizures. Cooling the child without bringing on hypothermia is an important care objective.

Should you find an infant or child with high fever, take the following steps:

1. Remove the child's clothing, but do not allow him to be exposed to conditions that may bring on hypothermia. If the child objects to having clothing removed, let the child keep on light clothing or underwear.

2. If the condition is a result of heat exposure, and if local protocols permit, cover the child with a towel soaked in tepid water. This will cool the child quickly.

3. Monitor for shivering and avoid hypothermia. This may develop quickly in children. If shivering develops, stop the cooling activities and cover the child with a light blanket.

4. If local protocols permit, give the child fluids by mouth or allow him to suck on chipped ice. This may not prevent dehydration but will increase comfort.

5. *Be aware that a mild fever can quickly turn into a high fever that may indicate a serious, if not life-threatening, problem. If the infant or child feels very warm-to-hot to the touch, then prepare the patient for transport. Transport all children who have suffered a seizure as quickly as possible, protecting the patient from temperature extremes.*

There are also some "do nots" in treating an infant or child with fever:

- Do not submerge the child in cold water, or cover with a towel soaked in ice water (which can cause hypothermia rapidly).
- DO NOT USE RUBBING ALCOHOL TO COOL THE PATIENT. (IT CAN BE ABSORBED IN TOXIC AMOUNTS AND IS A FIRE HAZARD.)

Diarrhea and Vomiting

Diarrhea and vomiting are common in childhood illness. Either one can cause dehydration that worsens whatever other condition the child may have and may lead to life-threatening shock. Infants are more susceptible to the effects of dehydration because, compared to adults, a greater percentage of their body is water and their fluid maintenance needs are greater.

● Patient ASSESSMENT

Diarrhea and Vomiting

For any pediatric patient with diarrhea or vomiting:

1. Monitor the airway.

2. Monitor respiration.

3. Be alert for signs of shock.

Diarrhea and Vomiting

Emergency care includes the following:

1. Maintain an open airway and be prepared to provide oral suctioning.

2. Provide oxygen if respirations are compromised.

3. If signs of shock are present, contact medical direction immediately and transport.

4. If your protocols or medical direction permits, offer the child sips of clear liquids or chipped ice if only diarrhea is present. Many physicians recommend nothing by mouth if there is nausea or vomiting.

5. Save a sample of vomitus and rectal discharge (e.g., a soiled diaper).

Seizures

Fever is the most common cause of seizures in infants and children. Epilepsy, infections, poisoning, hypoglycemia, trauma including head injury, or decreased levels of oxygen can also bring on seizures. Some seizures in children are idiopathic; that is, they have no known cause. They may be brief or prolonged. They are rarely life threatening in children who have them frequently. However, SEIZURES, INCLUDING THOSE CAUSED BY FEVER, SHOULD BE CONSIDERED LIFE THREATENING BY THE EMT-B.

Usually, you will arrive after the convulsion has passed.

● **Patient** *ASSESSMENT*

Seizures

Interview the patient as well as family members and bystanders who saw the convulsion. Ask them if the child has a history of seizures. Ask:

- Has the child had prior seizures?
- If yes, is this the child's normal seizure pattern? (How long did the seizure last? What part of the body was seizing?)
- Has the child had a fever?
- Has the child taken any anti-seizure medication? Other medication?

Assess the child for signs and symptoms of illness or injury, taking care to note any injuries sus-

tained during the convulsion. All infants and children who have undergone a seizure require medical evaluation. The seizure itself may not be serious but it may be a sign of an underlying condition. Be aware that seizures may be caused by a head injury.

● **Patient** *CARE*

Seizures

If the patient has a seizure in your presence, possibly during transport, provide the following care:

1. Maintain an open airway. Do not insert an oropharyngeal airway or bite stick.

2. Position the patient on his side if there is no possibility of spinal injury.

3. Be alert for vomiting. Suction as needed.

4. Provide oxygen. If the patient is in respiratory arrest, provide artificial ventilations with supplemental oxygen.

5. Transport.

6. Monitor for inadequate breathing and/or altered mental status, which may occur following a seizure.

Altered Mental Status

Altered mental status may be caused by a variety of conditions, including hypoglycemia, poisoning, infection, head injury, decreased oxygen levels, shock, or the aftermath of a seizure.

● **Patient** *ASSESSMENT*

Altered Mental Status

Assessment of the patient with altered mental status focuses on life-threatening problems discovered during the initial assessment.

- Be alert for a mechanism of injury that may have caused the altered mental status, such as head injury.
- Be alert for signs of shock.
- Look for evidence of poisoning by ingested, inhaled, or absorbed substances.
- Attempt to quickly obtain a history of any seizure disorder or diabetes.

Altered Mental Status

Emergency care of a pediatric patient with altered mental status includes the following:

1. Assure an open airway. Be prepared to suction.

2. Protect the spine while managing the airway if a head injury or other trauma is present.

3. Administer high-concentration oxygen by pediatric nonrebreather mask or blow-by technique. Be prepared to perform artificial ventilations by pediatric pocket mask or bag-valve mask with supplemental oxygen.

4. Treat for shock.

5. Transport.

Poisoning

Children are often the victims of accidental poisoning, often resulting from the ingestion of household products or medications. Certain poisons can quickly depress the respiratory system, cause respiratory arrest, and cause life-threatening conditions of the circulatory and nervous systems. The airway and gastrointestinal tract can also be burned by corrosive substances upon ingestion and with subsequent vomiting.

Review Chapter 21, "Poisoning and Overdose Emergencies," for information on ingested, inhaled, absorbed, and injected poisons. This information applies to children as well as to adults.

Poisoning

Some types of poisonings are not often associated with adult patients but are common to children. These special cases include:

- *Aspirin poisoning.* Look for hyperventilation, vomiting, and sweating. The skin may feel hot. Severe cases cause seizures, coma, or shock.

- *Acetaminophen poisoning.* Many medications have this compound, including Tylenol, Comtrex, Bancap, Excedrin PM, and Datril. Initially, the child may have no abnormal signs or symptoms. The child may be restless (early) or drowsy.

Nausea, vomiting, and heavy perspiration may occur. Loss of consciousness is possible.

- *Lead poisoning.* This usually comes from ingesting chips of lead-based paint. It is often chronic (building up over a long time). Look for nausea with abdominal pain and vomiting. Muscle cramps, headache, muscle weakness, and irritability are often present.

- *Iron poisoning.* Iron compounds such as ferrous sulfate are found in some vitamin tablets and liquids. As little as one gram of ferrous sulfate can be lethal to a child. Within 30 minutes to several hours, the child will show nausea and bloody vomiting, often accompanied by diarrhea. Typically the child will develop shock, but this may be delayed for up to 24 hours as the child appears to be getting better.

- *Petroleum product poisoning.* The patient will usually be vomiting with coughing or choking. In most cases, you will smell the distinctive odor of a petroleum distillate (e.g., gasoline, kerosene, heating fuel).

Poisoning

Emergency care for a responsive patient includes:

1. Contact medical direction or the poison control center.

2. Consider the need to administer activated charcoal.

3. Provide oxygen.

4. Transport.

5. Continue to monitor the patient. The patient may become unresponsive.

Emergency care for an unresponsive patient includes:

1. Assure an open airway.

2. Provide oxygen.

3. Be prepared to provide artificial ventilation.

4. Transport.

5. Contact medical direction or the poison control center.

6. Rule out trauma as a cause of altered mental status.

MENINGITIS

Meningitis is caused by either a bacterial or a viral infection of the lining of the brain and spinal cord (the meninges). The majority of meningitis cases occur between the ages of 1 month and 5 years.

● Patient ASSESSMENT

Meningitis

The following are signs and symptoms of meningitis:

- High fever
- Lethargy
- Irritability
- Headache
- Stiff neck
- Sensitivity to light
- In infants, the fontanelles may be bulging unless the child is dehydrated.
- Movement is painful and the child does not want to be touched or held.
- Sudden excitement may cause seizures.
- A rash may be present in the bacterial-type infection.

● Patient CARE

Meningitis

It is most important to carefully take appropriate BSI precautions. Wear a surgical mask, since this is an airborne disease. When meningitis is suspected, provide the following care:

1. Monitor airway, breathing, circulation, and vital signs.

2. Provide high-concentration oxygen by nonrebreather mask.

3. Ventilate with a pediatric pocket mask or bag-valve mask with supplemental oxygen if necessary.

4. Provide CPR if necessary.

5. Be alert for seizures.

6. Transport immediately. This is a TRUE EMERGENCY. Do not delay.

Safety Note

All EMS personnel should immediately get a follow-up evaluation by a physician after any call where meningitis is suspected.

Near-Drowning

Near-drowning means that a patient has been submerged in water and has suffered either a cardiac or a respiratory arrest. If heart and respiratory function are not restored, it is a drowning. However, if the patient has a return of pulse and/or breathing, even temporarily, it is a near-drowning. Patients who have been submerged in cold water have been revived 30 minutes or more after submersion.

● Patient ASSESSMENT

Near-Drowning

Assess as for any unresponsive patient:

1. Establish unresponsiveness, breathlessness, and pulselessness.

2. If alone, call for help after 1 minute of resuscitation.

3. If trauma may have been a cause or result of the submersion incident (such as, injury from a dive), maintain spinal stabilization and follow trauma assessment procedures. Remember, however, that resuscitation is your first priority.

4. Consider possible ingestion of alcohol as a cause of the near-drowning, especially in adolescents.

5. Consider the possibility of "secondary drowning syndrome"—deterioration after normal breathing resumes, minutes to hours after the event.

● Patient CARE

Near-Drowning

For the drowning or near-drowning patient, provide the following care:

1. Provide artificial ventilation or CPR as necessary. This is your first treatment priority.

2. Protect the airway. Suction if necessary.

3. Protect against possible hypothermia, especially if the patient has been in cool or cold water. As soon as practical, remove wet clothing, dry the skin, and cover with a blanket.

4. Treat any trauma.

5. Transport all near-drowning patients to the hospital, even if they seem to have recovered.

Sudden Infant Death Syndrome

In the United States, sudden infant death syndrome (SIDS)—the sudden unexplained death during sleep of an apparently healthy baby in its first year of life—occurs to between 6,500 and 7,500 babies each year. These babies were usually receiving proper care and frequently have passed physical examinations within days of their sudden death.

Many possible causes have been investigated but are not well understood. The problem is not caused by external methods of suffocation or by vomiting or choking. The problem may possibly be related to nerve cell development in the brain or the tissue chemistry of the respiratory system or the heart. Some relationships have been drawn to family history of SIDS and respiratory problems, but there is still no accepted reason why these babies die.

When asleep, the typical SIDS patient will show periods of cardiac slowdown and temporary cessation of breathing known as sleep apnea. Eventually, the infant will stop breathing and will not start again on its own. Unless reached in time, the episode can be fatal. The baby's condition is most commonly discovered in the early morning when the parents go to wake the baby.

It is not up to you, as an EMT-B, to diagnose SIDS. All you or the parents will know is that the baby is in respiratory and cardiac arrest. You will treat the baby as you would any patient in this condition:

1. Unless there is rigor mortis (stiffening of the body after death), provide resuscitation and transport to the hospital. Let the pronouncement of death come from hospital personnel, not from you.

2. Be certain that the parents receive emotional support and that they understand that everything possible is being done for the child at the scene and during transport.

Parents who lose a child to SIDS often suffer intense guilt feelings from the moment they find the child. Whether or not the parents express such guilt, remind them that SIDS occurs to apparently healthy babies who are receiving the best of parental care. Do not speak with a suspicious tone or ask inappropriate questions. Do not be embarrassed to express your sorrow for their loss, but be sure to do so only after a physician has officially informed them of the child's death.

TRAUMA

Trauma is the number one cause of death in infants and children. Blunt trauma far exceeds penetrating trauma in this age group. Much of this trauma occurs because they are curious and learning about their environment. Exploring often leads to injury from accidental falls or things falling on them, burns, entrapment, crushing, and other mechanisms of injury.

When providing emergency care for the injured child, always tell him what you are going to do before you do it. If the child cries, let him know this is all right and you know he is trying to be brave, but everyone gets scared when hurt. Carry brightly colored adhesive bandages to hold dressings in place, and let the child know these are especially for him as a reward for bravery. You can carry along other small rewards like sheets of peel-off stickers. (Be sure the rewards are not small items that can be swallowed.)

Injury Patterns

Injury management is basically the same for children as for adults (Figure 31-9). However, their anatomic

> ### HOW AND WHY?
>
> Most injuries to children are preventable. Knowledge about injury prevention will help you provide important information to the families you encounter on calls—as well as to your own family. Go to your Electronic Extras CD for more.

Figure 31-9 Infant receiving emergency care.

and physiological differences cause children to have different patterns of injury. During motor-vehicle collisions:

- Unrestrained child passengers (those without seatbelts or restraint in a child safety seat) tend to have head and neck injuries.
- Restrained passengers may have abdominal and lower spine injuries.

Children who are struck by autos while bicycle riding often have head, spinal, and abdominal injuries. The child who has been struck by a vehicle may present with the following triad of injuries:

- Head injury
- Abdominal injury with possible internal bleeding
- Lower extremity injury (possibly a fractured femur)

Other common injuries include diving injuries with associated head and neck injury, sports injuries, which also often involve the head and neck, and injuries from child abuse.

You will need to have a good understanding of pediatric anatomic and physiologic characteristics as they relate to trauma in order to deliver expert emergency care. These include features of the head, chest, abdomen, and extremities, as described below.

Head

Recall that the head is proportionately larger and heavier in the small child. This leads to head injury when the head is propelled forward in an accident. This is often combined with internal injuries. Suspect internal injuries whenever a child with a head injury presents with shock, since head injury itself is seldom a cause of shock. Respiratory arrest is a common secondary effect of head injury, so be alert to this possibility. Although the most frequent sign of head injury is an altered mental status, nausea and vomiting also often occur.

The most important common cause of hypoxia in the unconscious head-injury patient is the tongue falling back and blocking the airway. Use the jaw-thrust maneuver to reposition the tongue and open the airway.

An error to avoid in caring for the child with a head injury is using sandbags to stabilize the head. Should the patient begin to vomit, the backboard will need to be turned on its side, and the weight of the heavy sandbag on the child's head may cause further injury.

Chest

The less-developed respiratory muscles of the chest and the more elastic ribs make the pediatric chest more easily deformed. The immature respiratory muscles

may tire easily and cannot maintain rapid respiratory rates for long. The more elastic ribs rarely fracture; however there is more likely to be injury to the structures beneath the ribs. You must suspect internal chest injuries when the mechanism of injury is significant, despite the absence of external signs of chest injury.

Abdomen

Infants and young children are abdominal breathers, using their diaphragms for breathing. Thus they may not have significant movement of their chests while breathing. Watch the abdomen to evaluate breathing. In addition, other abdominal muscles are immature and therefore provide less protection to internal organs than do adult abdominal muscles.

The abdomen can be a site of "hidden" injuries. You must suspect an internal abdominal injury when the patient deteriorates even without evidence of external injury. In addition, air in the stomach can distend the abdomen and interfere with artificial ventilation. This may also lead to vomiting. Be prepared to suction the patient.

Extremities

Despite the more flexible bones in the pediatric patient, their extremity injuries are managed the same way as extremity injuries in adults.

Pneumatic Anti-Shock Garments

In some EMS systems, pneumatic anti-shock garments (PASG), may be employed for the treatment of shock and bleeding in pediatric patients. Some general principles for their use in pediatric patients include the following:

- Use them only if they fit the patient. Never place the infant in one leg of an adult garment.
- Do not inflate the abdominal compartment. This may compromise breathing.
- PASG are indicated for the treatment of the pediatric trauma patient with signs of severe hypoperfusion and pelvic instability.

Burns

Burns are a common pediatric injury. Review the "rule of nines" (in Chapter 27), as it applies to estimating the extent of burns in children and infants. Follow these guidelines when managing patients with burns:

- Identify candidates for transportation to burn centers. Local protocols should guide your determination.

- Cover the burn with sterile dressings. Non-adherent dressings are the best, but sterile sheets may be used.

Moist dressings should be used with caution in the pediatric patient. Remember that the child's body surface area is larger proportionately to their body mass, making them more prone to heat loss. Burned patients who become hypothermic have a higher death rate. You must keep the infant or child covered to prevent a drop in body temperature.

Patient *CARE*

Trauma

Emergency care steps for the pediatric trauma patient should include the following:

1. Assure an open airway. Use the jaw-thrust maneuver.

2. Suction as necessary, using a large bore suction catheter.

3. Provide high-concentration oxygen.

4. Ventilate with a pediatric pocket mask or bag-valve mask as needed.

5. Provide spinal immobilization, in the car seat if necessary (Figure 31-10).

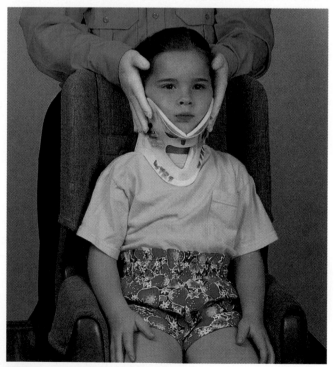

Figure 31-10 The child trauma patient may be immobilized in her car seat or extricated from the car seat to a spine board.

6. Transport immediately.

7. Continue to reassess en route.

8. Assess and treat other injuries en route if time permits.

CHILD ABUSE AND NEGLECT

The number of known child abuse cases is large but the real number may be even larger than the statistics indicate. Experts believe that for every abused child seen by the emergency department or family physician, there are many more unreported cases who never receive care.

Child abusers are mothers, fathers, sisters, brothers, grandparents, stepparents, baby-sitters and other care givers, white-collar workers, blue-collar workers, and those who are unemployed, rich, or poor. There is no distinction as to race, creed, ethnicity, or economic background.

Child abuse can take several different forms, often occurring in combination. These forms include:

- Psychological (emotional) abuse
- Neglect
- Physical abuse
- Sexual abuse

What constitutes neglect is a serious legal question. If a child goes without proper food, shelter, clothing, supervision, treatment of injuries and illnesses, a safe environment, and love, the effects surely will be seen but will seldom directly trigger an emergency call. Physical and sexual abuse are the problems likely to be seen by EMT-Bs. If signs of neglect are observed in the course of a call, they should also be reported to the proper authorities.

Physical and Sexual Abuse

Abusers inflict almost every imaginable kind of injury and maltreatment. Physically abused children—often called "battered" children—are beaten with fists, hair brushes, straps, electric cords, pool cues, razor straps, bottles, broom handles, baseball bats, pots and pans, and almost any other object that can be used as a weapon. They are intentionally burned by hot water, steam, open flames, cigarettes, and other thermal sources. Battered children may be severely shaken, thrown into their cribs or down steps, pushed out of windows and over railings, and even pushed from moving cars. Some are shot, stabbed, electrocuted, or suffocated.

Sexual abuse ranges from adults exposing themselves to children to sexual intercourse or sexual torture. Adults exposing themselves to children are often reported to the authorities. Cases in which sexual abuse results in serious physical injury also are typically reported. The cases in between, especially those in which emotional injury or minor physical injury were done, are usually not reported, and therefore are difficult to estimate.

Physical Abuse

In child physical abuse cases, you will find (Figure 31-11):

- Slap marks, bruises, abrasions, lacerations, and incisions of all sizes and with shapes matching the item used. You may see wide welts from belts, in a looped shape from cords, or in the shape of a hand from slapping. You may find swollen limbs, split lips, black eyes, and loose or broken teeth. Often the injuries are to the back, legs, and arms. The injuries may be in various stages of healing, as evidenced by different-colored bruises.

- Broken bones are common and all types of fractures are possible. Many battered children have multiple fractures, often in various stages of healing, or have fracture-associated complications.

- Head injuries are common, with concussions and skull fractures being reported. Closed head injuries occur to many infants and small children who have been severely shaken.

- Abdominal injuries include ruptured spleens, livers and lungs lacerated by broken ribs, internal bleeding from blunt trauma and punching, and lacerated and avulsed genitalia.

- Bite marks may be present showing the teeth size and pattern of the adult mouth.

- Burn marks that are small and round from cigarettes; "glove" or "stocking" burn marks from dipping in hot water; burns on buttocks and legs (creases behind the knees and at the thighs are protected when flexed); and demarcation burns in the shape of an iron, stove burner, or other hot utensil are frequently found.

- Indications of shaking an infant include a bulging fontanelle due to increased intracranial pressure from the bleeding of torn blood vessels in the brain, unconsciousness, and typical signs and symptoms of head and brain injury. Injuries to the central nervous system from "the shaken baby syndrome" are the most lethal child abuse injuries.

Sometimes you will treat an injured child and never think that he has been abused. The child relates well with the parents and there appears to be a strong bond between them. However, there can be certain indications that abuse may be occurring in or outside the home, with the family feeling they must not admit to the problem. Be on the alert for:

- Repeated responses to provide care for the same child or children in a family. Remember that in areas with many hospitals, you may see the child more frequently than any one hospital.

- Indications of past injuries. This is why you must do a physical examination and why you must remove articles of clothing. Pay special attention to the back and buttocks of the child.

- Poorly healing wounds or improperly healed fractures. It is extremely rare for a child to receive a fracture, be given proper orthopedic care, and then show angulations and large "bumps" and "knots" of bone at the "healed" injury site.

- Indications of past burns or fresh bilateral burns. Children seldom put both hands on a hot object or touch the same hot object again (true, some do . . . this is only an indication, not proof). Some types of burns are almost always linked to child abuse, such as cigarette burns to the body and burns to the buttocks and lower extremities that result from the child being dipped in hot water.

Figure 31-11 Examples of child abuse injuries.

- Many different types of injuries to both sides or the front and back of the body. This gains even more importance if the adults on the scene keep insisting that the child "falls a lot."
- Fear on the part of the child to tell you how the injury occurred. The child may seem to expect no comfort from the parents and may have little or no apparent reaction to pain.
- The parent or care giver at the scene who does not wish to leave you alone with the child, tells conflicting or changing stories, overwhelms you with explanations of the cause of the injury, or faults the child may rouse your suspicions and cause you to assess the situation more carefully.

Pay attention to the adults as you treat the child:

- Do they seem inappropriately unconcerned about the child?
- Do they have trouble controlling anger?
- Do you feel that at any moment there may be an emotional explosion?
- Do any of the adults appear to be in a deep state of depression?
- Are there indications of alcohol or drug abuse?
- Do any of the adults speak of suicide or seeking mercy for their unhappy children?

Parents or care givers may have called for help for the child, yet be reluctant to provide a history of the injury and refuse transport. Take note of any parent who refuses to have their child sent to the nearest hospital or to a hospital where the child has been seen before. This may indicate fear of the staff remembering or seeing a record of past injuries. (You cannot transport without parental consent; however, you may be able to convince the parents the child needs to be seen by a doctor because of certain signs and symptoms that are "difficult to determine" in the field.) Be the child's advocate, but do not accuse the parent.

Patient ASSESSMENT

Sexual Abuse

Rearrange or remove clothing only as necessary to determine and treat injuries. This will help preserve evidence where possible. Examine the genitalia only if there is obvious injury or the child tells you of a recent injury. The child may be hysterical, frightened, or withdrawn and unable to give you a history of the incident. Be calm and as reassuring as possible. Signs of sexual abuse include:

- Obvious results of sexual assault, including burns or wounds to the genitalia

- Any unexplained genital injury such as bruising, lacerations, or bloody discharge from genital orifices (openings)
- Seminal fluid on the body or clothes or other discharges associated with sexually transmitted diseases
- In rare cases, the child may tell you that he was sexually assaulted.

Remain professional and control your emotions. Protect the child from embarrassment. Say nothing that may make the child believe that he is to blame for the sexual assault. (Many believe that they are.)

Patient CARE

Physical or Sexual Abuse

Emergency care includes the following:

1. Dress and provide other appropriate care for injuries as necessary.

2. Preserve evidence of sexual abuse if it is suspected.

- Discourage the child from going to the bathroom (for both defecation and urination).
- Give nothing to the patient by mouth.
- Do not have the child wash or change clothes.

3. Transport the child.

Note

You must plainly and clearly report to the medical staff any finding or suspicion regarding possible physical or sexual abuse.

Role of the EMT-B in Cases of Suspected Abuse

Remember that you are charged with providing emergency care for an injured child. You are not a physician trained to detect abuse, a police officer, court investigator, social worker, judge, or one-person jury. Gather information from the parents or care giver away from the child without expression of disbelief or judgment. Talk with the child separately about how the injury occurred. As you assess the patient and provide appropriate care, control your emotions and hold back accusations. Do not indicate to the parents or other adults at the scene that you suspect child abuse. Do not ask the child if he has been abused. To do so when others are around could produce stress too great for the injured child to handle.

If you are suspicious about the mechanism of injury, transport the child even though the severity of injury may not warrant such action.

ALWAYS report your suspicions to the emergency department staff and in accordance with local policies. Every medical facility should take action to see if your fears are well founded. If you fear that the medical staff has not taken you seriously, then you must report your suspicions to the juvenile authorities of the local police department. In some states, EMT-Bs are mandatory reporters; that is, they are required by law to report suspicions of child abuse. Be familiar with your state laws. Even if reporting possible child abuse is not a legal requirement in your state, it is a professional obligation.

Documentation Tip—Suspected Child Abuse

Keep accurate records of possible child abuse. State all of your objective findings, but do not state a conclusion that there is abuse. Draw a picture to indicate the size and location of all the child's injuries. Do not assume the cause of an injury (e.g., a cigarette burn). Instead, provide a detailed description of the injury and injury site.

Maintain patient and family confidentiality. You cannot name the child or the family or give any details concerning the family to anyone other than the medical staff, the police, or your superior officer. Follow department requirements and state laws in reporting the problem.

Past responses can be checked and future responses noted in case a pattern develops to indicate possible abuse. However, even when talking to your partner, the hospital staff, the police, and your superiors, use the terms "suspicious" and "possible." Do not call someone a child abuser. If you break confidentiality, you could be sued. Keep in mind that the courts can deal harshly with those who provide patient care and then violate the confidentiality of the patient, the family, and the home. Keep in mind that rumors about abuse may, in the long run, cause mental or physical harm to your child patient.

It may be difficult, but keep in mind that the parent or care giver needs help also. Your actions, response, and concern directed toward the suspected abuser can help them recognize their problem and may encourage them to seek therapy and rehabilitation. Also bear in mind that your suspicions may be unfounded. Not every injury to a child is the result of child abuse. Suspicions should be aroused not by individual injuries but by patterns of injuries and behavior.

INFANTS AND CHILDREN WITH SPECIAL NEEDS

Over the years, medical expertise has improved significantly, allowing many children who would formerly have died to live. The group of children with special needs includes:

- Premature infants with lung disease
- Infants and children with heart disease
- Infants and children with neurological disease
- Children with chronic disease or altered function from birth

Often these children are able to live at home with their parents. This means that you may receive calls to care for children who have complicated medical problems and are dependent on various technologies (Figure 31-12). The children's parents will be familiar with the various devices and can serve as a valuable resource. Common devices include tracheostomy tubes, home artificial ventilators, central intravenous lines, gastrostomy tubes and gastric feeding tubes, and shunts.

Tracheostomy Tubes

Tracheostomy tubes are tubes that have been placed into the child's trachea to create an open airway. They are often used when a child has been on a ventilator for a prolonged time. Although

Figure 31-12 Child with spina bifida.

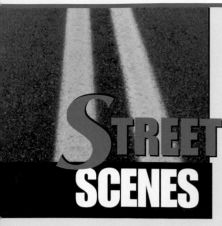

Shawna Simon is an active 2-year-old. She has been playing most of the afternoon since her nap. After dinner, her mother notices that her face seems flushed, her forehead is warm, and she is not her usual self. After getting Shawna ready for bed, the mother sits with her for a while. Just as she is about to leave the room, Shawna arches her back and starts to shake. The mother is frightened, and when she turns on the light, Shawna appears not to be breathing. The mother calls 9-1-1 immediately. The dispatcher has trouble calming her down, but he does hear her say, "My baby isn't breathing."

While one dispatcher continues to calm the mother, another dispatches you to 143 Pine Lane for "a child not breathing. More information to follow."

STREET SCENE QUESTIONS

1. What is your assessment plan for this patient?

2. What equipment should be brought into the house?

3. Should ALS be dispatched to the scene prior to your arrival?

Your response time is less than 5 minutes. Your partner radios the dispatcher and asks for an ALS response before arriving at the scene. Dispatch has informed you that the mother is still very upset and he has no additional information. About a minute before arriving, you discuss with your partner the equipment that needs to go into the house, and you both agree to take in the pediatric bag that contains the airway equipment, including the BVM, an oxygen tank, and suction.

You volunteer to get the equipment, while your partner goes to the patient. Your partner enters the house just before you and he sees the mother holding a limp child. He takes Shawna and places her on the couch.

Your partner immediately evaluates the airway and breathing. He then performs a head-tilt, chin-lift maneuver, which brings the tongue forward. He sees mucus around the mouth, so he clears the airway by suctioning. Shawna becomes more responsive and cries. Her respirations are deep and adequate. (They would have to be for her to cry that loudly.) You and your partner realize that it is a good sound.

STREET SCENE QUESTIONS

4. What care should be provided next?

5. What additional assessment needs to be done?

6. What information needs to be relayed to the ALS unit?

You administer blow-by oxygen to the patient, while your partner gets a full set of vital signs. You reassure the mother that Shawna is breathing and tell her that she can help by answering some questions. You proceed to ask all the SAMPLE questions. Shawna's mother describes what led up to this event. You radio the ALS unit with this information and are informed of a two-minute ETA, so you start to package the patient for transport to the hospital. As you are doing this, Shawna opens her eyes. She continues to cry and you ask her mother to hold her hand and talk to her. Although she is not fully

---

there are various types of tubes, the potential complications are identical. You may be called to help when there is:

- Obstruction
- Bleeding from the tube or around the tube
- Air leak around the tube
- Infection
- Dislodged tube

Your emergency care will consist of:

- Maintaining an open airway
- Suctioning the tube as needed

- Allowing the patient to remain in a position of comfort, perhaps on the parent's lap
- Transporting the patient to the hospital

Home Artificial Ventilators

Artificial ventilators in the home are becoming more common. The parents will be trained in its use but will call EMS when there is trouble. Regardless of the problem, your emergency care will include:

- Maintaining an open airway
- Artificially ventilating with a pocket mask or bag-valve mask with oxygen
- Transporting the patient

PATIENT NAME: Shawna Simon						PATIENT AGE: 2 years	

CHIEF COMPLAINT

"Isn't breathing"

PAST MEDICAL HISTORY

- ☒ None
- ☐ Allergy to _____
- ☐ Hypertension   ☐ Stroke
- ☐ Seizures   ☐ Diabetes
- ☐ COPD   ☐ Cardiac
- ☐ Other (List)   ☐ Asthma

Current Medications (List)

VITAL SIGNS	TIME	RESP	PULSE	B.P.	MENTAL STATUS	R PUPILS L	SKIN
	1905	Rate: 32 ☐ Regular ☒ Shallow ☐ Labored	Rate: 120 ☒ Regular ☐ Irregular		☐ Alert ☐ Voice ☐ Pain ☑ Unresp.	☑ Normal ☑ ☐ Dilated ☐ ☐ Constricted ☐ ☐ Sluggish ☐ ☐ No-Reaction ☐	☐ Unremarkable ☐ Cool ☐ Pale ☑ Warm ☐ Cyanotic ☑ Moist ☑ Flushed ☐ Dry ☐ Jaundiced
	1915	Rate: 30 ☒ Regular ☐ Shallow ☐ Labored	Rate: 110 ☒ Regular ☐ Irregular		☐ Alert ☑ Voice ☐ Pain ☐ Unresp.	☑ Normal ☑ ☐ Dilated ☐ ☐ Constricted ☐ ☐ Sluggish ☐ ☐ No-Reaction ☐	☐ Unremarkable ☐ Cool ☐ Pale ☑ Warm ☐ Cyanotic ☑ Moist ☐ Flushed ☐ Dry ☐ Jaundiced
	1925	Rate: 30 ☒ Regular ☐ Shallow ☐ Labored	Rate: 110 ☒ Regular ☐ Irregular		☐ Alert ☑ Voice ☐ Pain ☐ Unresp.	☑ Normal ☑ ☐ Dilated ☐ ☐ Constricted ☐ ☐ Sluggish ☐ ☐ No-Reaction ☐	☐ Unremarkable ☐ Cool ☐ Pale ☑ Warm ☐ Cyanotic ☐ Moist ☐ Flushed ☑ Dry ☐ Jaundiced

NARRATIVE On arrival, mom was holding the child, who was limp in her arms. Mother stated the patient became flushed, lethargic, and felt warm to the touch, and suddenly began to shake and appeared not to be breathing. The patient was unresponsive initially. While assessing the patient, she was noted to be breathing with mucus around her mouth. After suctioning, oxygen was initiated at 10 LPM with a pediatric nonrebreather via blow-by technique. Patient gradually became more responsive and was crying prior to transport. ALS arrived at the scene but did not come with us to the hospital. Both the paramedics and medical direction felt the patient was stable and appropriate for BLS transport.

alert, she is breathing well and her skin color is improving.

As you arrive at the ambulance, the ALS unit pulls up and a paramedic gets into your patient compartment. She does an assessment and is confident that a BLS transport is all that is required. She calls medical direction and provides a patient history with vital signs. Medical direction concurs that a BLS transport is appropriate. As she returns to her vehicle, the paramedic compliments you and your partner on a job well done.

Central Intravenous Lines

Central lines are intravenous lines that are placed close to the heart. Unlike most peripheral IV lines, central lines may be left in place for long-term use. Possible complications of central lines are:

- Infection
- Bleeding
- Clotting-off of the line
- Cracked line

Your emergency care will include:

- Applying pressure if there is bleeding
- Transporting the patient

Gastrostomy Tubes and Gastric Feeding

Gastrostomy tubes are tubes placed through the abdominal wall directly into the stomach. These are used when a patient is not able to be fed orally. The most dangerous potential problem involves respiratory distress. The emergency care will include:

- Being alert for altered mental status in diabetic patients. They may become hypoglycemic quickly when unable to eat.
- Assuring an open airway
- Suctioning the airway as needed
- Providing oxygen if needed

- Transporting the patient in either a sitting position or lying on the right side with the head elevated to reduce the risk of aspiration

Shunts

A shunt is a drainage device that runs from the brain to the abdomen to relieve excess cerebrospinal fluid. There will be a reservoir on the side of the skull. Should the shunt malfunction, pressure inside the skull will rise, causing an altered mental status. An altered mental status may also be caused by an infection. These patients are prone to respiratory arrest. Your emergency care will include:

- Maintaining an open airway
- Ventilating with a pocket mask or bag-valve mask and high concentration oxygen if needed
- Transporting the patient

THE EMT-B AND PEDIATRIC EMERGENCIES

Many types of pediatric illnesses and injuries have been discussed. The focus has been on the patient. Now we will look at the psychological responses of the EMT-B.

It is well known that pediatric calls can be among the most stressful for the EMT-B, even when they are uneventful. EMT-Bs who have children often identify their patients with their own children. Other EMT-Bs have no experience with children and feel anxiety about communicating with them and treating them—even about estimating their ages. However, the skills of communicating with and treating children can be learned and applied. Often the EMT-B who starts out "knowing nothing about children" turns out to have a real knack for dealing with them.

Most of the care of children consists of applying what you have learned about the care of adult patients with knowledge of the key differences in developmental characteristics, anatomy, and physiology of children.

Often the most serious stresses an EMT-B faces result from pediatric calls that involve a very sick, injured, or abused child, or a child who has died or who dies during or after emergency care. Such calls are, fortunately, rare, and can be prepared for with advance training.

When you have had an experience like this, talk with other EMT-Bs. If your squad or service has a counselor, see this person for advice. You may think that you can handle the stress or sorrow by yourself, but experienced EMT-Bs know better. Unless you resolve the impact of stressful events, the problems created may compound and could lead to "burnout." Contact your local Critical Incident Stress Management (CISM) team for assistance after incidents such as these.

CHAPTER REVIEW

SUMMARY

For the most part, treatment for the illnesses and injuries of infants and children is like the treatment for adults. However, children do have some special developmental characteristics and characteristics of anatomy and physiology. To treat infants and children effectively, you should know something about these special characteristics of children and the illnesses and injuries to which they are prone.

REVIEW QUESTIONS

1. Name one psychological/social characteristic that you would be likely to find in a patient of each of the following ages and explain how you would tailor your actions as an EMT-B to accommodate this characteristic: 2-year-old, 6-year-old, and 15-year-old. (p. 663)

2. For each of the following physical characteristics of pediatric patients, explain how it might affect assessment and care. (pp. 661, 664, 669, 677, 678)
   – Large, heavy head relative to neck and body
   – Large body surface relative to body mass

3. Explain how to differentiate between an upper airway obstruction and a lower airway disease or disorder. Explain how and why the two should be treated differently. (p. 669)

4. Explain the main steps of emergency treatment for any infant or child trauma patient. (p. 678)

5. Explain how suspicion of child abuse should or should not affect the care you provide for an infant or child patient. Explain the reporting requirements in your state or locality. (pp. 678–681)

APPLICATIONS

- You are called to the scene of a collision between a vehicle and a 5-year-old on a bicycle. The child is lying near the curb. Based on what you know about the developmental characteristics of children as well as common injury patterns in children, explain some of the special elements you should take into consideration as you proceed to assess and care for this patient.

WEB MEDIC

Visit Brady's *Emergency Care* website for direct weblinks. At **www.bradybooks.com/emergencycare**, you will find information related to the following Chapter 31 topics:

- Child development
- Children with tracheostomy tubes
- Pediatric respiratory issues

Chapter
Thirty-Two

AMBULANCE OPERATIONS

Your responsibilities may differ somewhat depending on the type of EMS agency you join. However most non-medical operational responsibilities include the following five phases:

- Preparing for the ambulance call
- Receiving and responding to a call
- Transferring the patient to the ambulance
- Transporting the patient to the hospital
- Terminating the call

PREPARING FOR THE AMBULANCE CALL

The modern ambulance has come a long way from its primitive beginnings. Far more than just a means of transport, today's ambulance is a well-equipped and efficiently organized mobile pre-hospital emergency department and communications unit.

The U. S. Department of Transportation has issued specifications for Type I, Type II, and Type III ambulances. Because of the extra equipment now placed on ambulances for specialty rescue, advanced life support, and hazardous materials operations, the gross vehicle weight has been easily exceeded in some communities. This has necessitated introduction of a medium-duty truck chassis built for rugged durability and large storage and work areas (Figure 32-1). As needs evolve, ambulance standards will also continue to evolve.

Ambulance Supplies and Equipment

If it does not have the proper equipment for patient care and transportation, an ambulance is just another truck. Following are lists of supplies and equipment that should be carried in an ambulance. The lists are based on recommendations of the American College of Surgeons and various ambulance services.

Patient Infection Control, Comfort, and Protection Supplies

The following supplies should be carried in the ambulance:

- Two pillows
- Four pillow cases
- Two spare sheets
- Four blankets
- Six disposable emesis (vomit) bags or basins
- Two boxes of facial tissues
- Disposable bedpan, urinal, and toilet paper
- One package of drinking cups
- One package of wet wipes
- Four liters of sterile water or saline
- Four soft restraining devices (upper and lower extremities)
- Packages of large and small red biohazard bags for waste or severed parts
- One package of large yellow bags for used linens or garbage (or otherwise color-coded or labeled according to your service's Exposure Control Plan)
- EPA-registered, intermediate-level disinfectant (which destroys mycobacterium tuberculosis)
- EPA-registered, low-level disinfectant such as Lysol

TOPIC OVERVIEW

In this chapter, you will learn about the following topics:

Phases of an ambulance call

Emergency driving laws and regulations

Operating an emergency vehicle

Preparation for a call

How to clean and disinfect EMS equipment

DOT OBJECTIVES

✔ Knowledge and Attitude

1. Discuss the medical and non-medical equipment needed to respond to a call. (pp. 687, 689–692)

2. List the phases of an ambulance call. (p. 687)

3. Describe the general provisions of state laws relating to the operation of the ambulance and privileges in any or all of the following categories: (pp. 695–698, 700) (Scan 32-2, p. 699)
- Speed
- Warning lights
- Sirens
- Right-of-way
- Parking
- Turning

4. List contributing factors to unsafe driving conditions. (p. 698)

5. Describe the considerations that should be given to: (pp. 697–698)
- Request for escorts
- Following an escort vehicle
- Intersections

6. Discuss "Due Regard For Safety of All Others" while operating an emergency vehicle. (p. 696)

7. State what information is essential in order to respond to a call. (pp. 693–694)

8. Discuss various situations that may affect response to a call (p. 698) (Scan 32-7, p. 713)

9. Differentiate between the various methods of moving a patient to the unit based upon injury or illness. (p. 698)

10. Apply the components of the essential patient information in a written report. (pp. 702, 704)

11. Summarize the importance of preparing the unit for the next response. (pp. 705–707, 711) (Scan 32-4, p. 706; Scan 32-5, pp. 708–709)

12. Identify what is essential for completion of a call. (pp. 703, 705, 707) (Scan 32-3, p. 704)

13. Distinguish among the terms cleaning, disinfection, high-level disinfection, and sterilization. (p. 710)

14. Describe how to clean or disinfect items following patient care. (pp. 707, 711) (Scan 32-6, p. 710)

15. Explain the rationale for appropriate report of patient information. (pp. 702, 704)

16. Explain the rationale for having the unit prepared to respond. (pp. 692, 694) (Scan 32-1, p. 693)

A

B

C

D

Figure 32-1 Four types of ambulances: (A) Type I, (B) Type II, (C) Type III, and (D) medium duty.

- An empty plastic spray bottle with lines at the 1:100 level, a plastic bottle of water, and a plastic bottle of bleach for cleaning up blood spills (Measure a fresh mixture of 1 part bleach to 100 parts water each day as needed.)
- Eye shields or other protective eyewear for each crew member
- Sharps container for the vehicle (BLS or ALS unit) and (for ALS unit) drug box
- Disposable latex, vinyl, or other synthetic gloves: a box of each size
- N-95 or HEPA respirator for each crew member

Initial and Focused Assessment Equipment

Portable first-in kits come in all shapes and sizes, in hard cases or soft bags. A first-in kit should include supplies for:

- *Airway.* Airways, suction, infection control, personal protective equipment; if permitted for EMT-B use by local protocols, equipment for adult and pediatric orotracheal intubation
- *Breathing.* Stethoscope, pocket mask with one way valve and oxygen inlet, bag-valve mask, oxygen, oxygen delivery devices
- *Circulation.* Blood pressure cuff, bandages and dressings, occlusive dressings, AED (automated external defibrillator)
- *Neck and spine stabilization.* Set of rigid cervical collars
- *Exposure.* Scissors and blankets to expose and deal with exposure
- *Vital signs:*
  - Sphygmomanometer kit with separate cuffs for average-size and obese adults as well as child sizes
  - Adult and a pediatric stethoscopes
  - Thermometer and a hypothermia thermometer that goes down to at least 82° Fahrenheit
  - One penlight
  - Many services carry a pocket guide with pediatric vitals and other quick resource information.

Equipment for Transfer of Patient

The following carrying devices should be included:

- Wheeled ambulance stretcher is designed so that a sick or injured person can be transported in the Fowler's (sitting), supine, or Trendelenberg position. Also called a cot or gurney, the wheeled stretcher should have a number of features. It should be adjustable in height and have detachable supports for intravenous fluid containers. Restraining devices should be provided so that a pa-

tient can be prevented from falling off the stretcher or sliding past the foot end or head end.
- Reeves stretcher for carrying a patient who must lie supine down stairs when a cot is too heavy or wide
- Folding stair chair for moving patients down stairs in a sitting position
- Scoop stretcher, also called an orthopedic stretcher, for picking up patients found in tight spaces with a minimum of movement
- Stokes or basket stretcher for long-distance carries, high-angle, or off-the-road rescues
- Child safety seat for transporting infants and small children in the ambulance (optional)

Equipment for Airway Maintenance, Ventilation, and Resuscitation

A number of devices should be carried for maintaining an open airway and assisting breathing:

- Oropharyngeal airways in sizes suitable for adults, children, and infants
- Soft rubber nasopharyngeal airways in sizes 14 through 30
- Two pocket face masks with one-way valves and filters for times when ventilation is necessary or when you are the only person ventilating a patient who does not have an endotracheal tube inserted
- Three manually operated, self-refilling bag-valve-mask units (infant, child, adult) capable of delivering 100% oxygen to a patient by the addition of a reservoir. Masks of various sizes should be designed to ensure a tight face seal and should have an air cushion. The masks should be clear so you can see vomitus and the clouding caused by exhalations.

Oxygen Therapy and Suction Equipment

An ambulance should have two oxygen supply systems (one fixed, one portable) so oxygen can be supplied to two patients at once:

- Fixed oxygen delivery system supplies oxygen to a patient in the ambulance. A typical installation consists of a minimum 3,000-liter reservoir, a two-stage regulator, plus yokes, reducing valve, and non-gravity-type flowmeter. Oxygen delivery tubes, transparent masks, and controls should all be located within easy reach when you are sitting at the patient's head. The system should be capable of delivering at least 15 liters of oxygen per minute and adaptable to the bag-valve-mask units carried on the ambulance.
- Two portable oxygen delivery systems that have a capacity of at least 350 liters. Each system should have a regulator capable of delivering at least 15

liters of oxygen per minute. Many ambulances are equipped with multiple function regulators that can be used for liter-flow oxygen, suctioning, and positive pressure ventilation.

In addition, an ambulance should have the following:

- Spare D, E, or jumbo D oxygen cylinders with a current hydrostat test date seal imprinted on the tank
- Six adult and four pediatric nonrebreather masks
- Six adult and four pediatric nasal cannulas
- One flow-restricted, oxygen-powered ventilation device
- One automatic transport ventilator (ATV) (optional)
- One plastic comic cup for administering blow-by oxygen to a child

The fixed suction system should be sufficient to provide an air flow of over 30 liters per minute at the end of the delivery tube. A vacuum of at least 300 mmHg should be reached within 4 seconds after the suction tube is clamped. The suction should be controllable. The installed system should have a large-diameter, non-kinking tube fitted with a rigid tip. There should be a spare non-breakable, disposable suction bottle and a container of water for rinsing the tubes. There should be an assortment of sterile catheters. The suction system should be usable by a person seated at the head of the patient.

The portable suction unit can be one of the many models powered by battery, hand or foot action, oxygen, or compressed air. The unit should be fitted with a non-kinking tube as well as a large-bore Yankauer tip.

Equipment for Assisting with Cardiac Resuscitation

The following equipment for assisting with cardiopulmonary resuscitation and defibrillation should be carried on the ambulance:

- Short or long spine board to provide rigid support during CPR efforts
- An automated external defibrillator (AED)
- A mechanical CPR compressor (e.g., Thumper)—especially helpful for doing CPR for services with transports over 15 minutes to the hospital (optional)

Supplies and Equipment for Immobilization of Suspected Bone Injuries

The ambulance should carry a variety of devices for immobilization of injured extremities and suspected spine injuries:

- Adult and pediatric traction splints (e.g., Sager or Hare) for the immobilization of a painful, swollen, or deformed thigh
- Padded board splints for the immobilization of upper and lower extremities. Recommended are two 3 × 54-inch splints, two 3 × 36-inch splints, and two 3 × 15-inch splints.
- Variety of splints: air-inflatable splints, vacuum splints, wire ladder splints, cardboard splints, soft rubberized splints with aluminum stays and Velcro fasteners, padded aluminum (SAM) splints, and splints that are inflated with cryogenic (cold) gas
- Tongue depressors to use to immobilize broken fingers
- Triangular bandages for use with splints and for making slings and swathes
- Several rolls of self-adhering roller bandage for securing the various splints
- Six chemical cold packs for use on injured extremities
- Two long spine boards for full-body immobilization, preferably with speed clips or Velcro straps. The long spine board can also be used for patient transfer
- Rigid cervical collars in a variety of adult and child sizes
- One KED, XP1, Kansas Board, or LSP halfback board for seated persons with possible spinal injuries
- Six 9-foot-by-2-inch web straps with air-craft-style buckles or D-rings for securing patients to carrying devices
- Head immobilizer device such as the Headbed, Bashaw CID, Ferno Head Immobilizer, or a rolled blanket

Supplies for Wound Care and Treatment of Shock

A variety of dressings and bandaging materials should be carried on the ambulance:

- Sterile gauze pads (2 × 2 inches and 4 × 4 inches)
- 5 × 9 inch combine dressings
- Sterile universal dressings (multi-trauma dressings) approximately 10 × 36 inches
- Self-adhering roller bandages in 4- and 6-inch width × 5 yards
- Occlusive dressings (Vaseline gauze) for sealing open (sucking) chest wounds and eviscerations
- Aluminum foil (sterilized in a separate package) for various uses such as occlusive dressings and also to maintain body heat or to form an oxygen tent for a newborn infant

- Sterile burn sheets or prepackaged burn kit
- Adhesive strip bandages for minor wound care (1 × ¾ inch and 1 × ½ inch), individually packaged
- Hypoallergenic adhesive tape (1- and 3-inch rolls)
- Large safety pins for the securing of slings and swathes
- Bandage scissors
- Pneumatic anti-shock garments (PASG) in sizes for adults and children
- Aluminum blankets (survival blankets) for maintaining body heat

Supplies for Childbirth

A sterile childbirth kit, either provided by a local medical facility or a commercially available disposable kit, as mandated by your system, should contain the following:

- Several pairs of sterile surgical gloves
- Four umbilical cord clamps or umbilical tape
- One pair of sterile surgical scissors
- One rubber bulb syringe (3 oz.)
- Twelve 4 × 4 inch gauze pads
- Four pairs of sterile disposable gloves
- Five towels
- One baby blanket (receiving blanket)
- Infant swaddler
- Sanitary napkins
- Two large plastic bags
- Two stockinette infant caps

Also carry items that you can wear to minimize contamination of or by the mother and baby during and after childbirth:

- Two surgical gowns
- Two surgical caps
- Two surgical masks
- Two pairs of goggles or eye shields

Supplies, Equipment, and Medications for the Treatment of Acute Poisoning, Snakebite, Chemical Burns, and Diabetic Emergencies

A number of poison control kits are available from emergency care equipment suppliers. Whether purchased intact or hand-made, a poison control kit should include these items:

- Drinking water to dilute poisons
- Activated charcoal
- Paper cups and other equipment for oral administration
- Equipment for irrigating a patient's eyes or skin with sterile water

- Constriction bands for snakebites
- Instant glucose paste

Special Equipment for Paramedics and Physicians

Depending on state laws and your medical director, some ambulances are provided with locked kits of supplies and equipment that can be used by paramedics or physicians, especially in rural areas. This equipment may include supplies for:

- Endotracheal intubation, orotracheal and endotracheal suctioning, and pediatric nasogastric intubation (In some areas EMT-Bs will be trained to perform these procedures.)
- Chest decompression
- Drug administration
- Advanced airways such as the esophageal obturator airway (EOA), esophageal gastric tube airway (EGTA), or Combitube® airway
- Cricothyrotomy
- Cardiac monitoring and defibrillation

Safety and Miscellaneous Equipment

Ambulances should also be provided with personal protective equipment for you; equipment for warning, signaling, and lighting; hazard control devices; and tools for gaining access and disentanglements including:

- *North American Emergency Response Guidebook*
- Binoculars
- Clipboard, prehospital care reports (PCRs), and other documentation forms
- Ring cutter
- Portable radio
- Multiple-casualty incident management logs
- Triage tags and destination logs
- Command vests
- Tarps in red, green, black, and yellow for multiple-casualty incident field treatment areas
- Disposable Tyvek jumpsuits
- Flares
- Jumper cables
- Set of turnout gear (coat, helmet, protective eyewear, gloves) for each crew member
- Large floodlight/spotlight
- Concentrated sports drink (e.g., Gatorade) and a cooler for rehabilitation sector (optional)
- Self-contained breathing apparatus (SCBA) (optional)
- Spring-loaded center punch
- Glas-Master or flathead ax

- Small sledge hammer, prybar, Biel tool, and other tools for gaining access
- Wheel chocks
- Utility rope
- Stuffed animal for child patients

Compare the items listed in this chapter with the inventory of your ambulance. Learn where each item is stored, what every item is for, and when it should be used. If the item is a mechanical device, also learn how it works and how it should be maintained.

Ensuring Ambulance Readiness for Service

The most modern, well-equipped ambulance is not worth the room it takes up in the garage unless it is ready to respond at the time of an emergency. A planned preventive maintenance program includes periodic servicing. Oil should be changed regularly, tires rotated, the vehicle lubricated, and so on.

Let us say that you and your partner have just reported for duty. As soon as it is practical, speak with the crew going off duty. Learn whether they experienced any problems with either the ambulance or its equipment during their shift. Make a thorough bumper-to-bumper inspection of the ambulance (Scan 32-1). Use the checklist provided by your service to do this.

Ambulance Inspection, Engine Off

Following are inspection steps that can be taken while the ambulance is in quarters:

1. Inspect the body of the vehicle. Look for damage that could interfere with safe operation. A crumpled fender, for example, may prevent the front wheels from turning the maximum distance.

2. Inspect the wheels and tires. The tires take a beating in normal operation. At collision scenes they may contact shards of glass and sharp pieces of metal and other debris. Check for damage or worn wheel rims and tire sidewalls. Check the tread depth. Use a pressure gauge to ensure that all tires are properly inflated. Do not forget to inspect the inside rear tires.

3. Inspect windows and mirrors. Look for broken glass and loose or missing parts. See that mirrors are clean and properly adjusted for maximum visibility.

4. Check the operation of every door and latches and locks.

5. Inspect the components of the cooling system. (**Warning:** Allow the engine to cool before removing any pressure caps.) Check the level of the coolant. Inspect the cooling system hoses for leaks and cracks.

6. Check the level of the other vehicle fluids, including the engine oil and the brake, power, and steering fluids.

7. Check the battery. If the battery has removable fill caps, check the level of the fluid. If the battery is the sealed type, determine its condition by checking the indicator port. Inspect the battery cable connections for tightness and signs of corrosion.

8. Inspect the interior surfaces and upholstery for damage and cleanliness.

9. Check the windows for operation. See that the interior surface of each window is clean.

10. Test the horn.

11. Test the siren for full range of operation.

12. Check the seat belts. Examine each belt to see that it is not damaged. Pull each belt from its storage spool to ensure that the retractor mechanisms work. Buckle each belt to ensure that latches work properly.

13. Adjust the driver's seat for comfort and optimum steering wheel and pedal operation.

14. Check the fuel level. Refuel after each call whenever practical.

Ambulance Inspection, Engine On

The next steps require you to start the engine. Pull the ambulance from quarters if engine exhaust fumes will be a problem. Set the parking brake, put the transmission in "park," and have your partner chock the wheels before undertaking the following steps:

1. Check the dash-mounted indicators to see if any light remains on to indicate a possible problem with oil pressure, engine temperature, or the vehicle's electrical system.

2. Check dash-mounted gauges for proper operation.

3. Depress the brake pedal. Note whether pedal travel seems correct or excessive. Check air pressure as needed.

4. Test the parking brake. Move the transmission level to a drive position. Replace the level to the "park" position as soon as you are sure that the parking brake is holding.

5. Turn the steering wheel from side to side.

6. Check the operation of the windshield wipers and washers. The glass should be wiped clean each time the blade moves.

7. Turn on the vehicle's warning lights. Have your partner walk around the ambulance and check each flashing and revolving light for operation. Turn off the warning lights.

8. Turn on the other vehicle lights. Have your partner walk around the ambulance again, this time checking the headlights (high and low beams), turn signals, four-way flashers, brake lights, side and rear scene illumination lights, and box marker lights.

INSPECTING THE AMBULANCE

▲ **1.** Check the ambulance body, wheels, tires, and windshield wipers.

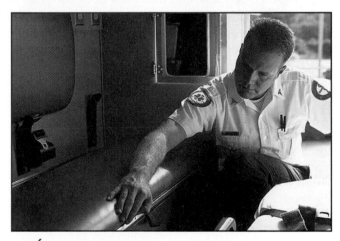

▲ **2.** Check windows, doors, and mirrors.

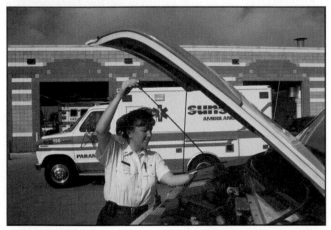

▲ **3.** Check under the hood.

▲ **4.** Check interior surfaces and upholstery.

▲ **5.** Check dash instruments and communications equipment.

▲ **6.** Check the fuel level and fill up.

693

9. Check the operation of the heating and air-conditioning equipment in both the driver's compartment and the patient compartment. This is also a good time to check the onboard suction if the engine is running.

10. Check transmission fluid.

11. Operate the communications equipment. Test portable as well as fixed radios and any radio-telephone communications.

Return the ambulance to quarters, and while you are backing up, have your partner note whether the backup alarm is operating (if the vehicle is so equipped).

Inspection of Patient Compartment Supplies and Equipment

Shut off the engine and complete your inspection by checking the patient compartment and all exterior cabinets:

1. Check the interior of the patient compartment. Look for damage to the interior surfaces and upholstery. Be certain that any needed decontamination has been completed and that the compartment is clean.

2. Check treatment supplies and equipment and rescue equipment. Items should not only be identified, they should also be checked for completeness, condition, and operation. Check the pressure of oxygen cylinders. Inflate air splints and examine them for leaks. Test oxygen and ventilation equipment for proper operation. Examine rescue tools for rust and dirt. Operate battery-powered devices to ensure that the batteries have a proper charge. Some equipment, such as the AED, may require additional testing. See that an item-by-item inspection of everything carried on the ambulance is done, with findings recorded on the inspection report.

3. When you are finished, complete the inspection report. Correct any deficiencies. Replace missing items. Make your supervisor aware of any deficiencies that cannot be immediately corrected.

4. Finally, clean the unit for infection control and appearance. Maintaining the ambulance's appearance enhances your organization's image in the public's eye. People who take pride in their work show it by taking pride in the appearance of their ambulance.

RECEIVING AND RESPONDING TO A CALL

In many areas of the country, a person needs only to dial 9-1-1 to access ambulance, fire, or police services 24 hours a day. A trained Emergency Medical Dispatcher (EMD) records information from callers, decides which service is needed, and alerts that service to respond. (Always say "nine-one-one" when talking to community or school groups. Children cannot find "eleven" on the phone dial or key pad.)

Role of the Emergency Medical Dispatcher

Many cities and communication centers train and certify Emergency Medical Dispatchers (EMDs) based on the medical priority card system, originated in 1979 through the leadership of Jeffrey Clawson, M.D. An EMD is trained to perform the following tasks:

- Interrogate the caller and assign a priority to the call
- Provide pre-arrival medical instructions to callers and information to crews
- Dispatch and coordinate EMS resources
- Coordinate with other public safety agencies

When answering a call for help, the EMD must obtain as much information as possible about the situation that may help the responding crew. The questions the EMD should ask are:

1. *What is the exact location of the patient?* The EMD must ask for the house or building number and the apartment number, if any. It is important to ask the street name with the direction designator (e.g., North, East), the nearest cross street, the name of the development or subdivision, and the exact location of the emergency.

2. *What is your call-back number?* (Enhanced 9-1-1 will show the number.) *Stay on the line. Do not hang up until I* (the EMD) *tell you to.* In life-threatening situations, the EMD will offer instruction to the caller, after the units have been dispatched, that the caller or others on the scene should follow until the units arrive. It is also important for the caller to stay on the line in case a question arises about the location that was given.

3. *What's the problem?* This will provide the chief complaint. It will help the EMD decide which line of questioning to follow and the priority of the response to send.

4. *How old is the patient?* Most ambulances are set up to respond to the scene with a pediatric kit if the patient is a child rather than an adult. If pre-arrival CPR instructions are given, it will be necessary to distinguish between an infant, a child, and an adult.

5. *What's the patient's sex?* (if not obvious from caller's voice or information)

6. *Is the patient conscious?* An unconscious patient is a higher response priority.

7. *Is the patient breathing?* If the patient is conscious and breathing, the EMD will often ask many additional questions relative to the chief complaint to determine the appropriate level of response; for example, First Responders, EMT-Paramedics, or ambulance responding COLD (at normal speed—sometimes called Priority 3) or HOT (an emergency, lights-and-siren mode—sometimes called Priority 1). If the patient is not breathing, or the caller is not sure, the EMD will dispatch the maximum response and begin the appropriate pre-arrival instructions for a non-breathing patient, which may also involve telephone CPR if the patient is pulseless.

If the call is for a traffic collision, a series of key questions must be asked to help determine the priority and amount of response. With good interrogation of the caller, it may be possible for the EMD to appropriately dispatch one unit HOT and backup units COLD, which in turn will help prevent emergency vehicle collisions.

1. *How many and what kinds of vehicles are involved?* The EMD should determine, if possible, how many vehicles are involved in the collision and if they are cars, trucks, or buses. Any injury resulting from a collision involving a bicycle, motorcycle, or pedestrian versus an automobile should receive the highest priority of response because of the mechanisms of injury involved. If the EMD learns that a truck is involved, he will try to determine if it is a vehicle that may be carrying a hazardous load.

2. *How many persons do you think are injured?* When the EMD learns from the caller that five people have been injured, he may send two or three ambulances at the same time. Time, and perhaps lives, may be saved by knowing the precise number of people injured in a collision.

3. *Do the victims appear trapped?* It may be necessary to dispatch a rescue unit also.

4. *What is the exact location of the collision?* You should be able to learn a street address or the name of the nearest cross street. If the collision has occurred in a rural or wilderness area, the EMD must try to pinpoint the location by asking questions about the nearest landmark visible from the caller's point of view (e.g. mile posts, water towers, large silos, or radio antennas). If the caller cannot pinpoint his location, the telephone company should be able to provide the location of the phone.

Next, the EMD should attempt to learn something about the scene. If the EMD learns that all lanes of a road leading to the collision scene are blocked, for example, operators can select alternative response routes.

1. Is traffic moving?
2. How many lanes are open?
3. How far is traffic backed up?
4. Are any of the vehicles on fire?
5. Are any of the vehicles leaking fuel?
6. Are any electrical wires down?
7. Do any of the vehicles appear unstable? Is any vehicle on its side or top?
8. Does a truck appear to be carrying a hazardous cargo?

This is how an EMD might dispatch an ambulance to the location of a sick person:

> MEDCOM to Ambulance 641 and Medic 640, respond priority one to a 60-year-old unconscious female with breathing difficulty. The location is the Boston Market on Route 9 with Kunker Road on the cross. Time now is 1745 hours.

The EMD will repeat the message to minimize any question as to its content and assure the ambulance has received the call.

Operating the Ambulance

If you will be driving an ambulance even occasionally, you should or may be mandated to attend emergency vehicle operator training, which has both classroom and in-vehicle road sessions.

Being a Safe Ambulance Operator
To be a safe ambulance operator, you must:

- Be physically fit. You should not have any impairment that prevents you from operating the ambulance or any medical condition that might disable you while driving.
- Be mentally fit, emotions under control. Driving an ambulance is not a job for someone who gets turned on by lights and sirens!
- Be able to perform under stress.
- Have a positive attitude about your ability as a driver but not be an overly confident risk taker.
- Be tolerant of other drivers. Always keep in mind that people react differently when they see an emergency vehicle. Accept and tolerate the bad habits of other drivers without flying into a rage.
- Never drive while under the influence of alcohol, illicit or "recreational" drugs such as marijuana or cocaine, medicines such as antihistamines, "pep pills," or tranquilizers.
- Never drive with a restricted license.
- Always wear your glasses or contact lenses if required for driving.
- Evaluate your ability to drive based on personal stress, illness, fatigue, or sleepiness.

Understanding the Law

Every state has statutes that regulate the operation of emergency vehicles. Emergency vehicle operators are generally granted certain exemptions with regard to speed, parking, passage through traffic signals, and direction of travel. However, the laws also state that if an emergency vehicle operator does not drive with due regard for the safety of others, he must be prepared to pay the consequences, such as tickets, law suits, or even time in jail.

Following are some points typically included in laws regulating ambulance operation:

- An ambulance operator must have a valid driver's license and may be required to have completed a training program.
- Privileges granted under the law to the operators of ambulances apply when the vehicle is responding to an emergency or is involved in the emergency transport of a sick or injured person. When the ambulance is not on an emergency call, the laws that apply to the operation of non-emergency vehicles also apply to the ambulance.
- Even though certain privileges are granted during an emergency, the exemptions granted do not provide immunity to the operator in cases of reckless driving or disregard for the safety of others.
- Privileges granted during emergency situations apply only if the operator uses warning devices in the manner prescribed by law.

Most statutes allow emergency vehicle operators to:

- Park the vehicle anywhere if it does not damage personal property or endanger lives.
- Proceed past red stop signals, flashing red stop signals, and stop signs. Some states require that emergency vehicle operators come to a full stop, then proceed with caution. Other states require only that an operator slow down and proceed with caution.
- Exceed the posted speed limit as long as life and property are not endangered.
- Pass other vehicles in no-passing zones after properly signaling, ensuring that the way is clear, and taking precautions to avoid endangering life and property. This does not include passing a school bus with its red lights blinking. Wait for the bus driver to clear the children and then turn off the red lights of the bus.
- With proper caution and signals, disregard regulations that govern direction of travel and turning in specific directions.

Should you ever become involved in an ambulance collision, the laws will be interpreted by the court based upon two key issues. *Did you use due regard for the safety of others?* and *Was it a true emergency?* The requirement of due regard actually sets a higher standard for drivers of emergency vehicles than for other drivers. This is why an investigation by the district attorney or grand jury, as well as your ambulance service, is not uncommon following a collision.

Most states reserve the emergency mode of operation for a *true emergency,* defined as one in which the best information available to you is that loss of life or limb is possible. When dispatched to a call, there is often not much information to go on, so a "collision" will get an emergency response. However, once you arrive and find that your patient is stable with no life-threatening injuries or conditions, it is no longer a true emergency. A lights-and-siren, high-speed response to the hospital in such a situation would be improper.

The exemptions described here are just examples of those often granted to ambulance operators. Do not assume that they are granted in your state. Obtain a copy of your state's rules and regulations and study them carefully.

Using the Warning Devices

Safe emergency vehicle operation can be achieved only when proper use of warning devices is coupled with sound emergency and defensive driving practices. Studies show that other drivers do not see or hear an ambulance until it is within 50 to 100 feet. So never let the lights and siren give you a false sense of security.

The Siren. Although the siren is the most commonly used audible warning device, it is also the most misused. Consider the effects that sirens have on other motorists, patients in ambulances, and ambulance operators themselves:

- Motorists are less inclined to give way to ambulances when sirens are continually sounded. Many feel that the right-of-way privileges granted to ambulances by law are being abused when sirens are sounded.
- Continuous sound of a siren may cause a sick or injured person to suffer increased fear and anxiety, and his condition may worsen as stress builds up.
- Ambulance operators themselves are affected by the continuous sound of a siren. Tests have shown that inexperienced ambulance operators tend to increase their driving speeds from 10 to 15 miles per hour while continually sounding the siren. In

some cases, operators using a siren were unable to negotiate curves that they could pass through easily when not sounding the siren. Sirens also affect hearing, especially if used for long periods with the siren speaker over the cab. The best placement for the speaker is in the vehicle grill.

Many states have laws that regulate the use of audible warning signals, and where there are no statutes, ambulance organizations usually create their own policies. If your organization does not, you may find the following suggestions helpful:

- Use the siren sparingly, and only when you must. Some states require use of the siren at all times when the ambulance is responding in the emergency mode. Others require it only when the operator is exercising any of the exemptions discussed earlier.
- Never assume that all motorists will hear your signal. Buildings, trees, and dense shrubbery may block siren sounds. Soundproofing keeps outside noises from entering vehicles, and radios or tape systems also decrease the likelihood that an outside sound will be heard.
- Always assume that some motorists will hear your siren but ignore it.
- Be prepared for the erratic maneuvers of other drivers. Some drivers panic when they hear a siren.
- Do not pull up close to a vehicle and then sound your siren. This may cause the driver to jam on his brakes and you may be unable to stop in time. Use the horn when you are close to a vehicle ahead.
- Never use the siren indiscriminately, and never use it to scare someone.

The Horn. The horn is standard equipment on all ambulances. Experienced operators find that often the judicious use of the horn clears traffic as quickly as the siren. The guidelines for using a siren apply to the horn as well.

Visual Warning Devices. Whenever the ambulance is on the road, night or day, the headlights should be on. This increases the visibility of the vehicle to other drivers. In some states headlights are now required of all vehicles in low visibility conditions or whenever the windshield wipers are in use. Alternating flashing headlights should be used only if they are attached to secondary head lamps. In most states it is illegal to drive at night with one headlight out.

The large lights on the outermost corners of the box should blink in tandem, or unison, rather than wigwagging or alternating. This helps the vehicle that is approaching from a distance identify the full size of your vehicle. There is a lot of controversy about the use of strobes on ambulances. When planning the lighting package of an ambulance, check the research before making your decision. In general, it is wisest for the package to combine single beam bulbs and strobes rather than just one type of lighting system.

Four-way flashers and directional signals should not be used as emergency lights. This is very confusing to the public, as well as being illegal in some states. Drivers expect a vehicle with four-way flashers on to be traveling at a very slow speed. Additionally, the flashers disrupt the function of the directional signals.

When the ambulance is in the emergency response mode, either en route to the scene or to the hospital with a high-priority patient, all the emergency lights should be used. The vehicle should be easily seen from 360 degrees.

In some communities, fire department ambulances still follow an old tradition of using their emergency lights when returning to the station. However, this practice is very confusing to the public. Do not be surprised if other drivers do not pull over when you are on an emergency run if they constantly see your ambulance with emergency lights on. SAVE THE USE OF LIGHTS AND SIREN FOR LIFE- OR LIMB-THREATENING EMERGENCIES.

Speed and Safety

You are often told to drive slowly and carefully. At this point you may be inclined to say something like, "How will I ever get a seriously ill or injured person to a hospital if I poke along?" We are not suggesting that you "poke along." But do drive with these facts in mind:

- Excessive speed increases the probability of a collision.
- Speed increases stopping distance, reducing the chance of avoiding a hazardous situation.

Remember that the laws in most states excuse you from obeying certain traffic laws only in a true emergency and only with due regard for the safety of others. Except in these circumstances, obey speed limits, stoplights and signs, yield signs, and other laws and posted limits. Approach intersections with caution, avoid sudden turns, and always properly signal lane changes and turns. Be sure that the ambulance driver and all passengers wear seat belts whenever the ambulance is in motion.

Escorted or Multiple-Vehicle Responses

When the police provide an escort for an ambulance, there are additional hazards. Too often, the inexperienced ambulance operator follows the escort vehicle too closely and is unable to stop when the lead vehicle(s) make an emergency stop. Also, the inexperienced operator may assume that other drivers know his vehicle is following the escort. In fact, other drivers will often pull out in front of the ambulance just after the escort vehicle passes.

Because of the dangers involved with escorts, most EMS systems recommend no escorts unless the operator is not familiar with the location of the patient (or hospital) and must be given assistance from the police.

In multiple-vehicle responses, the dangers can be the same as those generated by escorted responses, especially when the responding vehicles travel in the same direction, close together. A great danger also exists when two vehicles approach the same intersection at the same time. Not only may they fail to yield for each other; other drivers may yield for the first vehicle but not the second. Obviously, great care must be used at intersections during multiple-vehicle responses.

Factors That Affect Response

Most ambulance collisions take place in seemingly safe conditions. In New York State, 18 years of ambulance-collision statistics show that the typical collision happens on a dry road (60%) with clear weather (55%) during daylight hours (67%) in an intersection (72%). During this period, there were 5,782 ambulance collisions, which involved 7,267 injuries and 48 fatalities! Additionally, an ambulance response can be affected by several factors:

- *Day of the week.* Weekdays usually have the heaviest traffic because people are commuting to and from work. In resort areas, weekend traffic may be heavier.
- *Time of day.* In major employment centers, traffic over major arteries tends to be heavy in all directions during commuter hours.
- *Weather.* Adverse weather conditions reduce driving speeds and thus increase response times. A heavy snowfall can temporarily prevent any response at all. Be careful to lengthen your following distance whenever there is decreased road grip due to inclement weather.
- *Road maintenance and construction.* Traffic can be seriously impeded by road construction and maintenance activities. Be aware of area road construction and plan responses accordingly.
- *Railroads.* There are still more than a quarter-million grade crossings in the United States with traffic often blocked by long, slow freight trains. Some communities need a secondary response system on the other side of train tracks that split the town in half.

- *Bridges and tunnels.* Traffic over bridges and through tunnels slows during rush hours. Collisions—including ambulance collisions—tend to occur when drivers forget that bridges freeze before roadways.
- *Schools and school buses.* The reduced speed limits in force during school hours slow the flow of vehicles. An emergency vehicle should never pass a stopped school bus with its red lights flashing. Wait for the school bus driver to signal you to proceed by turning off the lights. In addition, emergency vehicles attract children, who often venture out into the street to see them. The operator of every emergency vehicle should slow down when approaching a school or playground. Obey the directions given by school crossing guards.

Selecting an Alternative Route

When it appears that an ambulance will be delayed in reaching a sick or injured person, the operator should consider taking an alternative route or requesting the response of another ambulance. Plan for times when changing conditions affect response. Obtain detailed maps of your service area. On the maps, indicate usually troublesome traffic spots such as schools, bridges, tunnels, railroad grade crossings, and heavily congested areas. Also indicate temporary problems such as road and building construction sites and long- and short-term detours. Using another color, indicate alternative routes, snow routes, and so on.

Hang one map in quarters and place another in the ambulance. Then when you encounter a problem area, you will be able to select an alternative route that will get you to your destination quickly and safely.

Positioning the Ambulance at the Scene of a Vehicle Collision

When responding to the scene of a vehicle collision, be sure to take all steps to size up the scene—assessing scene safety and establishing a danger zone. Park at least 100 feet from the wreckage, upwind, and uphill (if possible) to avoid fire or any escaping hazardous liquids or fumes. If there is no fire or escaping liquids or fumes, park at least 50 feet from the wreckage.

Park in front of the wreckage if you are the first emergency vehicle on the scene so your warning lights can warn approaching motorists before flares and other signals can be placed. If the scene has already been secured, park beyond the wreckage to prevent having your expensive ambulance struck by oncoming traffic. (See Scan 32-2.)

When backing up an ambulance, be aware that there are large blind spots in your mirrors and a danger of striking a pedestrian, object, or other vehicle.

PARKING THE AMBULANCE

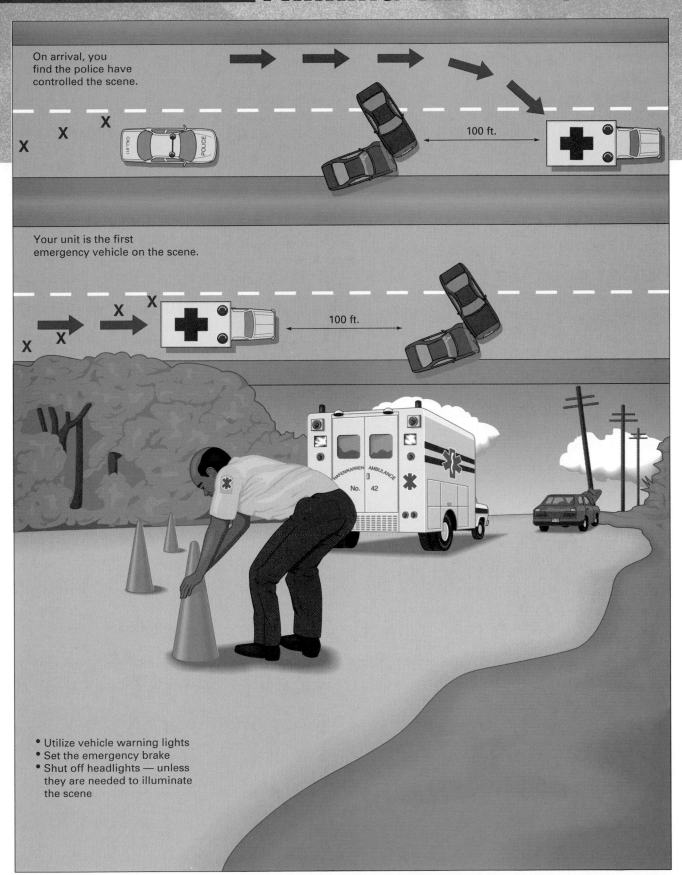

On arrival, you find the police have controlled the scene.

100 ft.

Your unit is the first emergency vehicle on the scene.

100 ft.

- Utilize vehicle warning lights
- Set the emergency brake
- Shut off headlights — unless they are needed to illuminate the scene

Figure 32-2 Use a spotter to help guide the ambulance when backing up.

When possible, position someone at the rear of the ambulance to act as a spotter and guide the backing process (Figure 32-2).

Studies show that red revolving beacons attract drunk or tired drivers. Consider pulling off the road, turning off your headlights, and using just amber rear sealed beam blinkers that blink in tandem or unison to identify the size of your vehicle. Once the ambulance is parked, set its parking brake and firmly wedge wheel chocks under the tires in such a way that forward movement will be retarded if the ambulance is struck.

Be sure to perform a scene size-up and take all necessary body substance isolation and hazardous materials precautions.

TRANSFERRING THE PATIENT TO THE AMBULANCE

On most ambulance runs you will be able to reach a sick or injured person without difficulty, assess his condition, carry out emergency care procedures where he lies, and then transfer him to the ambulance. At times, dangers at the scene or the priority of the patient will dictate moving the patient before assessment and emergency treatments can be completed. When a spinal injury is suspected, the patient's head must be manually stabilized, a cervical collar must be applied, and the patient must be immobilized on a spine board.

Transfer to the ambulance is accomplished in four steps, regardless of the complexity of the operation:

1. Select the proper patient-carrying device.
2. Package the patient for transfer.
3. Move the patient to the ambulance.
4. Load the patient into the ambulance.

The wheeled ambulance stretcher is the most commonly used device for transferring the patient to the ambulance.

The term *packaging* refers to the sequence of operations required to ready the patient to be moved and to combine the patient and the patient-carrying device into a unit ready for transfer. A sick or injured patient must be packaged so that his condition is not aggravated. Necessary care for wounds and other injuries should be completed, impaled objects must be stabilized, and all dressings and splints must be checked before the patient is placed on the patient-carrying device. The properly packaged patient is covered and secured to the patient-carrying device.

Do not spend too much time packaging a badly traumatized patient. Whenever a patient is categorized as high priority, transport quickly. A neatly packaged corpse has not received optimal care.

Covering a patient helps to maintain body temperature, prevents exposure to the elements, and helps assure privacy (Figure 32-3). A single blanket or perhaps just a sheet may be all that is required in warm weather. A sheet and blankets should be used in cold weather. When practical, cuff the blankets under the patient's chin, with the top sheet outside. Do not leave sheets and blankets hanging loose. Tuck them under the mattress at the foot and sides of the stretcher. In wet weather, a plastic cover should be placed over the blankets during transfer. Remove it once in the ambulance to prevent overheating. In cold or wet weather cover the patient's head, leaving the face exposed.

A patient-carrying device should have a minimum of three straps for holding the patient securely. The first should be at the chest level, the second at hip or waist level, and the third on the lower extremities. Sometimes there is a fourth strap if two are crossed at the chest.

Figure 32-3 A patient packaged for cold, wet conditions.

All patients, including those receiving CPR, must be secured to the patient-carrying device before transfer to the ambulance. If your patient is not on a carrying device such as a spine board but is just on the ambulance stretcher, some states, as a matter of policy, require shoulder harnesses that secure the patient to the stretcher to prevent him from sliding forward in case of a short stop.

TRANSPORTING THE PATIENT TO THE HOSPITAL

Transport involves more than just driving to the hospital. A series of tasks must be undertaken from the time a patient is loaded into the ambulance until he is handed over to hospital personnel.

Preparing the Patient for Transport

The following activities may be required to prepare the patient for transport once he is in the ambulance:

- *Perform ongoing assessment.* Make sure that a conscious patient is breathing without difficulty once you have positioned him on the stretcher. If the patient is unconscious with an airway in place, make sure he has an adequate air exchange once you have moved him into position for transport.

- *Secure the stretcher* in place in the ambulance. Always ensure that the patient is safe during the trip to the hospital. Before closing the door, and certainly before signaling the ambulance operator to move, make sure that the cot is securely in place. Patient compartments are equipped with a locking device that prevents the wheeled stretcher from moving about while the ambulance is in motion. Failure to fully engage the locking device at both ends of the stretcher can have disastrous consequences once the ambulance is in motion.

- *Position and secure the patient.* During transfer to the ambulance, the patient must be firmly secured to a stretcher. This does not mean that he must be transported in that position. Positioning in the ambulance should be dictated by the nature of his illness or injury.

  - If he was not transferred to the ambulance in that position, shift an unconscious patient who has no potential spine injury, or one with an altered mental status, into the recovery position (on his side) that will promote maintenance of an open airway and the drainage of fluids.

  - Remember that the head and foot ends of the ambulance stretcher can be raised. A patient with breathing difficulty and no possibility of spinal injury may be more comfortable being transported in a sitting position. A patient in shock can be transported with the legs raised 8 to 12 inches.

  - A patient with potential spinal injury must remain immobilized on the long spine board, patient and board together being secured to the stretcher. If resuscitation is required, he must remain supine with constant monitoring of the airway and suctioning equipment ready. If resuscitation is not required, the unresponsive patient and spine board can be rotated as a unit and the board propped on the stretcher so that the patient is on his side for drainage of fluids and vomitus from the mouth.

  - Adjust the security straps. Security straps applied when a patient is being prepared for transfer to the ambulance may tighten unnecessarily by the time he is loaded into the patient compartment. Adjust straps so they still hold the patient safely in place but are not so tight that they interfere with circulation or respiration or cause pain.

- *Prepare for respiratory or cardiac complications.* If the patient is likely to develop cardiac arrest, position a short spine board or CPR board underneath the mattress prior to starting on the trip. Then, if he does go into arrest, time will not be wasted locating and positioning the board. Riding on a hard board may not be comfortable, but temporary discomfort is better than permanent injury or even death from delayed resuscitation.

- *Loosen constricting clothing.* Clothing may interfere with circulation and breathing. Loosen ties and belts and open any clothing around the neck. Straighten clothing that is bunched under safety straps. Remember that clothing bunched at the crotch may be painful. Before you do anything to rearrange the patient's clothing, however, explain what you are going to do and why.

- *Check bandages.* Even properly applied bandages can loosen during transfer to the ambulance. Check each bandage to see that it is secure. Do not take a loosened bandage lightly. Severe bleeding can resume when pressure from a bandage is removed, and if the wound site is covered with a sheet or blanket, bleeding may go unnoticed until the patient develops shock or is delivered to the hospital.

- *Check splints.* Immobilizing devices can also loosen during transfer to the ambulance. Inspect the bandages or cravats that hold board splints in place. Test air splints with your fingertip to see that they have remained properly inflated. Inspect traction devices to ensure that proper traction is still maintained. Check the splinted limb for distal pulses, motor function, and sensation. Remember that the safe adjustment of splinting devices is virtually impossible when an ambulance is pitching about during the trip to a hospital, so complete this step before the ambulance moves unless immediate transport is required.

- *Load a relative or friend* who must accompany the patient. Consider the following guidelines if your service does not prohibit the transportation of a relative or friend with a patient: First, encourage the person to seek alternative transportation, if available. If there is just no other way the relative or friend can get to the hospital, allow him to ride in the operator's compartment—not in the patient's compartment where he may interfere with patient care. Make certain the person buckles his seat belt. If an uninjured child must come along, bring the family's child car seat and use it.

- *Load personal effects.* If a purse, briefcase, overnight bag, or other personal item is to accompany the patient, make sure it is properly secured in the ambulance. If you load personal effects at the scene of a collision, be sure to tell a police officer what you are taking. Follow policies and fill out forms, if any, required by your local system for safeguarding personal effects.

- *Reassure the patient.* Apprehension often mounts in a sick or injured person after he is loaded in an ambulance. Not only is he held down by straps in a strange, confined space, but he may also be suddenly separated from family members and friends. Say a few kind words and offer a reassuring hand in a compassionate manner.

When you are satisfied that the patient is ready, signal the operator to begin the trip to the hospital. If this is a high-priority patient, most of the preparation steps—loosening clothing, checking bandages and splints, reassuring the patient, even vital signs—can be done en route rather than delaying transport.

Pediatric Notes

Remember that a toy such as a teddy bear can do much to calm a frightened child. Many ambulance units carry a sanitized, soft or padded, brightly colored toy just for these occasions. It is difficult at best to get information from a young child whose parents may have been injured and transported in another ambulance. Small children do not, as a rule, carry identification and you are a complete stranger in a hostile environment.

The crash scene, confusion, noise, injuries, possible pain, disappearance of a parent, EMT-Bs caring for injuries and gathering information all create a ter-

rifying experience for a child. A female EMT-B or police officer may be helpful. Sometimes young children feel more comfortable talking to a woman. A smile and calm reassuring tone of voice are something that cannot be learned from a textbook, and they may be the most critical care needed by the frightened child.

Caring for the Patient en Route

At least one EMT-B in the patient compartment is minimum staffing for an ambulance, although two are preferred. Seldom will you be able to merely ride along with your patient. You may have to undertake a number of activities en route:

- *Notify the EMD* that you are departing the scene.

- *Continue to provide emergency care* as required. If life-support efforts were initiated prior to loading the patient into the ambulance, they must be continued during transportation to the hospital. Maintain an open airway, resuscitate, administer to the patient's needs, provide emotional support, and do whatever else is required, including updating your findings from the initial patient assessment effort.

- *Compile additional patient information.* If the patient is conscious and emergency care efforts will not be compromised, record patient information. Compiling information during the trip to the hospital serves two purposes. First, it allows you to complete your report. Second, supplying information temporarily takes your patient's mind off his problems. Remember, however, that this is not an interrogation session. Ask your questions in an informal manner.

- *Perform ongoing assessment* and monitor vital signs. Keep in mind that vital sign changes indicate a change in a patient's condition. For example, an unexplained increase in pulse rate may signify deepening shock. Record vital signs and be prepared to report changes to an emergency department staff member as soon as you reach the medical facility. Reassess vital signs every 5 minutes for an unstable patient, every 15 minutes for a stable patient.

- *Notify the receiving facility.* Transmit patient assessment and management information and provide your estimated time of arrival.

- *Recheck bandages and splints.* Even though you checked bandages after loading the patient into the ambulance, check them again while in transit.

- *Collect vomitus* if the patient becomes nauseated. If he is not already in position, arrange the patient so that the chance of his aspirating vomitus is minimized. Be prepared to apply suction. Place an emesis basin or bag by his mouth. When he has finished vomiting, place a towel over the container and deliver it to emergency department personnel when you hand over the patient. Examination of the vomitus may be important to treatment, especially in cases of poisoning. Wear a mask, protective eyewear, and disposable gloves if your patient is vomiting.

- *Talk to the patient*, but control your emotions. Continued conversation is often soothing to a frightened patient.

- *Advise the ambulance operator of changing conditions*. No one likes a "back-seat driver." However, sometimes you will need to ask the ambulance operator to adjust speed or alter his driving technique to suit the needs of your patient. On the one hand, if what began as a routine transport develops into an emergency call, you may have to ask the operator to accelerate. On the other hand, if you think that swaying because of high speeds and uneven streets is detrimental to a patient's condition, have the operator slow down or take an alternative route.

    While the operator of an ambulance is responsible for his vehicle and passengers, it is your responsibility to care for sick and injured persons; thus the operator should drive the ambulance according to your suggestions. The decision on use of lights and siren should always be made with the medical condition of the patient in mind.

- *If cardiac arrest develops*, have the operator stop the ambulance while you apply and operate the AED. Signal the operator to start up again once you have completed the shock sequence or determined that the patient does not have a shockable rhythm. Make certain that the emergency department is made aware of the arrest. If you routinely position a rigid device between the back of high-risk patients and the cot mattress, you have only to drop the cot back to a horizontal position and start CPR. If not, you must position an object like a short spine board or CPR board so that chest compression efforts will be effective.

    If the patient remains pulseless despite the AED, begin CPR. Local protocols may mandate intercept by an advanced life support (ALS) team. You may want the ambulance operator to assist you with CPR or AED while additional resources come to your aid. Use your judgment on this.

TRANSFERRING THE PATIENT TO THE EMERGENCY DEPARTMENT STAFF

The following are steps that you should take to see that the transfer of a patient to the care of emergency department personnel is accomplished smoothly and without incident. Brief as it may be, the transfer is a crucial step during which your primary concern must be the continuation of patient-care activities. The steps of the transfer are illustrated in Scan 32-3.

- In a routine admissions situation or when an illness or injury is not life-threatening, check first to see what is to be done with the patient. If emergency department activity is particularly hectic, it might be better to leave your patient in the relative security and comfort of the ambulance while your operator determines where he is to be taken. Otherwise the patient may be subjected to distressing sights and sounds and perhaps be in the way. (If you do this, make sure an EMT-B remains with the patient at all times.) UNDER NO CIRCUMSTANCES SHOULD YOU SIMPLY WHEEL A NON-EMERGENCY PATIENT INTO A HOSPITAL, PLACE HIM IN A BED, AND LEAVE HIM! This is an important point. Unless you transfer care of your patient directly to a member of the hospital staff, you may be open to a charge of abandonment.

    Staff members may be treating other seriously ill and injured persons, so suppress any urge to demand attention for your patient. Simply continue emergency care measures until someone can assume responsibility for the patient. When properly directed, transfer the patient to a hospital stretcher.

- Assist emergency department staff as required and provide a verbal report. Stress any changes in the condition of the patient that you have observed.

- As soon as you are free from patient-care activities, prepare the prehospital care report. Remember, the job is not over until the paperwork is complete. Find a quiet spot and complete your prehospital care report (PCR).

- Transfer the patient's personal effects. If a patient's valuables or other personal effects were entrusted to your care, transfer them to a responsible emergency department staff member. Some services have policies that involve obtaining a written receipt from emergency department personnel as protection from a charge of theft.

- Obtain your release from the hospital. This task is not as formal as it sounds. Simply ask the emergency department nurse or physician if your services are still needed. In rural areas where not all hospital services are available, it may be necessary to transfer a seriously ill or injured person to another medical facility. If you leave and have to be recalled, valuable time will be lost.

TRANSFERRING THE PATIENT

▲ **1.** Transfer the patient as soon as possible. Stay with the patient until transfer is complete.

▲ **2.** Assist the emergency department staff as required.

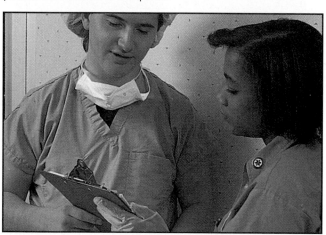

▲ **3.** Transfer patient information as a verbal report and in a written prehospital care report.

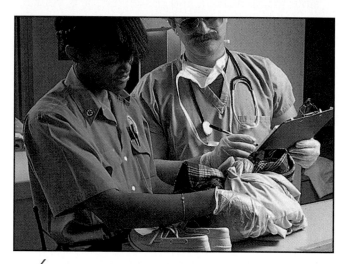

▲ **4.** Transfer the patient's personal effects.

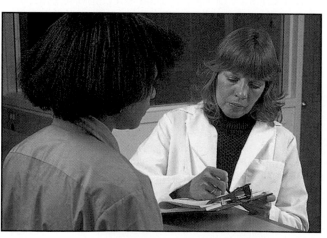

◄ **5.** Obtain your release from the hospital.

TERMINATING THE CALL

An ambulance run is not really over until the personnel and equipment that comprise the prehospital emergency care delivery system are ready for the next response. The functions of EMT-Bs in this final phase of activity include more than just changing the stretcher linen and cleaning the ambulance. A number of tasks must be accomplished at the hospital, during the return to quarters, and after arrival at the station.

At the Hospital

While still at the hospital, the ambulance crew should begin making the ambulance ready to respond to another call. Time, equipment, and space limitations sometimes preclude vigorous cleaning of the ambulance while it is parked at the hospital. However, you should make every effort to quickly prepare the vehicle for the next patient (Scan 32-4):

1. Quickly clean the patient compartment while wearing heavy-duty, dishwashing-style gloves. Follow biohazard disposal procedures according to your agency's OSHA exposure control plan. Examples of biohazards are contaminated dressings and used suction catheters.

- Clean up blood, vomitus, and other body fluids that may have soiled the floor. Wipe down any equipment that has been splashed. Place disposable towels used to clean up blood or body fluids directly in a red bag.
- Remove and dispose of trash such as bandage wrappings, open but unused dressings, and similar items.
- Sweep away caked dirt that may have been tracked into the patient compartment. When the weather is inclement, sponge up water and mud from the floor.
- Bag dirty linens or blankets to be appropriately laundered.
- Use a deodorizer to neutralize odors of vomit, urine, and feces. Various sprays and concentrates are available for this purpose.

2. Prepare respiratory equipment for service:

- Clean and then properly disinfect nondisposable, used bag-valve-mask units and other reusable parts of respiratory-assist and inhalation-therapy devices to keep them from becoming reservoirs of infectious agents that can easily contaminate the next patient. Disinfect the suction unit.
- Place used disposable items in a plastic bag and seal it. Replace the items with similar ones carried in the ambulance as spares.

3. Replace expendable items:

- If you have a supply replacement agreement with the hospital, replace expendable items from hospital storerooms on a one-for-one basis—such as sterile dressings, bandaging materials, towels, disposable oxygen masks, disposable gloves, sterile water, and oral airways.
- Do not abuse this exchange program. Keep in mind that the constant abuse of a supply-replacement program usually leads to its discontinuation. At the very least, abuse places a strain on ambulance-hospital relations.

4. Exchange equipment according to your local policy:

- Exchange items such as splints and spine boards. Several benefits are associated with an equipment exchange program: There is no need to subject patients to injury-aggravating movements just to recover equipment, crews are not delayed at the hospital, and ambulances can return to quarters fully equipped for the next response.
- When equipment is available for exchange, quickly inspect it for completeness and operability. Parts are sometimes lost or broken when an immobilizing device is removed from a patient.
- If you do find that a piece of equipment is broken or incomplete, notify someone in authority so the device can be repaired or replaced.

5. Make up the ambulance cot. The following procedure is one of many that can be used to make up a wheeled ambulance stretcher:

- Raise the stretcher to the high-level position, if possible; this makes the procedure easier. The stretcher should be flat with the side rails lowered and straps unfastened.
- Remove unsoiled blankets and pillow, and place them on a clean surface.
- Remove all soiled linen, and place it in the designated receptacle.
- Clean the mattress surface with an appropriate EPA-approved, low-level disinfectant unless there is visible blood, which should be cleaned up using a 1:100 bleach/water solution.
- Turn the mattress over; rotation adds to the life of the mattress.
- Center the bottom sheet on the mattress and open it fully. If a full-sized bed sheet is used, first fold it lengthwise.

ACTIVITIES AT THE HOSPITAL

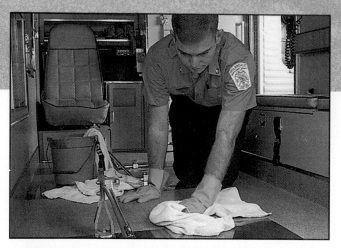

▲ **1.** Clean the ambulance interior as required.

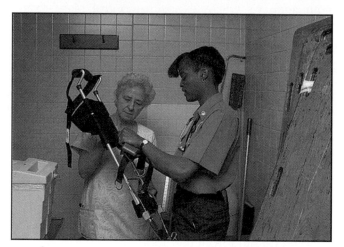

▲ **2.** Replace respiratory equipment as required.

▲ **3.** Replace expendable items per local policies.

▲ **4.** Exchange equipment per local policies.

◀ **5.** Make up the wheeled stretcher.

- Tuck the sheet under each end of the mattress; form square corners and then tuck under each side.
- Place a disposable pad, if one is used, on the center of the mattress.
- Fully open the blanket. If a second blanket is used, open it fully and match it to the first blanket. This task should be done with an EMT-B at each end of the stretcher.
- Open a top sheet in the same way, placing it on top of the blanket. Fold the blanket(s) and top sheet together lengthwise to match the width of the stretcher; fold one side first, then the other.
- Tuck the foot of the folded blanket(s) and sheet under the foot of the mattress.
- Tuck the head of the folded blanket(s) and sheet under the head of the mattress.
- Place the slip-covered pillow lengthwise at the head of the mattress and secure it with a strap.
- Buckle the safety straps and tuck in excess straps.
- Raise the side rails and foot rest.

The stretcher is now ready for the next patient. It must be re-emphasized that this is one of many techniques for preparing a wheeled ambulance stretcher for service. Whatever the method, it should meet the following objectives:

- Preparation for the next call should be done as soon and as quickly as possible.
- All linens, blankets, and pouches should be stored neatly on the stretcher.
- All linens and blankets should be folded or tucked so that they will be contained within the stretcher frame.
- The cot must be replaced in the ambulance.
- Any non-disposable patient-care items should be replaced.
- A check should be made for equipment left in the hospital.

Note: A neatly prepared stretcher inspires the patient's confidence. Do not use stained linen, even though it might be clean. Always make the presentation of your stretcher a matter of personal and professional pride.

En Route to Quarters

Emphasis should be on a safe return. An ambulance operator may practice every suggestion for safe vehicle operation while en route to the hospital and then totally disregard those suggestions during the return to quarters. Defensive driving must be a full-time effort. Do not forget that the driver and all passengers must wear seat belts.

1. *Radio the EMD* that you are returning to quarters and that you are available (or not available) for service. Valuable time is lost if an EMD has to locate and alert a back-up ambulance when he does not know that a ready-for-service unit is on the road. Be sure that you notify the EMD if you stop and leave the ambulance unattended for any reason during the return to quarters.

2. *Air the ambulance* if necessary. If the patient just delivered to the hospital has an airborne communicable disease, or if it was not possible to neutralize disagreeable odors while at the hospital, make the return trip with the windows of the patient compartment partially open, weather permitting. If the unit has sealed windows, use the air-conditioning or ventilating system (do not set on "recirculate") to air the patient compartment out.

3. *Refuel the ambulance.* Local policy usually dictates the frequency with which an ambulance is refueled. Some services require the operator to refuel after each call regardless of the distance traveled. In other services the policy is to refuel when the gauge reaches a certain level. At any rate, the fuel should be at such a level that the ambulance can respond to an emergency and then to the hospital without fear of running out.

In Quarters

When you return to quarters, there are a number of activities that need to be completed before the ambulance can be placed in service and before it is ready for another call (Scan 32-5).

With the emphasis today on protection from infectious diseases, you need to take every precaution to protect yourself. It is essential that you follow your agency's OSHA exposure control plan. Always wear gloves when handling contaminated linen, cleaning the equipment, handling the respiratory equipment, and cleaning the ambulance interior (where there may be many hidden nooks and crannies where the patient's blood or body fluids could be).

Once in quarters, you are ready to complete cleaning and disinfecting chores. Consult Scan 32-6 for the levels of reprocessing to be used for equipment.

1. Place badly contaminated linens in a biohazard container, non-contaminated linens in a regular hamper.

2. As necessary, clean any equipment that touched the patient. Brush stretcher covers and other rubber,

TERMINATING ACTIVITIES IN QUARTERS

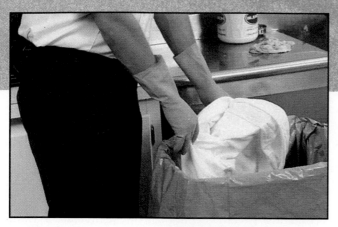

▲ **1.** Place contaminated linens in a biohazard container, noncontaminated linens in a regular hamper.

▲ **2.** Remove and clean patient-care equipment as required.

▲ **3.** Clean and sanitize respiratory equipment as required.

▲ **4.** Clean and sanitize the ambulance interior as required. Use germicide on devices or surfaces that were in contact with blood or other body fluids.

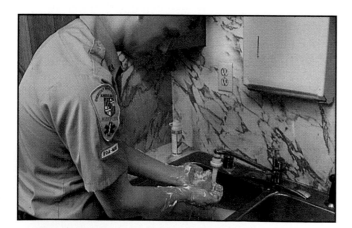

▲ **5.** Wash thoroughly, and change soiled clothing. Do this first if exposed to a communicable disease.

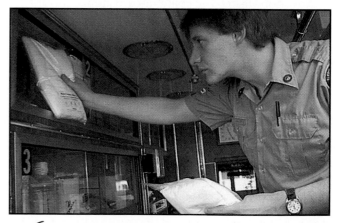

▲ **6.** Replace expendable items as required.

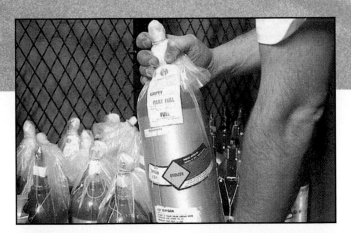

▲ **7.** Replace oxygen cylinders as necessary.

▲ **8.** Replace patient-care equipment as needed.

▲ **9.** Maintain the ambulance as required. Report problems that will take the vehicle out of service.

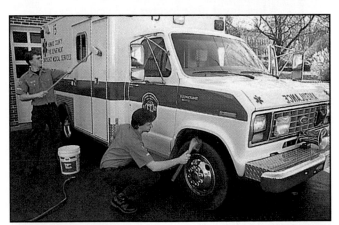

▲ **10.** Clean the ambulance exterior as needed.

▲ **11.** Report the unit ready for service.

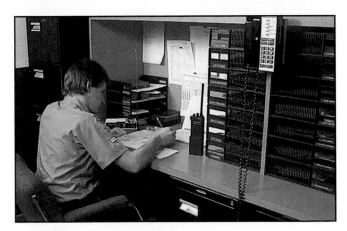

▲ **12.** Complete any unfinished report forms as soon as possible.

CLEANING AND DISINFECTING EQUIPMENT

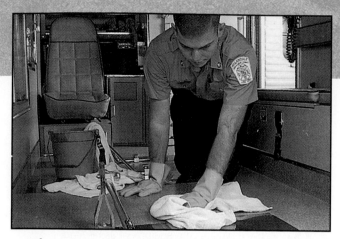

▲ **1.** A **low-level disinfectant** approved by the U.S. Environmental Protection Agency, for example a commercial product such as Lysol, will clean and kill germs on ambulance floors and walls.

▲ **2.** An **intermediate-level disinfectant,** such as a mixture of 1:100 bleach-to-water can be used to clean and kill germs on equipment surfaces.

▲ **3.** A **high-level disinfectant,** such as Cidex Plus, will destroy all forms of microbial life except high numbers of bacterial spores.

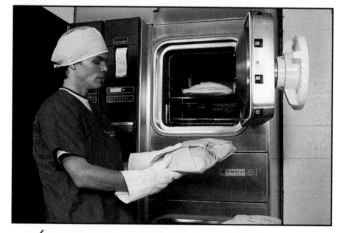

▲ **4.** **Sterilization** is required to destroy all possible sources of infection on equipment that will be used invasively.

vinyl, and canvas materials clean, then wash them with soap and water.

3. Clean and disinfect used non-disposable respiratory-assist and inhalation therapy equipment.
   - Disassemble the equipment so that all surfaces are exposed.
   - Fill a large plastic container with the cleaning solution outlined in your service's infection control plan.
   - Clean the inner and outer surfaces with a suitable brush. Inner surfaces can be cleaned with a small bottle brush, while outer surfaces can be cleaned with a hand or nail brush. Make sure all encrusted matter is removed.
   - Rinse the items with tap water.
   - Soak the items in an EPA-approved germicidal solution. An inhalation therapist at a local hospital can suggest a germicide suitable for respiratory equipment. Follow directions for dilution, safe handling, and soaking time. Gloves are recommended when using some germicides.
   - After the prescribed soaking period, hang the equipment in a well-ventilated clean area and allow it to dry for 12 to 24 hours.

4. Clean and sanitize the patient compartment. Use an EPA-approved germicide to clean any fixed equipment or surfaces contacted by the patient's body fluids.

5. Prepare yourself for service.
   - Wash thoroughly, paying attention to the areas under your fingernails. Remember that contaminants can collect there and become a source of infection not only to you but also to the persons whom you touch.
   - Change soiled clothes. Clean contaminated clothing as soon as possible, especially if you were exposed to someone with a communicable disease. It is a good policy to bring a spare uniform to work, and each EMS agency should have a washer and dryer. It is against OSHA regulations for blood or body fluid soiled clothes to be taken home to be washed.

6. Replace expendable items with items from the unit's storeroom.

7. Replace or refill oxygen cylinders in accordance with your service's procedures.

8. Replace patient-care equipment.

9. Carry out post-operation vehicle maintenance procedures as required. If you find something wrong with the vehicle, correct the problem or make someone in authority aware of it.

10. Clean the vehicle. A clean exterior lends a professional appearance to an ambulance. Check for broken lights, glass and body damage, door operation, and other parts that may need repair or replacement.

11. Complete any unfinished report forms as soon as possible, and report the unit ready for service.

AIR RESCUE

In some circumstances, it is best for a patient to be transported by an air rescue helicopter (Figure 32-4) or fixed-wing aircraft. The following are some considerations for use of this kind of transport. Since geographic and other circumstances and the availability of such transport will vary in different localities, follow your local protocols.

How AND Why?

Air medical transport is designed for patients in critical condition, but most air transport programs will not transport patients who are in cardiac arrest. Go to your Electronic Extras CD to find out more.

When to Call for Air Rescue

Air rescue may be required for any of the following reasons:

- *Operational reasons.* To speed transport to a distant trauma center or other special facility, or when extrication of a high-priority patient is prolonged

Figure 32-4 Patients are sometimes transported by air rescue helicopter.

and air rescue can speed transport, or when a patient must be rescued from a remote location that can only be reached by helicopter. Follow local protocols.

- *Medical reasons.* The patient is high priority for rapid transport (e.g., a patient in shock, a patient with a Glasgow Coma Scale total of 13 or less, a patient who has a head injury with altered mental status, a patient with chest trauma and respiratory distress, a patient with penetrating injuries to the body cavity, a patient with an amputation proximal to the hand or foot, a patient with extensive burns, or a patient with a serious mechanism of injury). Cardiac-arrest patients are usually not transported by air rescue unless hypothermic. Follow local protocols.

How to Call for Air Rescue

Air rescue may be called for by any law enforcement, fire, or EMS command officer at the scene of an incident, or you may radio dispatch for advice if you think such a service is needed. When calling an air rescue service, give your name and call-back number, your agency name, the nature of the situation, the exact location including crossroads and major landmarks, and the exact location of a safe landing zone. Follow local protocols.

How to Set up a Landing Zone

A helicopter requires a landing zone, or LZ, approximately 100-by-100 feet (approximately 30 large steps on each side) on ground with less than an 8-degree slope. The landing zone and approach/departure path should be clear of wires, towers, vehicles, people, and loose objects (Figure 32-5). The landing zone should be marked with one flare in an upwind position. During night operations, NEVER shine a

Figure 32-5 Helicopter landing zone.

light into the pilot's eyes during landing or takeoff or while the aircraft is running on the ground. Keep emergency red lights on.

Describe the landing zone to the air rescue service:

- *Terrain.* "The landing zone is located on top of a hill." "The landing zone is located in a valley."
- *Major landmarks.* "There is a river (major highway, factory, water tower) to the north (or other direction) of the landing zone."
- *Estimated distance to nearest town.* "The landing zone is approximately 12 miles west of Centerville."
- *Other pertinent information.* "There are wires on the east side of the landing zone." "There is a deep ditch to the west." "Winds are out of the north-northeast at about 10 mph."

How to Approach a Helicopter

Do not approach a helicopter unless escorted by the flight personnel. Allow the helicopter crew to direct the loading on board of the patient. Stay clear of the tail rotor at all times. Keep all traffic and vehicles 100 feet or more distant from the helicopter. Do not smoke within 200 feet of the aircraft. Be aware of the danger areas around helicopters, as shown in Scan 32-7. NEVER walk around the tail rotor area.

DANGER AREAS AROUND HELICOPTERS

◄A. Area around the tail rotor is extremely dangerous. A spinning rotor cannot be seen.

◄B. Sudden gust of wind can cause the main rotor of a helicopter to dip to a point as close as 4 feet from the ground. Always approach a helicopter in a crouch when the rotor is moving.

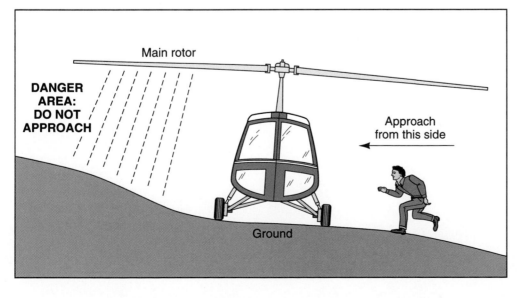

◄C. Approach the aircraft from the downhill side when a helicopter is parked on a hillside.

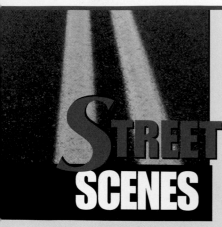

STREET SCENES

You receive a priority-1 call. "Ambulance 19, respond to 1901 Greentop Road for a report of a cardiac arrest." You acknowledge, get into the ambulance, and buckle up. Your partner does the same and turns on the red lights and siren. The dispatcher tells you that there is no additional information from the caller, and you will be the first unit to arrive. You know it will be a long response because the call is at the far end of your district, and you feel pressured to hurry. As you approach an intersection, your partner changes the siren from wail to yelp and goes through without slowing down. "That light was red," you tell him. He doesn't respond and keeps driving at the same speed. When he starts to weave through traffic, you suggest an alternative route to avoid the approaching rush-hour congestion.

STREET SCENE QUESTIONS

1. When operating an ambulance using the red lights and siren, what precautions do you need to take?

2. How can speed affect the safety of ambulance operation?

3. What driving techniques might be used to make driving to this scene safer?

All of a sudden, a car comes out of a driveway and into your path. Your partner hits the brakes, performs an evasive move, and just misses the other vehicle. You notice that a box of tissues and a stethoscope landed on the floor in the patient compartment. "What would have happened if I had been back there with a patient?" you ask. Your partner finally realizes he is driving too fast and slows down. At the next intersection, he slows down even more and makes sure that traffic has come to a stop before going through. During the rest of the response, you focus on preparing for your arrival on the scene.

You have decided to load all your equipment on the stretcher and wheel it to the front door as soon as the ambulance is parked. As you pull up to the scene, your partner finds a good spot to park where the ambulance will not create a hazard. He leaves the warning lights on for visibility.

STREET SCENE QUESTIONS

4. What should you do first for patient care?

5. What information should you provide to the dispatcher?

Your patient is in his bedroom, sitting on his bed, and greets you as you approach. You immediately ask him why EMS was called. "My wife called because I passed out. It's happened before, but my doctor isn't sure what causes it." Your partner radios dispatch that the patient is alert and that another unit is not needed. You assess the patient, obtain a patient history, and get a set of vital signs. The patient is alert and oriented, his pulse is 82 with a blood pressure of 130/82, respirations are 20, and skin is unremarkable. The patient says that he takes a medication because his cholesterol is "way up

| PATIENT NAME: *Faris Kazi* | | | | | | PATIENT AGE: *66* | | |

CHIEF COMPLAINT		TIME	RESP	PULSE	B.P.	MENTAL STATUS	R PUPILS L	SKIN
"I passed out"	V I T A L S I G N S	*1 7 3 0*	Rate: *20* ☒ Regular ☐ Shallow ☐ Labored	Rate: *82* ☒ Regular ☐ Irregular	*130* / *82*	☑ Alert ☐ Voice ☐ Pain ☐ Unresp.	☑ ☑ Normal ☐ ☐ Dilated ☐ ☐ Constricted ☐ ☐ Sluggish ☐ ☐ No-Reaction	☑ Unremarkable ☐ Cool ☐ Pale ☐ Warm ☐ Cyanotic ☐ Moist ☐ Flushed ☐ Dry ☐ Jaundiced
PAST MEDICAL HISTORY		*1 7 4 2*	Rate: *18* ☒ Regular ☐ Shallow ☐ Labored	Rate: *84* ☒ Regular ☐ Irregular	*130* / *80*	☑ Alert ☐ Voice ☐ Pain ☐ Unresp.	☑ ☑ Normal ☐ ☐ Dilated ☐ ☐ Constricted ☐ ☐ Sluggish ☐ ☐ No-Reaction	☑ Unremarkable ☐ Cool ☐ Pale ☐ Warm ☐ Cyanotic ☐ Moist ☐ Flushed ☐ Dry ☐ Jaundiced
☐ None ☐ Allergy to _____ ☐ Hypertension ☐ Stroke ☐ Seizures ☐ Diabetes ☐ COPD ☐ Cardiac ☒ Other (List) ☐ Asthma *Syncope* Current Medications (List) *Pravachol*			Rate: ☐ Regular ☐ Shallow ☐ Labored	Rate: ☐ Regular ☐ Irregular	/	☐ Alert ☐ Voice ☐ Pain ☐ Unresp.	☐ ☐ Normal ☐ ☐ Dilated ☐ ☐ Constricted ☐ ☐ Sluggish ☐ ☐ No-Reaction	☐ Unremarkable ☐ Cool ☐ Pale ☐ Warm ☐ Cyanotic ☐ Moist ☐ Flushed ☐ Dry ☐ Jaundiced

NARRATIVE *On arrival at a reported cardiac arrest, we are met by an alert male patient. His wife reports patient slumped over and "passed out" while sitting in a chair. She moved him to the floor, and he regained consciousness within 2 minutes. She did not observe any seizure activity. He appears to be in no obvious distress and denies complaint. He states a history of syncope, which is currently being assessed by his physician. Our patient assessment is unremarkable, and our plan is to transport patient for further evaluation of syncope.*

there." The patient's wife reports that he was sitting in a chair and slumped over. She did not see any seizure activity. He did not respond to verbal stimulus, so she moved him to the floor. He regained consciousness within two minutes.

The patient consents to transport to the hospital for further evaluation. You move him by stair chair from the bedroom to the stretcher. The patient is placed on the stretcher and all the safety straps are fastened. You place it into the ambulance compartment and, after it is in the bracket, you recheck to make sure it is secured properly. Your partner puts the stair chair away in its compartment and asks what the priority is to the hospital. "Priority 2," you answer. "Based on the assessment, there is no need to use the red light and siren."

CHAPTER REVIEW

SUMMARY

There are 5 phases to ambulance operations:

1. *Preparing for the call.* Make sure that all required equipment and supplies are on board, in good repair or operating order, and properly stored. Inspect the ambulance itself to make sure that it is ready for service.

2. *Receiving and responding to the call.* Receive call information from the EMD (Emergency Medical Dispatcher). Operate the ambulance safely. Understand the laws of your state and locality with regard to operation in an emergency situation, and always operate the ambulance with due regard for the safety of others. Park the ambulance outside the danger zone at a vehicle collision site.

3. *Transferring the patient to the ambulance.* Select a patient-carrying device suitable for the patient's injuries or medical condition. Make sure that the patient is properly packaged and secured to the device. Assure that the stretcher is secured within the ambulance before the ambulance begins to move.

4. *Transporting the patient to the hospital.* Perform and document ongoing assessment, needed treatments, and patient's condition. Notify dispatch, and transmit information to the receiving facility.

5. *Transferring the patient to the emergency department staff.* Do not leave the patient until emergency department personnel have taken over his care. Assist in transferring the patient to the hospital stretcher. Give a verbal report to emergency department personnel. Complete your prehospital care report. Transfer the patient's personal effects. Obtain your release from hospital personnel.

At the conclusion of the call, make up the ambulance stretcher, clean and restock the ambulance, and make sure that it is in good order for the next call.

On some occasions, your service may request that an air-rescue service transport the patient. Be aware of procedures for requesting this service, for setting up a landing zone, and for safety procedures around a helicopter.

REVIEW QUESTIONS

1. List five categories of equipment and supplies that should be carried on an ambulance. (pp. 687, 689–692)

2. Describe the laws (those described in this chapter or your local or state laws) with regard to operation of an ambulance in an emergency. Describe considerations for safe operation of an ambulance in emergency and non-emergency situations. (pp. 695–698, 700)

3. Describe the steps that must be followed in transferring a patient to an ambulance; for care of the patient en route; for transferring a patient to emergency department personnel. (pp. 700–703)

4. Describe the steps that should be followed when air rescue is required. (pp. 711–712)

APPLICATIONS

- What equipment should you include in a kit that you carry to the scene? How should the equipment be positioned so that you can reach urgently needed items quickly? What special items, if any, should be in the kit to meet local needs?

WEB MEDIC

Visit Brady's *Emergency Care* website for direct weblinks. At **www.bradybooks.com/emergencycare**, you will find information related to the following Chapter 32 topics:

- Air rescue

Chapter
Thirty-Three

GAINING ACCESS AND RESCUE OPERATIONS

*W*ord on the Street

"My partner and I had come on the scene of a motor-vehicle collision with the driver slumped over the wheel. The driver's door was locked, but the window on the passenger's side was broken, so we were able to unlock the passenger door and gain access. I was in the back seat manually stabilizing the patient's c-spine and my partner was beginning to examine the patient when another rescuer tried to pull the door open. When it refused to budge, he began working a tool into the door. Just then, my partner unlocked and opened the door from the inside—to the surprise of the rescuer who apparently never saw us. Remember: safe and simple."

Will Chapleau EMT-P, RN, TNS
Assistant EMSS Coordinator, Good Samaritan Hospital
Downers Grove, Illinois

There are at least 10 types of specialty rescue teams that may be available in various communities. Each specialty requires a significant amount of additional training over and above your EMT-Basic course. These specialties include vehicle rescue, water rescue, ice rescue, high-angle rescue, hazardous materials response, trench rescue, dive rescue, back country or wilderness rescue, farm rescue, and confined space rescue. Training that is available in each of these specialties often depends on the types of emergency responses that might be required in your community. If there is a gorge in the area, there often is a high-angle team. If there is a river with low-head dams running through your district, a water rescue team would be appropriate.

In this chapter, the focus is on the role of the EMT-B at a vehicle collision where extrication of the patient is required, since this is the most common type of rescue across the United States.

VEHICLE RESCUE

Extrication is the process by which entrapped patients are rescued from vehicles, buildings, tunnels, or other places. There are 10 phases of the extrication or rescue process that you, as an EMT-B, should understand:

1. Preparing for the rescue
2. Sizing up the situation
3. Recognizing and managing hazards
4. Stabilizing the vehicle prior to entering
5. Gaining access to the patient
6. Providing initial patient assessment and a rapid trauma exam
7. Disentangling the patient
8. Immobilizing and extricating the patient from the vehicle
9. Providing a detailed physical exam, ongoing assessment, treatment, and transport to the most appropriate hospital
10. Terminating the rescue

Every step of this process needs input from you, the EMT-B, acting as an advocate for the patient's medical needs. Attention to safety must be your highest priority—to help minimize the potential for injury to yourself, the other rescuers, or any additional injury to your patient. Although you may never personally perform disentanglement, since in many communities this is accomplished by a fire department rescue squad, it is important for you to understand the process so you can keep your patient informed and anticipate any dangerous steps in the extrication action plan.

You have already learned about some of the 10 phases of the extrication process (phases 2, 3, 6, 8, and 9) in the Assessment and Trauma modules, as well as in the chapter "Ambulance Operations." You will learn about phases 1–5 and 7 in this chapter.

Preparing for the Rescue

Vehicle rescue prior to the mid 1960s is best described as crude. So-called "rescue" trucks were usually small walk-in step vans that carried more equipment for fire suppression and salvage than for rescue. The inventory of rescue equipment might have

TOPIC OVERVIEW

In this chapter, you will learn about the following topics:

- Extrication and the extrication process

- What personal protective equipment to wear at the rescue scene

- How to determine the need for an extrication

- The need for personal safety at rescue scenes

DOT OBJECTIVES

✔ **Knowledge and Attitude**

1. Describe the purpose of extrication. (p. 719)

2. Discuss the role of the EMT-Basic in extrication. (pp. 719–720) (Scan 33-1, p. 723; Scan 33-2, p. 726)

3. Identify what equipment for personal safety is required for the EMT-Basic. (pp. 721–722)

4. Define the fundamental components of extrication. (p. 719) (Scan 33-3, p. 728; Scan 33-4, p. 733; Scan 33-5, p. 734; Scan 33-6, p. 735)

5. State the steps that should be taken to protect the patient during extrication. (p. 722)

6. Evaluate various methods of gaining access to the patient. (pp. 730–732)

7. Distinguish between simple and complex access. (pp. 730–731)

included some long pry bars, a few lengths of utility rope, a minimal hand tool kit, shovels and brooms, and—if the rescue unit was progressive—a four-ton hydraulic jack kit. Proper protective clothing and gear for rescue personnel were similarly lacking. Personnel were poorly trained for rescue and, more often than not, victims were simply pulled through openings created by the collision.

Modern rescue is a far more sophisticated process. It requires preparation that is a combination of training, practice, and the right protective gear and tools. As discussed above, training and practice for specific types of rescue, including vehicle rescue, will be above and beyond your EMT-B course. Availability of such training will depend to a great extent on the kinds of rescues most likely to be required in your area. The kinds of protective gear and tools that should be available for vehicle rescue will be discussed throughout this chapter.

Sizing Up the Situation

As you arrive on the scene of a collision, it is important to have a keen eye, because the first thing you need to do is evaluate hazards and calculate the need for additional BLS (basic life support—EMT-B level) or ALS (advanced life support—EMT-Paramedic level) backup, police, fire, or specialty rescue response, or services such as a power company representative. Quickly determine how many patients are involved, their priority, and the mechanisms of injury. If you think additional ambulances will be needed, call for them right away. You can always cancel them if they are not actually needed.

An important part of scene size-up is determining the extent of the patient's entrapment and the most appropriate means of getting the patient out. As soon as possible, evaluate if the patient is high or low priority. During scene size-up, you must be able to "read" a collision vehicle and develop a plan of action based on your knowledge of rescue operations and your estimate of the patient's condition and priority. During all of this, you will keep in mind that the most seriously injured patients have, at a maximum, a "golden hour" from the time of the injury until surgery at the hospital to control internal bleed-

ing and other life-threatening conditions. Beyond the golden hour, survival rates diminish drastically. As the patient advocate on the scene, you must plan how you can begin emergency care and initiate transport as rapidly as possible.

A low-priority patient can wait for rescue personnel to force open the doors, then remove the roof and/or displace the front end of the vehicle. For such a patient, there is time to do a short spine board or vest immobilization, then carefully transfer the patient to the stretcher using the long board. If the patient is a high priority, it may make more sense to use the rapid extrication technique, whether for a vertical removal through the opened roof or for a horizontal removal through a doorway. The principles of spinal immobilization remain the same whether the patient is low or high priority, but the requirements for speed of removal will dictate the specific technique you use.

During the scene size-up, check to see if the vehicle is equipped with air bags. A car with an air bag has a large, rectangular steering wheel hub. A passenger-side bag, if any, would be in the glove-compartment area. Special steps should be followed if the air bag or bags have not deployed. If an air bag has deployed, observers may have noticed "smoke" inside the vehicle during deployment. This actually is not smoke but dust from the cornstarch or talcum used to lubricate the bag, as well as from the seal and particles from within the bag. The powder may contain sodium hydroxide, which can irritate the skin. For this reason, it will be important to wear protective gloves and eyewear when you gain access to the passenger compartment. It also will be important to protect the patients from getting additional dust in their eyes or wounds. Air-bag manufacturers recommend that the EMT-B lift a deployed bag and examine the steering wheel and dash, which may reveal if the patients struck any of these areas with enough energy to damage them.

Recognizing and Managing Hazards

In some rural areas, fire departments have no rescue capabilities, and ambulance services are called upon to carry out vehicle rescue on their own. In areas where rescue and fire units are available, the ambulance may nevertheless arrive at the scene first. In this situation, time and lives can be saved if EMT-Bs—after sizing up the situation and calling for the appropriate additional help—are able to recognize and initiate hazard management, at least until personnel with more expertise arrive.

Hazards at a collision scene can range from nuisances—such as broken glass and debris, a slippery road, inclement weather, or darkness—to severe threats to safety—such as downed wires, spilled fuel, or fire. Also during scene size-up, watch out for loaded bumpers. Most cars are equipped with 5-mile-per-hour bumpers designed to absorb low-speed front and rear-end collision damage. If the bumpers were involved in the collision, you may notice that the bumper shock absorber system is compressed, or "loaded." Never stand in front of a loaded bumper. If it springs out and strikes your knees, it will likely break your legs. Some rescue teams are trained to unload or chain the shock absorber to prevent an uncontrolled release.

Traffic and spectators can become hazards if they are not controlled. A number of EMT-Bs have been killed at the scenes of collisions by oncoming traffic when drivers were watching the collision and not the EMT-B.

As explained below, some collision-related hazards must be managed, if not eliminated, before any attempt is made to reach injured persons in damaged vehicles.

Safeguarding Yourself from Hazards

Collision sites can be dangerous workplaces. Jagged edges, flying glass, and fire are only a few of the hazards you may need to deal with. Remember that you are no good to your patient and crew if you become a patient yourself. It is vital that you take the time to properly protect yourself before engaging in any rescue activities. The unsafe act that contributes most to collision scene injuries is failure to wear protective gear during rescue operations. The following human factors can increase the potential for an EMT-B to be injured at a collision site:

- Careless attitude toward personal safety
- Lack of skill in tool use
- Physical problems that impede strenuous effort

Unsafe and improper acts and omissions also cause injuries:

- Failure to eliminate or control hazards
- Failure to select the proper tool for the task
- Using unsafe tools
- Failure to recognize mechanisms of injury and unsafe surroundings
- Lifting heavy objects improperly

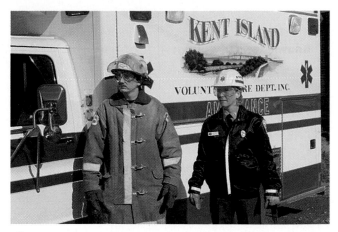

Figure 33-1   Two EMT-Bs dressed for vehicle operations.

- Deactivating safety devices designed to prevent injury
- Failure to wear highly visible outer clothing, especially when exposed to highway traffic

Figure 33-1 shows two EMT-Bs dressed for collision scene operations. The EMT-B on the left is dressed for a wide range of hazard management and extrication operations. At a collision scene any personnel who are allowed to work in the "inner circle," that is the area immediately around and including the vehicle, should wear full protective gear to avoid being injured. The EMT-B on the right is dressed for situations where hazards are minimal.

Learn the value of protective gear. Get your own if your service does not provide it (most states require it on ambulances), and use it! Consider reviewing the following National Fire Protection Association standards when purchasing protective gear and uniforms: NFPA 1972 (Helmets for Structural Firefighting), NFPA 1973 (Gloves for Structural Firefighting), and NFPA 1975 (Station/Work Uniforms). Following are descriptions of personal protective gear that EMT-Bs should use during rescue operations.

Headgear.   Good head protection is essential. Trendy baseball caps, uniform hats, and wool watch caps do little except protect against sunlight, identify the wearer as a member of an emergency service, or keep the head warm. Plastic "bump caps" worn by butchers and warehouse workers also do not provide adequate protection.

One good piece of headgear that does offer adequate protection is the rescue helmet. The model illustrated in Figure 33-1 does not have the firefighter's helmet rear brim, which can be awkward in tight spaces, although many EMT-Bs do prefer and use firefighters' helmets.

All helmets should be brightly colored with reflective stripes and lettering to make the wearer visible both day and night, and the Star of Life on each side to identify the wearer as an EMS provider. The level of training should also be indicated to make scene management easier when many EMS and rescue units are on hand.

Eye Protection. Eye protection is vital. Hinged plastic helmet shields do not provide adequate protection; flying particles can strike the eyes from underneath or from the side. Protection is best provided by safety goggles with a soft vinyl frame that conforms to the face and indirect venting to keep them fog-free, or safety glasses with large lenses and side shields.

Hand Protection. Because EMT-Bs stick their hands into all sorts of unfriendly places, every EMT-B should have optimal hand protection. Good protection is afforded by wearing disposable latex, vinyl, or other synthetic gloves underneath either firefighter's gloves or leather gloves.

Firefighter's gloves will protect an EMT-B's hands from a variety of sharp, hot, cold, and dangerous surfaces. They are bulky, but can be worn in most rescue situations. If greater dexterity is needed, intermediate weight leather gloves can be worn. Fabric garden or work gloves are too thin to offer adequate protection.

Body Protection. An EMT-B will often protect head, eyes, and hands and leave the body virtually unprotected. Light shirts or nylon jackets should never be allowed inside the inner circle because they do little to *protect from jagged metal, broken glass, or flash fires.*

Good upper body protection is offered by wearing either a short or mid-length turnout coat that meets Occupational Safety and Health Administration (OSHA) requirements. A heavy-duty EMS or rescue jacket can be used to protect you from weather and minor injury. As with helmets, bright colors and reflective material will help make your jacket more visible.

Good lower body protection can be provided by wearing either turnout pants with cuffs wide enough to pull over work shoes or fire-resistant trousers or jumpsuits. Serious consideration should be given to wearing high-top, steel toe, work shoes with extended tops to protect the ankles.

Safeguarding Your Patient from Hazards

When your patients have been injured in a collision, it is your responsibility to see to it that further injuries are not inflicted during the rescue operation. You can minimize the chance of such additional injuries by shielding the patient and exercising care. The following items can be used to protect the patient from heat, cold, flying particles, and other hazards:

- Aluminized rescue blanket offers protection from weather and, to a degree, from flying particles. A paper blanket does not afford this protection; it merely hides the patient's view of the debris that is about to strike him.
- Lightweight vinyl-coated paper tarpaulin can protect from weather.
- Wool blanket should be used to protect from cold. Cover the wool blanket with an aluminized blanket or a salvage cover whenever glass must be broken near a patient, since glass particles are just about impossible to remove from wool blankets.
- Short and long spine boards can shield a patient from contact with tools and debris.
- Hard hats, safety goggles, industrial hearing protectors, disposable dust masks, and thermal masks (in cold weather—and unless the patient has airway or breathing problems or is on oxygen) will protect a patient's head, eyes, ears, and respiratory passages.

Managing Traffic Hazards

Collisions almost always produce traffic problems. Often the wreckage blocks lanes of traffic. Even if it does not, backups are caused when curious drivers slow down to "rubberneck," or stare at the scene. Rescuers, firefighters, and police usually handle traffic control; but what if the ambulance EMT-Bs are responding alone or ahead of other emergency service units?

Obviously, personal safety, rescue, and emergency care have priority. However, an ambulance crew should still initiate basic traffic control, channeling vehicles past the scene. Remember to be extremely watchful and careful when you work to control traffic to be sure that you are not struck by an approaching or passing vehicle.

Your ambulance with its warning lights will serve as the first form of traffic control. However, you should position other warning devices as soon as possible. Bad weather, darkness, vegetation, and curved or hilly roadways may keep approaching motorists from seeing your ambulance soon enough to stop safely.

Using Flares for Traffic Control

Although some argue that flares are unsafe, when used properly they are still a good device for warning motorists of dangerous conditions. Moreover, several dozen flares can be carried behind the front seat of an ambulance, while battery-powered flashing lights—an alternative to flares—take up valuable compartment space.

Scan 33-1 shows the proper positioning of flares at collision scenes, including a straight road, a curved road, and a hill. Keep in mind that the stopping

POSITIONING FLARES TO CONTROL TRAFFIC

Posted speed (mph)	Stopping distance for that speed		Posted speed (in feet)		Distance of the farthest warning device
20 mph	50 feet	+	20 feet	=	70 feet
30 mph	75 feet	+	30 feet	=	105 feet
40 mph	125 feet	+	40 feet	=	165 feet
50 mph	175 feet	+	50 feet	=	225 feet
60 mph	275 feet	+	60 feet	=	335 feet
70 mph	375 feet	+	70 feet	=	445 feet

◀ Flares are positioned according to a formula that includes the stopping distance for the posted speed plus a margin of safety.

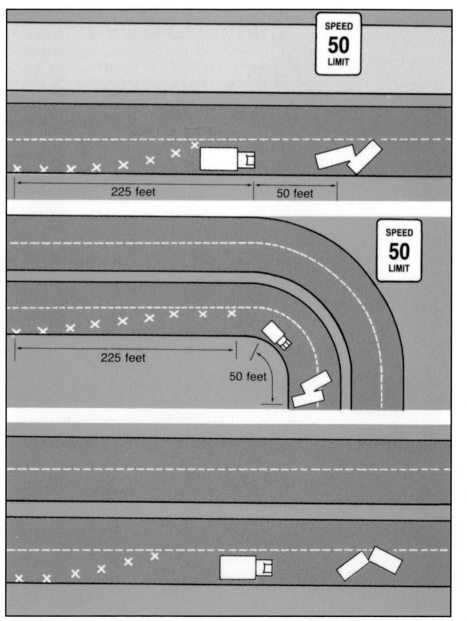

◀ Flares positioned on a straight road. Approaching vehicles are moved into the correct lane before they reach the edge of the danger zone.

◀ Flares positioned ahead of a curved section of road. The start of the curve is considered to be the edge of the danger zone.

◀ Flares positioned on a hill. The flares slow approaching vehicles and make them turn into the correct lane before they reach the top of the hill.

distance for large trucks is much greater than for cars. When the road carries truck traffic, extend the flare strings beyond the distances shown.

Remember the following points when you place flares:

- Look for and avoid spilled fuel, dry vegetation, and other combustibles before you ignite and position flares, especially at a road edge.
- Do not throw flares out of moving vehicles.
- Position a few flares at the edge of the danger zone as soon as the ambulance is parked. They will supplement the ambulance warning lights.
- Take a handful of flares and walk (carefully) toward oncoming traffic.
- Position the flares every 10 feet, if possible, to channel vehicles into an unblocked lane. (Do not turn your back to traffic while placing flares.)
- If the collision has occurred on a two-lane road, position flares in both directions.
- Never use a flare as a traffic wand; flares can spew molten phosphorous, which can cause third degree burns to the skin.

Controlling Spectators

Spectators do more than just create problems for passing motorists. If allowed to wander freely, they will close in on the wreckage just to get a better view. They may get so close that they interfere with rescue and emergency care efforts.

Rescue squads, police, and fire units have personnel and equipment for crowd control; ambulances usually do not. However, an EMT-B can usually initiate some crowd-control measures. If local policies permit it, ask for assistance from one or more responsible-looking bystanders. Ask the persons you recruit to keep the spectators away from the danger zone. Give them a roll of barricade tape if you have one. Be sure not to put the recruited personnel in unsafe positions such as near spilled fuel or an unstable vehicle.

Coping with Electrical Hazards

Electricity poses many dangers at vehicle-collision scenes. When there is an electrical hazard, establish a danger zone and a safe zone. The danger zone should only be entered by individuals responsible for controlling the hazard, such as power company personnel or specialty rescue. The safe zone should be sufficiently far away to assure that an arcing or moving wire could not possibly injure any of the rescue personnel or bystanders.

Keep in mind the safety points listed below. Many have to do with taking precautions around conductors. A conductor is a wire or any other object or material that will carry electricity.

- High voltages are not as uncommon on roadside utility poles as people often think. In some areas, wood poles support conductors of as much as 500,000 volts.
- Assume that the entire area is extremely dangerous. Conductors may have touched and energized any part of the system, including electrical, telephone, cable TV, and other wires supported by the utility pole, guy wires, ground wires, the pole itself, the ground surrounding the pole, and nearby guard rails and fences. Assume that severed or displaced conductors may be touching and energizing every wire and conductor at the highest voltage present. Dead wires may be re-energized at any moment. Energized conductors may arc to the ground.
- Ordinary protective clothing does not protect against electrocution.

Remembering these points and the following procedures may keep you alive at the scene of a collision where unconfined electricity is a hazard.

Broken Utility Pole with Wires Down. A broken utility pole with wires down is very dangerous. You probably cannot work safely in the area until a power company representative assures you that the power is off and the scene is safe. If you discover that a utility pole is broken and wires are down:

- Park the ambulance outside the danger zone.
- Before you leave the ambulance, be sure that no portion of the vehicle, including the radio antenna, is contacting any sagging conductors.
- Order spectators and nonessential emergency service personnel from the danger zone. Use perimeter tape to set up a large safety zone.
- Discourage occupants of the collision vehicle from leaving the wreckage.
- Prohibit traffic flow through the danger zone.
- Determine the number of the nearest pole you can safely approach, and ask your dispatcher to advise the power company of the pole number and location.
- Do not attempt to move downed wires. Metal implements will, of course, conduct electricity, but even implements that may not appear to be conductive, such as tools with wood handles or natural fiber ropes, may have a high moisture content that will conduct electricity and may cause a well-intentioned rescuer to become electrocuted.
- Stand in a safe place until the power company cuts the wires or disconnects the power.

Be especially careful when approaching a collision located in a dark area such as a rural roadside at night. As you walk from the ambulance, sweep the area ahead of you, to each side and overhead, with the beam of a powerful hand light. An energized conductor may be dangling just at head level. If you discover that a wire is down, leave the area immediately and notify the power company.

Sometimes, especially in wet weather, a phenomenon known as *ground gradient* may provide your first clue that a wire is down. Voltage is greatest at the point where a conductor touches the ground, then diminishes with distance from the point of contact. That distance may be several inches or many feet. Being able to recognize and respond properly to energized ground can save your life.

Stop your approach immediately if you feel a tingling sensation in your legs and lower torso. This sensation means that you are on energized ground. Current is entering one foot, passing through your lower body, and exiting through your other foot. If you continue on, you risk being electrocuted!

Turn 180 degrees and take one of two escape measures. Hop to a safe place on one foot. Or shuffle away from the danger area with both feet together, allowing no break in contact between your two feet or between your feet and the ground. Either technique helps prevent your body from completing a circuit with energized ground, which can cause electrocution. (A circuit is a circular path for electrical flow, such as up one leg, down the other, and through the ground. Hopping on one leg or keeping your feet together creates a straight path rather than a circular circuit, which may prevent electrocution.)

Broken Utility Pole with Wires Intact. Even if wires are intact, a broken utility pole is still dangerous. Wires that are still holding up the pole can break at any time, dropping pole and wires onto the scene. If you arrive to find such a situation:

- Park the ambulance outside the danger zone.
- Notify your dispatcher of the situation.
- Stay outside the danger zone until power company representatives can de-energize the conductors and stabilize the pole.
- Keep spectators and other emergency service personnel out of the danger zone.

Damaged Pad-Mounted Transformer. When electrical cables run underground, the transformer may be mounted on a pad above ground (Figure 33-2). When an above-ground pad-mounted electrical transformer is struck and damaged, it poses a serious threat. In such a situation:

- Request an immediate power company response.
- Do not touch either the transformer case or a vehicle touching it, and warn other emergency service personnel not to.

Figure 33-2 A pad-mounted transformer, if damaged, poses a serious threat.

- Stand in a safe place until the power company de-energizes the transformer.
- Keep spectators out of the danger zone.

Coping with Vehicle Fires

When you find a vehicle on fire, always request the response of firefighting apparatus. Do not assume that someone else has called the fire department. In fact, an engine should always stand by at a vehicle rescue.

Extinguishing a vehicle fire is the responsibility of persons who are trained and equipped for the job: firefighters. Nonetheless, there are some measures that trained EMT-Bs can take when they arrive before fire units (Scan 33-2).

For small fires, a 15- or 20-pound class A:B:C dry chemical fire extinguisher can extinguish virtually anything that may be burning in a vehicle, including upholstery, fuel, and electrical components. Only burning magnesium and other flammable metals cannot be extinguished by an A:B:C extinguisher. Before you try to put out a fire, always put on a full set of protective gear.

Fire in the Engine Compartment. If the hood is fully open, stand close to an A-post (front roof-supporting post) of the vehicle and, if possible, with your back to the wind to guard against the agent blowing back into your face or entering the passenger compartment. (Dry chemical extinguishing agent irritates respiratory passages and may contaminate open wounds.) Then sweep the extinguisher across the base of the fire with short bursts. Use no more than necessary to extinguish the fire. You will need what is left if there is a subsequent flare-up.

If the hood is open to the safety latch, do not raise the hood farther. This will help to restrict air flow and deprive the fire of oxygen. Then direct the agent through any opening to the engine compartment:

EXTINGUISHING FIRES IN COLLISION VEHICLES

▲ Markings that identify an extinguisher that can be used for Class A, B, and C fires.

▲ Extinguishing a fire in the engine compartment when the hood is fully open.

▲ Extinguishing a fire in the engine compartment when the hood is partially open.

▲ Extinguishing a fire under the dash. Care must be taken not to fill the vehicle's interior with a cloud of agent.

◄ Extinguishing fuel burning under a vehicle. Flames are swept away from the vehicle.

between hood and fender, around the grill, under a wheel well, or through a broken head lamp assembly. Again, use no more agent than is needed.

If the hood is closed tight, let the fire burn under the closed hood, leaving its extinguishment to the fire department, and continue to get the patients out of the vehicle. The firewall should protect the passenger area long enough to get the patients out of the vehicle, using emergency moves.

Fire in the Passenger Compartment or Trunk. If the fire is under the dash or in upholstery or other combustibles, carefully apply the agent directly to the burning material. Apply sparingly to avoid creating a cloud of powder that may be harmful to occupants. If there is fire in the trunk, as with fire under a closed hood, leave extinguishment to the fire department and continue working to get patients out of the vehicle.

Fire under the Vehicle. Using a portable unit to extinguish burning fuel under a vehicle may be an exercise in futility when the spill is large. But when people are trapped in the vehicle, you may feel you must try. Attempt to sweep the flames from under the passenger compartment as you apply the agent. If you do extinguish the fire, be sure that sources of ignition are then kept away. The vehicle's own catalytic converter (usually found in the area under the front passenger's feet) can be an ignition source since its temperature can reach over 1200 degrees.

Truck Fires. An A:B:C extinguisher can also be used to combat truck fires. Be aware, however, that burning truck tires are especially dangerous. Flames can quickly spread to the body of the vehicle and its cargo, or the tires can blow apart when heated by fire. NEVER stand directly in front of a truck wheel when there is a fire; approach from a 45-degree angle.

✋ Safety Note

At times you will find that fuel is leaking from a damaged vehicle but is not on fire. If you discover that a fuel tank is leaking, call for fire department response. The decision to continue the rescue effort should be governed by your perception of the danger. You should not be expected to continue rescue operations if gasoline is pooled under the vehicle or flowing toward a source of ignition. Warn spectators away from flowing fuel to minimize possible sources of ignition. Do not use flares near spilled fuel or in the path of flowing fuel. Watch where you park your vehicle, as your ambulance's catalytic converter can easily ignite spilled fuel or other combustibles.

Coping with a Vehicle's Electrical System

Many rescue units routinely disable the electrical system of every collision vehicle by cutting a battery cable. This was a reasonable practice years ago when vehicles had more combustible materials and when wiring did not have self-extinguishing insulation. Today, however, the situation is different. Unless gasoline is pooled under a vehicle or undeployed air bags need to be disabled, cutting the battery out of the electrical system may not only be a waste of time, it may actually hinder the rescue operation.

Remember that many cars have electrically powered door locks, window operators, and seat adjustment mechanisms. Being able to lower a window rather than breaking it eliminates the likelihood of spraying occupants with glass. Being able to operate door locks may eliminate the need to force doors open. And being able to operate a powered seat will create space in front of an injured driver.

If there is reason to disrupt the electrical system, disconnect the ground cable from the battery. In this way, you will not be likely to produce a spark that can drop onto spilled fuel or ignite battery gases. Such a spark can be created when the positive cable is pulled away from the battery terminal, or when a tool touches a metal component while in contact with the positive terminal or cable.

Stabilizing a Vehicle

Unstable collision vehicles pose a hazard to rescuers and patients alike. Scan 33-3 shows methods for stabilizing a vehicle on its wheels, a vehicle on its side, and a vehicle on its roof.

✋ Safety Note

Rescuers often fail to stabilize a collision vehicle because it appears to be stable. Rather than taking the chance of incorrectly "reading" a collision vehicle's stability—and having the vehicle move during rescue with disastrous results—you should consider any collision vehicle from which patients need to be extricated to be unstable and act accordingly.

If your ambulance is equipped with stabilization equipment, you should attend a formal vehicle rescue course that includes basic stabilization procedures taught by a qualified instructor. If the ambulance is not equipped for stabilization procedures, or if you are not trained, stand by until a rescue unit has stabilized the vehicle, even if roof posts are intact and the vehicle appears to be stable.

The information on vehicle stabilization that follows is intended only to help you, as an EMT-B, understand the process that trained personnel will be

STABILIZING COLLISION VEHICLES WITH CRIBBING

▲ A car on its wheels can be stabilized with cribbing under the rocker panels to minimize rescuer-produced movements that may be harmful to the occupants. Deflate the vehicle's tires for maximum stability.

▲ A car on its side can be stabilized by placing cribbing under the wheels, moving the car to the vertical position, and then . . .

▲ . . . placing cribbing under the A- and C-posts. Stabilizing in this manner allows rescuers to pull the roof down to expose the entire interior of the car.

▲ An overturned car can be stabilized by placing jacks and/or cribbing under the trunk, under the hood, or at both locations, depending on the position of the vehicle.

following. It is not a substitute for formal training in stabilization procedures.

Vehicle on Its Wheels

A collision vehicle that is upright on four inflated tires looks stable. However, it is easily rocked up and down, side to side, and back and forth as rescuers climb into and over it. These motions can seriously aggravate occupants' injuries. First, if rescuers have access to the inside of the vehicle, they should make sure the engine is turned off, the vehicle is in park, the keys are removed from the ignition, and the parking brake is set. Using three step chocks, one on each side and a third under the front or back of the vehicle, is the best method of stabilizing a vehicle on its wheels.

Then all the tires should be deflated. This can be accomplished by simply pulling the valve stems from their casing with pliers. A police officer should be told that this has been done so investigators will not think that the tires are flat as a result of the collision.

A listing of the equipment that can be carried to accomplish vehicle stabilization and gaining access is listed in Table 33-1. If the ambulance is not equipped with step chocks, a degree of stabilization can be accomplished by placing wheel chocks or 2 × 4-inch cribbing in front of and behind two tires on the same side.

If a car has rolled over several times and come to rest on its wheels, the roof may be crushed and access through windows precluded. The roof may need to be raised with heavy-duty jacks before doors can be opened or the roof removed.

Table 33-1 Supplies and Equipment for Vehicle Stabilization and Gaining Access

Quantity	Item
10	2 × 4 × 18-inch cribbing
10	4 × 4 × 18-inch cribbing
4	step chocks
6	wood wedges
2	vehicle wheel chocks
100 feet	nylon ½-inch utility rope
2	hi-lift heavy duty jacks

1	"door-and-window kit" with hand tools such as . . .
	  1 pair, battery pliers
	  1, 12-inch adjustable wrench
	  1, 3- or 4-pound drilling hammer
	  1, spring-loaded center punch
	  2, hacksaws with spare blades
	  1, 10-inch locking-type pliers
	  1, 10-inch water-pump pliers
	  several, 12- to 15-inch flat pry bars
	  1, 8-inch flat blade screwdriver
	  1, 12-inch flat blade screwdriver
	  1, spray container of power steering fluid as a lubricant

1	flathead ax
1	Glas-Master windshield saw
1	combination forcible entry tool such as a Halligan or Biel tool
500 feet	perimeter tape

Vehicle on Its Side

When a vehicle is on its side, spectators will often attempt to push it back onto its wheels. They fail to realize that this movement may injure, or more severely injure, occupants of the vehicle. Instead, the vehicle should be stabilized on its side. If the vehicle is on its side, do not attempt to gain access before it is stabilized using ropes, hi-lift jacks, and/or cribbing. While a car on its side may appear stable, simply climbing onto one side in an attempt to open a door may cause the vehicle to drop onto its roof or wheels. Moreover, you can be trapped under the vehicle when it topples.

A person who will act as a safety guide can be placed at each end of the vehicle to "feel" the movement of the vehicle and quickly warn the rescuers placing cribbing, jacks, or ropes to get back if the vehicle begins to fall over. Some services will deploy two ropes looped around the same wheel in both directions so that personnel can temporarily hold the vehicle stable while jacks and/or cribbing are placed. There are many ways to stabilize a vehicle on its side, from using manpower alone to using hydraulic rams and pneumatic jacks. The objective is to increase the number of contacts with the ground to make the vehicle on its side more stable.

Safety Note

When placing cribbing, NEVER kneel down. Always squat, staying on both feet so you can quickly move away from the vehicle if you have to. Once the vehicle is stabilized, if a door must be opened, tie it in the fully open position before you try to crawl inside.

Vehicle on Its Roof

If the vehicle is resting on its roof, roof posts are intact, and the vehicle appears stable, it may be tempting to try to reach the vehicle's occupants by gaining access through window or door openings—immediately, and without stabilizing the vehicle. However, if the posts collapse, as is often the case when the windshield integrity has been broken, the vehicle may come crashing down and injure the EMT-B who is attempting to climb into the vehicle or who has an arm in a window opening. You must wait to gain access until the rescue crew has stabilized the vehicle. This is usually accomplished by building a box crib with 4 × 4s under the vehicle.

A vehicle on its roof is likely to be in one of four positions:

- Horizontal, with the roof crushed flat against the body of the vehicle and both the trunk lid and hood contacting the ground

- Horizontal, resting entirely on the roof, with space between the hood and the ground and space between the trunk lid and the ground
- Front end down, with the front edge of the hood contacting the ground and the rear of the car supported by the C-posts (rear posts)
- Front end up, with the trunk lid contacting the ground and much of the weight of the vehicle supported by the A-posts (front posts)

If the vehicle is tilted with the engine, which is the heaviest part of the vehicle, on the ground and the trunk in the air, it can often be stabilized by using two step chocks upside down under the trunk.

When the roof is crushed flat against the body, as when all the roof posts have collapsed, the car is essentially a steel box resting on the ground with the occupants completely trapped inside. Unless the vehicle is on a hill or perched precariously on debris or another vehicle, this is the one time when stabilization is unnecessary. The structure is rigid. In such a situation it will, of course, be impossible to gain access through a window, door, or the roof. However, it may be possible to cut through the floor pan and have an EMT-B either crawl inside, if the opening is big enough or the EMT-B small enough, or to reach through the opening to touch and offer emotional support to the occupants until rescue personnel can lift or open the vehicle.

If the vehicle is unstable and cannot be safely approached by an EMT-B, get as close as you safely can so you can talk or signal to the occupants to reassure them that help is on its way and begin getting an idea of their condition.

Remember that when the vehicle is found in one of the positions described above, it should be considered unstable and must be stabilized by trained personnel prior to entry by an EMT-B.

Gaining Access

The National Highway Safety Act of 1966 required states to improve prehospital emergency care capabilities. It was recognized that EMS personnel could not do much for collision victims who could not be extricated from vehicles in time for live-saving efforts to be effective. So vehicle rescue training courses were developed, and bigger and better-equipped rescue units were placed in service.

Training courses began to prepare EMS personnel for a wide range of collision scene rescue activities aimed at gaining access to patients: unlocking and unlatching doors with commercially available and homemade tools, removing windshields intact, using hydraulic rescue tools to open vehicle doors one at a time, and so on.

Problems did not start to plague the rescue services until the mid 1980s. Suddenly extrications were taking longer, powerful rescue tools did not seem to be working properly, and procedures that had worked well for years were no longer successful. The reason for this apparent backslide? Improved vehicle construction.

For example, the Nader pin (named for Ralph Nader, the consumer advocate who lobbied for the device) is a case-hardened pin in an automobile door. In a collision, the cams in the door locks grasp the pin to keep the door from flying open. Prior to the Nader pin, rescue personnel could open a door with a crowbar. Subsequently, rescuers had to start using a hydraulic spreader to peel the cams off the pins. Safety features designed to keep occupants inside wrecked vehicles were keeping rescuers out! Each new safety improvement to vehicles created a new challenge to rescue personnel.

Vehicle rescue training was becoming a complicated business, and rescuers were being asked to learn dozens of techniques, some of which could be used only on certain models of cars. The need for effective but simplified procedures became evident. The next few pages will describe a three-step procedure that has been developed to meet this need.

Simple Access

First remember that, as an EMT-B, your responsibility is not the rescue of the vehicle but the rescue of the patient. You will usually assume that an occupant or occupants of the vehicle have sustained life-threatening injuries, and that at least one EMT-B needs to gain quick access to the patient, even while rescuers are working to gain a more wide-open access, create exitways, and disentangle occupants.

After the vehicle is stable enough for you to approach it safely, check to see if a door can be opened or if an occupant of the vehicle can roll down a window or unlock a door. (Try Before You Pry!) Such ordinary ways of getting into the vehicle are known as *simple access*.

Complex Access

If simple access fails, you may need to use tools or special equipment to break a window and gain access even while the rescue crew is dismantling the vehicle for extrication of the occupants. When tools or equipment are used for this purpose, the process is known as *complex access*.

All automotive glass is one of two types: laminated or tempered. Windshields and some side and rear van and truck windows are laminated safety glass—two sheets of plate glass bonded to a sheet of tough plastic like a glass-and-plastic sandwich. Most passenger car side and rear windows are tempered glass. They are very resilient, but when they do break, rather than shattering into sharp fragments they break into small, rounded pieces.

You will usually try to gain access through a side or rear window as far as possible from the passengers. Use a center punch against a lower corner to break the glass. Punch out finger holds in the top of the window and use your gloved fingers to pull fragments away from the window.

A flathead ax is usually required to break through a windshield. This can also be done very quickly using a Glas-Master saw (Figure 33-3). A windshield is usually not broken to gain access, but the rescue squad may need to remove it if they plan to displace the dash or steering column or remove the roof. Before the windshield is broken, passengers should be covered with aluminized rescue blankets or tarps, if possible.

Once an entry point is gained, at least one EMT-B, who is properly dressed, should crawl inside the vehicle and immediately begin the initial assessment and rapid trauma exam as well as manual cervical stabilization. Do not forget to explain what is going on and provide emotional support to the patient by talking and reassuring him that everything that can be done for him is being done. Access holes are usually small. So do not be tempted to pull a patient out of an access hole prior to spinal immobilization.

Disentanglement: A Three-Part Action Plan

In most instances, EMT-Bs will not be directly involved in disentanglement other than acting as the patient's advocate and being the EMT-B inside the vehicle. However, it is helpful to understand the plan for complex access that may be used by rescue personnel to free the trapped patient.

Figure 33-3 A Glas-Master saw can aid in windshield removal.

Following is a description of a three-part procedure that can be accomplished by fire, rescue, and EMS personnel with the appropriate equipment. The procedure is not vehicle specific; that is, it can be used on virtually any car or truck. The procedure does not include a lot of techniques that require special equipment. Personnel can be trained in a short course. And, most important to EMS personnel, there is no need to fill several compartments of the ambulance with rescue equipment.

Step One: Gain Access by Disposing of the Roof. For more than 20 years, emergency service personnel have been trained to carry out a progression of procedures to reach the occupants of a wrecked vehicle: first try the doors; if that fails, unlock and unlatch the doors by nondestructive or destructive means; when all else fails, gain access through window openings. This multi-part procedure is time-consuming and requires a number of tools.

A quicker and far more efficient procedure is to dispose of the roof of a collision vehicle as soon as hazards have been controlled and the vehicle is stable. Disposing of the roof has three benefits:

- It makes the entire interior of the vehicle accessible. EMS personnel can stand beside or climb into the vehicle and pursue emergency care efforts while rescuers carry out disentanglement procedures.
- It creates a large exitway through which an occupant can be quickly removed when he has a life-threatening injury or when fire or another hazard is threatening the operation.
- It provides fresh air and helps cool off the patient when heat is a problem.

Scan 33-4 illustrates the procedure for folding a collision vehicle's roof back like the roof of a convertible. While this is the most commonly used procedure, it is not the only way to dispose of a roof. A roof can be folded forward after cutting both C- and B-posts (rear and middle posts), folded to either side after cutting the posts of the opposite side, or removed altogether after severing all of the roof posts. Lacking a hydraulic rescue tool, you can accomplish all of these procedures with ordinary hacksaws and a spray container of lubricant.

Step Two: Create Exitways by Displacing Doors and Roof Posts. When rapid vertical extrication through the opened roof is not indicated, the next step is to open doors and displace roof posts. The benefits of this step are that EMS personnel can kneel beside the vehicle while carrying out patient care and immobilization procedures, and the immobilized

patients can be easily rotated onto a long spine board. Scan 33-5 shows a team of rescuers using a combination hydraulic rescue tool to open doors that cannot be unlatched and pulled open in the usual manner, as when doors are damaged or locks and latches jammed.

Step Three: Disentangle Occupants by Displacing the Front End. Most vehicle rescue training courses include procedures for displacing or removing seats, dash assemblies, steering wheels, steering columns, and pedals. A quicker and more efficient way to disentangle an injured driver and/or passenger from these mechanisms of entrapment is to displace the entire front end of the vehicle. While the task sounds difficult, it is not. Scan 33-6 illustrates the procedure for displacing the front end of a passenger car with a combination hydraulic rescue tool. A dash displacement can also be accomplished with heavy duty jacks and hacksaws.

If the steering wheel hub is large and rectangular, the car probably has an air bag or bags (the passenger-side bag being in the glove compartment area). If the bags have not deployed, they are not likely to deploy now unless extrication involves displacing the dash or steering wheel. If such displacement is to be done, air bag manufacturers recommend following these guidelines:

- Avoid placing your body or objects against an air bag module or in its path of deployment.
- Disconnect the battery cables.
- Do not displace or cut the steering column until the system has been fully deactivated.
- Do not cut or drill into an air bag module.
- Do not apply heat in the area of the steering wheel hub.

Must the three-part procedure just described be used for all extrication operations? Must the three procedures always be accomplished in the same order? Must all three procedures always be used? Not at all. In some cases, it may be necessary only to force a door open to reach a single patient and create an exitway for his removal. In other cases, it may be prudent to open doors before disposing of the roof. In still other situations, there may not be a need to displace the front end of a collision vehicle.

The extent to which you, as an EMT-B, will participate in vehicle rescue procedures depends on the role your EMS unit plays in vehicle rescue and whether or not your ambulance arrives ahead of fire and rescue units. The main purpose for the EMT-B to know extrication procedures is to incorporate them into the patient care plan.

DISPOSING OF THE ROOF OF A CAR

▲ Folding the roof forward can be accomplished quickly when the C-posts are narrow. The roof is hinged either on the top or the bottom of the windshield, depending on the need for working space.

▲ The traditional procedure for disposing of the roof is to sever the A- and B-posts, cut through the roof rails just ahead of the C-posts, and fold the roof back like the roof of a convertible. It is necessary either to remove or to cut the windshield, depending on the need for working space.

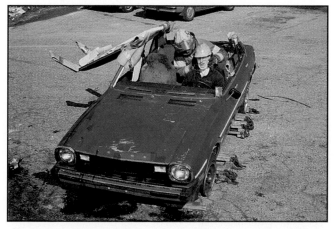

▲ When a car has only one occupant, the roof can be folded to one side after severing the A-, B-, and C-posts of the opposite side.

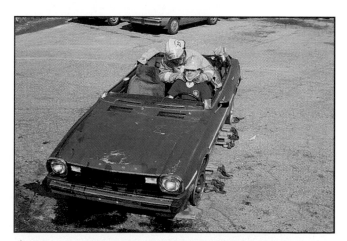

▲ When a car has narrow C-posts, removing the roof altogether provides maximum working space.

733

DISPLACING DOORS AND ROOF POSTS OF A CAR

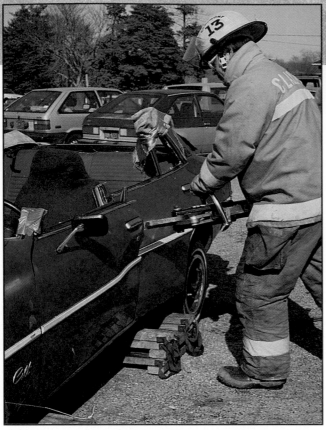

▲ **1.** A collision vehicle's doors can be opened quickly with a hydraulic rescue tool. Doors can be opened at the latch or by breaking the hinges.

▲ **2.** Once the front door has been opened, it can be moved beyond the normal range of motion by simply pushing on it. Seldom is there a need for removing a front door.

◄ **3.** When the front doors of a four-door car have been opened at the latch side, the roof post and rear door can be pulled down simultaneously to expose the entire side of the vehicle.

DISPLACING THE FRONT END OF A CAR

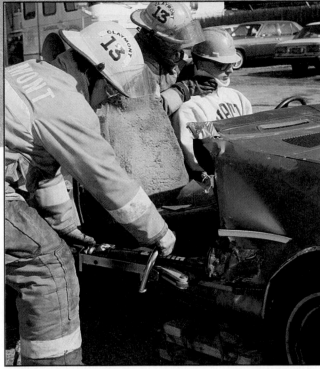

▲ **1.** Relief cuts are made at the junction of the A-post with the rocker panel, and in the A-post between the door hinges.

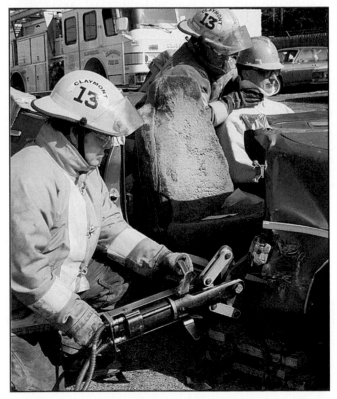

▲ **3.** The combination hydraulic tool can be used in the spreading mode to displace the front end.

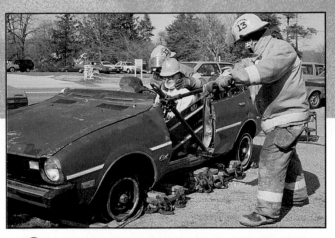

▲ **2.** Heavy-duty jacks can be used to pivot the front end of the vehicle away from the relief cuts.

▲ **4.** Displacing the front end will tend to lift the vehicle from the cribs. Cribbing must be added to the front cribs to prevent destabilization.

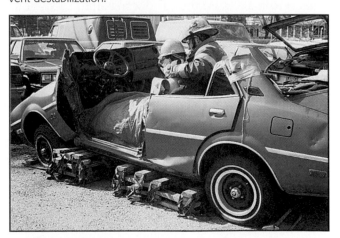

▲ **5.** Displacing the front end creates working space by moving a number of mechanisms of entrapment away from front-seat occupants.

735

STREET SCENES

You're on the scene of a one-car crash into a telephone pole. You position the ambulance about 50 feet behind the crash site with warning lights on, and both you and your partner put on full turnout gear including helmet, gloves, eye protection, and a reflective vest.

To control traffic, your partner places flares over a 200-foot section leading to the scene. You look around to make sure that there are no wires in the area and none on the vehicle. The scene appears to be safe. You go to the patient, notice the passenger side is intruded 2 feet, and see only one passenger, the driver. Two wheels of the vehicle are up on the sidewalk and the car appears to be unstable. You identify yourself to the occupant but don't get a response. Next, you try to open the door, but it is jammed. The car must have spun around as you observe there is more damage on the driver's side of the vehicle. You advise dispatch that heavy rescue is needed.

STREET SCENE QUESTIONS

1. What are the scene safety issues that you need to address?
2. What techniques should you consider for extrication?

Heavy rescue has an ETA of 10 minutes. The patient isn't responding, so you and your partner agree that entry is needed now. First, you put blocks at the wheels to make sure the car doesn't shift. Next, you pick a spot on the window that seems to place the patient at lowest risk, use a punch, and start removing glass. Once inside, you observe that your patient is a male about 30 years old with snoring respirations. You perform an initial assessment and find he is only responsive to painful stimuli. The snoring respirations stop when you move his jaw forward and manually stabilize his head and neck, but his breathing remains irregular. You administer O_2, and you suspect that you may need to start assisting respirations. At that moment, heavy rescue arrives and you report scene status and patient condition.

STREET SCENE QUESTIONS

3. Should rapid extrication be considered for this patient?
4. Describe assessment for this patient.

The lieutenant of heavy rescue tells you he will handle the battery disconnect and have his crew check to see if more cribbing is needed for vehicle stability. You maintain an airway and manual stabilization of the patient from inside the vehicle, while your partner applies a cervical collar and leaves to prepare the backboard. Rescue is able to pop a door open and allow full access to the patient. You are just about to say that the patient is clear when you see his foot is caught under a pedal. You tell the lieutenant from heavy rescue, and his crew sets up a small hydraulic jack. You make sure the patient is protected.

Once the foot is free, you and your partner decide that a rapid extrication is the best approach and move the patient to the board. When the patient is outside the vehicle, your partner is able to perform a rapid trauma assessment while you maintain manual stabilization. He checks the chest and it seems okay (the patient was wearing a seatbelt).

PATIENT NAME: Malik Cooper   **PATIENT AGE:** 30

CHIEF COMPLAINT								

CHIEF COMPLAINT
Unresponsiveness

PAST MEDICAL HISTORY
- [ ] None
- [ ] Allergy to _____
- [ ] Hypertension   [ ] Stroke
- [ ] Seizures   [ ] Diabetes
- [ ] COPD   [ ] Cardiac
- [ ] Other (List)   [ ] Asthma
  Unknown

Current Medications (List)
Unknown

VITAL SIGNS

TIME	RESP	PULSE	B.P.	MENTAL STATUS	R PUPILS L	SKIN
0010	Rate: 28 [ ] Regular [ ] Shallow [ ] Labored	Rate: 90 [x] Regular [ ] Irregular	120 / 76	[ ] Alert [ ] Voice [ ] Pain [x] Unresp.	[x] Normal [x] [ ] Dilated [ ] [ ] Constricted [ ] [ ] Sluggish [ ] [ ] No-Reaction [ ]	[ ] Unremarkable [ ] Cool [ ] Pale [x] Warm [ ] Cyanotic [ ] Moist [ ] Flushed [x] Dry [ ] Jaundiced
0015	Rate: 28 [ ] Regular [ ] Shallow [x] Labored	Rate: 90 [x] Regular [ ] Irregular	124 / 76	[ ] Alert [x] Voice [ ] Pain [ ] Unresp.	[x] Normal [x] [ ] Dilated [ ] [ ] Constricted [ ] [ ] Sluggish [ ] [ ] No-Reaction [ ]	[ ] Unremarkable [ ] Cool [ ] Pale [x] Warm [ ] Cyanotic [ ] Moist [ ] Flushed [x] Dry [ ] Jaundiced
	Rate: [ ] Regular [ ] Shallow [ ] Labored	Rate: [ ] Regular [ ] Irregular	/	[ ] Alert [ ] Voice [ ] Pain [ ] Unresp.	[ ] Normal [ ] [ ] Dilated [ ] [ ] Constricted [ ] [ ] Sluggish [ ] [ ] No-Reaction [ ]	[ ] Unremarkable [ ] Cool [ ] Pale [ ] Warm [ ] Cyanotic [ ] Moist [ ] Flushed [ ] Dry [ ] Jaundiced

NARRATIVE

Our patient is the victim of an apparent slow-moderate speed crash. He was restrained with a seatbelt. A witness reported the vehicle impacted on the driver's side door into a telephone pole. On our arrival, our patient is noted to be unresponsive with snoring respirations. Patient is accessed after forcible entry. We immediately maintained an airway, applied manual C-spine stabilization, and O_2 by nonrebreather mask. A rigid cervical collar is also applied prior to the arrival of heavy rescue. We determine this patient to be unstable. After a brief extrication, our patient is removed from the vehicle on a long backboard with appropriate manual stabilization. Patient has a bump on the left side of his head and a swollen left ankle, which was pinned down by the brake pedal. Once en route, we performed a quick reassessment. Patient's mental status improved to "verbal" during transport to the hospital.

The patient's respiration rate is about 28 and slightly irregular; ventilatory assistance is not needed yet. His pulse is 90 and regular. The patient is secured to the board and taken to the ambulance for further assessment and transport to the hospital. Considering the damage to the vehicle, the only injuries you find are a bump on the left side of the head and a swollen left ankle. By the time you get to the hospital, the patient is responding to verbal stimuli.

Later that day you are curious about this patient and call the hospital. The charge nurse tells you it was just a concussion and he will stay overnight for observation.

CHAPTER REVIEW

SUMMARY

As an EMT-B, you will not usually be responsible for vehicle or other kinds of rescue and extrication unless you undertake special training. However, it is important to understand how the process is done, how it may affect the patient, and how you can gain early access to the patient to begin care.

Vehicle extrication or rescue includes 10 phases: preparing for the rescue, sizing up the situation, recognizing and managing hazards, stabilizing the vehicle, gaining access to the patient, providing initial assessment and a rapid trauma exam, disentangling the patient, immobilizing and extricating the patient, providing ongoing assessment and transport, and terminating the rescue.

REVIEW QUESTIONS

1. Explain the role of the EMT-B in the size-up of a motor vehicle collision. (p. 720)
2. Discuss what the EMT-B should do upon arrival at a collision if a power pole is broken in half and the lines are down in the street. (pp. 724–725)
3. Explain whom you should call for assistance in your community if, on size-up of a collision, you observe a truck turned on its side and leaking fuel. (p. 727)

4. Discuss ways to stabilize a vehicle that is resting on its wheels, a vehicle that is resting on its side, and a vehicle that is resting on its roof. (pp. 727, 729–730)
5. Explain the difference between simple access and complex access to a patient in a vehicle. (pp. 730–731)

APPLICATIONS

• With knowledge of your own community, which of the 10 types of rescue specialty teams are needed and who provides the service?

• After considering safety of yourself and others, what should be your primary goal at the scene of a vehicle collision?

WEB MEDIC

Visit Brady's *Emergency Care* website for direct weblinks. At **www.bradybooks.com/emergencycare**, you will find information related to the following Chapter 33 topics:

- Hazardous materials
- Basic Incident Command System

Chapter
Thirty-Four

SPECIAL OPERATIONS

*W*ord on the Street

"EMS has always had to prepare for natural disasters, but who would have ever thought that we would need so much specialized education and training to respond to MCIs involving hazardous materials, terrorist attacks, and school shootings. These types of incidents place great demands on EMS personnel resources and equipment. My 25 years of experience warns that chaos can happen when other agencies aren't as well prepared as yours. In the past, when disasters would strike, we experienced total chaos and confusion during the first hour. Today we know that planning, practice, the Incident Command System, and CISM can help you better manage special operation incidents."

Ken Bouvier   Fire Chief, Monsanto Company, New Orleans, Louisiana

You have already learned how to deal with many situations in which an individual patient needs emergency care. However, you also need to know what to do if you are called to the scene of an explosion, an airline crash, a multiple vehicle pile-up, an earthquake, or other situation in which there may be many known or potential victims. Although you are not trained to deal with all the complexities of such emergencies, you must be able to recognize them and call for the appropriate assistance. This chapter offers the essentials that every EMT-Basic should know about special operations involving multiple patients and/or hazardous materials.

HAZARDOUS MATERIALS

Hazardous materials (hazmats) are everywhere, and EMS responds to incidents involving them frequently. Because many incidents begin as routine EMS calls, it will be up to you to recognize a hazmat early, be familiar with your local plan for management of a hazardous material incident, and understand your role in such an incident.

According to the U.S. Department of Transportation (DOT), a **hazardous material** is "any substance or material in a form which poses an unreasonable risk to health, safety, and property when transported in commerce." One of the undesirable aspects of our modern world is the growing number of such materials (Table 34-1). Hazardous materials are used for the manufacture of products and also can be the waste products of manufacturing. Even though safety procedures have been established and are followed for the most part, accidents involving hazardous materials do occur. Hazardous materials accidents are especially likely to take place at factories, along railroads, and on local, state, and federal highways.

As an EMT-Basic, you will be highly skilled in emergency care. However, without specialized training, you are still a lay person when it comes to hazardous materials. Special training is required to understand hazmats, to work at the scene of incidents involving these materials, and to render the scene safe. You cannot judge the state of a container or the probability of explosion without the benefit of such training. Do not believe that you can use safety equipment unless you are trained in the care, field testing, and use of the equipment. With hazmat accidents, you may be able to do nothing more than stay a safe distance away from the scene until expert help arrives.

Training Required by Law

Two federal agencies—the Occupational Safety and Health Administration (OSHA) and the Environmental Protection Agency (EPA)—have developed regulations to deal with the increasing frequency of hazmat emergencies. These regulations are meant to enhance the knowledge, skills, and safety of emergency response personnel, as well as to bring about a more effective response to hazmat emergencies. The regulations are described in the OSHA publication "29 CFR 1910.120—Hazardous Waste Operations and Emergency Response Standard."

According to the regulations, it is the responsibility of employers to determine, provide, and document the appropriate level of training for each employee. Training is required for "all employees who participate, or who are expected to participate, in

TOPIC OVERVIEW

In this chapter, you will learn about the following topics:

- How to identify and take appropriate action in a hazardous-materials incident

- How to identify a multiple-casualty incident

- The role of an EMT-B at a multiple-casualty incident

- The incident command system

emergency response to hazardous substance accidents."

The regulations identify four levels of training:

- *First Responder Awareness.* Rescuers at this level are likely to witness or discover a hazardous substance release. They are trained only to recognize the problem and initiate a response from the proper organizations. There are no minimum training hours required.

- *First Responder Operations.* This level of training is for those who initially respond to releases or potential releases of hazardous materials in order to protect people, property, and the environment. They stay at a safe distance, keep the incident from spreading, and protect from any exposures. A minimum of 8 hours of training is required.

- *Hazardous Materials Technician.* This level is for rescuers who actually plug, patch, or stop the release of a hazardous material. A minimum of 24 hours of training is required.

- *Hazardous Materials Specialist.* This level rescuer is expected to have advanced knowledge and skills and to command and support activities at the incident site. A minimum of 24 hours of additional training is required.

Most of the training levels outlined by OSHA have a fire-service focus. EMS responders should be trained to the awareness level and perhaps the operations level but in different skills. Responding to this difference, the National Fire Protection Association has published Standard #473, which deals with competencies for EMS personnel at hazardous materials incidents.

Regardless of agency affiliation, EMT-Bs play an important role. You are usually among the first on the scene for all types of hazmat calls. Your initial decisions and actions lay crucial groundwork for the remainder of the incident.

Responsibilities of the EMT-B

Recognize a Hazmat Incident

Whether hazmat incidents are very obvious or very subtle, you must quickly recognize one for what it is. It helps to be aware of the locations where hazmats are likely. They include highway accidents involving common carriers, trucking terminals, chemical plants or places where chemicals are used, delivery trucks, agriculture and garden centers, railway incidents, and laboratories.

Every community has chemical hazards. Identification starts with awareness and knowledge of what exists in the community. Spend some time with local police and fire agencies. Learn about or develop pre-incident plans for common hazardous materials.

When you arrive at a potential incident, as an EMT-B, you must restrain your natural impulse to take action. Never assume the scene is safe. After the initial victims, EMT-Bs are the most likely to become injured or killed because they tend to react quickly. So assess the situation first. Take a command position and stay a safe distance from the site before you take action. Once a hazmat is recognized, only those personnel trained to the technician level and equipped with the proper personal protective equipment should enter the immediate site. All victims leaving the site of the incident should be considered contaminated until proven otherwise.

Control the Scene

As a responding EMT-Basic, you may be the first to recognize that a hazardous material situation exists. For example, you may answer a call to a business where four employees are ill after being in the ware-

Table 34-1   Examples of Hazardous Materials

Material	Possible Hazard
Benzene (benzol)	Toxic vapors; can be absorbed through the skin; destroys bone marrow
Benzoyl peroxide	Fire and explosion
Carbon tetrachloride	Damages internal organs
Cychohexane	Explosive; eye and throat irritant
Diethyl ether	Flammable and can be explosive; irritant to eyes and respiratory tract; can cause drowsiness or unconsciousness
Ethyl acetate	Irritates eyes and respiratory tract
Ethylene chloride	Damages eyes
Ethylene dichloride	Strong irritant
Heptane	Respiratory irritant
Hydrochloric acid	Respiratory irritant; exposure to high concentration of vapors can produce pulmonary edema; can damage skin and eyes
Hydrogen cyanide	Highly flammable; toxic through inhalation or absorption
Methyl isobutyl ketone	Irritates eyes and mucous membranes
Nitric acid	Produces a toxic gas (nitrogen dioxide); skin irritant; can cause self-ignition of cellulose products (e.g., sawdust)
Organochloride (Chlordane, DDT, Dieldrin, Lindane, Methoxyclor)	Irritates eyes and skin; fumes and smoke toxic
Perchloroethylene	Toxic if inhaled or swallowed
Silicon tetrachloride	Water-reactive to form toxic hydrogen chloride fumes
Tetrahydrofuran (THF)	Damages eyes and mucous membranes
Toluol (toluene)	Toxic vapors; can cause organ damage
Vinyl chloride	Flammable and explosive; listed as a carcinogen

house. When there are multiple medical victims, "think hazmat."

Your primary concerns at the scene of a hazardous material incident are your safety and the safety of your crew, the patient, and the public. Should you arrive first at the scene of a hazardous material accident, establish a "danger zone" and a "safe zone." Keep all people out of the danger zone, and try to convince them to leave the immediate area. Stay in the safe zone until expert help arrives and makes other areas safe to enter.

The safe zone should be on the same level as, and upwind from, the hazardous material accident site. Avoid being downhill in case there are flowing liquids or gases that are burning or otherwise unsafe. Avoid low-lying areas in case fumes are escaping and hanging close to the ground. Avoid placing yourself higher than the accident scene so that you will not be in the path of escaping gases or heated air. Also be alert to the fact that a sewer system can rapidly spread hazardous materials over a large area.

Call for the help that you will need. The support services required at the scene of a hazardous material accident may include fire services, special rescue personnel, local or state hazardous materials experts, and law enforcement personnel for crowd control. If the accident has taken place at an industrial site or along a railway, the company experts in hazardous materials need to be notified. Much of this can be done by a single call to your dispatcher.

Implement your agency's Incident Management System. Establish and remain in command until you are relieved by someone higher in the chain of command.

The situation must be prevented from becoming worse. Establish a perimeter, evacuate people if necessary, and direct bystanders to a safe area. It cannot be overemphasized that EMT-Bs should not risk personal safety by initiating rescue attempts.

While help is on the way, establish control zones. Isolate the **hot zone** (the area of contamination or the area of danger). Establish a decontamination corridor (area where patients will be decontaminated) in the **warm zone**, an area immediately adjacent to the hot zone. Equipment and other emergency rescuers should be staged in the next adjacent area—the **cold zone.** Station yourself in the cold zone.

Identify the Substance

An attempt must be made to identify the hazardous material and assess the severity of the situation. Until that is done, it will be difficult to determine the risk to the public, rescuers, patients, and the environment. You must try to find out what the substance is and what its properties and dangers might be; whether or not there is imminent danger of the contamination spreading; what you can hear, see, and smell; how many victims are involved; and if there is any danger of secondary contamination from the victims. (Secondary contamination occurs when a contaminated person makes contact with someone who previously was "clean.")

Warning

Do not approach the scene to obtain this information.

Because it is not safe to approach the scene, you must obtain information indirectly or from a distance.

Figure 34-1   Binoculars will allow a visual inspection of the hot zone from a safe distance.

Ways of obtaining information safely may include the following:

- *Use binoculars to look for identifying signs, labels, or placards* from a safe distance (Figure 34-1). In many cases there will be a colored placard (Figure 34-2) on the storage container, vehicle, tank, or railroad car.
  - A commonly used placarding system is the National Fire Protection Association (NFPA) 704 System. It uses numerical and color coding to show the type and degree of health hazard, fire hazard, reactivity, and specific hazard contained within a fixed facility (Figure 34-3).
  - The U.S. Department of Transportation requires that packages, storage containers, and vehicles containing hazardous materials bear labels or placards with markings that identify the nature of the contents (Figure 34-4). Diamond-shaped placards used in the transportation of dangerous

Figure 34-2   Vehicles carrying hazardous materials are required to display placards that communicate the nature of their cargo.

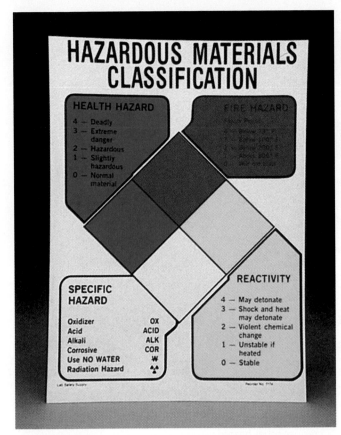

Figure 34-3 This is the key to the National Fire Protection Association (NFPA) 704 system of numeric and color codes to hazardous materials.

goods not only show the hazard class, such as "explosives," "flammable gas," "poison," or other, they also bear a division number which provides more specific information on the material as shown in Table 34-2. In addition, a four-digit identification number may appear on the placard itself or on a panel near the placard. Older placards are usually orange and have an identification number preceded by the letters UN or UA. Your dispatcher may have access to the name of the material through this identification number.

- *Invoices, bills of lading (trucks), and shipping manifests (trains),* if you can safely obtain them, will identify the exact substance being transported, the exact quantity, its place of origin, and its destination.

Warning

Recent studies by the Office of Technology Assessment have shown that some states report 25% to 50% of identification placards have been found to be incorrect. These same studies indicate that many shipping documents also are inaccurate or incomplete.

- *Material Safety Data Sheets (MSDS) on hazardous materials are required* to be provided by all manufacturers. These sheets must be maintained at the work site by the employer and available to all employees on the grounds that employees working with hazardous materials have a right to know about them. If you can safely obtain these sheets, they generally name the substance, its physical properties, fire and explosion hazard information, health hazard information, and emergency first aid treatment.

- *Interview workers or others leaving the hot zone* who may be good sources of information about the substance involved. Vehicle drivers, plant and railroad personnel, and perhaps even bystanders may be able to tell you the name of the hazardous material. Workers at a manufacturing site often understand very well what chemicals are used, the processes and reactions. However, note that workers may identify a substance by its trade name and not realize that it is a mixture of many chemicals.

Warning

Do not take hasty action because you think you have identified the nature of the substance. Seek and follow expert advice. Do only what you have been trained to do.

EMT-Bs are only expected to understand some of the common substance-identifying systems available and to make a preliminary identification based on this information. On the basis of this preliminary information, you can obtain advice about what initial actions should be taken at the scene from your dispatcher, a hazardous materials expert, or one of the sources listed below.

- *North American Emergency Response Guidebook (RSPA P 5800.7)* (Figure 34-5). This essential booklet, published by the U. S. Department of Transportation, Transport Canada, and the Secretariat of Communications and Transportation of Mexico, provides the names of chemicals and concise but thorough descriptions of the actions that should be taken in case of a hazmat emergency. Be sure to have the latest edition in your vehicle at all times.

- *Chemical Transportation Emergency Center (CHEMTREC)* has been established in Washington, D.C., as a service of the Chemical Manufacturers Association. They can provide your dispatcher or you with information about the hazardous material. They have a 24-hour toll-free telephone number for the United States and Canada, which is 800-424-9300. For calls originating elsewhere and for collect calls the number is 703-527-3887. When you call, keep the line open so that changes at the

Figure 34-4 The U.S. Department of Transportation (DOT) requires that hazard labels or placards be displayed on packages, storage containers, and vehicles containing hazardous materials.

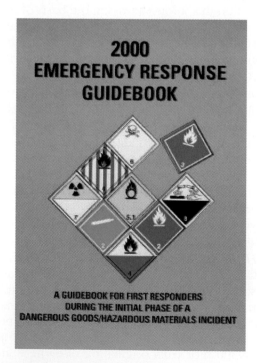

Figure 34-5 Have the latest edition of the *Emergency Response Guidebook* in your vehicle at all times.

scene can be reported to CHEMTREC and the center can confirm that they have contacted the shipper or manufacturer. CHEMTREC will be able to direct you as to your initial course of action.

- *CHEM-TEL, Inc.* is an emergency response communication service that can be reached 24 hours a day at 800-255-3924 in the U.S. and Canada. For calls originating elsewhere or collect calls, use 813-979-0626.
- *A current list of state and Federal radiation authorities* (who provide information and technical assistance on handling incidents involving radioactive materials) is maintained by both CHEMTREC and CHEM-TEL, Inc.
- *Regional poison control centers* are a source that is often overlooked during a hazardous material situation. Using their reference and medical resources, they can provide essential guidance in the decontamination and treatment of patients affected by hazardous materials.

When you call one of the above-named sources for advice, do the following:

Table 34-2   Hazard Classification System

Class 1—Explosives

Division 1.1	Explosives with a mass explosion hazard
Division 1.2	Explosives with a projection hazard
Division 1.3	Explosives with predominantly a fire hazard
Division 1.4	Explosives with no significant blast hazard
Division 1.5	Very insensitive explosives; blasting agents
Division 1.6	Extremely insensitive detonating articles

Class 2—Gases

Division 2.1	Flammable gases
Division 2.2	Non-flammable, non-toxic, compressed gases
Division 2.3	Gases toxic by inhalation
Division 2.4	Corrosive gases

Class 3—Flammable Liquids and Combustible Liquids
Class 4—Flammable Solids; Spontaneously Combustible Materials; and Dangerous-When-Wet Materials

Division 4.1	Flammable solids
Division 4.2	Spontaneously combustible materials
Division 4.3	Dangerous-when-wet materials

Class 5—Oxidizers and Organic Peroxides

Division 5.1	Oxidizers
Division 5.2	Organic peroxides

Class 6—Toxic Materials and Infectious Substances

Division 6.1	Toxic materials
Division 6.2	Infectious substances

Class 7—Radioactive Materials
Class 8—Corrosive Materials
Class 9—Miscellaneous Dangerous Goods

Division 9.1	Miscellaneous dangerous goods
Division 9.2	Environmentally hazardous substances
Division 9.3	Dangerous wastes

1. Give your name, your call-back number, and your FAX number.

2. Explain the nature and location of the problem.

3. Report the identification number(s) of the material(s) involved, if there is a safe way for you to obtain this information.

4. Give the name of the carrier, shipper, manufacturer, consignee, and point of origin.

5. Describe the container type and size.

6. Report if the container is on rail car, truck, open storage, or housed storage.

7. Estimate the quantity of material transported and released.

8. Report local conditions (e.g., the weather, terrain, and proximity to schools or hospitals).

9. Report injuries and exposures.

10. Report local emergency services that have been notified.

11. Keep line of communication open at all times.

If there is no identification number and no one knows what is being carried, you may have no other choice but to wait for experts to arrive at the scene. When a hazmat team arrives, they will identify and deal with unknown substances and the necessary computer and textbook resources.

ESTABLISH A TREATMENT SECTOR

All EMS personnel and equipment must be staged in the cold zone. EMS personnel have two responsibilities at a hazmat incident: *to monitor and rehabilitate the hazmat team members and to take care of the injured.*

Rehabilitation Operations

In order to safely enter the hot zone, the hazmat team members must wear chemical-protective clothing and breathing apparatus that both slows heat loss and prevents heat stress. Team members must be carefully monitored prior to, during, and after emergency operations. This is done to make sure that their condition does not deteriorate to a point where safety or the integrity of the operation is jeopardized. To address this need, a sector of operations called rehabilitation (rehab) should be established. While the rehab sector officer may not be an EMS provider, all rehab operations must include EMT-Bs or advanced-level EMTs.

The characteristics of the rehab sector must include the following:

• Located in the cold zone
• Protected from weather (shielded from rain or snow, a warm area in a cold environment, a cool area in a warm environment)

• Large enough to accommodate multiple rescue crews
• Easily accessible to EMS units
• Free from exhaust fumes
• Allows for rapid re-entry into the emergency operation

While suiting up in chemical-protective equipment, hazmat team members should have their baseline vital signs taken. When the hazmat team members show signs of fatigue or when they have had 45 minutes of work time, they are sent to rehab. As soon as possible after exit from the hot zone, reassess their vital signs. If heart rate exceeds 110 beats per minute, an oral temperature should be taken. If temperature exceeds 100.6°F, the rescuer must stay in rehab until pulse slows and temperature returns to normal. Always follow local protocols and consult medical direction. All pre-entry and exit vitals should be tracked on a flow sheet.

In addition to medical monitoring, rehab should be set up for pre-hydration and hydration, rest, and in some cases nourishment of hazmat team members. Proper hydration is an important element in preventing heat stress and promoting optimal physical performance. Heat injury is usually caused by imbalances of water and electrolytes during periods of high heat stress and physical exertion. During physical exertion, at least one quart of water per hour should be consumed. For short-duration emergency operations, electrolyte sport drinks usually are not necessary. However, if they are used they should be diluted to half strength. Coffee and caffeinated beverages should be avoided because they promote dehydration.

When incidents will be of extended duration, some type of nourishment may be provided in rehab. Foods low in salt and saturated fats are ideal. Bananas, apples, oranges, and other fruits are excellent for fast nourishment. In cold environments, soups and stews are more easily eaten and digested than sandwiches.

Care of Injured and Contaminated Patients

EMT-Bs must work with the Incident Manager and hazmat team members to determine the most appropriate course of action. The decision to stay at the scene and decontaminate or to begin evacuation must be made after careful consultation with CHEMTREC, the poison control center, and other reference sources.

EMS is responsible for setting up the medical treatment sector in the cold zone to receive decontaminated patients. In the decontamination (decon) corridor, the hazmat team will decontaminate hazmat team members and any patients rescued. Unless EMS personnel are trained to the hazmat technician level, they must remain in the cold zone.

The field decon process is designed to remove most of the poison and deliver a relatively "clean" patient to EMS personnel for care and transportation (Figure 34-6). However, there still may be some chance of secondary contamination from patients to EMS personnel. It is important that EMS personnel work closely with the

9-Station Decontamination Procedure

STEPS	

Station 1. Rescuers enter decon areas and mechanically remove contaminants from victims. Tools are dropped in tool drop area. Rescuers are in SCBA and protective clothing. **Proceed to Station 2.**

Remove Contaminants

Tool Drop

Station 2. *Gross Decontamination*: Victims and rescue personnel are showered and/or scrubbed by decon personnel. Dilution is conducted inside diked area. Victims may be transported directly to Station 6. **Proceed to Station 6.**

Gross Decon

Station 3. *Protective Clothing Removal*: Rescuers remove protective clothing, clothing is isolated and labeled for later disposal. Clothing is placed on contaminated side. **Proceed to Station 4.**

PPC Removal

Station 4. *SCBA Removal*: Rescue personnel remove and isolate their SCBA. If re-entry is necessary, personnel don new SCBA from non-contaminated side. **Proceed to Station 5.**

SCBA Removal

Station 5. *Personal Clothing Removal*: All clothing and personal items are removed. Victims who have not been undressed are undressed here. All clothing and personal items are isolated in plastic bags and labeled for later disposal. **Proceed to Station 6.**

Personal Clothing Removal

Station 6. *Body Washing*: Full body washing is performed using soft scrub brushes or sponges and soap or mild detergent. Cleaning tools are bagged for later disposal. **Proceed to Station 7.**

Body Washing

Station 7. *Dry Off*: Towels and sheets are used to dry off. Rescuers and victims are dressed in clean clothes. Towels/sheets are bagged for later disposal. **Proceed to Station 8.**

Dry Off

Station 8. *Medical Assessment*: Rapid patient assessment is conducted by rescuers. Necessary stabilization procedures are accomplished. **Proceed to Station 9.**

Medical Assessment

Station 9. *Transport*: Transfer of patient to hospital for medical attention or to recovery areas for rest and observation.

Transport

Figure 34-6 An example of a field decontamination process.

decon officer and consult with medical direction on both treatment and appropriate protection during transportation.

The following points must be kept in mind about treating and transporting hazmat patients:

• Field-decontaminated patients are not completely "clean." Chemicals that pose a risk of secondary contamination to rescuers sometimes settle in hard-to-clean areas of the body. These areas are typically the scalp/hair, groin, buttocks, between fingers and toes, and the arm pits.

• Personal protective equipment or clothing (PPE/PPC) is needed to prevent secondary contamination of rescuers. EMS personnel will need to wear Tyvek coveralls and booties to keep clothing from being contaminated. A double layer of gloves also may need to be worn. Often nitrile or neoprene is best, because these are more resistant to chemicals than standard latex or vinyl gloves. Work with the decon officer to determine if your supplies are appropriate or if they have items that might work better than yours.

• Vehicles must be protected from contamination. In the decon process, patients are washed and are usually dripping wet. Since they cannot be completely decontaminated in the field, some of their water runoff could contaminate an emergency vehicle. To prevent this, the water runoff must be contained by either placing the patient in a disposable decontamination pool or covering the inside of an ambulance vehicle with plastic.

• Consider any equipment used to be disposable. When an item such as a spine board, splint, blood-pressure cuff, or stethoscope is used, it may not be able to be decontaminated and may need to be disposed of.

When treating a contaminated patient is unavoidable, identification of the hazardous material is crucial. Follow the treatment instructions given in the *North American Emergency Response Guidebook* or by the poison control center.

There are four types of patients likely to be encountered by EMT-Bs:

- Uninjured and not contaminated
- Injured but not contaminated
- Uninjured but contaminated
- Injured and contaminated

Anyone who is not contaminated, whether injured or not, can be treated like any other patient. However, anyone who is contaminated—whether injured or not—poses a risk of secondary contamination and should be decontaminated prior to leaving the scene. Unfortunately, field decontamination is not always possible because of poor weather, because there is no one at the scene who is trained to perform the decon process, or because the patient is high priority for immediate care, and treatment and transport cannot be delayed for decontamination.

If you are confronted with patients at risk of causing secondary contamination prior to the arrival of the hazmat team, do the following:

1. Take precautions appropriate to the substance as listed in the *North American Emergency Response Guidebook*. This usually means isolation from the substance. Be sure to use personal protective equipment similar to what you would use for splash protection from blood-borne pathogens.

2. Follow the first aid measures listed in the *North American Emergency Response Guidebook.*

3. Be sure to manage the patient's critical needs, just as you would any other patient. Do not forget to manage the ABCs.

4. If treatment calls for irrigation with water, remember that water only dilutes most substances. It does not neutralize

them. Cut the patient's clothing off and irrigate with large amounts of water. Try to contain the runoff. If possible, use tepid or warm water to prevent hypothermia. If there are open wounds, try to avoid flushing contaminants directly into them. Pay particular attention to cleaning areas such as dense body hair, ear canals, navel, fingernails, crotch, arm pits, and so on. Also try to use as much disposable equipment as possible. Discard it later.

5. After treating the patient, decontaminate yourself. Some of your clothing may also need to be disposed of.

Remember that the severity of any poisoning depends on the substance, route of entry, dosage, and duration of contact. Immediate emergency care measures as listed in the *North American Emergency Response Guidebook* may decrease the severity of the poisoning and save lives. Whenever possible, the entire decontamination process should be carried out by qualified personnel from the hazmat team before the EMT-B touches the patient.

When this is not possible—when a contaminated patient who has been brought out of the hot zone requires immediate life-saving care but has not yet been decontaminated—provide the required care, taking as many precautions as possible to protect yourself. Use the proper personal protective clothing and equipment, and decontaminate yourself as soon as you can.

Patient ASSESSMENT

Hazardous Materials Injuries

Be sure that you are wearing full-body protective clothing and, if necessary, a self-contained breathing apparatus. Follow normal patient assessment procedures, including patient and bystander interviews, to assess injuries. Do not overlook medical conditions and injuries that may be present in addition to burns and other immediate effects of the hazardous material.

Patient CARE

Hazardous Materials Injuries

Emergency care of patients with hazardous materials injuries includes the following:

1. If patients are not already in the safe or cold zone, they must be moved away from the danger or hot zone. Note that this is the kind of situation in which an emergency move of patients may need to be executed before assessment and care can begin.

2. Provide basic life support. For artificial ventilations and CPR, use oxygen from a flow-restricted, oxygen-powered ventilation device or a bag-valve mask and oxygen reservoir so that you do not have to take off your own protective gear.

3. Administer a high concentration of oxygen to any patient having difficulty breathing.

4. Immediately flush with water the skin, clothing, and eyes of anyone who has come into contact with the hazardous material. Retain the runoff.

5. Remove clothing, shoes, and jewelry from all persons who have come into contact with the hazardous material. Place those items in a sealed, labeled container. Continue flushing the patient's skin with water for no less than 20 minutes. Continue to retain runoff.

6. Remove your protective gear only when and in the manner recommended by local guidelines.

7. Transport the patient as soon as possible, providing care for shock, administering oxygen, and taking all steps necessary to maintain normal body temperature.

Warning

Do not neglect to decontaminate or to be sure others with the proper training have decontaminated the patient prior to transport. Otherwise the ambulance crew may be overcome en route. A contaminated patient or EMT-Basic can contaminate and even shut down the hospital emergency department.

MULTIPLE-CASUALTY INCIDENTS

A **multiple-casualty incident (MCI)**—or in some areas, a multiple-casualty situation (MCS)—is an event that places a great demand on EMS equipment and personnel resources (Figure 34-7). The number of patients required before an MCI can be declared varies in practice. Some jurisdictions will declare an MCI for as few as three patients on the grounds that practice with smaller-scale incidents will help prepare for larger ones. Other jurisdictions reserve the MCI designation for five, seven, or more patients. The most common MCI is an automobile crash with three or more patients. You will likely respond to many incidents with three to fifteen potential patients. Incidents with large-scale casualties are rare and apt to be "once in a career" events.

The important ingredient in defining an MCI is that, for whatever reason, the ability of the EMS system to respond to the situation is challenged or hampered by the situation itself. For any MCI plan to be effective, it must be flexible and expandable enough to be used from small three-patient incidents to large scale in-cidents of fifteen or more patients. In other words, the plan for "the big one" should be a logical extension of the same plan used to manage smaller incidents.

Multiple-Casualty Incident Operations

Though the principles of managing small- and large-scale MCIs are generally the same, large-scale MCIs unfold over a longer period of time and require greater support from outside agencies. Well-trained and practiced EMT-Bs can usually cope with a small-scale MCI pretty well. However, experience has shown that even the best-trained EMT-Bs have a difficult time managing an incident of greater magnitude.

One way to minimize the operating difficulties of a large-scale MCI is for every EMT-B to be familiar with the local disaster plan. A **disaster plan** is a pre-defined set of instructions that tells a community's various emergency responders what to do in specific emergencies. While no disaster plan can address every problem that could arise, there are several features common to every good disaster plan. The disaster plan should be:

- *Written to address the events* that are conceivable for a particular location (e.g., Kansas needs to plan for tornadoes, not hurricanes).
- *Well publicized.* Each emergency responder should be familiar with the plan and how it is to be put into operation.
- *Realistic.* The plan must be based on the actual availability of resources.
- *Rehearsed.* Experience has proven that the only way to get a plan to work correctly is to exercise it and, in so doing, work out the unforeseen "bugs."

It is beyond the scope of this text to teach you how to write a disaster plan or even to impart enough knowledge for you to be in charge of a disaster operation. However, it is important to introduce basic information about your potential roles in such an incident.

Incident Command System

One of the most widely used systems in the country is the **Incident Management System (IMS)**—also known as the **Incident Command System (ICS).** While not specifically a plan designed for MCI management, it provides a clear management framework for all types of large-scale incidents. In addition, it is mandated by law for the management of some types of incidents, such as those involving hazardous materials.

ICS originated in California, where it was designed as a management plan to handle large-scale firefighting operations involving multiple agencies

Figure 34-7 A multiple-casualty incident.

and jurisdictions. A flexible tool for managing people and resources, the system components include Command, Operations, Logistics, Planning, and Finance. The most commonly used components are Command and Operations.

Command

Command, which must be established at all incidents, is the person who assumes responsibility for incident management. This individual stays in command unless that function is transferred to another person or until the incident is brought to a conclusion.

IMS systems recognize that the manageable span of control is six people. As the MCI escalates and becomes more complex, the number of people and span of control become too large for one person to manage effectively. It is at this point that Command designates sector officers to help. Command handles all functions except those that are delegated to a sector officer.

There are two methods of Command—singular and unified. In singular command, a single agency controls all resources and operations. In many communities, for example, EMS is managed by fire services. Accordingly, singular command is often used at fire and rescue incidents. However, if police agencies have major involvement, if there is a separate EMS provider, or if other agencies are involved, unified command is more appropriate (Figure 34-8). In unified command, several agencies work independently but cooperatively rather than one agency exercising control over the others. In most communities unified command is the best way to manage resources. It recognizes that large-scale incidents tend to be complex and that the right agency must take the lead at the right time, with command officers from all agencies cooperating.

Command Functions

Initially, **Incident Command** is assumed by the most senior member of the first service on the scene. Very often this will be an EMS unit, and the senior EMS person will assume both Incident Command and **EMS Command.**

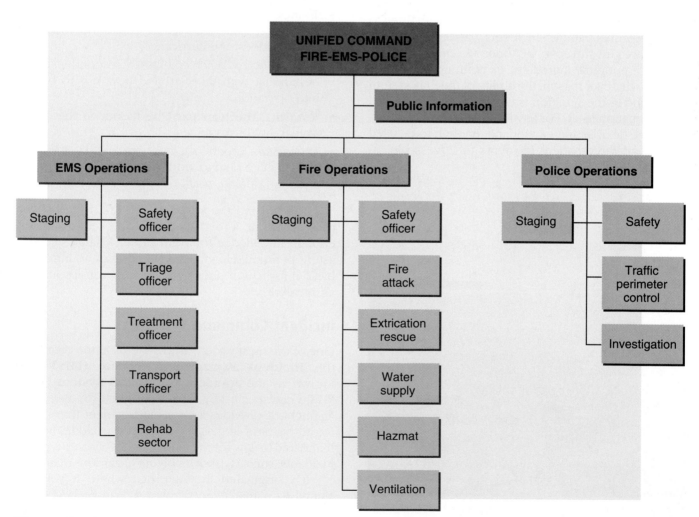

Figure 34-8 A unified command organization.

Two modes or phases of action must then be undertaken: scene size-up/triage and organization/delegation. First, Command and the crew do an initial scene size-up, start the triage process, and call for backup. While waiting for help, initial triage is completed and Command gets ready for arriving resources.

When reinforcements arrive, there are two options for the person who initially assumed command: Continue to be in command or transfer command to someone of higher rank. In a unified system, Incident Command would be assumed cooperatively by the Command of each service. Command is positioned at a location close enough to allow observation of the scene but secure enough to permit management of incoming resources and communication with others. In a unified command system, EMS, Police, and Fire Command establish one field command post together and stay there. Some plans call for the field command vehicle or command post to be designated by placing two traffic cones on top of the vehicle being used.

Scene Size-Up

Size up the scene by making a sweep to determine what needs must be met:

1. Arrive at the scene and establish EMS command. Put on the proper identification.

2. Do a quick walk through the scene (or, if it is a hazmat scene, observe from a safe distance) and assess the number of patients, hazards, and degree of entrapment. Identify the number of patients, including the "walking wounded," apparent priority of care, need for extrication, number of ambulances needed, other factors affecting the scene and corresponding resources needed to address them, and areas where resources can be staged.

3. Get as calm and composed as possible to radio in an initial scene report and call for additional resources.

Communications

Once scene size-up has been done, an initial scene report should be made to the communications center. Keep the report short and to the point, but give enough information for the communications center and other responders to understand the severity of the situation and react accordingly. Give yourself a unique Command name to distinguish yourself and your incident location from other personnel and incidents that may be using the same radio system. Example:

MEDCOM, this is Medic 640. We are on the scene of a two-car MVA with severe entrapment of four Priority 1 patients. Dispatch a rescue company and four paramedic ambulances. I will now be called Franklin Avenue Command. Police are needed at the scene to

assist with traffic and crowd control as soon as possible.

If the disaster plan is to be put into operation, it is critical that other responding units be informed of this fact. Your communications may also include telling other units what equipment to bring, what they should plan on doing once they arrive, how best to access the scene, and where to park.

As help begins to arrive, control of on-scene communication is important. Once units arrive, as much face-to-face communication as possible should be used, especially between Command and sector officers and between sector officers and subordinates. This will help to reduce radio channel crowding. If you feel you are getting too tied up in radio communications, designate a radio aide.

Basically, the flow of communications at the scene should correspond to the organizational chart being used. Accordingly, the only unit talking to the communications center and requesting resources is Command. The only ones who talk to Command are the sector officers. All others talk only to the sector officer they are assigned to.

Organization

Getting organized early and aggressively is very important. You must have a plan to deploy resources when they arrive. You must have decided what sector officers will be needed and where resources will be placed. A common mistake is to underestimate the resources that will be needed. Somehow new patients not found during size-up have a way of appearing. Think big. Order big. Put resources in the staging area if they are not needed right away. In urban/suburban incidents, backup can be fast and overwhelming. Think about supply and staging areas early or you take the chance of being overrun.

It is important to prevent "freelancing." Freelancing is uncoordinated or undirected activity at the scene. Given the opportunity, most rescuers will arrive on the scene and begin setting their own priorities. Command can prevent this problem. When established early, people and crews are assigned to tasks as they arrive.

Often it is helpful to have some personal tools to help to get organized. For example, many organizations have distilled the major points of their plans into a "tactical worksheet" they can use in the field. With enough use, the plan can become committed to memory. (See Figure 34-9.)

Scene Management

The senior person on the first arriving EMS unit, who will have assumed EMS Command, establishes an EMS command post to oversee the medical aspects

COLONIE EMS
Incident Tactical Worksheet

Location _____
Med. Command _____

___ Establish underlined command with fire & police
___ Place 2 cones on command vehicle
___ Put bib on
___ Designate triage office

___ Advise inbound units where to stage
___ Advise crews to stay with units until given instructions
___ Advise units to switch to EMS Admin., 265 or 715

LEVEL 1 (3-10 Patients)	LEVEL 2 (11-25 Patients)	LEVEL 3 (over 25 Patients)	FIRE	RESCUE
___ Declare MCI	___ Declare MCI	___ Declare MCI	___ Assess # of Units Needed	___ Establish Perimeter
___ EMS All Call	___ EMS All Call	___ EMS All Call	___ EMS All Call Req. 619	___ Request Speciality Units
___ Request # of Units Needed	___ Request # of Units Needed	___ Request # of Units Needed	___ Designate Triage	___ Triage Officer Handles Inner
___ Cover Town/Sr. Medic Act 615	___ Cover Town/Sr. Medic Act 615	___ Cover Town/Sr. Medic Act 615	___ Set up Rehab at Air Bank	___ Circle
___ Roll Call Hospitals	___ Roll Call Hospitals	___ Roll Call Hospitals	___ Use 619 as ALS Unit	
___ Transport Officer?	___ Get Mutual Aid Units	___ Get Mutual Aid Units		
	___ Designate Treatment Officer	___ Designate Treatment Officer	**HAZ-MAT**	
	___ Designate Transport Officer	___ Designate Transport Officer	___ Req. # of Units Needed	___ Medical Baseline Assess-
	___ Designate Staging Officer	___ Designate Staging Officer	___ EMS All Call	ment of Team
	___ REMO MD to Scene	___ REMO MD to Scene	___ Est. Command in Cold Zone	___ Don Protective Barriers
	___ Consider Rehab & CISD	___ Request Bus to Scene	___ Designate Triage	___ Assist With Decontamination
(2-5 Amb. Needed)	(6-13 Amb. Needed)	(over 13 Amb. Needed)	___ Identify Agent	___ Rehabilitate
			___ Research Decontamination	
			___ Research Med.	

HOSPITAL ROLL CALL	AMCH	St. PETERS	MEMORIAL	VA	ELLIS	St. CLARE'S	LEONARD	St. MARY'S	SAMARITAN
CAN TAKE									
# PATIENTS SENT									

UNITS RESPONDING

620	621	622
630	631	632
640	641	642
650	651	652
610	611	605

TSU-1 _____ TSU-2 _____
619 _____
Guild. _____
CPHM _____
Albany _____
Mohawk _____
Empire _____

UNITS IN STAGING

620	621	622
630	631	632
640	641	642
650	651	652
610	611	605

TSU-1 _____ TSU-2 _____
619 _____
Guild. _____
CPHM _____
Albany _____
Mohawk _____
Empire _____

 # OF PATIENTS BY PRIORITY

1 (Red)	2 (Yellow)	3 (Green)	0 (Black)	TOTALS

Figure 34-9 An example of an incident tactical worksheet.

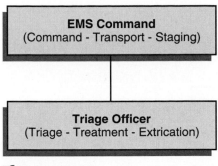

EMS Command
(Command - Transport - Staging)

Triage Officer
(Triage - Treatment - Extrication)

Figure 34-10 An organization for a smaller incident.

of the incident and the safety of all personnel, to designate sector officers, and to work closely with the fire and police commanders. On larger incidents, EMS Command may have an aide to assist with communications as well as a public information officer and a safety officer.

It is important to keep uninjured people from becoming injured. This will probably require restricting access to the scene to only those personnel performing triage (explained below), extrication from wreckage, and patient care. As resources arrive at the scene, police officers or safety officers may take over this function.

EMS Sector Functions

For smaller MCIs, EMS Command may be able to handle all aspects of management without delegating tasks to others. However, as an incident increases in size and complexity, additional staff and sector officers will be needed (Figures 34-10 through 34-12). EMS sectors generally include the following:

- Mobile command center
- Staging sector
- Supply sector
- Extrication sector (in cases of entrapment)
- Triage sector
- Treatment sector
- Transportation sector
- Rehabilitation sector (if hazardous materials are involved)

Individuals and agencies on the scene will be assigned particular roles in one or more sectors. Most systems use brightly colored reflective vests that can be worn over protective clothing to make each incident sector officer easy to identify. Any EMT-B arriving at the scene at this time would be expected to report to a sector officer for assignment of specific duties. Once assigned a specific task, the EMT-B should complete the task and report back to the sector officer.

Once EMS command has been established, the next task is to quickly assess all the patients and assign each a priority for receiving emergency care or transportation to definitive care. This process is called **triage,** which comes from a French word meaning "to sort." The most knowledgeable EMS provider becomes the **triage officer.** The triage officer calls for additional help if needed, assigns available personnel and equipment to patients, and remains at the scene to assign and coordinate personnel, supplies, and vehicles.

Initial Triage

When faced with more than one patient, your goal must be to afford the greatest number of people the greatest chance of survival. To accomplish this goal, you must provide care to patients according to the seriousness of illness or injury while keeping in mind that spending a lot of time trying to save one life may prevent a number of other patients from receiving the treatment they need.

To properly triage a group of patients, you should quickly classify each patient into one of four groups:

- *Priority 1: Treatable Life-Threatening Illness or Injuries.* Airway and breathing difficulties; uncontrolled or severe bleeding; decreased mental status; patients with severe medical problems; shock (hypoperfusion); severe burns

EMS Command

Triage Officer

Treatment Officer

Transportation Officer

Figure 34-11 An organization for a medium-size incident.

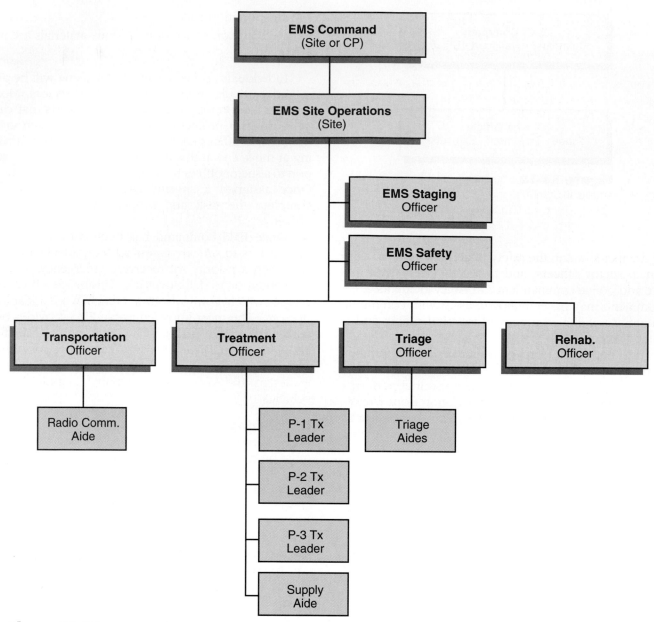

Figure 34-12 An organization for a major incident.

- *Priority 2: Serious But Not Life-Threatening Illness or Injuries.* Burns without airway problems; major or multiple bone or joint injuries; back injuries with or without spinal cord damage
- *Priority 3: "Walking Wounded."* Minor musculoskeletal injuries; minor soft-tissue injuries
- *Priority 4 (sometimes called Priority 0): Dead or Fatally Injured.* Examples include exposed brain matter, cardiac arrest (no pulse for over 20 minutes except with cold-water drowning or severe hypothermia), decapitation, severed trunk, and incineration.

Patients in arrest are considered Priority 4 (or 0) when resources are limited. The time that must be devoted to rescue breathing or CPR for one person is not justified when there are many patients needing attention. Once ample resources are available, patients in arrest become Priority 1.

How triage is performed depends on the number of injuries, the immediate hazards to personnel and patients, and the location of backup resources. Local operating procedures will give you more guidance on the exact method of triage for a given situation. Basic principles of triage are presented here.

The first triage cut can be done rapidly by using a bullhorn, PA system, or loud voice to direct all patients capable of walking (Priority 3) to move to a particular area. This has a two-fold purpose. It quickly identifies the individuals who have an airway and circulation, and it physically separates them from patients who will generally need more care.

You must rapidly assess each remaining patient, stopping only to secure an airway or stop profuse bleeding. It is important that you not develop "tunnel vision"—spending time rendering additional care to any one patient and thus failing to identify and correct life-threatening conditions of the remaining patients. If Priority 3 patients are nearby and well enough to help, they may be employed to assist you by maintaining an airway or direct pressure on bleeding wounds of other patients. Priority 3 patients who have been reluctant to leave ill or injured friends or relatives may be permitted to stay near them where they can be of possible help later.

Once all patients have been assessed and treated for airway and breathing problems and severe bleeding, more thorough treatment can be initiated. You will need to render care to the patients who are most seriously injured or ill but who stand the best chance of survival with proper treatment. This requires treating all the Priority 1 patients first, Priority 2 patients next, and Priority 3 patients last. Priority 4 patients do not receive treatment unless no other patients are believed to be at risk of dying or suffering long-term disability if their conditions go unattended.

. Usually patients will be immobilized on backboards if necessary and carried by "runners" to the appropriate secondary sector (as described below). Extensive treatment does not occur at the incident site since it is in a hazard zone and since it could impede rescue and initial treatment of other patients.

Patient Identification

By now it should be clear that a system will be required to group and identify patients by treatment priority. A widely used system is to color-code patients according to their priority. For example, Priority 1 = red, Priority 2 = yellow, Priority 3 = green, Priority 4 (if a separate category) = black or gray.

Different localities have different systems. It is important that you know and understand the system used in your area. It is equally important that different services in the same region use the same coding system. This is because many MCIs are multiple-agency events. If each agency were to use a different system, there would be no way to correctly coordinate the order in which patients are to receive care.

As you move among patients to conduct initial triage, you should affix a **triage tag** to each patient,

Figure 34-13 The triage tag indicates the priority group to which that patient has been assigned.

indicating the priority group to which that patient has been assigned. Triage tags are color-coded and may have space in which limited medical information can be recorded (Figures 34-13 and 34-14).

There are some local variations of the triage tag. Some use adhesive-backed colored shipping labels. Others use colored surveyor's tape or duct tape to classify patients. Surveyor's tape can be quickly tied on as an arm band. Duct tape will stick to just about anything in any kind of weather. For this reason it is particularly useful in an MCI setting. It is also useful to have a laundry marker or wax pencil handy for wet conditions when a standard pen or pencil will not write well.

Whatever system you use, it is vital that the color coding be easily located and identified. Properly done, this allows a later EMT-B to quickly identify which treatment group patients belong to and to institute treatment accordingly.

Secondary Triage and Treatment

As more personnel arrive at the incident scene, they should be directed to assist with the completion of initial triage. If triage has been completed, these EMT-Bs can initiate treatment.

Figure 34-14 Triage tag (front and back) used to identify Priority 1, 2, 3, and 0 patients.

Secondary triage generally begins at this point. In ideal triage systems, patients are gathered into a **triage sector** and, under the direction of the triage officer, are physically separated into treatment groups based on their priority level as designated by a triage tag. Some systems call for vehicles to carry red, yellow, and green tarps, which are used to designate these areas. An area to which patients are removed is referred to as a **treatment sector.** Each treatment sector should have its own **treatment officer,** an EMT responsible for overseeing the triage

and treatment within that sector. The treatment officer should again triage the patients in that sector to determine the order in which they will receive treatment.

During secondary triage, it may be necessary to re-categorize a patient whose condition has deteriorated or improved or who was incorrectly triaged to a higher or lower priority group than was medically warranted. This will necessitate moving the patient to the proper treatment sector as resources permit. Some systems use a different disaster tag during sec-

Figure 34-15 EMS disaster tag (front and back).

ondary triage on which more detailed information about the patient can be recorded (Figure 34-15).

The treatment-sector EMT-Bs will need supplies and equipment from the ambulances such as bandages, blood pressure cuffs, and oxygen.

Transportation and Staging Logistics

Once patients have been properly assessed and separated, and once treatment for the patients has been initiated according to their priority, consideration must be given to the order in which the patients will be transported to a hospital. Again, this is done according to triage priority.

It is advisable to have a **staging sector** from which ambulances can be called to transport patients. The staging sector will be the responsibility of the **staging officer.** This person must keep track of the ambulance vehicles and personnel. In large-scale incidents, the staging officer may need to arrange to meet human needs, such as rest rooms, meals, and rotation of crews.

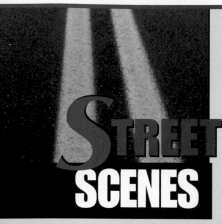

It's raining hard outside and there's a loud noise on the station PA system with the dispatcher saying: "Ambulances Alpha 2, Alpha 5, Bravo 1, and Charlie 10, respond to a three-car motor-vehicle crash at the intersection of Avenues A and B. Unknown how many occupants. Timeout of 1933 hours." You turn to your partner and say, "This call is only about 10 blocks away. We should be the first on scene." As you head toward the scene, you are notified by dispatch that the police are on scene and report a total of 9 occupants. Additional ambulances are being dispatched.

You and your partner agree that you will establish EMS command and he will do triage. "Dispatch, Bravo 1 is on scene and establishing EMS command." The first thing you do is put on the command bib for identification. Your partner puts on the triage bib and takes triage tags to check on the occupants. You briefly tell the police officer you are EMS command and he informs you that his captain is responding and has three units handling traffic control. He has also requested heavy rescue from the fire department in case extrication is needed.

With flashlight in hand and trying to keep the rain out of your eyes, you perform a scene size-up. You realize that you need a place to stage the other ambulances for easy access and so they don't get blocked in. You see a location and quickly share your idea with the police officer. He agrees. He will tell his units to make sure that area is accessible for the ambulances. You call dispatch on the radio using the identifier "EMS command" and ask that they instruct all responding ambulances to stage in the parking lot of the insurance company.

STREET SCENE QUESTIONS

1. As EMS command, what are some of the things you need to do?

2. What information do you expect first from the triage officer?

3. How will you decide what patients go to what hospitals?

Your partner advises you that 3 patients are priority-one, 5 are priority-two, and 1 is priority-three. You radio dispatch with this information. You are told that a canvass has already been done and the trauma center can handle all priority-one patients and the other patients can be divided between the other three area hospitals. You ask that they call the trauma center back and confirm that they will be getting 3 patients and the other hospitals will be getting 2 each.

You then ask dispatch to tell you how many ambulances have been dispatched. You are informed there is a total of five. Remembering that one of the ambulances is yours, you request two more ambulances. Two ambulances are on scene and parked in the staging area. You tell them to each take a priority-

No ambulance should proceed to a treatment sector without having been requested by the **transportation officer** and directed by the staging officer. The staging officer is responsible for communicating with each treatment sector the number and priority of the patients in that sector. This information can then be used by the transportation officer to arrange for transport of patients from the scene to the hospital in the most efficient way.

It is vital that no ambulance transport any patient without the approval of the transportation officer. This is because the transportation officer is responsible for maintaining a list of patients and the hospitals to which they are transported. This information is relayed from the transportation officer to each receiving hospital. (In a large-scale incident, the transportation officer may actually have an aide who does nothing but speak to hospitals.) In this way the hospitals know what to expect and receive only the patients they are capable of handling. It is critical that the EMT-Bs on the ambulance comply with the instructions of the transportation officer. Failure to do so may result in patients being transported to the wrong facilities.

Once an ambulance has completed a run to a hospital, it will probably be directed to return to the

SPECIAL INCIDENT REPORT *On arrival during a heavy rainstorm, we noticed 3-car motor-vehicle crash with a total of 9 patients. We activated our agency's MCI plan. I assumed EMS command, and my partner became the triage officer. I maintained unified command with police and fire command. As requested by triage, additional units were requested and staged as needed. We transported a total of 3 priority-one patients, 5 priority-two patients, and 1 priority-three. Total scene time was 30 minutes. We returned to service after restocking.*

one patient. The next ambulance is assigned to the last priority-one patient. You ask the triage officer if some of the priority twos or three can be doubled up, which seems appropriate for four of the patients.

STREET SCENE QUESTIONS

4. Is there a need for a safety officer on this scene?
5. How should patient information be transmitted to the hospitals?
6. What information should you be sharing with police command and fire command?

The fire captain tells you that his crew has disconnected the batteries of all the vehicles and will stand by to assist with extrication. Access has been gained to all patients using hand tools. You ask if his safety officer can continue in that role until all the patients are off the scene.

The first ambulance is loaded and en route to the trauma center. The second will be en route shortly. You advise these crews to notify the hospital directly but tell them to keep the transmission short.

The last priority-one patient is out of the car, and you tell the triage officer that the other hospitals get two patients each. He should coordinate this with crews and tell them to call the patient information to the hospital directly.

Within 30 minutes of the call notification, every patient is en route to a hospital. You let police and fire command know. Your partner looks at you and says "Not bad for someone who looks like a drowned rat."

staging area, perhaps bringing needed supplies, to await its next instructions from the staging officer.

Communicating with Hospitals

It is important that receiving hospitals be alerted to the nature of the MCI or disaster as soon as the magnitude of the incident is known. This allows the hospitals to call in additional personnel or to clear beds as necessary to accept the anticipated number of patients.

Because radio communication channels will be heavily used, the transportation officer, not individual EMT-Bs, should communicate with the hospitals. This will keep unnecessary radio usage to a minimum. It will also ensure that the proper information is recorded at both ends of the ambulance ride. In large-scale MCIs, it is not necessary to give a patient report for each patient. This is because the transporting and treating EMT-Bs will most likely be different and because there will generally be too many patients to allow EMT-Bs to give a good patient radio report under the circumstances. In these instances, the hospital may be told only that they are receiving a Priority 1 patient with respiratory problems, for example.

PSYCHOLOGICAL ASPECTS OF MCIs

During MCIs, EMT-Bs often encounter another, frequently overlooked condition: psychologically stressed patients. While they may outwardly exhibit few signs of injury or emotional stress, people involved in MCIs have been subjected to devastating circumstances with which they are normally unprepared to cope. Proper early management of the psychologically stressed patient can support later treatment and help ensure a faster recovery.

Adequately managing a patient during an MCI may require you to administer "psychological first aid." This may take the form of talking with a terrified parent, child, or witness. You should not attempt to engage in psychoanalysis and should not say things that are untrue in an attempt to calm a patient. However, a caring honest demeanor can reassure a patient, as will listening to the patient and acknowledging his fears and problems. Often this is all the patient will need.

Patients are not the only ones subject to emotional stress during a multiple-casualty incident; so are emergency responders. It is very important that you understand that large-scale or horrific MCIs (Figures 34-16 and 34-17) may affect rescuers as much as, if not more than, non-rescuers.

EMT-Bs who become emotionally incapacitated should be treated as patients and removed to an area where they can rest without viewing the scene. These patients must be monitored by an EMS provider until a clinically competent provider can take over. These EMT-Bs should not be allowed to return to duty without first being evaluated by someone professionally trained to do so.

Critical incident stress debriefing (CISD) teams are a resource that can provide the emotional and psychological support required by this type of incident. Intervention by a CISD team may help to prevent post-traumatic stress disorder.

Figure 34-16 A tornado can cause great devastation.

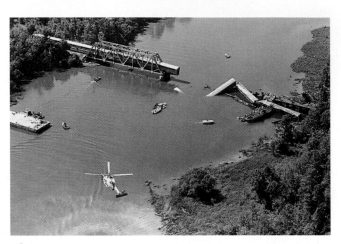

Figure 34-17 A train wreck can cause multiple casualties.

CHAPTER REVIEW

SUMMARY

Become familiar with your local plans for dealing with hazardous materials and multiple-casualty incidents. Practice every chance you get. Understand the management systems and triage systems used in your area, and be prepared to do your part. Also remember that hazardous materials accidents require specialized training beyond your expertise. However, you can learn to recognize them quickly, call for the appropriate assistance, and help to ensure the safety of rescuers, patients, and bystanders.

KEY TERMS

cold zone area where the incident command post and support functions are located.

disaster plan a predefined set of instructions for a community's emergency responders.

EMS Command the senior EMS person on scene who oversees medical aspects of an MCI.

hazardous material any substance or material in a form which poses an unreasonable risk to health, safety, and property when transported in commerce.

hot zone area immediately surrounding a hazmat incident; extends far enough to prevent adverse effects outside the zone.

Incident Command the person or persons who assume overall direction of a large-scale incident.

Incident Command System (ICS) see *Incident Management System*

Incident Management System (IMS) a system used for the management of a multiple-casualty incident.

multiple-casualty incident (MCI) any medical or trauma incident involving multiple patients.

staging officer person responsible for overseeing ambulances and ambulance personnel at an MCI.

staging sector the area where ambulances are parked and other resources are held until needed.

transportation officer person responsible for communicating with sector officers and hospitals to manage transportation of patients to hospitals from an MCI.

treatment officer person responsible for overseeing treatment of patients who have been triaged at an MCI.

treatment sector the area in which patients are treated at an MCI.

triage the process of quickly assessing MCI patients and assigning each a priority for receiving treatment; from a French word meaning "to sort."

triage officer the person responsible for overseeing triage at an MCI.

triage sector the area in which secondary triage takes place at an MCI.

triage tag color-coded tag indicating the priority group to which a patient has been assigned.

warm zone area where personnel and equipment decontamination and hot zone support take place; it includes control points for the access corridor and thus assists in reducing the spread of contamination.

REVIEW QUESTIONS

1. List the information in an initial report of a hazardous material incident. (pp. 746, 748)
2. Explain how to identify a hazardous material and how to obtain information about that material. (pp. 744–746)
3. Describe the general assessment and emergency care of a patient with a hazardous material injury. (pp. 748–750)
4. Describe the major components and benefits of an incident management system. (pp. 751–753)
5. Define the basic role of the EMT-B at a multiple-casualty incident. (pp. 755–759)
6. Explain why patients are assigned priorities during triage. (pp. 755–757)
7. Identify four priority categories of triage. (pp. 755–756)

APPLICATIONS

• Your call is to a motor-vehicle collision with an unknown number of injuries. As your unit approaches the scene, you see that three cars and downed wires are involved. You get a whiff of gasoline as you pass by. The drivers are visible in each vehicle—one appears to be conscious and the other two are bent forward or slumped back. There are passengers visible in two vehicles, one or more of whom may need extrication. How should you proceed?

WEB MEDIC

Visit Brady's *Emergency Care* website for direct weblinks. At **www.bradybooks.com/emergencycare**, you will find information related to the following Chapter 34 topics:

• Trench, water, and cave rescue training

Chapter
Thirty-Five

ADVANCED AIRWAY MANAGEMENT

irway control is the highest priority in managing any critically ill or injured patient, because without an adequate airway the patient will die no matter what other care you provide. Advanced airway management can only be effective and successful if you have already mastered the basic airway techniques discussed in Chapter 6, "Airway Management."

ANATOMY AND PHYSIOLOGY

The anatomy and physiology of the respiratory system have already been discussed at length in Chapters 4, "The Human Body;" 6, "Airway Management;" and 17, "Respiratory Emergencies." There are, however, specific aspects of both airway anatomy and physiology that the EMT-Basic who performs advanced airway skills must understand in greater depth in order to optimize the effectiveness and success of these advanced skills.

Anatomy

Air initially enters the respiratory tract via the nose and the mouth. Air that enters through the nose then passes through the **nasopharynx** and air that enters through the mouth passes through the **oropharynx.** The **hypopharynx** is the area directly above the openings of both the **trachea** (windpipe) and the **esophagus** (the tube to the stomach). The **epiglottis** is a leaf-shaped structure that acts as a covering to the opening of the trachea. The epiglottis protects the airway by covering the entrance to the trachea when food or liquids are being swallowed. Anterior to the epiglottis is a groove-like structure called the **vallecula.**

The epiglottis allows air to pass into the opening of the trachea and through the **larynx,** or voice box. The larynx contains the two **vocal cords.**

Giving support to the larynx and trachea are several rigid pieces of cartilage. The thyroid cartilage is a shield shaped structure that is at the anterior of the larynx. Multiple horseshoe-shaped cartilages give support to the trachea. The **cricoid cartilage** is a cartilage at the lower portion of the larynx. It is unique in that it is the only tracheal cartilage that completely surrounds the windpipe.

Once air has passed through the larynx, it proceeds through the trachea until the trachea bifurcates, or splits, into the two **mainstem bronchi** at the level of the **carina.** The right mainstem bronchus splits off the carina at less of an angle than the left mainstem bronchus. Because of the angle of the right mainstem bronchus, objects that pass all the way down the trachea (such as aspirated food) tend to lodge in the right rather than the left mainstem bronchus. The mainstem bronchi subsequently divide into smaller air passages until reaching the level of the **alveoli** where the exchange of oxygen and carbon dioxide takes place.

When trying to study and memorize the anatomy of the airway, remember that the majority of the time you are managing a critical airway problem the patient will be supine, or lying flat. For this reason it is important to visualize the anatomy in both the traditional upright "anatomical position" (Figure 35-1) and in the supine position (Figure 35-2).

Physiology

The most important aspect of respiratory physiology for the EMT-B who uses advanced airways is an understanding of what can cause the respiratory system to fail so severely that an advanced airway is necessary. When the respiratory system functions properly, adequate breathing is the result of many factors including the following:

- Functioning brainstem where the brain's centers of respiratory control are located

TOPIC OVERVIEW

In this chapter, you will learn about the following topics:

- The purpose and procedure for gastric tubes

- The purpose and procedure for orotracheal intubation

- How to perform Sellick's maneuver

✔ **Knowledge and Attitude**

1. Identify and describe the airway anatomy in the infant, child, and adult. (pp. 765–769)

2. Differentiate between the airway anatomy in the infant, child, and adult. (pp. 765–769)

3. Explain the pathophysiology of airway compromise. (pp. 765–769)

4. Describe the proper use of airway adjuncts. (p. 769)

5. Review the use of oxygen therapy in airway management. (p. 769)

6. Describe the indications, contraindications, and technique for insertion of nasal gastric tubes. (pp. 782–783) (Scan 35-2, p. 784)

7. Describe how to perform Sellick's maneuver (cricoid pressure). (pp. 777–778)

8. Describe the indications for advanced airway management. (pp. 765–769, 773)

9. List the equipment required for orotracheal intubation. (pp. 770–773)

10. Describe the proper use of the curved blade for orotracheal intubation. (p. 771)

11. Describe the proper use of the straight blade for orotracheal intubation. (pp. 772–773) (Scan 35-1, pp. 774–776)

12. State the reasons for and proper use of the stylet in orotracheal intubation. (pp. 772–773)

13. Describe the methods of choosing the appropriate size endotracheal tube in an adult patient. (pp. 771–772)

14. State the formula for sizing an infant or child endotracheal tube. (pp. 780–781)

15. List complications associated with advanced airway management. (pp. 769–770)

16. Define the various alternative methods for sizing the infant and child endotracheal tube. (p. 786)

17. Describe the skill of orotracheal intubation in the adult patient. (pp. 773, 777–780)

18. Describe the skill of orotracheal intubation in the infant and child patient. (pp. 780–783)

19. Describe the skill of confirming endotracheal tube placement in the adult, infant, and child patient. (pp. 778–779, 782)

- Open airway
- Intact chest wall
- Ability of gas exchange to take place at the alveoli

Injuries or illnesses that affect any of these components can result in inadequate breathing and respiratory failure. For example, a massive head injury could result in both brainstem injury and an airway obstructed by blood and broken teeth. Similarly, a patient with massive pulmonary edema from congestive heart failure can go into respiratory failure because edema prevents adequate gas exchange at the level of the alveoli.

Assessing the adequacy of a patient's breathing is an essential skill when making decisions about what basic and advanced airway management is indicated.

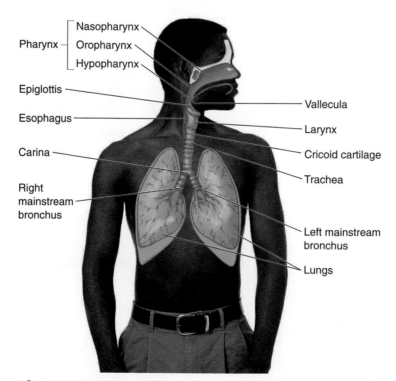

Figure 35-1   The airway.

20. State the consequence of and the need to recognize unintentional esophageal intubation. (pp. 769–770, 778–779, 782)

21. Describe the skill of securing the endotracheal tube in the adult, infant, and child patient. (pp. 779, 782)

22. Recognize and respect the feelings of the patient and family during advanced airway procedures. (p. 776)

23. Explain the value of performing advanced airway procedures. (pp. 765–766)

24. Defend the need for the EMT-Basic to perform advanced airway procedures. (pp. 765–766)

25. Explain the rationale for the use of a stylet. (pp. 772–773)

26. Explain the rationale for having a suction unit immediately available during intubation attempts. (pp. 783, 786) (Scan 35-3, p. 785)

27. Explain the rationale for confirming breath sounds. (pp. 778–780)

28. Explain the rationale for securing the endotracheal tube. (pp. 778–780)

✔ Skills

1. Demonstrate how to perform Sellick's maneuver (cricoid pressure).

2. Demonstrate the skill of orotracheal intubation in the adult patient.

3. Demonstrate the skill of orotracheal intubation in the infant and child patient.

4. Demonstrate the skill of confirming endotracheal tube placement in the adult patient.

5. Demonstrate the skill of confirming endotracheal tube placement in the infant and child patient.

6. Demonstrate the skill of securing the endotracheal tube in the adult patient.

7. Demonstrate the skill of securing the endotracheal tube in the infant and child patient.

A patient's respiratory status can range anywhere from normal, unlabored breathing to complete cessation of breathing or respiratory arrest. Recognition of adequate breathing or respiratory arrest is rarely a diagnostic challenge for the EMT-B. It is recognizing the more subtle signs and symptoms of inadequate breathing that is an essential skill for the EMT-B.

In general, when assessing the adequacy of breathing you should carefully observe the rate, rhythm, quality, and depth of the patient's respirations. The normal rate of breathing is dependent on the age of the patient (Table 35-1). An adequately breathing patient will normally be breathing in a regular rather than an irregular rhythm.

The quality of a patient's breathing should be assessed by listening for breath sounds and observing chest expansion and effort of breathing. The adequately breathing patient will have breath sounds that are equal and present bilaterally. In addition, when observing the patient's chest during normal breathing you will note equal and full expansion of the chest and a lack of any accessory muscle use in the chest or neck during inspiration.

Finally, the depth of breathing (tidal volume) will normally be sufficient not only to expand the lungs, but also to assure adequate delivery of oxygen and removal of carbon dioxide at the level of the alveoli.

When a patient is in respiratory distress because of inadequate breathing the following variations in rate, rhythm, quality, and depth will be noted:

- Rate—outside the normal range: either too fast or too slow
- Rhythm—irregular pattern of breathing

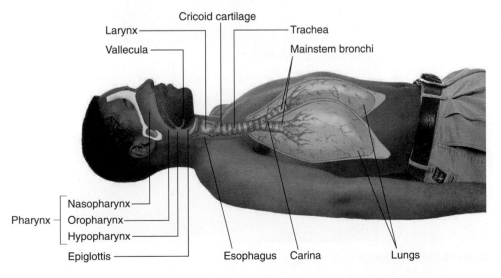

Larynx — Vallecula — Cricoid cartilage — Trachea — Mainstem bronchi

Pharynx — Nasopharynx — Oropharynx — Hypopharynx — Epiglottis — Esophagus — Carina — Lungs

Figure 35-2 The airway, supine position.

Table 35-1	Normal Rates of Breathing
Adult	12–20 breaths per minute
Child	15–30 breaths per minute
Infant	25–50 breaths per minute

- Quality—
  - Breath sounds: diminished, unequal, or absent
  - Chest expansion: unequal or inadequate
  - Effort of breathing: increased effort, use of accessory muscles, and inability to speak in full sentences
- Depth—shallow

In addition, you may also note the following signs and symptoms in the patient with inadequate breathing:

- Cyanosis in the lips, nailbeds, and finger-tips
- Cool and clammy skin
- Agonal breathing (gasping breaths just prior to respiratory arrest)

Pediatric Airway

The pediatric airway is not simply a miniature version of an adult airway. The anatomy and physiology of infants' and children's respiratory systems differ in important respects from those of adults (Figure 35-3).

Not surprisingly, these younger patients may also have different signs and symptoms of respiratory failure than adults.

Features that are unique to the anatomy and physiology of the infant and child versus the adult include the following:

- All structures in the mouth and nose are smaller in the child and can be more easily obstructed.
- Tongue is proportionately larger, occupying more of the mouth and pharynx.
- Trachea is softer and more flexible, allowing the airway to be closed off if the neck is too far extended when opening the airway.
- Trachea is narrower, allowing the airway to become more easily obstructed if swelling occurs.
- Narrowest area in the airway is at the level of the cricoid cartilage.
- Because the chest wall is softer, the diaphragm is relied on heavily for the work of breathing.

Although infants and children may manifest inadequate breathing with the signs and symptoms mentioned above for adults, they also frequently show respiratory distress in other ways, including:

- Slower than normal heart rate
- Weak or absent peripheral pulses
- Retractions between and below the ribs, above the clavicles, and at the sternal notch
- Nasal flaring, in which the nostrils "flare" open with exhalation and clamp almost shut with inhalation

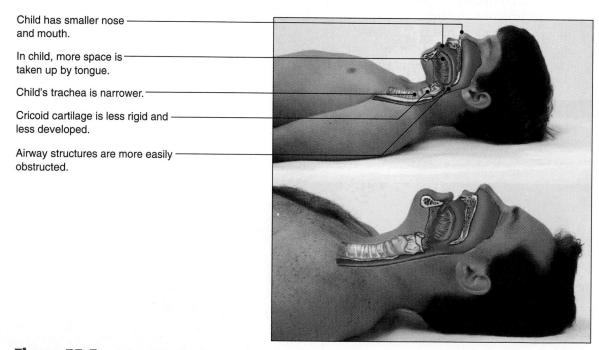

Child has smaller nose and mouth.

In child, more space is taken up by tongue.

Child's trachea is narrower.

Cricoid cartilage is less rigid and less developed.

Airway structures are more easily obstructed.

Figure 35-3 Comparison of child and adult respiratory passages.

- So-called "seesaw" breathing, in which the chest and abdomen move in opposite directions during breathing

Recognition of respiratory distress and inadequate breathing is especially critical in infants and children, since respiratory failure is the leading cause of cardiac arrest in this age group.

MANAGEMENT OF THE AIRWAY

Although this chapter is about advanced airway management, it cannot be over-emphasized that the primary management of any airway is with basic airway techniques such as opening and suctioning the airway, administration of supplemental oxygen, and using oro- and nasopharyngeal airways. You should review these skills (as taught in Chapter 6) prior to learning the techniques of advanced airway management.

Oropharyngeal Suctioning

The goal of airway management is keeping the airway open and free of obstructions. If the airway is obstructed with secretions, blood, or foreign materials, the airway will have to be suctioned. Suction equipment should always be within easy reach when managing any critically ill patient. If the patient is being managed outside the ambulance, either an electrical or hand-operated suction device should be brought to the patient's side. If the patient is in the ambulance, the on-board suction system should be set up and ready for immediate use. Nothing is more embarrassing for the EMT-B, or harmful for the patient, than fumbling around to get a suction unit working when the airway is filled with vomit or blood.

You will learn that a working rigid-tip suction catheter is an essential piece of equipment. In Chapter 6, "Airway Management," you learned the technique for oropharyngeal suctioning—suctioning the mouth and pharynx—with a rigid-tip catheter. This must be done before performing orotracheal intubation.

Orotracheal Intubation

An **endotracheal tube** is a tube designed to be inserted into the trachea (*endo* meaning "into," *tracheal* referring to the trachea). Oxygen, medication, or a suction catheter can be directed into the trachea through the endotracheal tube. **Intubation** means the insertion of a tube. **Orotracheal intubation** is the placement of an endotracheal tube orally, that is, by way of the mouth (*oro* means "mouth"), then through the vocal cords and into the trachea.

Orotracheal intubation allows direct ventilation of the lungs through the endotracheal tube, bypassing the entire upper airway. The endotracheal tube is placed through the vocal cords with direct visualization of the process (that is, seeing what you are doing). A **laryngoscope** is an illuminating instrument that is inserted into the pharynx and allows you to visualize the pharynx and larynx.

The advantages of orotracheal intubation of the apneic (nonbreathing) patient include:

- Complete control of the airway (the tube going directly into the trachea prevents the tongue, blood, or debris that may be present in the upper airway from interfering with the passage of air into the trachea and lungs)
- Minimizes the risk of aspiration (the tube blocks vomitus or foreign matter from being aspirated, or breathed into the lungs)
- Allows for better oxygen delivery (oxygen is fed directly to the lungs via the trachea)
- Allows for deeper suctioning of the airway (a flexible suction catheter can be passed through the endotracheal tube to suction the trachea to the level of the carina)

Complications

Although orotracheal intubation is frequently a life-saving procedure, it has many potential complications. Orotracheal intubation is considered an "invasive" technique because it requires placement of equipment inside the body cavity. Whenever you perform an invasive procedure, you must be aware of the potential complications and be prepared to recognize and treat them should they arise. These concerns about invasive procedures are never more critical than in orotracheal intubation, since improper placement of the endotracheal tube in the apneic patient can rapidly result in the patient's death if it is not immediately detected and corrected.

Specific complications of orotracheal intubation include:

- *Slowing of the heart rate.* Stimulation of the airway with the laryngoscope and the endotracheal tube can lead to a slowing of the heart. The patient's heart rate should be monitored throughout the intubation.
- *Soft-tissue trauma* to the teeth, lips, tongue, gums, and airway structures.
- *Hypoxia.* Prolonged attempts at intubation may lead to inadequate oxygenation, or oxygen starvation, known as hypoxia. To prevent this, you should hyperventilate the patient with high-concentration oxygen (ventilations provided at about double the normal rate, or 24 ventilations per minute) prior to

intubation. Any attempts to insert the endotracheal tube (during which ventilations cannot be provided) should be limited to no more than 30 seconds.

- *Vomiting.* Stimulation of the airway may cause the patient to gag and vomit.

- *Right main-stem intubation.* The endotracheal tube has to remain superior to the carina (before the point where the right and left mainstem bronchi branch off) in order to send air into both lungs. If the tube is advanced too far, the tube is likely to go down the steep right mainstem bronchus. Mainstem intubation results in only one lung being ventilated and the development of hypoxia.

- *Esophageal intubation.* This is the most serious complication. The unrecognized placement of the tube in the esophagus rather than the trachea prevents any ventilation of the lungs and will rapidly result in death.

- *Accidental extubation.* Even if the endotracheal tube is properly placed initially, the tube can become dislodged while moving the patient, or by the patient himself if he regains consciousness. Reassess chest wall movement and breath sounds after every major move with the intubated patient, such as down the stairs or from the floor to the stretcher.

Equipment

Orotracheal intubation requires specialized equipment.

BSI Precautions. Because of the high risk of splattering of sputum or blood during intubation, it is essential that body substance isolation precautions be taken. This means that a mask and goggles or other protective eyewear be worn in addition to gloves. This is mandatory since your face will be in direct line with the path of secretions, blood, and vomit coming from the mouth while you attempt to visualize the airway.

Laryngoscope. A **laryngoscope** is made up of two components: the handle that contains the batteries, and the blade that is inserted in the airway and illuminates the airway. In most laryngoscopes, the handle and the blades are two separate pieces that need to be assembled with each use. In these devices, the blade is placed parallel to the handle and the notch at the base of the blade is attached to the bar on the handle.

The blade is then lifted to a 90 degree angle with the handle and, as the blade locks into place, the light at the tip of the blade illuminates (Figure 35-4). Always check the light at the end of the blade to assure that it illuminates with a bright white color and

Align indentation with bar, press forward to lock   Press to lock

A

Elevate blade to a right angle

B

Figure 35-4 (A) Affix the laryngoscope blade and (B) then elevate it.

that the bulb is tightly secured to the blade. It should be noted that some disposable laryngoscopes are preassembled with the handle and blade as a single fixed unit.

No matter what type of laryngoscope you use, it is essential that you conduct a daily check of the device to assure that it is working properly. Spare batteries and bulbs should always be stored with the laryngoscope.

Laryngoscope blades are specifically designed to fit into the anatomy of the airway, providing optimal illumination of the vocal cords to enable you to pass

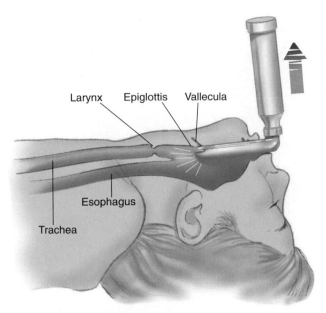

Figure 35-5 The straight blade lifts the epiglottis.

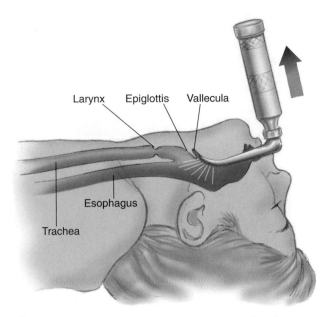

Figure 35-6 The curved blade lifts the vallecula.

the endotracheal tube between them. Most commercially available blades are designed with the light on the right side of the blade. This requires that the handle of the scope be held in the left hand to provide optimal illumination of the airway.

There are two general types of blades, straight and curved. Both types of blades come in assorted sizes ranging from the smallest size, 0, to the largest size, 4. The size of the blade used depends on the size of the patient. Most adult patients can be intubated using a size 2 or 3 straight blade or a size 3 curved blade. (Pediatric blade sizes will be discussed later in this chapter.) The decision as to whether to use a straight or curved blade depends on individual preference; however, straight blades are preferred for pediatric orotracheal intubations.

Each blade type is designed to enable you to visualize the cords by taking advantage of different anatomical mechanisms. The straight blade is designed so that the tip of the blade is placed under the epiglottis to lift the epiglottis upward and bring the **glottic opening** (the opening to the trachea) and the vocal cords into view (Figure 35-5). The curved blade is designed so that the tip of the blade is inserted into the vallecula so that lifting the laryngoscope handle upward brings the glottic opening and the vocal cords into view (Figure 35-6).

Endotracheal Tube. The **endotracheal tube** (Figure 35-7) consists of a single lumen tube through which air and supplemental oxygen are delivered. At the proximal end of the tube (the end that will remain outside the patient) is a standard 15 millimeter adapter for connection to the bag valve.

At the distal end of the tube (the end that will go into the patient) is a cuff. It is designed to be inflated after the tube is placed to prevent leakage of air and fluid around the tip of the tube. Usually 8 to 10 cc of air will obtain an adequate seal.

The cuff is filled with a 10 cc syringe at the inflation valve. Just below the inflation valve is the pilot balloon, which fills when the cuff is inflated. Since the cuff is inside the trachea, you will not be able to see if it is inflated, but the inflation of the pilot balloon will verify that there is air in the cuff. If the pilot balloon does not hold air, then you must assume that the cuff at the end of the tube has also failed.

Endotracheal tubes used on infants and children less than 8 years old do not have a cuff (see Orotracheal Intubation of an Infant or Child later in this chapter). Many endotracheal tubes have a small hole on the left side of the tube opposite the bevel, known as a Murphy eye. This feature is designed to lessen the chances of tube obstruction.

Endotracheal tubes come in various diameters, from 2.0 millimeters (used on premature infants) to 10.0 millimeters (used on very large adults). The diameter measured is the distance from one side of the internal wall of the tube to the other, called the internal diameter or "i.d." No matter what the internal diameter of the tube, the standard 15 millimeter adapter is affixed to the end of the tube.

When determining the proper size of the endotracheal tube for the adult patient, the rule of thumb is: In an emergency, use a 7.5 mm tube. For more precise sizing of the endotracheal tube, it is generally accepted that the adult male should receive either an 8.0 or an 8.5 mm tube and the adult female should receive from

Open end (top)

15mm adaptor

Inflation valve

Pilot balloon

10cc syringe

Open end
(bottom)

Cuff

Murphy Eye

A

B

Figure 35-7 (A) The endotracheal tube and (B) endotracheal tube with stylet in place.

a 7.0 to an 8.0 mm tube. The sizing of pediatric endotracheal tubes will be discussed later in this chapter.

The adult endotracheal tube has a standard length of 33 centimeters. The side of the tube is marked in centimeters starting from the tip of the tube. The most important number to remember is that, as a general rule, a properly placed endotracheal tube will have the 22 centimeter mark at the teeth of an adult. This position assures that the tip of the tube is in the trachea above the carina. (As you will learn, assuring proper placement of the tube is a critical skill, and checking the length marking is only a small part of this procedure.) It may be helpful to envision the depth of tube by reviewing the following distances in the average adult:

- 15 centimeters from the teeth to the vocal cords
- 20 centimeters from the teeth to the suprasternal notch
- 25 centimeters from the teeth to the carina

As you can see, there is very little room for error when placing the endotracheal tube, since only a few centimeters can mean the difference between proper placement and the tube being past the carina into the right main stem bronchus.

Accessories to the Endotracheal Tube. There are several accessories to the endotracheal tube with which you need to be familiar. These include the stylet, lubricant, a 10 cc syringe, devices for securing

the tube once it is placed, devices for assuring the proper placement of the tube, and a suction device.

Because the endotracheal tube is made of relatively flexible plastic, it is generally recommended that a **stylet** (Figure 35-8)—a long, thin, bendable metal probe—be inserted into the tube prior to intubation to help stiffen the tube and provide it with a shape that will ease its insertion through the vocal cords. It is recommended that the stylet be lubricated with water-soluble lubricant, such as K-Y® jelly, Lubrifax®, or Surgilube®, prior to insertion into the endotracheal tube to allow for a smooth withdrawal of the stylet once the tube is successfully placed. (A silicone-based lubricant or a petroleum-based lubricant such as Vaseline® must not be used.)

Once the lubricated stylet is inserted, the endotracheal tube should be shaped into a "hockey stick" configuration. To avoid trauma to the airway it is essential that the stylet should not be inserted past the tip of the tube. Since the stylet is longer than the endotracheal tube, it is easy to inadvertently allow the tip to extend beyond the end of the tube. Such an error, however, could cause a puncture of the trachea. To avoid this complication, the tip of the stylet should not be inserted beyond the proximal end of the Murphy eye and the excess length should be bent over the 15 mm adapter.

When performing orotracheal intubation, it is often a problem that excessive oral secretions obstruct an adequate view of the vocal cords. Paradoxically, airways are sometimes very dry, thus making

A

B

Figure 35-8 (A) Stylet and (B) stylet in place.

insertion of the tube difficult because of friction between the end of the tube and the patient's pharynx and glottis. For these reasons, it is important both that a wide bore suction device be operational and within easy reach during intubation attempts, and that water soluble lubricant be applied to the outside of the distal portion of the tube. The suction device should be turned on and placed by your right hand (since your left hand will be holding the laryngoscope). In general, you can use half a packet of lubricant on the stylet and the other half of the packet on the outside of the tube.

Another piece of essential equipment for use with the endotracheal tube is a 10 cc syringe. As mentioned above, the syringe is used to inflate the cuff through the inflation valve. The syringe should also be used to test that the cuff is intact and holds air prior to inserting the tube. Once the integrity of the cuff has been assured, the air should be withdrawn, but the syringe should remain attached to the tube so that it is easily found when it is time to reinflate the cuff after the patient is intubated. It should be noted that, following final inflation of the cuff, the 10 cc syringe should be detached from the inflation valve to prevent any subsequent leakage of air out of the cuff and back into the syringe.

One of the final steps in orotracheal intubation is securing the tube to the patient so that it does not move or become dislodged. This is especially important in the prehospital setting where the tube can easily be dislodged during patient movement. Prior to securing the endotracheal tube, an oral airway or similar device should be inserted as a bite block in case the patient becomes responsive and gnaws at the tube. There are a number of methods for securing endotracheal tubes. These range from cloth tape to commercially available devices. The manner in which tubes are secured is usually dictated by the medical direction of the EMS system you work in. Whatever system you use to secure the tube, make sure the tube is firmly secured in place and able to withstand the tugs and pulls that are routine during moves of critically ill patients.

Indications

When properly performed, orotracheal intubation is clearly a life-saving technique. It is essential, however, that you know under what conditions a patient needs to be intubated. The following is a list of indications:

• Inability to ventilate the apneic patient
• To protect the airway of a patient without a gag reflex or cough
• To protect the airway of a patient unresponsive to any painful stimuli
• Cardiac arrest

Technique of Insertion—Adult Patient

Orotracheal intubation is the most complicated and difficult procedure the EMT-B is expected to perform. Properly performed, it is truly a life-saving procedure. Incorrectly performed, the EMT-B's actions can easily result in the patient's death. Because many EMT-Bs will only rarely perform orotracheal intubation, it is essential that you not only learn and practice the technique extensively during your training but also practice the technique on a regular basis once you are a certified EMT-B.

The following is a step-by-step guide to orotracheal intubation of the adult patient (Scan 35-1):

Preparation

1. Assure body substance isolation precautions. This should include gloves, goggles or other protective eye wear, and a mask.

2. Assure that adequate ventilation with a bag-valve mask and high-concentration oxygen is being performed.

OROTRACHEAL INTUBATION—ADULT PATIENT

▲ **1.** Hyperventilate the patient.

▲ **2.** Assemble, prepare, and test all equipment.

▲ **3.** Position the patient's head.

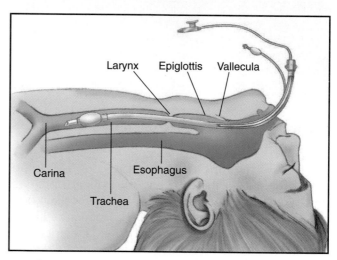

Larynx   Epiglottis   Vallecula

Carina

Esophagus

Trachea

▲ **4.** Make sure the airway is aligned. (If trauma is suspected, keep patient's head and neck in a neutral position. Endotracheal tube shown already in place.)

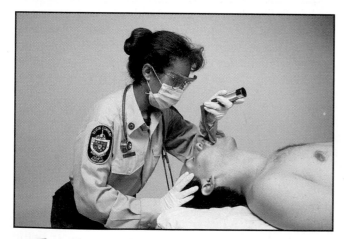

▲ **5.** Prepare to insert laryngoscope blade.

▲ **6.** Lift the tongue out of the way.

▲ **7.** Insert the blade (curved blade into vallecula; straight blade under epiglottis) and lift to bring glottic opening into view.

▲ **8.** A second rescuer may perform Sellick's maneuver (cricoid pressure) during intubation to suppress vomiting and aid visualization.

▲ **9.** Visualize the glottic opening.

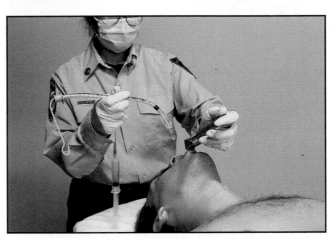

▲ **10.** Insert endotracheal tube with stylet.

▲ **11.** Remove laryngoscope and stylet. Inflate the cuff with 5–10 cc of air.

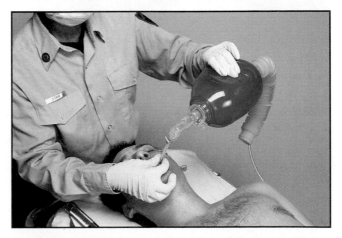

▲ **12.** Attach a bag-valve unit or other ventilation device to tube.

(continued)

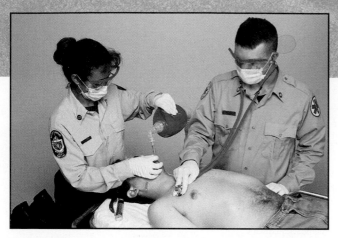

▲ **13.** Auscultate lung and epigastrium areas to confirm correct placement.

Confirm correct placement of tube:

*   If local protocol permits, use esophageal intubation detector device (EIDD) before ventilating the patient.

*   Ventilate.

*   Observe rise and fall of chest.

*   Auscultate epigastrium for absence of breath sounds.

*   Auscultate over both lungs for breath sounds. The sounds should be equal when comparing the left and right sides.

*   Observe the patient for signs of deterioration, e.g., cyanosis.

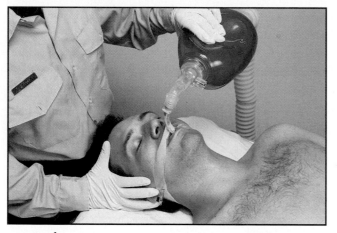

▲ **14.** If correct placement is confirmed, secure the tube in place.

Correct any incorrect placement of tube:

*   If air cannot be drawn into EIDD bulb or syringe and/or breath sounds are present in epigastrium—the esophagus has been intubated. Deflate cuff and withdraw tube. Hyperventilate 2–5 minutes.

*   If breath sounds are present on right, diminished or absent on left—the right mainstem bronchus has probably been intubated. Deflate cuff and gently withdraw tube (continue ventilation) until breath sounds are equal right and left.

Note: Make only two attempts at intubation. If both attempts fail, insert an oral airway and continue to ventilate with pocket mask or bag-valve mask. Aggressively suction the airway. If tube has been correctly placed and secured, reassess breath sounds and placement after every major move with patient. Offer reassurance and emotional support to the patient and family.

3. Hyperventilate the patient at a rate of 24 breaths per minute prior to any intubation attempts.

4. Assemble, prepare, and test all equipment including

- A suction unit with a large bore rigid tip—It should be functional and positioned so that it is within easy reach of the intubator's right hand should it be needed.
- The cuff on the endotracheal tube—It should be tested and then deflated, with the 10 cc syringe left attached to the inflation valve.
- The laryngoscope—Assemble and assure that the light is bright and constant.
- The stylet—Insert the stylet into the tube and form the tube into a hockey-stick shape.
- The device that will be used to secure the tube after successful intubation

5. Position yourself at the patient's head so that, during intubation, left and right are your left and right as well as the patient's left and right.

Visualizing the Glottic Opening and Vocal Cords

6. Position the patient's head to assure good visualization of the vocal cords. Remove the oral airway.

7. Hold the laryngoscope in your left hand and insert the laryngoscope into the right corner of the patient's mouth.

8. Use a sweeping motion to lift the tongue upward and to the left, out of the way, to enable visualization of the glottis.

9. Insert the blade into the proper anatomical location.

- Curved blade fits into the vallecula.
- Straight blade lifts the epiglottis.

10. Lift the scope up and away from the patient.

- If trauma is not suspected, tilt the head, lift the chin, and attempt visualization of the cords. If the cords cannot be seen, raise the patient's shoulders approximately one inch by placing a towel beneath them and attempt visualization again.
- If trauma is suspected, the patient will have to be intubated with the head and neck in a neutral position with a second rescuer maintaining in-line stabilization of the neck and head.

11. Avoid using the teeth as a fulcrum.

12. Application of cricoid pressure **(Sellick's maneuver)** during intubation attempts may be beneficial. Sellick's maneuver is performed by a second rescuer who uses his index finger and thumb to exert direct pressure on the patient's cricoid cartilage (Figures 35-9 and 35-10). Since the cricoid cartilage is the only cartilage in the neck that completely encircles the trachea, direct pressure helps to compress the esophagus, which is posterior to the trachea, reducing the risk of vomiting. In addition, the pressure often brings the vocal cords into better view. Cricoid pressure should be maintained until the patient is intubated.

13. Visualize the glottic opening and vocal cords. Once the cords come into view do not lose sight of them!

Inserting the Endotracheal Tube

14. With the right hand, carefully insert the endotracheal tube through the vocal cords. The tube should be inserted just deep enough so that the cuff is past the cords. Verify that the endotracheal tube is at about 22 cm at the gums and teeth.

15. Remove the laryngoscope and extinguish the lamp.

16. Remove the stylet, if used.

17. Inflate the cuff with 5 to 10 cc of air and remove the syringe.

18. Continue to hold onto the endotracheal tube. Never let go of the endotracheal tube until it is secured in place.

19. Have a partner attach the bag valve to the endotracheal tube and deliver artificial ventilations.

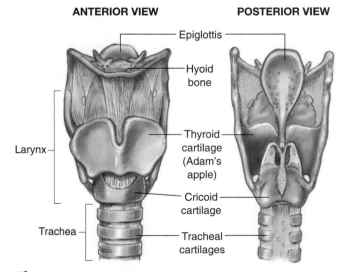

Figure 35-9 The tracheal cartilages are C-shaped, open at the posterior side next to the esophagus. The cricoid cartilage at the lower end of the larynx is the only cartilage that completely encircles the trachea.

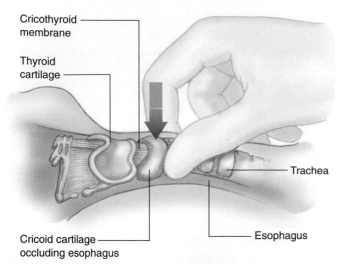

Cricothyroid membrane

Thyroid cartilage

Trachea

Cricoid cartilage occluding esophagus

Esophagus

A

B

Figure 35-10 In the Sellick's maneuver, pressure is placed on the crocoid cartilage, pushing it posteriorly against the esophagus. By closing off the esophagus, vomiting is suppressed. The maneuver also helps bring the vocal cords into view.

Assuring Correct Tube Placement

20. The single most accurate way of assuring proper tube placement in the trachea (Figure 35-11) is visualizing the endotracheal tube as it passes through the vocal cords. All the following methods are for verification of tube placement:

– Observe the patient's chest rise and fall with each ventilation.

– Auscultate for the presence of breath sounds. Begin over the epigastrium. Breath sounds heard here during ventilations indicate air entering the stomach rather than the lungs. Then listen over the left apex (top of the left lung area). Compare the breath sounds with those at the right apex. Breath sounds should be heard equally on both sides. Finally, listen over the left base (bottom of the

lung area). Compare the breath sounds with those at the right base. Breath sounds should be heard equally on both sides.

– Observe the patient for signs of deterioration after tube placement, for example becoming combative or developing cyanosis. Both are signs of hypoxia and probable incorrect tube placement.

– If allowed by local protocol, use other objective measures such as pulse oximetry or end tidal carbon dioxide detectors, to confirm correct placement.

Detecting and Correcting Incorrect Tube Placements

21. An incorrect tube placement must be detected and corrected without delay.

– If breath sounds are diminished or absent on the left but present on the right, it is likely the tube has advanced beyond the carina and intubated the right mainstem bronchus. If this occurs, deflate the cuff and gently withdraw the tube while artificially ventilating and while auscultating over the left apex of the chest. Take care not to completely remove the endotracheal tube. When the breath sounds become equal at both the left and right apex, reinflate the cuff and follow the directions in Step 22 for securing the tube.

– If breath sounds are only present in the epigastrium, the esophagus has been intubated

(A) RIGHT

(B) WRONG

Figure 35-11 (A) The endotracheal tube is correctly placed in the trachea. (B) The endotracheal tube is incorrectly placed in the esophagus—a life-threatening error.

and air is being sent into the stomach instead of the lungs (Figure 35-11). Since esophageal intubation is a fatal occurrence, immediately deflate the cuff and withdraw the tube. Hyperventilate for at least 2 to 5 minutes prior to your second attempt to intubate.

Note: If permitted by local protocol, an esophageal intubation detector device (EIDD) may be used to detect incorrect placement (or to verify correct placement). The EIDD is a disposable bulb or syringe (Figure 35-12). After the endotracheal tube has been placed and before any ventilation attempts, attach the EIDD to the endotracheal tube and squeeze the syringe. If the tube is in the esophagus, its soft, unsupported walls will collapse around the end of the tube. This will prevent air from being drawn into the EIDD. If it is a bulb device, the bulb will remain collapsed and will not refill; if it is a syringe device, you will not be able to draw the plunger out of the syringe reservoir. By contrast, if the tube is in the trachea, the rigid trachea remains patent, allowing an EIDD bulb to refill or the plunger of an EIDD syringe to be easily withdrawn from the syringe reservoir.

Warning

The EMT-B should make only two attempts at orotracheal intubation. If both attempts fail, insert an oral airway, continue to ventilate the patient with high-concentration oxygen via bag-valve mask, and aggressively suction the airway.

Securing the Tube

22. If breath sounds are heard bilaterally and no sounds are heard over the epigastrium, the endotracheal tube should be secured in place using tape or whatever system that is approved by your medical director. An oral airway may be inserted as a bite block to protect the tube. Note the depth of the tube at the teeth both before and after securing it to assure that the tube has not been dislodged during the procedure.

Ongoing Assessment

23. Be sure to assess and reassess the breath sounds following every major move with the patient.

Warning

Although the complications of orotracheal intubation have already been discussed, it cannot be over-emphasized that inadvertent esophageal intubation will likely result in the patient's death. Because of the magnitude of this complication, if at any time—despite your efforts to properly assess

A

B

C

Figure 35-12 (A) Esophageal intubation detector device, bulb style. (B) An esophageal intubation detector device—syringe style. (C) An esophageal detector device—capnography.

tube placement—you are in doubt of proper tube placement, immediately withdraw the tube and manage the airway with basic airway adjuncts.

Orotracheal Intubation of an Infant or Child

Although the goal of orotracheal intubation is identical in both adult and pediatric patients, intubation of the infant and child requires special training because of various considerations of anatomy, physiology, and size. The specific anatomy and physiology of the pediatric airway has been discussed earlier. The importance of these factors as they relate to orotracheal intubation are as follows:

- In an infant or child, it is often difficult to create a single clear visual plane from the mouth through the pharynx and into the glottis for orotracheal intubation because of such factors as the relatively large size of the tongue.
- Because of size differences among infants and children as well as the fact that the narrowest portion of the airway is at the level of the cricoid ring, the proper sizing of the endotracheal tube is crucial.
- Because infants and children tend to develop hypoxia and bradycardia (slowed heartbeat) easily during intubation attempts, pediatric intubations require careful monitoring coupled with swift and accurate technique.

The indications for orotracheal intubation of the infant and child are similar to those for the adult patient as follows:

- When prolonged artificial ventilation is required
- When adequate artificial ventilation cannot be achieved by other means
- To ventilate the clearly apneic patient
- To ventilate the cardiac arrest patient
- To control the airway of an unresponsive patient without a cough or gag reflex

The laryngoscope blades and the endotracheal tubes necessary for the orotracheal intubation of infants and children must be carefully sized to the patient. In general the straight blade, usually a size 1, is preferred in infants and small children because it provides for greater displacement of the tongue and better visualization of the glottis. As in adults, the blade lifts the epiglottis, bringing the vocal cords into view. In older children the curved blade is often preferred because the blade's broad base displaces the tongue better, allowing better visualization of the vocal cords once the blade is placed into the vallecula and lifted.

Assorted sizes of endotracheal tubes should always be stocked in the pediatric airway kit. As previously mentioned, the proper sizing of the tube is essential in children. Ideally a chart should be placed in the airway kit to assist the EMT-B in determining what size tube is generally used for a specific age patient. As an alternative a Broselow™ tape can be used to estimate tube size based on the height of the patient (Figure 35-13).

Figure 35-13 A Broselow™ tape can be used to estimate the tube size based on the height of a pediatric patient.

A formula—(patient's age in years + 16) ÷ 4 = tube size—can also be used to estimate the proper size. Finally, using the diameter of the patient's little finger or the diameter of the nasal opening are alternative techniques for estimating correct tube size.

Because infants are often the pediatric patients who require orotracheal intubation, it is helpful to simply memorize that newborns and small infants generally require a 3.0 to a 3.5 tube, and a 4.0 tube can be used for older infants up to the age of 1 year. No matter what system you use in determining tube size, it is always prudent to have one half-size larger tube and one half-size smaller tube on stand-by, since the size of the glottic structure does vary in infants and children.

Endotracheal tubes come in both cuffed and uncuffed versions. Cuffed tubes are always used in adult patients. In the pediatric population, cuffed tubes are reserved for children 8 years of age and older. For younger children and infants, uncuffed tubes are used since the narrowing at the level of the cricoid cartilage serves as a functional cuff, snugging the tube in the airway. Uncuffed tubes (Figure 35-14) should display a vocal cord marker to assure proper placement of the tube. This marker is designed so that the vocal cords are at the level of the translucent marker in the tube. If the child is old enough to get a cuffed tube it should be inserted, like the adult tube, just deep enough that the cuff material is inferior to the cords.

Proper depth of tube placement can also be approximated by age (Table 35-2). However, direct visualization of the tube being placed at the proper depth is the best measure of tube depth.

The step-by-step procedure for orotracheal intubation of infants and children is very similar to the procedure outlined for adults (earlier and Scan 35-1).

Table 35-2 Infant/Child Endotracheal Tubes

Measurement of Endotracheal Tube at the Teeth

6 months to 1 year	12 cm teeth to mid-trachea
2 years	14 cm teeth to mid-trachea
4–6 years	16 cm teeth to mid-trachea
6–10 years	18 cm teeth to mid-trachea
10–12 years	20 cm teeth to mid-trachea

There are, however, some important differences that you must keep in mind when performing a pediatric intubation:

1. The rate of hyperventilation both before and after intubation must be adjusted to the patient's age.

2. The patient's heart rate must be continuously monitored during intubation attempts, since mechanical stimulation of the airway and hypoxia can both slow the heart rate. If the heart rate is noted to slow during intubation, the blade should immediately be withdrawn and the infant or child reventilated with high-concentration oxygen.

3. The optimal manner of positioning the patient's head is to gently tilt the head forward and lift the chin into the "sniffing position" (Figure 35-15).

4. Very little force is needed to intubate the infant or child. Gentle finesse is the rule, not the exception.

Figure 35-14 An uncuffed endotracheal tube is used for patients under eight years of age.

Figure 35-15 Place the pediatric patient's head in the "sniffing" position for intubation.

5. Sellick's maneuver is also often beneficial, but the landmarks may be difficult to locate in the infant and child. In addition, excessive pressure on the relatively soft cartilage may cause tracheal obstruction.

6. When using a straight blade, realize that the epiglottis in infants and children is not as stiff as in adults and may partially obscure a clear view of the vocal cords.

7. Since distances in the infant and child are small, be certain to hold onto the tube until you are assured that it is well secured. As with adults, reassess tube placement every time you move the patient.

8. In infants and children, the best indicator of tube placement is symmetrical rise and fall of the chest during ventilation.

9. Breath sounds in infants and children can often be misleading since the chest is small and sounds are easily transmitted from one area to another.

10. Observe the patient for increase in heart rate and improving color after intubation. An infant or child who becomes dusky in color and slows his heart rate after intubation is likely not to be properly intubated.

11. Once tube placement is confirmed, the patient should be secured to an appropriate device to prevent any head movement from dislodging the tube.

12. If the tube is properly placed but there is inadequate chest expansion, seek out one of the following causes:

- The tube is too small and there is an air leak around the tube at the glottic opening. This is detected by auscultating over the neck. The tube should be replaced by a larger tube.
- The pop-off valve on the bag-valve device has not been deactivated.
- There is a leak in the bag-valve device.
- The ventilator is delivering an inadequate volume of air/oxygen.
- The tube is blocked with secretions. This can be treated initially with endotracheal suctioning (see later in this chapter). If suctioning fails, the tube should be removed.

13. Infants and children are at risk for the same complications of orotracheal intubation as adult patients. Inadvertent esophageal intubation is perhaps even more rapidly fatal in infants and children than adults. In addition, barotrauma from over inflation of the lungs can result in collapse of the lung, which can further compromise your ability to ventilate the patient.

Nasogastric Intubation of an Infant or Child

An additional procedure the EMT-B may have to master in conjunction with orotracheal intubation of an infant or child is the placement of a **nasogastric tube (NG tube).** A nasogastric tube is inserted through the nose into the infant's or child's stomach. The most common use of the NG tube in regard to advanced airway management is that the tube is used to decompress the stomach and proximal bowel of air. In infants and children, air frequently fills the stomach and bowel after overly aggressive artificial ventilation or as a result of air swallowing. The NG tube provides a route for escape of the excess air. The NG tube can also be used to drain the stomach of blood or other substances. In the hospital setting, NG tubes can be used to give medication and provide a route for nutrition as well.

The indications for insertion of the NG tube in pediatric patients are as follows:

- Inability to adequately ventilate the patient because of distention of the stomach
- Unresponsive patient with gastric distention

Many experts believe that the NG tube should only be inserted after the trachea has been secured with an endotracheal tube to prevent incorrectly placing the NG tube into the trachea instead of the esophagus. Other possible complications of NG intubation include trauma to the nose, triggering vomiting, and—in very rare cases—passing the tube into the cranium through a basilar skull fracture. *Because of the risk of cranial intubation with the NG tube, the presence of major facial trauma or head trauma is considered a contraindication to the nasogastric tube.* In such cases, the insertion of the tube through the mouth (orogastric technique) is preferred.

The equipment required for nasogastric tube insertion is listed in Table 35-3. The procedure for insertion of the nasogastric tube as illustrated in Scan 35-2 is:

1. Prepare and assemble all equipment.

2. Assure that the patient is well oxygenated prior to the procedure.

3. Measure the tube from the tip of the nose and around the ear to below the xiphoid process. (If the tube will be inserted by the orogastric technique, measure from the lips.) This length will determine the depth the tube will be inserted (Figure 35-16).

4. Lubricate the end of the tube.

5. Pass the tube gently downward along the nasal floor.

Table 35-3 Nasogastric Intubation Equipment

Equipment for Nasogastric Intubation

Nasogastric tubes of various sizes:

Newborn/infant:	8.0 French
Toddler/preschool:	10.0 French
School age:	12.0 French
Adolescent:	14.0–16.0 French

20 cc syringe

Water-soluble lubricant

Emesis basin

Tape

Stethoscope

Suction unit with connecting tube

(a)

(b)

Figure 35-16 (A) Measure the nasogastric tube from the tip of the nose around the ear, to below the xiphoid process. (B) The nasogastric tube in position, ready to attach to suction.

6. Confirm that the tube is in the stomach by
   – Aspirating stomach contents
   – Auscultating a rush of air over the epigastrium while injecting 10–20 cc of air into the tube
7. Aspirate gastric contents.
8. Secure the tube in place with tape.

Orotracheal Suctioning

In conjunction with your training in advanced airway management, you may also be trained in the techniques of orotracheal suctioning. For this procedure, a flexible soft suction catheter is used to suction the trachea, usually down to the level of the carina in the artificially ventilated patient. This procedure is sometimes referred to as "deep suctioning" to set it apart from the basic airway management procedure, suctioning of the oropharynx, in which suctioning does not advance as far as the trachea.

The indications for orotracheal suctioning are as follows:

• Obvious secretions in the airway—This may be detected by either moist bubbling sounds during ventilation with the bag-valve mask or by visible secretions inside the endotracheal tube after the patient has been intubated.

• Poor compliance with bag-valve-mask ventilation—Resistance to ventilation may be caused by secretions below the level of the larynx in the trachea.

The technique for orotracheal suctioning is shown in Scan 35-3. (Note: Although orotracheal suctioning can be performed on an unintubated patient, the procedure is by far most commonly performed through an endotracheal tube.) Specific steps in the procedure include:

1. Pre-oxygenate the patient with high-concentration oxygen prior to attempting suction.
2. Hyperventilate the patient prior to suctioning.
3. Check that all equipment is operating correctly.
4. Use sterile technique.
5. Observe body substance isolation precautions. Be especially mindful to have eye protection, as splattering during deep suctioning is common.
6. Approximate the desired length of the catheter to be inserted by measuring from the lips to the ear to the nipple line. This will approximate the level of the carina.
7. Advance the catheter to the desired location.
8. Apply suction and withdraw the catheter in a twisting motion.

NASOGASTRIC INTUBATION—INFANT OR CHILD

▲ **1.** Oxygenate the patient.

▲ **2.** Measure tube from tip of nose, over ear, to below xiphoid process.

▲ **3.** Pass lubricated tube gently downward along nasal floor to stomach.

▲ **4.** To confirm correct placement, auscultate over epigastrium. Listen for bubbling while injecting 10–20 cc air into tube.

▲ **5.** Use suction to aspirate stomach contents.

▲ **6.** Secure tube in place.

OROTRACHEAL SUCTIONING

▲ **1.** Hyperventilate the patient.

▲ **2.** Carefully check equipment.

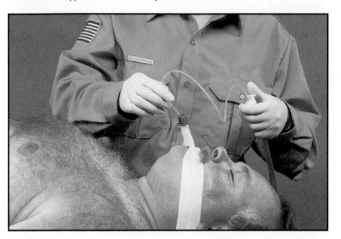

▲ **3.** Insert catheter without applying suction.

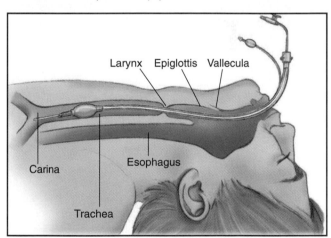

Larynx Epiglottis Vallecula

Carina

Esophagus

Trachea

▲ **4.** Advance catheter to desired level, which may be as far as carina.

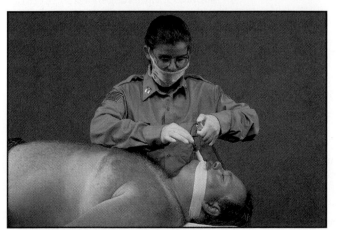

▲ **5.** Then apply suction and withdraw catheter with a twisting motion.

6. Resume ventilation. Suctioning procedure should interrupt ventilation for no more than 15 seconds.

9. Resume ventilations.

10. Attempts at deep suctioning should not exceed 15 seconds to prevent hypoxia.

Deep suctioning is not without potential complications. Most of the serious complications relate to the fact that the ventilated patient is deprived of oxygen during suctioning. Hyperventilation prior to suctioning, careful technique, and limiting suctioning to 15 seconds can help prevent the following complications of deep suctioning:

- Cardiac dysrhythmias
- Hypoxia
- Coughing
- Damage to the lining (mucosa) of the airway
- Spasm of the bronchioles (bronchospasm) if catheter extends past the carina
- Spasm of the vocal cords (laryngospasm) during orotracheal suctioning

ADDITIONAL ADVANCED AIRWAY TECHNIQUES

Esophageal and Multilumen Airways

In some EMS systems medical direction may elect to allow the EMT-B to use esophageal and/or multilumen airways such as the Combitube®. Although these devices do not provide the definitive airway control of an endotracheal tube, when properly used they provide superior ventilation of the apneic patient as compared with a simple oral airway adjunct.

EOA and EGTA

For over 20 years, alternative methods of intubating the patient using the esophageal obturator airway (EOA) (Figure 35-17) and its close cousin the esophageal gastric tube airway (EGTA) have been available. They can be passed "blindly" into the pharynx, eliminating the need to use a laryngoscope to visualize the process as it is happening, and they do not need to be maneuvered between the vocal cords into the trachea, so many of the problems of improper placement are eliminated.

The ease of use and simplicity of both these devices have probably been overemphasized. It is true that they are easier to insert than the endotracheal tube. Nevertheless, they are invasive procedures, and the EMT using either device must be well versed in its complications, indications, and contraindications.

The major feature of the EOA or EGTA is an inflatable cuff that allows the trachea to be open but closes off the esophagus. The device is usually used during CPR or rescue breathing to "seal the meal," or prevent regurgitation (bringing up stomach contents that can be aspirated into the lungs) and prevent gastric distention (blowing air meant for the lungs into the stomach, which in turn tends to cause vomiting or regurgitation).

Both the EOA and the EGTA are usually connected to a bag-valve-mask unit, which blows air or oxygen through the mask port. (As noted above, the EOA or EGTA tube does not go into the trachea, but since the inflatable cuff seals off the esophagus, the only place for the ventilation to go is into the trachea and the lungs.)

Although the EOA or EGTA is less often misplaced than an endotracheal tube, it does sometimes get pushed into the trachea instead of the esophagus. When this happens—if the error is not quickly recognized through listening for lung sounds—it can be fatal.

There are certain contraindications to the use of the EOA or the EGTA. Neither should be used in:

- A patient who is alert, verbally responsive, or who responds to painful stimuli and still has a gag reflex. Vomiting and aspiration are likely.

- A patient who is under the age of 16 or who is less than 5 feet tall. The devices come in only one size and are too long for the anatomy of a small patient.

- A patient who has ingested a corrosive substance. A corrosive could perforate the tip of the device, or may weaken the esophagus so that the device could perforate the esophagus wall.

- A patient with a known esophageal disease such as cancer or esophageal varices, which weaken the wall of the esophagus and increase the chance for a ruptured esophagus.

- A patient with significant upper airway bleeding. Blood flowing from the nose or mouth will pass directly into the lungs once the inflated cuff has closed off the esophagus.

Although the EOA and EGTA have much in common, the differences are important to learn. Both have an air-cushion-inflatable mask and a 16-inch tube with a 30–35 cc inflatable air cuff on the distal end. The EOA has a closed distal end and a series of air holes on the proximal end of the tube. As air is ventilated into the tube with the mask sealed against the face, the air exits the holes into the pharynx. Since the tube has a blind end and the cuff is inflated after insertion, no air gets into the esophagus.

The EGTA has an open end to the tube, or a valve at the end through which a tube can be inserted into the esophagus and the stomach. In this way, stomach contents can be suctioned or medications administered to the stomach. Ventilations are not blown through the tube port (indeed, this port is designed so that a BVM coupling will not fit, thus avoiding ventilating the stomach by mistake). Instead, the ventilations enter through a second port which, like the first and only EOA port, is a standard 15 mm ventilation device adapter. These ventilations, of course, do not travel through the tube at all but flow freely under the mask and into the mouth and pharynx on the outside of the tube. In other words, the EGTA provides access to the stomach while still protecting the trachea, while the EOA only protects the trachea.

To attach the mask to the tube of either device, insert the tube into the port 180 degrees from the desired normal

A

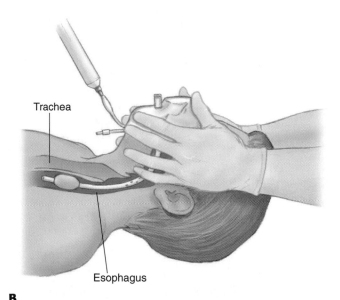

Trachea

Esophagus

B

Figure 35-17 (A) The esophageal obturator airway, or EOA and (B) the EOA in place.

anatomical position, then twist the tube 180 degrees until it snaps into place in the mask. To detach the mask from the tube, simply squeeze the plastic tips that protrude through the mask and pull out the tube from the opposite direction from which it was inserted. Both devices should be stored in the position of function. They should never be stored flat or rolled into a coil as the shape of the tube will be lost and will decrease your chances of correctly intubating the esophagus.

To insert either device, you will first need to assemble all the correct supplies:

• An EOA or EGTA tube with the proper mask (the masks are not interchangeable and will fit only the correct tube)
• A water-soluble lubricant
• A BVM with reservoir
• A stethoscope
• A suction unit and rigid Yankauer tip
• A few 4 × 4 gauze pads
• A 35 cc syringe
• Gloves, mask, and protective eye wear

Then perform the following procedures:

1. Another EMT hyperventilates the patient with the BVM. Meanwhile . . .

2. Lubricate the tip of the tube with the water-soluble lubricant.

3. Stop the resuscitation momentarily and lift the jaw and tongue straight upward without hyperextending the neck. This is best accomplished with the neck in the neutral or slightly flexed position.

4. Pass the tube following the pharyngeal curvature until the mask is seated against the face (Figure 35-18).

5. Give one ventilation with the BVM and watch for the chest to rise. This is the

way to check that the tube has been correctly placed in the esophagus and has not been incorrectly inserted into the trachea (which would block off the trachea and air pathway into the lungs). Once you are certain that the tube is correctly placed in the esophagus . . .

6. Inflate the cuff using the 35 cc syringe. (You must be certain the tube is in the esophagus. Inflation of the cuff in the trachea could cause serious damage.)

Figure 35-18 Advance the EOA or EGTA tube carefully behind the tongue into the pharynx and esophagus.

7. Use the stethoscope to listen to both lung fields (sounds of air intake into the lungs should be present) and the epigastrium. Having assured correct placement of the device . . .

8. Ventilate the patient using the BVM or a flow-restricted, oxygen-powered ventilation device.

Note: An extremely important point to remember is that the EOA or EGTA mask must be sealed in the same manner as a BVM mask. The American Heart Association Emergency Cardiac Care Guidelines recommend that ventilation with a mask is a two-person, four-handed skill: two hands on the mask attending to the seal, two hands squeezing the bag. Otherwise, a sufficient ventilation is unlikely to be delivered.

When working with the EOA or EGTA, keep the following considerations in mind:

• Remove the bag from the mask prior to each defibrillation attempt to prevent its weight from pulling out the tube.

• Be alert for vomitus in the airway and the need for suction, since regurgitation can occur even with the EOA or EGTA in place. If you need to suction, temporarily remove the mask from the tube.

• If a CPR board is used, which has an indentation to hyperextend the neck, be especially careful as hyperextension can increase the chances of misplacing the EOA or EGTA in the trachea. To guard against this possibility it is wise to place a towel in the indentation where the patient's head rests. This places the head in a neutral position. Remove the towel after EOA insertion. The importance of listening to lung sounds to confirm correct placement cannot be over-emphasized.

If the patient becomes conscious, you must remove the tube. Remember that extubation is likely to be followed by vomiting. Follow these guidelines for removing the EOA or EGTA:

• Always have the suction unit with a rigid Yankauer tip standing by.

• Do not deflate the EOA or EGTA cuff until the patient has resumed breathing or an endotracheal tube has been inserted and its cuff is inflated in the trachea. If you are using an EGTA, a gastric tube can be inserted through it to decompress the stomach or evacuate its contents to reduce the chances of regurgitation or vomiting.

• Provided there is no possibility of a spinal injury, or if the patient is secured to a spine board, turn the patient on his side, insert the syringe into the one-way valve, and withdraw air slowly from the EOA or EGTA cuff.

• Carefully remove the tube, staying alert for vomiting.

⚠ Warning

Whenever an EOA or EGTA is inserted or extubated, gloves, mask, and protective eye wear should be worn to protect the EMT-B from the potential spraying of body fluids.

Esophageal Tracheal Combitube®

The most recent alternative to the EOA and EGTA airways is called the esophageal tracheal combitube or, more commonly, "Combitube®" (Figure 35-19). The Combitube® is a double lumen airway where the two lumens are separated by a partition wall.

In one lumen of the Combitube®, the distal end is sealed and there are perforations in the area that would be in the pharynx. When the tube is in the esophagus, ventilations are delivered through this tube. The sealed end prevents the ventilations from entering the esophagus and stomach and diverts them through the perforations into the pharynx from which they flow into the trachea and the lungs.

In the other lumen of the Combitube®, the distal end is open. When the tube is in the trachea, ventilations are delivered through this tube. The Combitube® has a distal cuff that inflates to seal the esophagus or trachea, depending on which passageway it is in. (When the trachea is sealed, the cuff prevents stomach contents from being aspirated, but does not prevent ventilations from entering the trachea via the tube that passes through the cuff.)

There is also a pharyngeal balloon that seals the pharynx, preventing air from escaping the mouth and nose, and blood and debris from entering the airway.

As with the EOA or EGTA, the Combitube® should not be used on:

• Conscious patient or one with a gag reflex

• Patient under the age of 16
• Patient who has swallowed a corrosive substance
• Patient with a known esophageal disease

Follow these steps to insert the Combitube®:

1. Insert the device blindly, watching for the two black rings on the Combitube® that are used for measuring the depth of insertion. The teeth, or their bony cavities if the teeth are missing, should be positioned between these rings.

2. Use the large syringe to inflate the pharyngeal cuff with 100 cc of air. On inflation, the device will seat itself in the posterior pharynx behind the hard palate.

3. Use the smaller syringe to fill the distal cuff with 10 cc to 15 cc of air.

4. Usually the tube will have been placed in the esophagus. On this assumption, ventilate through the esophageal connector. It is the external tube that is the longer of the two and is marked #1. You must listen for the presence of breath sounds in the lungs and the absence of sounds from the epigastrium in order to be sure that the tube is, in fact, placed in the esophagus.

5. If there is an absence of lung sounds and presence of sounds in the epigastrium, the tube has been placed in the trachea. In this case, change the ventilator to the shorter tracheal connector, which is marked #2. Listen again to be sure of proper placement of the tube.

An advantage of the Combitube® over the EOA or EGTA is the automatic seating of the pharyngeal cuff. The biggest advantage of the Combitube® is that rapid intubation is possible independent of the position of the patient, which is helpful for trauma patients requiring limited cervical spine movement.

As with the EOA or EGTA, if the patient becomes conscious, you must remove the Combitube®. Remember that extubation is likely to be followed by vomiting. Have suction equipment ready. Follow the same guidelines as for removal of the other airway devices.

⚠ Warning

Whenever a Combitube® is inserted or extubated, gloves, mask, and protective eyewear should be

A

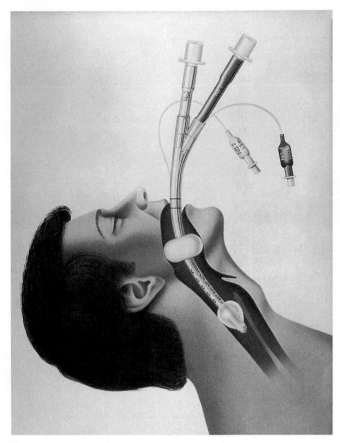

B

Figure 35-19 (A) The esophageal tracheal Combitube® and (B) the Combitube® in place.

Automatic Transport Ventilators

Automatic transport ventilators (ATVs) have been used extensively in Europe for a number of years (Figure 35-20). The devices are rapidly gaining popularity in the United States as recent studies have demonstrated them to be superior in some respects to manual ventilation with the bag-valve mask.

ATVs are compact devices that have controls that set both the rate of ventilation and the tidal volume. Tidal volumes are determined by the patient's weight. A number of different ATV models are commercially available. The American Heart Association recommends that ATVs should meet certain minimum standards. They should:

• Have the ability to deliver 100% oxygen

worn to protect the EMT-B from the potential spraying of body fluids.

• Be able to provide at least two rates of ventilation: 10 breaths per minute for adults and 20 breaths per minute for children

• Be lightweight (2 to 5 kg) and rugged

• Be equipped with an audible alarm to alert the user to problems in ventilation

• Have a standard 15 mm/22 mm coupling to connect with a mask or endotracheal tube

Although some units are marketed for pediatric use with controls for lower tidal volumes, the device is not suitable for children less than 5 years of age.

Because ATVs do require some additional training for safe use, the decision to use ATVs in an EMS system and the establishment of ATV protocols should be done by the medical director.

Figure 35-20 The automatic transport ventilator (ATV). The coin is shown for scale.

STREET SCENES

You and your partner are asked to standby for your community's annual Memorial Day parade. As the first floats and bands begin passing the reviewing stand, you hear a lady scream for help. Turning to your left, you see three people standing over a man lying on the ground. Grabbing your medical gear, you hurry to the victim. Someone identifying himself as a doctor states the man does not have a pulse.

STREET SCENE QUESTIONS

1. What priority would you assign this patient?
2. What definitive treatment do pulseless patients require?

While taking BSI precautions, your general impression is of an unconscious elderly male. Jan, your partner, performs an initial assessment, verifies pulselessness, and calls for the AED. You proceed to the head of the patient to manage his airway, while Jan opens the AED and applies the pads. The patient has a patent airway, with no signs of foreign objects or fluids. You grab an oropharyngeal airway, size it, and insert it into the patient's oropharynx. Simultaneously, the doctor hands you the bag-valve mask, which he has already hooked up to your oxygen bottle. You begin ventilating the patient while Jan finishes applying the AED.

Jan clears the patient and presses "analyze." The AED advises "shock." After one shock, reassessment verifies the patient has a pulse. However, he is not breathing. You also now observe secretions in the patient's oropharynx. Jan hands you the portable suction with the rigid catheter attached. Slipping your protective eyewear over your eyes, you insert the catheter into the patient's oropharynx. After clearing the patient's airway, the patient is still in respiratory arrest.

STREET SCENE QUESTIONS

3. What alternatives for managing the airway might you consider?
4. What assessment procedures should be performed at this time?

Since your EMS system allows you to use advanced airway maneuvers, the decision is made to orally intubate the patient. While you prepare your equipment, it is determined the patient has a pulse of 80 and regular with a BP of 80/46. The patient is loaded into the ambulance on a backboard.

Grabbing a curved laryngoscope blade and an 8.0 endotracheal tube, you ensure that the lighted blade is functioning. Jan places the patient's head into a sniffing position, and you insert the blade into the vallecula and lift to visualize the glottic opening. While you do this, Jan presses downward on the cricoid cartilage, which helps you better visualize the opening. You insert the endotracheal tube with a stylet and observe it pass through the vocal cords. Removing the laryngoscope and stylet, you inflate the cuff and attach the bag-valve mask. Jan listens to the lungs and epigastrium, and tells you that the tube is placed correctly. You double check with an esophageal intubation detector device.

STREET SCENE QUESTIONS

5. How often should this patient be reassessed?

PATIENT NAME: Rafael Gomez   **PATIENT AGE:** 67

CHIEF COMPLAINT		TIME	RESP	PULSE	B.P.	MENTAL STATUS	R PUPILS L	SKIN
Cardiac arrest	V I T A L	1005	Rate: 0 ☐ Regular ☐ Shallow ☐ Labored	Rate: 0 ☐ Regular ☐ Irregular	0 / 0 / 0	☐ Alert ☐ Voice ☐ Pain ☑ Unresp.	☑ Normal ☑ / ☐ Dilated ☐ / ☐ Constricted ☐ / ☐ Sluggish ☐ / ☐ No-Reaction ☐	☐ Unremarkable / ☐ Cool ☐ Pale / ☐ Warm ☐ Cyanotic / ☐ Moist ☐ Flushed / ☐ Dry ☐ Jaundiced
PAST MEDICAL HISTORY	S I G N S	1010	Rate: 0 ☐ Regular ☐ Shallow ☐ Labored	Rate: 80 ☒ Regular ☐ Irregular	80 / 46	☐ Alert ☐ Voice ☐ Pain ☑ Unresp.	☑ Normal ☑ / ☐ Dilated ☐ / ☐ Constricted ☐ / ☐ Sluggish ☐ / ☐ No-Reaction ☐	☐ Unremarkable / ☐ Cool ☐ Pale / ☐ Warm ☐ Cyanotic / ☐ Moist ☐ Flushed / ☐ Dry ☐ Jaundiced
☐ None ☐ Allergy to____ ☐ Hypertension ☐ Stroke ☐ Seizures ☐ Diabetes ☐ COPD ☐ Cardiac ☐ Other (List) ☐ Asthma Unknown Current Medications (List) Unknown			Rate: ☐ Regular ☐ Shallow ☐ Labored	Rate: ☐ Regular ☐ Irregular	/	☐ Alert ☐ Voice ☐ Pain ☐ Unresp.	☐ Normal ☐ / ☐ Dilated ☐ / ☐ Constricted ☐ / ☐ Sluggish ☐ / ☐ No-Reaction ☐	☐ Unremarkable / ☐ Cool ☐ Pale / ☐ Warm ☐ Cyanotic / ☐ Moist ☐ Flushed / ☐ Dry ☐ Jaundiced

NARRATIVE Patient was a bystander-witnessed cardiac arrest. Physician on scene stated patient had no pulse; verified by EMS crew. CPR ongoing while AED attached and detected shockable rhythm (see AED printout attached). One shock delivered with patient's pulse returning. No respirations, and with airway secretions noted. Patient suctioned with rigid catheter and decision to intubate with #8.0 ET tube x 1 attempt = successful. Prior to intubation, patient oxygenated with BVM and OPA. Lung sounds equal bilaterally and negative findings over epigastric area. Patient reassessed throughout with no changes noted other than patient seemed to respond to verbal stimuli as we neared the hospital. On-line medical direction established.

Securing the tube, you quickly reassess vitals and then recheck the tube in case it has become misplaced. You inform medical direction of your actions, and tell them you will be at their facility in 3 minutes. En route, you continually assess lung sounds. You observe the patient's eyes open, and he responds to your commands to keep his hands away from the tube. At the hospital, you quickly transfer the patient to a bed in the emergency department.

Later that day, you learn that the patient is doing well. He had suffered a myocardial infarction.

CHAPTER REVIEW

SUMMARY

Airway control is the highest priority in managing any critically ill or injured patient, because without an adequate airway the patient will die no matter what other care you provide. Control of a patient's airway is recognized as so crucial a skill that advanced airway skills are now included as an elective in the EMT-Basic curriculum.

Advanced airway management centers on the skill of orotracheal intubation, the placement of an endotracheal tube through the mouth and into the patient's trachea. This permits complete control of the airway, minimizes the risk of aspiration, allows for better oxygen delivery, and allows for deep suctioning of the trachea.

Endotracheal intubation of infants and children is similar to the procedure for adults with these exceptions: All structures in the mouth and nose are smaller, the tongue is proportionately larger, the trachea is softer, more flexible, and narrower, the airway is especially narrow at the cricoid cartilage, and the chest wall is softer.

These differences result in the airways of infants and children being more easily obstructed, in the use of uncuffed endotracheal tubes under the age of 8 because the narrow cricoid acts as a cuff, and in distinctive breathing patterns. Infants and children are more susceptible to damage from incorrect placement of a tube and to interruptions of the supply of oxygen and must be monitored especially carefully during intubation and suctioning procedures.

Nasogastric intubation is performed on infants and children to relieve the pressure of swallowed air in the stomach.

Endotracheal suctioning is performed by inserting a suction catheter—usually through an endotracheal tube—to the level of the carina.

KEY TERMS

alveoli (al-VE-o-li) the microscopic sacs of the lungs where gas exchange with the bloodstream takes place.

bronchi (BRONG-ki) the two large sets of branches that come off the trachea and enter the lungs. There are right and left mainstem bronchi. The singular is *bronchus.*

carina (kah-RI-nah) the fork at the lower end of the trachea where the two mainstem bronchi branch.

cricoid (KRIK-oid) **cartilage** the ring-shaped structure that circles the trachea at the lower edge of the larynx.

cricoid pressure pressure applied to the cricoid cartilage to suppress vomiting and bring the vocal cords into view. Also called *Sellick's maneuver.*

endotracheal (EN-do-TRAY-ke-ul) **tube** a tube designed to be inserted into the trachea. Oxygen, medication, or a suction catheter can be directed into the trachea through an endotracheal tube.

epiglottis (EP-i-GLOT-is) a leaf-shaped structure that prevents food and foreign matter from entering the trachea.

esophagus (eh-SOF-uh-gus) the tube that leads from the pharynx to the stomach.

glottic opening the opening to the trachea.

hyperventilate (HI-per-VEN-ti-late) to provide ventilations at a higher rate to compensate for oxygen not delivered during intubation or suctioning.

hypopharynx (HI-po-FAIR-inks) the area directly above the openings of both the trachea and the esophagus.

hypoxia (hi-POK-se-uh) inadequate oxygenation, or oxygen starvation.

intubation (IN-tu-BAY-shun) insertion of a tube.

laryngoscope (lair-ING-uh-skope) an illuminating instrument that is inserted into the pharynx to permit visualization of the pharynx and larynx.

larynx (LAIR-inks) the voice box.

mainstem bronchi See *bronchi.*

nasogastric (NAY-zo-GAS-trik) **tube (NG tube)** a tube designed to be passed through the nose, nasopharynx, and esophagus. It is used to relieve distention of the stomach in an infant or child patient.

nasopharynx (NAY-zo-FAIR-inks) the area directly posterior to the nose.

oropharynx (OR-o-FAIR-inks) the area directly posterior to the mouth.

orotracheal (OR-o-TRAY-ke-ul) intubation placement of an endotracheal tube through the mouth and into the trachea.

Sellick's maneuver See *cricoid pressure*.

stylet a long, thin, flexible metal probe.

trachea (TRAY-ke-uh) the "windpipe"; the structure that connects the pharynx to the lungs.

vallecula (val-EK-yuh-luh) a groove-like structure anterior to the epiglottis.

vocal cords two thin folds of tissue within the larynx that vibrate as air passes between them, producing sounds.

REVIEW QUESTIONS

1. Explain why it is important for EMT-Bs to be able to perform orotracheal intubation. (pp. 772–773)
2. List and explain the errors in intubation that can lead to a patient's death. (p. 770)
3. Explain the procedures for assuring correct placement of an endotracheal tube. (pp. 769–770, 778–779, 782–783)
4. Explain reasons and describe the procedure for insertion of a nasogastric tube in an infant or child. (pp. 782–783)
5. Explain how orotracheal suctioning differs from oropharyngeal suctioning. Explain reasons why orotracheal suctioning may be advisable. (p. 783)

APPLICATIONS

• You have successfully intubated a non-breathing patient and transferred him to the ambulance. During your ongoing assessment you auscultate the chest and find that there are breath sounds on the right, but not the left. What does this indicate? What should you do in this situation?

WEB MEDIC

Visit Brady's *Emergency Care* website for direct weblinks. At **www.bradybooks.com/ emergencycare**, you will find information related to the following Chapter 35 topics:

• Prehospital airway management devices

Photograph: HMC(SW/FMF) Les Painter

Chapter
Thirty-Six

MILITARY EMERGENCY CARE

*W*ord on the Street

Emergency Medical Services as we know it today has deep roots in the military. Due to the significant numbers of soldiers who have died from wounds received in combat, never having reached a medical treatment facility, minimal prehospital medical care has been moved closer to the battlefield. Injured soldiers with life-threatening injuries are treated before transport to a rear treatment facility. Casualty evacuation by aircraft is another step initiated by the military to decrease the time from injury to definitive medical treatment. During the Vietnam War, civilian emergency medical services developed from the funeral home patient transportation hearse to the efficient system of advanced life-support vehicles. Many things taken for granted in the civilian sector today, such as interstate highways and air ambulances, all came from military applications, and we as a country are richer for it.

*MSG **William Breshears**,* NREMT-B
Course Coordinator for EMT Education
10th Battalion (PN/HS)
Houston, Texas

Wars and other tactical operations occur in all corners of the globe and in all possible conditions. This chapter focuses on the emergency care provided in these unique environments by specialized military medical personnel, which is different from civilian EMS. Patients in these environments require special access and have different priorities for care. The information in this chapter is not a substitute for the U.S. DOT National Standard Curriculum. Rather, it is additional information to meet the needs of our military medical personnel who are or may be in these situations.

—James Miller, NREMT-P
US Army EMT Program Manager

HISTORY

The EMS System we know today dates back to the late 1960s and the White Paper ("Accidental Death and Disability: The Neglected Disease of Modern Society") written by the National Research Council. However, this modern-day delivery of prehospital emergency medical care has come about as the result of the lessons learned and expertise gathered through a long history of medical support to military operations.

Prior to the eighteenth century, the medical support of armies was usually limited to surgeons who served only the nobility. Ordinary wounded soldiers were left on the battlefield to depend upon comrades or family for care. The first recorded use of an ambulance by the military was in 1487, at the siege of

Malaga (Spain). Queen Isabella of Spain had her armies carry wounded soldiers in bedded wagons to tent hospitals miles from the battlefield. The wagons required up to 40 horses to pull them and were stationed near the distant hospitals. Surgeons waited hours to provide what little care was possible.

In 1797, Baron Dominique-Jean Larrey, chief physician in Napoleon's army, designed the first prehospital system of triage and transport to field aid stations. The horse-drawn carts that he introduced became known as the "flying ambulances." This concept actually addressed all of the early EMS issues such as the training of persons who ride on the ambulances, rapid response into the battlefield, and rapid transportation back to the hospital. Treatment

Figure 36-1   The Civil War was the first test of the United States military emergency medical care system. *Photograph: Mathew Brady Collection (Army)*

1. Define the key events in military history that have influenced the development of modern Emergency Medical Services.

2. Discuss the role that aeromedical evacuation played in reducing the time from injury to arrival at a hospital unit.

3. Compare the levels of training provided to military medics of each branch of the services.

4. Define the military levels of care.

5. Identify the stages of care associated with casualty care in a hostile environment.

---

of the wounded soldiers in the field was not considered during Larrey's time.

The first test of the US military's emergency medical care system came during the Civil War. The first battle of the war, Bull Run (1861), was a disaster for the Union Army by most military and medical standards. They had few ambulances or medical personnel. The most unfit soldiers were detailed as litter bearers, and they were little better as medical assistants. They often drank the alcohol in their medicine chests and stayed near the battlefield only long enough to rob the wounded. In the Union Army's retreat, not a single casualty was taken to safety. Three thousand wounded soldiers lay on the battlefield without food or water three days after the battle of Bull Run. Some were without care for as long as six to seven days.

As a result of Bull Run, the Union Army restructured its wartime medical care. Jonathan Letterman, surgeon of the Army of the Potomac, is credited with developing the first Army-wide ambulance service in 1862 (Letterman Ambulance Plan). In this system, the ambulances of a division moved together. Under the direction of a mounted line sergeant, two stretcher-bearers and one driver per ambulance collected the wounded from the field, brought them to the dressing stations, and then took them to the field hospital. Men who volunteered were given training in first aid and litter bearing. After a one-year apprenticeship, candidates were eligible for selection as privates in the Hospital Corps. After an additional year of probationary training and passing an examination, they could be appointed as Hospital Stewards.

The first reported use of air transportation in support of medical activities occurred during the siege of Paris (Franco-Prussian War) in 1870 when a total of 160 patients were said to have been removed from that city by means of an observation balloon. However, most modern aeromedical historians believe that this was a bogus report. In 1912 the Association of Military Surgeons of the US Committee on Air Transportation of Wounded in War recommended that airplanes transport surgical cases from the battlefield to the hospital. These recommendations were squashed by the contemporary press [". . . *the use of the airplane for evacuation is, for the moment, in the*

realm of fiction," Le Caducee, *French medical journal].* However, in November 1915, 13 injured French Army soldiers in Serbia were air evacuated from the battlefield in an open cockpit biplane.

During World War I, Letterman's ambulance concept, now motorized, added a new level of mobility to the evacuation techniques—significantly reducing the time from injury to arrival at a treatment facility. At the end of WWI, the mortality rate for casualties reaching treatment facilities had been reduced to 8 percent.

World War II saw the mortality rate reduced to 4 percent for wounded soldiers reaching a treatment facility. Drugs such as sulfa (Sulfanilamide) and penicillin were widely utilized, and advanced surgical techniques helped make this improvement possible. But the primary reason for such success was the speed with which the wounded men were treated. This began with the frontline combat medic.

Figure 36-2 Wounded American soldiers are given medical treatment at a first aid station in Korea, July 25, 1950. *Pfc. Tom Nebbia (Army)*

The objective of the medic was to get the wounded away from the front lines to a point of safety. There the medic would do a brief examination, evaluate the wound, apply a tourniquet if necessary, sometimes inject a vial of morphine, clean up the wound as well as possible, and sprinkle sulfa powder on the wound followed by a bandage. Then he would drag or carry the patient out of harm's way. Many times this was done under enemy fire or artillery shelling. However, in most cases, the enemy respected the Red Cross armband that by the **Geneva Convention** identified medical personnel exclusively engaged in the search for, collection, transport, or treatment of the wounded.

During the Korean War in 1951, the first helicopter ambulance unit began operations. A wounded soldier could reach a sterile, fully equipped hospital in minutes. By the cease-fire in 1953, over 17,000 casualties had been airlifted by helicopter, and the mortality rate for those reaching treatment facilities was reduced to 2.5 percent. In 1961 the Army Medical Department started formal aviation medicine training at Fort Rucker, Alabama.

In Vietnam, the efficiency and speed of casualty care and evacuation were enhanced with the use of the UH-1 helicopter and its "Dustoff" crews. The UH-1 could carry up to 6 litter or 9 ambulatory patients and was equipped with an internal rescue hoist. The combat medics supported by the "Dustoff" crews were able to significantly reduce the time from injury to arrival at the hospital to 30 to 60 minutes (modern EMS's "**Golden Hour**") and further reduced the **mortality rate** to 2 percent.

Lessons learned and expertise gained continue to be brought back to the United States by returning military care providers from Bosnia, Somalia, Iraq, and numerous other locations.

Contributing to today's modern EMS system are military influences in aeromedical evacuation, centers specializing in the care of trauma victims, advanced life-support care, and multiple levels of providers. EMS has grown tremendously due to the role the military has played.

CURRENT MILITARY EMS

Today's modern military EMS system supports both military wartime and peacetime requirements. The end goal is to accomplish the mission. The military medical system's mission is to *conserve the fighting strength*. The peacetime mission is accomplished much in the same manner as it is in the civilian community. However, during wartime, the means to accomplishing the mission are drastically modified.

Levels of Training

A wide variety of trained medical personnel exist within the military prehospital emergency medical system. From the front-line health care specialist with

Figure 36-3 Medical personnel are assembled with lifesaving equipment at HQs of the 8225th Mobile Army Surgical Hospital, Korea, October 14, 1951. *Photograph: Cpl. Charles Abrahamson (Army)*

Table 36-1   Mortality Rates and Evacuation Times

Mortality Rates

War	Mortality (%)*
World War I	8.0%
World War II	4.5%
Korea	2.5%
Vietnam	2.0%

* Mortality of battle casualties reaching treatment facilities

Evacuation Times to a Hospital Unit

War	Evacuation Time*
19th Century	Days
WW I	Up to a day
World War II	10 hours
Korea	5 hours
Vietnam	30–60 minutes

* Time from injury to arrival at hospital

basic skills to the highly flexible independent duty technician are individuals assigned specific jobs divided into different levels of care providers.

Self-Aid/Buddy-Aid or Care

Each service member is trained to be proficient in a variety of specific first aid procedures such as bleeding control and simple splinting. (These procedures include aid for chemical casualties with particular emphasis on lifesaving tasks.) This training enables immediate care to alleviate life-threatening conditions. Self-aid/buddy-aid or care compares to bystanders trained in first aid in the civilian EMS system.

Combat Lifesaver

In the Army, selected nonmedical soldiers (typically one individual per squad, crew, team or equivalent sized unit) are trained beyond basic first aid procedures. This additional training includes intravenous insertions, advanced splinting, and other more advanced measures, approximating the civilian first responder program with an expanded scope of practice.

The primary duty of this individual does not change. The combat lifesaver duties are performed when the situation permits.

Combat Medic/Corpsman/Medical Technician

The Army Military Occupational Specialty (MOS) 91B Medical Specialist ("combat medic") receives 10 weeks of training that includes Emergency Medical Technician Basic (EMT-B) training. Additional training is provided in intravenous insertion, medication administration, and the care of patients with wartime related injuries (such as nuclear, biological, and

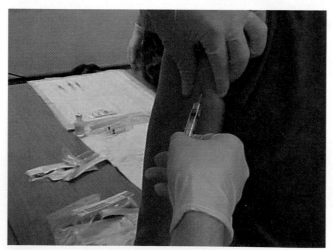

Figure 36-4   Combat Lifesavers receive training in IV insertions and other advanced life saving measures. *Photograph: SFC Allen Bala*

Figure 36-5   A wide variety of trained prehospital medical personnel exists within the military. *Photograph: SFC Allen Bala*

Figure 36-6 The first medical care a casualty will receive may be at an aid station. *Photograph: HMC(SW/FMF) Les Painter*

chemical warfare). Beginning in 2001, the Army is expanding this training to 16 weeks to facilitate an expansion of skills with increased emphasis on preventive medicine and weapons of mass destruction casualty management. Increased medical oversight, clinical practicums in initial training, and a minimum requirement to maintain National Registry EMT-B certification will become the standard. This increased standard will bring the expanded scope of practice of the "combat medic" to near that of the civilian EMT-Intermediate. These individuals will be assigned the MOS of 91W Health Care Specialist.

The Air Force's version of the Army MOS is the Air Force Specialty Code (AFSC). The 4N0X1 Medical Service Technician receives 16 weeks of training including an EMT-B curriculum and additional training similar to that of the Army 91W.

Navy corps personnel receive didactic and practical skills training containing the majority of the EMT-B National Standard Curriculum, operational medicine, and basic nursing care procedures as part of the Hospital Corpsman Basic "A" School. Following completion of "A" School, corpsmen are classified as general duty, or 0000. Corpsmen assigned to deployable Fleet Marine Force Units are provided further training as Field Medical Technicians (8404). This training is approximately 12 weeks long and includes the civilian equivalent of Prehospital Trauma Life Support, treatment of chemical, biological, and nuclear agent casualties, and other medical skills.

Independent Duty Medical Technician
Within the US Military exists another level of prehospital care providers with no real civilian counterpart. They are the Navy Independent Duty Hospital Corpsman, Air Force Independent Duty Technician, and Army Special Operation Medic.

These medics are trained to provide medical care in remote areas where an on-site physician is not available. Each shares a common experience of extensive (1,000–2,000+ hours) training. This training includes diagnosis and treatment of minor ailments and limited laboratory and radiographic interpretation. Specialty training is slightly different for each service. Independent duty medics are registered with the National Registry of EMTs as intermediates or paramedics and have special authorizations to provide supervised primary care.

Levels of Care

The military Levels of Care [formerly referred to as "Echelons of Care"] describe the system of combat medical care and facilities. Treatment capabilities are approximately the same for each level across the branches of service, in compliance with Joint Chiefs of Staff doctrinal directives.

Level I
The first medical care a soldier receives is provided at this level and includes (1) self- and buddy-aid; (2) combat lifesaver care; (3) combat medic care; and (4) "aid station" care. For the US Army and Marines, the aid station is the first medical "facility" a casualty will encounter. The physician and/or the physician assistant in the aid station are trained and equipped to provide advanced trauma management to the battlefield casualty including endotracheal intubation, tube thoracostomy, intravenous medication, and other physician-directed medical care. Navy ships have an approximate equivalent in their "battle

Figure 36-7 Emergency medical treatment including resuscitation procedures is provided at a divisional clearing station, Level II. *Photograph: HMC(SW/FMF) Les Painter*

Figure 36-8 An Army combat support hospital provides care for all categories of casualties. *Photograph: HMC(SW/FMF) Les Painter*

dressing stations," a satellite of the primary shipboard medical department.

Level II

Level II is a divisional clearing station or, in the Air Force, air transportable clinic operated by a medical staff of physicians, nurses, and medics to evacuate casualties received from Level I. Emergency medical treatment including resuscitation procedures is provided at this level; however, it does not go beyond the measures dictated by immediate need. Those patients who can return to duty within 24 to 72 hours are held for treatment. Support duplicates Level I and expands services available by adding dental, laboratory, x-ray, and patient-holding capabilities. Navy ship medical departments approximate this capability, as do the Marine Fleet Surgical Support Groups.

Figure 36-9 Level V represents a fixed hospital located outside a theater of operations. *Photograph: HMC(SW/FMF) Les Painter*

Patients with injuries or illnesses beyond the capabilities of the ship's sick bay are evacuated to a rear area facility or major hospital ship.

Level III

Level III is the first true medical facility a casualty sees on the battlefield. This is a US Army combat support hospital, Air Force air transportable hospital/Air Force theater hospital, or Navy fleet hospital. Level III hospitals provide care for all categories of casualties with comprehensive resuscitative surgery and medical care. Casualties who are unlikely to return to duty are evacuated as soon as possible after stabilization.

Table 36-2 Levels of Military Medical Care

Level	Personnel/Facility	Type of Care
I	Self-, Buddy-Aid Combat Lifesaver Combat Medic Small Portable Expeditionary Aeromedical Rapid Response (SPEAR) Aid station	• First aid • Early emergency treatment • Emergency medical treatment • Advanced trauma and medical management
II	Medical company (Clearing station) Air transportable clinic/Expeditionary Medical Support System (EMEDS) Field surgical support group	• Initial surgical resuscitation
III	Combat support hospital Air transportable hospital/Air Force theater hospital Fleet hospital	• Resuscitative surgery and medical care
IV	Combat support hospital Host nation hospitals USAF contingency hospital Hospital ships	• Definitive care
V	Fixed medical facilities	• Restorative and rehabilitative care

Level IV

Level IV care is represented by treating a casualty in a general or field hospital staffed and equipped for general and specialized medical and surgical care. This level of care provides further treatment to stabilize those patients requiring evacuation to the Continental United States (CONUS). The Navy's two 1,000-bed hospital ships (*USNS Mercy* and *USNS Comfort*) are Level IV facilities. Both were in use and in theater during Operation Desert Storm.

Level V

Level V represents a fixed hospital located outside the theater of operations. Definitive and rehabilitative care of all types is available in Level V facilities.

TACTICAL CASUALTY CARE

Rapid responses, advanced life support, focus on the individual patient's medical needs, and rapid transports characterize civilian EMS. The potential for a delayed response, access to basic life support only, delayed transport, penetrating trauma, limited equipment, and an austere environment characterize EMS for the military medic.

The military medic has a responsibility to protect the Constitution, defend the nation, and obey all lawful orders. Implied is the obligation to carry out the mission to the best of his or her abilities. *The military medic gives first priority to the mission and places his or her own welfare after it.* Our country's history is full of examples of medics who, despite overwhelming odds, risked their lives to accomplish their sworn duty.

In a hostile situation, emergency medical care takes on new meaning. Factors such as enemy fire, medical equipment limitations, a widely variable evacuation time, tactical considerations, and the unique problems of transporting casualties all must be addressed. The remaining sections discuss the principles of casualty care in a hostile environment.

Stages of Care

Casualty care provided in a hostile environment can be divided into three distinct phases.

1. Care Under Fire is the care rendered by the medic at the scene of the injury while he and the casualty are still under effective hostile fire. The available medical equipment is limited to that carried in his medical pack.

Figure 36-10 Recruits from the Woman Recruit Training Command conduct first-aid exercises during basic training. *Photograph: DOD Photo*

2. Tactical Field Care is the care rendered by the medic once he and the casualty are no longer under effective hostile fire. This phase also applies to situations in which an injury has occurred on a mission but there has not been hostile fire. Available medical equipment is limited and evacuation times to a Medical Treatment Facility (MTF) may vary considerably.

3. Combat Casualty Evacuation Care is the care provided while the casualty is being transported by a ground vehicle, aircraft or marine vehicle. Additional medical personnel and equipment may be pre-staged to support this phase of casualty management.

Care Under Fire

Casualty care under fire will typically take place in the middle of an active engagement with hostile forces. Military medics carry small arms with which to defend themselves in the field. In small unit operations, additional firepower provided by the special operations medic may be required to obtain tactical superiority. As a result, the special operations medic may need to assist in returning fire before stopping to care for a casualty. *The best medicine on any battlefield is fire superiority.* As soon as the medic is able to render care, *preventing a casualty from further injury is his first objective.*

Table 36-3 General Approach to Patient Management in the Tactical Environment: Initial Assessment and Management

- **Airway**
  Manual maneuvers
  Airway adjuncts
  Advanced airway adjuncts
  > Dual lumen airway
  > Endotracheal intubation
  > Cricothyrotomy or cricothyrostomy

- **Breathing**
  Artificial ventilation
  > Bag-valve-mask ventilation
  Needle thoracostomy for tension pneumothorax

- **Circulation**
  Control bleeding with direct pressure or
  > tourniquet
  Start large bore IV
  Fluid resuscitation with normal saline or Lactated
  > Ringer's

- **Focused and Detailed Assessment and Management**

- **Disability**
  Rapid head-to-toe assessment
  Splint suspected fractures
  Dress open wounds as indicated
  Analgesia
  Antibiotics

- **Evacuation**

Table 36-4 Care Under Fire

- Return fire as directed or required

- Protect self

- Protect casualty from hostile fire

- Stop any life-threatening bleeding with a tourniquet

- Evacuate the casualty to cover

If the casualty is conscious, the medic may be able to lead the casualty to cover. If the casualty is unable to move, the medic may need to provide transportation utilizing a drag, a shoulder carry, or an improvised litter.

Tactical Field Care

In this phase there is more time in which to render care, and the threat of hostile fire is reduced. In some cases the tactical field care will consist only of rapid treatment of wounds due to the possibility of the return of hostile fire at any moment. At other times, intensive care may be provided to the casualty once an anticipated **extraction** or **evacuation** point has been reached. In this instance, there may be time to provide all necessary interventions, without haste, in the field. The time prior to extraction or evacuation can range from less than a half-hour to many hours.

In the Tactical Field Care phase the injury may occur prior to engagement with hostile forces. In this case, the mission commander must make a decision regarding the continuance of the operation and what to do with the casualty prior to extraction or evacuation.

The general approach to patient management in the Tactical Field Care phase is described in Table 36-5a. Unlike Care Under Fire, the medic and the casualty are not under effective hostile fire. This affords the benefit of providing more intensive emergency treatment. Tactical Field Care focuses on management of airway and breathing, dressing of wounds, and splinting of fractures. Because there remains some risk of hostile fire, care may need to be adjusted accordingly.

Combat Casualty Evacuation Care

Combat Casualty Evacuation Care is a continuation of the Tactical Field Care phase except that the casualty

Because of the need to remove the casualty to cover as soon as possible, no immediate management of the airway is provided while under fire. It is extremely important, however, to control any major bleeding as soon as possible since injury to a major vessel may result in the very rapid onset of hypovolemic shock. Hemorrhage from extremity wounds was the cause of death in more than 2,500 casualties in Vietnam who had no other injuries. Due to the need to move the casualty and the resultant inability of the medic to maintain direct pressure, the tourniquet is the initial choice to stop major bleeding. Both the medic and the casualty are in extreme danger while a tourniquet is being applied, and treatment of non-life-threatening bleeding should be delayed until the Tactical Field Care phase.

Removing the casualty to cover will often be the most difficult aspect of providing care in this phase.

Table 36-5a   Tactical Field Care

Airway management
Manual maneuvers
Airway adjuncts
Advanced airway adjuncts
　Dual lumen airway
　Endotracheal intubation
　Cricothyrotomy or cricothyrostomy

Breathing
Artificial ventilation
Needle thoracostomy for tension pneumothorax

Circulation
Control remaining bleeding with tourniquet or
　direct pressure
Start large bore IV
Fluid resuscitation with normal saline or Lactated
　Ringer's

Detailed assessment and management
Inspect and dress wounds
Check for additional wounds
Analgesia (as necessary)
　Morphine: 5mg IV
Splint fractures and recheck pulses

Cardiopulmonary Resuscitation

Note
Resuscitation in a hostile environment for
victims of blast or penetrating trauma who
have no pulse, no respirations, and no other signs of
life will not be successful and should not be
attempted.

Table 36-5b   Airway Management in the Tactical Field Care Phase

- Casualty conscious, alert, and talking
  No interventions indicated

- Casualty unconscious or with altered mental status
  Open airway
  　Chin-lift or jaw-thrust maneuver
  Airway Adjuncts
  　Naso- or oro-pharyngeal airway, if tolerated

- Casualty unconscious—advanced management
  Without airway obstruction
  　Dual lumen airway
  　Endotracheal intubation
  Complete unrelieved upper airway obstruction
  　Needle cricothyrostomy or cricothyrotomy
  Light-restricted environment
  　Digital intubation

Table 36-5c   Cervical Immobilization in the Tactical Field Care Phase

- Cervical spine immobilization not indicated:
  Penetrating head or neck trauma
  Falls from standing or off low (3 to 5 feet) objects

- Indications for cervical spine immobilization
  *If feasible for unconscious or conscious casualties
  with neck pain and:*
  High speed (> 30 mph) vehicle collision
  Falls from significant height
  Direct blunt neck trauma
  Blast injury
  Any casualty with neurological signs of a cervical
  　spine injury

and the medic are on the move. The casualty and medic move toward the rear for additional care. The usual means of evacuation is by ground or air ambulance, but may be accomplished by any means at hand including many carry and marine vehicles. As mentioned previously, the time to extraction or evacuation varies. The general casualty management plan outline for Combat Casualty Evacuation Care is outlined in Table 36-6 following.

Table 36-6   Combat Casualty Evacuation Care

Airway management
Same as tactical field care

Breathing
Same as tactical field care
Oxygen therapy

Circulation
Same as tactical field care
Consider removing tourniquets and using direct
　pressure to control bleeding if possible
Large bore IV with saline if not already done

Monitoring
Initiate electronic monitoring of heart rate, blood
　pressure and hemoglobin oxygen saturation (if
　available)

Continued Assessment
Inspect and dress wounds if not already done
Check for additional wounds
Analgesia as necessary
　Morphine: 5mg IV
Splint fractures and recheck pulses
Antibiotics

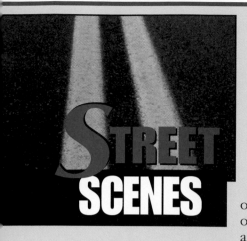

Fort Bragg, NC 0015 hours—A military medic receives an alert to report to his unit, Charlie Company, Second Platoon. As he arrives he sees that all the soldiers assigned to his unit are loading essential equipment onto a C-5 aircraft. Another group of soldiers are loading a second C-5 aircraft. At 0200 hours both aircraft are in the air. This medic carries with him a trauma pack (Aid Bag) and other essential survival equipment. The Platoon Leader explains the mission: Objective one is to secure the airport near the drop zone. Objective two is to stop drug traffic transportation occurring at that airport.

0500 hours—While it is still nightfall, the C-5s arrive at the designated drop zone. Due to weather conditions, the unit initiates the jump at 500 feet above ground level. Security forces at the airport had been increased due to prior civilian riots a few days earlier. Avenues of approach are open flat terrain with minimal cover, with a few aircraft on the airstrip and two buildings. Additional security forces are identified in roving.

As the unit hits the drop zone, the security force's roving patrols begin small arms fire. Four soldiers are wounded, one with a GSW to the chest, two with GSW to the lower extremities, and three others with suspected fractures from the jump. After a firefight, the security forces are overwhelmed with casualties and limited supplies, and they surrender.

MSG Kim Travella
NCOIC, 91W Sustainment/Transition
Army Medical Department Center and School
Fort Sam Houston, Texas

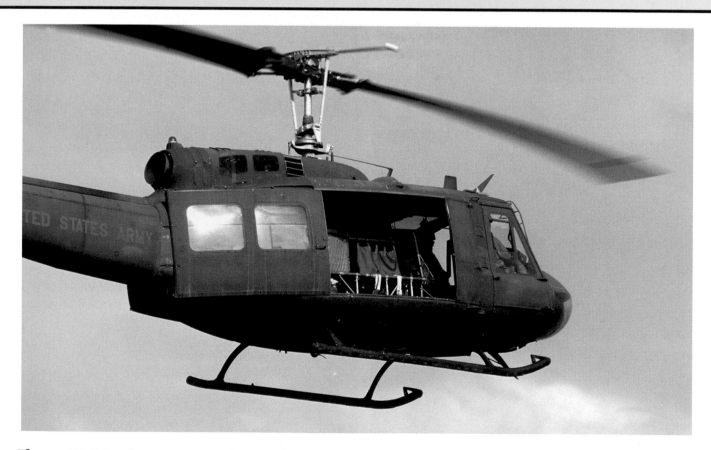

Figure 36-11 The UH-1 (Huey) is the oldest member of the helicopter fleet in the Department of Defense inventory. The first one was delivered in 1958. The Huey transports troops and equipment into combat and flies command and control, combat resupply, and aeromedical evacuation missions. It has a crew of three—two pilots and a crew chief—and can carry a 3,000 pound (1,350 kg) payload, eight combat troops or a 4,000 pound (1,800 kg) sling load. In the Marine Corps, the Huey provides utility combat helicopter support to the landing force commander during ship-to-shore movement. *Photograph: DOD Photo*

STREET SCENE QUESTIONS

1. What are the stages of care for this scenario?

Care Under Fire is the care rendered by the medic at the scene of injury while he and the casualty are still receiving hostile fire. Available medical equipment is limited to that carried by the soldier medic.

Tactical Field Care is the care rendered by the medic once he and the casualty are no longer under hostile fire. This also applies to situations in which an injury has occurred on a mission independent of hostile fire. Available medical equipment is still limited to that carried by the medic. The time prior to medical evacuation to a Medical Treatment Facility (MTF) is considerable.

Combat Casualty Evacuation Care (CASEVAC) is the care rendered once the casualty (and usually the rest of the mission personnel) have been picked up by aircraft, vehicle, or boat. Additional medical personnel and equipment that have been pre-staged assets should be available at this stage of casualty management.

2. How would the tactical field care of these casualties differ if there were expectations of re-engagement of hostile forces?

Tactical field care of these casualties focuses on management of airway and breathing, dressing of wounds, and splinting of fractures. Because of expectations of re-engagement of hostile forces the care should be adjusted to facilitate rapid evacuation of the casualty or movement of the casualty to cover.

CHAPTER REVIEW

SUMMARY

The world's military has pioneered today's system of systematic emergency medical care. Our civilian and military EMS systems have both adapted wartime lessons to peacetime missions. Today's military medics are trained to function in small tactical units, on board ships or aircraft, and to perform a wide variety of duties. In addition to emergency care these duties include ambulatory care, preventive medicine, field sanitation, and psychological stress control.

The tactical field environment poses significant challenges to the military medic. With limited equipment, harsh weather, darkness, and hostile fire, the military medic needs to adapt his approach to combat casualty care and focus priorities to the immediate tactical situation.

KEY TERMS

evacuation movement of casualties toward a care facility (i.e., aid station). Emergency medical care provided enroute.

extraction removal from a hostile location (a tactical extrication). Little or no emergency medical care is provided enroute.

Geneva Convention Collectively, the treaties and conventions pertinent to warfare on land are referred to as The Hague and Geneva Conventions. The Geneva Conventions concern the victims of war or armed conflict. The Geneva Conventions are four separate international treaties signed in 1949.

Golden Hour the optimum limit of one hour between the time of injury and surgery at the hospital. See also *platinum ten minutes.*

Military Occupational Specialty (MOS) primary job code description for enlisted military personnel, i.e., 91W (US Army Health Care Specialist); 11B (US Army Combat Infantryman); etc.

mortality rate the death rate, noted as the number of deaths per unit of population for a specific group.

REVIEW QUESTIONS

1. Historically, what army is credited with the first recorded use of ambulances?
2. What is surgeon Jonathan Letterman credited with developing?
3. What are the civilian EMS sytem equivalents to the following military levels of training?
   Self-Aid/Buddy-Aid or Care
   Combat Lifesaver
   Combat Medic/Corpsman
4. Care provided in a divisional clearing station is considered what level of care according to the Joint Chiefs of Staff doctrinal directives?
5. What is the first priority of care in the Care Under Fire phase of tactical casualty care?

APPLICATIONS

- As a military medic, how would you balance the need for appropriate on-scene assessment and treatment with the need to evacuate casualties?

- One of the casualties is unresponsive and not breathing. What would be the appropriate on-scene triage steps?

WEB MEDIC

US Army EMT Program:
http://www.cs.amedd.army.mil/91W

US Navy EMT Program:
http://bumed.med.navy.mil

US Air Force EMT Program:
http://sg-www.satx.disa.mil/school/emthome.html

Additional Military EMT training information:
http://www.medtrng.com

SUGGESTED FURTHER READING

1. *Tactical Emergency Care: Military and Operational Out-of-Hospital Medicine*, 1999, De Lorenzo, R., Porter, R., Brady/Prentice Hall.

2. *EMT-Tactical Provider Program, Student Manual*, 15th Edition, February 2001, Heck J. J., Kepp J. J., Walos G., Vayer J. S., Uniformed Services University.

3. *Combat Casualty Care in Special Operations*, Military Medicine, 1996, Suppl: 3–15, Butler F. K., Hagmann J., Butler E. J.

4. *FM 8-10, Health Service Support in a Theater of Operations*, March 1991, Headquarters, Department of the Army.

5. *Prehospital Systems and Medical Oversight*, 2001, Kuehl A., Mosby/Harcourt.

APPENDIX A

ALS-ASSIST SKILLS

Local protocol may require you to assist more highly trained EMS personnel in the administration of advanced life support (ALS) procedures. There are several new skills you can learn to enhance your capability as a "team player" on such calls. Your instructor will discuss the skills that are authorized by your medical director. However, the most common are:

- Assisting in the endotracheal intubation of a patient
- Applying ECG/defibrillator electrodes
- Assisting in intravenous (IV) fluid therapy

Note: The following information is intended as a summary of ALS-assist skills. More detailed information and additional in-service training may be required. Consult with your instructor on local protocols.

ASSISTING WITH ENDOTRACHEAL INTUBATION

Among the highest priorities of patient care is to assure a patient airway and to prevent aspiration. The "gold standard" for airway care is the endotracheal tube. Other airway devices, such as the EOA, EGTA, and Combitube®, are at best secondary. This is because the endotracheal tube is directly inserted into the trachea, forming an open pathway for air, oxygen, or medications to be blown into the lungs. In addition, adult sizes have an inflatable cuff that seals off the trachea to prevent aspiration. (In an infant or young child, the narrow trachea creates a seal.)

Patients who typically need to have an endotracheal tube inserted are those in pulmonary or cardiopulmonary arrest, trauma patients in need of airway control or supplemental oxygen, and those in respiratory distress or failure due to overdose, fluid in the lungs, asthma, asphyxia, or allergic reaction.

In some areas, EMT-Basics will be trained to perform endotracheal intubation of a patient. The skill is taught as an elective in Chapter 35, "Advanced Airway Management." In other areas, only EMT-Intermediates or EMT-Paramedics will perform endotracheal intubation, but EMT-Basics may be asked to assist with the

procedure. The skills of assisting with endotracheal intubation are presented below.

Preparing the Patient for Intubation

Before the paramedic inserts the endotracheal tube, you may be asked to give the patient an extra amount of oxygen. This can easily be accomplished by ventilating with a bag-valve-mask device once every 2 seconds. Then the paramedic will position the patient's head to align the mouth, pharynx, and trachea. The paramedic will remove the oral airway and pass the endotracheal tube through the mouth (sometimes through the nose) into the throat past the vocal cords and into the trachea. This procedure usually requires a laryngoscope to move the tongue and other obstructions out of the way.

In order to maneuver the tube past the vocal cords correctly, the paramedic will need to see them. You may be asked to gently press on the throat to push the vocal cords into the paramedic's view. You will do this by pressing your thumb and index finger just to either side of the medial throat over the cricoid cartilage, the ring-shaped cartilage just below the thyroid cartilage, or Adam's apple. This procedure is known as cricoid pressure, or Sellick's maneuver (Figure A–1).

Once the tube is properly placed, the cuff is inflated with air from a 10 cc syringe. While holding the tube, the paramedic assures proper tube placement by using an esophageal intubation detector device and then listens with a stethoscope for lung sounds on both sides and over the epigastrium (the area of the upper abdomen just under the xiphoid

Figure A–1 In Sellick's maneuver, press your thumb and index finger on either side of the medial throat over the cricoid cartilage.

process). If the tube has been correctly placed, there will be sounds of air entering the lungs but no sounds of air in the epigastrium. Air sounds in the epigastrium indicate that the tube has been incorrectly placed in the esophagus instead of the trachea so that air is entering the stomach instead of the lungs. The tube position must be corrected immediately by removing the tube, re-oxygenating the patient, and repeating the process of intubation.

The correctly positioned tube is anchored in place with tape or a commercially made tube restraint. The entire procedure—including the last ventilation, passing the tube, and the next ventilation—should take less than 30 seconds.

Ventilating the Tubed Patient

When asked to ventilate a tubed patient, keep in mind that very little movement can displace the endotracheal tube. Look at the gradations on the side of the tube. In the typical adult male, for example, the 22 cm mark will be at the teeth when the tube is properly placed. If the tube moves, report this to the paramedic immediately.

Warning

Be especially careful NOT to disturb the endotracheal tube. If the tube is pushed in, it will most likely enter the right mainstem bronchus, preventing oxygen from entering the patient's left lung. If the tube is pulled out, it can easily slip into the esophagus and send all the ventilations directly to the stomach, denying the patient oxygen. *This is a fatal complication if it goes unnoticed.*

Hold the tube against the patient's teeth with two fingers of one hand (Figure A–2). Use the other hand to work the bag-valve-mask unit. A patient with an endotracheal tube offers less resistance to ventilations, so you may not need two hands to work the bag. If you are ventilating a breathing patient, be sure to provide ventilations that are timed with the respiratory effort as much as possible so the patient can take full breaths. It is also possible to help the patient increase respiratory rate, if needed, by interposing extra ventilations. There are some cautions to remember:

- Pay close attention to what the ventilations feel like. Report any change in resistance. Increased resistance when ventilating with the bag-valve mask is one of the first signs of air escaping through a hole in the lungs and filling the space around the lungs, an extremely serious problem. A change in resistance can also indicate that the tube has slipped into the esophagus.

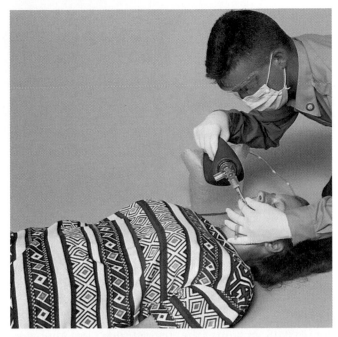

Figure A–2   Make sure the endotracheal tube does not move. Hold it with two fingers against the patient's teeth.

- With each defibrillation attempt, carefully remove the bag from the tube. If you do not, the weight of the unsupported bag may accidentally displace the tube.
- Watch for any change in the patient's mental status. A patient who becomes more alert may need to be restrained from pulling out the tube. In addition, an oral airway generally is used as a bite block (a device that prevents the patient from biting the endotracheal tube). If the patient's gag reflex returns along with increased consciousness, you may need to pull the bite block out a bit.

Finally, during a cardiac arrest in the absence of an IV line for administering medications, you may be asked to stop ventilating and remove the BVM. The paramedic may then inject a medication such as epinephrine down the tube. To increase the rate at which medication enters the blood stream through the respiratory system, you then may be asked to hyperventilate the patient for a few minutes (give ventilations at a faster-than-normal rate).

Assisting with a Trauma Intubation

Occasionally you will be asked to assist in the endotracheal intubation of a patient with a suspected cervical-spine injury. Since using the "sniffing position," which involves elevating the neck, risks worsening cervical spine injury, some modifications are necessary. Your role will change as well. You may be required to provide manual in-line stabilization during the whole procedure.

Figure A–3 To assist in the intubation of a patient with suspected cervical-spine injury, maintain manual stabilization throughout the procedure.

To accomplish this the paramedic will hold manual stabilization while you apply a cervical collar. In some EMS systems, the patient may be intubated without a cervical collar in place but with attention to manual stabilization during and after intubation. Since the paramedic must stay at the patient's head, it will be necessary for you to stabilize the head and neck from the patient's side (Figure A–3). Once you are in position, the paramedic will lean back and use the laryngoscope, which will bring the vocal cords into view. The patient can then be tubed.

After intubation, you will hold the tube against the teeth until placement is confirmed with both an esophageal intubation detector device and auscultation of both lungs and the epigastrium. Then the tube is anchored. At that time you can change your position to a more comfortable one. However, until the patient is immobilized on a long backboard, it will be necessary to assign another EMS worker to maintain manual stabilization while you ventilate the patient. Never assume that a collar provides adequate immobilization by itself. Manual stabilization must be used in addition to a collar until the head is taped in place on the backboard.

APPLYING ECG/DEFIBRILLATOR ELECTRODES

An electrocardiogram (ECG) provides data on the electrical activity of the heart. In the field, it is used to alert EMS personnel to life-threatening rhythm disturbances. Interpretation of an ECG has traditionally been a paramedic skill. However, to save time on calls you may be asked to assist. Make sure that you review the ECG equipment (Figure A–4). You should know how to turn on the monitor, how to record an ECG strip, how to change the battery, and how to change the roll of ECG paper. (These are the things

Figure A–4 An ECG monitor/defibrillator.

that most often need to be done while the paramedic is involved with the patient.)

You also may be asked to carry out four steps in the process of applying the electrodes:

1. Turn on the ECG monitor.
2. Plug in the monitoring cables or "leads."
3. Attach the monitoring cables to the electrodes.
4. Apply the electrodes to the patient's body.

Become familiar with the electrodes used by the paramedics with whom you work. There are two types: monitoring electrodes (with smaller pads) and combination monitoring/defibrillator electrodes (with larger pads). The one most commonly used by paramedics is the monitoring electrode.

If you are asked to apply monitoring electrodes to the patient's body, you will need three—each one giving a different "view" of the heart's electrical activity. First prepare the patient's skin. The best connection is on dry, bare skin, so it may be necessary to dry the area and shave excessive hair. Use a wash cloth to remove oil from the skin and consider using an antiperspirant on patients with very sweaty skin. Become familiar with the monitoring configuration (where to place the electrodes) used by ALS personnel in your system. The most common setup is placing the negative (white) electrode under the center of the right clavicle, the positive (red) electrode on the left lower chest, and the ground (black or green) electrode under the center of the left clavicle or the right lower chest (Figure A–5).

Some ALS systems have moved toward the routine use of a 12-lead ECG in the field. These machines usually provide a computerized interpretation of the patient's cardiogram that can easily be transmitted to the emergency department via cellular phone. A 12-lead ECG is used to assist in the diagnosis of an acute myocardial infarction (AMI). As the saying goes, in the case of an AMI "time is muscle."

Figure A–5 The most common positioning of electrodes for an ECG is shown here. Become familiar with the monitoring configuration used by ALS personnel in your system.

As the clock ticks, more and more heart muscle becomes dysfunctional and finally dies in the absence of oxygenated blood. With field diagnosis of AMI made possible by the 12-lead ECG, the time from MI to the administration of "clotbuster" drugs, which break up the clots causing the AMI, can be reduced.

If 12-lead ECG monitors are used in your system, ask the paramedics to review the lead placement with you as this is slightly more complex than the simple three electrodes you may be used to.

ASSISTING IN IV THERAPY

Setting Up an IV Fluid Administration Set

IV therapy is an advanced life support procedure. An intravenous (IV) line is inserted into a vein so that blood, fluids, or medications can be administered directly into the patient's circulation. A blood transfusion is almost always given at the hospital. An infusion of other fluids or medications can usually be done in the field.

The bag of fluid that feeds the IV is usually a clear plastic bag that collapses as it empties. The administration set is the clear plastic tubing that connects the fluid bag to the needle, or catheter. There are three important parts to this tubing:

- The *drip chamber* is near the fluid bag. There are two basic types: the mini drip and the macro drip. The mini drip is used when minimal flow of fluid is needed (with children, for example). Sixty small drops from the tiny metal barrel in the drip chamber equal one cubic centimeter (cc) or one milliliter (ml). The macro drip is used when a higher flow of fluid is needed (for a multi-trauma victim in shock, for example). There is no little barrel in

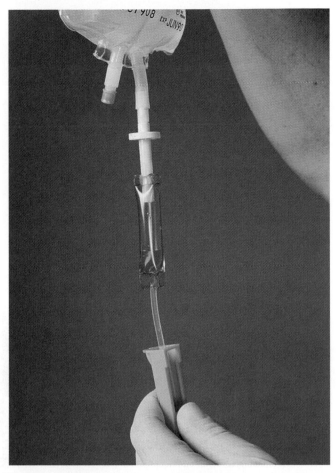

Figure A–6 Located below the drip chamber, the flow regulator is a stopcock that can be pushed up or down to start, stop, or control the rate of flow.

the drip chamber of the macro drip, and only 10 to 15 large drops equal one cc or one ml.

- The *flow regulator* is located below the drip chamber. It is a device that can be pushed up or down to start, stop, or control the rate of flow (Figure A–6).
- The *drug or needle port* is below the flow regulator. The paramedic can inject medication into this opening.

An extension set includes an extra length of tubing, which can make it easier to carry or disrobe the patient without accidentally pulling out the IV. Extension sets are sometimes not used with the macro drip set because lengthening tubing reduces the flow rate.

In most cases, a paramedic will insert the IV into the patient's vein. However, you may be enlisted to help set up the IV administration set. You will need to:

1. Take out and inspect the fluid bag. The bags come in a protective wrapping to keep them clean. If you are setting up the IV, you must remove the wrapper, then inspect the bag to be sure it contains

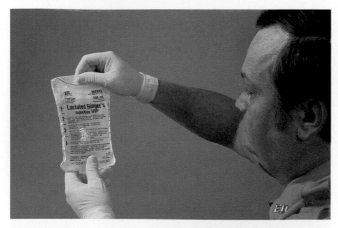

Figure A–7 Inspect the IV bag to be sure it contains the solution that was ordered, for clarity, leaks, and to be sure it has not expired.

Figure A–8 Setting up the IV administration set includes removing the protective coverings from the port of the fluid bag and the spiked end of the tubing.

the fluid that has been ordered. Check the expiration date to make sure the fluid is usable, and look to see that the fluid is clear and free of particles. Squeeze the bag to check for leaks. Occasionally, the fluid comes in a bottle. If so, be sure it is free of cracks. If anything is wrong, report the problem and inspect another bag or bottle (Figure A–7).

2. Select the proper administration set. Uncoil the tubing, and do not let the ends touch the ground.

3. Connect the extension set to the administration set, if an extension set is to be used.

4. Make sure the flow regulator is closed. To do this, roll the stopcock away from the fluid bag.

5. Remove the protective covering from the port of the fluid bag and the protective covering from the spiked end of the tubing (Figure A–8). Insert the spiked end of the tubing into the fluid bag with a quick twist. Do this carefully. *Maintain sterility. If these parts touch the ground, they must not be used. Running germs or dirt directly into a patient's bloodstream can be extremely serious, even fatal.*

6. Hold the fluid bag higher than the drip chamber. Squeeze the drip chamber a time or two to start the flow. Fill the chamber to the marker line (approximately one-third full).

7. Open the flow regulator and allow the fluid to flush all the air from the tubing. You may need to loosen the cap at the lower end to get the fluid to flow. Maintain the sterility of the tubing end and replace the cap when you are finished. Most sets can be flushed without removing the cap. Be sure that all air bubbles have been flushed from the tubing to avoid introducing a dangerous air embolism into the patient's vein.

8. Turn off the flow.

Make certain that the setup stays clean until the paramedic removes the needle and connects the IV tubing to the catheter inside the patient's vein. Occasionally, the paramedic will draw blood from the vein to obtain samples before inserting the IV. You may be asked to assist by placing the blood in sample tubes and labeling the tubes with the patient's name and any other information that your hospital requires. Remember that they are potential carriers of pathogens. Be sure to take BSI precautions. Carry the blood tubes to a safe place where they will not be in danger of breaking.

Do not be surprised if you are asked to hold up the arm for a few minutes during a cardiac arrest. During cardiac arrest, medications can be more effective if the patient's arm is temporarily raised after a drug is injected into the IV.

Maintaining an IV

An IV must continue to flow at the proper rate once it has been inserted into the patient's vein. However, a number of things may interrupt the flow. If you are charged with maintaining an IV, be sure to check for and correct the following problems:

- Flow regulator may be closed.
- Clamp may be closed on the tubing.
- Tubing may kink.
- Tubing may get caught under the patient or the backboard.
- Constricting band used to raise the vein for insertion of the needle may have been mistakenly left on the patient's arm, perhaps covered by a sleeve.
- Tubing may have pulled out of the catheter.

The position of the IV or of the patient's arm also may need to be adjusted. Some IVs only flow when the patient's arm or IV site is in a certain position. Adjusting or even splinting the arm may be helpful as long as the splint is not too tight. Since the IV flow usually depends on gravity, be sure that the bag is held well above the IV site and the patient's heart.

Insufficient flow can cause blood to clot in the catheter. This can be prevented by adjusting the flow to an adequate "keep the vein open" or KVO rate. The KVO rate varies, but it is usually about 30 drops per minute for a micro drip and 10 drops per minute for a macro drip set. If the drip chamber is overfilled, clamp the tubing, invert the drip chamber, and pump some fluid back into the bag.

An IV with a flow rate that is too fast is called a "runaway IV." It can rapidly overload the patient with fluid and cause serious problems, especially in an infant or child.

An infiltrated IV is one where the needle has either punctured the vein and exited the other side or has pulled out of the vein. In either case, the fluid is flowing into the surrounding tissues instead of into the vein. An unnoticed infiltrated IV can be very dangerous. Certain high-concentration medications (such as 50% dextrose) can cause the death of the surrounding tissue. In addition to complaining of pain, the patient will show swelling at the site (noticeable in all but some obese patients). The person in charge of maintaining the IV must stop the flow and discontinue the IV according to local protocol. If you are not authorized to do this, report the problem immediately to the paramedic or medical direction.

If you learn how to help advanced life support personnel start an IV, run through an administration set, label blood tubes, and maintain an IV, valuable time can be saved at the scene and during transport.

STRESS IN EMS

Take a minute to think about the last time you told someone that you felt "stressed out." How did you feel? Did you feel tense, as if every muscle was tight, every nerve on edge? Were your palms sweaty and your stomach in knots? Was your heart pounding and did you have a lump in your throat? Did you have trouble sleeping or always feel exhausted no matter how much sleep you had the previous night? What was going on in your life at that time? Were you preparing for a big exam? Was a family member's illness causing you to worry? Did you feel torn between the demands of family, work, and school? Were you worried about your financial state, wondering how you would cover some large unexpected expense? Were you about to change jobs or were you going through a divorce? How you manage these and other stressors is critical to your well-being.

PHYSIOLOGIC ASPECTS OF STRESS

During the Middle Ages and for much of the next two or three hundred years, people viewed the mind and body as separate entities. In the last third of the twentieth century, however, medical science began to give increasing scrutiny to how the mind and body work together and influence each other. In fact, today it would be hard to find anyone who denies that there is a connection between mind and body or that stress plays a role in illness.

Stress is a widely used term in today's society. It is derived from a word used in the 1600s (*stresse,* a variation of *distresse*), which meant acute anxiety, pain, or sorrow. Today, doctors and psychologists generally define stress as a state of physical and/or psychological arousal to a stimulus. Any stimulus is capable of being a stressor for someone, and stressors vary from individual to individual and from time to time.

Many agree that stress poses a potential hazard for EMS personnel; however, it is important to recognize that stress is a normal part of life and, when managed appropriately, does not have to pose a threat to your well-being. As an EMT-B you will be routinely exposed to stress-producing agents or situations. These stressors may be environmental factors (e.g., noise, inclement weather, unstable wreckage), your dealings with other people (e.g., unpleasant family or work relationships, abusive patients or bystanders), or your own self-image or performance expectations (e.g., worry over your expertise at specific skills or guilt over poor patient outcomes).

Ironically these stress-causing factors may be some of the same things that first attracted you to EMS, such as an atypical work environment, an unpredictable but varied work load, dealing with people in crisis, or the opportunity to work somewhat independently. How you manage these stressors is critical to your survival as an EMS provider as well as in life.

Dr. Hans Selye (a Canadian physician and educator who was born in Austria) did a great deal of research in this area and found that the body's response to stress (*general adaptation syndrome*) has three stages.

During the first stage (*alarm reaction*), your sympathetic nervous system increases its activity in what is known as the "fight or flight" syndrome. Your pupils dilate, your heart rate increases, your bronchial passages dilate. In addition, your blood sugar increases, your digestive system slows, your blood pressure rises, and blood flow to your skeletal muscles increases. At the same time, the endocrine system produces more cortisol, a hormone that influences your metabolism and your immune response. Cortisol is critical to your body's ability to adapt to and cope with stress.

In the second stage (*stage of resistance*), your body systems return to normal functioning. The physiologic effects of sympathetic nervous system stimulation and the excess cortisol are gone. You have adapted to the stimulus and it no longer produces stress for you. You are coping. Many factors contribute to your ability to cope; these include your physical and mental health, education, experiences, and support systems, such as family, friends, and coworkers.

Exhaustion, the third stage of the general adaptation syndrome, occurs when exposure to a stressor is prolonged or the stressor is particularly severe. During this stage, the physiologic effects described by Selye include what he called the stress triad: enlargement (hypertrophy) of the adrenal glands which produce adrenaline, wasting (atrophy) of lymph nodes, and bleeding gastric ulcers. At this point the individual has lost the ability to resist or adapt to the stressor and may become seriously ill as a consequence. Fortunately, most individuals do not reach this stage.

TYPES OF STRESS REACTIONS

Three types of stress reactions are commonly encountered: acute stress reactions, delayed stress reactions, and cumulative stress reactions. Any of these may occur as a result of a *critical incident,* which is any situation that triggers a strong emotional response. An *acute stress reaction* occurs simultaneously with or shortly after the critical incident. A *delayed stress reaction* (also known as *post-traumatic stress disorder*) may occur at any time, days to years, following a critical incident. A *cumulative stress reaction* (also known as *burnout*) occurs as a result of prolonged recurring stressors in our work or private lives.

Acute Stress Reaction

Acute stress reactions are often linked to catastrophes, such as a large-scale natural disaster, a plane crash, or a coworker's line-of-duty death or injury. Signs and symptoms of an acute stress reaction will develop simultaneously or within a very short time following the incident. They may involve any one or a combination of the following areas of function: physical, cognitive (the ability to think), emotional, or behavioral. These are signs that this particular situation is overwhelming your usual ability to cope and to perform effectively. It is important to keep in mind that they are ordinary reactions to extraordinary situations. They reflect the process of adapting to challenge. They are normal and are not a sign of weakness or mental illness.

Some of these signs and symptoms require immediate intervention from a physician or mental health professional, while others do not. As a rule, any sign or symptom that indicates an acute medical problem (such as chest pain, difficulty breathing, or abnormal heart rhythms) or an acute psychological problem (such as uncontrollable crying, inappropriate behavior, or a disruption in normal, rational thinking) are the kinds of problems that demand immediate corrective action. These are the same kinds of problems that alert us to a potentially dangerous situation when we see them in a patient, and they should trigger the same response when exhibited by us or our coworkers. Helping people is not just about taking care of your patient; it is also always about taking care of each other and yourself.

As previously mentioned, some signs and symptoms associated with an acute stress reaction may not require intervention. For instance, you may feel nauseated, tremulous, or numb after working a cardiopulmonary arrest, particularly if your patient is close to your age. You may feel confused or have trouble concentrating or difficulty sleeping after working at a particularly bloody crash scene or a prolonged extrication. You may find that you have no appetite for food or cannot get enough to eat. If not too severe or long-lasting, these responses are uncomfortable but probably not dangerous, since they pose no immediate threat to your health, safety, or well-being.

Remember that you are not losing your mind if you exhibit signs and symptoms of stress after a critical incident. You are merely reacting to an extraordinary situation. Remember, too, that there is nothing wrong with you if you do not experience any symptoms after such an incident. This, too, is common. In other words, a wide range of responses is normal and to be expected.

Delayed Stress Reaction

Like an acute stress reaction, a delayed stress reaction, also known as post-traumatic stress disorder (PTSD), can be triggered by a specific incident; however the signs and symptoms may not become evident until days, months, or even years later. This delay in presentation may make it harder to deal with the stress reaction since the individual has seemingly put the incident behind him and moved on with his life. Signs and symptoms may include flashbacks, nightmares, feelings of detachment, irritability, sleep difficulties, or problems with concentration or interpersonal relationships.

It is not uncommon for persons suffering from PTSD to seek solace through drug and alcohol abuse. Because of the delay and the apparent disconnect between the triggering event and the response, the victim of PTSD may not understand what is causing the problems. PTSD requires intervention by a mental health professional.

Cumulative Stress Reaction

Cumulative stress reaction, or burnout, is not triggered by a single critical incident, but instead results from sustained, recurring low-level stressors—possibly in more than one aspect of one's life—and develops over a period of years.

The earliest signs are subtle. They may present as a vague anxiety, progressing to boredom and apathy and a feeling of emotional exhaustion. If problems are not identified and managed at this point, the progression will continue. Now the individual will develop physical complaints (such as headaches or stomach ailments), significant sleep disturbances, loss of emotional control, irritability, withdrawal from others, and increasing depression. Without appropriate intervention, the person's physical, emotional, and behavioral condition will continue to deteriorate, with manifestations such as migraines, increased smoking or alcohol intake, loss of sexual drive, poor interpersonal relationships, deterioration in work performance, limited self control, and significant depression.

At its worst, cumulative stress may present as physical illness, uncontrollable emotions, overwhelming physical and emotional fatigue, severe withdrawal, paranoia, or suicidal thoughts. Long-term psychological intervention is critical at this stage if the individual is to recover.

The ultimate key to preventing or managing cumulative stress lies in seeking balance in our lives.

STRESS MANAGEMENT

How should critical incident stress reactions be managed? Dr. Jeff Mitchell of the University of Maryland developed an approach called Critical Incident Stress Debriefing (CISD) which many people have found to be helpful. Using the CISD model, an EMS system or region establishes a team of mental health professionals and peer support personnel from all components of the EMS team (dispatch, police, fire, EMS, hospital personnel) who work together to assist individuals who are experiencing acute stress reactions. CISD teams also help EMS personnel to learn to manage day-to-day job-related stress, as well as serving as an educational resource and functioning as a referral network for individuals who need longer-term intervention.

Personnel who are not mental health professionals but who wish to become peer support members of a CISD team must undergo a screening process and special training to prepare them for this role. During training, they learn about all aspects of stress as well as communication techniques, group dynamics, and facilitation skills.

CISD may take one of two forms, a defusing or a debriefing. A *defusing,* a shorter and less structured form of a debriefing (see below), is usually led by a peer support member of the CISD team and should occur within a relatively short time (1 to 4 hours) after the incident. The primary purpose of a defusing is to reduce tensions, allowing those most affected by an incident to vent their feelings, work through their initial stress, and return to duty. It should be noted that in well-run, well-led units where honest, open communication is the rule, defusings occur routinely following each call for service.

A *debriefing* is led jointly by a team of mental health professionals and peer support members. It includes all of the personnel (from dispatch to the

Figure B–1 A critical incident stress debriefing is led jointly by a team of mental health professionals and peer support members.

hospital) who were involved in a critical incident (Figure B–1). The debriefing is a formal, highly structured process which includes six phases: fact, thought, reaction, symptom, teaching, and re-entry. Each phase must be completed in order. The process is intended to reconstruct the incident and work through the associated thoughts, reactions, and symptoms. In doing so, the debriefing can help the participants to put a critical incident in perspective by talking through it and by learning about stress reactions and their management.

The work of others, such as Vicki Harris Taylor from Prince William County, Virginia, and Richard Gist from Kansas City, Missouri, suggests that while CISD may be helpful, it is even more important that organizations recognize the need to create a prevention mindset prior to incidents, adopting the viewpoint that critical incidents can be developmental and need not be pathogenic. This school of thought supports the idea that people come out of incidents just as they were going into them, which is to say that if you were already feeling overwhelmed in your life prior to an incident, you will feel more overwhelmed afterward. It recognizes that the best prevention for critical incident stress is a well-grounded life on and off duty. It focuses on developing healthy life styles, balancing our work and non-work lives, plus creating and maintaining a humane organization that is supportive of its members.

A corollary concept is that crisis is a matter of context, not content; thus it requires a proactive perspective, not a reactive one. For instance, almost every emergency situation carries with it the potential to become a critical incident if poorly managed. Conversely, many critical incidents could be avoided by implementing a sound incident command structure that is utilized routinely. Critiques should follow every call (or incident). Ideally these should be done informally, as part of the day-to-day job. This allows the veteran provider to share information and "lessons learned" with the rookie, as well as enhancing the sense, and the reality, of being a member of a team. It recognizes that in times of stress we all tend to look at our response in terms of "How am I doing compared to others?"—particularly compared to those whom we respect.

Investigation of job-related stress reveals that oftentimes it is not the job itself that is the stressor, but rather organizational and functional factors. The use of positive management practices (sensible, humane) goes a long way to alleviating job-related stress. Individuals need information that is consistent and factual. It is the responsibility of the leader to know his or her personnel and their limits. It is the responsibility of the leader to create an environment in which it is acceptable for an individual to ask for help in working through a situation without losing face.

Certainly, organizations have a role to play in stress management and prevention. There is no denying that personnel who are well-trained, well-conditioned, and well-equipped will perform their jobs effectively and efficiently. In the end, however, responsibility for stress management lies with each of us, for the organization can do only so much. Ultimately, you are responsible for yourself. Remember that you are the most important "thing" that you bring to your job. Listed below are several ways in which we can ensure our readiness to deal with and adapt effectively to stress:

- *Eat a balanced diet.* Have a diet that is high in complex carbohydrates, fruits, and vegetables. Avoid fatty foods, as well as those that have high levels of refined sugar, salt, and caffeine. Limit your intake of alcohol.
- *Exercise regularly.* Exercise is essential to physical and mental well-being. Its benefits include enhanced cardiopulmonary efficiency, decreased cholesterol levels, and improved self-esteem.
- *Stop smoking.* Nicotine is a stimulant that triggers the same chemical and physiologic effects as stress. It also depletes vitamins C and E, which can decrease your ability to cope with stress.
- *Get enough sleep.* Sleep deprivation saps your ability to meet the demands of daily life.
- *Make time for yourself.* Seek balance in your life. You have heard the saying about "all work and no play." It is true. Remember that it is important to relax. Spend time away from the job with family and friends. Get involved in hobbies or sports. Create and maintain a life off-duty.

GRIEF AND MOURNING

One of the realities about the business of EMS is that even when care is provided promptly and appropriately, some of our patients will die. It is an inescapable truth that as an EMS provider you will encounter death. To prepare yourself for that eventuality you should come to terms with your own thoughts and feelings about death and dying, for they will determine how you react toward these patients and their loved ones. This is particularly important since, in many situations, the death may be sudden and to some degree unexpected, so we may initially be the only professionals present to help the grieving family and friends.

Grief is the emotional reaction to a loss and includes the process of recovery and adjustment to the loss. Every individual reacts to loss differently and each loss is unique unto itself. As EMS providers, our job is not to judge those who are grieving, but rather to offer support as they begin the process of mourning the loss of their loved one.

Dr. Elizabeth Kübler-Ross is known for her studies of the grief process from the perspective of the dying patient and the family. She describes grief as a process of five stages: denial and isolation, anger, bargaining, depression, and acceptance. For some, the process may include a steady progression through all phases, while others may skip some phases altogether or move back and forth between the phases several times. The process may be affected by one's spiritual beliefs, education, experience, and cultural or ethnic background:

- *Denial and isolation.* The majority of individuals react to news of a terminal illness (or event) with the statement, "No! It can't be true! Not me!" Denial functions as a buffer between receiving shocking news and beginning to mobilize resources to deal with it.
- *Anger.* As denial gives way to realization of the reality of the news, "Not me" is often replaced by "Why me?" The anger is often displaced and projected onto anything and everything in the patient's path. This phase tends to be very difficult for family and caregivers to deal with since they are often unwittingly the targets of the patient's anger. However, the anger is usually more about the inequity of the situation (life ending before its time) than about some concrete action someone has taken.
- *Bargaining.* Bargaining is an attempt to negotiate one's departure, by postponing it until after some selected event, such as the birth of a grandchild or a son's wedding. This strategy is often helpful in prolonging life, at least for the short term.
- *Depression.* Once the terminally ill person can no longer deny the illness, or when the pain of the

therapy or the reality of the end is in sight, depression is common. Reactive depression is seen as patients come to terms with the results of body-modifying surgery or changes in their ability to manage their life due to their illness. Preparatory depression helps the individual prepare for the ultimate loss. It is important to remember that depression is normal. These patients may wish to talk little, if at all, as they process the events of their life and legacy.

- *Acceptance.* During this phase, the person has come to peace with impending death. The patient typically becomes withdrawn and prefers companionship without conversation. During this phase the family often needs more support than the patient does.

While we have focused this discussion of the grief process on the patient, we would be remiss if we did not remind you that this process can apply to anyone (patient, family, friends, or in fact, you the provider) who must come to terms with a loss or significant event. For instance, it is not uncommon to see similar responses in people who have been diagnosed with a life-altering illness, such as heart disease, diabetes, or multiple sclerosis, or who have been forced into a career change due to a severe injury.

When caring for a patient who is critically ill or injured, you should not be surprised if they bring up the subject of their death. This is often true even when the terminal nature of their (perhaps chronic) illness may have been intentionally kept from them, as in the case of small children. Answer their questions honestly, but kindly. Do not give false hope or lie to the patient or family members. Offer to summon clergy or other family members if they would like you to do so. You may find it easier and more appropriate to provide nonverbal communication rather than words to convey your feelings.

When you are dealing with a sudden death, it is important to remember that the survivors have not had the luxury of time to prepare for this loss. As a result, they are often overcome with a sense of unreality and helplessness. They may have feelings of guilt or rage, and the need to place blame is extremely strong. Ultimately, most survivors will cope with this event by accepting the reality of their loss, experiencing the pain of grief, and adjusting to an environment without their loved one. However, at this moment they may be overwhelmed and will rely on your professionalism and kindness to see them through.

YOUR FUTURE IN EMS

You are embarking on a rewarding and demanding career that will bring you in contact with people at moments of crisis in their life. Remember that your patients and their families are your "customers" and that they deserve your personal and professional best. Remember that it is their emergency, not yours. Treat them with kindness and respect, and in return they will provide you with a greater education than any course you might take. Remember that providing patient care is a rare and respected privilege that is based on art and science. Remember to take care of yourself too.

REFERENCES AND FURTHER READING

Bledsoe, Brian E., Robert S. Porter, and Bruce R. Shade. *Paramedic Emergency Care,* Third Edition, 110–121. Upper Saddle River, NJ: Brady Prentice Hall, 1997.

Brunacini, Alan V. *Phoenix Fire Department: The Wellness Challenge,* 1996. Presented at the Annual Leadership, Change, and Survival Conference, Big Sky, Montana, 1996.

Dernocoeur, Kate. *Streetsense: Communication, Safety and Control, Third Edition.* St. Louis: Mosby, 1996.

Doka, Kenneth J. *Living with Grief After Sudden Loss.* Hospice Foundation of America. Bristol, PA: Taylor & Foster, 1996.

Kübler-Ross, Elizabeth. *On Death and Dying.* New York: Macmillan Publishing Co., Inc., 1969.

Mitchell, Jeff, and Grady Bray. *Emergency Services Stress: Guidelines for Preserving the Health and Careers of Emergency Services Personnel.* Englewood Cliffs, NJ: Brady Regents/Prentice Hall, 1990.

Pelletier, Kenneth R. *Mind as Healer, Mind as Slayer: A Holistic Approach to Preventing Stress Disorders.* New York: Delta Book/Dell Publishing Co., Inc., 1977.

Taylor, Vickie Harris. *Critical Incident Management Development Program.* Presented at the Annual Leadership, Change, and Survival Conference, Big Sky, Montana, 1995.

Taylor, Vickie Harris. *Personal, Organizational and Agency Development: The Psychological Dimension.* Community Response Associates, 1994. Presented at the Annual Leadership, Change, and Survival Conference, Big Sky, Montana, 1994.

Thibodeau, Gary A., and Kevin T. Patton. *Anatomy and Physiology, Third Edition,* 744–755. St. Louis: Mosby-Year Book, Inc., 1996.

Wolin, Steve, Sybil Wolin, and Vickie Harris Taylor. *Qualities of a Winner.* Project Resilience, Washington, DC, 1996. Presented at the Annual Leadership, Change, and Survival Conference, Big Sky, Montana, 1996.

APPENDIX C

NATIONAL REGISTRY SKILL SHEETS

The National Registry of Emergency Medical Technicians is an organization founded in 1970, one of whose goals is to establish nationwide professional standards for EMTs. Many state EMS systems use examinations developed by the National Registry to establish certification of EMTs.

NATIONAL REGISTRY EXAMINATIONS

The National Registry has prepared a certification examination correlated to the 1994 U.S. Department of Transportation's "Emergency Medical Technician-Basic: National Standard Curriculum." The National Registry's examination includes both a written portion and a practical portion that consists of a series of performance-based skill stations.

To assist students in preparing for the skill stations that are part of the EMT-Basic examination, as well as to establish guidelines for those who will evaluate student performance at the skill stations, the National Registry has developed a series of skill sheets. Each skill sheet contains a set of directions, the skill criteria, and the critical criteria that result in immediate failure of the station.

In studying for the National Registry examination, these skill sheets should be used in conjunction with the material presented in the textbook and not as the sole means of learning the individual skills. The skill sheets will aid you in organizing the steps necessary to perform each skill and in identifying the criteria that will be used to evaluate your performance. You can use these sheets to evaluate your own performance when practicing these skills and preparing for your practical skills evaluation.

Note: Three skill sheets regarding advanced airway management are included. The use of these skills will vary based on your medical director, training program, and local protocol.

Organization of the National Registry Examination

The practical examination consists of six stations—five mandatory stations and one random basic skill station—consisting of both skill-based and scenario-based testing. The random skill station is conducted so the candidate is totally unaware of the skill to be tested until he arrives at the test site.

The candidate will be tested individually in each station and will be expected to direct the actions of any assistant EMTs who may be present in the station. The candidate should pass or fail the examination based solely on his actions and decisions.

Table C-1 on page 822 offers a list of the stations and their established time limits. The maximum time is determined by the number and difficulty of tasks to be completed. Examples of instructions that would be given to a candidate at the start of each skill station exam follow.

Instructions to the Candidate:
Patient Assessment/Management—Trauma
This station is designed to test your ability to perform a patient assessment of a victim of multi-system trauma and voice-treat all conditions and injuries discovered. You must conduct your assessment as you would in the field, including communicating with your patient. You may remove the patient's clothing down to shorts or swimsuit if you feel it is necessary. As you conduct your assessment, you should state everything you are assessing. Clinical information not obtainable by visual or physical inspection—such as blood pressure—will be given to you after you demonstrate how you would normally gain that information. You may assume that you have two EMTs working with you and that they are correctly carrying out the verbal treatments you indicate. You have (10) ten minutes to complete this skill station. Do you have any questions?

Instructions to the Candidate:
Patient Assessment/Management—Medical
This station is designed to test your ability to perform a patient assessment of a victim with a chief complaint of a medical nature and voice-treat all conditions and injuries discovered. You must conduct your assessment as you would in the field, including communicating with your patient. As you conduct your assessment, you should state everything you are assessing. Clinical information not obtainable by visual or physical inspection, for example, blood pressure, will be given to you after

819

you demonstrate how you would normally gain that information. You may assume that you have two EMTs working with you and that they are correctly carrying out the verbal treatments you indicate. You have (10) ten minutes to complete this skill station. Do you have any questions?

Instructions to the Candidate:
Cardiac Arrest Management
This station is designed to test your ability to manage a prehospital cardiac arrest by integrating CPR skills, defibrillation, airway adjuncts, and patient/scene management skills. There will be an EMT assistant in this station. The EMT assistant will only do as you instruct him. As you arrive on the scene, you will encounter a patient in cardiac arrest. A First Responder will be present performing single rescuer CPR. You must immediately establish control of the scene and begin resuscitation of the patient with an automated external defibrillator. At the appropriate time, you must control the airway and ventilate the victim using adjunctive equipment. You may not delegate this action to the EMT assistant. You may use any of the supplies available in this room. You have (15) fifteen minutes to complete this skill station. Do you have any questions?

Instructions to the Candidate:
Airway, Oxygen, Ventilation Skills—
Bag-Valve Mask for Apneic Patient with Pulse
This station is designed to test your ability to ventilate a patient using a bag-valve mask. As you enter the station, you will find an apneic patient with a palpable central pulse. There are no bystanders and artificial ventilation has not been initiated. The only patient intervention required is airway management and ventilatory support using a bag-valve mask. You must initially ventilate the patient for a minimum of 30 seconds. You will be evaluated on the appropriateness of ventilator volumes. I will inform you that a second rescuer has arrived and will instruct you that you must control the airway and the mask seal while the second rescuer provides ventilation. You may use only the equipment available in this room. Do you have any questions?

Instructions to the Candidate:
Spinal Immobilization–Supine Patient
This station is designed to test your ability to provide spinal immobilization on a patient using a long spine immobilization device. You arrive on the scene with an EMT assistant. The assistant EMT has completed the scene size-up as well as the initial and focused assessments. As you begin the station, there are no airway, breathing, or circulatory problems. You are required to treat the specific, isolated problem of an unstable spine using a long spine immobilization de-

vice. When moving the patient to the device, you should use the help of the assistant EMT and the evaluator. The assistant EMT should control the head and cervical spine of the patient while you and the evaluator move the patient to the immobilization device. You are responsible for the direction and subsequent action of the EMT assistant. You may use any equipment available in this room. You have (10) ten minutes to complete this procedure. Do you have any questions?

Instructions to the Candidate:
Spinal Immobilization Skills—Seated Patient
This station is designed to test your ability to provide spinal immobilization on a patient using a half spinal immobilization device. You arrive on the scene with an EMT assistant. The assistant EMT has completed the scene size-up, and initial and focused assessments. As you begin the station, there are no airway, breathing, or circulatory problems. You are required to treat the specific, isolated problem of an unstable spine using a half spinal immobilization device. Continued assessment of airway, breathing, and central circulation is not necessary. You are responsible for the direction and subsequent actions of the EMT assistant.

Transferring the patient to the long spine board should be accomplished verbally. You may use any equipment available in this room. You have (10) ten minutes to complete this procedure. Do you have any questions?

Instructions to the Candidate:
Immobilization Skills—Long Bone
This station is designed to test your ability to properly immobilize a closed, non-angulated long bone injury. You are required to treat only the specific, isolated injury. The scene size-up and initial assessment have been completed and during the focused assessment a closed, non-angulated injury of the _____ (radius, ulna, tibia, fibula) was detected. Ongoing assessment of the patient's airway, breathing, and central circulation is not necessary. You may use any equipment available in this room. You have (5) five minutes to complete this procedure. Do you have any questions?

Instructions to the Candidate:
Immobilization Skills—Joint Injury
This station is designed to test your ability to properly immobilize a non-complicated shoulder injury. You are required to treat only the specific, isolated injury. The scene size-up and initial assessment have been accomplished on the victim and during the focused assessment a shoulder injury was detected. Ongoing assessment of the patient's airway, breathing, and central circulation is not necessary. You may

use any equipment available in this room. You have (5) five minutes to complete this procedure. Do you have any questions?

Instructions to the Candidate:
Immobilization Skills—Traction Splinting

This station is designed to test your ability to properly immobilize a mid-shaft femur injury with a traction splint. You will have an EMT assistant to help you in the application of the device by applying manual traction when directed to do so. You are required to treat only the specific, isolated injury. The scene size-up and initial assessment have been accomplished on the victim and during the focused assessment a mid-shaft femur deformity was detected. Ongoing assessment of the patient's airway, breathing, and central circulation is not necessary. You may use any equipment available in this room. You have (10) ten minutes to complete this procedure. Do you have any questions?

Instructions to the Candidate:
Bleeding Control/Shock Management

This station is designed to test your ability to control hemorrhage. This is a scenario-based testing station. As you progress through the scenario, you will be offered various signs and symptoms appropriate for the patient's condition. You will be required to manage the patient based on these signs and symptoms. A scenario will be read aloud to you and you will be given an opportunity to ask clarifying questions about the scenario; however, you will not receive answers to any questions about the actual steps of the procedures to be performed. You may use any of the supplies and equipment available in this room. You have (10) ten minutes to complete this skill station. Do you have any questions?

Instructions to the Candidate: Airway, Oxygen, Ventilation Skills—Upper Airway Adjuncts and Suction

This station is designed to test your ability to properly measure, insert, and remove an oropharyngeal and a nasopharyngeal airway as well as suction a patient's upper airway. This is an isolated skills test comprised of three separate skills. You may use any equipment available in this room. Do you have any questions?

Instructions to the Candidate:
Airway, Oxygen, Ventilation Skills—
Mouth-to-Mask with Supplemental Oxygen

This station is designed to test your ability to ventilate a patient with supplemental oxygen using a mouth-to-mask technique. This is an isolated skills test. You may assume that mouth-to-mouth ventilation is in progress and that the patient has a central pulse. The only patient management required is ventilator support using a mouth-to-mask technique with supplemental oxygen. You must ventilate the patient for at least 30 seconds. You will be evaluated on the appropriateness of ventilatory volumes. You may use any equipment available in this room. Do you have any questions?

Instructions to the Candidate:
Airway, Oxygen, Ventilation Skills—
Supplemental Oxygen Administration

This station is designed to test your ability to correctly assemble the equipment needed to administer supplemental oxygen in the prehospital setting. This is an isolated skills test. You will be required to assemble an oxygen tank and regulator and administer oxygen to a patient using a nonrebreather mask. Because the patient cannot tolerate the mask, at this point, you will be instructed to discontinue oxygen administration by the nonrebreather mask and start oxygen administration using a nasal cannula. Once you have initiated oxygen administration using a nasal cannula, you will be instructed to discontinue oxygen administration completely. You may use only the equipment available in this room. Do you have any questions?

See Table C–1 on the next page for a list of stations and their established time limits.

TABLE C–1 Stations and Time Limit for Each One

	Stations	Time Limit
Station 1	Patient Assessment/Management—Trauma	10 min.
Station 2	Patient Assessment/Management—Medical	10 min.
Station 3	Cardiac Arrest Management/AED	15 min.
Station 4	Bag-Valve Mask—Apneic Patient	10 min.
Station 5	Spinal Immobilization Station	
	Spinal Immobilization—Supine Patient	10 min.
	Spinal Immobilization—Seated Patient	10 min.
Station 6	Random Basic Skill Verification:	
	Long Bone Injury	5 min.
	Joint Injury	5 min.
	Traction Splint	10 min.
	Bleeding Control/Shock Management	10 min.
	Upper Airway Adjuncts and Suction	5 min.
	Mouth-to-Mask with Supplemental Oxygen	5 min.
	Supplemental Oxygen Administration	5 min.

PATIENT ASSESSMENT/MANAGEMENT
TRAUMA

	Points Possible	Points Awarded
Takes or verbalizes body substance isolation precautions	1	
SCENE SIZE-UP		
Determines the scene is safe	1	
Determines the mechanism of injury	1	
Determines the number of patients	1	
Requests additional help if necessary	1	
Considers stabilization of spine	1	
INITIAL ASSESSMENT		
Verbalizes general impression of patient	1	
Determines responsiveness	1	
Determines chief complaint/apparent life threats	1	
Assesses airway and breathing — Assessment	1	
Initiates appropriate oxygen therapy	1	
Assures adequate ventilation	1	
Injury management	1	
Assesses Circulation — Assesses for and controls major bleeding	1	
Assesses pulse	1	
Assesses skin (color, temperature and condition)	1	
Identifies priority patients/makes transport decision	1	
FOCUSED HISTORY AND PHYSICAL EXAM/RAPID TRAUMA ASSESSMENT		
Selects appropriate assessment (focused or rapid assessment)	1	
Obtains or directs assistant to obtain baseline vital signs	1	
Obtains SAMPLE history	1	
DETAILED PHYSICAL EXAMINATION		
Assesses the head — Inspects and palpates the scalp and ears	1	
Assesses the eyes	1	
Assesses the facial area including oral and nasal area	1	
Assesses the neck — Inspects and palpates the neck	1	
Assesses for JVD	1	
Assesses for tracheal deviation	1	
Assesses the chest — Inspects	1	
Palpates	1	
Auscultates the chest	1	
Assesses the abdomen/pelvis — Assesses the abdomen	1	
Assesses the pelvis	1	
Verbalizes assessment of genitalia/perineum as needed	1	
Assesses the extremities — 1 point for each extremity	4	
includes inspection, palpation, and assessment of pulses, sensory and motor activities		
Assesses the posterior — Assesses thorax	1	
Assesses lumbar	1	
Manages secondary injuries and wounds appropriately		
1 point for appropriate management of secondary injury/wound	1	
Verbalizes reassessment of the vital signs	1	
TOTAL:	40	

CRITICAL CRITERIA

___ Did not take or verbalize body substance isolation precautions
___ Did not assess for spinal protection
___ Did not provide for spinal protection when indicated
___ Did not provide high concentration of oxygen
___ Did not find or manage problems associated with airway, breathing, hemorrhage or shock (hypoperfusion)
___ Does other detailed physical examination before assessing airway, breathing and circulation
___ Did not transport patient within ten (10) minute time limit

---

PATIENT ASSESSMENT/MANAGEMENT
MEDICAL

	Points Possible	Points Awarded
Takes or verbalizes body substance isolation precautions	1	
SCENE SIZE-UP		
Determines the scene is safe	1	
Determines the mechanism of injury/nature of illness	1	
Determines the number of patients	1	
Requests additional help if necessary	1	
Considers stabilization of spine	1	
INITIAL ASSESSMENT		
Verbalizes general impression of patient	1	
Determines responsiveness/level of consciousness	1	
Determines chief complaint/apparent life threats	1	
Assesses airway and breathing — Assessment	1	
Initiates appropriate oxygen therapy	1	
Assures adequate ventilation	1	
Assesses Circulation — Assesses/controls major bleeding	1	
Assesses pulse	1	
Assesses skin (color, temperature and condition)	1	
Identifies priority patients/makes transport decision	1	
FOCUSED HISTORY AND PHYSICAL EXAM/RAPID ASSESSMENT		
Signs and Symptoms (Assess history of present illness)	4	

Respiratory	Cardiac	Altered Mental Status	Allergic Reaction	Poisoning/Overdose	Environmental Emergency	Obstetrics	Behavioral
•Onset?	•Onset?	•Description of the episode	•History of allergies?	•Substance?	•Source?	•Are you pregnant?	•How do you feel?
•Provokes?	•Provokes?	•Onset?	•What were you exposed to?	•When did you ingest/become exposed?	•Environment?	•How long have you been pregnant?	•Determine suicidal tendencies
•Quality?	•Quality?	•Duration?	•How were you exposed?	•How much did you ingest?	•Duration?	•Pain or contractions?	•Is the patient a threat to self or others?
•Radiates?	•Radiates?	•Associated symptoms?	•Effects?	•Over what time period?	•Loss of consciousness?	•Bleeding or discharge?	•Is there a medical problem?
•Severity?	•Severity?	•Evidence of trauma?	•Progression?	•Interventions?	•Effects - General or local?	•Do you feel the need to push?	•Interventions?
•Time?	•Time?	•Interventions?	•Interventions?	•Estimated weight?		•Last menstrual period?	
•Interventions?	•Interventions?	•Seizures?		•Effects?		•Crowning?	
		•Fever?					

	Points Possible	Points Awarded
Allergies	1	
Medications	1	
Past medical history	1	
Last Meal	1	
Events leading to present illness (rule out trauma)	1	
Performs focused physical examination		
Assesses affected body part/system or, if indicated, completes rapid assessment	1	
Vitals (Obtains baseline vital signs)	1	
Interventions Obtains medical direction or verbalizes standing order for medication interventions and verbalizes proper additional intervention/treatment	1	
Transport (Re-evaluates transport decision)	1	
Verbalizes the consideration for completing a detailed physical examination	1	
Ongoing assessment (verbalized)		
Repeats initial assessment	1	
Repeats vital signs	1	
Repeats focused assessment regarding patient complaint or injuries	1	
Checks interventions	1	
TOTAL:	34	

CRITICAL CRITERIA

___ Did not take or verbalize body substance isolation precautions if necessary
___ Did not determine scene safety
___ Did not obtain medical direction or verbalize standing orders for medication interventions
___ Did not provide high concentration of oxygen
___ Did not evaluate and find conditions of airway, breathing, circulation
___ Did not find or manage problems associated with airway, breathing, hemorrhage or shock (hypoperfusion)
___ Did not differentiate patient's needing transportation versus continued assessment at the scene
___ Does detailed or focused history/physical examination before assessing airway, breathing and circulation
___ Did not ask questions about the present illness
___ Administered a dangerous or inappropriate intervention

BAG-VALVE-MASK APNEIC PATIENT

	Points Possible	Points Awarded
Takes or verbalizes body substance isolation precautions	1	
Voices opening the airway	1	
Voices inserting an airway adjunct	1	
Selects appropriate size mask	1	
Creates a proper mask-to-face seal	1	
Ventilates patient at no less than 800 ml volume *(The examiner must witness for at least 30 seconds)*	1	
Connects reservoir and oxygen	1	
Adjust liter flow to 15 liters/minute or greater	1	
The examiner indicates the arrival of second EMT. The second EMT is instructed to ventilate the patient while the candidate controls the mask and the airway.		
Voices re-opening the airway	1	
Creates a proper mask-to-face seal	1	
Instructs assistant to resume ventilation at proper volume per breath *(The examiner must witness for at least 30 seconds)*	1	
TOTAL:	11	

CRITICAL CRITERIA

___ Did not take or verbalize body substance isolation precautions

___ Did not immediately ventilate the patient

___ Interrupted ventilations for more than 20 seconds

___ Did not provide high concentration of oxygen

___ Did not provide or direct assistant to provide proper volume/breath *(more than 2 ventilations per minute are below 800 ml)*

___ Did not allow adequate exhalation

CARDIAC ARREST MANAGEMENT/AED

	Points Possible	Points Awarded
ASSESSMENT		
Takes or verbalizes body substances isolation precautions	1	
Briefly questions rescuer about events	1	
Directs rescuer to stop CPR	1	
Verifies absence of spontaneous pulse *(skill station examiner states "no pulse")*	1	
Turns on defibrillator power	1	
Attaches automated defibrillator to patient	1	
Ensures all individuals are standing clear of the patient	1	
Initiates analysis of rhythm	1	
Delivers shock (up to three successive shocks)	1	
Verifies absence of spontaneous pulse *(skill station examiner states "no pulse")*	1	
TRANSITION		
Directs resumption of CPR	1	
Gathers additional information on arrest event	1	
Confirms effectiveness of CPR (ventilation and compressions)	1	
INTEGRATION		
Directs insertion of a simple airway adjunct (oropharyngeal/nasopharyngeal)	1	
Directs ventilation of patient	1	
Assures high concentration of oxygen connected to the ventilatory adjunct	1	
Assures CPR continues without unnecessary/prolonged interruption	1	
Re-evaluates patient/CPR in approximately one minute	1	
Repeats defibrillator sequence	1	
TRANSPORTATION		
Verbalizes transportation of patient	1	
TOTAL:	20	

CRITICAL CRITERIA

___ Did not take or verbalize body substance isolation precautions

___ Did not evaluate the need for immediate use of the AED

___ Did not direct initiation/resumption of ventilation/compressions at appropriate times

___ Did not assure all individuals were clear of patient before delivering each shock

___ Did not operate the AED properly (inability to deliver shock)

SPINAL IMMOBILIZATION
SEATED PATIENT

	Points Possible	Points Awarded
Takes or verbalizes body substance isolation precautions	1	
Directs assistant to place/maintain head in neutral in-line position	1	
Directs assistant to maintain manual immobilization of the head	1	
Assesses motor, sensory, and distal circulation in extremities	1	
Applies appropriate size extrication collar	1	
Positions the immobilization device behind the patient	1	
Secures the device to the patient's torso	1	
Evaluates torso fixation and adjusts as necessary	1	
Evaluates and pads behind the patient's head as necessary	1	
Secures the patient's head to the device	1	
Verbalizes moving the patient to a long board	1	
Reassesses motor, sensory, and distal circulation in extremities	1	
TOTAL:	12	

CRITICAL CRITERIA

____ Did not immediately direct or take manual immobilization of the head

____ Releases or orders release of manual immobilization before it was maintained mechanically

____ Patient manipulated or moved excessively, causing potential spinal compromise

____ Device moves excessively up, down, left, or right on patient's torso.

____ Head immobilization allows for excessive movement

____ Torso fixation inhibits chest rise, resulting in respiratory compromise

____ Upon completion of immobilization, head is not in the neutral position

____ Did not reassess motor, sensory, and distal circulation after voicing immobilization to the long board

____ Immobilized head to the board before securing the torso

SPINAL IMMOBILIZATION
SUPINE PATIENT

	Points Possible	Points Awarded
Takes or verbalizes body substance isolation precautions	1	
Directs assistant to place/maintain head in neutral in-line position	1	
Directs assistant to maintain manual immobilization of the head	1	
Assesses motor, sensory, and distal circulation in extremities	1	
Applies appropriate size extrication collar	1	
Positions the immobilization device appropriately	1	
Directs movement of the patient into device without compromising the integrity of the spine	1	
Applies padding to voids between the torso and the boards as necessary	1	
Immobilizes the patient's torso to the device	1	
Evaluates the pads behind the patient's head as necessary	1	
Immobilizes the patient's head to the device	1	
Secures the patient's legs to the device	1	
Secures the patient's arms to the device	1	
Reassesses motor, sensory, and distal circulation in extremities	1	
TOTAL:	14	

CRITICAL CRITERIA

____ Did not immediately direct or take manual immobilization of the head

____ Releases or orders release of manual immobilization before it was maintained mechanically

____ Patient manipulated or moved excessively, causing potential spinal compromise

____ Patient moves excessively up, down, left, or right on the device.

____ Head immobilization allows for excessive movement

____ Upon completion of immobilization, head is not in the neutral in-line position

____ Did not reassess motor, sensory, and distal circulation after immobilization to the device

____ Immobilized head to the board before securing torso

IMMOBILIZATION SKILLS
JOINT INJURY

	Points Possible	Points Awarded
Takes or verbalizes body substance isolation precautions	1	
Directs application of manual stabilization of the injury	1	
Assesses motor, sensory, and distal circulation	1	
NOTE: The examiner acknowledges present and normal		
Selects proper splinting material	1	
Immobilizes the site of the injury	1	
Immobilizes bone above injured joint	1	
Immobilizes bone below injured joint	1	
Reassesses motor, sensory, and distal circulation	1	
NOTE: The examiner acknowledges present and normal		
TOTAL:	8	

CRITICAL CRITERIA

___ Did not support the joint so that the joint did not bear distal weight

___ Did not immobilize bone above and below injured joint

___ Did not reassess motor, sensory and distal circulation before and after splinting

IMMOBILIZATION SKILLS
LONG BONE

	Points Possible	Points Awarded
Takes or verbalizes body substance isolation precautions	1	
Directs application of manual stabilization	1	
Assesses motor, sensory, and distal circulation	1	
NOTE: The examiner acknowledges present and normal		
Measures splint	1	
Applies splint	1	
Immobilizes the joint above the injury site	1	
Immobilizes the joint below the injury site	1	
Secures the entire injured extremity	1	
Immobilizes hand/foot in the position of function	1	
Reassesses motor, sensory, and distal circulation	1	
NOTE: The examiner acknowledges present and normal		
TOTAL:	10	

CRITICAL CRITERIA

___ Grossly moves injured extremity

___ Did not immobilize adjacent joints

___ Did not assess motor, sensory, and distal circulation before and after splinting

IMMOBILIZATION SKILLS
TRACTION SPLINTING

	Points Possible	Points Awarded
Takes or verbalizes body substance isolation precautions	1	
Directs application of manual stabilization of the injured leg	1	
Directs the application of manual traction	1	
Assesses motor, sensory, and distal circulation	1	
NOTE: The examiner acknowledges present and normal.		
Prepares/adjusts splint to the proper length	1	
Positions the splint at the injured leg	1	
Applies the proximal securing device (e.g., ischial strap)	1	
Applies the distal securing device (e.g., ankle hitch)	1	
Applies mechanical traction	1	
Positions/secures the support straps	1	
Re-evaluates the proximal/distal securing devices	1	
Reassesses motor, sensory, and distal circulation	1	
NOTE: The examiner acknowledges present and normal		
NOTE: The examiner must ask candidate how he/she would prepare the patient for transportation.		
Verbalizes securing the torso to the long board to immobilize the hip	1	
Verbalizes securing the splint to the long board to prevent movement of the splint	1	
TOTAL:	14	

CRITICAL CRITERIA

___ Loss of traction at any point after it is assumed

___ Did not reassess motor, sensory, and distal circulation before and after splinting

___ The foot is excessively rotated or extended after splinting

___ Did not secure the ischial strap before taking traction

___ Final immobilization failed to support the femur or prevent rotation of the injured leg

___ Secures leg to splint before applying mechanical traction

NOTE: If the Sager splint or Kendrick Traction Device is used without elevating the patient's leg, application of manual traction is not necessary. The candidate should be awarded 1 point as if manual traction were applied.

NOTE: If the leg is elevated at all, manual traction must be applied before elevating the leg. The ankle hitch may be applied before elevating the leg and used to provide manual traction.

BLEEDING CONTROL/SHOCK MANAGEMENT

	Points Possible	Points Awarded
Takes or verbalizes body substance isolation precautions	1	
Applies direct pressure to the wound	1	
Elevates the extremity	1	
NOTE: The examiner must now inform the candidate that the wound continues to bleed.		
Applies an additional dressing to the wound	1	
NOTE: The examiner must now inform the candidate that the wound still continues to bleed. The second dressing does not control the bleeding.		
Locates and applies pressure to appropriate arterial pressure point	1	
NOTE: The examiner must now inform the candidate that the bleeding is controlled.		
Bandages the wound	1	
NOTE: The examiner must now inform the candidate that the patient is showing signs and symptoms indicative of hypoperfusion.		
Properly positions the patient	1	
Applies high concentration oxygen	1	
Initiates steps to prevent heat loss from the patient	1	
Indicates need for immediate transportation	1	
TOTAL:	10	

CRITICAL CRITERIA

___ Did not take or verbalize body substance isolation precautions.

___ Did not apply high concentration of oxygen

___ Applies tourniquet before attempting other methods of bleeding control

___ Did not control hemorrhage in a timely manner

___ Did not indicate a need for immediate transportation

MOUTH-TO-MASK WITH SUPPLEMENTAL OXYGEN

	Points Possible	Points Awarded
Takes or verbalizes body substance isolation precautions	1	
Connects one-way valve to mask	1	
Opens patient's airway or confirms patient's airway is open (manually or with adjunct)	1	
Establishes and maintains a proper mask to face seal	1	
Ventilates the patient at the proper volume and rate *(800–1200 ml per breath/10–20 breaths per minute)*	1	
Connects mask to high concentration oxygen	1	
Adjusts flow rate to 15 liters/minute or greater	1	
Continues ventilation at proper volume and rate *(800–1200 ml per breath/10–20 breaths per minute)*	1	
NOTE: The examiner must witness ventilations for at least 30 seconds.		
TOTAL:	8	

CRITICAL CRITERIA

___ Did not take or verbalize body substance isolation precautions

___ Did not adjust liter flow to 15 L/min or greater

___ Did not provide proper volume per breath *(more than 2 ventilations per minute are below 800 ml)*

___ Did not ventilate the patient at 10–20 breaths per minute

___ Did not allow for complete exhalation

AIRWAY, OXYGEN, AND VENTILATION SKILLS
UPPER AIRWAY ADJUNCTS AND SUCTION

OROPHARYNGEAL AIRWAY

	Points Possible	Points Awarded
Takes or verbalizes body substance isolation precautions	1	
Selects appropriate size airway	1	
Measures airway	1	
Inserts airway without pushing the tongue posteriorly	1	
NOTE: The examiner must advise the candidate that the patient is gagging and becoming conscious.		
Removes oropharyngeal airway	1	

SUCTION

NOTE: The examiner must advise the candidate to suction the patient's oropharynx/nasopharynx		
Turns on/prepares suction device	1	
Assures presence of mechanical suction	1	
Inserts suction tip without suction	1	
Applies suction to the oropharynx/nasopharynx	1	

NASOPHARYNGEAL AIRWAY

NOTE: The examiner must advise the candidate to insert a nasopharyngeal airway.		
Selects appropriate airway	1	
Measures airway	1	
Verbalizes lubrication of the nasal airway	1	
Fully inserts the airway with the bevel facing toward the septum	1	
TOTAL:	13	

CRITICAL CRITERIA

___ Did not take or verbalize body substance isolation precautions

___ Did not obtain a patent airway with the oropharyngeal airway

___ Did not obtain a patent airway with the nasopharyngeal airway

___ Did not demonstrate an acceptable suction technique

___ Inserts any adjunct in a manner dangerous to the patient

VENTILATORY MANAGEMENT
ENDOTRACHEAL INTUBATION

NOTE: If a candidate elects to initially ventilate with a BVM attached to a reservoir and oxygen, full credit must be awarded for steps denoted by "**" if the first ventilation is delivered within the initial 30 seconds

	Points Possible	Points Awarded
Takes or verbalizes body substance isolation precautions	1	
Opens airway manually	1	
Elevates tongue and inserts simple airway adjunct (oropharyngeal or nasopharyngeal airway)	1	
NOTE: The examiner now informs the candidate no gag reflex is present and the patient accepts the adjunct.		
**Ventilates the patient immediately using a BVM device unattached to oxygen	1	
**Hyperventilates the patient with room air	1	
NOTE: The examiner now informs the candidate that ventilation is being performed without difficulty.		
Attaches the oxygen reservoir to the BVM	1	
Attaches BVM to high-flow oxygen	1	
Ventilates the patient at the proper volume and rate (800–1200 ml per breath/10–20 breaths per minute)	1	
NOTE: After 30 seconds, the examiner auscultates and reports breath sounds are present and equal bilaterally and medical control has ordered intubation. The examiner must now take over ventilation.		
Directs assistant to hyperventilate patient	1	
Identifies/selects proper equipment for intubation	1	
Checks equipment — Checks for cuff leaks — Checks laryngoscope operation and bulb tightness	1 1	
NOTE: The examiner must remove the OPA and move out of the way when the candidate is prepared to intubate.		
Positions the head properly	1	
Inserts the laryngoscope blade while displacing the tongue	1	
Elevates the mandible with the laryngoscope	1	
Introduces the ET tube and advances it to the proper depth	1	
Inflates the cuff to the proper pressure	1	
Disconnects the syringe from the cuff inlet port	1	
Directs ventilation of the patient	1	
Confirms proper placement by auscultation bilaterally and over the epigastrium	1	
NOTE: The examiner must ask, "If you had proper placement, what would you expect to hear?"		
Secures the ET tube (may be verbalized)	1	
TOTAL:	21	

CRITICAL CRITERIA

_____ Did not take or verbalize body substance isolation precautions
_____ Did not initiate ventilations within 30 seconds after applying gloves or interrupts ventilations for greater than 30 seconds at any time
_____ Did not voice or provide high oxygen concentrations (15 L/min or greater)
_____ Did not ventilate patient at a rate of at least 10/minute
_____ Did not provide adequate volume per breath (maximum of 2 errors/minute permissible)
_____ Did not hyperventilate the patient prior to intubation
_____ Did not successfully intubate within 3 attempts
_____ Used the patient's teeth as a fulcrum
_____ Did not assure proper tube placement by auscultation bilaterally and over the epigastrium
_____ If used, the stylette extended beyond the end of the ET tube
_____ Inserts any adjunct in a manner that would be dangerous to the patient
_____ Did not disconnect syringe from cuff inlet port

OXYGEN ADMINISTRATION

	Points Possible	Points Awarded
Takes or verbalizes body substance isolation precautions	1	
Assembles regulator to tank	1	
Opens tank	1	
Checks for leaks	1	
Checks tank pressure	1	
Attaches non-rebreather mask	1	
Prefills reservoir	1	
Adjusts liter flow to 12 liters/minute or greater	1	
Applies and adjusts mask to the patient's face	1	
NOTE: The examiner must advise the candidate that the patient is not tolerating the non-rebreather mask. Medical direction has ordered you to apply a nasal cannula to the patient.		
Attaches nasal cannula to oxygen	1	
Adjusts liter flow up to 6 liters/minute or less	1	
Applies nasal cannula to the patient	1	
NOTE: The examiner must advise the candidate to discontinue oxygen therapy.		
Removes the nasal cannula	1	
Shuts off the regulator	1	
Relieves the pressure within the regulator	1	
TOTAL:	15	

CRITICAL CRITERIA

_____ Did not take or verbalize body substance isolation precautions
_____ Did not assemble the tank and regulator without leaks
_____ Did not prefill the reservoir bag
_____ Did not adjust the device to the correct liter flow for the non-rebreather mask (12 L/min or greater)
_____ Did not adjust the device to the correct liter flow for the nasal cannula (up to 6 L/min)

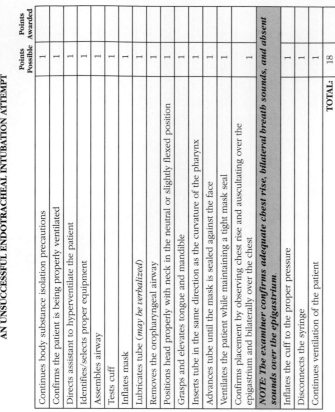

VENTILATORY MANAGEMENT
ESOPHAGEAL OBTURATOR AIRWAY INSERTION FOLLOWING AN UNSUCCESSFUL ENDOTRACHEAL INTUBATION ATTEMPT

	Points Possible	Points Awarded
Continues body substance isolation precautions	1	
Confirms the patient is being properly ventilated	1	
Directs assistant to hyperventilate the patient	1	
Identifies/selects proper equipment	1	
Assembles airway	1	
Tests cuff	1	
Inflates mask	1	
Lubricates tube (may be verbalized)	1	
Removes the oropharyngeal airway	1	
Positions head properly with neck in the neutral or slightly flexed position	1	
Grasps and elevates tongue and mandible	1	
Inserts tube in the same direction as the curvature of the pharynx	1	
Advances tube until the mask is sealed against the face	1	
Ventilates the patient while maintaining a tight mask seal	1	
Confirms placement by observing chest rise and auscultating over the epigastrium and bilaterally over the chest	1	
NOTE: The examiner confirms adequate chest rise, bilateral breath sounds, and absent sounds over the epigastrium.		
Inflates the cuff to the proper pressure	1	
Disconnects the syringe	1	
Continues ventilation of the patient	1	
TOTAL:	18	

CRITICAL CRITERIA

____ Did not take or verbalize body substance isolation precautions

____ Interrupted ventilation for more than 30 seconds

____ Did not direct hyperventilation of the patient prior to placement of the device

____ Did not assure proper placement of the device

____ Did not successfully ventilate the patient

____ Did not provide high-flow oxygen (15 L/min or greater)

____ Inserted any adjunct in a manner that would be dangerous to the patient

---

VENTILATORY MANAGEMENT
DUAL LUMEN AIRWAY DEVICE (PTL OR COMBI-TUBE) INSERTION FOLLOWING AN UNSUCCESSFUL ENDOTRACHEAL INTUBATION ATTEMPT

	Points Possible	Points Awarded
Continues body substance isolation precautions	1	
Confirms the patient is being properly ventilated with high percentage oxygen	1	
Directs assistant to hyperventilate the patient	1	
Checks/prepares airway device	1	
Lubricates distal tip of the device (may be verbalized)	1	
Removes the oropharyngeal airway	1	
Positions the head properly	1	
Performs a tongue-jaw lift	1	
Inserts airway device to proper depth	1	

COMBI-TUBE	**PTL**	
Inflates pharyngeal cuff and removes syringe	Secures strap	1
Inflates distal cuff and removes syringe	Blows into tube #1 to inflate both cuffs	1

	Points Possible	Points Awarded
Ventilates through proper first lumen	1	
Confirms placement by observing chest rise and auscultating over the epigastrium and bilaterally over the chest	1	
NOTE: The examiner states: "You do not see rise and fall of the chest and hear sounds only over the epigastrium."		
Ventilates through the alternate lumen	1	
Confirms placement by observing chest rise and auscultating over the epigastrium and bilaterally over the chest	1	
NOTE: The examiner confirms adequate chest rise, bilateral breath sounds, and absent sounds over the epigastrium		
Secures tube at appropriate step in sequence	1	
TOTAL:	16	

CRITICAL CRITERIA

____ Did not take or verbalize body substance isolation precautions.

____ Interrupts ventilation for greater than 30 seconds.

____ Did not direct hyperventilation of the patient prior to placement of the device.

____ Did not assure proper placement of the device.

____ Did not successfully ventilate patient.

____ Did not provide high flow oxygen (15 L/min or greater).

____ Inserts any adjunct in a manner that would be dangerous to the patient.

BASIC CARDIAC LIFE SUPPORT REVIEW

Before beginning your EMT-Basic course, you are required to have completed a course in cardiopulmonary resuscitation (CPR). The elements of CPR are reviewed here.

BEFORE BEGINNING RESUSCITATION

When a patient's breathing and heartbeat stop, *clinical death* occurs. This condition may be reversible through CPR and other treatments. However, when the brain cells die, *biological death* occurs. This usually happens within 10 minutes of clinical death, and it is not reversible. In fact, brain cells will begin to die after 4 to 6 minutes without fresh oxygen supplied from air breathed in and carried to the brain by circu-

lating blood. *Cardiopulmonary resuscitation (CPR)* consists of the actions you take to revive a person—or at least temporarily prevent biological death—by keeping the person's heart and lungs working.

Before you begin resuscitation (rescue breathing or CPR), you must take certain steps, including assessing the patient, activating EMS, positioning the patient, and assuring an open airway. These first steps are listed in Table BCLS–1.

Assessing the Patient

Patient assessment is crucial. Never initiate resuscitation without first establishing that the patient needs it. The required assessments are often categorized in two ways: (1) determining unresponsiveness, breathlessness, and pulselessness; and (2) assessing the ABCs (airway, breathing, and circulation). As Table BCLS–1 shows, these categories overlap.

Determining Unresponsiveness

When you encounter a patient who has collapsed, your first action is to determine unresponsiveness. Tap or gently shake the patient (being careful not to

---

TABLE BCLS–1   Basic Life Support Sequence

ABCs	Assessment	Actions	Special Considerations
	Determine unresponsiveness ("Are you okay?")	*If unresponsive:* • Activate EMS. • Position patient.	*For child/infant:* Activate EMS after 1 minute of resuscitation.
Airway	**Airway open?**	*If unresponsive, assume airway is or may become compromised.* • Open the airway.	*If no trauma, use head-tilt, chin-lift.* *If trauma suspected, use jaw thrust.*
Breathing	**Determine breathlessness** (Look, listen, feel)	*If no breathing:* • Provide 2 ventilations.	*If breathing is present:* Continue care as necessary. *If first ventilation is unsuccessful:* Reposition head and try again. *If ventilations are still unsuccessful:* Follow airway obstruction clearance procedures.
Circulation	**Determine pulselessness** Check for pulse and other signs of circulation (breathing, cough, movement)	*If no pulse:* Begin chest compressions (CPR).	*In an infant:* Feel for brachial pulse. *If pulse is present but breathing is absent:* Continue rescue breathing. *In infants and children with pulse less than 60/min and poor perfusion:* Begin chest compressions.

move a patient with possible spinal injury) and shout, "Are you okay?" The patient who is able to respond does not require resuscitation.

If the patient is unresponsive, immediately activate EMS (but if the patient is a child or an infant, activate EMS after 1 minute of resuscitation). Then position the patient and open the airway with the head-tilt, chin-lift or the jaw-thrust maneuver.

Determining Breathlessness

Determine breathlessness by the look-listen-feel method. Place your ear beside the patient's nose and mouth with your face turned toward the patient's chest. Look for chest rise and fall. Listen and feel for escape of air from the mouth or nose. The patient who is breathing adequately does not require resuscitation.

If the patient is not breathing, provide 2 ventilations (as explained later).

Determining Pulselessness

Determine pulselessness by feeling for the carotid artery in an adult or a child, by feeling for the brachial artery in an infant. Also observe the patient for breathing, movement, coughing, or other signs of circulation. The adult who has a pulse does not require chest compressions.

If the patient has a pulse but is not breathing, provide rescue breathing (artificial ventilations). If the patient is pulseless, begin CPR (ventilations and chest compressions).

Assessing the ABCs

Assessments of the ABCs are included in the steps described above. Keep the ABCs in mind throughout every patient encounter, whether or not resuscitation is underway. If the answer to any of the ABC questions is *no,* take the appropriate steps to correct the situation.

- Is the patient's *airway* open?
- Is the patient *breathing?*
- Does the patient have *circulation* of blood (a pulse)?

Activating EMS

If you have assistance, the other person should call 9-1-1 or otherwise activate the EMS system as soon as a patient collapses or is discovered in collapse. The quicker a defibrillator can reach the patient, the greater the patient's chances of survival.

If you are alone, and the patient is an adult, first determine unresponsiveness (as described earlier) and then activate EMS before returning to the patient to initiate the next steps. If the patient is a child or an infant, perform 1 minute of resuscitation before activating EMS.

The reason for the difference in timing of EMS activation is that cardiac arrest in an adult is likely to be the result of a disturbance of the heart's electrical activity that will require defibrillation; so getting defibrillation equipment to the patient takes precedence over starting CPR. Children and infants generally have healthy hearts, and cardiac arrest is likely to have resulted from respiratory arrest. In this situation, rescue breathing is more likely to be helpful in a child than in an adult, and defibrillation will not help. So 1 minute of resuscitation before activating EMS is recommended for children and infants, but immediate activation of EMS is recommended for adults.

Positioning the Patient

As soon as you have determined unresponsiveness and activated EMS, make sure that the patient is lying supine (on his back) before attempting to open the airway and assess breathing and circulation. If you find the patient in some other position, help him to the floor or stretcher. If the patient is already lying on the floor, move him onto his back. If you suspect that the patient may have been injured, you or a helper must support the patient's neck and hold the head still and in line with his spine while you are moving, assessing, and caring for him.

Opening the Airway

Most airway problems are caused by the tongue. As the head tips forward, especially when the patient is lying on his back, the tongue may slide into the airway. When the patient is unconscious, the risk of airway problems is worsened because unconsciousness causes the tongue to lose muscle tone and the muscles of the lower jaw (to which the tongue is attached) to relax.

Two procedures can help to correct the position of the tongue and thus open the airway. These procedures are the head-tilt, chin-lift maneuver and the jaw-thrust maneuver.

Head-Tilt, Chin-Lift Maneuver

The head-tilt, chin-lift maneuver (Figure BCLS–1) provides for maximum opening of the airway. It is useful on all patients who need assistance in maintaining an airway or breathing. It is one of the best methods for correcting obstructions caused by the tongue. However, since it involves changing the position of the head, the head-tilt, chin-lift maneuver should be used only on a patient who you can be quite sure has not suffered a spinal injury.

Follow these steps to perform the head-tilt, chin-lift maneuver:

1. Once the patient is supine, place one hand on the forehead and the fingertips of the other hand under the bony area at the center of the patient's lower jaw.

Figure BCLS–1   The head-tilt, chin-lift maneuver, side view. Insert show EMT's fingertips under boney area at center of patient's lower jaw.

2. Tilt the head by applying gentle pressure to the patient's forehead.

3. Use your fingertips to lift the chin and support the lower jaw. Move the jaw forward to a point where the lower teeth are almost touching the upper teeth. Do not compress the soft tissues under the lower jaw, which can press and close off the airway.

4. Do not allow the patient's mouth to close. To provide an adequate opening at the mouth, you may need to use the thumb of the hand supporting the chin to pull back the patient's lower lip. For your own safety (to prevent being bitten), do not insert your thumb into the patient's mouth.

Jaw-Thrust Maneuver

The jaw-thrust maneuver (Figure BCLS–2) is most commonly used to open the airway of an unconscious patient or one with suspected head, neck, or spinal injuries.

Note

THE JAW-THRUST MANEUVER IS THE ONLY WIDELY RECOMMENDED PROCEDURE FOR USE ON PATIENTS WITH POSSIBLE HEAD, NECK, OR SPINAL INJURIES.

Follow these steps to perform the jaw-thrust maneuver.

1. Carefully keep the patient's head, neck, and spine aligned, moving him as a unit, as you place him in the supine position.

2. Kneel at the top of the patient's head, resting your elbows on the same surface the patient is lying on.

3. Reach forward and gently place one hand on each side of the patient's lower jaw, at the angles of the jaw below the ears.

4. Stabilize the patient's head with your forearms.

5. Using your index fingers, push the angles of the patient's lower jaw forward.

6. You may need to retract the patient's lower lip with your thumb to keep the mouth open.

7. Do not tilt or rotate the patient's head. REMEMBER, THE PURPOSE OF THE JAW-THRUST MANEUVER IS TO OPEN THE AIRWAY WITHOUT MOVING THE HEAD OR NECK.

Initial Ventilations and Pulse Check

Deliver 2 slow breaths of sufficient volume to make the chest rise (Table BCLS–2). If the first breath is

Figure BCLS–2 The jaw-thrust maneuver, side view. Insert shows EMT's finger position at angle of jaw just below the ears.

unsuccessful, reposition the patient's head before attempting the second breath. If the second ventilation is unsuccessful, assume that there is a foreign-body airway obstruction and perform airway clearance techniques (as described later).

If the initial ventilations are successful, you have confirmed an open airway and should feel for a pulse. If the patient has no pulse, begin chest compressions with ventilations (as described later under CPR). If the patient has a pulse but breathing is absent or inadequate, perform rescue breathing.

RESCUE BREATHING

Mouth-to-Mask Ventilation

Mouth-to-mask ventilation is performed using a pocket face mask with one-way valve. The pocket face mask is made of soft, collapsible material and can be carried in your pocket, jacket, or purse. The steps of mouth-to-mask ventilation are illustrated in Scan BCLS–1 and summarized in Table BCLS–2.

Gastric Distention

Rescue breathing can force some air into the patient's stomach, causing the stomach to become distended. This may indicate that the airway is blocked, that there is improper head position, or that the ventilations being provided are too large or too quick to be accommodated by the lungs or the trachea. This problem is seen more frequently in infants and children but can occur with any patient.

A slight bulge is of little worry, but major distention can cause two serious problems. First, the air-filled stomach reduces lung volume by forcing the diaphragm upward. Second, *regurgitation* (the passive

TABLE BCLS–2 Rescue Breathing			
	Adult	**Child**	**Infant**
Age	8 yrs and older	1-8 yrs	birth–1 yr
Ventilation duration	2 sec	1 to 1½ sec	1 to 1½ sec
Ventilation rate	10–12 breaths/min	20 breaths/min	20 breaths/min

MOUTH-TO-MASK VENTILATION

▲**1** Position the patient and prepare to place the mask.

▲ **2** Seat the mask firmly on the patient's face.

▲ **3** Open the patient's airway and watch the chest rise as you ventilate through the one-way valve.

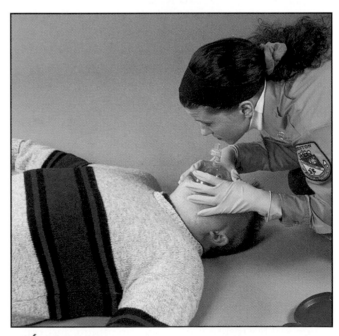

▲**4** Watch the patient's chest fall during exhalation. Ventilate the adult patient 10 to 12 times a minute, a child or infant 20 times a minute. If the pocket mask has an oxygen inlet, provide supplemental oxygen.

Figure BCLS–3   Be prepared for vomiting when attempting to relieve gastric distention.

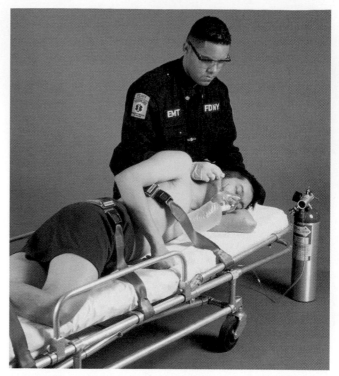

Figure BCLS–4   Place the breathing but unresponsive patient who has no head, neck, or spine injury in the recovery position (on his side) to protect the airway.

expulsion of fluids and partially digested foods from the stomach into the throat) or *vomiting* (the forceful expulsion of the stomach's contents) are strong possibilities. This could lead to additional airway obstruction or aspiration of vomitus into the patient's lungs. When this happens, lung damage can occur and a lethal form of pneumonia may develop.

The best way to avoid gastric distention, or to avoid making it worse once it develops, is to position the patient's head properly, avoid too forceful and too quickly delivered ventilations, and limit the volume of ventilations delivered. The volume delivered should be limited to the size breath that causes the chest to rise. This is why it is so important to watch the patient's chest rise as each ventilation is delivered and to feel for resistance to your breaths.

When gastric distention is present, be prepared for vomiting (Figure BCLS–3). If the patient does vomit, roll the entire patient onto his side. (Turning just the head may allow for aspiration of vomitus as well as aggravation of any possible neck injury.) Manually stabilize the head and neck of the patient as you roll him. Be prepared to clear the patient's mouth and throat of vomitus with gauze and gloved fingers. Apply suction if you are trained and equipped to do so.

Recovery Position

Patients who resume adequate breathing and pulse after rescue breathing or CPR, and who do not require immobilization for possible spinal injury, are placed in the recovery position (Figure BCLS–4). This position is also suitable for patients who are uncon-

scious, but with adequate pulse and respirations. The recovery position allows for drainage from the mouth and prevents the tongue from falling backward and causing an airway obstruction.

The patient should be rolled onto his side. This should be done moving the patient as a unit, not twisting the head, shoulders, or torso. The patient may be rolled onto either side; however, it is preferable to have the patient facing you so that monitoring and suctioning may be more easily performed.

If the patient does not have respirations that are sufficient to support life, the recovery position must not be used. The patient should be placed supine and his ventilations assisted.

CPR

Checking the Pulse

Before beginning CPR, you must confirm that the patient is pulseless. In an adult or child (not infant), check the carotid pulse (Figure BCLS–5). While stabilizing the patient's head and maintaining the proper head tilt, use your hand that is closest to the patient's neck to locate his "Adam's apple" (the prominent bulge in the front of the neck). Place the tips of your index and middle fingers directly over the midline of this structure. (Do not use your thumb. It has a pulse

Figure BCLS–5   Check the carotid pulse to confirm circulation.

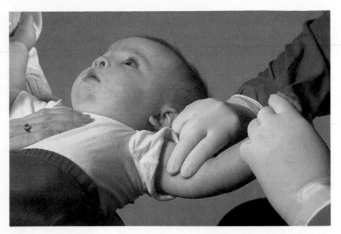

Figure BCLS–6   For infants, determine circulation by feeling for a brachial pulse.

that you may feel instead of the patient's pulse.) Slide your fingertips to the side of the patient's neck closest to you. Keep the palm side of your fingertips against the patient's neck. (*Do not* slide your fingertips to the opposite side of the patient's neck, which may cause you to put pressure on the trachea and interfere with the patient's airway.) Feel for a groove between the Adam's apple and the muscles located along the side of the neck. Very little pressure needs to be applied to the neck to feel the carotid pulse. Be sure to look for breathing, coughing, and movement as additional signs that circulation is present.

In an infant, check for a brachial pulse (Figure BCLS–6).

If the patient is pulseless, begin CPR.

How CPR Works

CPR is a method of artificial breathing and circulation. When natural heart action and breathing have stopped, we must provide an artificial means to oxygenate the blood and keep it in circulation. This is accomplished by providing *chest compressions* and *ventilations*:

- To provide *chest compressions,* place the patient supine on a hard surface and compress the chest by applying downward pressure with your hands. This action causes an increase of pressure inside the chest and possible actual compression of the heart itself, one or both of which force the blood out of the heart and into circulation. When pres-

sure is released, the heart refills with blood. The next compression sends this fresh blood into circulation and the cycle continues.

- To provide *ventilations,* use mouth-to-mask, mouth-to-mouth, mouth-to-nose, mouth-to-stoma methods, or a bag-valve-mask if you are qualified to use it. IT IS HIGHLY RECOMMENDED THAT CPR BE PERFORMED USING A POCKET FACE MASK WITH ONE-WAY VALVE OR OTHER BARRIER DEVICE AS PROTECTION AGAINST INFECTIOUS DISEASES.

Both compressions and ventilations are necessary in CPR. Compressions without ventilations would circulate blood without enough oxygen in it to sustain brain or heart function. Ventilations without compressions would force oxygen into the lungs without circulating the blood to pick up the oxygen and deliver it to the body.

 Remember

DO NOT INITIATE CPR ON ANY ADULT PATIENT WHO HAS A PULSE.

How to Perform CPR

CPR can be done by one or by two rescuers. All of the information under "Providing Chest Compressions," and "Providing Ventilations" applies to both one-rescuer and two-rescuer CPR. Specific information about each type of CPR follows under "One-Rescuer CPR" and "Two-Rescuer CPR." Scans BCLS–2 and BCLS–3 can help you follow and review these procedures as they are described below. These procedures are for an adult patient. Procedures for infants and children will be described later.

LOCATING THE CPR COMPRESSION SITE

▲ **1** Use the index and middle fingers of the hand that is closer to the patient's feet to locate the lower border of the rib cage.

▲ **2** Move your fingers along the rib cage to the point where the ribs meet the sternum, the substernal notch. Keep your middle finger at the notch and your index finger resting on the lower tip of the sternum.

▲ **3** Move your hand to the midline. Place its thumb side against the index finger of the lower hand.

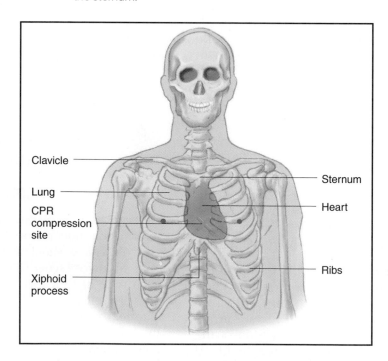

Clavicle

Sternum

Lung

Heart

CPR compression site

Xiphoid process

Ribs

Locate the compression site for CPR using the steps outlined above. This is the preferred method for professional rescuers.
Note: The American Heart Association has identified an alternative method which involves placing the heel of the hand on the sternum between the nipples. This correlates with the lower half of the sternum.

CPR SUMMARY—ADULT PATIENT

ONE RESCUER	FUNCTIONS		TWO RESCUERS
	• Establish unresponsiveness • If there's no response, call 9-1-1 • Position patient • Open airway • Look, listen, and feel (for 3–5 seconds)		
	• Deliver 2 breaths (2 sec/ ventilation). If unsuccessful, reposition head and try again. Clear airway if necessary.		
	• Check carotid pulse. . . (5–10 seconds) If no pulse. . . • Begin chest compressions		
	DELIVER COMPRESSIONS		
	1½–2 inches 100/min	1½–2 inches 100/min	
	DELIVER VENTILATIONS **10–12 breaths/min**		
	15:2	15:2	
	• Do 4 cycles • Check pulse	• Ventilator checks effective- ness	
	CONTINUE PERIODIC ASSESSMENT		

Changing Positions

• Compressor—signal to change; provide 15 compressions • Ventilator—2 ventilations	New ventilator checks pulse If no pulse, instructs compressor to begin CPR	Continue CPR sequence

NOTE: Wear gloves and use either a pocket mask with one-way valve or bag-valve mask

Providing Chest Compressions

After your hands are properly positioned on the CPR compression site:

1. Straighten your arms and lock your elbows. You must not bend the elbows when delivering or releasing compressions.

2. Make certain that your shoulders are directly over your hands (directly over the patient's sternum). This will allow you to deliver compressions straight down onto the site. Keep both of your knees on the ground or floor.

3. Deliver compressions STRAIGHT DOWN, with enough force to depress the sternum of a typical adult 1½ to 2 inches.

Note

Monitoring the depth of your compressions is one way to determine if they are adequate—the *only* way if you are working alone. Another method for determining whether your compressions are adequate is to have someone else feel for a carotid pulse while you perform compressions. When CPR compressions are being performed properly, they should produce a carotid pulse. Never try to feel for a carotid pulse during compressions if

you are by yourself; rather, perform compressions at 1½ to 2 inches until help arrives.

4. Fully release pressure on the patient's sternum, but *do not* bend your elbows and *do not* lift your hands from the sternum, which can cause you to lose correct positioning of your hands. Your movement should be from your hips, which act as a fulcrum. Compressions should be delivered in a rhythmic, not a "jabbing," fashion. THE AMOUNT OF TIME YOU SPEND COMPRESSING SHOULD BE THE SAME AS THE TIME FOR THE RELEASE. This is known as the 50:50 rule: 50% compression, 50% release.

Providing Ventilations

Ventilations are given between sets of compressions. The mouth-to-mask techniques described earlier for rescue breathing are used.

One-Rescuer CPR

Scan BCLS–3 shows the techniques of one-rescuer CPR for the adult patient.

Compressions and Ventilations: Rates and Ratios

Table BCLS–3 describes compression rates and ratios for CPR on adults, children, and infants.

TABLE BCLS–3   CPR for Adults, Children, and Infants

	Adult	**Child**	**Infant**
Age	8 yrs and older	1–8 yrs	birth–1 yr
Compression depth	1½ to 2 inches	1 to 1½ inches	½ to 1 inch (newborn approx. ⅓ the depth of the chest)
Compression rate	100/min	100/min	at least 100/min (newborn 120/min)
Each ventilation	2 seconds	1 to 1½ seconds	1 to 1½ seconds
Pulse check location	carotid artery (throat)	carotid artery (throat)	brachial artery (upper arm)
One-rescuer CPR compressions-to-ventilations ratio	15:2	5:1	5:1 (newborn 3:1)
Two-rescuer CPR compressions-to-ventilations ratio	15:2 (5:1 if patient is endotracheally intubated)	5:1	5:1 (newborn 3:1)
When working alone: Call 9-1-1 or emergency dispatcher	After establishing unresponsiveness—before beginning resuscitation	After establishing unresponsiveness and 1 minute of resuscitation	After establishing unresponsiveness and 1 minute of resuscitation

Checking for Pulse and Breathing

CPR should be carried out for approximately ONE MINUTE, or FOUR CYCLES of 15 compressions and 2 ventilations. At this point, you should check for a carotid pulse (no more than 10 seconds). At the same time, you should look, listen, and feel for breathing. If there is no pulse, return to CPR. If there is a pulse but no breathing, perform rescue breathing. If there are both pulse and breathing, move the patient into the recovery position and continue to monitor carefully, taking care to check every few minutes for a carotid pulse.

CPR should not be delayed for more than a few seconds for a pulse-and-breathing check. If CPR is continued after the first check, break to check for a carotid pulse and the return of spontaneous breathing every few minutes thereafter. After breaking for the pulse-and-breathing check, resume CPR, beginning with chest compressions rather than ventilations.

Two-Rescuer CPR

Scan BCLS–3 shows the technique of two-rescuer CPR for the adult patient.

How to Join CPR in Progress

If CPR has been started by someone who is trained to perform CPR but is not part of the EMS system, and you join this person to perform CPR:

1. Identify yourself as someone who knows CPR and ask to help.
2. Ensure that EMS has been activated.
3. Allow the first rescuer to complete a cycle of 15 compressions and 2 ventilations.
4. Check for a pulse. If there is no pulse, start one-rescuer CPR. If you tire before EMS arrives, let the other rescuer perform CPR. Alternate until EMS arrives.

If you wish to join another member of the EMS system who has initiated CPR, you should:

1. Identify yourself and your training, and state that you are ready to perform two-rescuer CPR.
2. While the first rescuer is providing compressions, spend 5 seconds checking for a carotid pulse produced by each compression. This is to determine if the compressions being delivered are effective. Inform the first rescuer if there is or is not a pulse being produced. (If the first rescuer cannot deliver effective compressions, you will have to take over for him when CPR is resumed.)
3. You should say, "Stop compressions," and check for spontaneous pulse and breathing. This should take only a few seconds.

4. If there is no pulse, you should state, "No pulse. Continue CPR."
5. The switch from one-rescuer to two-rescuer CPR should take place after the first rescuer has completed a cycle of 15 compressions and 2 ventilations.
6. The first rescuer resumes compressions, and the second rescuer provides 2 ventilations during a pause after every 15th compression. If desired, the second rescuer can start compressions and allow the first rescuer to provide the ventilations.

How to Change Positions

When two rescuers are performing CPR, one of the rescuers may wish to change positions (Scan BCLS–3). Often the compressor is the one who becomes fatigued, but the ventilator also may request a change. The most important factor in the change is that it is done in as little time as possible. The compressor controls the change and will signal the pending change at the beginning of a series of compressions as follows: "CHANGE. One and two and three and four and five, BREATHE." The ventilator will provide one full breath, and the two rescuers will quickly change positions.

The rescuer who was previously providing compressions is now the ventilator. This rescuer opens the airway immediately upon reaching the patient's head and checks for a carotid pulse and respirations. These checks should take no more than 5 seconds. If a change takes place every 2 minutes or less, a check of pulse and breathing does not need to be done on every change.

For a review of CPR for the adult patient, see the summary in Scan BCLS–3.

CPR Techniques for Children and Infants

The techniques of CPR for children and infants are essentially the same as those used for adults. However, some procedures and rates differ when the patient is a child or an infant. (If younger than 1 year of age, the patient is considered an infant. Between 1 and 8 years of age, the patient is considered a child. Over the age of 8 years, adult procedures apply to the patient. Keep in mind that the size of the patient can also be an important factor. A very small 9-year-old may have to be treated as a child.)

The techniques of CPR for an infant are shown in Scan BCLS–4. For a child, CPR is conducted as for an adult, the chief difference in procedure being the hand position—using the heel of one hand—for chest compressions (Figure BCLS–7). To compare adult, child, and infant CPR, review Table BCLS–3.

INFANT CPR

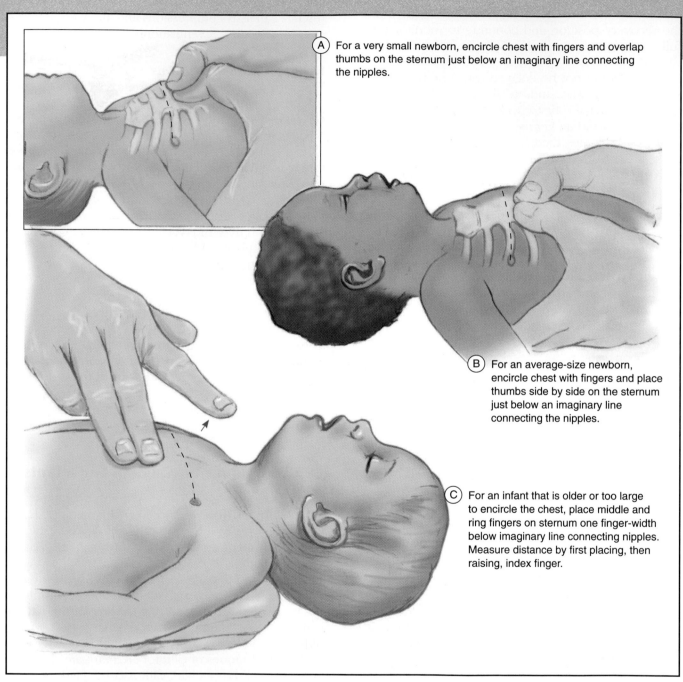

A For a very small newborn, encircle chest with fingers and overlap thumbs on the sternum just below an imaginary line connecting the nipples.

B For an average-size newborn, encircle chest with fingers and place thumbs side by side on the sternum just below an imaginary line connecting the nipples.

C For an infant that is older or too large to encircle the chest, place middle and ring fingers on sternum one finger-width below imaginary line connecting nipples. Measure distance by first placing, then raising, index finger.

Position fingers for chest compressions according to the age and size of the infant. The two thumb–encircling hands method is preferred when two rescuers are present.

Figure BCLS-7 Performing chest compressions on a child

Positioning the Patient

When CPR must be performed, adults, children, and infants are placed on their backs on a hard surface. For an infant, the hard surface can be the rescuer's hand or forearm.

Opening the Airway

For an infant or a child, use the head-tilt, chin-lift or the jaw-thrust maneuver, but apply only a slight tilt for an infant. Too great a tilt may close off the infant's airway; however, make certain that the opening is adequate (note chest rise during ventilation). Always be sure to support an infant's head.

Establishing a Pulse

Take these steps to establish a pulse in an infant or a child:

*   INFANT. For infants, you should use the brachial pulse.
*   CHILD. Determine circulation in the same manner as for an adult.

Special Considerations in CPR

How to Know if CPR Is Effective

To determine if CPR is effective, *if possible have someone else feel for a carotid pulse* during compressions and watch to see the patient's chest rise during ventilations. *Listen for exhalation of air,* either naturally or during compressions, as additional verification that air has entered the lungs.

In addition, any of the following indications of effective CPR may be noticed:

*   Pupils constrict.
*   Skin color improves.
*   Heartbeat returns spontaneously.
*   Spontaneous, gasping respirations are made.
*   Arms and legs move.
*   Swallowing is attempted.
*   Consciousness returns.

Interrupting CPR

Once you begin CPR, you may interrupt the process for no more than a few seconds to check for pulse and breathing or to reposition yourself and the patient. The first recommended pulse and breathing check is after the first minute of CPR. You should continue to check for these vital signs every few minutes.

In addition to these built-in interruptions, you may interrupt CPR to:

*   Move a patient onto a stretcher.
*   Move a patient down a flight of stairs or through a narrow doorway or hallway.
*   Move a patient on or off the ambulance.
*   Suction to clear vomitus or airway obstructions.
*   Allow for defibrillation or advanced cardiac life support measures to be initiated.

When CPR is resumed, begin with chest compressions rather than with ventilations.

When Not to Begin or to Terminate CPR

As discussed earlier in this chapter, CPR should not be initiated when you find that the patient—even though unresponsive and perhaps not breathing—does have a pulse. Usually, of course, you will perform CPR when the patient has no pulse. However, there are special circumstances in which CPR should not be initiated *even though the patient has no pulse:*

*   *Obvious mortal wounds.* These include decapitation, incineration, a severed body, and injuries that are so extensive that CPR cannot be effectively performed (e.g., severe crush injuries to the head, neck, and chest).
*   *Rigor mortis.* This is the stiffening of the body and its limbs that occurs after death, usually within 4 to 10 hours.
*   *Obvious decomposition.*
*   *A line of lividity.* Lividity is a red or purple skin discoloration that occurs when gravity causes the

blood to sink to the lowest parts of the body and collect there. Lividity usually indicates that the patient has been dead for more than 15 minutes unless the patient has been exposed to cold temperatures. Using lividity as a sign requires special training.

- *Stillbirth.* CPR should not be initiated for a stillborn infant who has died hours prior to birth. This infant may be recognized by blisters on the skin, a very soft head, and a strong disagreeable odor.

In all cases, if you are in doubt, seek a physician's advice. Once you have started CPR, you must continue to provide CPR until:

- Spontaneous circulation occurs . . . then provide rescue breathing as needed.
- Spontaneous circulation and breathing occur.
- Another trained rescuer can take over for you.
- You turn care of the patient over to a person with a higher level of training.
- You are too exhausted to continue.
- You receive a "no CPR" order from a physician or other authority per local protocols.

If you turn the patient over to another rescuer, this person must be trained in basic cardiac life support.

CLEARING AIRWAY OBSTRUCTIONS

Not every airway problem is caused by the tongue (the situation in which you would use the head-tilt, chin-lift maneuver or the jaw-thrust maneuver, described earlier, to open the airway). The airway can also be blocked by foreign objects or materials. These can include pieces of food, ice, toys, or vomitus. This problem is often seen with children and with patients who have abused alcohol or other drugs. It also happens when an injured person's airway becomes blocked by blood or broken teeth or dentures or when a person chokes on food.

Airway obstructions are either partial or complete. Partial and complete obstructions have different characteristics that may be noted during assessment, and each type has a different procedure of care. It is important to understand the differences between partial and complete obstruction and the correct care for each.

Partial Airway Obstruction

A conscious patient trying to indicate an airway problem will usually point to his mouth or hold his neck. Many do this even when a partial obstruction does not prevent speech. Ask the patient if he is choking, or ask if he can speak or cough. If he can, then the obstruction is partial.

For the conscious patient with an apparent partial airway obstruction, have him cough. A strong and forceful cough indicates he is exchanging enough air. Continue to encourage the patient to cough in the hope that such action will dislodge and expel the foreign object. *Do not* interfere with the patient's efforts to clear the partial obstruction by means of forceful coughing.

In cases where the patient has an apparent partial airway obstruction but he cannot cough or has a very weak cough, or the patient is blue or gray or shows other signs of poor air exchange, treat the patient as if there is a complete airway obstruction, as described below.

Complete Airway Obstruction

Be alert for signs of a complete airway obstruction in the conscious or unconscious patient:

- *The conscious patient* with a complete airway obstruction will try to speak but will not be able to. He will also not be able to breathe or cough. Usually, he will display the distress signal for choking by clutching the neck between thumb and fingers.
- *The unconscious patient* with a complete airway obstruction will be in respiratory arrest. When ventilation attempts are unsuccessful, it becomes apparent that there is an obstruction.

Procedures for Clearing the Airway

When you have determined that the airway is obstructed, you must take appropriate measures to clear it:

1. Open the airway. Since so many obstructions are caused by the tongue, you must first try to open the airway by using a head-tilt, chin-lift or a jaw-thrust maneuver.

2. If the patient is unconscious and not breathing, attempt to provide ventilations (rescue breathing). If the first ventilation is unsuccessful, re-adjust head position and attempt another ventilation. If still unsuccessful, then assume that there is foreign matter in the airway that must be cleared. *If the patient is conscious and indicating that he is choking, do not attempt artificial ventilations, but instead move right to step 3.*

3. Remove any foreign object. If the patient is choking or, for the unconscious patient (if you have already opened the airway and unsuccessfully tried ventilation), two techniques are recommended for removal of a foreign object:

- Manual thrusts (abdominal or chest thrusts)
- Finger sweeps

On any given patient, you may have to use both manual thrusts and finger sweeps.

Abdominal Thrusts. The use of abdominal thrusts (the Heimlich maneuver) to clear a foreign body from the airway of an adult or child (not infant) patient is shown in Scan BCLS–5, and described on the following page.

CLEARING THE AIRWAY—ADULT

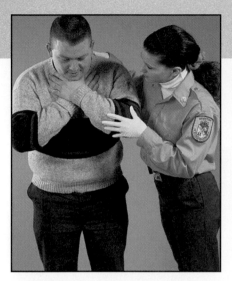

▲ **1** Recognize and assess for choking.

▲ **2** Position yourself to perform the Heimlich maneuver.

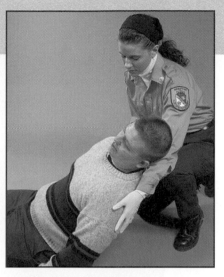

▲ **3** If the patient becomes weak or unconscious, assist him to the floor. If you are working alone, activate the EMS system.

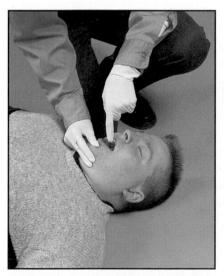

▲ **4** Do a tongue-jaw lift and a finger sweep.

▲ **5** Attempt to ventilate. If this fails, reposition head and try again. If you are not successful . . .

▲ **6** Perform the Heimlich maneuver. Repeat steps 4 through 6 if necessary.

Figure BCLS–8 The chest thrust applied to a pregnant patient

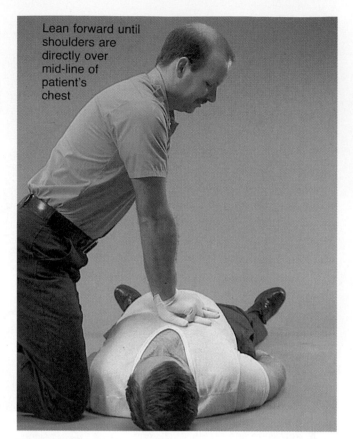

Lean forward until shoulders are directly over mid-line of patient's chest

Figure BCLS–9 The chest thrust applied to a supine patient

For the conscious adult or child (not infant) who is standing or sitting

1. Make a fist, and place the thumb side of this fist against the midline of the patient's abdomen between waist and rib cage. Avoid touching the chest, especially the area immediately below the sternum.

2. Grasp your properly positioned fist with your other hand and apply pressure inward and up toward the patient's head in a smooth, quick movement. Deliver 5 rapid thrusts.

For the unconscious adult or child (not infant) or for a conscious patient who cannot sit or stand, or if you are too short to reach around the patient to deliver thrusts

1. Place the patient in a supine position.

2. Kneel and straddle the patient at the level of the thighs, facing his chest.

3. Place the heel of your hand on the midline of his abdomen, slightly above the navel and well below the sternum.

4. Now place your free hand over the positioned hand, shoulders directly over the patient's abdomen. Be sure that you are positioned over the midline so that thrusts will be delivered straight up, not off to one side.

5. Deliver 5 rapid thrusts by pressing your hands inward and upward toward the patient's diaphragm.

If the obstruction is not relieved after a series of 5 thrusts, reassess your position and the patient's airway (if the patient is unconscious, also attempt finger sweeps to attempt to remove the obstruction). Attempt to ventilate the patient and, if unsuccessful, repeat the series of thrusts. Repeat the sequence until the obstruction is relieved.

Chest Thrusts. Chest thrusts are used in place of abdominal thrusts when the patient is in the late stages of pregnancy, or when the patient is too obese for abdominal thrusts to be effective. The use of chest thrusts to relieve an airway obstruction is shown in Figures BCLS–8 and BCLS–9 and described below.

For the conscious adult who is standing or sitting

1. Position yourself behind the patient and slide your arms under his armpits, so that you encircle his chest.

2. Form a fist with one hand, and place the thumb side of this fist on the midline of the sternum about 2 to 3 finger widths above the xiphoid process. This places your fist on the lower half of the sternum but not in contact with the edge of the rib cage.

TABLE BCLS–4 Airway Clearance Sequences

	Adult	Child	Infant
Age	8 yrs and older	1–8 yrs	Birth–1 yr
Conscious	Ask, "Are you choking?" Heimlich maneuver until obstruction is relieved or patient loses consciousness	Ask, "Are you choking?" Heimlich maneuver until obstruction is relieved or patient loses consciousness	Observe signs of choking (small objects or food, wheezing, agitation, blue color, not breathing). Series of: 5 back blows and 5 chest thrusts
Loses consciousness during procedure	Assist patient to floor. Establish unresponsiveness (ask, "Are you OK?") If alone, call for help, then . . . Open airway. Perform finger sweeps. Attempt to ventilate. If unsuccessful, reposition head and attempt to ventilate again. If unsuccessful, perform Heimlich maneuver. (Repeat as needed.)	Assist patient to floor. Establish unresponsiveness (ask, "Are you OK?") Open airway. Remove visible objects (NO blind sweeps). Attempt to ventilate. If unsuccessful, reposition head and attempt to ventilate again. If unsuccessful, perform Heimlich maneuver. (Repeat as needed.) After 1 minute, call for help if alone.	Establish unresponsiveness (tap or speak loudly). Open airway. Remove visible objects. (NO blind sweeps). Attempt to ventilate. If unsuccessful, reposition head and attempt to ventilate again. If unsuccessful, perform back blows and chest thrusts. (Repeat as needed.) After 1 minute, call for help if alone.
Unconscious when found	Establish unresponsiveness. If alone, call for help, then . . . Open airway. Attempt to ventilate. If unsuccessful, reposition head and attempt to ventilate again. If unsuccessful, Heimlich maneuver, finger sweeps. (Repeat as needed.)	Establish unresponsiveness. Open airway. Attempt to ventilate. If unsuccessful, reposition head and attempt to ventilate again. If unsuccessful, Heimlich maneuver. Remove visible objects (NO blind sweeps). (Repeat as needed.) After 1 minute, call for help if alone.	Establish unresponsiveness. Open airway. Attempt to ventilate. If unsuccessful, reposition head and attempt to ventilate again. If unsuccessful, back blows and chest thrusts. Remove visible objects (NO blind sweeps). (Repeat as needed.) After 1 minute, call for help if alone.

3. Grasp the fist with your other hand and deliver 5 chest thrusts directly backward toward the spine.

For the unconscious adult

1. Place the patient in a supine position.
2. Perform 5 chest thrusts as you would for CPR.

If the obstruction is not relieved after a series of 5 thrusts, reassess your position and the patient's airway (if the patient is unconscious, also attempt finger sweeps to attempt to remove the obstruction). Attempt to ventilate the patient and, if unsuccessful, repeat the series of thrusts. Repeat the sequence until the obstruction is relieved.

Airway Clearance Sequences. Table BCLS–4 lists sequences of procedures to use in the event of a complete airway obstruction or a partial airway obstruction with poor air exchange. Note that, as discussed earlier, you should activate the EMS system as soon as unresponsiveness is determined, before carrying out the remainder of the airway clearance procedures.

Airway clearance procedures are considered to have been effective if any of the following happens:

- Patient re-establishes good air exchange or spontaneous breathing.
- Foreign object is expelled from the mouth.

- Foreign object is expelled into the mouth where it can be removed by the rescuer.
- Unconscious patient regains consciousness.
- Patient's skin color improves.

If a person has only a partial airway obstruction and is still able to speak and cough forcefully, do not interfere with his attempts to expel the foreign body. Carefully watch him, however, so that you can immediately provide help if this partial obstruction becomes a complete one.

Procedures for a Child or an Infant

The procedure for clearing a foreign body from the airway of a child is very similar to that used for an adult. The airway clearance procedure for an infant uses a combination of back blows and chest compressions as shown in Scan BCLS–6.

For both a child and an infant, two major differences from adult procedures are:

- If the child or infant becomes unconscious, send someone else to activate the EMS system. If no one else is available, wait until you have either relieved the obstruction or you have attempted the airway obstruction sequence for 1 minute.
- Do not perform blind finger sweeps. Instead, look in the mouth and perform a finger sweep only if you see a foreign body.

Note

As an EMT-Basic you will be trained as a "professional rescuer" in CPR. The training you will receive will be more in-depth than a lay rescuer or bystander would receive. The course for people who wish to learn CPR and have no medical background differs from the training you receive in the following ways:

- Lay rescuers are not trained to check for a pulse before beginning compressions in CPR. If the patient is not breathing and does not otherwise respond (breathing, coughing, or movement), it is acceptable for the lay rescuer to begin compressions.
- Lay rescuers who are treating an unresponsive person with a foreign body airway obstruction will perform CPR compressions instead of abdominal thrusts.
- As an EMT you will be taught additional techniques that are not taught to lay rescuers, such as the two thumb–encircling hands technique for two-rescuer compression on infants.

It is possible for you to come upon a bystander performing CPR and see some of these differences in practice. If you ask the bystander "Does the patient have a pulse?" they might not have checked, nor were they required to do so.

Remember that performing CPR is quite stressful for the bystander. In many cases this CPR will be performed by one family member on another. It is important to be supportive and use a non-judgmental tone about the efforts taken by the bystander.

CLEARING THE AIRWAY—INFANT

▲ **1** Recognize and assess for choking. Look for breathing difficulty, ineffective cough, and lack of strong cry.

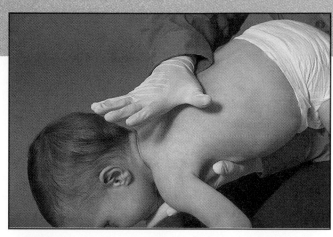

▲ **2** Give up to 5 back blows and . . .

▲ **3** 5 chest thrusts.

▲ **4** If the infant becomes unresponsive, perform a tongue-jaw lift and look for a foreign body. If you see one, use a finger sweep to remove it. (Never do blind finger sweeps in an infant or child.) Attempt to ventilate. If this fails, reposition the head and try again. If you are not successful, repeat the sequence shown above. If you are working alone, after 1 minute activate the EMS system and continue airway clearance and ventilation efforts. Transport as quickly as possible.

NOTE: For realism, the photo sequence above shows airway clearance procedures being performed on a real baby. The baby is awake. In practice, of course, a baby with an airway obstruction is likely to be unresponsive.

REFERENCE SECTION

MUSCULOSKELETAL SYSTEM

Skeleton

The skeleton is a living framework made by the joining of bones. It serves to provide support, body movement powered by muscular contractions, protection for the vital organs and other soft structures, blood cell production, and storage for essential minerals. There are 206 bones in the adult body, forming the two divisions of the skeletal system. The axial skeleton is comprised of skull, vertebrae, rib cage, and sternum. The upper and lower extremities and the shoulder and pelvic girdles form the appendicular skeleton.

Skull (Cranium)
Orbit (Eye Socket)
Zygomatic Bone
Cervical Vertebra (Neck)
Sternum (Breast Bone)
Xiphoid Process
Costal Cartilage
Lumbar Vertebra
Iliac Crest
Ilium (Hip)
Pelvic Girdle
Greater Trochanter
Lesser Trochanter
Symphysis Pubis

Frontal Bone
Parietal Bone
Occipital Bone
Temporal Bone
Temporomandibular Joint
Maxilla
Mandible
Acromioclavicular Joint
Glenohumeral Joint
Scapula (Shoulder Blade)
Ribs
Humerus (Arm Bone)
Elbow
Forearm
Ulna
Radius
Sacrum

Clavicle (Collarbone)

Ischium
Coccyx (Tail Bone)
Carpals (Wrist)
Metacarpals (Hand)
Phalanges (Fingers)
Femur (Thigh Bone)
Patella (Knee Cap)
Lower Leg Bones
Tibia
Fibula

Tarsals (Ankle)
Metatarsals (Foot)
Phalanges (Toes)
Calcaneus (Heel)

The Skeleton
- Axial
- Appendicular

The Vertebral Column (Spine)

Atlas
Axis

Cervical
Thoracic
Lumbar

Sacrum

Small Intestine

Duodenum
Ascending Colon
Cecum

Descending Colon
Jejunum
Ileum

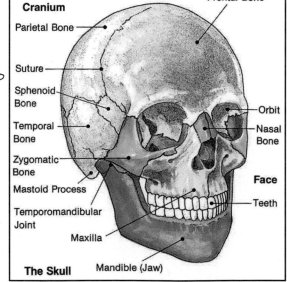

Cranium

Parietal Bone
Suture
Sphenoid Bone
Temporal Bone
Zygomatic Bone
Mastoid Process
Temporomandibular Joint
Maxilla

Frontal Bone
Orbit
Nasal Bone
Face
Teeth
Mandible (Jaw)

The Skull

Muscles

The tissues of the muscular system comprise 40% to 50% of the body's weight. The skeletal muscles of the body are voluntary muscles, subject to conscious control. They exhibit the properties of excitability; that is, they will react to nerve stimulus. Once stimulated, skeleton muscles are quick to contract and can relax and very quickly be ready for another contraction. There are 501 separate skeletal muscles that provide contractions for movement, coordinated support for posture, and heat production. Muscles connect to bones by way of tendons.

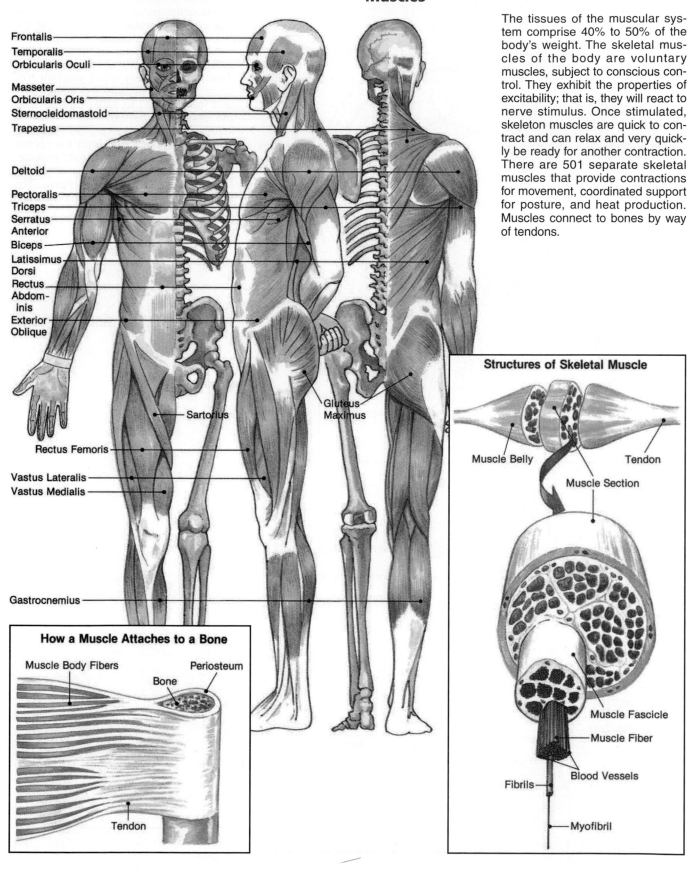

Frontalis
Temporalis
Orbicularis Oculi
Masseter
Orbicularis Oris
Sternocleidomastoid
Trapezius
Deltoid
Pectoralis
Triceps
Serratus Anterior
Biceps
Latissimus Dorsi
Rectus Abdominis
Exterior Oblique
Sartorius
Rectus Femoris
Vastus Lateralis
Vastus Medialis
Gastrocnemius
Gluteus Maximus

Structures of Skeletal Muscle

Muscle Belly
Tendon
Muscle Section
Muscle Fascicle
Muscle Fiber
Blood Vessels
Fibrils
Myofibril

How a Muscle Attaches to a Bone

Muscle Body Fibers
Periosteum
Bone
Tendon

NERVOUS SYSTEM

Brain and Spine

The Brain

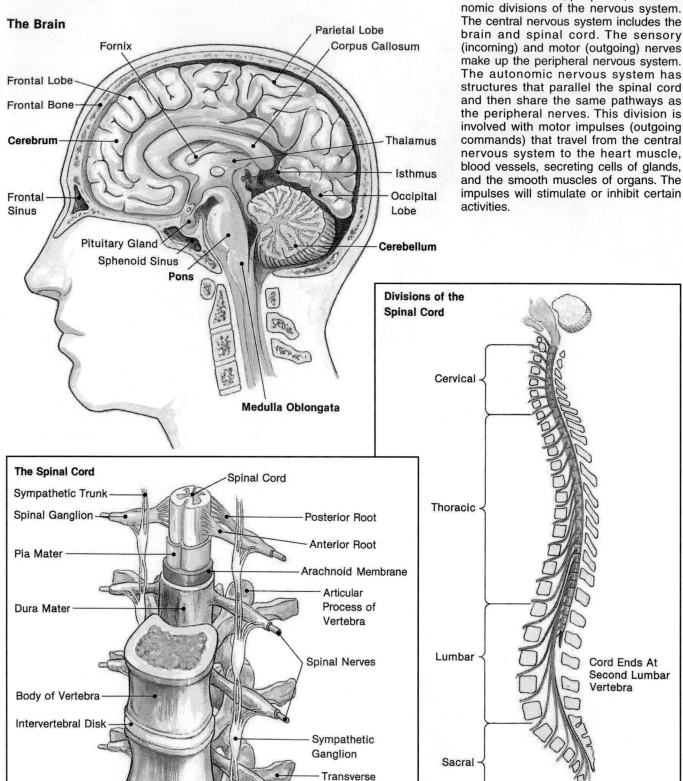

Fornix

Parietal Lobe

Corpus Callosum

Frontal Lobe

Frontal Bone

Cerebrum

Thalamus

Isthmus

Frontal Sinus

Occipital Lobe

Pituitary Gland

Sphenoid Sinus

Pons

Cerebellum

Medulla Oblongata

The Spinal Cord

Sympathetic Trunk

Spinal Ganglion

Pia Mater

Dura Mater

Body of Vertebra

Intervertebral Disk

Spinal Cord

Posterior Root

Anterior Root

Arachnoid Membrane

Articular Process of Vertebra

Spinal Nerves

Sympathetic Ganglion

Transverse Process of Vertebra

Divisions of the Spinal Cord

Cervical

Thoracic

Lumbar

Sacral

Cord Ends At Second Lumbar Vertebra

Coccyx

The nervous system includes the brain, spinal cord, and nerves. Structures within the system may be classified according to divisions: central, peripheral, and autonomic divisions of the nervous system. The central nervous system includes the brain and spinal cord. The sensory (incoming) and motor (outgoing) nerves make up the peripheral nervous system. The autonomic nervous system has structures that parallel the spinal cord and then share the same pathways as the peripheral nerves. This division is involved with motor impulses (outgoing commands) that travel from the central nervous system to the heart muscle, blood vessels, secreting cells of glands, and the smooth muscles of organs. The impulses will stimulate or inhibit certain activities.

NERVOUS SYSTEM

Nerves

- Brain (in Cranial Cavity)
- Brachial Plexus
- Axillary
- Ulnar
- Musculo Cutaneous
- Radial
- Median
- Phrenic
- Spinal Cord (in Spinal Cavity)
- Lateral Femoral Cutaneous
- Femoral
- Sciatic
- Common Peroneal
- Superficial Peroneal
- Deep Peroneal
- Tibial
- Saphenous
- Sural

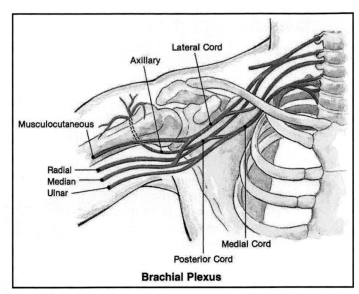

- Lateral Cord
- Axillary
- Musculocutaneous
- Radial
- Median
- Ulnar
- Medial Cord
- Posterior Cord

Brachial Plexus

Autonomic Nervous System

The autonomic nervous system affects the heart, blood vessels, digestive tract, salivary and digestive glands, pancreas, liver, spleen, anal sphincter, kidneys, urinary bladder, urinary sphincter, adrenal glands, thyroid gland, gonads, genitalia, nasal lining, larynx, bronchi, lungs, iris and ciliary muscles of the eyes, tear glands, and hair muscles. Impulses can increase or slow heart rate, stimulate dilation or constriction of blood vessels, cause glands to secrete or decrease secretion, initiate or inhibit contractions in the bladder, stimulate or decrease a wave of muscle contraction along the digestive tract, and many other essential body activities.

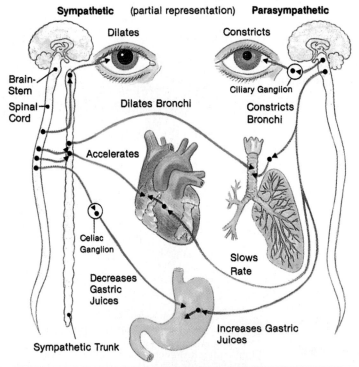

Sympathetic (partial representation) **Parasympathetic**

- Dilates
- Constricts
- Brain-Stem
- Spinal Cord
- Ciliary Ganglion
- Dilates Bronchi
- Constricts Bronchi
- Accelerates
- Celiac Ganglion
- Slows Rate
- Decreases Gastric Juices
- Increases Gastric Juices
- Sympathetic Trunk

CARDIOVASCULAR SYSTEM

Heart

The heart is a hollow, muscular organ that pumps 450 million pints of blood in the average lifetime. Its superior chambers, the atria, receive blood. Both atria fill and then contract at the same time. The inferior chambers are the ventricles. They pump blood out of the heart. Both ventricles fill and then contract at the same time. When the atria are relaxing, the ventricles are contracting.

The right side of the heart receives blood from the body and sends it to the lungs (pulmonic circulation). The heart's left side receives oxygenated blood from the lungs and sends it out to the body (systemic circulation).

The heartbeat originates at the sinoatrial note (pacemaker) and spreads across the atria to stimulate contraction. After a slight delay, the impulse is sent from the atrioventricular node, down the bundles of His, and out across the ventricles. This stimulates the ventricles to contract while the atria are relaxing.

The heart muscle (myocardium) receives its blood supply by way of the right and left coronary arteries. These vessels are the first branches of the aorta.

From Body
Superior Vena Cava

Aorta

To Lung
Right Pulmonary Artery (Branches)

To Lung
Left Pulmonary Artery (Branches)

Pulmonary Valve

From Lung
Left Pulmonary Vein (Branches)

From Lung
Right Pulmonary Vein (Branches)

Left Atrium

Aortic Valve

Mitral Valve

Right Atrium

Coronary Sinus

Tricuspid Valve

Left Ventricle

Right Ventricle

Interventricular Septum

Epicardium (Outer Layer)

Myocardium (Heart Muscle)

Inferior Vena Cava

Apex

Descending Aorta

From Body

To Body

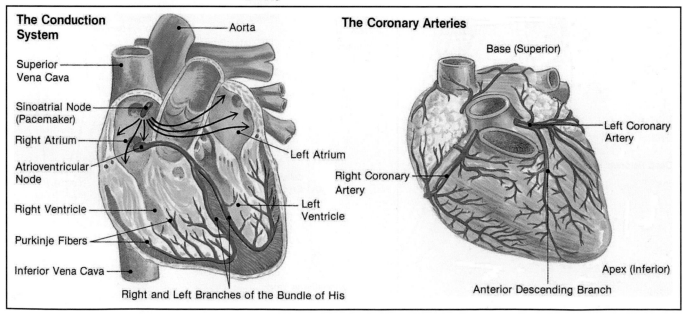

The Conduction System

Aorta

Superior Vena Cava

Sinoatrial Node (Pacemaker)

Right Atrium

Atrioventricular Node

Right Ventricle

Purkinje Fibers

Inferior Vena Cava

Left Atrium

Left Ventricle

Right and Left Branches of the Bundle of His

The Coronary Arteries

Base (Superior)

Left Coronary Artery

Right Coronary Artery

Apex (Inferior)

Anterior Descending Branch

CIRCULATORY SYSTEM
Blood Vessels

Major Arteries

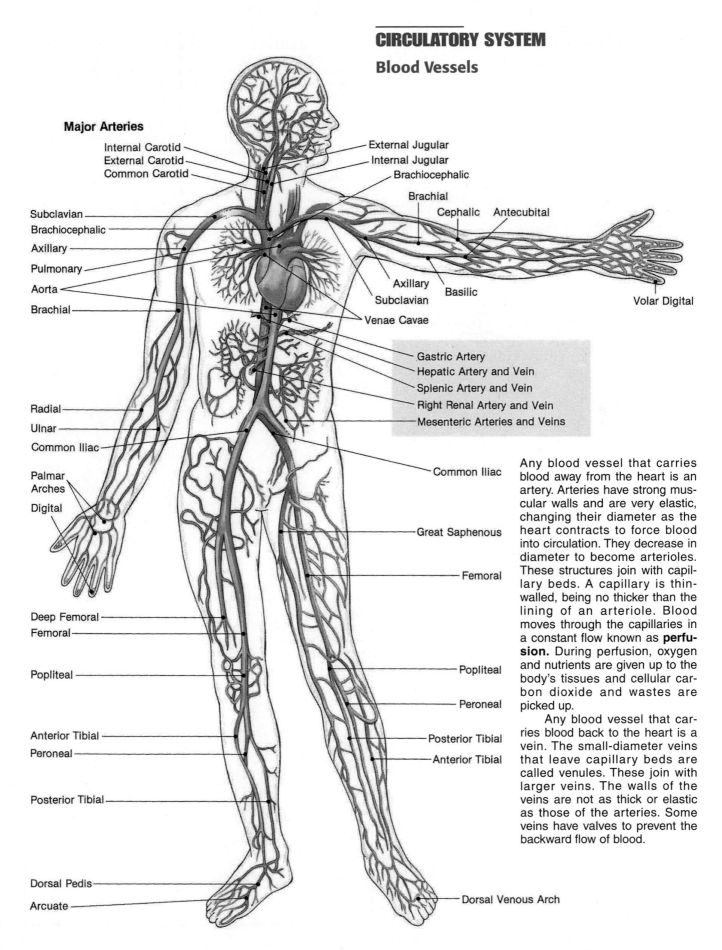

Internal Carotid
External Carotid
Common Carotid

External Jugular
Internal Jugular
Brachiocephalic

Brachial
Cephalic Antecubital

Subclavian
Brachiocephalic
Axillary
Pulmonary
Aorta
Brachial

Axillary
Subclavian
Basilic

Venae Cavae

Volar Digital

Gastric Artery
Hepatic Artery and Vein
Splenic Artery and Vein
Right Renal Artery and Vein
Mesenteric Arteries and Veins

Radial
Ulnar
Common Iliac

Palmar Arches
Digital

Common Iliac

Great Saphenous

Femoral

Deep Femoral
Femoral

Popliteal

Popliteal

Peroneal

Anterior Tibial
Peroneal

Posterior Tibial
Anterior Tibial

Posterior Tibial

Dorsal Pedis
Arcuate

Dorsal Venous Arch

Any blood vessel that carries blood away from the heart is an artery. Arteries have strong muscular walls and are very elastic, changing their diameter as the heart contracts to force blood into circulation. They decrease in diameter to become arterioles. These structures join with capillary beds. A capillary is thin-walled, being no thicker than the lining of an arteriole. Blood moves through the capillaries in a constant flow known as **perfusion.** During perfusion, oxygen and nutrients are given up to the body's tissues and cellular carbon dioxide and wastes are picked up.

Any blood vessel that carries blood back to the heart is a vein. The small-diameter veins that leave capillary beds are called venules. These join with larger veins. The walls of the veins are not as thick or elastic as those of the arteries. Some veins have valves to prevent the backward flow of blood.

RESPIRATORY SYSTEM

The airway consists of structures involved with the conduction and exchange of air. Conduction is the movement of air to and from the exchange levels of the lungs. Air enters through the nose (primary) and mouth (secondary) and travels down the pharynx to enter the larynx. After passing through the larynx, air enters the trachea. At its distal end, the trachea branches into the left and right primary bronchi. These bronchi branch into secondary bronchi, which then branch into the bronchioles. Some of the bronchioles end as closed tubes. Air movement in them helps the lungs expand. The rest of the bronchioles carry the air to the exchange levels of the lungs.

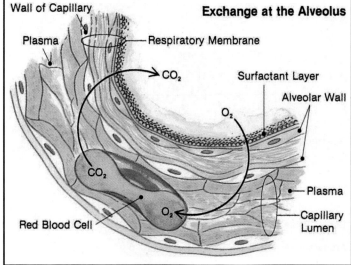

Alveolar Sacs

The respiratory bronchioles turn into alveolar ducts. These form alveolar sacs that are made up of the alveoli. Gas exchange takes place between the alveoli and the capillaries in the lungs.

DIGESTIVE SYSTEM

The digestive system includes the digestive tract and various supportive structures and accessory glands. The tract begins at the oral cavity with the teeth and tongue. The salivary glands release saliva into the mouth to moisten food for swallowing. The tract continues down the throat to the esophagus, through the cardiac sphincter, and into the stomach. Acid and digestive enzymes are added to the food to produce chyme. The chyme passes through the pyloric sphincter to enter the small intestine. Digestive enzymes from the pancreas and bile from the liver are added to the chyme. The processes of digestion and absorption are completed in the small intestine. Wastes are carried through the ileoceccal valve into the large intestine. The wastes are moved to the rectum, from where they can be expelled through the anus.

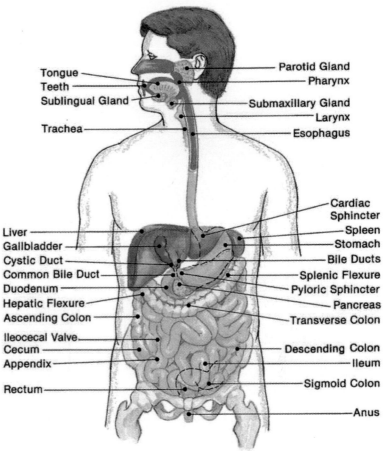

Organs of the Digestive System

Liver, Stomach, and Pancreas

Small Intestine

Large Intestine

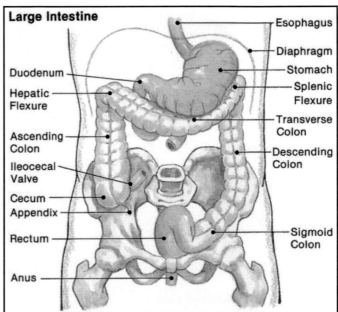

URINARY SYSTEM

The urinary system is part of the body's excretory structures (urinary system, lungs, sweat glands, and intestine). The kidneys remove the wastes of chemical activities (metabolism) in the body. These wastes are removed from the blood to produce urine. At the same time, the kidneys remove certain excess compounds, regulate the blood pH (acid-base balance), and the concentration of sodium, potassium, chlorine, glucose, and other important chemicals.

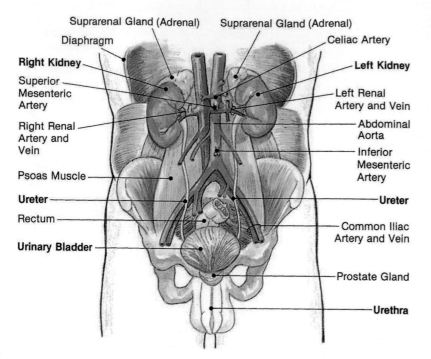

Suprarenal Gland (Adrenal)
Diaphragm
Right Kidney
Superior Mesenteric Artery
Right Renal Artery and Vein
Psoas Muscle
Ureter
Rectum
Urinary Bladder

Suprarenal Gland (Adrenal)
Celiac Artery
Left Kidney
Left Renal Artery and Vein
Abdominal Aorta
Inferior Mesenteric Artery
Ureter
Common Iliac Artery and Vein
Prostate Gland
Urethra

The Nephron

Each kidney is made up of microscopic nephrons. Both wastes and needed chemicals are filtered from the blood. As these materials are passed through the nephron, the needed compounds (including water) are sent back into the blood. Wastes are collected as urine.

Cortex
Renal Column
Papilla
Calyx
Medulla
Pelvis
Pyramid
Renal Capsule
Ureter

Sectioned Kidney

Bowman's Capsule
Peritubular Capillaries
Distal Convoluted Tubule
H_2O
Sodium
Glomerulus
Potassium
Circulatory System
H_2O
Sodium
Proximal Convoluted Tubule
Glucose
NH_3
H^+
Collecting Tubule
(Osmosis)
(Active Transport)
Loop of Henle

Microscopic Nephron

REPRODUCTIVE SYSTEM

The reproductive system consists of the organs, glands, and supportive structures that are involved with human sexuality and procreation. In the male, spermatozoa and the hormone testosterone are produced in the testes. The female produces ova (eggs) and the hormones estrogen and progesterone in her ovaries. The union of ovum and sperm produce a single cell called a zygote. Through growth, cell division, and cellular differentiation (the formulation of specialized cells) the new individual develops and matures.

Female

- Fundus
- Ovary
- Uterus
- Cervix
- Vagina
- Rectum
- Fallopian (Uterine) Tube
- Urinary Bladder
- Symphysis Pubis
- Urethra
- Labium Minus
- Clitoris
- Labium Majus

Labium Minus (singular), Labia Minora (plural)
Labium Majus (singular), Labia Majora (plural)

Male

- Ductus (Vas) Deferens
- Urinary Bladder
- Seminal Vesicle
- Rectum
- Ejaculatory Duct
- Bulb of Penis
- Symphysis Pubis
- Prostate Gland
- Urethra
- Corpus Cavernosum
- Corpus Spongiosum
- Testis
- Epididymis
- Duct of Bulbourethral Gland

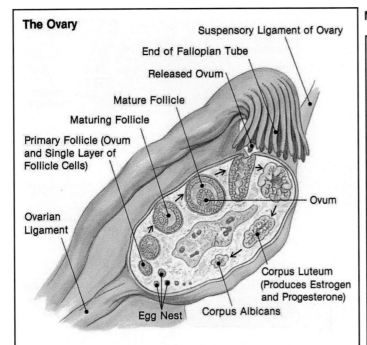

The Ovary

- Suspensory Ligament of Ovary
- End of Fallopian Tube
- Released Ovum
- Mature Follicle
- Maturing Follicle
- Primary Follicle (Ovum and Single Layer of Follicle Cells)
- Ovarian Ligament
- Ovum
- Corpus Luteum (Produces Estrogen and Progesterone)
- Egg Nest
- Corpus Albicans

The developing ovum and its supportive cells are called a follicle. Each month, follicle-stimulating hormone (FSH) from the pituitary gland starts the growth of several follicles. Usually, only one will mature and release an ovum (ovulation). During its growth, the follicle produces estrogen. After ovulation, the remaining cells of the follicle form a specialized structure that produces both estrogen and progesterone.

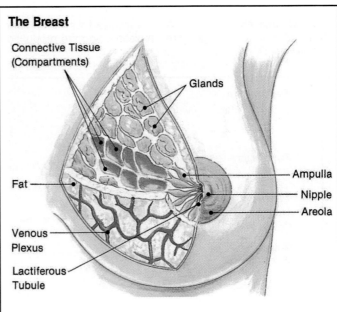

The Breast

- Connective Tissue (Compartments)
- Glands
- Fat
- Ampulla
- Nipple
- Areola
- Venous Plexus
- Lactiferous Tubule

The breasts contain the mammary glands that produce milk (lactation). A mammary gland is a highly modified form of sweat gland. Estrogen stimulates the growth of the ducts, while progesterone stimulates the development of the secreting (milk-producing) cells. Lactic hormone from the pituitary stimulates milk production. Another pituitary hormone, oxytocin, stimulates the milk-producing cells to eject their milk into the ducts.

Anatomy and Physiology Illustrations **861**

INTEGUMENTARY SYSTEM

Membranes

The Skin

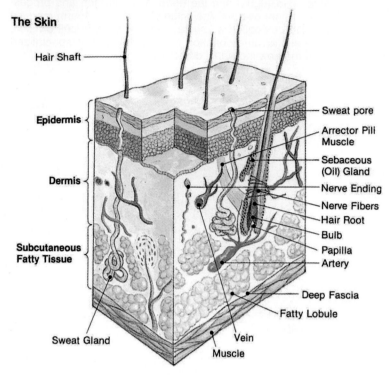

- Hair Shaft
- Epidermis
- Dermis
- Subcutaneous Fatty Tissue
- Sweat Gland
- Sweat pore
- Arrector Pili Muscle
- Sebaceous (Oil) Gland
- Nerve Ending
- Nerve Fibers
- Hair Root
- Bulb
- Papilla
- Artery
- Deep Fascia
- Fatty Lobule
- Vein
- Muscle

The skin is the largest organ of the body. In the adult the skin covers about 3,000 square inches (1.75 square meters) and weighs about 6 pounds. It is involved with protection, insulation, thermal regulation, excretion, and the production of vitamin D.

Membranes

Membranes cover or line body structures to provide protection from injury and infection. There are four major classes of membranes. Mucous membranes line those structures that open to the outside world (for example, the mouth, the airway, digestive tract, urinary tract, and vagina). Serous membranes line the closed body cavities and cover the outsides of organs. The cutaneous membrane is the skin. Synovial membranes line joints to reduce friction during movement.

A serous membrane that covers an organ is called a visceral layer. The term parietal layer is used for the part of the serous membrane that lines a cavity. The serous membrane in the thoracic cavity is called pleura (for example, the parietal pleura lines the chest cavity). In the abdominal cavity, it is called peritoneum (for example, the parietal peritoneum). A double layer of peritoneum is called mesentery. The membrane that lines the sac surrounding the heart is pericardium.

The Peritoneum

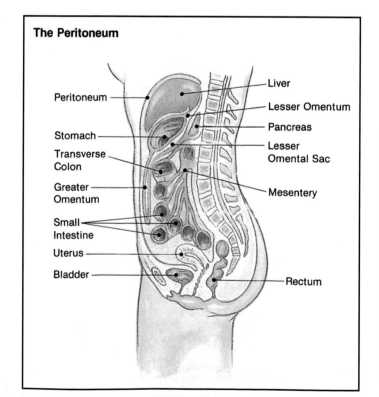

- Peritoneum
- Stomach
- Transverse Colon
- Greater Omentum
- Small Intestine
- Uterus
- Bladder
- Liver
- Lesser Omentum
- Pancreas
- Lesser Omental Sac
- Mesentery
- Rectum

Synovial Joint

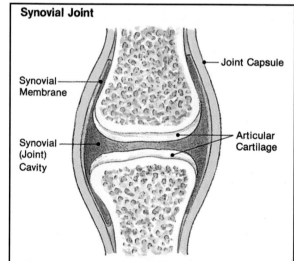

- Synovial Membrane
- Synovial (Joint) Cavity
- Joint Capsule
- Articular Cartilage

The Pleura

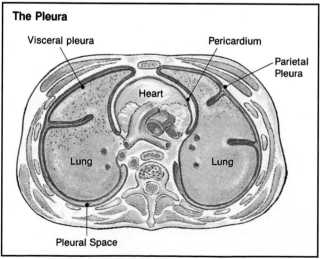

- Visceral pleura
- Heart
- Lung
- Lung
- Pericardium
- Parietal Pleura
- Pleural Space

SENSES

Eye and Ear

The body has the sense of vision, hearing, balance and equilibrium, touch, pain, heat, cold, pressure, taste, and smell.

The eye can receive and focus light and then convert this energy into nerve impulses to be sent to the brain. The nerve impulses originate from the retina. Visual receptors in the retina called rods can work in low intensity light. They have no color function. The visual receptors called cones operate in high intensity light and do receive colors.

The Eye

The ear's functions include hearing, static equilibrium (balance while standing still), and dynamic equilibrium (balance when moving). The outer and middle ear are responsible for sound gathering and its transmission. The inner ear has the nerve endings for hearing and equilibrium.

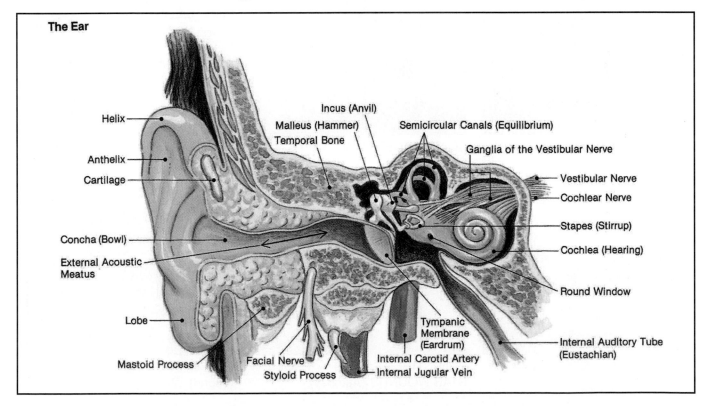

Anatomy and Physiology Illustrations 863

Atlas of Injuries

ABRASION (Gravel Roadway)

ABRASION (Rope or Cord)

PITTED ABRASION

INCISION

INCISION

LACERATION (Jagged Margins)

LACERATION (Tendons Still Intact)

SCALP LACERATION (With Skin Separation)

SCALP LACERATION (Minor)

PUNCTURE WOUNDS (Stab Wounds)

PUNCTURED LUNGS — FROM STAB WOUNDS (Autopsy)

PERFORATED HEART (Bullet Wound)

Atlas of Injuries

ENTRANCE WOUND (Bullet)

ENTRANCE WOUND (Bullet — Close Range)

EXIT WOUND (Bullet)

SHOTGUN WOUND

FACIAL AVULSION

SKIN AVULSION (All Layers)

CONTUSIONS

CONTUSION (Opened to Show Blood Accumulation)

LACERATED LIVER (Abdominal Trauma)

LACERATED SPLEEN

FRACTURED RIBS (Death due to Blood Loss from Lacerated Lungs)

PERFORATED CHEST (Sucking Chest Wound)

ALL PHOTOGRAPHS ON THIS PAGE ARE FROM:
DR. LEE J. ABBOTT, PO BOX 1285, LAXAHATCHEE, FL 33470

Atlas of Injuries

BLUNT TRAUMA TO CHEST

OPEN HEAD WOUND — SKULL FRACTURE

RADIATING SKULL FRACTURE (Blunt Trauma)

MULTIPLE SKULL FRACTURES (X-ray)

DEPRESSED SKULL FRACTURE (Force from Small Object)

BLEEDING FROM EAR (Possible Skull Fracture)

BLEEDING FROM NOSE (Possible Skull Fracture)

EPIDURAL HEMATOMA (D = Dura, B = Bone Fragment)

EXTENSIVE BILATERAL INJURY — LOWER EXTREMITIES (Impact with Car)

SUPERFICIAL BURN

PARTIAL THICKNESS BURN

FULL THICKNESS BURN

ALL PHOTOGRAPHS ON THIS PAGE ARE FROM:
DR. LEE J. ABBOTT, PO BOX 1285, LAXAHATCHEE, FL 33470

Atlas of Injuries

ELECTRICAL BURN
(Contact with Source)
   LJA

ELECTRICAL BURN (Exit)
   LJA

OPEN FRACTURE (Femur)
   UT

FROSTBITE

SNAKEBITE
   UT

BOWEL EVISCERATION

ORBITAL EDEMA

HIVES
   AFIP Neg. No. 65-6982-4

DOG BITE (Leg)
   AFIP Neg. No. 62-12291

AMPUTATION (Fingers)
   AFIP Neg. No. 75-20914

LACERATED LEG
   AFIP Neg. No. 68-15269

BURN (Hot Water)
   AFIP Neg. No. 64-8320

LJA = Dr. Lee J. Abbott   AFIP = Armed Forces Institute of Pathology
UT = University of Tennessee, Memphis, Division of Forensic Pathology

MEDICAL TERMINOLOGY

As an EMT, you will probably never have to use more than a few medical terms in the course of your prehospital emergency care activities, and most of them will probably deal with parts of the body. Physicians and nurses prefer EMTs to speak in other than medical terms. But if you are an avid reader, much of what you read is likely to be freely sprinkled with medical terms, and if you cannot translate them, you may not understand what you are reading.

Medical terms are comprised of words, word roots, combining forms, prefixes, and suffixes—all little words, if you will, and each with its own definition.

Sometimes medical terms are made up of two whole words. For example, the word SMALL, is joined with the word POX to form the medical term SMALLPOX, the name of a disease. Would that it were all so simple!

Word roots are the foundations of words and are not used by themselves. THERM is a word root that means heat; to use it alone would make no sense. But when a vowel is added to the end of the word root to make it the combining form THERM/O, it can be joined with other words or word roots to form a compound term. THERM/O and METER (an instrument for measuring) combine to form THERMOMETER, an instrument for measuring heat or temperature.

More than one word root or combining form can be joined to form medical terms; ELECTROCARDIOGRAM is a good example. ELECTR/O (electric) is joined to CARDI (heart) and the suffix -GRAM (a written record) to form the medical term that means a written record of the heart's electrical activity.

Prefixes are used to modify or qualify the meaning of word roots. They usually tell the reader what kind of, where (or in what direction), or how many.

The term -PNEA relates to breathing, but it says nothing about the quality or kind of breathing. Adding the prefix DYS- qualifies it as difficult breathing.

ABDOMINAL PAIN is a rather broad term; it gives the reader no clue as to exactly where the pain is located either inside or outside the abdomen. Adding the prefix -INTRA to ABDOMINAL pinpoints the location of the pain, for INTRA-ABDOMINAL PAIN means pain within the abdomen. -PLEGIA refers to paralysis of the limbs. The prefix QUADRI informs the reader as to how many limbs are paralyzed. QUADRIPLEGIA means paralysis of all four limbs.

Suffixes are word endings that form nouns, adjectives, or verbs. Medical terms can have more than one suffix, and a suffix can appear in the middle of a compound term affixed to a combining form. A number of suffixes have specialized meanings. -ITIS means inflammation; thus ARTHRITIS means inflammation of a joint. -IAC forms a noun indicating a person afflicted with a certain disease, as for example, HEMOPHILIAC.

Some suffixes are joined to word roots to form terms that indicate a state, quality, condition, procedure, or process. PNEUMO<u>NIA</u> and PSORI<u>ASIS</u> are examples of medical conditions, while APPENDEC-TOM<u>Y</u> and ARTHROSCOP<u>Y</u> are examples of medical procedures. The suffixes in each case are underlined.

Some suffixes combine with word roots to form adjectives, words that modify nouns by indicating quality or quantity or by distinguishing one thing from another. GAST<u>RIC</u>, CARDI<u>AC</u>, FIBR<u>OUS</u>, ARTH<u>RITIC</u>, and DIAPHO<u>RETIC</u> are all examples of adjectives formed by adding suffixes (underlined) to word roots.

Some suffixes are added to word roots to express reduction in size, -OLE and -ULE, for example. An ARTERI<u>OLE</u> is smaller than an ARTERY, and a VEN<u>ULE</u> is smaller than a vein.

When added to word roots, -E and -IZE form verbs. EXCIS<u>E</u> and CATHETER<u>IZE</u> are examples.

Finally, some of what are commonly accepted as suffixes are actually the combination of a word root and a suffix. -MEGALY (enlargement) results from the combination of the word root MEGAL (large) and the suffix -Y (which forms the term into a noun). CARDIOMEGALY means enlargement of the heart.

STANDARD TERMS

The following terms are used to denote direction of movement, position, and anatomical posture.

abduction: movement away from the body's midline.
adduction: movement toward the body's midline.
afferent: conducting toward a structure.
anterior: the front surface of the body.
anterior to: in front of.
caudad: toward the tail.
cephalad: toward the head.
circumduction: circular movement of a part.
craniad: toward the cranium.
deep: situated remote from the surface.
distal: situated away from the point of origin.
dorsal: pertaining to the back surface of the body.
dorsiflexion: bending backward.
efferent: conducting away from a structure.
elevation: raising a body part.
extension: stretching, or moving jointed parts into or toward a straight condition.
external: situated outside.
flexion: bending, or moving jointed parts closer together.
inferior: situated below.
internal: situated inside.

laterad: toward the side of the body.

lateral: situated away from the body's midline.

lateral rotation: rotating outward away from the body's midline.

left lateral recumbent: lying horizontal on the left side.

mediad: toward the midline of the body.

medial: situated toward the body's midline.

medial rotation: rotating inward toward the body's midline.

palmar: concerning the inner surface of the hand.

peripheral: away from a central structure.

plantar: concerning the sole of the foot.

posterior: pertaining to the back surface of the body.

posterior to: situated behind.

pronation: lying face downward or turning the hand so the palm faces downward or backward.

prone: lying horizontal, face down and flat.

protraction: a pushing forward, as the mandible.

proximal: situated nearest the point of origin.

recumbent: lying horizontal, generally speaking.

retraction: a drawing back, as the tongue.

right lateral recumbent: lying horizontal on the right side.

rotation: turning around an axis.

superficial: situated near the surface.

superior: situated above.

supination: lying face upward or turning the hand so the palm faces forward or upward.

supine: lying horizontal, flat on the back and face up.

ventral: the front surface of the body.

PLANES

A plane is an imaginary flat surface that divides the body into sections.

coronal or frontal plane: an imaginary plane that passes through the body from side to side and divides it into front and back sections.

midsagittal plane: an imaginary plane that passes through the body from front to back and divides it into right and left halves.

sagittal plane: an imaginary plane parallel to the median plane. It passes through the body from front to back and divides the body into right and left sections.

transverse plane: an imaginary plane that passes through the body and divides it into upper and lower sections.

WORD PARTS

Prefixes are generally identified by a following dash (AMBI-). Combining forms have a slash and a vowel following the word root (ARTHR/O). Suffixes are generally identified by a preceding dash (-EMIA).

a- (not, without, lacking, deficient); *afebrile,* without fever.

ab- (away from); *abduct,* to draw away from the midline.

-able, -ible (capable of); *reducible,* capable of being reduced (as a fracture).

abdomin/o (abdomen); *abdominal,* pertaining to the abdomen.

ac- (to); *acclimate,* to become accustomed to.

acou (hear); *acoustic,* pertaining to sound or hearing.

acr/o (extremity, top, peak); *acrodermatitis,* inflammation of the skin of the extremities.

acu (needle); *acupuncture,* the Chinese practice of piercing specific peripheral nerves with needles to relieve the discomfort associated with painful disorders.

ad- (to, toward); *adduct,* to draw toward the midline.

aden/o (gland); *adenitis,* inflammation of a gland.

adip/o (fat); *adipose,* fatty; fat (in size).

aer/o (air); *aerobic,* requiring the presence of oxygen to live and grow.

af- (to); *afferent,* conveying toward.

ag- (to); *aggregate,* to crowd or cluster together.

-algesia (painful); *hyperalgesia,* overly sensitive to pain.

-algia (painful condition); *neuralgia,* pain that extends along the course of one or more nerves.

ambi- (both sides); *ambidextrous,* able to perform manual skills with both hands.

ambl/y (dim, dull, lazy); *amblyopia,* lazy eye.

amphi-, ampho- (on both sides, around both); *amphigonadism,* having both testicular and ovarian tissues.

amyl/o (starch); *amyloid,* starchlike.

an- (without); *anemia,* a reduced volume of blood cells.

ana- (upward, again, backward, excess); *anaphylaxis,* an unusual or exaggerated reaction of an organism to a substance to which it becomes sensitized.

andr/o (man, male); *android,* resembling a man.

angi/o (blood vessel, duct); *angioplasty,* surgery of blood vessels.

ankyl/o (stiff); *ankylosis,* stiffness.

ant-, anti- (against, opposed to, preventing, relieving); *antidote,* a substance for counteracting a poison.

ante- (before, forward); *antecubital,* situated in front of the elbow.

antero- (front); *anterolateral,* situated in front and to one side.

ap- (to); *approximate,* to bring together; to place close to.

apo- (separation, derivation from); *apoplexy,* sudden neurologic impairment due to a cardiovascular disorder.

-arium, -orium (place for something); *solarium,* a place for the sun.

arteri/o (artery); *arteriosclerosis,* thickening of the walls of the smaller arteries.

arthrio (joint, articulation); *arthritis,* inflammation of a joint or joints.

articul/o (joint); *articulated,* united by joints.

as- (to); *assimilate,* to take into.

at- (to); *attract,* to draw toward.

audi/o (hearing); *audiometer,* an instrument to test the power of hearing.

aur/o (ear); *auricle,* the flap of the ear.

aut/o (self); *autistic,* self-centered

bi- (two, twice, double, both); *bilateral,* having two sides; pertaining to two sides.

bi/o (life); *biology,* the study of life.

blephario (eyelid); *blepharitis,* inflammation of the eyelid.

brachi/o (upper arm); *brachialgia,* pain in the upper arm.

brady- (slow); *bradycardia,* an abnormally slow heart rate.

bronch/o (larger air passages of the lungs); *bronchitis,* inflammation of the larger air passages of the lungs.

bucc/o (cheek); *buccal,* pertaining to the cheek.

cac/o (bad); *cacosmis,* a bad odor.

calc/o (bad); *calculus,* an abnormal hard inorganic mass such as a gallstone.

calcane/o (heel); *calcaneus,* the heel bone.

calor/o (heat); *caloric,* pertaining to heat.

cancr/o (cancer); *cancroid,* resembling cancer.

capit/o (head); *capitate,* head-shaped.

caps/o (container); *capsulation,* enclosed in a capsule or container.

carcin/o (cancer); *carcinogen,* a substance that causes cancer.

cardi/o (heart); *cardiogenic,* originating in the heart.

carp/o (wrist bone); *carpal,* pertaining to the wrist bone.

cat-, cata- (down, lower, under, against, along with); *catabasis,* the stage of decline of a disease.

-cele (tumor, hernia); *hydrocele,* a confined collection of water.

celi/o (abdomen); *celiomyalgia,* a pain in the muscles of the abdomen.

-centesis (perforation or tapping, as with a needle); *abdominocentesis,* surgical puncture of the abdominal cavity.

cephal/o (head); *electroencephalogram,* a recording of the electrical activity of the brain.

cerebr/o (cerebrum); *cerebrospinal,* pertaining to the brain and spinal fluid.

cervic/o (neck, cervix); *cervical,* pertaining to the neck (or cervix).

cheil/o, chil/o (lip); *cheilitis,* inflammation of the lips.

cheirio, chir/o (hand); *cheiralgia,* pain in the hand.

chlor/o (green); *chloroma,* green cancer, a greenish tumor associated with myelogenous leukemia.

chol/e (bile, gall); *choledochitis,* inflammation of the common bile duct.

chondr/o (cartilage); *chondrodynia,* pain in a cartilage.

chrom/o, chromat/o (color); *monochromatic,* being of one color.

chron/o (time); *chronic,* persisting for a long time.

-cid- (cut, kill, fall); *insecticide,* an agent that kills insects.

circum- (around); *circumscribed,* confined to a limited space.

-cis- (cut, kill, fall); *excise,* to cut out.

-clysis (irrigation); *enteroclysis,* irrigation of the small intestine.

co- (with); *cohesion,* the force that causes various particles to unite.

col- (with); *collateral,* secondary or accessory; a small side branch such as a blood vessel or nerve.

col/o (colon, large intestine); *colitis,* inflammation of the colon.

colp/o (vagina); *colporrhagia,* bleeding from the vagma.

com- (with); *comminuted,* broken or crushed into small pieces.

con- (with); *congenital,* existing from the time of birth.

contra- (against, opposite); *contraindicated,* inadvisable.

cor/e, core/o (pupil); *corectopia,* abnormal location of the pupil of the eye.

cost/o (rib); *intercostal,* between the ribs.

crani/o (skull); *cranial,* pertaining to the skull.

cry/o (eold); *cryogenic,* that which produces low temperature.

crypt/o (hide, cover, conceal); *cryptogenic,* of doubtful origin.

cyan/o (blue); *cyanosis,* bluish discoloration of the skin and mucous membranes.

cyst/o (urinary bladder, cyst, sac of fluid); *cystitis,* inflammation of the bladder.

-cyte (cell); *leukocyte,* white cell.

cyt/o (cell); *cytoma,* tumor of the cell.

dacry/o (tear); *dacryorrhea,* excessive flow of tears.

dactyl/o (finger, toe); *dactylomegaly,* abnormally large fingers or toes.

de- (down); *descending,* coming down from.

dent/o (tooth); *dental,* pertaining to the teeth.

derm/o, dermat/o (skin); *dermatitis,* inflammation of the skin.

dextr/o (right); *dextrad,* toward the right side.

di- (twice, double); *diplegia,* paralysis affecting like parts on both sides of the body.

dia- (through, across, apart); *diaphragm,* the partition that separates the abdominal and thoracic cavities.

dipl/o (double, twin, twice); *diplopia,* double vision.

dips/o (thirst); *dipsomania,* alcoholism.

dis- (to free, to undo); *dissect,* to cut apart.

dors/o (back); *dorsal,* pertaining to the back.

-dynia (painful condition); *cephalodynia,* headache.

dys- (bad, difficult, abnormal, incomplete); *dyspnea,* labored breathing.

-ectasia (dilation or enlargement of an organ or part); *gastrectasia,* dilation (stretching) of the stomach.

ecto- (outer, outside of); *ectopic,* located away from the normal position.

-ectomy (the surgical removal of an organ or part); *appendectomy,* surgical removal of the appendix.

electr/o (electric); *electrocardiogram,* the written record of the heart's electrical activity.

-emia (condition of the blood); *anemia,* a deficiency of red blood cells.

en- (in, into, within); *encapsulate,* to enclose within a container.

encephal/o (brain); *encephalitis,* inflammation of the brain.

end-, endo- (within); *endotracheal,* within the trachea.

ent-, ento- (within, inner); *entopic,* occurring in the proper place.

enter/o (small intestine); *enteritis,* inflammation of the intestine.

ep-, epi- (over, on, upon); *epidermis,* the outermost layer of skin.

erythr/o (red); *erythrocyte,* a red blood cell.

esthesia (feeling); *anesthesia,* without feeling.

eu (good, well, normal, healthy); *euphoria,* an abnormal or exaggerated feeling of well-being.

ex- (out of, away from); *excrement,* waste material discharged from the body.

exo- (outside, outward); *exophytic,* to grow outward or on the surface.

extra- (on the outside, beyond, in addition to); *extracorporeal,* outside the body.

faci/o (face, surface); *facial,* pertaining to the face.

febr/i (fever); *febrile,* feverish.

-ferent (bear, carry); *efferent,* carrying away from a center.

fibr/o (fiber, filament); *fibrillation,* muscular contractions due to the activity of muscle fibers.

-form (shape); *deformed,* abnormally shaped.

-fugal (moving away); *centrifugal,* moving away from a center.

galact/o (milk); *galactopyria,* milk fever.

gangli/o (knot); *ganglion,* a knotlike mass.

gastr/o (stomach); *gastritis,* inflammation of the stomach.

gen/o (come into being, originate); *genetic,* inherited.

-genesis (production or origin); *pathogenesis,* the development of a disease.

-genic (giving rise to, originating in); *cardiogenic,* originating in the heart.

gloss/o (tongue); *glossal,* pertaining to the tongue.

glyc/o (sweet); *glycemia,* the presence of sugar in the blood.

gnath/o (jaw); *gnathitis,* inflammation of the jaw.

-gram (drawing, written record); *electrocardiogram,* a recording of the heart's electrical activity.

-graph (an instrument for recording the activity of an organ); *electrocardiograph,* an instrument for measuring the heart's electrical activity.

-graphy (the recording of the activity of an organ); *electrocardiography,* the method of recording the heart's electrical activity.

gynec/o (woman); *gynecologist,* a specialist in diseases of the female genital tract.

gnos/o (knowledge); *prognosis,* a prediction of the outcome of a disease.

hem/a, hem/o, hemat/o (blood); *hematoma,* a localized collection of blood.

hemi- (one-half); *hemiplegia,* paralysis of one side of the body.

hepat/o (liver); *hepatitis,* inflammation of the liver.

heter/o (other); *heterogeneous,* from a different source.

hidr/o, hidrot/o (sweat); *hidrosis,* cxcessive sweating.

hist/o (tissue); *histodialysis,* the breaking down of tissue.

hom/o, home/o (same, similar, unchanging, constant); *homeostasis,* stability in an organism's normal physiological states.

hydr/o (water, fluid); *hydrocephalus,* an accumulation of cerebrospinal fluid in the skull with resulting enlargement of the head.

hypn/o (sleep); *hypnotic,* that which induces sleep.

hyal/o (glass); *hyaline,* glassy, transparent.

hyper- (beyond normal, excessive); *hypertension,* abnormally high blood pressure.

hypo- (below normal, deficient, under, beneath); *hypotension,* abnormally low blood pressure.

hyster/o (uterus, womb); *hysterectomy,* surgical removal of the uterus.

-iasis (condition); *psoriasis,* a chronic skin condition characterized by lesions.

iatr/o (healer, physician); *pediatrician,* a physician that specializes in children's disorders.

-id (in a state, condition of); *gravid,* pregnant.

idio (peculiar, separate, distinct); *idiopathic,* occurring without a known cause.

il- (negative prefix); *illegible,* cannot be read.

ile/o (ileum); *ileitis,* inflammation of the ileum.

ili/o (ilium); *iliac,* pertaining to the ilium.

im- (negative prefix); *immature,* not mature.

in- (in, into, within); *incise,* to cut into.

infra- (beneath, below); *infracostal,* below a rib, or below the ribs.

inter- (between); *intercostal,* between two ribs.

intra- (within); *intraoral,* within the mouth.

intro- (within, into); *introspection,* the contemplation of one's own thoughts and feelings; self-analysis.

ir/o, irid/o (iris); *iridotomy,* incision of the iris.

ischi/o (ischium); *ischialgia,* pain in the ischium.

-ismus (abnormal condition); *strabismus,* deviation of the eye that a person cannot overcome.

iso- (same, equal, alike); *isometric,* of equal dimensions.

-itis (inflammation); *endocarditis,* inflammation within the heart.

kerat/o (cornea); *keratitis,* inflammation of the cornea.

kinesi/o (movement); *kinesialgia,* pain upon movement.

labi/o (lip); *labiodental,* pertaining to the lip and teeth.

lact/o (milk); *lactation,* the secretion of milk.

lal/o (talk); *lalopathy,* any speech disorder.

lapar/o (flank, abdomen, abdominal wall); *laparotomy,* an incision through the abdominal wall.

laryng/o (larynx); *laryngoscope,* an instrument for examining the larynx.

lept/o (thin); *leptodactylous,* having slender fingers.

leuc/o, leuk/o (white); *leukemia,* a malignant disease characterized by the increased development of white blood cells.

lingu/o (tongue); *sublingual,* under the tongue.

lip/o (fat); *lipoma,* fatty tumor.

lith/o (stone); *lithotriptor,* an instrument for crushing stones in the bladder.

-logist (a person who studies); *pathologist,* a person who studies diseases.

log/o (speak), give an account; *logospasms,* spasmodic speech.

-logy (study of); *pathology,* the study of disease.

lumb/o (loin); *lumbago,* pain in the lumbar region.

lymph/o (lymph); *lymphoduct,* a vessel of the lymph system.

-lysis (destruction); *electrolysis,* destruction (of hair, for example) by passage of an electric current.

macr/o (large, long); *macrocephalous,* having an abnormally large head.

malac/o (a softening); *malacia,* the morbid softening of a body part or tissue.

mamm/o (breast); *mammary,* pertaining to the breast.

-mania (mental aberration); *kleptomania,* the compulsion to steal.

mast/o (breast); *mastectomy,* surgical removal of the breast.

medi/o (middle); *mediastinum,* middle partition of the thoracic cavity.

mega- (large); *megacolon,* an abnormally large colon.

megal/o (large); *megalomaniac,* a person impressed with his own greatness.

-megaly (an enlargement); *cardiomegaly,* enlargement of the heart.

melan/o (dark, black); *melanoma,* a tumor comprised of darkly pigmented cells.

men/o (month); *menopause,* cessation of menstruation.

mes/o (middle); *mesiad,* toward the center.

meta- (change, transformation, exchange); *metabolism,* the sum of the physical and chemical processes by which an organism survives.

metr/o (uterus); *metralgia,* pain in the uterus.

micr/o (small); *microscope,* an instrument for magnifying small objects.

mon/o (single, only, sole); *monoplegia,* paralysis of a single part.

morph/o (form); *morphology,* the study of form and shape.

multi- (many, much); *multipara,* a woman who has given two or more live births.

myc/o, mycet/o (fungus); *mycosis,* any disease caused by a fungus.

my/o (muscle); *myasthenia,* muscular weakness.

myel/o (marrow, also often refers to spinal cord); *myelocele,* protrusion of the spinal cord through a defect in the spinal column.

myx/o (mucous, slimelike); *myxoid,* resembling mucous.

narc/o (stupor, numbness); *narcotic,* an agent that induces sleep.

nas/o (nose); *oronasal,* pertaining to the nose and mouth.

ne/o (new); *neonate,* a newborn infant.

necr/o (corpse); *necrotic,* dead (when referring to tissue).

nephr/o (kidney); *nephralgia,* pain in the kidneys.

neur/o (nerve); *neuritis,* inflammation of nerve pathways.

noct/i (night); *noctambulism,* sleep walking.

norm/o (rule, order, normal); *normotension,* normal blood pressure.

null/i (none); *nullipara,* a woman who has never given birth to a child.

nyct/o (night); *nycturia,* excessive urination at night.

ob- (against, in front of, toward); *obturator,* a device that closes an opening.

oc- (against, in front of, toward); *occlude,* to obstruct.

ocul/o (eye); *ocular,* pertaining to the eye.

odont/o (tooth); *odontalgia,* toothache.

-oid (shape, form, resemblance); *ovoid,* egg-shaped.

olig/o (few, deficient, scanty); *oligemia,* lacking in blood volume.

-oma (tumor, swelling); *adenoma,* tumor of a gland.

o/o- (egg); *ooblast,* a primitive cell from which an ovum develops.

onych/o (nail); *onychoma,* tumor of a nail or nail bed.

oophor/o (ovary); *oophorectomy,* a surgical removal of one or both ovaries.

-opsy (a viewing); *autopsy,* postmortem examination of a body.

opthalm/o (eye); *opthalmic,* pertaining to the eyes.

opt/o, optic/o (sight, vision); *optometrist,* a specialist in adapting lenses for the correcting of visual defects.

or/o (mouth); *oral,* pertaining to the mouth.

orch/o, orchid/o (testicle); *orchitis,* inflammation of the testicles.

orth/o (straight, upright); *orthopedic,* pertaining to the correction of skeletal defects.

-osis (process, an abnormal condition); *dermatosis,* any skin condition.

oste/o (bone); *osteomyelitis,* inflammation of bone or bone marrow.

ot/o (ear); *otalgia,* earache.

ovari/o (ovary); *ovariocele,* hernia of an ovary.

ov/i, ov/o (egg); *oviduct,* a passage through which an egg passes.

pachy- (thicken); *pachyderma,* abnormal thickening of the skin.

palat/o (palate); *palatitis,* inflammation of the palate.

pan- (all, entire, every); *panacea,* a remedy for all diseases, a "cure-all."

para- (beside, beyond, accessory to, apart from, against); *paranormal,* beyond the natural or normal.

path/o (disease); *pathogen,* any disease-producing agent.

-pathy (disease of a part); *osteopathy,* disease of a bone.

-penia (an abnormal reduction); *leukopenia,* deficiency in white blood cells.

peps/o, pept/o (digestion); *dyspepsia,* poor digestion.

per- (throughout, completely, extremely); *perfusion,* the passage of fluid through the vessels of an organ.

peri- (around, surrounding); *pericardium,* the sac that surrounds the heart and the roots of the great vessels.

-pexy (fixation); *splendopexy,* surgical fixation of the spleen.

phag/o (eat); *phagomania,* an insatiable craving for food.

pharyng/o (throat); *pharyngospasms,* spasms of the muscles of the pharynx.

phas/o (speech); *aphasic,* unable to speak.

phil/o (like, have an affinity for); *necrophilia,* an abnormal interest in death.

phleb/o (vein); *phlebotomy,* surgical incision of a vein.

-phobia (fear, dread); *claustrophobia,* a fear of closed spaces.

phon/o (sound); *phonetic,* pertaining to the voice.

phor/o (bear, carry); *diaphoresis,* profuse sweating.

phot/o (light); *photosensitivity,* abnormal reactivity of the skin to sunlight.

phren/o (diaphragm); *phrenic nerve,* a nerve that carries messages to the diaphragm.

physi/o (nature); *physiology,* the science that studies the function of living things.

pil/o (hair); *pilose,* hairy.

-plasia (development, formation); *dysplasia,* poor or abnormal formation.

-plasty (surgical repair); *arthroplasty,* surgical repair of a joint.

-plegia (paralysis); *paraplegia,* paralysis of the lower body, including the legs.

pleur/o (rib, side, pleura); *pleurisy,* inflammation of the pleura.

-pnea (breath, breathing); *orthopnea,* difficult breathing except in an upright position.

pneum/o, pneumat/o (air, breath); *pneumatic,* pertaining to the air.

pneum/o, pneumon/o (lung); *pneumonia,* inflammation of the lungs with the escape of fluid.

pod/o (foot); *podiatrist,* a specialist in the care of feet.

-poiesis (formation); *hematopoiesis,* formation of blood.

poly- (much, many); *polychromatic,* multicolored.

post- (after, behind); *postmortem,* after death.

pre- (before); *premature,* occurring before the proper time.

pro- (before, in front of); *prolapse,* the falling down, or sinking of a part.

proct/o (anus); *proctitis,* inflammation of the rectum.

pseud/o (false); *pseudoplegia,* hysterical paralysis.

psych/o (mind, soul); *psychopath,* one who displays aggressive antisocial behavior.

-ptosis (abnormal dropping or sagging of a part); *hysteroptosis,* sagging of the uterus.

pulmon/o (lung); *pulmonary,* pertaining to the lungs.

py/o (pus); *pyorrhea,* copious discharge of pus.

pyel/o (renal pelvis); *pyelitis,* inflammation of the renal pelvis.

pyr/o (fire, fever); *pyromaniac,* compulsive fire setter.

quadri- (four); *quadriplegia,* paralysis of all four limbs.

rach/i (spine); *rachialgia,* pain in the spine.

radi/o (ray, radiation); *radiology,* the use of ionizing radiation in diagnosis and treatment.

re- (back, against, contrary); *recurrence,* the return of symptoms after remission.

rect/o (rectum); *rectal,* pertaining to the rectum.

ren/o (the kidneys); *renal,* pertaining to the kidneys.

retro- (located behind, backward); *retroperineal,* behind the perineum.

rhin/o (nose); *rhinitis,* inflammation of the mucus membranes of the nose.

-rrhage (abnormal discharge); *hemorrhage,* abnormal discharge of blood.

-rrhagia (hemorrhage from an organ or body part); *menorrhea,* excessive uterine bleeding.

-rrhea (flowing or discharge); *diarrhea,* abnormal frequency and liquidity of fecal discharges.

sanguin/o (blood); *exsanguinate,* to lose a large volume of blood either internally or externally.

sarc/o (flesh); *sarcoma,* a malignant tumor.

schiz/o (split); *schizophrenia,* any of a group of emotional disorders characterized by bizarre behavior (erroneously called split personality).

scler/o (hardening); *scleroderma,* hardening of connective tissues of the body, including the skin.

-sclerosis (hardened condition); *arteriosclerosis,* hardening of the arteries.

scoli/o (twisted, crooked); *scoliosis,* sideward deviation of the spine.

-scope (an instrument for observing); *endoscope,* an instrument for the examination of a hollow body, such as the bladder.

-sect (cut); *transsect,* to cut across.

semi- (one-half, partly); *semisupine,* partly, but not completely, supine.

sept/o, seps/o (infection); *aseptic,* free from infection.

somat/o (body); *psychosomatic,* both psychological and physiological.

son/o (sound); *sonogram,* a recording produced by the passage of sound waves through the body.

spermat/o (sperm, semen); *spermacide,* an agent that kills sperm.

sphygm/o (pulse); *sphygmomanometer,* a device for measuring blood pressure in the arteries.

splen/o (spleen); *splenectomy,* surgical removal of the spleen.

-stasis (stopping, controlling); *hemostasis,* the control of bleeding.

sten/o (narrow); *stenosis,* a narrowing of a passage or opening.

stere/o (solid, three-dimensional); *stereoscopic,* a three-dimensional appearance.

steth/o (chest); *stethoscope,* an instrument for listening to chest sounds.

sthen/o (strength); *myasthenia,* muscular weakness.

-stomy (surgically creating a new opening); *colostomy,* surgical creation of an opening between the colon and the surface of the body.

sub- (under, near, almost, moderately); *subclavian,* situated under the clavicle.

super- (above, excess); *superficial,* lying on or near the surface.

supra- (above, over); *suprapubic,* situated above the pubic arch.

sym-, syn- (joined together, with); *syndrome,* a set of symptoms that occur together.

tachy- (fast); *tachycardia,* a very fast heart rate.

-therapy (treatment); *hydrotherapy,* treatment with water.

therm/o (heat); *thermogenesis,* the production of heat.

thorac/o (chest cavity); *thoracic,* pertaining to the chest.

thromb/o (clot, lump); *thrombophlebitis,* inflammation of a vein.

-tome (a surgical instrument for cutting); *microtome,* an instrument for cutting thin slices of tissue.

-tomy (a surgical operation on an organ or body part); *thoracotomy,* surgical incision of the chest wall.

top/o (place); *topographic,* pertaining to special regions (of the body)

trache/o (trachea); *tracheostomy,* an opening in the neck that passes to the trachea.

trans- (through, across, beyond); *transfusion,* the introduction of whole blood or blood components directly into the bloodstream.

tri- (three); *trimester,* a period of three months.

trich/o (hair); *trichosis,* any disease of the hair.

-tripsy (surgical crushing); *lithotripsy,* surgical crushing of stones.

troph/o (nourish); *hypertrophic,* enlargement of an organ or body part due to the increase in the size of cells.

ultra- (beyond, excess); *ultrasonic,* beyond the audible range.

uni- (one); *unilateral,* affecting one side.

ur/o (urine); *urinalysis,* examination of urine.

ureter/o (ureter); *ureteritis,* inflammation of a ureter.

urethr/o (urethra); *urethritis,* inflammation of the urethra.

vas/o (vessel, duct); *vasodilator,* an agent that causes dilation of blood vessels.

ven/o (vein); *venipuncture,* surgical puncture of a vein.

ventr/o (belly, cavity); *ventral,* relating to the belly or abdomen.

vesic/o (blister, bladder); *vesicle,* a small fluid-filled blister.

viscer/o (internal organ); *visceral,* pertaining to the viscera (abdominal organs).

xanth/o (yellow); *xanthroma,* a yellow nodule in the skin.

xen/o (stranger); *xenophobia,* abnormal fear of strangers.

xer/o (dry); *xerosis,* abnormal dryness (as of the mouth or eyes).

zo/o (animal life); *zoogenous,* acquired from an animal.

GLOSSARY

abandonment leaving a patient after care has been initiated and before the patient has been transferred to someone with equal or greater medical training.

abdominal quadrants four divisions of the abdomen used to pinpoint the location of a pain or injury: the right upper quadrant, the left upper quadrant, the right lower quadrant, and the left lower quadrant.

abortion spontaneous (miscarriage) or induced termination of pregnancy.

abrasion (ab-RAY-zhun) a scratch or scrape.

abruptio placentae (ab-RUPT-si-o plah-SENT-ta) a condition in which the placenta separates from the uterine wall; a cause of prebirth bleeding.

absorbed poisons poisons that are taken into the body through unbroken skin.

acetabulum (AS-uh-TAB-yuh-lum) the pelvic socket into which the ball at the proximal end of the femur fits to form the hip joint.

acromioclavicular (ah-KRO-me-o-klav-IK-yuh-ler) **joint** the joint where the acromion and the clavicle meet.

acromion (ah-KRO-me-on) **process** the highest portion of the shoulder.

activated charcoal a powder, usually pre-mixed with water, that will adsorb some poisons and help prevent them from being absorbed by the body.

active rewarming application of an external heat source to rewarm the body of a hypothermic patient. See also central rewarming.

acute myocardial infarction (ah-KUTE MY-o-KARD-e-ul in-FARK-shun) **(AMI)** the condition in which a portion of the myocardium dies as a result of oxygen starvation; a heart attack.

afterbirth the placenta, membranes of the amniotic sac, part of the umbilical cord, and some tissues from the lining of the uterus that are delivered after the birth of the baby.

air embolism gas bubble in the bloodstream. The plural is *air emboli*. The more accurate term is *arterial gas embolism (AGE)*.

airway the passageway by which air enters or leaves the body. The structures of the airway are the nose, mouth, pharynx, larynx, trachea, bronchi, and lungs.

allergen something that causes an allergic reaction.

allergic reaction an exaggerated immune response.

alveoli (al-VE-o-li) the microscopic sacs of the lungs where gas exchange with the bloodstream takes place.

amniotic (am-ne-OT-ik) **sac** the "bag of waters" that surrounds the developing fetus.

amputation (am-pyu-TAY-shun) the surgical removal or traumatic severing of a body part, usually an extremity.

anaphylaxis (an-ah-fi-LAK-sis) a severe or life-threatening allergic reaction in which the blood vessels dilate, causing a drop in blood pressure, and the tissues lining the respiratory system swell, interfering with the airway. Also called *anaphylactic shock*.

anatomical position the standard reference position for the body in the study of anatomy. The body is standing erect, facing the observer. The arms are down at the sides and the palms of the hands are forward.

anatomy the study of body structure.

aneurysm (AN-u-rizm) the dilation, or ballooning, of a weakened section of the wall of an artery.

angina pectoris (AN-ji-nah [or an-JI-nah] PEK-to-ris) pain in the chest, occurring when blood supply to the heart is reduced and a portion of the heart muscle is not receiving enough oxygen.

anterior the front of the body or body part. Opposite of *posterior*.

antidote a substance that will neutralize a poison or its effects.

aorta (ay-OR-tah) the largest artery in the body. It transports blood from the left ventricle to begin systemic circulation.

apnea (ap-ne-ah) absence of breathing.

arrhythmia (ah-RITH-me-ah) a disturbance in heart rate and rhythm.

arterial bleeding bleeding from an artery, which is characterized by bright red blood and as rapid, profuse, and difficult to control.

arteriole (ar-TE-re-ol) the smallest kind of artery.

arteriosclerosis (ar-TE-re-o-skle-RO-sis) a condition in which artery walls become hard and stiff due to calcium deposits.

artery any blood vessel carrying blood away from the heart.

artificial ventilation forcing air or oxygen into the lungs when a patient has stopped breathing or has inadequate breathing.

asystole (ay-SIS-to-le) when the heart has ceased generating electrical impulses.

atherosclerosis (ATH-er-o-skle-RO-sis) a buildup of fatty deposits on the inner walls of arteries.

atria (AY-tree-ah) the two upper chambers of the heart. There is a right atrium (which receives unoxygenated blood returning from the body) and a left atrium (which receives oxygenated blood returning from the lungs).

auscultation (os-skul-TAY-shun) istening. A stethoscope is used to auscultate for characteristic body sounds.

auto-injector a syringe pre-loaded with medication that has a spring-loaded device that pushes the needle through the skin when the tip of the device is pressed firmly against the body.

automaticity (AW-to-muh-TISS-it-e) the ability of the heart to generate and conduct electrical impulses on its own.

876

autonomic (AW-to-NOM-ik) **nervous system** the division of the peripheral nervous system that controls involuntary motor functions.

AVPU a memory aid for *alert, verbal response, painful response, unresponsive* as a classification of a patient's level of responsiveness. See also *mental status*.

avulsion (ah-VUL-shun) the tearing away or tearing off of a piece or flap of skin or other soft tissue. This term also may be used for an eye pulled from its socket or a tooth dislodged from its socket.

bag-valve mask (BVM) a hand-held device with a face mask and self-refilling bag that can be squeezed to provide artificial ventilations to a patient. Can deliver air from the atmosphere or oxygen from a supplemental oxygen supply system.

bandage any material used to hold a dressing in place.

base station a two-way radio at a fixed site such as a hospital or dispatch center.

behavior the manner in which a person acts.

behavioral emergency when a patient's behavior is not typical for the situation; when the patient's behavior is unacceptable or intolerable to the patient, his family, or the community, or when the patient may harm himself or others.

bilateral on both sides.

blood pressure the force of blood against the walls of the blood vessels. Usually arterial blood pressure (the pressure in an artery) is measured. See also *diastolic blood presasure; systolic blood pressure.*

blunt-force trauma injury caused by a blow that does not penetrate through the skin or other body tissues.

body mechanics the proper use of the body to facilitate lifting and moving and prevent injury.

body substance isolation (BSI) a form of infection control based on the presumption that all body fluids are infectious. BSI calls for always using appropriate barriers to infection at the emergency scene, such as gloves, masks, gowns, and protective eyewear.

bones hard but flexible living structures that provide support for the body and protection to vital organs.

brachial (BRAY-ke-al) **artery** artery of the upper arm.

brachial pulse the pulse felt in the upper arm; the pulse checked during infant CPR.

bradycardia (BRAY-duh-KAR-de-uh) a slow heart rate; any pulse rate below 60 beats per minute.

breech presentation when the baby appears buttocks or both legs first during birth.

bronchi (BRONG-ki) the two large sets of branches that come off the trachea and enter the lungs. There are right and left bronchi. The singular is *bronchus*.

bronchoconstriction constriction, or blockage, of the bronchi that lead from the trachea to the lungs.

calcaneus (kal-KAY-ne-us) the heel bone.

capillary (KAP-i-lair-e) a thin-walled, microscopic blood vessel where oxygen/carbon dioxide and nutrient/waste exchange with the body's cells takes place.

capillary bleeding bleeding from capillaries, which is characterized by a slow, oozing flow of blood.

cardiac compromise a blanket term for any heart problem.

cardiac conduction system a system of specialized muscle tissues that conduct electrical impulses that stimulate the heart to beat.

cardiac muscle specialized involuntary muscle found only in the heart.

cardiogenic shock shock, or lack of perfusion, brought on not by blood loss but by inadequate pumping action of the heart. It is often the result of a heart attack or congestive heart failure.

cardiovascular system the heart and the blood vessels; the circulatory system.

carina (kah-RI-nah) the fork at the lower end of the trachea where the two mainstem bronchi branch.

carotid (kah-ROT-id) **arteries** the large neck arteries, one on each side of the neck, that carry blood from the heart to the head.

carotid (kah-ROT-id) **pulse** the pulse felt along the large carotid artery on either side of the neck.

carpals (KAR-pulz) the wrist bones.

cartilage tough tissue that covers the joint ends of bones and helps to form certain body parts such as the ear.

cellular phone a phone that transmits through the air instead of over wires so that the phone can be transported and used over a wide area.

central nervous system (CNS) the brain and spinal cord.

central pulses the carotid and femoral pulses, which can be felt in the central part of the body.

central rewarming application of heat to the lateral chest, neck, armpits, and groin of a hypothermic patient.

cephalic (se-FAL-ik) **presentation** when the baby appears head first during birth. This is the normal presentation.

cerebrospinal (suh-RE-bro-SPI-nal) **fluid (CSF)** the fluid that surrounds the brain and spinal cord.

cerebrovascular (suh-RE-bro VAS-ku-ler) **accident (CVA)** See *stroke*.

cervix (SUR-viks) the neck of the uterus at the entrance to the birth canal.

chief complaint in emergency medicine, the reason EMS was called, usually in the patient's own words.

circulatory system See *cardiovascular system*.

clavicle (KLAV-i-kul) the collarbone.

closed extremity injury an injury to an extremity with no associated opening in the skin.

closed wound an internal injury with no open pathway from the outside.

cold zone area where the command post and support functions that are necessary to control a hazardous material incident are located.

colostomy [ko-LOS-to-me] like an ileostomy, a surgical opening in the wall of the abdomen with a bag in place to collect excretions from the digestive system.

compensated shock when the patient is developing shock but the body is still able to maintain perfusion. See *decompensated shock; shock.*

concussion mild closed head injury without detectable damage to the brain. Complete recovery is usually expected.

conduction the direct transfer of heat from one material to another through direct contact.

confidentiality the obligation not to reveal information obtained about a patient except to other health care professionals involved in the patient's care, or under subpoena, or in a court of law, or when the patient has signed a release of confidentiality.

congestive heart failure (CHF) the failure of the heart to pump efficiently, leading to excessive blood or fluids in the lungs, the body, or both.

consent permission from the patient for care or other action by the EMT-B. See also *expressed consent; implied consent.*

constrict (kon-STRIKT) get smaller.

contamination the introduction of dangerous chemicals, disease, or infectious materials. See also *decontamination.*

contraindications (KON-truh-in-duh-KAY-shunz) specific signs or circumstances under which it is not appropriate and may be harmful to administer a particular drug to a patient.

contusion (kun-TU-zhun) a bruise; in brain injuries, a bruised brain caused when the force of a blow to the head is great enough to rupture blood vessels.

convection carrying away of heat by currents of air or water or other gases or liquids.

coronary (KOR-o-nar-e) **arteries** blood vessels that supply the muscle of the heart (myocardium).

coronary artery disease (CAD) diseases that affect the arteries of the heart.

cranium (KRAY-ne-um) the bony structure making up the forehead, top, back, and upper sides of the skull.

crepitation (krep-uh-TAY-shun) the grating sound or feeling of broken bones rubbing together; also called *crepitus.*

cricoid (KRIK-oid) **cartilage** the ring-shaped structure that circles the trachea at the lower edge of the larynx.

cricoid pressure pressure applied to the cricoid cartilage to suppress vomiting and bring the vocal cords into view. Also called *Sellick's maneuver.*

critical incident stress debriefing (CISD) a process in which teams of professional and peer counselors provide emotional and psychological support to EMS personnel who are or have been involved in a critical (highly stressful) incident.

crowning when part of the baby is visible through the vaginal opening.

crush injury an injury caused when force is transmitted from the body's exterior to its internal structures. Bones can be broken, muscles, nerves, and tissues damaged, and internal organs ruptured, causing internal bleeding.

cyanosis (SIGH-uh-NO-sis) a blue or gray color resulting from lack of oxygen in the body (see *hypoxia*).

danger zone the area around the wreckage of a vehicle collision or other accident within which special safety precautions should be taken.

DCAP-BTLS A memory aid to remember deformities, contusions, abrasions, punctures/penetrations, burns, tenderness, lacerations, and swelling—signs and symptoms of injury found by inspection or palpation during patient assessment.

decompensated shock occurs when the body can no longer compensate for low blood volume or lack of perfusion. Late signs such as decreasing blood pressure become evident. See *compensated shock; shock.*

decompression sickness a condition resulting from nitrogen trapped in the body's tissues caused by coming up too quickly from a deep, prolonged dive. A symptom of decompression sickness is "the bends," or deep pain in the muscles and joints.

decontamination the removal or cleansing of dangerous chemicals and other dangerous or infectious materials. See also *contamination.*

delirium tremens (duh-LEER-e-um TREM-uns) **(DTs)** a severe reaction that can be part of alcohol withdrawal, characterized by sweating, trembling, anxiety, and hallucinations. Severe alcohol withdrawal with the DTs can lead to death if untreated.

dermis (DER-mis) the inner (second) layer of skin found beneath the epidermis. It is rich in blood vessels and nerves.

designated agent an EMT-B or other person authorized by a Medical Director to give medications and provide emergency care. The transfer of such authorization to a designated agent is an extension of the Medical Director's license to practice medicine.

detailed physical exam an assessment of the head, neck, chest, abdomen, pelvis, extremities, and posterior of the body to detect signs and symptoms of injury. The examination of the head includes detailed examination of the face, ears, eyes, nose, and mouth. It may be done en route to the hospital after earlier on-scene assessments and interventions are completed.

diabetes mellitus (di-ah-BEE-tez MEL-i-tus) also called "sugar diabetes" or just "diabetes," the condition brought about by decreased insulin production. The person with this condition is a diabetic.

diaphragm (DI-uh-fram) the muscular structure that divides the chest cavity from the abdominal cavity. A major muscle of respiration.

diastolic (di-as-TOL-ik) **blood pressure** the pressure remaining in the arteries when the heart is relaxed and refilling.

dilate (DI-late) get larger.

dilution (di-LU-shun) thinning down or weakening by mixing with something else. Ingested poisons are sometimes diluted by drinking water or milk.

direct carry a method of transferring a patient from bed to stretcher in which two or more rescuers curl the patient to their chests, then reverse the process to lower the patient to the stretcher.

direct ground lift a method of lifting and carrying a patient from ground level to a stretcher in which two or more rescuers kneel, curl the patient to their chests, stand, then reverse the process to lower the patient to the stretcher.

disaster plan a predefined set of instructions that tells a community's various emergency responders what to do in specific emergencies.

dislocation the disruption or "coming apart" of a joint.

distal farther away from the torso. Opposite of *proximal*.

distention (dis-TEN-shun) a condition of being stretched, inflated, or larger than normal.

do not resuscitate (DNR) order a legal document, usually signed by the patient and his physician, which states that the patient has a terminal illness and does not wish to prolong life through resuscitative efforts.

dorsal referring to the back of the body or the back of the hand or foot. A synonym for *posterior*.

dorsalis pedis (dor-sal-is PEED-is) **artery** artery supplying the foot, lateral to the large tendon of the big toe.

downers depressants, such as barbiturates, that depress the central nervous system, often used to bring on a more relaxed state of mind.

draw sheet method a method of transferring a patient from bed to stretcher by grasping and pulling the loosened bottom sheet of the bed.

dressing any material (preferably sterile) used to cover a wound that will help control bleeding and help prevent additional contamination.

drowning death caused by changes in the lungs resulting from immersion in water. See also *near-drowning*.

duty to act an obligation to provide care to a patient.

dyspnea (DISP-ne-ah) shortness of breath; labored or difficult breathing.

eclampsia (e-KLAMP-se-ah) a severe complication of pregnancy that produces seizures and coma.

ectopic (ek-TOP-ik) **pregnancy** when implantation of the fertilized egg is not in the body of the uterus, occurring instead in the oviduct (fallopian tube), cervix, or abdominopelvic cavity.

edema (eh-DEEM-uh) swelling resulting from a buildup of fluid in the tissues.

embolism (EM-bo-lizm) a thrombus, or clot of blood and plaque, that has broken loose from the wall of an artery.

EMS Command the senior EMS person on the scene who establishes an EMS command post and oversees the medical aspects of a multiple-casualty incident.

endotracheal (EN-do-TRAY-ke-ul) **tube** a tube designed to be inserted into the trachea. Oxygen, medication, or a suction catheter can be directed into the trachea through an endotracheal tube.

epidermis (ep-i-DER-mis) the outer layer of skin.

epiglottis (EP-i-GLOT-is) a leaf-shaped structure that prevents food and foreign matter from entering the trachea.

epilepsy (EP-uh-lep-see) a medical condition that sometimes causes seizures.

epinephrine (EP-uh-NEF-rin) a hormone produced by the body. As a medication it dilates respiratory passages and is used to relieve severe allergic reactions.

esophagus (eh-SOF-uh-gus) the tube that leads from the pharynx to the stomach.

evacuation movement of casualties toward a care facility (i.e. aid station). Emergency medical care provided enroute.

evaporation the change from liquid to gas. When the body perspires or gets wet, evaporation of the perspiration or other liquid into the air has a cooling effect on the body.

evisceration (e-VIS-er-AY-shun) an intestine or other internal organ protruding through a wound in the abdomen.

exhalation (EX-huh-LAY-shun) a passive process in which the intercostal (rib) muscles and the diaphragm relax, causing the chest cavity to decrease in size and causing air to flow out of the lungs. Also called *expiration*.

expiration (EK-spuh-RAY-shun) See *exhalation*.

expressed consent consent given by adults who are of legal age and mentally competent to make a rational decision in regard to their medical well-being. See also *consent; implied consent*.

extraction removal from a hostile location (a tactical extrication). Little or no emergency medical care is provided enroute.

extremities (ex-TREM-i-teez) the portions of the skeleton that include the clavicles, scapulae, arms, wrists, and hands (upper extremities) and the pelvis, thighs, legs, ankles, and feet (lower extremities).

extremity lift a method of lifting and carrying a patient in which one rescuer slips hands under the patient's armpits and grasps the wrists, while another rescuer grasps the patient's knees.

femoral (FEM-or-al) **artery** the major artery supplying the thigh and leg.

femur (FEE-mer) the large bone of the thigh.

fetus (FE-tus) the baby as it develops in the womb.

fibula (FIB-yuh-luh) the lateral and smaller bone of the lower leg.

flow-restricted, oxygen-powered ventilation device (FROPVD) a device that uses oxygen under pressure to deliver artificial ventilations. Has automatic flow restriction to prevent over-delivery of oxygen to the patient.

flowmeter a valve that indicates the flow of oxygen in liters per minute.

focused history and physical exam the step of patient assessment that follows the initial assessment and includes the patient history, physical exam, and vital signs.

Fowler's position   a sitting position.

fracture (FRAK-cher)   any break in a bone.

full-thickness burn   a burn in which all the layers of the skin are damaged. There are usually areas that are charred black or areas that are dry and white. Also called a third degree burn.

gag reflex   vomiting or retching that results when something is placed in the back of the pharynx. This is tied to the swallow reflex.

Geneva Convention   Collectively, the treaties and conventions pertinent to warfare on land are referred to as The Hague and Geneva Conventions. The Geneva Conventions concern the victims of war or armed conflict. The Geneva Conventions are four separate international treaties signed in 1949.

glottic opening   the opening to the trachea.

glucose (GLU-kos)   a form of sugar, the body's basic source of energy.

golden hour   the optimum limit of one hour between the time of injury and surgery at the hospital. See also *platinum ten minutes.*

Good Samaritan laws   a series of laws, varying in each state, designed to provide limited legal protection for citizens and some health care personnel when they are administering emergency care.

hallucinogens (huh-LOO-sin-uh-jens)   mind-affecting or -altering drugs that act on the central nervous system to produce excitement and distortion of perceptions.

hazardous material   according to the U.S. Department of Transportation, "any substance or material in a form which poses an unreasonable risk to health, safety, and property when transported in commerce."

hazardous material incident   the release of a harmful substance into the environment.

head-tilt, chin-lift maneuver   a means of correcting blockage of the airway by the tongue by tilting the head back and lifting the chin. Used when no trauma, or injury, is suspected. See also *jaw-thrust maneuver.*

hematoma (hem-ah-TO-mah)   a swelling caused by the collection of blood under the skin or in damaged tissues as a result of an injured or broken blood vessel; in a head injury, a collection of blood within the skull or brain.

hemorrhage (HEM-o-rej)   bleeding, especially severe bleeding.

hemorrhagic (HEM-or-AJ-ik) **shock**   shock resulting from blood loss.

hives   red, itchy, possibly raised blotches on the skin that often result from allergic reactions.

hot zone   area immediately surrounding a hazardous material incident which extends far enough to prevent adverse effects from the released hazardous material to personnel outside the zone.

humerus (HYU-mer-us)   the bone of the upper arm, between the shoulder and the elbow.

humidifier   a device connected to the flowmeter to add moisture to the dry oxygen coming from an oxygen cylinder.

hyperglycemia (HI-per-gli-SEE-me-ah)   high blood sugar.

hyperthermia (HI-per-THURM-e-ah)   an increase in body temperature above normal.

hyperventilate (HI-per-VEN-ti-late)   to provide ventilations at a higher rate than normal.

hypoglycemia (HI-po-gli-SEE-me-ah)   low blood sugar.

hypoperfusion (HI-po-per-FEW-zhun)   inadequate perfusion of the cells and tissues of the body caused by insufficient flow of blood through the capillaries. Also called *shock.* See also *perfusion.*

hypopharynx (HI-po-FAIR-inks)   the area directly above the openings of both the trachea and the esophagus.

hypothermia (HI-po-THURM-e-ah)   a generalized cooling that reduces body temperature below normal.

hypovolemic (HI-po-vo-LE-mik) **shock**   shock resulting from blood or fluid loss.

hypoxia (hi-POK-se-uh)   an insufficiency of oxygen in the body's tissues.

ileostomy (il-e-OS-to-me)   See *colostomy.*

ilium (IL-e-um)   the superior and widest portion of the pelvis.

implied consent   the consent it is presumed a patient or patient's parent or guardian would give if they could, for example an unconscious patient or a parent who cannot be contacted when care is needed. See also *consent; expressed consent.*

Incident Command   the person or persons who assume overall direction of a large-scale incident.

Incident Command System (ICS)   See *Incident Management System.*

Incident Management System (IMS)   a system used for the management of a multiple-casualty incident, involving assumption of responsibility for command and designation and coordination of such elements as triage, treatment, transport, and staging.

index of suspicion   awareness, often based on the mechanism of injury, that a patient may have suffered injuries.

indications   specific signs or circumstances under which it is appropriate to administer a drug to a patient.

induced abortion   expulsion of a fetus as a result of deliberate actions taken to stop the pregnancy.

inferior   away from the head; usually compared with another structure that is closer to the head (e.g., the lips are inferior to the nose). Opposite of *superior.*

ingested poisons   poisons that are swallowed.

inhalation (IN-huh-LAY-shun)   an active process in which the intercostal (rib) muscles and the diaphragm contract, expanding the size of the chest cavity and causing air to flow into the lungs. Also called *inspiration.*

inhaled poisons   poisons that are breathed in.

inhaler a spray device with a mouthpiece that contains an aerosol form of a medication that a patient can spray into his airway.

initial assessment the first element in assessment of a patient; steps taken for the purpose of discovering and dealing with any life-threatening problems. The six parts of initial assessment are: forming a general impression, assessing mental status, assessing airway, assessing breathing, assessing circulation, and determining the priority of the patient for treatment and transport to the hospital.

injected poisons poisons that are inserted through the skin, for example by needle, snake fangs, or insect stinger.

inspiration (IN-spuh-RAY-shun) See *inhalation*.

insulin (IN-suh-lin) a hormone produced by the pancreas or taken as a medication by many diabetics.

interventions actions taken to correct a patient's problems.

intubation (IN-tu-BAY-shun) insertion of a tube. See also *endotracheal tube; nasogastric tube; orotracheal intubation*.

involuntary muscle muscle that responds automatically to brain signals but cannot be consciously controlled.

irreversible shock when the body has lost the battle to maintain perfusion to vital organs. Cell and tissue damage occur, especially to the liver and kidneys. Even if adequate vital signs return, the patient may die days later due to organ failure.

ischium (ISH-e-um) the lower, posterior portions of the pelvis.

jaw-thrust maneuver a means of correcting blockage of the airway by moving the jaw forward without tilting the head or neck. Used when trauma, or injury, is suspected to open the airway without causing further injury to the spinal cord in the neck. See also *head-tilt, chin-lift maneuver*.

joints places where bones articulate, or meet.

jugular (JUG-yuh-ler) **vein distention (JVD)** bulging of the neck veins.

labor the stages of the delivery of a baby that begin with the contractions of the uterus and end with the expulsion of the placenta.

laceration (las-er-AY-shun) a cut.

laryngoscope (lair-ING-uh-skope) an illuminating instrument that is inserted into the pharynx to permit visualization of the pharynx and larynx.

larynx (LAIR-inks) the voicebox.

lateral to the side, away from the midline of the body.

lateral recumbent (re-KUM-bunt) **position** lying on the side. See *recovery position*.

liability being held legally responsible.

ligaments connective tissues that connect bone to bone.

limb presentation when an infant's limb protrudes from the vagina before the appearance of any other body part.

local cooling cooling or freezing of particular (local) parts of the body.

lungs the organs where exchange of atmospheric oxygen and waste carbon dioxide take place.

mainstem bronchi See *bronchi*.

malar (MAY-lar) the cheek bone, also called the *zygomatic bone*.

malleolus (mal-E-o-lus) protrusion on the side of the ankle. The *lateral malleolus*, at the lower end of the fibula, is seen on the outer ankle; the *medial malleolus*, at the lower end of the tibia, is seen on the inner ankle.

mandible (MAN-di-bl) the lower jaw bone.

manual traction the process of applying tension to straighten and realign a fractured limb before splinting. Also called *tension*.

manubrium (man-OO-bre-um) the superior portion of the sternum.

maxillae (mak-SIL-e) the two fused bones forming the upper jaw.

mechanism of injury a force or forces that may have caused injury.

meconium staining amniotic fluid that is greenish or brownish-yellow rather than clear as a result of fetal defecation; an indication of possible maternal or fetal distress during labor.

medial toward the midline of the body.

medical direction oversight of the patient care aspects of an EMS system by the Medical Director. *Off-line medical direction* consists of standing orders and protocols issued by the Medical Director that allow EMTs to give certain medications or perform certain procedures without speaking to the Medical Director or another physician. *On-line medical direction* consists of orders from the on-duty physician given directly to an EMT-B in the field by radio or telephone.

Medical Director a physician who assumes the ultimate responsibility for the patient care aspects of the EMS system.

mental status level of responsiveness. See also *AVPU*.

metacarpals (MET-uh-KAR-pulz) the hand bones.

metatarsals (MET-uh-TAR-sulz) the foot bones.

mid-axillary (mid-AX-uh-lair-e) **line** a line drawn vertically from the middle of the armpit to the ankle.

mid-clavicular (mid-clah-VIK-yuh-ler) **line** a vertical line through the center of each clavicle.

midline an imaginary line drawn down the center of the body, dividing it into right and left halves.

Military Occupational Specialty (MOS) primary job code description for enlisted military personnel, i.e. 91W (US Army Health Care Specialist); 11B (US Army Combat Infantryman); etc.

miscarriage See *spontaneous abortion*.

mobile radio a two-way radio that is used or affixed in a vehicle.

mortality rate the death rate, noted as the number of deaths per unit of population for a specific group.

multiple birth when more than one baby is born during a single delivery.

multiple casualty incident (MCI) any medical or trauma incident involving multiple patients.

muscles tissues or fibers that cause movement of body parts and organs.

musculoskeletal (MUS-kyu-lo-SKEL-e-tal) **system** the system of bones and skeletal muscles that support and protect the body and permit movement.

narcotics a class of drugs that affect the nervous system and change many normal body activities. Their legal use is for the relief of pain. Illicit use is to produce an intense state of relaxation.

nasal (NAY-zul) **bones** the bones that form the upper third, or bridge, of the nose.

nasal cannula (NAY-zul KAN-yuh-luh) a device that delivers low concentrations of oxygen through two prongs that rest in the patient's nostrils.

nasogastric (NAY-zo-GAS-trik) **tube (NG tube)** a tube designed to be passed through the nose, nasopharynx, and esophagus. It is used to relieve distention of the stomach in an infant or child patient.

nasopharyngeal (NAY-zo-fah-RIN-jul) **airway** a flexible breathing tube inserted through the patient's nose into the pharynx to help maintain an open airway.

nasopharynx (NAY-zo-FAIR-inks) the area directly posterior to the nose.

nature of illness what is medically wrong with a patient.

near-drowning the condition of having begun to drown, but still able to be resuscitated.

negligence a finding of failure to act properly in a situation in which there was a duty to act, needed care as would reasonably be expected of the EMT-B was not provided, and harm was caused to the patient as a result.

nervous system the system of brain, spinal cord, and nerves that govern sensation, movement, and thought. See also *central nervous system; peripheral nervous system; autonomic nervous system*.

neurogenic shock hypoperfusion due to nerve paralysis (sometimes caused by spinal cord injuries) resulting in the dilation of blood vessels that increases the volume of the circulatory system beyond the point where it can be filled.

9-1-1 system a system for telephone access to report emergencies. A dispatcher takes the information, and alerts EMS or the fire or police departments as needed. *Enhanced 9-1-1* has the additional capability of automatically identifying the caller's phone number and location.

nitroglycerin a medication that dilates the blood vessels.

nonrebreather mask a face mask and reservoir bag device that delivers high concentrations of oxygen. The patient's exhaled air escapes through a valve and is not rebreathed.

occlusion (uh-KLU-zhun) blockage, as of an artery by fatty deposits.

occlusive dressing any dressing that forms an airtight seal.

ongoing assessment a procedure for detecting changes in a patient's condition. It involves four steps: repeating the initial assessment, reassessing and recording vital signs, repeating the focused assessment, and checking interventions.

open extremity injury an extremity injury in which the skin has been broken or torn through from the inside by an injured bone or from the outside by something that has caused a penetrating wound with associated injury to the bone.

open wound an injury in which the skin is interrupted, exposing the tissue beneath.

OPQRST a memory device for the questions asked to get a description of the present illness: Onset, Provokes, Quality, Radiation, Severity, Time.

oral glucose (GLU-kos) a form of glucose (a kind of sugar) given by mouth to treat an awake patient (who is able to swallow) with an altered mental status and a history of diabetes.

orbits the bony structures around the eyes; the eye sockets.

organ donor a person who has completed a legal document that allows for donation of organs and tissues in the event of death.

oropharyngeal (OR-o-fah-RIN-jul) **airway** a curved device inserted through the patient's mouth into the pharynx to help maintain an open airway.

oropharynx (OR-o-FAIR-inks) the area directly posterior to the mouth.

orotracheal (OR-o-TRAY-ke-ul) **intubation** placement of an endotracheal tube through the mouth and into the trachea. See also *endotracheal tube*.

oxygen a gas commonly found in the atmosphere. Pure oxygen is used as a drug to treat any patient whose medical or traumatic condition may cause them to be hypoxic, or low in oxygen.

oxygen cylinder a cylinder filled with oxygen under pressure.

palmar referring to the palm of the hand.

palpation touching or feeling. A pulse or blood pressure may be palpated with the fingertips.

paradoxical (pair-uh-DOCK-si-kal) **motion** movement of a part of the chest in the opposite direction to the rest of the chest during respiration.

partial-thickness burn a burn in which the epidermis (outer layer of skin) is burned through and the dermis (second layer) is damaged. Burns of this type cause reddening, blistering, and a mottled appearance. Also called a second degree burn.

passive rewarming covering a hypothermic patient and taking other steps to prevent further heat loss and help the body rewarm itself.

patella (pah-TEL-uh) the kneecap.

pathogens the organisms that cause infection, such as viruses and bacteria.

pedal edema accumulation of fluid in the feet or ankles.

penetrating trauma injury caused by an object that passes through the skin or other body tissues.

perfusion the supply of oxygen to and removal of wastes from the cells and tissues of the body as a result of the flow of blood through the capillaries.

perineum (per-i-NE-um) the surface area between the vagina and anus.

peripheral nervous system (PNS) the nerves that enter and leave the spinal cord and that travel between the brain and organs without passing through the spinal cord.

peripheral pulses the radial, brachial, posterior tibial, and dorsalis pedis pulses, which can be felt at peripheral (outlying) points of the body.

personal protective equipment (PPE) equipment such as eyewear, mask, gloves, gown, or turnout gear or helmet that protect the EMS worker from infection and/or from exposure to hazardous materials and the dangers of rescue operations.

phalanges (fuh-LAN-jiz) the toe bones and finger bones.

pharmacology (FARM-uh-KOL-uh-je) the study of drugs, their sources, characteristics, and effects.

pharynx (FAIR-inks) the area directly posterior to the mouth and nose. It is made up of the oropharynx and the nasopharynx.

physiology the study of body function.

placenta (plah-SEN-tah) the organ of pregnancy where exchange of oxygen, foods, and wastes occurs between a mother and fetus.

placenta previa (plah-SEN-tah PRE-vi-ah) a condition in which the placenta is formed in an abnormal location (low in the uterus and close to or over the cervical opening) that will not allow for a normal delivery of the fetus; a cause of prebirth bleeding.

plane a flat surface formed when slicing through a solid object.

plantar referring to the sole of the foot.

plasma (PLAZ-mah) the fluid portion of the blood.

platelets components of the blood; membrane-enclosed fragments of specialized cells.

platinum ten minutes the optimum limit of ten minutes at the scene with a serious trauma patient. See also *golden hour*.

pocket face mask a device, usually with a one-way valve, to aid in artificial ventilation. A rescuer breathes through the valve when the mask is placed over the patient's face. Also acts as a barrier to prevent contact with a patient's breath or body fluids. Can be used with supplemental oxygen when fitted with an oxygen inlet.

poison any substance that can harm the body by altering cell structure or functions.

portable radio a hand-held two-way radio.

positional asphyxia death of a person due to a body position that restricts breathing for a prolonged time.

positive pressure ventilation See *artificial ventilation*.

posterior the back of the body or body part. Opposite of *anterior*.

posterior tibial (TIB-ee-ul) **artery** artery supplying the foot, behind the medial ankle.

power grip gripping with as much hand surface as possible in contact with object being lifted, all fingers bent at the same angle, hands at least 10 inches apart.

power lift also called the *squat lift position*. It is a lift from a squatting position with weight to be lifted close to the body, feet apart and flat on the ground, body weight on or just behind balls of feet, back locked in. The upper body is raised before the hips.

preeclampsia (pre-e-KLAMP-se-ah) a complication of pregnancy where the woman retains large amounts of fluid and has hypertension (high blood pressure). She may also experience seizures and/or coma during birth, which is very dangerous to the infant.

premature infant any newborn weighing less than 5½ pounds or born before the 37th week of pregnancy.

pressure dressing a bulky dressing held in position with a tightly wrapped bandage to apply pressure to help control bleeding.

pressure point a site where a main artery lies near the surface of the body and directly over a bone. Pressure on such a point can stop distal bleeding.

pressure regulator a device connected to an oxygen cylinder to reduce cylinder pressure to a safe pressure for delivery of oxygen to a patient.

priapism (PRY-ah-pizm) persistent erection of the penis that may result from spinal injury and some medical problems.

prolapsed umbilical cord when the umbilical cord presents first and is squeezed between the vaginal wall and the baby's head.

prone lying face down.

protocols lists of steps, such as assessment and interventions, to be taken in different situations. Protocols are developed by the Medical Director of an EMS system.

proximal closer to the torso. Opposite of *distal*.

pubis (PYOO-bis) the medial anterior portion of the pelvis.

pulmonary (PUL-mo-nar-e) **arteries** the vessels that carry blood from the right ventricle of the heart to the lungs.

pulmonary edema accumulation of fluid in the lungs.

pulmonary veins the vessels that carry oxygenated blood from the lungs to the left atrium of the heart.

pulse the rhythmic beats felt as the heart pumps blood through the arteries.

pulse quality the rhythm (regular or irregular) and force (strong or weak) of the pulse.

pulse rate the number of pulse beats per minute.

pulseless electrical activity (PEA) a condition in which the heart's electrical rhythm remains relatively normal, yet the mechanical pumping activity fails to follow the electrical activity, causing cardiac arrest.

puncture wound an open wound that tears through the skin and destroys underlying tissues. A *penetrating puncture wound* can be shallow or deep. A *perforating puncture wound* has both an entrance and an exit wound.

pupil the black center of the eye.

quality improvement a process of continuous self-review with the purpose of identifying and correcting aspects of the system that require improvement.

radial artery artery of the lower arm. It is felt when taking the pulse at the wrist.

radial pulse the pulse felt at the wrist.

radiation sending out energy, such as heat, in waves into space.

radius (RAY-de-us) the lateral bone of the forearm.

rapid trauma assessment a rapid assessment of the head, neck, chest, abdomen, pelvis, extremities, and posterior of the body to detect signs and symptoms of injury.

reactivity (re-ak-TIV-uh-te) in the pupils of the eyes, reacting to light by changing size.

recovery position lying on the side. Also called *lateral recumbent position*.

red blood cells components of the blood. They carry oxygen to and carbon dioxide away from the cells.

repeater a device that picks up signals from lower-power radio units such as mobile and portable radios and retransmits them at a higher power. It allows low-power radio signals to be transmitted over longer distances.

respiration (RES-pir-AY-shun) breathing.

respiratory arrest when breathing completely stops.

respiratory failure the reduction of breathing to the point where oxygen intake is not sufficient to support life.

respiratory quality the normal or abnormal (shallow, labored, or noisy) character of breathing.

respiratory rate the number of breaths taken in one minute.

respiratory rhythm the regular or irregular spacing of breaths.

respiratory (RES-pir-uh-tor-e) **system** the system of nose, mouth, throat, lungs, and muscles that brings oxygen into the body and expels carbon dioxide.

rule of nines a method for estimating the extent of a burn. For an adult, each of the following areas represents 9% of the body surface: the head and neck, each upper extremity, the chest, the abdomen, the upper back, the lower back and buttocks, the front of each lower extremity, and the back of each lower extremity. The remaining 1% is assigned to the genital region. For an infant or child the percentages are modified so that 18% is assigned to the head, 14% to each lower extremity.

rule of palm a method for estimating the extent of a burn. The palm of the patient's hand, which equals about 1% of the body's surface area, is compared with the patient's burn to estimate its size.

SAMPLE history the present and past medical history of a patient, so called because the elements of the history begin with the letters of the word *sample*: signs/symptoms, allergies, medications, pertinent past history, last oral intake, events leading to the injury or illness.

scapula (SKAP-yuh-luh) the shoulder blade.

scene size-up steps taken by an ambulance crew when approaching the scene of an emergency call: checking scene safety, taking body substance isolation precautions, noting the mechanism of injury or nature of the patient's illness, determining the number of patients, and deciding what, if any, additional resources to call for.

scope of practice a set of regulations and ethical considerations that define the scope, or extent and limits, of the EMT-B's job.

seizure (SEE-zher) a sudden change in sensation, behavior, or movement. The most severe form of seizure produces violent muscle contractions called convulsions.

Sellick's maneuver See *cricoid pressure.*

shock See *hypoperfusion*. See also *cardiogenic shock; compensated shock; decompensated shock; irreversible shock; hemorrhagic shock; hypovolemic shock; neurogenic shock.*

shock position See *Trendelenburg position.*

side effect any action of a drug other than the desired action.

sign an indication of a patient's condition that is objective, or can be observed by another person; an indication that can be seen, heard, smelled, or felt by the EMT-B or others.

sphygmomanometer (SFIG-mo-mah-NOM-uh-ter) the cuff and gauge used to measure blood pressure.

spinous (SPI-nus) **process** the bony bump on a vertebra.

spontaneous abortion when the fetus and placenta deliver before the 28th week of pregnancy; commonly called a *miscarriage.*

sprain the stretching and tearing of ligaments.

staging officer the person responsible for overseeing and keeping track of ambulances and ambulance personnel at a multiple-casualty incident. The staging officer will direct ambulances to treatment areas at the request of the transportation officer.

staging sector the area where ambulances are parked and other resources are held until needed.

standing orders a policy or protocol that is issued by a Medical Director that authorizes EMT-Bs and others to perform particular skills in certain situations.

status epilepticus (STAY-tus or STAT-us ep-i-LEP-ti-kus) a prolonged seizure or when a person suffers two or more convulsive seizures without regaining full consciousness.

sternum (STER-num) the breastbone.

stillborn born dead.

stoma (STO-mah) a permanent surgical opening in the neck through which the patient breathes. See also *tracheostomy.*

strain muscle injury resulting from over-stretching or over-exertion of the muscle.

stroke a condition of altered function caused when an artery in the brain is blocked or ruptured, disrupting the supply of oxygenated blood or causing bleeding into the brain. Also called a *cerebrovascular accident (CVA).*

stylet (STI-let) a long, thin, flexible metal probe.

subcutaneous (SUB-ku-TAY-ne-us) **layers** the layers of fat and soft tissues found below the dermis.

sucking chest wound an open chest wound through which air is "sucked" into the chest cavity.

suctioning (SUK-shun-ing) use of a vacuum device to remove blood, vomitus, and other secretions or foreign materials from the airway.

sudden death a cardiac arrest that occurs within two hours of the onset of symptoms. The patient may have no prior symptoms of coronary artery disease.

superficial burn a burn that involves only the epidermis, the outer layer of the skin. It is characterized by reddening of the skin and perhaps some swelling. An example is a sunburn. Also called a first degree burn.

superior toward the head (e.g., the chest is superior to the abdomen). Opposite of *inferior.*

supine lying on the back.

supine hypotensive syndrome dizziness and a drop in blood pressure caused when the woman in advanced pregnancy is in a supine position and the weight of the uterus, infant, placenta, and amniotic fluid compress the inferior vena cava, reducing return of blood to the heart and cardiac output.

symptom an indication of a patient's condition that cannot be observed by another person but rather is subjective, or felt and reported by the patient.

systolic (sis-TOL-ik) **blood pressure** the pressure created when the heart contracts and forces blood out into the arteries.

tachycardia (TAK-uh-KAR-de-uh) a rapid heart rate; any pulse rate above 100 beats per minute.

tarsals (TAR-sulz) the ankle bones.

temporal (TEM-po-ral) **bone** bone that forms part of the side of the skull and floor of the cranial cavity. There are a right and a left temporal bone.

temporomandibular (TEM-po-ro-mand-DIB-yuh-lar) **joint** the movable joint formed between the mandible and the temporal bone, also called the TM joint.

tendons tissues that connect muscle to bone.

thorax (THOR-ax) the chest.

thrombus (THROM-bus) a clot formed of blood and plaque attached to the inner wall of an artery.

tibia (TIB-e-uh) the medial and larger bone of the lower leg.

torso the trunk of the body; the body without the head and the extremities.

tourniquet (TURN-i-ket) a device used for bleeding control that constricts all blood flow to and from an extremity.

toxin a poisonous substance secreted by bacteria, plants, or animals.

trachea (TRAY-ke-uh) the "windpipe"; the structure that connects the pharynx to the lungs.

tracheostomy (TRAY-ke-OS-to-me) a surgical incision in the neck held open by a metal or plastic tube. See also *stoma.*

traction splint a special splint that applies constant pull along the length of a lower extremity to help stabilize the fractured bone and to reduce muscle spasms in limb. Traction splints are used primarily on femoral shaft fractures.

transportation officer the person responsible for managing transportation of patients to hospitals from the scene of a multiple-casualty incident.

treatment officer the person responsible for overseeing treatment of patients who have been triaged at a multiple-casualty incident.

treatment sector the area in which patients are treated at a multiple-casualty incident.

Trendelenburg (trend-EL-un-berg) **position** a position in which the patient's feet and legs are higher than the head. Also called *shock position.*

trending the changes in a patient's condition over time, such as slowing respirations or rising pulse rate, that may show improvement or deterioration, and that can be shown by documenting repeated assessments.

triage the process of quickly assessing patients in a multiple-casualty incident and assigning each a priority for receiving treatment according to the severity of their illness or injuries. From a French word meaning "to sort."

triage officer the person responsible for overseeing triage at a multiple-casualty incident.

triage sector the area in which secondary triage takes place at a multiple casualty incident.

triage tag color coded tag indicating the priority group to which a patient has been assigned.

ulna (UL-nah) the medial bone of the forearm.

umbilical (um-BIL-i-kal) **cord** the fetal structure containing the blood vessels that carry blood to and from the placenta.

universal dressing a bulky dressing.

uppers stimulants such as amphetamines that affect the central nervous system to excite the user.

uterus (U-ter-us) the muscular abdominal organ where the fetus develops; the womb.

vagina (vah-JI-nah) the birth canal.

vallecula (val-EK-yuh-luh) a groove-like structure anterior to the epiglottis.

vein any blood vessel returning blood to the heart.

venae cavae (VE-ne KA-ve) the superior vena cava and the inferior vena cava. These two major veins return blood from the body to the right atrium. (*Venae cavae* is plural, *vena cava* singular.)

venom a toxin (poison) produced by certain animals such as snakes, spiders, and some marine life forms.

venous bleeding bleeding from a vein, which is characterized by dark red or maroon blood and as a steady flow, easy to control.

ventilation the breathing in of air or oxygen or providing breaths artificially. See also *artificial ventilation*.

ventral referring to the front of the body. A synonym for *anterior*.

ventricles (VEN-tri-kulz) the two lower chambers of the heart. There is a right ventricle (which sends oxygen-poor blood to the lungs) and a left ventricle (which sends oxygen-rich blood to the body).

ventricular fibrillation (ven-TRIK-u-ler fib-ri-LAY-shun) **(VF)** a condition in which the heart's electrical impulses are disorganized, preventing the heart muscle from contracting normally.

ventricular tachycardia (ven-TRIK-u-ler tak-i-KAR-de-uh) **(V-Tach)** a condition in which the heartbeat is quite rapid; if rapid enough, ventricular tachycardia will not allow the heart's chambers to fill with enough blood between beats to produce blood flow sufficient to meet the body's needs.

venule (VEN-yul) the smallest kind of vein.

vertebrae (VER-te-bray) the 33 bones of the spinal column (singular *vertebra*).

vital signs outward signs of what is going on inside the body, including respiration; pulse; skin color, temperature, and condition (plus capillary refill in infants and children); pupils; and blood pressure.

vocal cords two thin folds of tissue within the larynx that vibrate as air passes between them, producing sounds.

volatile chemicals vaporizing compounds, such as cleaning fluid, that are breathed in by the abuser to produce a "high."

voluntary muscle muscle that can be consciously controlled.

warm zone area at a hazardous material incident where personnel and equipment decontamination and hot-zone support take place.

water chill chilling caused by conduction of heat from the body when the body or clothing is wet.

watt the unit of measurement of the output power of a radio.

white blood cells components of the blood. They produce substances that help the body fight infection.

wind chill chilling caused by convection of heat from the body in the presence of air currents.

withdrawal referring to alcohol or drug withdrawal in which the patient's body reacts severely when deprived of the abused substance.

xiphoid (ZI-foid) **process** the inferior portion of the sternum.

zygomatic (ZI-go-MAT-ik) **bones** the cheekbones.

INDEX